Healthcare Politics and Policy in America

Health policy in the United States has been shaped by the political, socioeconomic, and ideological environment, with important roles played by public and private actors, as well as institutional and individual entities, in designing the contemporary American healthcare system. Now in a fully updated fifth edition, this book gives expanded attention to pressing issues for our policymakers, including the aging American population, physician shortages, gene therapy, specialty drugs, and the opioid crisis. A new chapter has been added on the Trump administration's failed attempts at repealing and replacing the Affordable Care Act and subsequent attempts at undermining it via executive orders.

Authors Kant Patel and Mark Rushefsky address the key problems of healthcare cost, access, and quality through analyses of Medicare, Medicaid, the Veterans Health Administration, and other programs, and the ethical and cost implications of advances in healthcare technology. Each chapter concludes with discussion questions and a comprehensive reference list. This textbook will be required reading for courses on health and healthcare policy, as well as all those interested in the ways in which American healthcare has evolved over time.

Kant Patel is Emeritus Professor of Political Science at Missouri State University, USA.

Mark Rushefsky is Emeritus Professor of Political Science at Missouri State University, USA.

Healthcare Politics and Policy in America

Fifth Edition

Kant Patel and

Mark Rushefsky

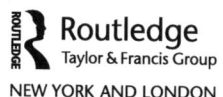
Routledge
Taylor & Francis Group
NEW YORK AND LONDON

To the memory of Marc Cooper.—Kant Patel

To my grandchildren, Echo, Damian, and Gabriel. You bring us joy and we hope that you can help make a better future for us all.—Mark Rushefsky

Fifth edition published 2020

by Routledge
52 Vanderbilt Avenue, New York, NY 10017

and by Routledge
2 Park Square, Milton Park, Abingdon, Oxon, OX14 4RN

Routledge is an imprint of the Taylor & Francis Group, an informa business

© 2020 Taylor & Francis

The right of Kant Patel and Mark Rushefsky to be identified as authors of this work has been asserted by them in accordance with sections 77 and 78 of the Copyright, Designs and Patents Act 1988.

All rights reserved. No part of this book may be reprinted or reproduced or utilized in any form or by any electronic, mechanical, or other means, now known or hereafter invented, including photocopying and recording, or in any information storage or retrieval system, without permission in writing from the publishers.

Trademark notice: Product or corporate names may be trademarks or registered trademarks, and are used only for identification and explanation without intent to infringe.

Library of Congress Cataloging-in-Publication Data
A catalog record for this title has been requested

First edition published by M.E. Sharpe 2005
Fifth edition published by Routledge 2019

ISBN: 978-0-8153-7633-0 (hbk)
ISBN: 978-0-367-02774-2 (pbk)
ISBN: 978-0-429-39787-5 (ebk)

Typeset in Times New Roman
by Swales & Willis, Exeter, Devon, UK
Visit the eResources: www.routledge.com/9780367027742

CONTENTS

List of tables and figures	xiii
Preface	xv
Foreword	xvii
List of Acronyms	xxiii
Acknowledgments	xxv

I
Healthcare Politics and Policy

1. Healthcare Politics 3
    Health Policymaking in the United States 3
    The Health Policy Environment 5
        The Constitutional Environment 5
        The Institutional Environment 8
        The Political Environment 12
        The Changing Political Environment 16
        The Economic Environment 21
        The Technological Environment 22
    Key Health Policy Actors 22
        Healthcare Providers 22
        Third-Party Payers 25
        Employers 28
        Consumers 28
        Interest Groups 30
    Conclusion 33
    Study Questions 33
    References 34

2. Healthcare Policy in the United States 41
    The US Healthcare System in a Comparative Context 42
    Healthcare in Colonial Times 43
    Healthcare in the Nineteenth Century 43
    The Transformation of US Medicine: 1900–1935 44
    The Role of the Federal Government in Healthcare 45
        Limited Federal Role: 1900s–1930s 45
        Expanded Federal Role: 1930s–1960s 46
        Efforts at Healthcare Cost Containment: 1970s–1980s 49
        Controlling Costs by Planning 50
    The Political Transformation of the US Healthcare System: 1981–2018 51
        The Reagan Administration: 1981–1989 52
        The George H. W. Bush Administration: 1989–1993 53
        The Clinton Administration: 1993–2001 54
        The George W. Bush Administration: 2001–2009 56
        The Barack Obama Administration: 2009–2017 60
        The Trump Administration: 2017– 61
    The Evolution of Public Health in the United States 63

    The Seventeenth Century 63
    The Eighteenth Century 63
    The Nineteenth Century 64
    The Twentieth Century 65
    The Twenty-First Century 66
    Organization and Functions of Public Health 67
    Public Health Spending and Financing 70
    Public Health Accomplishments and Challenges 70
  Conclusion 71
  Study Questions 73
  References 73

II
Government Health Programs

3. The Affordable Care Act: Stumbling Toward Universal Health Insurance? 81
  The Road to the Affordable Care Act (2006–2008) 81
    Kingdon's Multiple Streams Model 81
    The Political Stream 87
  The Legislative Process: An Ordeal by Fire (2008–2010) 87
    The Opening Moves 87
    The Legislative Process: Ideal versus Real 88
    Political Parties at War 89
    Moving Through Congress 90
    The Affordable Care Act Clears the Obstacles 95
  The Patient Protection and Affordable Care Act 96
    Goals and Purposes 96
    Major Provisions 96
  Challenging the Affordable Care Act 101
    The Affordable Care Act on Trial 101
    Electoral Challenges 105
    Public Opinion 105
  Implementing the Affordable Care Act 106
  Federalism and the Affordable Care Act 108
    Health Insurance Exchanges 108
    Medicaid Expansion and the States 109
  Legislative Challenges 111
  Administrative Challenges 113
  Evaluating the Affordable Care Act 115
    Insurance Coverage 115
    Affordable Care 117
    Criticisms of the Affordable Care Act 118
  Conclusion 120
  Study Questions 124
  References 124

4. Medicaid and the Children's Health Insurance Program: Healthcare for the Poor and the Disabled 130
  Important Facts about the Current Medicaid Program 131
  Program Objective and Structure 132
  Medicaid Eligibility and Coverage, Services and Benefits 132
    Eligibility and Coverage 132
    Benefits and Services 135
  Medicaid Financing 135
    Federal Financing 135
    State Financing 135
  The Children's Health Insurance Program (CHIP) 137

The Origins and Evolution of the CHIP 137
The Struggle over the Renewal of the CHIP 138
CHIP Eligibility, Benefits, Financing, and Cost-Sharing 139
The Affordable Care Act of 2010 and Medicaid Expansion 140
The Implementation of Medicaid Expansion under the ACA 141
What Factors Explain States' Decisions to Expand or Not to Expand? 142
Justifications for Expansion and Consequences 145
Justifications for Non-Expansion and Consequences 146
Changes in Medicaid Enrollees, Enrollment, and Expenditures 147
Characteristics of Program Enrollees 147
Medicaid Enrollment and Expenditures 147
Medicaid Waivers 148
What are Medicaid Waivers? 148
Types of Medicaid Waivers 148
Medicaid Waivers and State Medicaid Reforms, 1980s–2010s 149
The Current State of Medicaid Waivers and Reforms 150
Broad Overview of Approved and Pending Waivers 150
Trends in Medicaid Reforms and Experiments: Private-Sector Approaches 151
Long-Term Care: Transition from Institutional to Community-Based/Home Care 155
Medicaid Pay-For-Performance 157
Conclusion 158
Study Questions 159
References 159

5. Medicare: Healthcare for the Elderly **165**
The Origins of Medicare 165
Program Objectives and Structure 166
Objectives 166
Structure 167
Financing Medicare 168
Supplementing Medicare 169
Medicaid Buy-In 169
Medigap 170
Employment Retiree Benefits 170
Transforming Medicare 170
The Medicare Prescription Drug, Improvement, and Modernization Act of 2003 171
Medicare Advantage 175
Lessons from the Medicare Modernization Act 176
Controlling Costs 177
Prospective Payment System 179
Controlling Physician Costs 180
Reorganizing Payment Mechanisms and Service Delivery 182
The Problem of Long-Term Care 182
Long-Term Care Insurance 184
Policy Options: Transforming Medicare 185
Incremental Policy Alternatives 185
Comprehensive Policy Alternatives 187
Medicare and the Affordable Care Act 189
Conclusion: The Politics and Policy of Medicare 190
Study Questions 191
References 191

6. Healthcare for American Indians, Alaska Natives, and Veterans **196**
American Indians and Alaska Natives 196
Population Characteristics and Trends 197

Historical Background 198
The Legal and Constitutional Status of American Indians and Alaska Natives 198
   American Indians 198
   Alaska Natives 199
The Evolution of Health Policy 199
   The Nineteenth Century 199
   The Twentieth Century 200
   The Twenty-First Century 202
The Indian Health Service: Organization and Structure 203
   Organization and Delivery of Health Services 204
   Urban Indian Health Programs 204
   The Indian Health Service and Funding 205
Health Status and Trends 206
Accomplishments of the IHS 210
Challenges Confronting the IHS and Healthcare Policy for AIs/ANs 210
   Increasing Funding for the IHS 211
   Increasing Access to Healthcare Services 211
   Providing Culturally Competent Care 212
   Conclusion 213
Healthcare for Veterans 214
   Population Characteristics and Trends 214
Historical Background: The Development of Veterans' Benefits 214
Veterans' Health Policy Development 216
The Veterans Health Administration 219
   Mission 219
   Organization and Structure 219
Transitioning from Tricare to VA Healthcare 220
The VA Healthcare System 220
   Eligibility and Enrollment 220
   Benefits and Services 221
   Health Benefits for Family Members of Veterans 222
The Health Status of Veterans 222
Funding and Expenditures of the VA and VHA 225
Veterans' Use of Benefits and Services 226
A History of Scandals at the Veterans Administration 228
Challenges Confronting the VA Healthcare System 230
Conclusion 231
Study Questions 232
References 232

III
Problems of the Healthcare System

7. Falling Through the Safety Net: The Disadvantaged 243
Equality and Equity 243
Important Considerations 245
   Social Determinants of Health 246
   Geography is Destiny 247
   Addressing Social Determinants 248
The Uninsured and Underinsured 249
Consequences of Uninsurance and Underinsurance 253
Insurance and the Idea of Community 256
A Closer Look: The Poor, Minorities, and Women 257
   Minorities and Low-Income Groups 258
   Women 262
Immigrants and Healthcare 270

Lawful Noncitizen Immigrants and Healthcare 271
Undocumented Immigrants and Healthcare 272
Conclusion: The Problems of the Disadvantaged Remain 274
Study Questions 275
References 275

8. The Problem of Rising Healthcare Costs and Spending 283
Rising Healthcare Costs/Expenditures 283
Expenditures by Type of Health Service 286
Growth in Public-Sector Expenditures and Decline in Out-of-Pocket Expenditures 288
Concentration of Expenditures 290
Healthcare Expenditures in the United States Compared to Other Countries 294
Who is Affected by High and Increasing Healthcare Costs? 294
Households 294
Businesses 297
Government 297
Americans' Views about Healthcare Costs/Expenditures 299
Factors Responsible for Rising Healthcare Costs/Expenditures 299
The Role and Growth of Medical Technology 300
Medical Errors and Costs 304
Costs of Waste, Fraud, and Abuse in the US Healthcare System 308
Lifestyle Choices and Costs/Expenditures 310
Administration 311
The Overpriced American Healthcare System 312
Prescription Drugs and Costs/Expenditures 314
Cost Drivers 322
Healthcare Cost-Containment: Bending the Cost Curve 323
Theoretical Framework: Government Regulation and Market Competition 323
The Regulatory Strategy 323
The Market Strategy 324
Past Efforts at Controlling Healthcare Costs 327
Healthcare Planning and Cost-Containment 327
Professional Standards Review 327
Price Regulation 328
The Special Case of Maryland 329
Controlling Drug Prices 329
Health Maintenance Organizations, Healthcare Rationing, Managed Care, and Cost-Containment 331
Health Maintenance Organizations 331
Healthcare Rationing 332
Managed Competition 333
Managed Care 334
Wellness Programs 336
Cost-Sharing 336
Cost-Containment in the Twenty-First Century 337
Fraud, Waste, and Cost Control 338
The Affordable Care Act and Cost Control 341
The Federal Budget and Healthcare Costs 341
A Strategy for Controlling Costs 342
Conclusion 343
Study Questions 343
References 344

IV
Contemporary Challenges in American Healthcare

9. The Role of Biomedical Technology: The Beginning and the End of Life 361
   Medical Technologies: Law, Politics, Religion, and Ethics 361
   The Beginning of Life 363
      What are Assisted Reproductive Technologies? 363
      Types of ARTs 363
      The Role of Consent and Contracts in ARTs 364
      New Developments in ARTs 365
      Infertility and ARTs 367
      Government Regulation of ARTs and Surrogacy 367
      Courts and the Right to Conceive and Bear Children 368
   Preventing Unintended Pregnancies, Births, and Abortions 372
      Contraceptive Use, Unintended Pregnancies, and Abortions 372
      Abortions in the United States 373
      Federal and State Regulation of Abortions 374
   Emergency Contraception 375
      Background 375
      Use of Emergency Contraception 377
      State Governments and Emergency Contraception 377
      Emergency Contraception and the Courts 378
      The Politics of Emergency Contraception 378
   RU-486 and Medication Abortion 378
      State Governments and Medication Abortion 379
      Medication Abortion and the Courts 379
      The Politics of RU-486 380
   Courts and Abortion: The Right to Prevent Unwanted Pregnancies and Births 380
      ARTs, Religion, and Politics 382
      ARTs, Ethics, and Law 383
   The End of Life: The Right to Die and Physician-Assisted Suicide 384
      The Right-to-Die Movement 384
      The Right to Die and Physician-Assisted Suicide in Other Countries 385
   The Right to Die in the United States 386
      Courts and the Right to Refuse Life-Sustaining Treatments 386
      Courts and Physician-Assisted Suicide 390
      States and Physician-Assisted Suicide 391
      Physician-Assisted Suicide Statistics 392
      Public Opinion and the Right to Die 395
      Living Wills and Durable Power of Attorney 396
      Physician-Assisted Suicide: Religion, Morality, and Ethics 397
   Conclusion 398
   Study Questions 398
   References 399

10. Challenges Facing the American Healthcare System **407**
   The Opioid Crisis 407
      What Are Opioids? 408
      The Nature and Scope of the Opioid Epidemic 409
      The Demographics and Geography of the Opioid Epidemic 410
      The Economic and Social Costs of the Opioid Epidemic 412
      What is Responsible for the Opioid Epidemic? The Blame Game 413
      Government's Response to the Opioid Crisis 416
   Specialty Drugs/Pharmaceuticals 420
      What are Specialty Drugs? 421

The Management of Specialty Drugs 421
The Role of the FDA in Specialty Drugs 422
The Cost of Specialty Drugs and Price Increases 423
The Benefits and Effectiveness of Specialty Drugs 426
Policy Dilemma: Balancing the Costs and Benefits of Specialty Drugs 427
Gene Therapy: The Future of Medicine? 427
The Evolution of Gene Therapy 427
What are Gene Editing and Gene Therapy? 430
The Pros and Cons of Gene Therapy 431
The Cost of Gene Therapy 432
Controversy over Germline Human Gene Editing 433
Germline Human Gene Editing and Ethical Concerns 435
The Regulation of Gene Editing and Gene Therapy 436
The Role of the Healthcare Workforce 437
The Profile of the Healthcare Workforce 437
The Healthcare Workforce and Challenges Facing the American Healthcare System 439
Conclusion 443
Study Questions 443
References 444

V
The Continuing Struggle for Healthcare Reform in the United States

11. Healthcare Politics and Policy in America: Moving Toward Reform? 453
Healthcare System Goals and Values 453
Goals 453
Values 455
Fixing the Affordable Care Act 455
Liberal/Democratic Reform Proposals 457
Medicaid-Based Plans 457
Medicare-Based Plans 458
Conservative/Republican Proposals 462
Conclusion: Healthcare Reform Choices 469
Study Questions 471
References 471

Appendix A. Important Health Policy-Related Websites and Resources 473
Appendix B. Chronology of Significant Events and Legislation in US Healthcare 479
Appendix C. Important Concepts 489
Appendix D. Important Research Reports 493
Appendix E. Healthcare-Related Documentaries and Films 496
About the Authors 506
Index 507

TABLES AND FIGURES

TABLES

1.1	Occurrences of Unified and Divided Governments in the United States, 1900–2020	17
3.1	Ideological Change in Congress, Selected Years	90
3.2	Affordable Care Act (ACA) Timeline	95
4.1	Medicaid Benefits	134
4.2	State Action on Medicaid Expansion under the ACA, December 2018	143
4.3	Expenditures for Medicaid and CHIP Programs, Selected Calendar Years	144
5.1	Medicare Part A: Hospital Insurance-Covered Services, 2019	167
5.2	Medicare Part B: Medical Insurance-Covered Services, 2019	168
5.3	Sources of Prescription Drug Coverage for the Elderly, 2015	172
5.4	Medicare Expenditures, Selected Years, 1970–2016 (in $ billions)	178
5.5	Medicare Beneficiaries, Selected Years, 1970–2017 (in millions)	178
6.1	Indian Health Service Funding History and Budget Request, 2014–2019 (in $ millions)	206
6.2	Comparison of Selective Health Status Indicators for American Indians/Alaska Natives and the General Population, 2014–2015	207
6.3	Leading Causes of Death for American Indians and Alaska Natives, 1980 and 2015	208
6.4	The VA's Budget, FY 2015–2019 (in $ billions)	226
6.5	Veterans Administration Utilization Profile, 2016	227
7.1	Social Determinants of Health	246
7.2	Sources of Health Insurance Coverage, 1999–2016	250
8.1	Selected National Healthcare Expenditures by Sources of Funds and Types of Services, 1960–2016 (in $ billions)	284
8.2	Selected National Healthcare Expenditures by Sources of Funds and Types of Services, 2007–2016 (in $ billions)	287
8.3	National Healthcare Expenditures and the Economy, 1960–2016	289
8.4	National Healthcare Expenditures, 2001–2016	291
8.5	Federal Spending on Healthcare (in $ billions)	298
8.6	Estimates of the Cost of Waste, Fraud, and Abuse in Healthcare in the United States, 2009	309
8.7	National Retail Prescription Drug Expenditures by Sources of Funds, 1965–2016 (in $ billions)	317
8.8	National Retail Prescription Drug Expenditures by Sources of Funds, 2000–2016 (in $ billions)	319
9.1	Physician-Assisted Suicide Laws in American States, October 2018	392
9.2	Physician-Assisted Suicide Statistics in Oregon and Washington, 2009–2017	394

FIGURES

3.1	Healthcare Reform Implementation Timeline	97
3.2	Uninsured Rate Among the Nonelderly Population, 1972–2018	116
8.1	Bending the Cost Curve	324

PREFACE

We are gratified by the reception *Healthcare Politics and Policy in America* has received since publication of the first edition. It has been well reviewed, it has sold well, and it has been adopted by many colleges and universities. We thank all those who have adopted it for their courses. The first edition was the first joint research project between Patel and Rushefsky. Since that time, we have published several books on healthcare with M.E. Sharpe: *Politics, Power, and Policy Making: The Case of Health Care Reform in the 1990s; Health Care Policy in an Age of New Technologies; The Politics of Public Health in the United States*; and *Health Care in America: Separate and Unequal*. We are grateful that Routledge has picked up this project as part of its purchase of M.E. Sharpe. We appreciate the support and enthusiasm with which Routledge has allowed us to continue our work. The staff, from editor Laura Stearns to the copy-editors, have been wonderful to work with.

Patel began working on the first edition of the book while on a sabbatical in the spring of 1991. Rushefsky joined the project in 1994. It continues to be an interesting experience for both of us. We do not have the same kind of work habits. One of us (we won't tell you which one) is very meticulous and organized; the other is considerably more scattered and sloppy. This has sometimes led to noisy discussions and scampering to find things. This is the kind of book Felix and Oscar, the Odd Couple, might have written! One adjustment we did make was that the neat, meticulous one kept all the papers and files because the other misplaced his. That we remain close friends who share common interests in professional basketball (and computer games) helped the relationship. Patel, who is from Houston, roots for the Houston Rockets. Rushefsky, from New York, is a lifelong, avid, irrational Knicks fan. Patel retired from Missouri State University in 2011, and Rushefsky retired in 2014.

Both of us have had a long involvement in healthcare, dating back to the 1970s. Rushefsky first became interested in healthcare when his wife, Cynthia, began teaching childbirth classes in rural Rocky Mount, Virginia. She trained some of the nurses and the wife of the administrator of the local rural hospital (about ten miles along winding mountain roads from where they lived), and that hospital maintained its maternity ward rather than closing it. That was fortunate for the Rushefskys when their second child, Leah, was born shortly after midnight on Halloween. They just made it those ten miles to the hospital. Had that hospital not maintained its birthing facilities, they would have had to go another 25 miles to Roanoke. Given the speed with which Leah was born (so fast that she beat the doctor to the delivery room!), Rushefsky half-jokingly says she would have been born in Boones Mill (about halfway between Rocky Mount and Roanoke), which had no hospital. Updating from the first edition of this book, Leah is now married and has given Rushefsky and his wife three grandchildren, Echo, Damian, and Gabriel, to whom he has dedicated this book. Echo and Damian were born prematurely, so the Rushefsky clan has had some close encounters with the American healthcare system.

Patel's interest in healthcare was developed more conventionally, as an academic. He has a lifelong belief that access to good healthcare is a right. The two of us agree that the healthcare system has problems; before publication of the first edition of this book, there was no text that addressed those problems from a political perspective.

This fifth edition has been considerably updated and reconceptualized. The first two chapters of the book remain basically the same (with updates), providing background material. We have moved the discussion of the Affordable Care Act to Chapter 3. That chapter looks at the implementation of the legislation as well as the many challenges it faces. Chapters 4 and 5 examine Medicaid and Medicare, providing an update and pointing out how they have been affected by the Affordable Care Act. Chapter 6 focuses on veterans and Native Americans and Alaska Natives, as well as the Indian Health Service and the Department of Veterans Affairs. Chapter 7 discusses the safety net and focuses on access issues. Chapter 8 combines two chapters from the previous edition, looking at cost issues. Chapter 9 has been reconfigured, focusing on the legal, political, and ethical issues raised by biotechnology related to the beginning of life (reproductive rights) and the end of life (the right to die). Chapter 10 examines four challenges facing the US healthcare system: the opioid crisis, specialty drugs, gene therapy, and the healthcare workforce. Chapter 11, new to this edition, examines reform proposals: to the Affordable Care Act and from conservative and liberal perspectives.

Patel and Rushefsky, as noted above, have different lifestyles. Patel spends the colder months in southwestern Florida, lounging on the beach, venturing to various festivals, reading, etc. Rushefsky still teaches a bit, spends time with his family, and is an aspiring (if not altogether successful) musician (guitar and keyboard). Despite these differences and our retirement, we have, at this time anyway, agreed that we should do a sixth edition, if our health permits, after the 2020 elections.

FOREWORD

For some two decades or so, Kant Patel and Mark Rushefsky have been conducting studies of America's health delivery systems. The numerous articles and books resulting from the studies of these two political scientists have enriched the literature. It is thus heartening to be able to welcome this, their new study, and also to know that they intend to prepare another, after the outcomes of the 2020 elections are clear.

As one would expect from political scientists in view of the overwhelming pressure today throughout the discipline to be scrupulously objective, Patel and Rushefsky go to extraordinary lengths to be even-handed. They examine the alternate value structures that motivate various approaches to healthcare—approaches that generate different conclusions from consideration of the same facts. They are careful not to take sides in the political controversies that—one is tempted to think uniquely—swirl around questions of healthcare in the United States. They work diligently to present the facts, and the varied arguments involved. They deserve praise for daring to delve into public policy, a field that many political scientists avoid in their quest for unquestionable objectivity.

This does not mean that a thorough reading of this comprehensive work will produce a sense in the informed reader that the media are correct when they stress that "all sides do it," or that all sides take positions that are to be equally respected. In the current situation in the United States, a completely objective presentation of the facts frequently can appear partisan, especially when considerations of public policy are involved. Patel and Rushefsky generally succeed in the difficult task they set for themselves.

The current outlook for healthcare somewhat past the half-way moment of the Trump presidential term—as for social policies across the spectrum—is murky, at best. In a foreword, perhaps it is excusable to demonstrate less concern for even-handedness in an unbalanced situation than for speaking truth to power. Hence, this observation: One may hope that the forthcoming elections will produce more enlightened policies after 2020. At a minimum, such policies would introduce more rationality into the system, policies that could increase both the amount and the quality of social services in general, and of healthcare in particular.

Today's political world is certainly chaotic, but that only makes sound planning all the more important. In the best of possible worlds, healthcare costs would no longer burden citizens (or other residents), no one would go without needed care, the quality of care rendered would be uniformly excellent, and society as a whole would benefit.

Patel and Rushefsky present a sound portrait of the complexity of this country's entire healthcare delivery system, and of the ills that plague it. Such a system could hardly have evolved from careful planning, and indeed it did not. It emerged in hit-or-miss fashion.

Thomas Paine was perhaps the first to suggest public provision for citizens. As the eighteenth century was coming to a close, he had written highly relevant statements, *The Rights of Man*, and *Agrarian Justice*. The visionary nature of his social thought is astonishing. These works not only contained suggestions that foreshadowed, or at the least hinted at, the development of Social Security and similar programs, but even reflected ideas so advanced that they are hardly considered even today. For example, he recommended that, to serve as a nest egg of sorts and to assist in alleviating poverty, the government bestow a payment upon everyone reaching the age of 21. It is highly significant that he recommended the grant be paid both to men and women.

Such visionary thought, however, is hardly characteristic of Americans. To be fair, throughout the nineteenth and very early twentieth centuries, the state of medical science remained primitive. If there had been public provision for healthcare, it might have done as much harm as good.

Nevertheless, as the twentieth century progressed, so did the quality of medical science in America. Also, suggestions for social insurance began to be heard, and they often included healthcare. With the passage of years, they became more frequent. Bismarck's Germany in 1883 had implemented the world's first modern social welfare system, and in 1915, the American Medical Association signaled some interest in compulsory government health insurance, forming its own Social Insurance Committee. Three of the committee members, all physicians—Alexander Lambert, I. M. Rubinow, and S. S. Goldwater—were also members of a similar committee that the American Association for Labor Legislation, a progressive group, had formed earlier.

The very idea that the AMA ever had given thought to any kind of government health program will likely be astonishing to those who know the history of the bitter resistance that the AMA later directed at any such suggestion. The open-minded attitude was brief, and the receptive attitude from the AMA vanished quickly, and completely. By 1918, many insurance companies, pharmaceutical houses, and the AMA itself had begun to work vigorously against any suggestion of government assistance in paying for healthcare, let alone any consideration of providing health services directly (Skidmore 1970, 2).

It was the AMA, in fact, that succeeded in denying the country its first significant chance to move in the direction of government support for healthcare. Social Security became law with passage of the Social Security Act in 1935, as the jewel in the crown of Franklin D. Roosevelt's New Deal. FDR had hoped to include health coverage in the program, but the AMA let it be known that if the proposed program provided health benefits, the organization would mobilize its formidable lobbying powers against the bill. If there were no provision for healthcare, the AMA would sit out the fight, and take no position on Social Security. In view of the enormous political influence organized medicine possessed, it is likely that Social Security would never have been adopted if the AMA chose to oppose it. FDR concluded, prudently, that it would be better to have a program of social insurance with no healthcare provisions than to have no program at all. Thus, he supported the Social Security bill without any such benefit (Witte 1962).

Ironically, there was a development beginning in the early twentieth century that could potentially have evolved into a comprehensive system of healthcare outside of government. The discussion here of necessity is brief and incomplete, but it is sufficient to reveal both an opportunity lost, and the dynamics that make a successful program unlikely in the American setting without government involvement.

It began in Texas, shortly after the beginning of the twentieth century. Dallas teachers and Baylor University hospital worked out a plan to provide hospitalization to teachers for a small annual fee. Early in the 1930s, the plan expanded, in order both to benefit the community and to shore up the troubled finances of the hospital, by helping keep its beds filled.

Other states seized upon the idea, and they too expanded it. Quickly it grew to include multiple hospitals in a given location. With the cooperation of the American Hospital Association, plans spread across the country, and became Blue Cross. They incorporated several features that became nearly universal: they were voluntary and non-profit; they became available to anyone, regardless of health or risk; they were "community rated," charging a flat fee that was uniform throughout the service area; they operated as charitable associations, and they sought to provide service to the greatest number, at minimum cost consistent with the amounts needed to maintain the hospitals.

As could have been anticipated, physicians were more resistant to prepaid plans than were hospitals, but before long they began to form their own plans as well. Prepaid medical plans began in California. Like Blue Cross, they soon spread across the country. These became Blue Shield. For some time, Blue Cross/Blue Shield thrived as prepaid, non-profit, community-rated plans.

Blue Cross/Blue Shield emerged to employ the insurance principle to protect against rising healthcare costs, and to stabilize the finances of healthcare providers during the Great Depression. In the American economy, however, such a worthwhile arrangement could not prevail unless protected by regulation.

Insurance companies in the private market exist to make profits. Their executives recognized the potential for huge gains to be made by offering policies to the most healthy segments of the population. By covering only those that presented the least risk, they could offer the same benefits as Blue Cross, but at much lower rates. With profit-making companies cherry-picking their most profitable customers, the Blues were left with the highest-risk, thus highest-cost, parts of the population. Thus, to survive, the Blues ultimately were forced to abandon their most praiseworthy feature, community rating; they had to shift to the risk-rating practices of the profit-making insurance companies (Skidmore 2008).

The failure of the Blue Cross non-profit, community-rated experiment was a tragedy for healthcare in the United States. Along with other developments, it led to erecting the bulk of American healthcare upon a solid foundation of profits, thus ensuring that American healthcare would be enormously expensive—as it turned out, soon it was by far the most expensive in the world.

There were other dynamics at work as well that encouraged the growth of profit-making health insurance as the foundation for healthcare. For many reasons, employer-provided health insurance as a fringe benefit grew. Large groups can negotiate lower rates. Tax policies permitted employers to provide health insurance as a business expense—thus as a tax write-off—without subjecting employees to tax on the benefits. This connection meant that many Americans found it their only affordable source of coverage; it meant, also, that many were left without access to benefits. That worsened with tax policies redistributing wealth upward under Reagan and most of his Republican successors, with the decline of labor unions (the policies of the Reagan administration and subsequent Republican presidencies were influential here, also), and with the advent of business philosophies that saw maximum profits, astronomical executive salaries, and generous distributions to shareholders as the prime obligations of business ethics with little or no thought to civic obligation or workers' welfare.

The striking differences in this regard reflected between the two generations of prominent Romneys in politics are telling. Mitt Romney, the son, certainly is among the more moderate Republicans of his era. Nevertheless, he became notorious for having suggested, during his 2012 presidential campaign (aggravated, of course, by his having been surreptitiously caught on video making the criticism), that 47 percent of the people were "takers," in contrast, apparently, to good Republican producers. As Romney himself conceded to Chris Wallace of Fox News (reported by Chris Cillizza of *The Washington Post*), the comment was damaging, and made him look out of touch (Cillizza 2013).

Contrast this with George Romney, the father, another Republican governor (Michigan, for George; Massachusetts, for Mitt—where he pioneered a program of widespread health insurance), who was another would-be Republican candidate for the presidency (Mitt received the nomination; George did not). Before becoming governor, George was the highly successful CEO of American Motors, a major automobile company that manufactured an automobile, the Rambler, that for several years was extremely popular. As a corporate CEO George Romney did what today might seem unthinkable, either in politics or in economics: he rejected extra salary.

David Leonhardt looked back at earlier times in an interesting piece, "When the Rich Said No to Getting Richer," in *The New York Times*, in 2017. George Romney, he said, after turning down several large bonuses, told his board that he did so "because he believed that no executive should make more than $225,000 a year (which translates into almost $2 million today)." Romney's restraint came from his Mormon heritage, but also from a "culture of financial restraint that was once commonplace in this country." He did not try to make every dollar possible, nor did many other corporate peers. The CEO of a large American company, then, said Leonhardt, "made only 20 times as much as the average worker, rather than the current 271-to-1 ratio. Today, some CEOs make $2 million in a single month" (Leonhardt 2017).

In politics, consider whether it likely would have been possible for later politicians to be elected if they had echoed John F. Kennedy's stirring inaugural address of 1961. "Ask not what your country can do for you, ask what you can do for your country," he admonished. Following the "Reagan Revolution," one would have been far more likely to hear stark appeals to selfishness, as, "vote for me—I'll let you keep more of your hard-earned money. You can spend it better than government can!" Leonhardt pointed out the obvious: the tax structure had much to do with this. Now, it encourages concentration of wealth upward; then, it discouraged such upward skewing. Billionaires, non-existent then, are seen in the corporate world with increasing frequency because of a tax structure that explicitly encourages their creation. This phenomenon has as much to do with access to healthcare, and ultimately also with the quality of the care that is received, as it does with cultivation of the class of the ultra-wealthy.

Consider, also, in this regard, a great medical pioneer and humanitarian, Jonas Salk, the originator of the polio vaccine, a killed-virus vaccine that cannot itself cause polio. Today, polio is almost extinct. Virtually the only cases in the world are those caused—in extremely rare cases—by the live-virus Sabin vaccine, itself, which is no longer used in the US for that reason. Those of us of a certain age can all remember knowing someone who died from, or who was severely disabled from, polio (the disabled included a former president of the United States, Franklin D. Roosevelt). Perhaps equally horrible was the spectacle of the "iron lung." It was a coffin-like device in which those sufferers who had their breathing ability destroyed by the disease had to stay, literally in order to keep alive. Only the victim's head was outside the structure, which alternated pressure and release inside to provide an artificial respiration to permit the patient to breathe.

In the 1950s, those who today would be billionaires were "only" multi-millionaires. Considering the enormous scourge of polio, Salk could almost assuredly have been, literally, a billionaire in 1950s dollars, if he had patented his vaccine. "He did not even consider doing it, though, because he believed the vaccine should belong to the people" (Skidmore 2016, 9). By "the people," he meant not those cloistered and frightened behind a wall, but the people of the world. As the Salk Institute put it in a brief biographical statement, "hailed as a miracle worker, Salk never patented the vaccine or earned any money from his discovery, preferring it be distributed as widely as possible" (Salk Institute N.D.)

Blue Cross continues to exist, but it competes with profit-making companies in the insurance market and behaves accordingly. Many plans have openly shed their non-profit status; others ostensibly remain non-profit, but in most respects now function in a manner little different from their competitors who are openly profit-oriented.

When Franklin D. Roosevelt gave his State of the Union message in 1944, he called boldly for an "Economic Bill of Rights." He argued that many things should be added to the list of items considered as rights of citizenship. Among others, these included a well-paying job; decent housing; a good education; and comprehensive healthcare. He reiterated these in his next, and final, annual message, in 1945. Shortly thereafter, the great New Deal president died.

With no apparent recognition of the irony involved, Ronald Reagan a generation later called for his own "Economic Bill of Rights." Rather than implementing the rights of the people, Reagan's version would have made protecting the people even more difficult than it already was; he sought, instead, to secure the rights of the most privileged. His proposal attempted to counter what conservatives deemed to be "excesses of government budget policy." It would have required "a balanced federal budget every year," line-item veto authority on appropriations bills, a "super-majority vote for passing tax increases," and the like (see Boskin 1987 for a statement lauding Reagan's proposals from the point of view of an economic conservative). Reagan (and his supporters) erroneously equated the national government's budgetary policy with that of a family. Families, however, cannot create their own currency, paying their bills with money of their own creation; the government of the United States can, and in fact does so regularly. Moreover, by definition, super-majority requirements are explicitly undemocratic in that they empower a minority to thwart the will of the majority—in Reagan's case, this would have been a privileged minority formally endowed with permanent power to overrule the "will of the people."

FDR's successor as president, Harry Truman, was thwarted in his effort to implement FDR's second Bill of Rights, by a Republican takeover of both houses of Congress following the elections of 1946. Now, nearly three-quarters of a century later, FDR's bold plan has remained almost entirely beyond reach. Truman tried valiantly to secure universal healthcare, but in the face of enormous advertising campaigns and strong political propaganda on the part of the American Medical Association and other parts of the health community, he was unable to succeed.

Although he was prevented from expanding the New Deal, Truman fought back vigorously. He did succeed in holding the line against Republican efforts to roll back, or eliminate, New Deal programs. The Economic Bill of Rights, though, including its call for universal healthcare, got nowhere.

The far more conservative Eisenhower administration that followed Truman's made no effort to move toward healthcare for all. Significantly, however, Eisenhower did adopt what he called "Modern Republicanism," which meant an acceptance of basic New Deal programs. They had, Ike believed, become part of the "American Way of Life," and thus he halted efforts to curtail or eliminate them. He also, in 1956, signed into law a huge new benefit through Social Security: Disability benefits.

In contrast to Eisenhower, John F. Kennedy made healthcare his number-one domestic priority. By that time, the Democrats had more or less given up on universal healthcare as unrealistic at the moment, so the Kennedy Administration concentrated on healthcare for the most needy group, the aged. He worked diligently to secure what ultimately became "Medicare," embarking upon a furious battle with the American Medical Association and conservative forces in general, but by the time of his tragic assassination had made little headway.

Then came Lyndon Johnson, an acknowledged legislative genius, who succeeded. Medicare and Medicaid became law. They, along with environmental protections, fostering the arts, establishing public broadcasting, adopting the Freedom of Information Act, and many others, became part of LBJ's Great Society, along with its crown jewels: the Civil Rights Act of 1964 and the Voting Rights Act of 1965 (the latter, now, sadly, emasculated by the Supreme Court). Medicare's opponents had worked furiously to keep it from being enacted, but as then was customary among both Democrats and Republicans, once it was adopted, they worked for the good of the country to accept it, and improve it as time passed. No serious officeholder would have worked to make the program fail.

Subsequently, Richard Nixon proposed a plan to make health insurance more affordable for workers, but it failed. President Clinton, decades later, proposed a broad plan, somewhat similar to what later became the Affordable Care Act. Initially, large numbers of Republicans joined with Democrats to support the Clinton plan, but there also was formidable opposition from such activists as Newt Gingrich. Bill Kristol (1993), who had been chief of staff to the former vice president, Dan Quayle, sent a memorandum, in 1993, to all congressional Republicans—all Republican senators and all Republican representatives—urging them not to support such a bill so long as Clinton was in office. If it were to come, a Republican president should receive the credit. This memo was perhaps the coup de grace. All Republicans withdrew their support, and the bill died without even coming up for a vote.

The opponents had feared that Medicare would be "a foot in the door for socialized medicine." The supporters had hoped that it could be expanded until ultimately it became healthcare for all. Both were wrong.

The only truly substantial expansion of Medicare itself—despite the fears of opponents and the hopes of supporters—came under the administration of George W. Bush. Over the objections of many Republican conservatives—and most Democrats, who objected to the proposal's lack of a funding mechanism—Bush and his party succeeded in securing approval in both houses of Congress for Medicare Part D, the prescription-drug benefit. The inauguration of Part D was clumsy, awkward, and difficult but ultimately it began to function smoothly, and now provides a much-needed benefit for the people. It also provided, by design, an enormous boon for the pharmaceutical industry, which actually had supervised the Republican writing of the original bill, and it included an irrational "doughnut hole" in benefit coverage. The law is therefore flawed, but its flaws could easily be corrected, if the political climate permits it. At the moment, the flaws are worth enduring because of the good Part D accomplishes. In fact, the Affordable Care Act is gradually closing that infamous doughnut hole.

In 1997, President Clinton signed into law a joint federal-state program, SCHIP, to provide health services for children. President George W. Bush twice vetoed expansions of the plan on the grounds that the expanded plan would cover those who had sufficient resources to pay for healthcare. Expanding the plan, he thought, would point in the direction of healthcare for all.

President Obama, though, came to office in 2009 eager to make his mark on healthcare. During his first month in office, he signed expansions of SCHIP, and worked to move the country in the direction of universal health coverage. The next year, with strong efforts on the part of many Democrats—especially the enormously effective work by the leading Democrat in the House, Nancy Pelosi—Obama signed into law his signature accomplishment, the Affordable Care Act. Republicans soon sought to demonize it by referring constantly to it as the dreaded "Obamacare." After some resistance, President Obama actually accepted the term. Since then, despite virtually universal resistance from Republicans, persistent failed efforts to repeal it, and numerous attempts to sabotage the law and keep it from performing well, it has become increasingly popular.

Thus, even from this brief, incomplete summary, it is obvious that many ironies exist with regard to the evolutionary process that brought the complex, and often irrational, system that dominates healthcare delivery today in the United States. For instance, those on the American right, including much of the business community, tend to be ideologically opposed to government programs, with many exceptions for the exercise of police power over less-favored groups, or military programs. In most other countries, though, business has tended to be strong supporters of universal healthcare. They recognize that it is generally to their advantage to have the costs of healthcare spread widely throughout the economy, rather than falling especially upon the business community.

In America, by contrast, there has been such strong resistance on the right that complete opposition to universal healthcare, once supported by many in both parties, became a prominent feature of the Republican Party. Congressional Republicans all campaigned on a platform of "repealing Obamacare." Such resistance led to opposition even to the expansion of Medicaid, as provided by the Affordable Care Act, despite it being clearly to the advantage of states. Expansion would reduce the numbers of their people who lack health benefits, it would cause considerably more money to flow into the state, and the costs to the state would be minimal, because the federal government pays for nearly all the added expense. The opposition was both ideological, and personal: There was resistance to any expansion of government benefits, and also opposition to any program that President Obama had supported. The benefits of expansion were such, though, that many Republican governors and legislatures found ways to accomplish it, leaving only the most rigidly ideological states in the opposition.

This is the situation as it stands after the Obama presidency, and past the mid-point of Donald Trump's term in office. This is the chaotic reality with regard to America's healthcare delivery systems that Patel and Rushefsky scrutinize carefully. They admirably identify the patterns, presenting them in a manner that makes them accessible. They put their findings in readable form for the benefit of us all. Their work benefits citizens who seek to understand the complexity, scholars who attempt to make sense of what seems nonsensical, and especially—perhaps most important of all—for reformers who seek to bring improvements.

Reform ultimately may become Medicare for all, Medicaid for all, some other form of single-payer system, or another approach that helps to rationalize what exists by making care of high quality available to all who need it without huge financial demands. However it comes, and whatever form it takes, a prerequisite to improvement will be understanding of all the voluminous issues, not all of which will be immediately apparent. Patel and Rushefsky, with their keen appreciation of the nuances of the system have made signal contributions to the process. This book continues their important work, and promises to be the precursor of yet another study following the results of the forthcoming elections of 2020. It is an especially valuable contribution to the literature of healthcare in America.

Boskin, Michael J. 1987. "Reagan's Economic Bill of Rights," *Los Angeles Times*, July 14.
Cillizza, Chris. 2013. "Why Mitt Romney's '47 Percent' Comment Was so Bad." *Washington Post*, March 4.

Kristol, William. 1993. "Memorandum to Republican Leaders, Subject: Defeating President Clinton's Health Care Proposal." Online at www.scribd.com/doc/12926608/William-Kristols-1993-Memo-DefeatingpPresident-Clintons-Health-Care-Proposal.

Leonhardt, David. 2017. "When the Rich Said No to Getting Richer." *The New York Times*, September 17.

Salk Institute. n.d. "History of Salk: About Jonas Salk." Online at www.salk.edu/about/history-of-salk/jonas-salk/.

Skidmore, Max J. 1970. *Medicare and the American Rhetoric of Reconciliation*. Tuscaloosa, AL: University of Alabama Press.

Skidmore, Max J. 2008. *Securing America's Future: A Bold Plan to Secure, and Expand, Social Security*. Lanham, MD: Rowman and Littlefield.

Skidmore, Max J. 2016. *Presidents, Pandemics, and Politics*. New York: Palgrave Macmillan.

Witte, Edwin. 1962. *The Development of the Social Security Act*. Madison, WI: University of Wisconsin Press.

Max Skidmore
University of Missouri Curators' Distinguished Professor of Political Science and

Thomas Jefferson Fellow
University of Missouri at Kansas City

ACRONYMS

AAFP	American Academy of Family Physicians
AEI	American Enterprise Institute
ASRM	American Society for Reproductive Medicine
BLS	Bureau of Labor Statistics
CHIPRA	Children's Health Insurance Program Reauthorization Act
DEA	Drug Enforcement Agency
ECPs	emergency contraceptive pills
EPA	Environmental Protection Agency
GMO	genetically modified organisms
GWOT	Global War on Terror
HCBS	home- and community-based services
LTSS	long-term care services and support
MAGI	modified adjusted gross income
MAs	medical assistants
MLTSS	Medicaid long-term services and supports
MRT	mitochondrial replacement therapy
MST	military sexual trauma
NCCPA	National Commission on Certification of Physician Assistants
NPS	National Pharmaceutical Services
OSHA	Occupational Safety and Health Administration
PAs	physician assistants
PAS	physician-assisted suicide
PBMs	pharmacy benefit managers
PDMD	Prescription Drug Monitoring Program
UIHP	Urban Indian Health Program
UIOs	urban Indian organizations
USDA	United States Department of Agriculture
VSL	value of statistical life

ACKNOWLEDGMENTS

As is typical of any book, this text is not the product of its authors only. Patel would like to thank the Faculty Leave Committee at (Southwest) Missouri State University for the spring 1991 sabbatical that made the initial research for this project possible. We express our gratitude to Max Skidmore for his gracious offer to write the Foreword. We would also like to thank Laura Stearns, editor at Routledge, for her insightful judgment in continuing to support this project, and Katie Horsfall, along with the staff at Routledge. Of course, any remaining errors are the co-authors'.

Kant Patel
Mark Rushefsky

Section I
HEALTHCARE POLITICS AND POLICY

1

HEALTHCARE POLITICS

Healthcare is one of the more difficult areas of policymaking. Healthcare policymakers and providers must deal with a host of issues, ranging from jurisdictional authority, financing, organization, and administration of health policy and delivery to issues of vested interests, ideological and partisan conflicts, value conflicts, equity, and justice, access to healthcare and quality of care, and questions of life and death (Gauld 2001). Policymakers must address a host of difficult questions: what are the goals of the healthcare system? What do we hope to accomplish with a particular healthcare policy? Should patient participation be voluntary or mandatory? Should there be intermediaries (organizations that accept funds from sponsors to coordinate benefits and provider activities) between healthcare sponsors and healthcare providers? If there are intermediaries, how many should there be, and should they be for-profit or not-for-profit? How many sponsors should there be, and should they be governmental or private organizations? How should healthcare be funded, organized, and administered (Dudley and Luft 1999)? In addition, policymaking itself can be influenced by decision-making structures, that is, by the ways in which policymaking institutions like the executive, legislative, and judicial branches of government are organized and the rules by which they operate. It is very difficult to question and dramatically change decision-making structures and processes in healthcare, as in many other policy areas, because those with the greatest means and resources but not necessarily the best scientific evidence often are able to control the definition of "problem" and what the "truth" is. Thus, we must recognize the power of money/resources in influencing decision-making and policymaking processes in the field of healthcare (Tuulonen 2005).

Policymaking in healthcare is often more art than science since policymaking involves struggles over ideas and values (Stone 2011). This is illustrated by how numbers—statistics—are used by various actors in health policymaking. Statistics are an important tool for policymakers. They often serve as a warning signal indicating the existence or worsening of a problem, and they may be used to measure and evaluate policy outcomes. However, numbers can also be strategically used to further particular political agendas. It is often not the magnitude of numbers but rather the *interpretation* of the numbers that influences policymaking (Schlesinger 2004), while a great deal of the debate about healthcare policy is framed in terms of scientific, evidence-based medicine as if policy decisions are always driven by only facts and not societal values. This assumes that one can separate facts and values, that evidence is free of context and can be objectively weighed, and that health policymaking is essentially an exercise in scientific decision-making (Russell et al. 2008). In the real world, however, policymaking involves struggles over ideas and values. Debates over health policy are played out through the rhetorical use of language and the strategic portrayal of social situations. Policymaking revolves around the naming and framing of a problem (problem definition), the specification of problem boundaries, and the definition and negotiation of the ideas and values that guide the ways citizens create a shared meaning that motivates them to act (Russell et al. 2008).

It is also important to remember that health policymakers' decisions are also influenced by the underlying "politics." Thus, to understand health policy it is important to understand the underlying politics surrounding various health policy issues. Awareness of political factors such as partisanship, voters' views, public opinion, political ideology, values and belief systems, the power of entrenched interest groups, and the nature of media coverage, along with constitutional requirements and institutional arrangements, is essential to understanding health policymaking (Blendon and SteelFisher 2009; Theodoulou and Kofinis 2004; Weissert and Weissert 1996).

HEALTH POLICYMAKING IN THE UNITED STATES

Healthcare is the largest single industry in the United States (Skeen 2003). In 2016, the United States spent over $3.3 trillion on healthcare, which amounted to 17.9 percent of the gross domestic product (GDP) (Hartman et al. 2018). If spending on healthcare alone guaranteed physical well-being, Americans would be the healthiest people in the world. Unfortunately, spending alone does not ensure a high level of care, as witnessed by the fact that the American healthcare system does not fare well compared to other countries on several indicators such as infant mortality rates and average lifespan (see next chapter). It is not too surprising that the American healthcare system is often described as inefficient and ineffective (Freddi 2009) or as scandalous and wasteful (Dentzer 1990; Taylor 1990).

Health policymaking in the United States involves a complex web of decisions made by various institutions and political actors across a broad spectrum of public and private sectors. These institutions and actors include federal, state, and local governments in the public sector. In the private sector they include healthcare providers such as hospitals and nursing homes; healthcare professionals such as physicians; and healthcare purchasers such as insurance companies, industries, and consumers. In addition, a wide variety of interest groups and health-related professional associations influence and shape healthcare politics and policymaking.

These institutions and actors are involved throughout the policy cycle. This cycle includes getting problems to the government and agenda-setting; policy formulation and legitimation; budgeting, implementation and evaluation of policy, and decisions about policy continuation; and modifications and/or termination (Jones 1978; Rushefsky 2007). These institutions and actors interact at every stage of the policy cycle. No one institution or actor dominates any one stage of policy development. Each contributes to the process by providing input that often is designed to promote the individual institutions or the actor's own interests (Brown, Lawrence D. 1978).

Some of the problems in healthcare policymaking are rooted in this diversity of institutions and actors. Any decision designed to affect the healthcare system generates immediate and heated responses. Any attempt to regulate the healthcare system also produces pressures from opponents of regulation who favor market-oriented approaches to the delivery of healthcare. Government regulations have often been thwarted by those being regulated as well as by actors in the system who oppose a strong government role in the field of healthcare (Brown, J.H.A. 1978).

The development of a comprehensive and consistent healthcare policy is made difficult, if not impossible, by the shotgun approach followed by many policymakers, such as the president and Congress. For example, Congress deals with the most pressing problems one at a time and not in the framework of overall healthcare policy. Such an approach is often necessitated by the political realities of producing tangible results on a short-term basis for the purpose of reelection. Consequently, healthcare policy in the United States is in a constant state of fluidity. It lacks consistency and often encompasses a mishmash of programs involving conflicting values. Policymakers' discretion is often limited by a wide variety of restraints imposed by the policy environment. Just as a policy environment can help facilitate policymaking, it can also hinder policy development by the number and types of constraints it imposes on policymakers. The constraints imposed by the policy environment make it difficult for the government to resolve issues in a new or innovative manner (Rosenbaum 1985). The health policy environment can be thought of as a total matrix of factors that influence and shape the health policy cycle. These factors include constitutional or legal requirements, institutional settings, shared understandings about the rules of the game, cultural values of a society, political ideology, economic resources, and technological innovations and their impact on the cost and delivery of healthcare services.

Section I of this book examines the healthcare politics and policy in the United States. Chapter 1 has two goals: to provide a detailed and systematic analysis of the health policy environment that shapes healthcare policymaking and to examine the role played by key actors. Chapter 2 provides a historical perspective on the development of healthcare policy and the underlying politics in the United States.

Section II of the book examines government's healthcare programs created to provide healthcare services to those who for one reason or another are not covered by the private health insurance market. Thus, such government health programs are intended to supplement the largely private US healthcare system. Chapter 3 provides a detailed analysis of the enactment, main provisions, and implementation of the Affordable Care Act (ACA) of 2010, intended to overhaul the American healthcare system. Also examined are Republican efforts to defund and/or repeal, and repeal and replace ACA. Chapters 4 and 5 respectively examine the Medicaid and Medicare programs. Chapter 6 examines the role of the Indian Health Service and Veterans Health Administration (VHA) in meeting the healthcare needs of the American Indians and Alaska Natives (AI/AN) and veterans of the American wars. Chapter 7 examines the problem of the uninsured and the underinsured and healthcare disparities based on gender, race/ethnicity, and immigration status and equality and quality of care. It also examines social determinants of health.

Section III examines the problem of healthcare costs. In Chapter 8 we examine the high cost of care and factors contributing to escalating healthcare costs and provide an analysis of efforts to contain rising healthcare costs by the public and private sectors. In Section IV, we examine contemporary issues in the American healthcare system. Chapter 9 examines the role of biomedical technology, and the ethical dilemmas raised by such technologies with dealing with the beginning and end of life, and emergency contraceptives. Chapter 10 examines the current challenges confronting the American healthcare system such as the opioid crisis, the promise and pitfall of gene therapy, specialty drugs, the aging population and caring for the elderly, and the healthcare workforce.

Section V discusses the future of the American healthcare system. In Chapter 11 we discuss the potential implications and consequences of the election results of the November 2018 election and how it might influence future healthcare policy in the United States. We also discuss Republican/conservative and Democratic/liberal approaches to reforming American healthcare and reemphasize how health policy environment influences health policymaking in the United States.

THE HEALTH POLICY ENVIRONMENT

The Constitutional Environment

More than 200 years ago, the Founding Fathers established a constitutional system of government that had two purposes. First, it established a government with powers to act. But second, it also attempted to prevent a tyranny of the majority by creating a national government of limited powers. Having experienced the repressive measures of concentrated power under British rule, the Founding Fathers opted for a decentralized structure of government. The major features of the American system of government discussed next reflect these two conflicting objectives.

Separation of Powers, and Checks and Balances

The US Constitution created a system that disperses political power and decision-making authority among various branches of government. The powers of the national government are divided among the legislative, executive, and judicial branches of government. This is known as the separation of powers. The powers of the three branches are not totally separated, however, and thus it is more accurate to describe this arrangement as three coequal branches of government sharing powers. For example, "war powers" are shared by the president and Congress. The Constitution makes the president the commander-in-chief of the armed forces and gives him the power to wage a war, but the power to declare war is given to Congress. Similarly, the Constitution gives Congress the power to make laws but the president is given to power to veto laws. However, Congress can override a presidential veto by both houses of Congress passing the same legislation by a two-thirds vote in each house. The underlying principle behind such a sharing of powers was that it would lead to checks and balances among the three branches of government (Manning 2011). It is based on the assumption that other branches would check an attempt by one branch of government to assume too much power or abuse its powers. James Madison, one of the most influential delegates at the Constitutional Convention, argued in *The Federalist Papers* (No. 51) that "ambition must be made to counteract ambition" (Madison 1961a, 322).

A constitutional system of separation of powers and checks and balances with some exceptions creates constant competition among the three branches of government for preeminence in various policy areas. It necessitates lengthy negotiation, bargaining, and compromises in policymaking between the president and Congress. This makes it difficult to formulate a consistent and comprehensive set of policies. The result often is a government of deadlock and inaction. A period of unified government in which the same party controls the White House and both houses of Congress provides the party in power an opportunity to adopt its legislative agenda into policy assuming a comfortable Congressional majority and agreement on legislative agenda and priorities. Policymaking becomes more problematic during the periods of divided government when different political parties control the White House and Congress. This includes divided control of the Congress itself. We discuss the increased frequency of divided government in more detail under the section on "changing political environment" later in this chapter.

Federalism

A federal system of government is one in which the powers of the government are divided up between the national (central) government and its constituent units, that is, states. The national government and state governments share sovereignty. The Constitution gives exclusive authority over certain matters to the national government and over others to the states. Both levels of government are free to act in their areas of authority. Certain powers are shared by both levels of government. The residual or leftover powers are given to either the national government or the states. In a federal system, state government enjoys a considerable amount of autonomy and freedom. The actual balance of powers between the national and state governments may vary from one federal system to another. Examples of a federal system of government include the United States, Canada, and India. The advantages claimed for the federal system include regional autonomy and freedom, policy flexibility, innovations, and experimentation.

In a unitary system of government, the national government possesses all the power and is sovereign in all matters. It may delegate some of its powers to the states and may take them back. The state government enjoys only those powers that the national government delegates to it. The national government creates and is free to abolish them. Examples of a unitary system of government include Great Britain, Israel, France, and Finland. The advantages claimed for a unitary system include uniformity of laws and policies throughout the country, promotion of equality, and ability to act quickly and decisively. The reasons for a country to adopt a federal or unitary system of government depend on historical developments, shared experiences, practicality, and views about the use of governmental power.

The US Constitution, without even mentioning the word "federalism," created a federal system of government. An examination of various provisions in the Constitution reveals that it gives exclusive authority over certain subjects to the national government (e.g., foreign and defense matters), and state governments have the authority to legislate on all matters within their jurisdiction. States' "police power" does not derive from the Constitution but is viewed as an inherent characteristic of the states' territorial sovereignty (Thomas 2008). Certain powers, such as the power to tax, are shared by all levels of government. The Tenth Amendment to the Constitution specifies that powers not specifically given to the national government nor denied to the states are reserved for the states and their people. The Fourteenth Amendment to the Constitution also provides for the notion of dual citizenship, national and state.

Why did the Founding Fathers opt for a federal system of government? Some of the Founding Fathers held a conflicting view about the powers of and the relationship between different levels of governments. Alexander Hamilton believed in a powerful national government centered around a strong executive. In contrast, Thomas Jefferson believed in a decentralized system of government in which the federal government would focus mainly on foreign affairs while state and local government would set domestic policy. James Madison believed that the only way to limit the arbitrary use and exercise of excessive power by different levels governments should be through dividing up political power between different levels of government and creating a system of checks and balances (Sparer 2009a). The US federal system of government came about as a result of the Founding Fathers' desire to reconcile two strong but opposing views of Hamilton and Jefferson: the need to give the national government more authority and at the same time distrust of a single sovereign power. The US Constitution created a federal system of government that reflected Madison's approach to limiting powers of government. The Founders realized that the Articles of Confederation had failed because under it, the state government had too much authority and the national government was too weak to be effective in governing a new nation. On the other hand, the Founders feared too strong and powerful a national government as a threat to individual liberty and freedom. Their solution was a federal system. The new Constitution gave the national government stronger powers and at the same time created a government of limited powers, protecting individual liberty and states' rights (Bovbjerg, Wiener, and Houseman 2003). The hope was that such a division of powers between the national and state government, like the idea of the separation of powers, would create a system of checks and balances between the two levels (Nathan 2006). Despite the best efforts to divide up the power and authority between the national and state governments, some ambiguity in the allocation of power remained, creating a built-in tension between the levels of government.

Bovbjerg, Wiener, and Houseman (2003) provide an excellent analysis of arguments in favor of giving national or state government more powers. Those who advocate that state governments should be given more powers argue that geographically smaller governments know and represent citizens' values more, they know the unique nature of citizens' problems, and they can offer better solutions to those problems. In addition, they argue that interstate competition pressures states to improve their performance and attract and keep citizens and businesses. State governments can act as laboratories of democracy by experimenting with different policies, and such policies work better when implemented from the bottom up rather than the top down. On the other hand, proponents of giving more powers to the national government argue that national citizenship enjoys constitutional primacy and only the national government can provide uniformity and equality in areas such as Civil Rights because certain rights and responsibilities should not vary across states. Further, they argue that interstate competition promotes a race to the bottom rather than a race to the top among states. Interstate competition can also lead to a flight to the top, resulting in lower tax rates and revenue. Finally, proponents of giving more powers to the national government argue that certain problems are inherently national in scope and solving them requires the greater fiscal capacity of the national government (Bovbjerg, Wiener, and Houseman 2003).

How does the federal structure of government impact policymaking? Some have argued that a federal system of government has several negative consequences for policymaking. One, it adds to the fragmentation of authority and increases complexity, jurisdictional competition, delays, duplication, finger-pointing, and often the dodging of responsibilities by different levels of government. Second, attempts to reconcile many different geographical interests become problematic and tend to perpetuate a belief in organized chaos and flexible rules over central policymaking authority. The problem of regionalism and localism is accentuated by the need to satisfy the demands of a diverse and heterogeneous society. Thus, no single institution representing the nation as a whole defines the public interest and serves the public good. The result is a healthcare system made up of multiple "little governments" and "little empires" that pursue their own goals and interests. This, in turn, generates health policies that are vaguely defined and designed to serve "special publics" (Altenstetter 1974, 26–27). Third, the federal structure makes government slow to respond to new challenges because of the cumbersome nature of decision-making and policymaking as well as implementation structures (Nathan 2005).

Others have argued that the federal structure has several positive impacts on policymaking and implementation. First, it allows states to act as laboratories for policy innovation and experimentation. Second, it provides needed flexibility to state governments to adapt and implement national policies to fit local conditions. Third, it leads to cooperation and establishment of a partnership between different levels of governments in the area of policymaking and implementation (Balducchi and Wander 2008).

The continuing debate in US politics for over 200 years about the nature and meaning of American federalism suggests the tension and struggle between the national and state governments over power and authority to make and implement policies is likely to continue into the future. After examining the historical account of the founding of the federal system, Purcell (2009) observed that the Founders disagreed more and settled less with regard to federalism.

To what extent do the constitutional arrangements such as the federal structure of government influence the type of public policies in general and health policy in particular that are produced? Does federalism make a difference? Of course, as Banting and Corbett (2002) have suggested, political institutions alone are never determinative. Constitutional and institutional factors interact with other factors in shaping health policies. Thus, one can never assert that the federal structure of government leads to policy X. On the other hand, structures of governments are never completely neutral, because they make some outcomes easier than others. Experts and scholars are divided about whether the national or state government should have more powers and whether the federal structure of government has positive or negative effects on policymaking. The arguments range from philosophical to practical. What is clear is that health policymaking in the United States is a very complex process involving the private and public sectors and including multiple levels of government, and the distribution of authority and responsibility within the federal system does impact the making and implementation of health policymaking (Lee and Estes 1983).

Given that the Constitution was written and put into effect in the eighteenth century, it is not surprising that it is silent with respect to the national government's power/authority in the area of healthcare. However, two enumerated powers granted to the national government in the Constitution—Congress's power to tax and spend for the general welfare (James Madison viewed the "general welfare" clause as tied directly to national government's enumerated powers), and Congress's power to regulate interstate commerce—significantly influenced the development of health policy in the United States. The national government's power and responsibilities in the health area grew and expanded through various intergovernmental mechanisms such as grants-in-aid and healthcare financing, federal emergency relief to states, funded and unfunded mandates and regulations, and the creation of national government's health programs such as Medicare, Medicaid, and SCHIP (Colby 2002).

The controversy over whether power and authority should be more centralized in the national government or more decentralized in state and local governments has been a perennial question in US politics. In addition, both the national and the state governments have often delegated important functions to thousands of units of local government. As a result, it is difficult to find many governmental activities that do not, to some extent, involve all three levels of government. Thus, despite the increased role of the federal government in the healthcare field during the 1960s, overall authority over health policy remains divided and shared among the national, state, and local governments.

Federalism has played a major role in the piecemeal evolution of healthcare policy in the United States (Moncrieff and Lawless 2017). The controversy over the role of the state versus the national government in health policy, finance, and reform has been a steady staple of scholarly debate in American politics (Adler 2011; Beland and Vergniolle de

Chantal 2004; DiIulio and Nathan 1994; France 2008; Greer and Jacobson 2010; Hackey and Rochefort 2001; Holahan, Weil, and Wiener 2003; Nathan 2005; Peterson 2001; Plein 2010; Rich and White 1996; Stanek 2014).

Many of the federal health policies and programs are implemented by the state and local governments. The federal government has used a variety of carrot-and-stick approaches to encourage state government participation in adoption, expansion, and implementation of federal health programs. Some of these tactics include pre-empting state action, imposing federal mandates, threating withdrawal of federal funds for non-compliance, giving states more flexibility in the implementation of federal programs through waivers and giving states different options for participating in federal health programs and providing financial incentives.

The following examples illustrate the use of such tactics by the federal government. Following scandals involving private defined-benefit pension plans that left employees without their expected retirement income when their firms went bankrupt, Congress passed the Employee Retirement Income Security Act of 1974, a federal law that pre-empted state policy actions by setting minimum standards for most voluntary pension and health benefit plans in private industry in order to protect individuals in such plans (Pope 2013). The law superseded any and all state laws related to any employee benefit plan covered by the law. From the time Medicaid program was created in 1965 to the mid-1980s, the federal government had granted states broad decision-making authority with very few detailed federal requirements. However, starting in the mid-1980s federal government imposed a series of mandates forcing states to expand eligibility standards especially for pregnant women and children (Sparer 2009b). Almost all recent administrations from Ronald Reagan to Donald Trump have granted state governments waivers to allow them to experiment with Medicaid program. The original Medicaid program also provided states with financial incentives to encourage their participation in the program by providing federal matching funds ranging from 50 to 77 percent of the total cost of the program. Similarly, to encourage states to expand their Medicaid program, under the Affordable Care Act (ACA) of 2010 the federal government agreed to pay 100 percent of the cost of Medicaid expansion from 2014 to 2016 and then 90 percent of the cost (Callaghan and Jacobs 2013). ACA also gave states the option to create and manage their own insurance exchanges, partner with the federal government, or to let the federal government create exchanges. In summary, many of the federal health programs, such as the Medicaid program, the Children's Health Insurance Program (CHIP), and the ACA, are an experiment in federalism with respect to policy adoption and implementation (Bagley 2017; Dinan 2008; Doonan 2013; Dropp, Jackman, and Jackman 2013; Thompson 1986, 2012; Thompson and DiIulio 1998).

The Institutional Environment

The institutional environment consists of the rules, structures, and settings within which major institutions involved in policymaking and implementation operate. These include the legislative, executive, and judicial branches of government. Congress is the primary policymaking institution, while the executive is primarily responsible for implementing policies. The judiciary's principal responsibility is to resolve constitutional and legal conflicts. Since the beginning of the twentieth century, however, these areas of responsibility have become increasingly blurred, with all three branches of government sharing powers in the areas of policymaking, implementation, and adjudication.

Congress

Policymaking in Congress takes place in an environment of a decentralized and fragmented power structure where political power is dispersed among numerous committees and subcommittees in both chambers. This decentralization of power and authority in the committee structure has led some to describe Congress as a "kind of confederation of little legislatures" (Huitt 1970, 410). One of the consequences of this in health policymaking is competition among committees within and between the Senate and the House. The second consequence for health policymaking is bargaining and compromises. Thus, health policy formulation in Congress occurs in numerous subsystems with little coordination (Brown, Lawrence D. 1978). Both the House and the Senate operate by their own unique set of rules established by each body.

Under the leadership of Speaker Newt Gingrich (1995–1999), the Republican majority attempted to coordinate committee action under tight leadership control. House Speaker Newt Gingrich brought about more centralization of power in the House. He often stepped in and overruled committee chairmen on a range of significant legislation. This shift of power in the Speaker's office led at times to some loss of autonomy of committee chairs. However, in general, the ability of an individual to maintain discipline over party members and use policy expertise is often found only in chairs of committees and subcommittees (Koszczuk 1995). Since the mid-1990s, Republican speakers' attempts to limit the power of the minority party also followed an informal rule that the speaker would not allow a floor vote on a bill unless a majority of the majority party supported the bill. Republican Speaker of the House Dennis Hastert (1999–2007) explicitly adopted this rule and thus it came to be known as the Hastert Rule, also referred to as "the majority of the majority rule," even though Newt Gingrich, who preceded Hastert in the speakership role, had followed the same rule. The rule is essentially intended to prevent the minority party from passing a bill with the support of the minority members of the majority party. Thus, even if a bill has a majority support of the full House, it is prevented from becoming a law unless majority members of the majority party are in favor of it. Since it is an informal rule the speaker is free to use his/her discretion to invoke the rule. Republican speakers have frequently followed this rule when they are in the majority. Needless to say, such a rule makes bipartisan policymaking very difficult in the House.

Some of the rules of the United States Senate also make it difficult for the majority to prevail when it comes to policymaking. The most well-known rule is the "cloture." The Senate cloture rule originally required a supermajority of two-thirds of senators present and voting to prevent a filibuster of a bill. In 1975, the Democratic majority in the Senate reduced the necessary supermajority to three-fifths of the Senate, i.e., 60 votes out of 100. To prevent a minority of senators from filibustering a bill (killing a bill), 60 senators must vote to stop the floor debate on the bill and proceed to take a final vote on the bill. The cloture is justified on the ground that it is designed to prevent a "tyranny of the majority" by allowing a minority of senators who feel intensely about a bill to prevent its passage. Another additional factor that makes policymaking problematic in Congress is the fact that Senators and representatives are elected to represent their respective states and smaller congressional districts. This creates a tendency to promote state and local interests and makes members of Congress less sensitive to national interests and needs in healthcare policymaking.

A relatively new phenomenon that has become a critical feature of the Congressional policymaking landscape is the role of caucuses. A caucus refers to members of Congress who form themselves into small groups because of shared interests and meet regularly to promote causes they believe in. For example, Burgin (2003), after examining the important role played by the Diabetes Caucus in successfully pushing diabetes-related legislation through Congress, suggests that the role of caucuses in policymaking in Congress is unappreciated. Such caucuses may be based on race/ethnicity, such as a "Hispanic" or "African American" caucus, or gender, such as a "Women's Caucus," or a specific issue, such as the Diabetes Caucus. She further argues that a caucus often acts as a "policy entrepreneur" waiting for a window of opportunity to open in order to push their legislative agenda through Congress (Burgin 2003).

Research also suggests that policymaking in Congress has become more problematic because of increased partisanship and ideological polarization, making it difficult to engage in bargaining, compromises, and consensus building. Members who are elected from safe congressional districts (districts with very little two-party competition) are more likely to engage in partisan conflict even though partisanship damages the collective reputation of the Congress as an institution (Harbridge and Malhotra 2011). Ramirez (2009), after examining the quarterly congressional-approval data from 1974 to 2000 to determine the consequences of partisan conflict on congressional approval, concluded that over time changes in partisan conflict within the legislature have a direct and lasting effect on how citizens think about Congress. The increased ideological polarization and partisanship is also often accompanied by what Uslaner (1993) calls the decline of comity in Congress, that is, of the adherence to a set of norms including courtesy and reciprocity. In September 2009, during President Obama's speech to the joint session of Congress explaining his healthcare reform legislation, Republican Congressman Joe Wilson from South Carolina shouted, "You lie!", shocking many members of Congress and viewers. This is a perfect example of the decline in comity in Congress. This issue of partisanship and ideological polarization is discussed further in the section on the changing political environment later in the chapter.

One of the consequences of the unwillingness to compromise and bargain due to increased partisanship and ideological polarization is that Congress has come to rely on a full range of unusual special procedures and processes, such as filling the amendment tree (Senate), fewer conferences, more formal amendments, and earmarks and changes in the appropriation process. Sinclair (2012) refers to it as making nonincremental policy changes through hyper-unorthodox procedures. She cites the Bush-Pelosi-Boehner Stimulus Bill of 2008, the America Recovery and Reinvestment Act (ARRA) of 2009, and the Patient Protection and Affordability Care Act (PPACA) of 2010, also known as the Affordable Care Act (ACA), as recent examples of nonincremental policy changes made through hyper-unorthodox procedures.

The Executive

The Constitution assigns the president and the executive branch agencies (i.e., the bureaucracy) the role of implementing policies approved by Congress. In contrast to Congress, at least in theory, power in the executive branch is more centralized because the Constitution makes the president the chief executive. The executive branch is headed by one person, and the president is the highest official in the executive branch. Yet he does not directly control about 85 percent of the civil servants who work in the executive branch, because they are hired and promoted through a competitive civil service exam, and firing a civil servant is a slow and cumbersome process. The president appoints only about 15 percent of the top "political executives"—executive department heads and the like who serve at the pleasure of the president. This institutional feature is designed to make bureaucracy provide continuity from one administration to the next and to make bureaucracy semi-independent and impartial and not subject to the whims of political bosses who are elected to office for a fixed term and do not hold their office permanently. Even though the president is the chief executive, there are constraints on his ability to significantly influence the executive branch. He can accomplish some changes through executive orders, but any major reorganization of the executive branch requires congressional approval.

When it comes to presidential policymaking, it is said that the president proposes and Congress disposes; that is, the president proposes major policy initiatives and Congress acts on them by either accepting, modifying, or rejecting presidential initiatives. Presidents have been making policy since the time of George Washington and have become increasingly active in agenda-setting, decision-making, coalition-building, and the implementation of government policies (Light 2000). However, as Jones (1994) reminds us, the United States does not have a presidential system, and the president's impact on domestic policy is shaped by resources, advantages, and strategic position.

Increased partisanship, ideological and issue polarization, and divided government have made it difficult for the president and Congress to compromise and work together. The resulting legislative gridlock has led presidents to use techniques such as making recess appointments as a way to bypass the Senate's advice and consent role (Black et al. 2007), adopting new "interpretations" of statutes to further their policy goals and agenda (Luton 2009), and making frequent use of signing statements (Biller 2008). Presidents have used signing statements as a way to construe the intent of the bill passed by Congress they sign including claiming authority to disobey the laws passed by Congress. The practice of presidents using signing statements as a tool to shape policy agenda started with President Reagan but intensified during the administration of George W. Bush. The American Bar Association in 2006 issued a report decrying the misuse of presidential signing statements (Kennedy 2014). Presidents have also occasionally used signing statements as a way of rewarding specific members of Congress by giving them credit for the legislation (Evans and Marshall 2016). One of the consequences of the Congressional gridlock is the expansion of presidential power because the president and the executive branch are forced to act alone. This in turn has given rise to the administrative state (Bulman-Pozen 2016).

Another tool a president has to influence policymaking is the threat of and use of presidential veto and pocket veto. The Constitution gives the president the power to veto legislation passed by Congress. This is a major tool the president can use to prevent the passage of legislation that he does not like or disagrees with. It is difficult to override a presidential veto since it requires both houses of Congress to pass the same legislation with a two-thirds vote, which is not easy. The pocket veto is an absolute veto that cannot be overridden by Congress. Normally a president has a ten-day window to sign a bill into law. However, if the president refuses to sign a bill and Congress adjourns before the ten-day window has passed, the bill is dead since Congress is not in session to override the veto (Lewallen 2017; "Presidential Vetoes" 2017; Tenpas 2006). It is also important to recognize the important role played by bureaucratic agencies in health policymaking. Congress routinely delegates the authority for making many decisions to bureaucratic agencies. For example, Congress created the Occupational Safety and Health Administration (OSHA) and gave it the authority to write regulations concerning workers' health, safety, and privacy in the workplace. In addition, Congress often passes laws that are vague, very broad, or both, leaving bureaucratic agencies a significant amount of discretionary power to fill in the details of the law. Congress uses its legislative oversight and budgetary powers to exercise control over bureaucratic agencies. Nevertheless, the fact remains that congressional delegation of authority and discretionary power enjoyed by bureaucratic agencies gives them a significant role in health policymaking and implementation.

As with Congress, power and authority in the bureaucracy is highly dispersed and fragmented. Various health policies are under the jurisdiction of many different federal agencies, which in turn creates overlapping jurisdictions, authority, and responsibilities. In addition, as we discussed earlier, in a federal system of government, state bureaucracies implement many federal programs either partially or totally. Such dispersal and fragmentation of authority creates competition and conflicts along both vertical and horizontal planes throughout the health policy cycle. Turf fighting over program implementation, authority, and resources becomes the name of the game. The health policy cycle operates in a dynamic environment of constantly changing alignments of bureaucratic agencies, congressional committees, policymakers, and various interest groups shaping and reshaping health policy.

The Judiciary

The standard and general explanation of American government and policymaking is that Congress makes the law, the executive branch agencies implement the law, and the courts apply the law as written, as long as such laws are constitutional. In this explanation, courts and judges are viewed as influencing policymaking and implementation only indirectly and only to a limited extent.

Courts and judges influence health policymaking and implementation by the way in which they interpret the Constitution and laws. They make sure that implementation of laws meets constitutional standards and that administrative agencies discharge their assigned responsibilities. Federal courts are also responsible for enforcement of the Administrative Procedures Act, which governs administrative procedures in all federal agencies. In addition, individuals and groups who feel that the executive and legislative branches have failed to redress their grievances often resort to seeking help from the courts.

Miller and Barnes (2004) challenge this standard explanation of American government and policymaking. They argue that no one dominant institution or even a consistent pattern of relationships exists among various players in the federal policymaking process. They argue that at different times and under different circumstances, all branches of government play a role not only in making public policy but also in enforcing and legitimizing public policies as well. Epstein and Knight (1998) suggest that justices realize that their ability to achieve their policy and other goals depends on the preferences of other actors and choices they expect others to make as well as the institutional context in which they act. Thus, they take such factors into account in their decision-making. In fact, the judicial process operates at the intersection of law and politics, and courts not only enforce norms and resolve disputes but also engage in policymaking and shape the fundamental power relationships between various institutions in American politics (Porto 2009).

Thus, the view that American courts and judges are policymakers has become accepted wisdom among political scientists (Bloom 2001). In fact, Malcolm and Rubin (2000) argue that policymaking is a standard and legitimate function of the modern courts. They provide a detailed analysis of how between 1965 and 1990, federal judges in almost all of the states handed down sweeping rulings that affected virtually every prison and jail in the United States. The federal courts formulated and implemented major prison reform policies. Law (2010) provides an analysis of the federal judiciary's role in the nation's immigration policy. Similarly, after examining the active role played by the courts in Medicaid nursing facility reimbursement, Miller (2008) concludes that neither the executive nor the judiciary acts in isolation, but instead, they often serve as tandem institutions in guiding federal oversight of state policymaking.

The federal courts in general and the US Supreme Court in particular have come to play a significant role in policymaking in many aspects of the healthcare field because decisions of the Supreme Court become the law of the land. The Supreme Court's 1973 decision in *Roe v. Wade,* effectively legalizing abortion, was a major policy decision and a victory for groups supporting a woman's right to have an abortion. Similarly, the impact of healthcare technology on the treatment and delivery of health services and the ethical concerns raised by medical technology have drawn state and federal courts into such varied topics as reproductive rights, organ transplants, stem cell research, healthcare surrogacy, quality of life, and the right to die with dignity, among others. The role of the federal courts and the Supreme Court in particular in policymaking in these areas is examined in more detailed in Chapter 9 of the book (also see Patel and Rushefsky 2002).

The US Supreme Court has also played a major role in policymaking in the areas of Medicaid and the Affordable Care Act. In 2010, the Supreme Court in *National Federation of Independent Business v. Sebelius* ruled that the ACA was constitutional because Congress had the authority to mandate individuals to purchase health insurance and to impose a tax penalty under its power to tax on individuals who failed to purchase health insurance. In the same case, the Supreme Court also ruled that Congress cannot force the state to expand its Medicaid program under the ACA or face losing federal funds. This gave states the option of deciding for themselves whether they wanted to expand their Medicaid program under the ACA. In subsequent decisions dealing with ACA, the Supreme Court has added additional restrictions on some of the provisions of the Act (Brown-Nagin 2014; Hall 2013; Nichols 2012; Parmet 2016).

The discussion above points to the interconnection of federal judiciary and politics. Federal judges are appointed by the president and confirmed or rejected by the US Senate. Among the many criteria considered by the president in his selection of candidates for the federal judiciary are nominee's party affiliation, political ideology, and judicial philosophy. That is why, historically, Democratic presidents have largely nominated Democrats to the judiciary, and Republican presidents have largely nominated Republicans. Similarly, senators' own party affiliations and ideologies play a role in their decision to confirm or reject a nominee. Supreme Court nominations have failed to be confirmed by the Senate through the use of filibuster with some regularity since the early days of the Republic, but in recent years, increased partisan and ideological polarization has led to more gridlock between the president and the Senate over nominations to the federal judiciary.

In the past, the Senate used the same cloture rule (requiring 60 votes) for the confirmation of federal court nominees as it did for the passage of a major law. However, in 2013, when Republicans in the Senate blocked confirmation of several of President Obama's nominees to the US Courts of Appeal, the Democratic majority leader Harry Reid revised the Senate rule to eliminate filibuster of nominees to the federal courts except for the Supreme Court. In 2017, facing strong opposition from Democrats to President Trump's nomination of conservative Neil Gorsuch to the Supreme Court, the Republican majority eliminated the filibuster for the Supreme Court nominees. Thus, today, a simple majority vote is required to confirm nominees to the federal courts, including the Supreme Court, of the United States.

The Political Environment

The political environment includes a shared understanding among policymakers about how policy decisions should be made and of underlying values, political feasibility, electoral cycles, influence of organized interest groups, and political ideologies. The political environment itself is influenced and shaped by the constitutional, legal, institutional, economic, and technological environment of a given policy area.

Consensus-Building

The constitutional and institutional environments create diffused and fragmented systems of authority and responsibility in the health policy cycle. This, in turn, produces a political environment that is conducive to constant bargaining and compromises among major institutions and key actors in policymaking. Since no single institution or actor is in a position to dominate the process, coalition-building becomes inevitable. It also injects logrolling (trading votes to secure favors) into the policy process. One of the consequences of this environment is that the policymaking process is invariably driven toward consensus-building among diverse and conflicting interests, which often results in contradictory policies or policies that contain conflicting values (Allison 1971). Thus, the policymaking process, instead of being a science of creating a policy that solves a problem, becomes an art of creating a consensus that holds conflicting and diverse interests together in order to create majority support for that policy. The political logic of coalition-building in order to create a consensus creates a situation in which any measure that is successful, be it congressional or presidential, will have been changed in ways its proponents did not foresee or desire (Brown, Lawrence D. 1978). Attempts at comprehensive and major policy change often fail.

Political compromises and consensus-building between political parties in Congress and between the president and Congress have become more difficult in recent years due to increased political polarization in American society.

Incrementalism and Punctuated Equilibrium

Policymakers also share decision-making values that favor incremental policymaking, that is, relatively small or incremental changes and modifications in existing policies. Thus, rather than consider all possible alternatives in a comprehensive manner, policymakers concentrate only on marginal values or relatively few alternatives that bring about marginal changes in existing policies, that is, incrementalism (Lindblom 1959). The incremental theory of policymaking posits that the policymaking process should involve bargaining, delay, and compromises that lead to an incremental change in public policies. Incrementalism itself is viewed as a natural by-product of a system of checks and balances in which policymakers disagree over policy goals and how best to achieve them (Hayes 2001, 2006).

Incremental policymaking is politically attractive to policymakers because small policy adjustments reduce the impact of negative and politically risky consequences. Nevertheless, incremental policymaking can also inhibit imagination, innovation, and fresh new approaches to the solution of problems (Rosenbaum 1985). Policymakers end up creating policies aimed at "satisfying" diverse interests, rather than problem-solving. Herbert Simon (1957) first introduced the term "satisficing" to describe an outcome that is good enough. In other words, "satisficing" involves behavior that attempts to achieve some minimum level of a particular variable but does not strive to achieve its maximum possible value. He called this "bounded rationality."

While it is true that policymaking in the United States largely follows a pattern of incremental changes, major and significant policy changes have occurred from time to time in American history, such as the creation of

Social Security and welfare programs, Medicare and Medicaid, and the prescription drug coverage program. The incremental theory fails to explain such major policy changes. Recent research has suggested that the punctuated equilibrium theory better explains policymaking and policy outcomes (Robinson and Carver 2006).

The theory of punctuated equilibrium was first presented by Baumgartner and Jones (1993, 2009) in their book *Agendas and Instability in American Politics* and further refined in the second edition. They draw our attention to forces in politics that create stability as well as forces that make dramatic changes and innovations in public policy possible. According to them, such punctuations come rarely, but they can produce long-lasting consequences. The political system, at times, creates opportunities and makes it possible for dramatic policy changes to occur occasionally. However, such changes are rare because most efforts to produce significant changes fail, and no single policy actor's behavior determines the outcome. Rather, the policy process depends on interaction and expectation of several players in the process. A sluggish political system can act suddenly if outside pressure becomes strong enough and reaches a tipping point, forcing a political system to act (Baumgartner 2006). For example, the Great Depression and resulting economic crisis led to the election of Franklin Roosevelt and created a receptive climate for the adoption of the New Deal programs. Determinants of policy change are characterized by positive and negative feedback. Since negative feedback threatens existing policies, entrenched interests that favor the status quo rise up to beat back the forces demanding change. Sources of negative feedback include structural and institutional as well as behavioral factors, such as division of powers between national and state governments in a federal system; separation and diffusion of power between and within political institutions such as the executive, legislative, and judicial branches of government; and the tendency of entrenched interests to mobilize to support the status quo and oppose policy change. This negative feedback must be counterbalanced with positive feedback. Sources of positive feedback include factors such as the bandwagon effect for change, social learning, strong public opinion demanding change, and intense media attention paid to a policy issue. When a positive feedback force reaches a critical mass or tipping point, forces of entrenched interests can be defeated, making a major policy change and innovation possible (Repetto 2006).

Static, cross-sectional theory of incrementalism is challenged by punctuated equilibrium theory, which involves time-series analysis of dynamic processes in which an extended period of stability (incrementalism) is punctuated by short periods of instability during which major policy changes can take place, bypassing entrenched interests. In other words, public policies alternate between stasis and punctuation. The punctuated equilibrium theory itself has led to an examination of the role of information processing in policymaking (Breunig and Koski 2006; Givel 2010; Pump 2011; Robinson et al. 2007; Wood 2006; Workman and Jochim 2009).

Political Feasibility

Policymakers are also influenced and guided in their policy deliberations by political feasibility (Huitt 1970). This involves judgment about whether it is possible to enact a policy given the political realities and the political environment. One of the major political realities that policymakers face is the potential public reaction to a proposed policy. Members of Congress are more apt to support and vote for a policy that is likely to be popular with their constituents than a policy that may produce a strong negative reaction from them. For example, members are more likely to support tax cuts over increased taxes. Throughout the book, we have discussed how public opinion has shaped healthcare politics and policy. All the major institutions and actors involved in policymaking are influenced by considerations of political feasibility. This is especially true of elected public officials.

Electoral Cycle

Policymakers are influenced in their deliberations by the electoral cycle and the necessity of reelection. Thus, policy decisions are viewed from the perspective of potential electoral consequences. This is all the more true near election time. The policymaking process is driven by the need to produce short-term tangible benefits. The fact that the president, senators, and representatives not only have different constituencies to serve but different term lengths in office makes electoral calculations a permanent fixture of the political environment. For example, after the failure of healthcare reform during the Clinton administration in the 1990s, healthcare reform reemerged on the national agenda in 2008 presidential election. The Democratic presidential candidate Barack Obama campaigned on the platform of healthcare reform to make health insurance more affordable, reduce the number of the uninsured, and to contain rising healthcare costs. His victory paved the way for the passage of the ACA in 2010.

Public Philosophy

The term "public philosophy" can be defined as an outlook on public affairs shared by a wide coalition in a nation (Beer 1965). A public philosophy often may not be explicit, but the ideological debate on issues takes place within its confines.

The underlying principle in American public philosophy, resulting from constitutional guarantees of freedom of speech, expression, and petition, is that organized interests should have an important role in influencing public policies. The public philosophy in the United States was influenced greatly by the writing of John Locke, a seventeenth-century English philosopher. A central feature of Locke's argument is the belief that ultimate authority resides in the individual's inalienable right to seek his or her own self-preservation. According to Locke, people form a government to protect their natural right of self-preservation. For Locke, this right is closely associated with the right to acquire property, an idea that pervades American political thought and institutions (Bayes 1982).

The clearest integration of this Lockean idea is found in James Madison's "Federalist 10." According to Madison, a faction constitutes a number of citizens united by a common passion or interest adverse to the rights of other citizens or to the permanent and aggregate interests of the community. Madison argued that factions were evil and could lead to tyranny. Yet, elimination of the causes of factions was not a solution, because it could also destroy liberty. Therefore, Madison advocated controlling the effects of factions. Since American society is composed of a large number of geographic, ethnic, racial, economic, and religious groups, the way to control the negative effects of factions, according to Madison, was to create a representative form of government. In such a representative government, public views can be refined and enlarged by passing them through the medium of a chosen body of citizens (the legislature) whose wisdom can help determine the true interest of the country. Madison also asserted that a large republic was less susceptible to tyranny than a small one because in a large republic many different interests will exist, making it difficult for any single interest to regularly dominate all others (Madison 1961b).

This, in turn, helped to create a philosophy of liberalism, which argues that all interests should be able to penetrate the political arena. Theodore Lowi describes this philosophy as interest-group liberalism (Lowi 1967). This is called a pluralistic system, which is characterized by many channels of access, with various interest groups exercising countervailing veto power. This system is justified in terms of equality and the openness that guarantees political freedom, which in turn can be used to achieve social and economic freedoms (Wilsford 1991).

The decentralized governmental structure based on separation of powers, checks and balances, and federalism is designed to give interest groups access throughout the policy cycle. Thus, ironically, a Madisonian system designed to prevent a tyranny of the majority and control the mischiefs of factions (interest groups) also gives these factions many opportunities for devilment. To formulate a public policy under such a system requires public officials and institutions to reconcile the conflicting interests of many organized groups. In theory, the role of the government becomes one of neutral arbitrator resolving conflicts among organized groups. The broad and diffused distribution of political influences across numerous and diverse interest groups blurs the distinction between public and private power (Truman 1951).

Private interests battle with one another and define themselves in terms of the public interest. But because all interest groups do not have equal resources, those with more economic resources have greater access to channels of influence and thus more opportunities for engaging in mischief. As McConnell (1966) has persuasively argued, small groups monopolize political power by successfully defining their own narrow interests as the general public interest. In a pluralistic system, the public philosophy of interest-group liberalism makes possible private economic, regional, and constituency interests to be justified as public interests by appealing to values of individualism, constitution, democracy, freedom, and equality, which make up an important part of American culture and belief systems. Private interests, as well as public officials, often justify their narrow parochial interests as public interest. The consensus created from compromises and bargaining among competing interests gets defined as the public interest. The role of the government, according to the pluralistic formulation, becomes one of protecting these diverse and competing interests by creating a consensus through the give-and-take of politics.

The framework of pluralism assumes that multiple elites rule specific areas of public policy as a "subgovernment" or an "iron triangle." The concept of subgovernment or iron triangle presumes a small circle of participants, such as a couple of congressional committees (a few legislators), executive agencies (a few bureaucrats), and interest groups that become semiautonomous in policymaking in a particular policy area (Mawhinney 2001). However, others have argued that while this scenario is true in explaining policymaking prior to the 1970s, these concepts of rigid subgovernment or iron triangle no longer capture the role of interest groups in policymaking (Heclo 1978). The interest group explosion of the 1970s has replaced the subgovernment or iron triangle model of policymaking with the issue networks model of policymaking. Issue networks are composed of a large number of participants with variable degrees of mutual commitment or dependence on others in the environment (Heclo 1978). Interest groups form networks and alliances with other groups for the purpose of working together to act as policy advocacy groups to achieve mutual objectives. This idea of issue networks has become widely accepted as an empirical description of how policymaking takes place in the United States (Heaney 2004; Tichenor and Harris 2002/2003).

Reforming the present American healthcare system is difficult because every reform proposal gets trapped in pluralistic processes designed to safeguard all existing professional and organizational interests.

Interest Groups, Lobbying, and Policymaking

Interest groups try to influence policy process by endorsing and/or giving a campaign contribution to candidates for public office and through the dissemination of information on subject matters they claim to have the expertise or specialize in. The campaign contributions are used as a tool to get attention and to gain "access" to relevant policymakers. Dissemination of specialized information is seen as a way to influence the legislative policymaking process. In addition, interest groups use their economic resources to lobby for or against specific issues. Interest groups also sometimes fund policy research and use the research to influence policy process (Stone 2011).

The rise and active participation of interest groups in policymaking have been traced to government mobilization of interest groups during World War I because of the government's need to coordinate industry to meet wartime production needs (Herring 1967). However, Truman (1951) has argued that the group mobilization that occurred during the Great Depression is an example of how the economic crisis and social disturbances can give rise to interest groups and lobbying organizations. During the 1950s and 1960s, the Civil Rights movement, Women's Rights movement, and consumer and environmental activism also served as a catalyst for the rise of organized interests in American society (Walker 1991). However, prior to the 1950s, the lobbying community of organized interests in Washington, DC was relatively small. The immense growth in the number of interest groups and their lobbying activities with the national government happened during the post-World War II period. These organized interests represented trade associations, business organizations, professional associations, and labor unions as well as citizens groups (Walker 1991). The 1960s saw a dramatic increase in citizens groups, often referred to as "public interest groups." The distinction that is often made between private interest groups and public interest groups is that the former represent/promote solely the private interest of their members (e.g., the National Rifle Association [NRA]), while the latter represent/promote the interest of the public at large (e.g., Common Cause). Interest groups often lobby on their own behalf or hire lobbyists/lobbying firms to represent their interests in the political arena.

How effective are interest groups in having their voices heard and in influencing the policymaking process? Heinz et al. (1993) have argued interest groups are more successful in obstructing than in promoting new policy initiatives (Heinz et al. 1993). Negative lobbying is more effective than positive lobbying, and negative lobbying is a more powerful predictor of policy outcome than the level of conflict, the preferences of the majority of lobbyists, or the differences in interest-group resources (McKay 2012). Also, the proliferation of interest groups makes it difficult for any one group to yield tremendous power. Baumgartner and Leech (2001) have argued that despite the proliferation of interest groups, the number of them actively involved in a specific policy area remains relatively small. Interest groups' competition often can lead to conflicts or cooperation in the form of coalition-building with other interest groups in order to be effective and successful in influencing policy process (Holyoke 2009). When advocates of a given issue finally succeed, the policy can change significantly (Baumgartner et al. 2009).

Some have argued that during the early twentieth century, lobbyists began to use propaganda techniques, including false and misleading information, to assert a more prominent role in the policymaking process (Loomis 2009). Critics of interested groups have argued that interest group membership represents upper-class bias because research shows that people with more income and education are more likely to join interest groups, and the interests of the poor and less educated, and thus unorganized, are not represented in the policy process. Also, citizens' groups often cannot match the resources of business groups (Mills 1956; Schattschneider 1960). Lowi (1969) has described this as socialism for the organized and capitalism for the unorganized. Skopol (2004) has pointed to the demise of mass-membership organizations and voluntary organizations after the 1960s and the rise of professional lobby organizations that are divorced from regular citizens. Trevor (2006) has argued that contrary to conventional wisdom, a vast majority of groups, especially the poorest groups, simply do not have the resources to make noise, make news, and have their voices heard. Only the largest and well-funded groups have a place in the public debate. Thus, instead of a marketplace of pluralistic ideas in which every group's voice is heard, only the voice of a few powerful groups in each policy niche gets heard through the news media. The role played by interest groups in the health policy area can be seen in the MPDIMA of 2003, which added prescription drug coverage for Medicare, and the ACA of 2010, which overhauled the American healthcare system (Frakt, Pizer, and Hendricks 2008; Heaney 2006; Quadango 2011).

The Changing Political Environment

In the previous section we discussed how the constitutional and institutional environment in American politics has shaped the political environment that emphasized consensus-building through bargaining and compromises, political feasibility, electoral calculation, public philosophy of interest-group liberalism, and incrementalism in policymaking. However, the political environment is always dynamic and rarely constant. Sometimes political environment may change slowly and incrementally over a period of time while at other times it may undergo rapid changes. Here we discuss how the American political environment has changed over a period of time. We focus our discussion largely on some significant changes that have taken place since the 1970s. These changes have made it very difficult to achieve consensus in policymaking to address major societal problems and have led to more legislative gridlock. This is also reflected in health policymaking.

From Unified to Divided Government

Unified government is characterized by the same political party controlling the presidency and both houses of Congress. In contrast, divided government refers to a condition in which one party controls the presidency but one or both houses of Congress are controlled by the other political party. During a period of unified government policymaking is easier if there is a consensus on policy agenda and the party in power enjoys a comfortable majority in both houses of Congress. Policymaking becomes more problematic during a period of divided government since the president's party's policy agenda may differ significantly from the political party that controls one or both houses of Congress.

Prior to World War II, unified government was the norm. However, post-World War II divided government has become the norm. As Table 1.1 demonstrates, between 1901 and 1947, we had a unified government 87 percent of the time and a divided government only 13 percent of the time. However, post-World War II, the situation was dramatically reversed. Between 1947 and 2017, we had a unified government only 37 percent of the time and a divided government 63 percent of the time. In other words, since the end of World War II, divided government has become the norm in American politics.

When we further examine the post-World War II time period it becomes clear that the trend of divided government has become dominant since the 1970s. Between 1947 and 1969, 63 percent of the time unified government was still the norm. Things changed dramatically beginning in the 1970s. Between 1969 and 1991, divided government had increased to 82 percent of the time with unified government decreasing to only 18 percent of the time. Between 1991 and 2017 we had divided government 79 percent of the time.

Can presidents hope to be effective in policymaking when Congress is controlled by the other party, that is, during a period of divided government? Some have tended to blame the divided government for policy gridlock within Congress and between the executive and legislative branches of government (Galderisi, Herzberg, and McNamara 1996). Edwards, Barrett, and Peake (1997, 545) have argued that presidents oppose significant legislation more often under a divided government, and much more important legislation fails to pass under a divided government than under a unified government. Furthermore, they suggest that the odds of important legislation failing to pass are greater under a divided government. According to Badger (2010), divided government causes gridlock because political parties are less likely to compromise through bargaining and negotiations (Unekis 2011).

Some have argued that a divided government may work better because it requires the president to reach out to members of the other party to create majority support for his programs. For example, Niskanen (2003) points to the fact that the Reagan tax laws of 1981 and 1986 were both approved by a House of Representatives controlled by the Democrats. Similarly, some of the policy successes of President Clinton, such as the North Atlantic Free Trade Agreement (NAFTA) and welfare reform, were the result of his success in getting support from Republicans in Congress (Galderisi, Herzberg, and McNamara 1996; Niskanen 2003). In the health policy area, the passage of the State Children's Health Insurance Program (SCHIP) in 1997 and the Health Insurance and

Table 1.1

Occurrences of Unified and Divided Governments in the United States, 1900–2020

	Total Congressional Sessions	Unified	Divided
Pre-World War II, 1901–1947	23	20	3
	(100%)	(87%)	(13%)
Post-World War II, 1947–2017	35	13	22
	(100%)	(37%)	(63%)
1947–1969	11	7	4
	(100%)	(64%)	(36%)
1969–1991	11	2	9
	(100%)	(18%)	(82%)
1991–2020	14	3	11
	(100%)	(21%)	(79%)

Portability and Accountability Act (HIPAA) in 1996 are examples of policy accomplishments during a period of divided government between a Republican-controlled Congress and a Democratic president. Similarly, the passage of the Medicare Prescription Drug, Improvement, and Modernization Act (MPDIMA) of 2003 stands as an example of bipartisan cooperation between a Republican president, George W. Bush, and a Democrat-controlled Congress. Clearly, divided government in the past has produced some big policy accomplishments. However, it is also important to remember that during the 1960s and 1970s, 30 to 40 percent of the members of Congress were ideological moderates, which often made a compromise on major important legislation possible. Increased partisanship in Congress had made such compromises more difficult.

Conley (2003) makes a very persuasive argument that the conditions of "divided government" have changed significantly in recent years because of changes in electoral politics that have reduced presidential coattails, lack of presidents' popularity in opposition members' districts, changes in an institutional setting in Congress such as more assertive legislative majorities, changes in leadership structure, and increased party cohesion in voting. These changes have made it more difficult for the president to achieve his policy agenda in Congress. In response, to overcome such obstacles, presidents have come to rely on the use of presidential signing statements—written documents issued contemporaneously with the signing of a law in which the president states his objections to the law, including the reservation of the right not to enforce or comply with the law. Under the administration of George W. Bush, we witnessed a massive proliferation in the number of such presidential signing statements (Biller 2008; Evans and Marshall 2016; Kennedy 2014). During periods of divided governments, presidents have also used veto threats and/or exercised their veto power more frequently. Presidents under unified governments, on average, veto two bills per year while under divided governments (Reagan, Bush Sr. and Clinton) vetoed six bills annually on average (Tenpas 2006).

Some scholars have taken a middle approach on the questions of divided government and its impact on legislative gridlock. For example, Ewing and Kysar (2011) have argued that, ironically, the constitutional division of authority between the three branches of government and the system of checks and balances it creates can constrain collective political action on the one hand, while on the other hand creating a system of "prods and pleas" in which policy-makers in different branches of government can push each other to entertain collective political action when necessary. They further argue that the prods and pleas are a fail-safe mechanism for a limited government. Pandich (2007) has argued that the constitutional separation of powers and the resulting checks and balances do not always result in conflict and competition because occasionally one branch of government shows considerable deference to another branch even in matters on which they might be expected to conflict. Nzelibe and Stephenson (2010) also suggest that separation of powers does not necessarily induce gridlock or reduce the likelihood of policy change.

From Coalition- and Consensus-Building to Political Polarization and Tribalism

Another major change that has occurred in the political environment since the 1970s is a significant increase in polarization in American politics. Many politicians, journalists, and scholars have argued that polarization has become the defining characteristic of contemporary American politics and had led to congressional gridlock and dysfunction. While the term polarization has several meanings the most commonly used definition refers to polarization as a sharp division into opposing groups or factions (Wood and Jordan 2011). Such a sharp division has occurred in American politics along a partisan, ideological, electoral, and public opinion landscape.

What factors have contributed to polarization in American politics? A study by the Brookings Institution (Nivola 2005) examines the exogenous and endogenous factors that have contributed to polarization. The *exogenous factors* include historical circumstances; sectional realignment of the electorate (the Democratic Party's loss of the Southern base and the diminished Republican Party stronghold in the New England region); political party parity causing a quarrelsome atmosphere, distrust, and resentment; the role of religion leading to polarization on social issues such as abortion, same-sex marriage, gay and lesbian rights, among others; the media's role in exaggerating the "culture war" in American society; and the revolution in communication technology such as direct mail, cable TV, and the Internet, enabling individuals to congregate along partisan and ideological lines. The *endogenous factors* include Congressional redistricting and gerrymandering producing more "safe districts" and less need to compromise and appear moderate; the dominance of party primaries, forcing candidates to protect their flanks by moving away from the political center; the Electoral College system, which has produced presidential victors who lost the popular vote, generating more political animus (e.g., George W. Bush in 2000 and Donald Trump in 2016); new institutional norms producing abrasive adversarial and slash-and-burn tactics in both houses of Congress; and divided government (see also Berman 2016; Cohn 2014; Davis and Dunaway 2016; Jacobson 2013; Rosen 2016).

Partisan Polarization

The partisan polarization is reflected in increased partisan differences in congressional voting behavior (voting along party lines) and low-level or lack of party competition in congressional districts (McCarty, Poole, and Rosenthal 2009). The polarization of the Democratic and Republican parties has been at its highest since the end of the Civil War and partisan conflict has grown sharper and unrelenting (Hare and Poole 2014). In the 112th Congress (2011–2012), 91 percent of the Democrats and 93.5 percent of the Republicans voted with their fellow party members on roll calls, leaving very little room for compromise and coalition-building (Campbell 2016). Analysis of party unity votes within specific issues also suggest that the parties are instrumental in the polarization process and have played a role in the transformation of policy issues from multidimensional arenas to ideological and unidimensional ones (Jochim and Jones 2013). While more Americans identify themselves as independents instead of expressing loyalty to a particular party, suggesting a decline in partisanship, the voting behavior data suggest the opposite is happening. Straight-ticket voting has continued to increase while split-ticket voting has continued to decline (Chait 2015).

Partisan gerrymandering, in which congressional districts are drawn and redrawn by the majority party in state legislatures for partisan advantage, has led to increasing partisanship. As congressional districts become less competitive and it becomes easy to get reelected, representatives no longer feel the need to reach out to moderate and independent voters. However, it is important to note that the US Senate has also experienced partisan polarization, and gerrymandering is not an issue in the US Senate elections (McCarty, Poole, and Rosenthal 2009).

Political parties in Congress have assumed an "uncompromising mindset" marked by mutual distrust (Gutmann and Thompson 2010). An example of such an uncompromising mindset was the passage of the ACA of 2010. The debate surrounding the bill was one of the most intensely partisan legislative battles in many years. Very little, if any, compromises were made in the bill between Democrats and Republicans in Congress as it went through the legislative process and became law on a strict party-line vote (Frakes 2012). The hopes of less partisanship following Barack Obama's election in 2008 were quickly dashed as his policy agenda was met with almost universal Republican Party opposition in Congress, emboldened by the rise of the conservative Tea Party movement (Milkis, Rhodes, and Charnock 2012). To govern a nation effectively, what is required is a compromising mindset and mutual respect, and for policymakers to find ways to reach an agreement with their political opponents across ideological and party lines (*ibid.*).

Others have argued that partisan bickering is highlighted more today than in the past through traditional and nontraditional media outlets in the forms of radio and TV talk shows, blogs, newspapers, and magazines. In the television world, for example, FOX and MSNBC act respectively as a conservative and progressive/liberal voice. Some have blamed the increased political polarization on increased partisan and ideological news coverage by American media outlets (Frakes 2012).

Political parties in Congress have come to represent an increasingly divergent electoral constituency. Partisan disputes over large as well as small matters over personnel and policy have become the norm almost on a daily basis in Congress (Jacobson 2013). This has become particularly acute during the periods of divided government.

Ideological Polarization

The increase in partisan polarization is also associated with an increase in ideological polarization between the two political parties. Democrats and Republicans are ideologically further apart today than in the past (Hibbing, Hays, and Deol 2017.) This is reflected in the fact that from 2005 to 2012, every Democrat in Congress was ideologically to the left of every Republican. Also, in 2013, only 1 percent of Republicans in the House and 4 percent of Republicans in the Senate were moderate while the corresponding numbers for Democrats were 13 percent in the House and 9 percent in the Senate (Altschuler 2017).

Both political parties have moved away from the ideological center. Since the 1970s, the Republican and Democratic caucuses in Congress have become more homogeneous and have moved further apart (Farina 2015). However, most scholars seem to be in agreement that ideological polarization is asymmetric in that the Republican Party has moved further to the to the ideological right than the Democratic Party has moved to the ideological left (Thompsen 2014). Compared to the Republican Party in Congress, the Democratic Party has remained relatively more ideologically diverse. For example, the moderate "Blue Dog" Democrats have retained their presence in Congress. In contrast, Republicans have lost most of their moderates. For example, in the 1980s, only 10–20 percent of the Republicans in Congress belonged to the party's right-wing caucus, but in 2012, almost 70 percent were members of this caucus (Bonica 2013; Mann and Ornstein 2012).

Thompsen (2014) attributes the increased ideological polarization of parties to an ideological shift in the electorate in which the electoral bases of the two parties changed from being more diverse to more uniform, changes that have occurred within Congress such as reliance on extreme parliamentary procedures to pass legislation. He argues that the consequence of such ideological polarization between parties is that ideological moderates do not run for public office. Others have blamed the current system of campaign finance that makes candidates more reliant on the most ideological elements in both parties for campaign contributions. Current campaign finance laws impose constraints on party organizations giving outside non-party groups such as Super Political Action Committees (S-PACs) giving an advantage to extreme ideological partisans (La Raja 2014).

Increased partisan and ideological polarization is also strongly correlated with increased polarization of the American electorate.

Electoral and Public Opinion Polarization

Wood and Jordan (2011) define electoral ideological polarization as a condition in which Americans align themselves with respect to a set of liberal and conservative poles on a left-right continuum.

Quirk (2011) has argued that political polarization in America is more a function of what he calls "polarized populism," a condition of politics in which elected officials accord a great deal of deference to regular citizens, especially those who hold relatively extreme ideological views. In other words, increased partisan voting and ideological polarization in Congress simply reflects the increased partisan and ideological polarization of the American electorate. The public's evaluation of political officials and policies they endorse also has become more polarized. According to Cohn (2014) voters of both political parties have become more ideologically homogeneous than in the past. Ninety-nine percent of politically engaged Republican voters are more conservative than the median Democratic voter. Similarly, 98 percent of Democratic voters are more liberal than the median Republican voters. In 2004, the percentages were 88 percent and 84 percent, respectively.

The Pew Research Center conducted a major political survey of 10,000 adult Americans between January and March of 2014. The results of the study found that not only have Americans become more ideological but also that such ideological polarization is also reflected in their personal lives and lifestyles (Doherty 2014). The seven major findings of the survey were the following. In the last 20 years, first, the share of Americans who express consistently conservative or consistently liberal opinion has doubled from 10 percent to 21 percent. Second, the share of Republicans and Democrats who view the other political party unfavorably has also increased. Republicans who view the Democratic Party negatively has jumped from 17 to 43 percent while the percentage of Democrats who view the Republican Party negatively has increased from 16 percent to 38 percent. Third, about 63 percent of consistent conservatives and 49 percent of consistent liberals say that most of their close friends share their political views. Fourth, the differences between the right and the left go beyond politics and extend to social life and lifestyle choices. Fifth, the number of Americans who view themselves as moderate or close to the center of the ideological continuum has decreased. Sixth, the most ideologically oriented Americans engage in greater political participation in every stage of the political process and thus have their voices heard. Seventh, most Americans on the ideological left or right view or define "compromise" as their side getting more of what it wants and not as both sides getting something of equal value.

The question is whether the American public itself is polarized along the same ideological line as political officials or whether the population is simply responding to ideologically driven policy choices that are provided to them by politicians? Some have argued that the American electorate is increasingly ideologically polarized along the same lines as the political parties, while others have argued that most Americans tend to be ideologically moderate or centrist but view political officials as polarized (Rogowski and Sutherland 2016). In other words, Americans perceive more polarization with regards to policy issues than actually exists (Levendusky and Malhotra 2016). Similarly, Ahler (2014) also argues that the notion that the American electorate is divided into two deeply committed ideological factions does not match with the reality because citizens believe that their peers are more polarized than they actually are.

Finally, Americans have increasingly come to view and evaluate, from policy issues to institutions of government, through partisan and ideological lenses.

The Rise of Tribalism

Barber and Pope (2017) in their research ask an important question: which of the two identities—party affiliation and political ideology—do Americans give higher priority? Does party identity trump political ideology or ideology trump party identification? They conclude that to most Americans group loyalty and social identity are more important than any professed ideology in influencing their opinions. Another term for social identity is tribalism (Adler 2017). Some other synonyms for tribe include clique and pack. James Madison in "Federalist 10" referred to groups as factions (Fallows 2017). Madison viewed political parties as factions and argued that the only way to curb their mischief was through the division of power and a large republic. A democracy requires that different political groups view each other as valid, equal, and legitimate, even though they may disagree on specific issues. The absence of such conditions results in tribalism and conflict (Gibian 2012).

Humans are social species and tribal by nature, who need a sense of belonging and capacity for empathy and compassion. However, tribal humans also have a dark side, at times exhibiting belligerence, hostility, and a capacity for destruction (Levine 2018). Andrew Sullivan (2017), in a thought-provoking essay, argues that tribalism is a default human experience and healthy tribalism can exist in a civil society in benign ways because it provides individuals a sense of belonging, to one's neighborhood and community. However, benign and healthy tribalism become dangerous when they calcify into something bigger and more intense, turning tribes into enemies. Such forms of tribalism can destabilize democracy. He further argues that over the last few decades the complex divides of party, ideology, geography, class, religion, and race have mutated into two coherent tribes (the Democratic and Republican parties), fighting not just to advance their own interests but to condemn and defeat each other at any cost. One tribe (the Democratic Party) contains mostly racial minorities, lives on the coast and in the cities, is less tolerant of religion, and is globalist in its outlook, while the other tribe (the Republican Party) is disproportionately white, lives in rural areas, values traditional faith and religion, and is nationalist in its outlook. The incomprehension and hatred of each other have been further fueled by the arrival of partisan and ideologically based talk radio, Fox News, and MSNBC, and the Internet—making bargaining, compromises, and coalition-building between opposing tribes impossible. Under such conditions, politics becomes a zero-sum game where the goal of each side is to obliterate the other side. One of the great attractions of such tribalism is that one does not actually have to think for oneself since one's opinion on any subject is based on what side of the tribe one belongs to (Sullivan 2017). Kornacki (2018) traces the origins of tribalism in American politics to the early 1990s and the bare-knuckle brawls between President Bill Clinton and Speaker of the House Newt Gingrich that brought about major policy shifts and had far-reaching political consequences.

Congressional Gridlock and Dysfunction

The trend toward political polarization started in the 1970s and became more pronounced in the early 1980s (McCarty 2016). One of the most significant consequences of this changed political environment is legislative gridlock and Congressional dysfunction. In this atmosphere, neither political party can fully implement its policy agenda. The president and the Congress seem incapable of agreeing on policy agenda and proposals to address the challenges facing the country (Abramowitz 2013). The Madisonian principle of separation of powers and checks and balances was designed to encourage cooperation, bargaining, and compromises between different branches of government. However, in an environment of divided government and intense political polarization, the separation of powers and checks and balances have produced a stalemate, legislative gridlock, and government dysfunction (*ibid.ibid.*) and have led reform advocates, journalists, and disaffected voters to describe government in Washington as "broken" (Berman 2016). One of the clear indicators of legislative dysfunction is the decline in Congressional legislative output (McCarty 2016).

The Economic Environment

Decisions about healthcare policies are invariably intertwined with economics. The economic environment consists of a network of institutions, laws, and rules that deal with primary questions such as what goods and services to produce, how to produce them, and for whom (Samuelson 1970). The economic point of view is also rooted in three fundamental assumptions: (1) resources are limited or scarce in relation to human wants; (2) resources have alternative uses; and (3) people have different wants and do not attach the same importance to them (Fuchs 1995). Because economic resources are limited and have alternative uses, decisions must be made with regard to how and for what purposes to use these resources. The concept of opportunity cost suggests that when deciding to use resources in a certain way, one loses the opportunity to obtain benefits of using resources in some other way.

The field of economics offers several analytic tools that can be useful in health policymaking/decision-making as well as evaluation of health programs to determine its impact, effectiveness, and efficiency. Some of these tools include the following: *cost–benefit analysis* in the healthcare field can provide an analysis of expenditure of health resources relative to benefits. Such analysis can help determine whether the cost of a given program can be justified compared to the benefit it provides. It can also help in setting priorities when decisions or choices must be made in the face of limited resources. *Risk–benefit analysis* can allow policymakers to weigh the potential for undesirable outcomes and side-effects against the potential positive outcome of a policy/program or a medical treatment. *Cost-effectiveness analysis* involves comparing several different intervention strategies using common units of costs and benefits. The Center for Disease Control and Prevention (CDC) utilizes cost analysis, economic evaluation, regulatory and budget impact analysis, and health impact assessment in public health programs ("Public Health Economics and Methods" n.d.). Almost all state governments conduct cost–benefit analysis but the quality and impact of such analysis vary. At the federal level, the use of cost–benefit analysis is required in many federal agencies particularly with respect to regulatory decision-making (White and Silloway 2016).

Economic tools such as the ones mentioned above are designed to make policymaking a rational process in which decisions are based on available evidence. However, as we mentioned earlier, policymaking is more an art than a science and several other political and other considerations come into play in policymakers' calculations when making health policy. The economic environment affects policy decisions in healthcare in a number of ways. At any given point in time, health policymakers are influenced in their decisions by the notion of economic feasibility. When an economy is growing at a healthy rate, making economic resources available, policymakers find it economically feasible to establish new programs. Such was the case during the 1960s and to an extent in the early 1970s, when a number of new programs designed to increase access to healthcare were created. But corresponding increases in healthcare costs, a slower rate of economic growth, massive federal budget deficits, and an executive branch dominated by a conservative political philosophy during the 1980s not only made it economically difficult to establish new healthcare programs but also made it possible to cut expenditures on federal health programs (Sorkin 1986). If one accepts the assumptions of the scarcity of resources and the existence of competing goals, then the question faced by health policymakers becomes how to bring about the optimum distribution of healthcare resources. What is needed is not simply cost containment but a cost-effective healthcare system (Fuchs 1986). One of the major problems with the American healthcare system is that it is less cost-effective than healthcare systems in other industrialized countries. In a constrained economic environment, health policymakers are confronted with making choices and establishing priorities that are not easy to make.

An environment of limited resources and constantly changing healthcare needs requires policymakers to make value judgments about priorities. How much of society's resources should be devoted to healthcare? What priorities should be assigned to different groups competing for the same healthcare resources? Should more priority be given to the healthcare needs of the elderly or to those of infants and children? Should everyone be entitled to an organ transplant, regardless of cost or the ability to pay? In recent years, a constrained economic environment has increased concerns about the values of cost-effectiveness and efficiency. It has prompted some states to attempt healthcare rationing. This has generated significant controversy and public debate over the conflicting values of efficiency, access, and equality.

The interplay of economics and healthcare can be seen in the debate surrounding the ACA of 2010. One of the criticisms leveled by Republicans against the healthcare reform was that creating such a major and costly reform during a recession was a bad policy and it would only add to the federal government's deficit, while the defenders of healthcare reform argued that dramatically escalating healthcare costs were partly responsible for the deficits. They also stated that without the reform, the healthcare costs would rise even more, adding to the deficit, and the costs of the reform would be paid by savings in the Medicare program and added revenues. Thus, healthcare reform would actually help reduce deficits in the long run by controlling rising healthcare costs.

The Technological Environment

Dramatic advances in biomedical technology in the past 30 years have revolutionized the nature and delivery of health services in the United States. The rapid growth and adoption of new biomedical technologies have transformed many hospitals into very complex and resource-intensive institutions and have changed the very nature of medical practice. The new medical technologies are not only revalorizing the field of healthcare by providing earlier diagnosis, personalized treatment, and a wide range of other benefits to patients as well as a health professionals (Morrissey 2015). A high-tech sensor can monitor a patient's heart 24/7. A new type of computer chip embedded in a pill can be activated at the precise time the pill reaches a patient's stomach and confirm that the patient is taking his medication. Wearable medical technologies can monitor a patient's heart rate, blood pressure, and other vital signs continuously (*ibid.*; Topol 2012). Medical technologies can be classified as instrumental technology or transformative technology. Instrumental technology acts as a tool that serves an existing aspect of healthcare while a transformative technology can be viewed as pioneering, creating a new form of care. It is also important to remember that depending on the cost, medical technology can be available universally or it can be exclusionary (Huberfeld 2017).

Thus, many new biomedical technologies have also generated debate in society about problems of access, cost, and effectiveness of such technologies and its relationship to quality-of-life issues. Since every change in technology involves costs and benefits, the formulation of a good public policy depends on an accurate assessment of the relative magnitudes of costs and benefits.

The technological revolution in biomedicine also highlights questions about what medical technology should be developed and what is the proper and appropriate level of medical intervention to treat an illness. Since healthcare costs make up an increasing part of the government budget, the role of the government becomes crucial with respect to the allocation of healthcare resources. Should healthcare technologies be available to all persons on an equal basis? If not, what criteria should be used to decide who gets scarce health resources and who does not? Should the government be involved in technology assessment and play a role in encouraging or discouraging the development of particular technology through its funding? Should the government establish legal and ethical guidelines not only with respect to biomedical research but also regarding the application of biomedical technology?

Medical technology has not only revolutionized the field of healthcare but has also created a variety of legal and ethical issues in many areas of healthcare. We examine the legal, constitutional, and ethic issues raised by certain biomedical technologies in the areas of right to die and reproductive rights in Chapter 9 of the book.

KEY HEALTH POLICY ACTORS

The key policy actors in the healthcare system include a variety of public and private institutions and groups such as healthcare providers, healthcare practitioners, healthcare purchasers, and health insurers. The remainder of this chapter examines the role of the key health policy actors.

Healthcare Providers

The major healthcare providers include institutions such as hospitals, nursing homes, and pharmacies, as well as professionals such as physicians, nurses, and dentists. They are important actors in the healthcare system because they not only deliver healthcare services but also influence the way in which services are delivered and the type of services that are delivered. The major feature of the US healthcare system is its entrepreneurial nature.

Pharmacies and manufacturers of pharmaceutical and medical equipment and suppliers are private, profit-making enterprises. Similarly, many nursing homes are for-profit institutions.

Physicians

Physicians are key actors in the healthcare system because they are the primary caregivers. They enjoy considerable professional autonomy. In 2015 in the United States, there were 860,917 active physicians, including 65,070 with a Doctor of Osteopathic Medicine (DO) degree. DOs constituted about 7.6 percent of the total number of active physicians. There was one physician for every 373 Americans (Association of American Medical Colleges 2017).

With respect to specialties, the largest number of active physicians were in the specialty of internal medicine (114,089), family medicine/general practice (111,295), and pediatrics (57,543).

Thirty-Four percent of the active physician workforce was female. The percentage of females in the top specialties ranged from a high of 61.9 percent in pediatrics a low of 5 percent in orthopedic surgery (Association of American Medical Colleges 2016).

The average annual compensation for physicians in 2017 was $294,000, with specialists earning 46 percent higher ($316,000) than the primary care physicians ($217,000). The top three earners among all physicians were orthopedists ($489,000), plastic surgeons ($440,000), and cardiologists ($410,000), while the lowest earners were family physicians and pediatrics with average annual earnings of $209,000 and $202,000. Among primary care physicians as well as specialists, men earn more than women (Medscape 2017).

Physicians play a pivotal role and occupy a unique position in the healthcare system. Since they not only diagnose an illness but also prescribe treatment, they control both the supply of and the demand for healthcare services. In the process, they exert substantial influence over the pattern of health resources utilization in general and hospital resources in particular. Doctors conduct their practices in private offices, hospitals, and federal, state, and local governments, and a variety of other settings. Some work in outpatient care centers or educational services.

In 2016, for the first time less than half of practicing physicians (47.1 percent) owned their medical practice—down from 53.2 percent in 2012. This trend is more pronounced among young doctors who are shifting from owning their own practice to join larger group practices. Independent physicians are moving their practices to larger systems due to increased compliance costs and new payment models such as accountable care organization. Also, large health systems are aggressively acquiring physician practices. Consequently, the percentage of physicians in hospital-owned practices or who were employed directly by a hospital has jumped from 29 percent in 2012 to 32.8 percent in 2016 (Kane 2017).

In addition to physicians, in 2016, there were a total of 114,994 certified physician assistants (PAs), of which 67.8 percent were women and 32.2 percent were men; 86.8 percent were white and 13.2 percent were of minority ethnicity. The top PA practice areas are family medicine/general practice, surgical subspecialties, and emergency medicine. About 42 percent worked in office-based private practice, while another 39 percent worked in a hospital setting. The median salary for PAs was about $105,000 (National Commission on Certification of Physician Assistants 2018).

Nurses

Nurses play a critical role as intermediaries between physicians and patients. They manage patient care on a daily basis and make sure that doctors' instructions for patient care are carried out. The essential core functions of nursing are to deliver holistic, patient-centered care. This involves assessment, diagnostics, outcome planning, and implementation of a healthcare plan for a patient ("The Nursing Process" n.d.).

Licensed practical nurses (LPNs) or licensed vocational nurses (LVN) are some of the lowest-paid workers and they perform a number of different tasks such as administering medicine, checking patients' vital signs, and giving injections, under the supervision of a registered nurse. Practicing as an LPN/LVN does not require a college degree and some jobs require only a high school diploma with some minimal additional training.

Registered nurses (RNs) are nurses who have an associate or bachelor's degree in nursing. They constitute the largest part of the nurse workforce. They work in a variety of specialties and work environments. RNs who obtain an advanced nursing degree can earn more income and hold a more advanced nursing position with more clinical authority. Registered nurses constitute the largest healthcare occupation. In 2016, 2.9 million registered nurses were employed in the United States. Between 2016 and 2026 the employment of registered nurses is projected to grow by 15 percent, for a variety of reasons, such as aging of the population, increased inpatient population at long-term nursing facilities and outpatient care centers, as well as the anticipated greater need for home healthcare and residential care facilities. In 2016, the median annual salary for registered nurses was $68,450, with the lowest 10 percent earning less than $47,120 and the highest 10 percent earning more than $102,990 (Bureau of Labor Statistics 2018).

Advanced practice nurses are carving out a new role in healthcare delivery. The advanced practice nurse is an umbrella term given to a registered nurse who has at least a master's degree in educational and clinical practice requirements beyond the years of basic nursing education required of all RNs. Advanced practice nurses can be classified into four types: nurse practitioner (NP), certified nurse midwife (CNM), clinical nurse specialist (CNS), and certified registered nurse anesthetist (CRNA). NPs are qualified to handle a wide range of basic health problems, and most of them have specialties, such as adult, family, or pediatric care. CNMs provide well-woman gynecological and low-risk obstetrical care. CNSs are qualified to handle a wide range of physical and mental health problems, and they provide primary care and psychotherapy. CRNAs administer anesthetics given to patients each year (Santiago 2017a, 2017b).

Hospital nurses form the largest group of nurses. Most of them are staff nurses who provide bedside nursing care and carry out medical regimens. Office nurses care for outpatients in physicians' offices, clinics, and ambulatory surgical centers. Home healthcare nurses provide nursing services to patients at home, while nursing care facility nurses work in long-term care operations such as nursing homes. Public health nurses work in government and private agencies, including clinics, schools, and community settings, to improve the overall health of the community. Occupational health nurses (industrial nurses) provide nursing care at worksites.

Hospitals

The role of the hospital has changed dramatically from early America to the present day. In early America, hospitals were founded to shelter older adults, the dying, orphans, the contagiously sick, vagrants, and the insane. The main goal was to protect members of the community. All of the early hospitals were focused on an unfortunate segment of the population with physical and mental illness. The transformation of hospitals from charitable institutions to modern organizations began with the start of private health insurance in the 1940s and was given further impetus with the establishment of the Medicare and Medicaid programs in 1965. Today's hospitals are complex, technical organizations that provide the most advanced form of medical and surgical treatment to their patients (Sultz and Young 2011).

According to a 2015 survey by the American Hospital Association (AHA), there were a total of 5,564 registered hospitals in the United States, with a total of 897,961 staffed beds. Registered hospitals are those that meet the AHA's criteria for accreditation as a hospital (American Hospital Association 2017). Of the total registered hospitals, 4,862 are community hospitals, of which 2,845 are nongovernmental not-for-profit hospitals, 1,034 are investor-owned for-profit hospitals, and 983 are state and local government hospitals. The remainder is made up of federal government hospitals, nonfederal psychiatric hospitals, nonfederal long-term care hospitals, and hospital units of institutions such as prison hospitals and college infirmaries. Also, of the 4,862 community hospitals, 1,829 are rural and 3,033 are urban community hospitals (American Hospital Association 2017). Hospitals have become the primary setting for the delivery of healthcare services because most of the sophisticated medical technology and equipment is located there. Hospitals vary by purpose and ownership.

An acute-care hospital provides short-term care while a long-term-care hospital typically provides care for chronic illness, rehabilitation, or psychiatric care. Community hospitals are generally all nonfederal, short-term general and other special hospitals. The basic definition of a community hospital is a hospital that serves the community, is run by local leaders, and that provides financial opportunities for the local economy. A community hospital can be either rural or urban. A majority of community hospitals are urban, vary in size (under 100 to over 500 beds), and serve a densely populated area, while rural hospitals are located outside of a metropolitan area and are smaller (100 beds or less) with small budgets. Rural hospitals tend to serve more Medicare, Medicaid, and uninsured patients. Consequently, the Center for Medicare and Medicaid (CMS) often designates such hospitals as Critical Access Hospitals. Teaching hospitals are generally affiliated with a medical school and thus they serve the purpose of education and training of medical students, residents, and interns. They also are involved in ongoing research projects and trials. Federal hospitals include hospitals and clinics run by the Veteran's Administration, Department of Defense, and Department of Health and Human Services. State and local hospitals are run by state or local governments. Public hospitals can also be teaching hospitals. For-profit hospitals are investor-owned hospitals, designed to make a profit, and funnel excess profits to shareholders. Not-for-profit hospitals retain excess funds in the hospitals (American Medical Association 2017; Mitchell 2017).

Paul Starr (1982), in his classic work *The Social Transformation of American Medicine*, warned about the coming of corporate medicine as it relates to hospitals. He argued that corporatization of American medicine was reflected in the hospitals being increasingly viewed as "profit centers" instead of "health centers." Similarly, Poduval and Poduval (2008) have argued that the medical-industrial complex has led to commercialization of healthcare that treats medicine as a business concern and is motivated by cost curtailments and profit margins. Two recent trends with respect to hospitals seem to lend some credence to this argument. First, even though a majority of hospitals today are still not-for-profit (59 percent), the number of investor-owned for-profit hospitals are on the rise. However, it should be noted that the trend is a very modest one. Non-profit hospitals faced with cash flow problems and that unable to improve and upgrade their facilities have eagerly sought to change from non-profit to for-profit status by looking for profit suitors for mergers and acquisitions (Gold 2010). A second trend is that mergers and acquisitions in the healthcare sector have soared. The consequence of these two trends is that a growing number of hospitals are becoming part of a "health system" of "healthcare networks." In a health system, multiple facilities are administered from a central office. Such a health system can include one hospital and many separate specialized facilities or several hospitals and their related satellite facilities. In a healthcare network, groups of healthcare facilities, physicians, insurers, agencies, and others work together to coordinate patient services (Mitchell 2017).

Skilled Nursing Care Centers

A Skilled Nursing Care Center (SNCC) is the same as a Skilled Nursing Facility (SNF). A typical SNCC provides health services to patients who have complex medical conditions and need care and support with activities of daily living. There are 15, 655 SNCCs in the United States with 1.7 million beds. They serve 3.9 million individuals, ranging from short stays of less than 100 days (22 percent) to long stays of 100 days or more (78 percent). Of the total, 44 percent received post-acute rehabilitative care. These centers are located throughout the United States from major cities to small cities, towns, and rural areas. SNCCs employed about 1.7 million staff, of which 1.2 million were healthcare practitioners and support workers, 387,000 were ancillary staff, and 162,00 were administrative staff. SNCCs are largely staffed by registered nurses, and physical, occupational, and speech therapists with a small number of physicians. The overwhelming majority of workers tend to be women (85 percent) with persons of color making up about 37 percent (American Health Care Association n.d.).

Seventy percent of SNCCs are operated by for-profit companies, 24 percent are operated by not-for-profit companies, and the remaining 6 percent are operated by government agencies. Fifty-seven percent of the patient care cost in SNCCs is paid by Medicaid, 14 percent by Medicare, and 29 percent is paid by private insurance plans, other payers, and private individuals (American Health Care Association n.d.).

Other Healthcare Providers

Besides hospitals and SNCCs, residential and adult day services centers also provide health services to individuals. Persons living in state-regulated residential care facilities (RCFs) such as residents of assisted-living facilities receive housing and supportive services since they cannot live independently (Caffrey et al. 2012).

In 2016, an estimated 286,300 individuals were enrolled in adult day services centers. An adult day services center is a community-based center that is generally open on weekdays and provides services such as health monitoring, assistance with activities of daily living, and assistance to adults with disabilities. Home healthcare services provide similar assistance with assisted daily living such as bathing, eating, and the like at residents' homes (Lendon and Rome 2018). Both Medicare and Medicaid cover certain eligible home health services. Individuals with private long-term care insurance can also obtain certain home health services.

Finally, many basic and primary care services are provided by doctors' offices, urgent care centers, clinics at public schools, colleges, and universities, as well local public health centers.

Third-Party Payers

Third-party payers include organizations/institutions or companies that reimburse healthcare providers for health services rendered to a third party, i.e., patients. Third-party payers can include public organizations such as government or private businesses or companies.

Private Sector: Private Health Insurance

In 2016, total spending on private health insurance amounted to 1.1 trillion of the total national health expenditures of 3.3 trillion, 34 percent of the total national spending on health. Private insurance was the largest payer of healthcare goods and services. Slightly over 60 percent of the insured population was covered by some form of private insurance (Hartman et al. 2018). Also, 173 million individuals were enrolled in employer-sponsored health insurance ("National Health Care Spending in 2016" n.d.).

The US healthcare system over the years has undergone dramatic changes. Before the rise of the modern health insurance system, financial transactions between patient and healthcare provider were largely one-on-one in nature. Under this system, the patient paid for health services directly to the healthcare provider out of his or her own pocket. In the 1920s, the increased cost of hospital care caused by major investment in facilities, equipment, and physician training drove up the cost of medical care for patients, creating a need for health insurance (Anderson 2010).

The birth of the modern health insurance system can be traced to Baylor University in Texas, which in 1929 introduced the first prepaid hospital insurance plan for a small group of teachers, in which insurance paid for the cost of care in exchange for enrollees agreeing to a monthly premium. This came to be known as the "Blue Cross" hospital Plan. It became very popular and was soon expanded to include other workers. In fact, by the late 1930s, almost 3 million Americans were enrolled in the plan. This followed in 1939 with the introduction of the "Blue Shield" plans, initiated by physicians, to cover the cost of major medical services. The federal government gave a major boost to the development of such plans by declaring that premiums paid for such plans were exempted from federal taxes (Anderson 2010). This led to not only an increase in the number of private health insurance plans, but also an increase in the number of insurance companies offering private health insurance plans. Between 1930 and 1950, health insurance companies not only continued to cover more and more people under such plans but also expanded the scope of coverage. In 1960, the Blue Cross and the Blue Shield plans merged in what today we know as the Blue Cross-Blue Shield Plan. In 1965 the federal government entered the insurance market by creating two major insurance programs—Medicare for the elderly and Medicaid for the poor.

Despite the establishment of the government Medicare and Medicaid programs, employer-sponsored health insurance remains the dominant form of health insurance coverage in the United States (Graves and Mishra 2016). Employer-sponsored health coverage is likely to continue to dominate the market with a majority of Americans receiving insurance coverage as an employment benefit since all attempts by the federal government to establish a universal health insurance system have failed.

The private health insurance market can be divided into four categories. The first category is the large group market where large employers provide health benefits to their workers either through "self- funded" plans, which may be administered by a third party, or "fully insured" plans provided by an insurance carrier. The second category is the small-business-group insurance market. However, this market is relatively limited because small businesses (2–50 employees) often cannot get affordable insurance coverage because of the number of their employees. The third category is the individual insurance market. However, since individual insurance is not subsidized by an employer or through the tax code, each consumer is forced to pay the entire cost of the premium, which can be very expensive and often unaffordable. The fourth category contains health savings accounts (HSAs) and consumer-directed plans. Under this option, individuals, families, or employers are provided a comprehensive health insurance plan through an opportunity to save tax-deferred funds for qualified medical expenses ("Private-Market Health Insurance" n.d.).

Cost increases and pressure from employers have led insurance companies to look for ways to cut costs as well as increase the premiums they charge. Many insurance companies have developed managed care systems. The role of health insurers has changed considerably since the advent of managed care and managed competition in the 1990s, and it will change even more dramatically under the ACA of 2010. It will also have a considerable impact on the private health insurance market by expanding access to private health insurance to millions of people and employees of small businesses through the establishment of insurance exchanges, subsidizing insurance premiums for the poor, and by providing tax incentives to small businesses to encourage them to provide health insurance coverage to their workers ("Establishing Health Insurance Exchanges" 2012). In fact, the ACA has reduced the number of uninsured Americans to a historic low (Sommers et al. 2017).

Insurance companies have also come under increased criticisms in recent years for a variety of reasons. A recent report by the US Department of Health and Human Services (2016) shows that premiums on policies sold under the Healthcare.gov exchanges are expected to rise at a national average of 25 percent in 2017. The insurance companies have justified such increases on the grounds that they have suffered financial losses under Obamacare. For example, UnitedHealth, the country's largest health insurer, claimed that it was leaving the marketplace because the company suffered a financial loss of $850 million. However, despite this loss, the company's profits have soared. In 2016, the company recorded a revenue of $46.5 billion, which was an increase of $10 billion on 2015. Similarly, Aetna claimed a pretax loss of about $350 million in 2016 but in 2015 it reported annual operating revenue of $60.3 billion, a record for the company (Martyn 2016). Others blame the insurance companies for continuing to discriminate against the sick, providing less coverage while increasing costs, gaming the ACA for profit rather than servicing the patients, and for their exorbitant administrative costs (Geyman 2015).

Public Sector: Government Health Insurance Programs

The simple fact that the federal, state, and local governments are involved in the development of health policy, funding healthcare, maintaining and improving public health, and delivery of health services makes them important policy actors in the healthcare field. The federal and state governments spend a significant amount of money for a variety of government health insurance programs such as Medicare, Medicaid, and the Children's Health Insurance Program (CHIP). However, it is important to note that both the federal and state governments contract with private insurers to offer Medicare Advantage and Medicaid Managed plans. Medicare is the federal government insurance program for people aged 65 years and over. In addition, the federal government also pays for the health services provided to veterans and American Indians and Alaska Natives due to its statutory and/or treaty obligations. Medicaid and the CHIP provide health insurance coverage to the poor, disabled, and children who meet certain eligibility requirements, and are financed jointly by the federal and state governments.

In 2016, total national healthcare expenditures amounted to $3.3 trillion, about 17.9 percent of the gross domestic product (GDP) (Hartman et al. 2018). The majority of federal health spending is for the Medicare program for the elderly (65+) and the Medicaid program for the poor and disabled. Medicare is a federal program financed and administered by the federal government while Medicaid is a federal-state program financed jointly but administered by the state governments. Each state sets its own eligibility and benefit standards within certain constraints imposed by the federal government.

The total Medicare expenditures reached $672 million in 2016 and constituted 20 percent of the total healthcare spending by the federal government. The total combined federal-state spending for the Medicaid program in 2016 was $565.5 million, of which the federal share was $358 million and the state share was $207.5 million (Hartman et al. 2018). The combined federal and state government expenditures for the Medicare, Medicaid, and CHIP programs amounted to $1.3 trillion. In addition, the Department of Defense and the Department of Veterans Affairs spent around $109 million on veterans' healthcare while the Indian Health Service spent $3.9 million on providing health services to the American Indians and Alaska Natives ("National Health Expenditures by Types of Services and Sources of Funds: Calendar Years 1960 to 2016." n.d.).

In summary, in 2016, Medicare and Medicaid accounted for 37 percent and private health insurance amounted to 34 percent of the total national health expenditures (Centers for Medicare and Medicaid Services n.d.). A total of about 127 million individuals were enrolled in Medicare (55.8 million) and Medicaid (71.2 million) programs ("National Health Care Spending in 2016" n.d.).

At the federal level, the Department of Health and Human Services (DHHS) is the principal government agency responsible for carrying out federal health policies and programs. The DHHS is headed by a secretary who is appointed by the president with Senate confirmation. The secretary is responsible for administering federal healthcare programs and activities and for advising the president on health, welfare, and income security programs and policies of the federal government. Some of the most important agencies within the DHHS include the Centers for Medicare and Medicaid Services (CMS) (www.cms.hhs.gov/), which is responsible for the Medicare, Medicaid, and CHIP programs. The Indian Health Service (www.ihs.gov/) is responsible for administering healthcare services for American Indians and Alaska Natives. The Centers for Disease Control and Prevention (CDC) (www.cdc.gov/) are charged with the responsibility for protecting the public's health, preventing and controlling diseases, and responding to public health emergencies.

At the state level, each state has a health department (the name varies from state to state) that is led by a secretary of health or a state health commissioner who is typically appointed by the governor and is responsible for establishing and administering the state's health agenda. State health departments perform policy regulatory and administrative responsibilities and work closely with city and county health departments.

Local governments, that is, cities and counties, often play a critical role in administering state health programs and delivering health services. There are thousands of local health departments throughout the United States. They perform the important functions of health assessment, tracking population health, disease prevention, and development of community health services. In many communities, local health departments also provide primary and specialty services for mental health and sexually transmitted diseases.

The Department of Health and Human Services is the federal government's principal agency for carrying out federal health policies and programs.

Employers

Many major companies and firms in the private sector provide health insurance coverage to their employees as part of a benefits package. Today a majority of workers in the United States are employed by firms that offer health insurance. Whether employers provide health insurance benefits or not often depends on employer size, nature and type of industry/business, and full-time work status of employees. The health insurance coverage provided by employer group insurance plans also varies widely with respect to the scope of covered services, conditions of eligibility, and the share of employees' contribution to the plan. Many employers do not provide health benefits to part-time workers.

According to the Kaiser Family Foundation's annual health benefits survey of employers, in 2017, 53 percent of companies offered health benefits to at least some of their employees. Eighty-nine percent of employees worked in a firm that offered health benefits to at least some of its workers. The likelihood of an employer offering health benefits varied by size of the company. For example, only 40 percent of companies with three to nine workers offered health benefits. In contrast, virtually all companies with 1,000 or more workers offered health benefits. Of the large firms, 25 percent also offered health benefits to retired workers ("Employer Health Benefits: 2017 Summary of Findings" 2017).

Major industries and businesses have become key actors in the healthcare system because of the cost they incur in providing health insurance for their workers. In 2017, the average annual premium for employer-sponsored health insurance was $6,690 for single coverage and $18,764 for family coverage. The average single premium increased 4 percent and the average family premium increased 3 percent in 2017 ("Employer Health Benefits: 2017 Summary of Findings" 2017). Most covered workers do make a contribution toward the cost of premiums for their coverage. Employees paid about 31 percent of the premium for a family plan in 2017 (Shumsky 2017).

Employers expect healthcare costs to increase by 5.5 percent in 2018 according to the 22nd annual Best Practices in Health Care Employer Survey by Willis Towers Watson ("U.S. Employers Expect Health Care Costs to Rise by 5.5 percent in 2018, up from 4.6 percent in 2017" 2017). Such increases in healthcare premiums have made businesses more conscious of their costs and have led them to use a variety of cost-cutting measures. In the early 1990s companies tried to contain costs by moving their employees into tightly managed insurance plans such as Health Maintenance Organizations (HMOs). But, the so-called managed care revolution came to a halt as doctors, as well as patients, rebelled against restrictions on health services imposed by such plans (Tracer 2017). Employers are pursuing a variety of approaches to reduce their healthcare costs and risks. They include encouraging employees to use preferred healthcare delivery options, choosing carriers and vendors based on competitiveness of provider discounts and total cost of care, curbing the pharmacy and utilization costs, putting greater emphasis on consumer-driven plans, promoting employee health and wellness plans, increasing employee costs of deductibles and out-of-pocket maximum, contracting directly with specific providers for high-cost, high-risk procedures such as joint replacement and back surgery (PWC Health Research Institute 2017; "Employer Strategies for Combating Rising Health Care Costs," n.d.; "U.S. Employers Expect Health Care Costs to Rise by 5.5 percent in 2018, up from 4.6 percent in 2017" 2017). In Chapter 7 we provide a detailed analysis of the problems of rising healthcare costs and efforts by both the public and private sector to contain costs.

The cost of health insurance is a more serious problem for small businesses, which in turn contributes to the problem of wage stagnation. A survey of 20,000 its members conducted by the National Federation of Independent Business (NFIB) found that cost of health insurance was listed as the top problem by all respondents while 52 percent of the respondents listed it as a critical problem (Dunkelberg 2016). The Affordable Care Act attempted to help small businesses in a number of different ways. In Chapter 3 we provide a detailed analysis of the Affordable Care Act.

Consumers

The public can exert influence on policymakers and health policies not only as consumers of health products and services but also by their voting behavior and by expressing their opinions on various healthcare issues, including their level of satisfaction/dissatisfaction with respect to the American healthcare system.

In 2016, 91.1 percent of Americans were covered by some form of health insurance; 197 million Americans were covered by private health insurance, of which 173 million were covered by employer-sponsored health insurance. Medicare and Medicaid provided health insurance coverage to another 127 million Americans, of which 55.8 million were enrolled in Medicare and 71.1 million were enrolled in the Medicaid program. In addition, another 24.8 million Americans were covered (had bought insurance) through the individual marketplace ("National Health Care Spending in 2016" n.d.). Thus, a large majority of the healthcare cost of insured Americans was paid by public or private insurance. Despite this fact, many Americans feel the financial burden of paying out-of-pocket expenses for things such as coinsurance, deductibles, co-payments, and for services not covered by insurance, which have been rising annually.

In 2016, total out-of-pocket expenses amounted to $352.5 million (11 percent) of the total national health expenditures of $3.3 trillion. The out-of-pocket spending increased 3.8 percent from 2015. This was the fastest rate of growth since 2007 (Hartman et al. 2018; "National Health Expenditures 2016 Highlights." n.d.). Out-of-pocket expenses are expected to continue their upward trend because employers are increasingly shifting costs to employees. Also, per-capita spending on national health expenditures amounted to $10,348 (Hartman et al. 2018).

Some have argued that consumers should bear some of the responsibility for controlling the cost of their own healthcare. However, this is highly problematic. Consumers are generally aware of their co-payments, coinsurance, and deductibles but they are often unaware of the true price of health care the third party, i.e., insurance company, reimburses the healthcare provider directly. In addition, what the consumer and the insurance company pay is different than the listed price. Healthcare prices for the same health services also vary considerably by a patient's geographic location. Under such conditions, it is almost impossible for consumers to do comparative shopping for health services. It is estimated that only about 7 percent of spending on health services is subject to comparative shopping (Dolan 2017). Information asymmetry puts the consumer at a severe disadvantage (Nakhjiri 2017). Evidence also suggests even when price comparison and rating tools are available, very few consumers (about 3 percent) use such tools and hospital rating systems lead to more confusion and not less because there is no clear agreement on what is a "good" hospital (Dolan 2017). Many reforms have called for more price transparency in healthcare where consumers can clearly see the price of a particular treatment and how much their out-of-pocket cost will be (Robert Wood Johnson Foundation 2016).

What opinions do Americans as consumers of healthcare express about the American healthcare system, their level of satisfaction, and on other healthcare issues? Almost nine out of ten Americans (88 percent) agree that healthcare costs are too high, with 33 percent putting the blame on insurance companies, 22 percent on government, and another 13 percent on pharmaceutical companies. Others put the blame on hospitals (11 percent), lawyers (7 percent), doctors (7 percent), patients (6 percent), and employers (1 percent) (Lynch, Perosino, and Slover 2014). Similarly, 72 percent of Americans believe that pharmaceutical companies have too much influence in Washington, DC and 66 percent believe the same of insurance companies ("Poll: Public Says Drug Companies have More Influence in Washington than the NRA" 2018).

In a Gallup poll conducted in 2016, 65 percent of Americans stated they were satisfied with the way the healthcare system works for them (Auter 2016). However, in a 2017 Gallup poll, 71 percent of American expressed the belief that American healthcare system is in a state of crisis or has major problems. This percentage has stayed within a seven-percentage-point range (67 percent–74 percent) over the last ten years ("Americans Still Hold Dim View of U.S. Healthcare System" 2017). In another 2017 Gallup poll, 56 percent of Americans expressed the view that the federal government should be responsible for making sure that all Americans have health insurance coverage (Newport 2017).

However, when it comes to the national health insurance system, often called a "single-payer plan" or "Medicare-for-all" plan, Americans are very divided, with 53 percent favoring having a national health plan while 44 percent oppose such a plan. This opinion is heavily divided along political party affiliation, with 73 percent of Democrats favoring such a plan while 71 percent of Republicans express opposition to such a plan (Kirzinger et al. 2017). Finally, while the support for the ACA has increased over the years, with 52 percent holding a favorable opinion in 2017, the partisan divide remains. Sixty-one percent of Democrats expressed a very favorable opinion of the ACA, while 54 percent of Republicans had a very unfavorable opinion (Hamel et al. 2017). A great deal of the divide on healthcare issues also splits along partisan and ideological lines.

It is important to remember that simply because the public responds to questions asked in the opinion polls, it does not mean that their opinions are based on having accurate information, knowledge, and understanding of the topic on which they express an opinion. Polls also tend to show that the public is often confused and lacks a clear understanding of the subject matter on which they express an opinion. Thus, the opinions they express may be based on lack of information/understanding or on misinformation and are influenced more by partisan and ideological feelings and attitudes. An "interest" in a subject does not necessarily translate to "understanding" of the subject. When public opinion is very divided, confused, or diffused and lacks clarity and intensity, it provides interest groups, i.e., factions with a vested interest in exploiting the situation and exercising a disproportionate amount of influence in health policymaking.

Interest Groups

The role of interest groups in US politics has been debated intensely from the time of the founding of the Republic. The public philosophy of interest-group liberalism has accorded interest groups a dominant role in US politics. Proponents have praised the role of interest groups in American democracy. In his seminal work, *The Process of Government*, Arthur Bentley (1908) argued that all politics and government results from activities of interest groups and politics are a never-ending struggle for advantage among constantly shifting coalition of interest groups. Since there is no such thing as the "public," or "public interest," or "public opinion," or "popular will," the only way to influence politics is to organize and get involved in politics. In contrast, one of the most influential Founding Fathers, James Madison (1961b) called groups united by common passion and/or interest as "factions," capable of devilment, viewing them as negative. Health-related interest groups have been blamed for defeating efforts at major healthcare reforms in the twentieth century.

Regardless of how one views the role of interest groups in American politics, the fact is that since healthcare affects everyone in society, a wide variety of "interests" are affected by what happens in healthcare and health policymaking. Interest groups try to influence the political process and policymaking using a variety of tactics such as endorsing candidates, making campaign contributions to political parties and candidates running for public office, testifying before congressional committees, endorsing candidates, and engaging in political persuasion through advertisement and other communication channels.

In this section, we discuss the role of some of the most important and influential health-related professional groups in the healthcare field. It is important to note that these groups are not strictly "interest groups" in the traditional sense. Their sole purpose is not lobbying and engaging in political activities. Professional associations have a broader purpose and perform multiple functions compared to traditional interest groups. However, one of the functions they perform is political lobbying. They do so through their Political Action Committees (PACs). Federal campaign finance laws and rules limit the amount of campaign contributions PACs can make to candidates' political campaign committees as well as national political party committees. All PACs are required to register with the Federal Election Commission (FEC). Following a court decision, new forms of PACs, called Super PACs, emerged after 2010. Super PACs do not make a contribution to candidates or parties. But, they can make independent expenditures in federal races for things such as running political ads, and communicate via mails and other means to advocate election or defeat of specific candidates.

In 2018, the health sector as a whole employed 2,841 lobbyists and spent a total of $558 million on lobbying. The top spender within the health sector was the pharmaceuticals/health products industry, to the tune of $279 million (Center for Responsive Politics n.d.). In the 2016 election cycle, health sector PACs contributed $55 million to federal candidates, of which 40 percent ($22 million) went to Democrats and 60 percent ($33 million) went to Republicans (Center for Responsive Politics n.d.).

The American Medical Association

The American Medical Association (AMA) was established in 1847, and today it is one of the largest and most influential health-related groups. It is a professional association of physicians, the voice of organized medicine, and as such, it acts as an umbrella organization of US medicine. Its main functions include representing the interests of its members; providing scientific and socioeconomic information; keeping data on the profession; and developing and maintaining standards of professional education, training, and performance. The association is active at both national and state level in advocating reducing regulatory burden and promoting healthcare delivery models that support physicians. The AMA has played a major role in the development of medicine in America ("Founding of the AMA" n.d.).

The AMA has acted as a voice of free enterprise and has successfully argued against a national health insurance program because of the fear of losing its professional autonomy and of a decline in physicians' income. But the organization has articulated its opposition to national health insurance not on the ground of protecting self-interest but by using the rhetoric of defending free enterprise and patients' freedom to choose their own doctors. It has argued that adoption of national health insurance would lead to lower quality of healthcare and services. The AMA has not been above using scare tactics to achieve its objectives, but over the years it has softened its stand toward major healthcare reform.

The AMA has grassroots political power and is very active in lobbying Congress on health-related issues. It is very well financed. It has one of the largest political action committees. The mission of the American Medical Association Political Action Committee (AMPAC) is to find and support candidates for congressional office, whether a new candidate for office who will make physicians and patients a top priority or a candidate running for reelection who has proved to be a friend of medicine. In the 2016 election cycle, working with state medical society PACs, AMPAC spent nearly $2 million in direct campaign contributions to physician-friendly candidates for the US House and Senate. Sixty-one percent of the contribution went to Republican candidates and 39 percent was spent on Democratic candidates ("The 2016 Cycle AMPAC Election Report" n.d.).

The AMA is not the only physician group that has attempted to influence the political process. PACs representing groups such as physician assistants, clinical urologists, orthopedic surgeons, and emergency physicians have also contributed funds to political campaigns. In the 2016 election cycle, PACs representing health professionals contributed $9.9 million to federal candidates, of which 39 percent went to Democratic candidates and 61 percent went to Republican candidates (Center for Responsive Politics n.d.).

The American Nurses Association

The American Nurses Association (ANA) is a professional organization that represents the interests of the country's 3.6 million registered nurses through its state organizations and organizational affiliates. It is the strongest voice of the nursing profession. Besides promoting advances in the nursing professions by fostering high standards of nursing practice, the ANA lobbies Congress and regulatory agencies on healthcare issues affecting nurses and the general public. Through its legislative and political program, the ANA has taken positions on issues such as Medicare reform, patient rights, whistle-blower protection for healthcare workers, and access to healthcare. The association has advocated for an expanded role for RNs and APNs in the delivery of basic and primary healthcare ("About ANA" n.d.).

The ANA's political action committee ANA-PAC was formed in1970s. The voluntary contributions received from ANA members are used by the ANA-PAC for political purposes. The ANA-PAC endorses a handful of candidates in each election cycle ("About US" n.d.). The ANA-PAC is not as big a player in the area of lobbying and campaign contributions as some of the other groups. In 2016, the ANA-PAC spent only about $458,218 on political activities, an overwhelming majority of which went to Democratic candidates (Center for Responsive Politics n.d.).

The American Hospital Association

The National Hospital Superintendents' Association was created in 1899. Membership in this organization was limited to chief executive officers of hospitals. A few years after the organization's founding, its name was changed to the American Hospital Association (AHA). In 1917 it changed from an individual-membership organization to an organization of institutions (Weeks and Berman 1985). Today, the AHA represents and serves a variety of hospitals, healthcare networks, and individual members. In addition to conducting research and education projects, it acts as the voice of hospitals and represents their interests in national health policy development. Its advocacy efforts have included lobbying executive and legislative branches of government (American Hospital Association n.d.).

The American Hospital Association's political action committee, the AHA-PAC, spent slightly $3 million on political activities in the 2016 election cycle. It spent $1.4 million in campaign contributions to federal candidates, of which 55 percent went to Republican and 45 percent to Democratic candidates (Center for Responsive Politics n.d.).

America's Health Insurance Plans

America's Health Insurance Plans (AHIP) is the voice of US health insurers. AHIP is the national association that represents companies that provide health insurance coverage to millions of Americans. The association represents the interests of its members on legislative and regulatory issues at the federal and state levels (America's Health Insurance Plans n.d.).

In the 2016 election cycle, the AHIP-PAC spent close to $400,000 on lobbying, of which $262,500 went for campaign contributions to federal candidates, with Republican candidates receiving 61 percent and Democratic candidates receiving 41 percent (Center for Responsive Politics n.d.).

The largest five insurance companies are WellPoint Inc, Cigna, Aetna, Humana, and United Healthcare. WellPoint Inc has 34 million insured members in its affiliated health plans and the number increases to 70 million if one includes all its subsidiaries, making it the largest health insurance company in terms of its membership (Baltazar 2018).

Pharmaceutical Research and Manufacturers of America (PhRMA)

PhRMA represents the nation's major pharmaceutical research and biotechnology companies. Originally it started out as the Pharmaceutical Manufacturers of America (PMA) in 1958. In 1994, its name was changed to Pharmaceutical Research and Manufacturers of American (PhRMA) to emphasize the research aspect of its work. The pharmaceutical and biotechnological research sector in America is the global leader in medical innovation. Since the year 2000, the Food and Drug Administration has approved over 550 new medicines. In 2015, it spent close to $58 million in Research and Development (R&D) (Pharmaceutical Research and Manufacturers of America 2016).

PhRMA has consistently ranked among the biggest spenders on lobbying in the nation's capital over the last several years. In 2016 it spent $11.8 million on lobbying, making it the fourth-largest in lobbying (Karlin-Smith and Palmer 2017). In the 2016 election cycle, pharmaceuticals and health product companies' PACs contributed $18 million to federal candidates, with 62 percent of it going to Republican candidates and 38 percent going to Democratic candidates (Center for Responsive Politics n.d.).

The Medical Device Manufacturers of America

Created in 1992, the MDMA is a national trade organization based in Washington, DC. It represents the interests of smaller medical technology companies. The organization is active in representing its members' interests before Congress, the FDA, CMS, and other federal agencies. It provides its members with educational and advocacy assistance. The MDMA is relatively new and thus not as big a player as some other groups in the health policy fields (Medical Device Manufacturers of America n.d.).

Consumer Advocacy Groups

There has been significant growth in consumer/public interest groups in the field of healthcare. These groups essentially act as a voice and advocate for protecting and advancing consumers' interest in healthcare, including interest groups focused on patient interests. However, it is important to note that such groups are vastly outnumbered by occupationally based interest groups (Keller and Packel 2014). Some of the prominent consumer interest groups in the healthcare field include groups such as the Consumer Health Alliance (www.consumerhealthalliance.org), Families USA (www.familiesusa.org/), the American Health Care Association (www.ahcancal.org/Pages/Default.aspx), the Center for Health Care Strategies (www.chcs.org/), and the Children's Defense Fund (www.childrensdefense.org/).

Some patient advocacy groups are very specific and center around specific diseases. For example, the Lung Cancer Alliance (https://lungcanceralliance.org/) is a non-profit organization that provides information about lung cancer and support services. Aplastic Anemia and MDS International Foundation (www.aamds.org/) not only provides patient services but also funds research in the private sector and lobbies Congress for federal research dollars earmarked specifically for the disease the group represents. The disease-specific patient interest groups generally do not form coalitions across diseases (Keller and Packel 2014).

Non-Partisan Health Foundations

Two of the most important private, non-partisan foundations in the field of health are the Robert Wood Johnson Foundation (RWJF) (www.rwjf.org/) and the Kaiser Family Foundation (KFF) (www.kff.org/). The RWJF is the largest private philanthropic foundation devoted solely to the public's health and dedicated to the mission of improving the health and healthcare of all Americans. It does research as well as provides grants in the healthcare field. The KFF serves as a non-partisan source of information about health policy issues, and, unlike grant-making foundations, KFF runs its own research program, sometimes in partnership with other non-profit organizations. Both are excellent sources of information on healthcare issues for policymakers, administrators, educators, students, and consumers.

Examples of other private research foundations include the Glaucoma Research Foundation (www.glaucoma.org/), the Desmoid Tumor Research Foundation (http://dtrf.org/), the Children's Health and Research Foundation, Inc., (http://chrfoundation.net/), and the Mental Health Research Foundation (www.mentalhealthexcellence.org/), among others.

CONCLUSION

Healthcare politics and policies in the United States are shaped by a variety of factors. Health policy reflects a combination of initiatives taken by institutions and actors in the public and private sectors. The health policy cycle is influenced and shaped by the constitutional, institutional, political, economic, ideological, and technological environment within which it operates. The public philosophy of interest-group liberalism combined with constitutionally guaranteed freedom of speech, association, and petition allows a variety of interest groups to promote policies for private profit and to successfully defeat policies they perceive as harmful to their interests. Interest groups promote their narrow private interests using the rhetoric of the common good. The consensus created through compromise and bargaining between narrow private interests is often defined as the public interest. Such a policy process makes the establishment of a comprehensive national health policy highly improbable, if not impossible. The result is a mishmash of public- and private-sector healthcare programs and policies that often reflect conflicting values of access, equality, quality of care, and efficiency.

Effective health policy often requires formulating policies based on research, scientific evidence, facts, and rational public debate about the nature of the problem, available policy alternatives, and the best way to address a problem. However, this may become problematic because the scientific evidence is: (a) nonexistent; (b) weak; (c) inconclusive or contradictory; and (d) there is a disagreement over the nature and type of scientific evidence. Even when the scientific evidence is conclusive and strong, it may fail to inform policymaking because it conflicts with other societal, cultural, moral, religious, or political values. Thus, it may be ignored or twisted with misinformation and/or falsehood for partisan, ideological, and electoral calculations. The political environment has undergone a significant change since the 1970s from the environment of compromise, bargaining, consensus, and coalition-building to one characterized by divided government and partisan, ideological, and electorate polarization and tribalism. Congress has found it increasingly difficult to arrive at any type of bipartisan compromise on major policy issues, including healthcare. This has led to more concentration of power and authority in the presidency and the executive branch as Congress has often failed to act or has abdicated its responsibility to the executive branch, raising the specter of an "imperial presidency." Thus, more often than not, the science of policymaking is substituted by the art of deal-making. Health policies resulting from such deal-making may turn out to be ineffective. However, to understand health policy in the United States, one must understand the health policy environment, including the underlying politics. Further, it is important to keep in mind that no one single factor in the health policy environment influences and shapes health policymaking, but rather health policymaking in the United States is often a product of a variety of complex but interrelated factors.

STUDY QUESTIONS

1. How does "politics" influence health policymaking in the United States? What does one generally mean by politics? Give at least two specific examples where politics influenced health policymaking.
2. What constitutes the health policy environment? What are some of the major factors in the health policy environment that influence health policymaking in the United States?
3. Write an essay in which you discuss how some of the unique features of the American constitutional environment shape health policymaking in the United States. Be sure to give specific examples.
4. How do some of the unique features of American institutions—Congress, the presidency, and the judiciary—shape health policymaking in the United States? Give some specific examples.
5. What do the authors mean by "political environment," and what are major elements of this environment that help explain policymaking in the United States? How has the US political environment changed since the 1970s?
6. What is the theory of incrementalism, and how does the theory of punctuated equilibrium advance our understanding of incremental and major policy changes?
7. Should health policymaking in the United States be based solely on the best available scientific evidence, or should factors such as public opinion and cultural/social/political values also play a role in health policymaking? Why?
8. Discuss who some of the major public/government-sector health policy actors are in the United States. What makes them major policy actors?
9. Who are some of the major private-sector health policy actors in the United States? What makes them major policy actors?
10. Who are some of the major interest groups, and how do they exercise their influence in health policymaking?

REFERENCES

Abramowitz, Alan I. 2013. "The Electoral Roots of America's Dysfunctional Government." *Presidential Studies Quarterly*, 43, no. 4 (December): 709–731.
"About ANA." n.d. Silver Spring, MD: American Nurses Association. Online at www.nursingworld.org/.
"About Us." n.d. Aristotle. Online at http://aristotle.com/.
Adler, Jerry. 2017. "In 2017, the Tug of Tribalism Grew Stronger." Yahoo. Online at www.yahoo.com/news/2017-tug-tribalism-grew-stronger-100004695.html.
Adler, Jonathan H. 2011. "Cooperation, Commandeering, or Crowding Out? Federal Intervention and State Choices in Health Care Policy." *Kansas Journal of Law and Public Policy*, 20, no. 2: 199–221.
Ahler, Douglas. 2014. "Self-Fulfilling Misperceptions of Public Polarization." *Journal of Politics*, 76, no. 3: 607–620.
Allison, Graham. 1971. *The Essence of Decision*. Boston, MA: Little, Brown.
Altenstetter, Christa. 1974. *Health Policy-Making and Administration in West Germany and the United States*. Beverly Hills, CA: Sage.
Altschuler, Glenn C. 2017. "Partisanship, Polarization and the Future of American Politics." *The Huffington Post*. Online at www.huffingtonpost.com/.
"America Still Holds Dim View of U.S. Healthcare System." 2017. *Gallup Poll*. Online at http://news.gallup.com/.
America's Health Insurance Plans. n.d. "About Us." Washington, DC: America's Health Insurance Plans. Online at www.ahip.org/about/.
American Health Care Association. n.d. *Fast Facts*. Online at https://ahcancal.org/.
American Hospital Association. 2017. "Fast Facts on U.S. Hospitals." Chicago, IL: American Hospital Association. Online at www.aha.org/.
Anderson, Steve. 2010. "The American Way for Nearly 100 Years." Healthinsurance.org. Online at www.healthinsurance.org/.
Association of American Medical Colleges. 2016. "2016 Physician Specialty date Report: Executive Summary." Washington, DC: Association of American Medical Colleges. Online at www.aamc.org/.
Association of American Medical Colleges. 2017. "Active Physicians with a U.S. Doctor of Osteopathic Medicine (DO) by Specialty, 2015." Washington, DC: Association of American Medical Colleges. Online at www.aamc.org/.
Auter, Zac. 2016. "Americans' Satisfaction with Healthcare System Edges Down." *Gallup Poll*. Online at http://news.gallup.com/.
Badger, Emily. 2010. "Divided Government Usually Means Gridlock." Miller-McCune, *Idea Lobby*. Online at www.miller.mccune.com/.
Bagley, Nicholas. 2017. "Federalism and the End of Obamacare." *Yale Law Journal*, 127, no. 1: 1–26.
Balducchi, David E. and Stephen A. Wander. 2008. "Work Sharing Policy: Power Sharing and Stalemate in American Federalism." *Publius*, 38, no. 1: 111–136.
Baltazar, Amanda. 2018. "The Big Five Health Insurance Companies." Very Well Health. Online at www.verywellhealth.com/the-big-five-health-insurance-companies-2663838/.
Banting, Keith G. and Stan Corbett. 2002. "Health Policy and Federalism: An Introduction." In *Health Policy and Federalism: An Introduction*, eds. Keith G. Banting and Stan Corbett, 1–38. School of Policy Studies, Institute of Intergovernmental Relations, Social Union Series. Kingston, ON: Queens University.
Barber, Michael and Jeremy C. Pope. 2017. "Does Party Trump Ideology? Disentangling Party and Ideology in America." Brigham Young University Scholar Archives. Online at https://drive.google.com/file/d/0B6-zXaKeceR4dXJnMGhpblRFNjQ/preview.
Baumgartner, Frank R. 2006. "Punctuated Equilibrium Theory and Environmental Policy." In *Punctuated Equilibrium and the Dynamics of U.S. Environmental Policy*, ed. Robert C. Repetto, 24–46. New Haven, CT: Yale University Press.
Baumgartner, Frank R., Jeffrey M. Berry, Marie Hojnacki, David C. Kimball, and Beth L. Leech. 2009. *Lobbying and Policy Change: Who Wins, Who Loses, and Why*. Chicago, IL: University of Chicago Press.
Baumgartner, Frank R. and Bryan D. Jones. 1993. *Agendas and Instability in American Politics*. Chicago, IL: University of Chicago Press.
Baumgartner, Frank R. and Bryan D. Jones. 2009. *Agendas and Instability in American Politics*, 2d edn. Chicago, IL: University of Chicago Press.
Baumgartner, Frank R. and Beth L. Leech. 2001. "Interest Niches and Policy Bandwagons: Patterns of Interest Group Involvement in National Politics." *Journal of Politics*, 63, no. 4: 1191–1213.
Bayes, Jane H. 1982. *Ideologies and Interest-Group Politics*. Novato, CA: Chandler and Sharp.
Beer, S.H. 1965. *Modern British Politics*. London: Faber and Faber.
Beland, Daniel and Francois Vergniolle de Chantal. 2004. "Fighting 'Big Government': Frames, Federalism, and Social Policy Reform in the United States." *Canadian Journal of Sociology*, 29, no. 2: 241–264.
Bentley, Arthur F. 1908. *The Process of Government*. Chicago, IL: University of Chicago Press.
Berman, Russell. 2016. "What is the Answer to Political Polarization in the U. S.?" *The Atlantic*. Online at www.theatlantic.com/.
Biller, Sofia E. 2008. "Flooded by the Lowest Ebb: Congressional Response to Presidential Signing Statements and Executive Hostility to the Operation of Checks and Balances." *Iowa Law Review*, 93, no. 3: 1067–1133.
Black, Ryan C., Anthony J. Madonna, Ryan J. Owens, and Michael S. Lynch. 2007. "Adding Recess Appointment to the President's 'Tool Chest' of Unilateral Powers." *Political Research Quarterly*, 60, no. 4: 645–654.
Blendon, Robert J. and Gillian K. SteelFisher. 2009. "Commentary: Understanding the Underlying Politics of Health Care Policy Decision Making." *Health Services Research*, 44, no. 4: 1137–1143.

Bloom, Anne. 2001. "The Post-Attitudinal Moment: Judicial Policy Making Through the Lens of New Institutionalism." *Law & Society Review*, 35, no. 1: 219–231.

Bonica, Adam. 2013. "Mapping the Ideological Marketplace." *American Journal of Political Science*, 58, no. 2: 367–386.

Bovbjerg, Randall R., Joshua M. Wiener, and Michael Houseman. 2003. "State and Federal Role in Health Care: Rationale for Allocating Responsibilities." In *Federalism and Health Policy*, ed. John Holahan, Allan Weil, and Joshua Weiner, 25–57. Washington, DC: Urban Institute Press.

Breunig, Christian and Chris Koski. 2006. "Punctuated Equilibria and Budgets in the American States." *Policy Studies Journal*, 34, no. 3: 363–379.

Brown, J.H.A. 1978. *The Politics of Health Care*. Cambridge, MA: Ballinger.

Brown, Lawrence D. 1978. "The Formulation of Federal Health Care Policy." *Bulletin of the New York Academy of Medicine*, 54, no. 1 (January): 45–58.

Brown-Nagin, Tomiko. 2014. "Two America's In Healthcare: Federalism and Wars Over Poverty–From the New Deal–Great Society to Obamacare." *Drake Law Review*, 62, 981–1015.

Bulman-Pozen, Jessica. 2016. "Executive Federalism Comes to America." *Virginia Law Review*, 102, 953–1030.

Bureau of Labor Statistics. 2018. US Department of Labor, *Occupational Outlook Handbook, Registered Nurses*. Online at www.bls.gov/.

Burgin, Eileen. 2003. "Congress, Health Care, and Congressional Caucuses: An Examination of the Diabetes Caucus." *Journal of Health Politics, Policy and Law*, 28, no. 5: 789–821.

Caffrey, Christine, Manisha Sengupta, Eunice Park-Lee, Abigail Moss, Emily Rosenoff, and Lauren Harris-Kojetin. 2012. "Residents living in Residential Care Facilities: United States, 2010." NCHS Data Brief, no. 91. Hyattsville, MD: National Center for Health Statistics.

Callaghan, Timothy H. and Lawrence Jacobs. 2013. "Dynamic Federalism and the Implementation of the Affordable Care Act." *Paper delivered at the 2013 Annual Meeting of the American Political Science Association*, August 29–September 1, 2013.

Campbell, James E. 2016. *Polarized: Making Sense of a Divided America Princeton*. Princeton, NJ: Princeton University Press.

Center for Responsive Politics. n.d. "Health Sector." Online at www.opensecrets.org/.

Centers for Medicare and Medicaid Services. n.d. "Historical." Online at www.cms.gov/Research-Statistics-Data-and-Systems/Statistics-Trends-and-Reports/NationalHealthExpendData/NationalHealthAccountsHistorical.html.

Chait, Jonathan. 2015. "How 'Negative Partisanship' has Transformed American Politics." *New York Magazine*. Online at http://nymag.com/.

Cohn, Nate. 2014. "Polarization is Dividing American Society, Not Just Politics." *The New York Times*. Online at www.nytimes.com/.

Colby, David C. 2002. "Federal State Relations in United States Health Policy." In *Health Policy and Federalism: An Introduction*, eds Keith G. Banting and Stan Corbett, 143–172. School of Policy Studies, Institute of Intergovernmental Relations, Social Union Series. Kingston, ON: Queens University. Online. www.queensu.ca/iigr/pub/archive/socialunionseries.html.

Conley, Richard S. 2003. *The Presidency, Congress, and Divided Government: A Postwar Assessment*. College Station, TX: Texas A&M University Press.

Davis, Nicholas T. and Johanna L. Dunaway. 2016. "Party Polarization, Media Choice, and Mass Partisan-Ideological Sorting." *Public Opinion Quarterly*, 80, Special Issue: 272–297.

Dentzer, Susan. 1990. "America's Scandalous Health Care." *U.S. News and World Report*, March 12, 25–30.

DiIulio, John J., Jr. and Richard R. Nathan, eds. 1994. *Making Health Reform Work: The View from the States*. Washington, DC: Brookings Institution.

Dinan, John. 2008. "The State of American Federalism 2007–2008: Resurgent State Influence in the National Policy Process and Continued State Policy Innovation." *Publius*, 38, no. 3: 415–435.

Doherty, Carroll. 2014. "7 Things to Know about Polarization in America." Pew Research Center. Online at www.pewresearch.org/. The full PDF report is available at www.people-press.org/.

Dolan, Rachel. 2017. "From the Archives: Prices and Consumer Shopping." *Health Affairs Blog*, July 19. Online at www.healthaffairs.org/do/10.1377/hblog20170719.061105/full/.

Doonan, Michael. 2013. *American Federalism in Practice: The Formulation and Implementation of Contemporary Health Policy*. Washington, DC: Brookings Institution Press.

Dropp, Kyle A., Molly C. Jackman, and Saul P. Jackman. 2013. *The Affordable Care Act: An Experiment in Federalism?* Washington, DC: Center for Effective Public Management at The Brookings Institution. Online at www.brookings.edu/Dudley.

Dudley, R. Adam and Harold S. Luft. 1999. "Goals, Targets, and Tactics: Making Health Care Policy Decisions Explicit." *Journal of Health Politics, Policy, and Law*, 24, no. 4: 705–713.

Dunkelberg, William. 2016. "The Cost of Health Insurance is a Big Problem for Small Business." *Forbes*. Online at www.forbes.com/.

Edwards, George C., III, Andrew Barrett, and Jeffrey Peake. 1997. "The Legislative Impact of Divided Government." *American Journal of Political Science*, 41, no. 2: 545–563.

"Employer Health Benefits: 2017 Summary of Findings." 2017. Henry J. Kaiser Family Foundation and Health Research and Education Trust. Online at http://files.kff.org/.

"Employer Strategies for Combating Rising Health Care Costs." n.d. G&A Partners. Online at www.gnapartners.com/.

Epstein, Lee and Jack Knight. 1998. *The Choices Justices Make*. Washington, DC: Congressional Quarterly Press.

"Establishing Health Insurance Exchanges: An Overview of State Efforts." 2012. Washington, DC: Kaiser Family Foundation. Online at http://healthreform.kff.org/.

Evans, Kevin and Bryan Marshall. 2016. "Presidential Signing Statements and Lawmaking Credit." *Political Science Quarterly*, 131, no. 4: 749–778.

Ewing, Benjamin and Douglas A. Kysar. 2011. "Prods and Pleas: Limited Government in an Era of Unlimited Harm." *Yale Law Review*, 121, no. 2: 350–424.

Fallows, James. 2017. "The Animal Instincts at the Heart of Human Nature." *The Atlantic*. Online at www.theatlantic.com/.

Farina, Cynthia R. 2015. "Congressional Polarization: Terminal Constitutional Dysfunction?" *Columbia Law Review*, 115, no. 7: 1689–1738.

Feeley, Malcolm and Edward L. Rubin. 2000. *Judicial Policy Making and the Modern State: How the Courts Reformed America's Prisons*. Cambridge, MA: Cambridge University Press.

"Founding of AMA." n.d. Online at www.ama-assn.org/.

Frakes, Vincent L. 2012. "Partisanship and (Un)compromise: A Study of the Patient Protection and Affordable Care Act." *Harvard Journal on Legislation*, 49, no. 1: 135–149.

Frakt, Austin B., Steven D. Pizer, and Ann M. Hendricks. 2008. "Controlling Prescription Drug Costs: Regulation and the Role of Interest Groups in Medicare and the Veterans Health Administration." *Journal of Health Politics, Policy and Law*, 33, no. 6: 1079–1106.

France, George. 2008. "The Form and Context of Federalism: Meanings for Health Care Financing." *Journal of Health Politics, Policy and Law*, 33, no. 4: 649–705.

Freddi, Giorgio. 2009. "Health Care as the Central Civic and Political Problem of the United States: A Comparative Perspective." *European Political Science*, 8, 330–344.

Fuchs, Victor R. 1986. *The Health Economy*. Cambridge, MA: Harvard University Press.

Fuchs, Victor R. 1995. *Who Shall Live? Health, Economics and Social Choice*. New York: Basic Books.

Galderisi, Peter, Roberta Q. Herzberg, and Peter McNamara, eds. 1996. *Divided Government: Change, Uncertainty, and the Constitutional Order*. New York: Rowman and Littlefield.

Gauld, Robin. 2001. "Contextual Pressures on Health–Implications for Policy Making and Service Provision." *Policy Studies*, 22, no. 3–4: 167–179.

Geyman, Jon. 2015. "Why the Private Health Insurance Industry has to Go." *Huffington Post*. April 9. Online at www.huffingtonpost.com/.

Gibian, T.C. 2012. "Political Tribalism in the USA." *Daily Kos*. Online at www.dailykos.com/stories/2012/4/3/1079564/-Political-Tribalism-in-the-USA.

Givel, Michael. 2010. "The Evolution of the Theoretical Foundations of Punctuated Equilibrium Theory in Public Policy." *Review of Policy Research*, 27, no. 2: 187–198.

Gold, Jenny. 2010. "Mergers of Profit, Non-Profit Hospitals: Who Does It Help?" *USA Today*, July 13. Online at www.usatoday.com/money/.

Graves, John A. and Pranita Mishra. 2016. "The Evolving Dynamics of Employer-Sponsored Health Insurance." *Milbank Quarterly*, 94, no. 4: 736–767.

Greer, Scott L. and Peter D. Jacobson. 2010. "Health Care Reform and Federalism." *Journal of Health Politics, Policy and Law*, 35, no. 2: 203–226.

Gutmann, Amy and Dennis Thompson. 2010. "The Mindset of Political Compromise." *Perspectives on Politics*, 8, no. 4: 1125–1143.

Hackey, Robert B. and David A. Rochefort, eds. 2001. *The New Politics of State Health Policy*. Lawrence, KS: University of Kansas Press.

Hall, Mark A. 2013. "The Supreme Court's PPACA Decision: Healthcare Law versus Constitutional Law." *Journal of Health Politics, Policy and Law*, 38, no. 2: 267–272.

Hamel, Liz, Wu Bryan, Calley Munana, and Mollyann Brodie. 2017. "Data Note: Strongly Held Views on the ACA." Kaiser Family Foundation. Online at www.kff.org/.

Harbridge, Laurel and Neil Malhotra. 2011. "Electoral Incentives and Partisan Conflict in Congress: Evidence from Survey Experiments." *American Journal of Political Science*, 55, no. 3: 494–510.

Hare, Christopher and Keith T. Poole. 2014. "The Polarization of Contemporary American Politics." *Polity*, 43, no. 3: 411–429.

Hartman, Micah, Anne B. Martin, Nathan Espinosa, and Aaron Catlin. 2018. "National Health Care Spending in 2016." *Health Affairs*, 37, no. 1: 150–160.

Hayes, Michael T. 2001. *The Limits of Policy Change: Incrementalism, Worldview, and the Rule of Law*. Washington, DC: Georgetown University Press.

Hayes, Michael T. 2006. *Incrementalism and Public Policy*. Lanham, MD: University Press of America.

Heaney, Michael T. 2004. "Issue Networks, Information, and Interest Group Alliances: The Case of Wisconsin Welfare Politics, 1993–99." *State Politics and Policy Quarterly*, 4, no. 3 (Fall): 237–270.

Heaney, Michael T. 2006. "Brokering Health Policy Coalition, Parties, and Interest Group Influence." *Journal of Health Politics, Policy, and Law*, 31, no. 5: 887–944.

Heclo, Hugh. 1978. "Issues Networks and the Executive Establishment." In *The New American Political System*, ed. Anthony King, 87–124. Washington, DC: American Enterprise Institute Press.

Heinz, John P., Edward O. Laumann, Robert L. Nelson, and Robert H. Salisbury. 1993. *The Hollow Core: Private Interests in National Policy Making*. Cambridge, MA: Harvard University Press.

Herring, Pendleton. 1967. *Group Representation Before Congress*. New York: Russell and Russell.

Hibbing, Matthew V., Matthew Hays, and Raman Deol. 2017. "Nostalgia Isn't What it Used to Be: Partisan Polarization in Views on the Past." *Social Science Quarterly*, 98, no. 1: 230–243.

Holahan, John, Alan Weil, and Joshua M. Wiener. 2003. *Federalism and Health Policy*. Washington, DC: Urban Institute Press.

Holyoke, Thomas T. 2009. "Interest Group Competition and Coalition Formation." *American Journal of Political Science*, 53, no. 2: 360–375.

Huberfeld, Nicole. 2017. "Instrumental and Transformative Medical Technology." *Vanderbilt Journal of Entertainment and Technology Law*, 19, no. 2: 267–283.

Huitt, Ralph. 1970. "Political Feasibility." In *Policy Analysis in Political Science*, ed. Ira Sharkansky, 399–412. Chicago, IL: Markham.

Jacobson, Gary C. 2013. "Partisan Polarization in American Politics: A Background Paper." *Presidential Studies Quarterly*, 43, no. 4: 688–706.

Jochim, Ashely E. and Bryan D. Jones. 2013. "Issue Politics in a Polarized Congress." *Political Research Quarterly*, 66, no. 2: 352–369.

Jones, Charles O. 1978. *An Introduction to the Study of Public Policy*. North Scituate, MA: Duxbury Press.

Jones, Charles O. 1994. *The Presidency as a Separated System*. Washington, DC: Brookings Institution.

Kane, Carol K. 2017. *Updated Data on Physician Practice Arrangements: Physician Ownership Drops Below 50 Percent*. Chicago, IL: American Medical Association. Online at www.ama-assn.org/.

Karlin-Smith, Sarah and Anna Palmer. 2017. "Drug Lobby Adds $100 to War Chest Ahead of Pricing Battle." Politico. Online at www.politico.com/.

Keller, Ann C. and Laura Packel. 2014. "Going for the Cure: Patient Interest groups and Health Advocacy in the United States." *Journal of Health Politics, Policy and Law*, 39, no. 2: 331–367.

Kennedy, Joshua B. 2014. "Signing Statements, Gridlock, and Presidential Strategy." *Presidential Studies Quarterly*, 44, no. 4: 602–622.

Kirzinger, Ashley, Liz Hamel, Blanca DiJullio, Cailey Munana, and Mollyann Brodie. 2017. "Data Note: Public's Views of a National Health Plan." Kaiser Family Foundation. www.kff.org/health-reform/.

Kornacki, Steve. 2018. *The Red and the Blue: The 1990s and the Birth of Political Tribalism*. New York: Ecco Imprint; HarperCollins Publishers.

Koszczuk, Jackie. 1995. "Gingrich Puts More Power into Speaker's Hands." *Congressional Quarterly Weekly Report*, 53, no. 39 (October 7): 3049–3051.

La Raja, Raymond J. 2014. "Campaign Finance and Partisan Polarization in the United States Congress." *Duke Journal of Constitutional Law and Public Policy*, 9, 223–258.

Law, Anna O. 2010. "Making Policy in the Margins: The Federal Judiciary's Role in Immigration Policy." *Juniata Voices*, 10, 92–98.

Lee, Philip R. and Carroll L. Estes. 1983. "New Federalism and Health Policy." *Annals of the American Academy of Political and Social Science*, 468 (July): 88–102.

Lendon, Jessica P. and Vincent Rome. 2018. *Variation in Adult Day Services Center Participant Characteristics, by Center Ownership: United States, 2016*. NCHS Data Brief, no. 296. Hyattsville, MD: National Center for Health Statistics.

Levendusky, Matthew S. and Neil Malhotra 2016. "(Mis)perception of Partisan Polarization in the American Public." *Public Opinion Quarterly*, 80, no. 1: 378–391.

Levine, Saul. 2018. "Belonging is Our Blessing, Tribalism is Our Burden." *Psychology Today*. Online at www.psychologytoday.com/.

Lewallen, Jonathan. 2017. "The Issue Politics of Presidential Veto Threats." *Presidential Studies Quarterly*, 47, no. 2: 277–292.

Light, Paul C. 2000. "Domestic Policy Making." *Presidential Studies Quarterly*, 30, no. 1: 109–132.

Lindblom, Charles E. 1959. "The Science of Muddling Through." *Public Administration Review*, 19 (Spring): 79–88.

Loomis, Christopher M. 2009. "The Politics of Uncertainty: Lobbyists and Propaganda in Early Twentieth-Century in America." *Journal of Policy History*, 21, no. 2: 187–227.

Lowi, Theodore J. 1967. "The Public Philosophy: Interest Group Liberalism." *American Political Science Review*, 61, no. 1 (March): 5–24.

Lowi, Theodore J. 1969. *The End of Liberalism*. New York: Norton.

Luton, Larry S. 2009. "Administrative 'Interpretation' as Policy-Making." *Administrative Theory & Praxis*, 31, no. 4: 556–576.

Lynch, Wendy, Kristen Perosino, and Michael Slover. 2014. "Altarum Institute Survey of Consumer Health Care Opinions." Ann Arbor, MI: Altarum Institute. Online at https://altarum.org/.

Madison, James. 1961a. "Federalist 51." In *The Federalist Papers*, ed. Clinton Rossiter, 320–325. New York: New American Library.

Madison, James. 1961b. "Federalist 10." In *The Federalist Papers*, ed. Clinton Rossiter, 77–84. New York: New American Library.

Mann, Thomas E. and Norman J. Ornstein. 2012. *It's Even Worse Than It Looks: How the American Constitutional System Collided with the New Politics of Extremism*. New York: Basic Books.

Manning, John F. 2011. "Separation of Powers as Ordinary Interpretation." *Harvard Law Review*, 124, no. 8: 1941–2040.

Martyn, Amy. 2016. "Health Industry Rakes in Billions While Blaming Obamacare for Losses." *Consumer Affairs*. Online at www.consumeraffairs.com/.

Mawhinney, Hanne B. 2001. "Theoretical Approaches to Understanding Interest Groups." *Educational Policy*, 15, no. 1 (January/March): 187–214.

McCarty, Nolan. 2016. "Polarization, Congressional Dysfunction, and Constitutional Change." *Indiana Law Review*, 50, no. 1: 223–245.

McCarty, Nolan, Keith T. Poole, and Howard Rosenthal. 2009. "Does Gerrymandering Cause Polarization?" *American Journal of Political Science*, 53, no. 3: 666–680.

McConnell, Grant. 1966. *Private Power and American Democracy*. New York: Knopf.

McKay, Amy. 2012. "Negative Lobbying and Policy Outcomes." *American Politics Research*, 40, no. 1: 116–146.

Medical Device Manufacturers of America. n.d. "About MDMA." Washington, DC: Medical Device Manufacturers of America. Online at www.medicaldevices.org/

Medscape. 2017. *Physician Compensation Report 2017*. Medscape, LLC. New York. Online at www.medscape.com/.
Milkis, Sidney M., Jesse H. Rhodes, and Emily J. Charnock. 2012. "What Happened to Post-Partisanship Barack Obama and the New American Party System." *Perspectives on Politics*, 10, no. 1: 57–76.
Miller, Edward Alan. 2008. "Federal Administrative and Judicial Oversight of Medicaid: Policy Legacies and Tandem Institutions Under the Boren Amendment." *Publius*, 38, no. 2: 315–342.
Miller, Marc C. and Jeb Barnes, eds. 2004. *Making Policy, Making Laws: An Interbranch Perspective*. Washington, DC: Georgetown University Press.
Mills, Charles W. 1956. *The Power Elite*. New York: Oxford University Press.
Mitchell, Erica. 2017. "Types of Hospitals in the US." EOSCU. Online at http://blog.eoscu.com/blog/types-of-hospitals-in-the-us.
Moncrieff, Abigail and Joseph F. Lawless. 2017. "Chapter 5: Healthcare Federalism." In *Oxford Handbook of U.S. Health Law*, eds Glenn Cohen, Allison K. Hoffman, and William M. Sage, 93–113. New York: Oxford University Press.
Morrissey, John. 2015. "The Medical Technologies that are Changing Health Care." Hospitals & Health Networks. Online at www.hhnmag.com/.
Nakhjiri, Anahita. 2017. "If Prices are Kept Hidden, Consumers Can't Take More Responsibility for Their Health Care Costs." *Stat*. Online at www.statnews.com/.
Nathan, Richard P. 2005. "Federalism and Health Policy." *Health Affairs*, 24, no. 6: 1458–1466.
Nathan, Richard P. 2006. "Updating Theories of American Federalism." Conference Papers. *American Political Science Association Annual Meeting*. August 31–September 3. Philadelphia, PA.
National Commission on Certification of Physician Assistants. 2018. *Statistical Profile of Certified Physician Assistants by State*. Johns Creek, GA: National Commission on Certification of Physician Assistants. Online at www.nccpa.net/.
"National Health Care Spending in 2016" n.d. Center for Medicare and Medicaid Services, Office of the Actuary, National Health Statistics Group. Department of Health and Human Services. Online at www.cms.gov/.
"National Health Expenditures 2016 Highlights." n.d. Center for Medicare and Medicaid Services, Office of the Actuary, National Health Statistics Group. Department of Health and Human Services. Online at www.cms.gov/.
"National Health Expenditures by Types of Services and Sources of Funds: Calendar Years 1960 to 2016." n.d. Center for Medicare and Medicaid Services. Office of Actuary, National Health Statistics Group. Department of Health and Human Services. Online at www.cms.gov/.
Newport, Frank. 2017. "Majority Want Government to Ensure Healthcare Coverage." *Gallup Poll*. Online at http://news.gallup.com/.
Nichols, Len M. 2012. "Justice Robert's Health Care Stewardship." *Hastings Center Report*, 42, no. 5: 17–18.
Niskanen, William A. 2003. "A Case for Divided Government." *Cato Policy Report*, 25, no. 2 (March/April): 2.
Nivola, Pietro S. 2005. *Thinking About Political Polarization*. Policy Brief #139. Washington, DC: The Brookings Institution. Online at www.brookings.edu/.
Nzelibe, Jide O. and Matthew C. Stephenson. 2010. "Complementary Constraints: Separation of Powers, Rational Voting, and Constitutional Design." *Harvard Law Review*, 123, no. 3: 618–654.
Pandich, Scott C. 2007. "Six Out of Seven: The Missing Sin of Federalist 51." *Perspectives on Political Science*, 36, no. 3: 148–152.
Parmet, Wendy E. 2016. "Health: Policy or Law? A Population-Based Analysis of the Supreme Court's ACA Cases." *Journal of Health, Politics, Policy and Law*, 41, no. 6: 1061–1081.
Patel, Kant and Mark Rushefsky. 2002. *Health Care Policy in an Age of New Technologies*. Armonk, NY: M.E. Sharpe.
Peterson, Mark A. 2001. "Health Politics and Policy in a Federal System." *Journal of Health Politics, Policy and Law*, 26, no. 6: 1217–1222.
Pharmaceutical Research and Manufacturers of America. 2016. "2016 Biopharmaceutical Research Industry Profile." Phrma. Online at www.phrma.org/.
Plein, Christopher L. 2010. "Federalism, Intergovernmental Relations, and the Challenge of the Medically Uninsurable: A Retrospective on High Risk Pools in the States." *Journal of Health and Human Services Administration*, 33, no. 2: 135–157.
Poduval, Murali and Jayita Poduval. 2008. "Medicine as a Corporate Enterprise: A Welcome Step?" *Mens Sana Monograph*, 6, no. 1: 157–174.
"Poll: Public Says Drug Companies Have More Influenced in Washington than the NRA." 2018. Kaiser Family Foundation. Online at www.kff.org/.
Pope, Chris. 2013. "The Perils of Health-Care Federalism." *National Affairs* no. 16. Online at www.nationalaffairs.com/.
Porto, Brian L. 2009. *May It Please the Court: Judicial Processes and Politics in America*. Boca Raton, FL: CRC Press/Taylor Frances Group.
"Presidential Vetoes." 2017. United States House of Representatives. Online at http://history.house.gov/.
"Private-Market Health Insurance." n.d. Washington, DC: America's Health Insurance Plans. Online at www.ahip.org/.
"Public Health Economics and Methods." n.d. Centers for Disease Control and Prevention. Online at www.cdc.gov/.
Pump, Barry. 2011. "Beyond Metaphors: New Research on Agendas in the Policy Process." *Policy Studies Journal*, 39, no. 12: 1–12.
Purcell, Edward A. 2009. *Originalism, Federalism, and the American Constitution: A Historical Inquiry*. New Haven, CT: Yale University Press.
PWC Health Research Institute. 2017. *Medical Cost Trends: Behind the Numbers 2018*. PWC Health Research Institute. Online at www.pwc.com.
Quadango, Jill. 2011. "Interest-Group Influence on the Patient Protection and Affordable Care Act of 2010: Winners and Losers in the Health Care Reform Debate." *Journal of Health Policy, Policy and Law*, 36, no. 3: 449–453.
Quirk, Paul J. 2011. "Polarized Populism: Masses, Elites, and Partisan Conflict." *Forum*, 9, no. 1: 1–16.
Ramirez, Mark D. 2009. "The Dynamics of Partisan Conflict on Congressional Approval." *American Journal of Political Science*, 53, no. 3: 681–694.

Repetto, Robert C. 2006. "Introduction." In *Punctuated Equilibrium and the Dynamics of U.S. Environmental Policy*, ed. Robert C. Repetto, 1–23. New Haven, CT: Yale University Press.

Rich, Robert F. and William D. White. 1996. *Health Policy, Federalism, and the American States*. Washington, DC: Urban Institute Press.

Robert Wood Johnson Foundation. 2016. "How Price Transparency Can Control the Cost of Health Care." *Health Policy Snapshot Series*. Online at www.rwjf.org/.

Robinson, Scott E. and Floun'say R. Carver. 2006. "Punctuated Equilibrium and Congressional Budgeting." *Political Research Quarterly*, 59, no. 1: 161–166.

Robinson, Scott E., Floun'say R. Carver, Kenneth J. Meier, and Laurence J. O'Toole. 2007. "Explaining Policy Punctuations: Bureaucratization and Budget Change." *American Journal of Political Science*, 51, no. 1: 140–150.

Rogowski, Jon C. and Joseph L. Sutherland. 2016. "How Ideology Fuels Affective Polarization." *Political Behavior*, 38, no. 2: 485–508.

Rosen, Mark D. 2016. "Can Congress Play a Role in Remedying Dysfunctional Political Partisanship?" *Indiana Law Review*, 50, 265–279.

Rosenbaum, Walter A. 1985. *Environmental Politics and Policy*. Washington, DC: CQ Press.

Rushefsky, Mark. 2007. *Public Policy in the United States: At the Dawn of the Twenty-First Century*. Armonk, NY: M.E. Sharpe.

Russell, Jill, Trisha Greenhalgh, Emma Byrne, and Janet McDonnell. 2008. "Recognizing Rhetoric in Health Care Policy Analysis." *Journal of Health Services Research and Policy*, 13, no. 1: 40–46.

Samuelson, Paul. 1970. *Economics*. New York: McGraw-Hill.

Santiago, Andrea C. 2017a. "Average Nurse Salaries by Type of Nursing Career and Role." Verywell Health. Online www.verywell.com/.

Santiago, Andrea C. 2017b. "Different Types and Role of Nurses." Verywell Health. Online at https://verywell.com/.

Schattschneider, E.E. 1960. *The Semi-Sovereign People*. New York: Holt, Rinehart, and Winston.

Schlesinger, Mark. 2004. "Health Policy by the Numbers." *Journal of Health Politics, Policy and Law*, 29, no. 3: 347–357.

Shumsky, Tatyana. 2017. "The Morning Ledger: Cost of Health-Insurance Provided by U.S. Employers Keeps Rising." *Wall Street Journal*. Online at https://blogs.wsj.com/.

Simon, Herbert A. 1957. *Models of Man: Social and Rational; Mathematical Essays on Rational Behavior in Society Setting*. New York: Wiley.

Sinclair, Barbara. 2012. *Unorthodox Lawmaking: New Legislative Processes in the U.S. Congress*. Washington, DC: Congressional Quarterly Press.

Skeen, James W. 2003. "Health Care Fraud and Industry Structure in the United States." *Social Policy & Administration*, 37, no. 5: 516–529.

Skopol, T. 2004. *The Diminished Democracy: From Membership to Management in American Civic Life*. Norman, OK: University of Oklahoma Press.

Sommers, Benjamin D, Caitlin L. McMurtry, Robert J. Blendon, John M. Benson, and Justin M. Sayde. 2017. "Beyond Health Insurance: Remaining Disparities in US Health Care in the Post-ACA Era." *Milbank Quarterly*, 95, no. 1: 43–69.

Sorkin, Alan L. 1986. *Health Care and the Changing Economic Environment*. Lexington, MA: DC Heath.

Sparer, Michael. 2009a. *Healthcare Reform and American Federalism*. Washington, DC: Robert Wood Johnson Foundation.

Sparer, Michael S. 2009b. "Federalism and the Patient Protection and Affordable Care Act of 2010: The Founding Fathers Would Not Be Surprised." *Journal of Health Politics, Policy and Law*, 36, no. 3: 461–468.

Stanek, Mike. 2014. Federalism in Health Care: Identifying Role for Federal and State Partners." The Commonwealth Fund. Online at www.commonwealthfund.org/.

Starr, Paul. 1982. *The Social Transformation of American Medicine*. New York: Basic Books.

Stone, Daniel. 2011. "A Signal-Jamming Model of Persuasion: Interest Group Funded Policy Research." *Social Choice and Welfare*, 37, no. 3: 397–424.

Stone, Deborah A. 2011. *The Policy Paradox: The Art of Political Decision Making*, 3rd edn. New York: W.W. Norton.

Sullivan, Andrew. 2017. "Can Our Democracy Survive TTribalism?" *NY Mag*. Online at http://nymag.com/intelligencer/2017/09/can-democracy-survive-tribalism.html.

Sultz, Harry A. and Kristina M. Young. 2011. "Hospitals: Origin, Organization, and Performance." In *Healthcare USA: Understanding its Organization and Delivery*, 7th edn, eds Harry A. Sultz and Kristina M. Young, 65–112. Sudbury: MASS, Joes and Bartlett.

Taylor, Humphrey. 1990. "U.S. Health Care Built for Waste." *The New York Times*, April 17.

Tenpas, Kathryn D. 2006. "The Veto-Free Presidency: George W. Bush (2001-Present)." *Issues in Governance Studies*, no. 4: 1–8.

"The 2016 Cycle AMPAC Election Report." n.d. AMPAC. Online at www.ampaconline.org/.

"The Nursing Process." n.d. Silver Spring, MD: American Nurses Association. Online at http://nursingworld.org/.

Theodoulou, Stella Z. and Chris Kofinis. 2004. *The Art of the Game: Understanding American Public Policy Making*. Belmont, CA: Thomson/Wadsworth.

Thomas, Kenneth R. 2008. *Federalism, State Sovereignty, and the Constitution: Basis and Limits of Congressional Power*. Congressional Research Service Report. Washington, DC: Federation of American Scientists.

Thompson, Frank J. 1986. "New Federalism and Health Care Policy: States and the Old Questions." *Journal of Health Politics, Policy and Law*, 11, no. 4 (Tenth Anniversary Issue): 647–669.

Thompsen, Danielle M. 2014. "Ideological Moderates Won't Run: How Party Fits Matters for Partisan Polarization in Congress." *Journal of Politics*, 76, no. 3 (July): 786–797.

Thompson, Frank J. 2012. *Medicaid Politics: Federalism, Policy Durability, and Health Reform*. Washington, DC: Georgetown University Press.

Thompson, Frank J. and John J. DiIulio, Jr. 1998. *Medicaid and Devolution: A View from the States.* Washington, DC: Brookings Institution Press.

Tichenor, Daniel J. and Richard A. Harris. 2002/2003. "Organized Interests and American Political Development." *Political Science Quarterly*, 117, no. 4 (Winter): 587–612.

Topol, Eric. 2012. *The Creative Destruction of Medicine.* New York: Basic Books.

Tracer, Zachary. 2017. "Rising Health-Insurance Costs are Eating into Employers' Paycheck gains." *Bloomberg.* Online at www.bloomberg.com/.

Trevor, Thrall A. 2006. "The Myth of Outside Strategy: Mass Media News Coverage of Interest Groups." *Political Communication*, 23, no. 4: 407–420.

Truman, David B. 1951. *Governmental Process, Political Interests and Public Opinion.* New York: Knopf.

Tuulonen, Anja. 2005. "The Effects of Structures on Decision-Making Politics in Health Care." *Acta Ophthalmologica Scandanavia*, 83, no. 5: 611–617.

US Department of Health and Human Services. 2016. "Health Plan Choices and Premiums in the 2017 Health Insurance Marketplace." *ASPA Research Brief* (October 24). Online at https://aspe.hhs.gov/.

"U.S. Employers Expect Health Care Costs to Rise by 5.5% in 2018, up from 4.6% in 2017." 2017. Willis Towers Watson. Online at www.willistowerswatson.com/.

Unekis, Joseph. 2011. "Divided Government May Mean Gridlock Rules, Says Congressional Expert." Kansas State University. Online at www.k.state.edu/.

Uslaner, Eric M. 1993. *The Decline of Comity in Congress.* Ann Arbor, MI: University of Michigan Press.

Walker, J.L., Jr. 1991. *Mobilizing Interest Groups in America.* Ann Arbor, MI: University of Michigan Press.

Weeks, Lewis E. and Howard J. Berman. 1985. *Shapers of American Health Care Policy: An Oral History.* Ann Arbor, MI: Health Administration Press.

Weissert, Carol S. and William G. Weissert. 1996. *Governing Health: The Politics of Health Policy.* Baltimore, MD: Johns Hopkins University Press.

White, Darcy and Torey Silloway. 2016. "Cost-Benefit Analysis." Evidence-Based Policymaking Collaborative. Online at www.evidencecollaborative.org/.

Wilsford, David. 1991. *Doctors and the State: The Politics of Health Care in France and the United States.* Durham, NC: Duke University Press.

Wood, Robert S. 2006. "The Dynamics of Incrementalism: Subsystems, Politics, and Public Lands." *Policy Studies Journal*, 34, no. 1: 1–16.

Wood, Dan B. and Soren Jordan. 2011. *Electoral Polarization: Definition, Measurement, and Evaluation* (August 9). Online at SSRN: https://ssrn.com/.

Workman, Samuel and Ashley E. Jochim. 2009. "Information Processing and Policy Dynamics." *Policy Studies Journal*, 37, no. 1: 75–92.

2

HEALTHCARE POLICY IN THE UNITED STATES

There are substantial differences in the healthcare systems of various countries. They differ with respect to financing, delivery of healthcare, and the role of the government. Today there are three primary models of healthcare. In a mostly private healthcare system, workers and their dependents are covered by private insurance, even though the insurance is generally bought through employers. The government provides public insurance programs for those not covered by private insurance. Mostly private hospitals and doctors deliver healthcare. The United States is an example of such a system (Hacker 2002).

Other countries have a healthcare system that is mostly public. Healthcare is paid out of general taxation or through payroll taxes. It is provided by publicly owned hospitals and salaried doctors. Examples of countries with such a system include the United Kingdom, Sweden, and Italy.

The third model of the healthcare system is a hybrid model. In such a system, healthcare is mostly publicly financed, generally through payroll taxes, but is delivered by private hospitals and doctors. Germany, Japan, Canada, France, and Holland exhibit variants of this model. Most countries incorporate some public and private elements in their healthcare systems. No country follows one of these three models in its purest form. As mentioned, the US healthcare system follows the model of the mostly private healthcare system. A majority of Americans are covered by private insurance, usually bought through their employers. The government provides public health insurance programs to cover the healthcare needs of groups such as the retired elderly, the poor, the disabled, veterans, and children who are not covered by the private insurance market. Nevertheless, public health insurance programs in the United States do not cover all uninsured Americans. Thus, a sizable number of Americans remain uninsured because they either cannot afford private health insurance or are not eligible to receive coverage under public health insurance programs for one reason or another.

The American healthcare system is a highly complex and fragmented system in which healthcare is financed, administered, and delivered by a mix of public- and private-sector institutions and healthcare providers—a system that is very expensive and yet fails to produce the best healthcare outcomes and still leave millions of Americans without any health insurance coverage. It is not surprising that scholarly and journalistic literature has described the US healthcare system as "broken" (Brill 2015; Davidson 2010; "The Health Care System Is Broken" 1991), "sick" (Cohn 2008; Lewis 1991; Lynn 2004), "a disgrace" (Ehrenreich 1990), "wasteful" (Terris 1990), "built for waste" (Taylor 1990), "scandalous" (Dentzer 1990), "in crisis" (Ropes 1991), "deadly" (Moore 1995), "mismanaged" (Makover 1998), "accidental" (Reagan 1999), "licensed to steal" (Sparrow 2000), "an oxymoron" (Kleinke 2001), "in financial crisis" (Clark and McEldowney 2001), "fragmented" (Elhauge 2010; McCarthy 2001), "ailing" (Geyman 2002), "a mess" (Richmond 2005), "disorganized and irrational" (Mechanic 2004), "one nation, uninsured" (Quadagno 2005), in "critical condition" or "critical" (Barlett and Steele 2006; Daschle, Greenberger, and Lambrew 2008; Taurel 2005), "unsystematic" (Budrys 2011), "big business" (Rosenthal 2017), and in need of "healing" (Cortese 2006; Downing 2006; Reid 2010), "shock therapy" (Levine 2009), "reinventing" (Emanuel 2014), and "fixing" (Rangel 2009).

The patients in the American healthcare system are often described as "suffering" (Downing 2006), "worried sick" (Hadler 2008), "falling through the safety net" (Geyman 2005), "stuck in the waiting room" (Smerd 2006), "overdosed" (Abramson 2004), "overtreated" (Brownlee 2007; Hadler 2008), "overdiagnosed" (Welch, Swartz, and Woloshin 2011), "suffering from too much medicine" (Gottfried 2009), and surrounded by the "wall of silence" (Gibson 2003) in which they are left to "heal themselves" (Veatch 2009).

According to some analysts, the truth is that the American healthcare system puts health against wealth, in which corporate production of health goods for profit leads to multimillion-dollar PR campaigns designed to engage in "deadly spin" to mislead the press and the public and skew political debate, making true healthcare reform difficult (Anders 1997; Geyman 2010; Herzlinger 2007; Mechanic 2008; Potter 2010; Singer and Baer 2009; Starr 2011).

THE US HEALTHCARE SYSTEM IN A COMPARATIVE CONTEXT

Not only is the American healthcare system the most expensive in the world but it also spends more money on healthcare than any other country in the world. Americans pay more for their healthcare but receive less value compared with other industrialized countries. For example, hospital cost per day in the US is about $18,000, while in Japan it is about $2,000, Australia $765, Germany $632, and Spain $424. Yet, the length of average hospital stay in Japan is 16.9 days compared to 5.5 days in the US, 7.6 in Germany, 5.9 in Spain, and 4.7 in Australia (Powell 2017). The average cost of an angiogram in the US is $1,164, compared to $270 in Australia, $240 in Spain, and $204 in Germany. The average cost of MRI in the US is about $2,611, compared to $599 in Germany, $455 South Africa, $215 in Australia, $177 in Japan, and $130 in Spain (Powell 2017). In 2015, among members of the Organization for Economic Cooperation and Development (OECD), the United States ranked first in the number of CT exams performed and third in the number of MRI exams performed per 1,000 population. The United States ranked second with respect to the number of MRI units and third with respect to CT scanners housed in hospitals per 1 million population (Organization for Economic Cooperation and Development 2017).

It is not uncommon for wealthy countries to spend more per person on healthcare and related expenses than poorer countries. However, even among high-income countries, the US spends more per capita compared to other countries. For example, in 2016, the US spent $10,348 per person, which was 31 percent higher than Switzerland, the next highest per-capita spender, which spent $7,919 per capita. The average amount spent on health per person among the OECD countries was $4,908 (Sawyer and Cox 2018).

In 1970, the United States was relatively on pace with comparable wealthy OCED countries with respect to the percent of GDP spent on healthcare. In 1970, the US spent about 6 percent of its GDP on healthcare, which was similar to the average of 5 percent of GDP spent by wealthy OECD countries. However, the 1980s witnessed significantly accelerated growth in healthcare spending per capita in the United States, averaging 10.1 percent average annual growth rate—the highest among comparable countries. The average annual growth rate in comparable wealthy countries during the 1980s was about 7 percent (Sawyer and Cox 2018). Consequently, in 2016, the United States spent almost 18 percent of its GDP on health—the highest among OCED countries. The next-highest comparable country was Switzerland, which spent about 13 percent of its GDP on health. Over the last three decades, the US has increased spending on healthcare by both the public and private sectors (Sawyer and Cox 2018). Despite more spending on healthcare by the US compared to other OCED countries, in 2015, it ranked 34th among the 35 member countries, with 9.1 percent of its population lacking health insurance. Greece was ranked 35th, with 14 percent of its population lacking any health insurance coverage (Organization for Economic Cooperation and Development 2017). The United States trails behind many other OCED countries in access-to-healthcare indicators. However, it should be noted that the Affordable Care Act of 2010 has helped reduce the number of uninsured Americans.

Despite the fact that the United States spends more money on healthcare per capita as well as the percent of its GDP spent on healthcare, it does not rank high with respect to overall health system rating, and a variety of healthcare indicators and health outcomes. According to a study of 11 countries conducted by the Commonwealth Fund (2014), the US healthcare system consistently underperformed relative to other countries on most dimensions of performance. In fact, the US ranked last among the 11 countries on overall healthcare system performance ranking. The United States ranked last or near-last on dimensions of access to healthcare, health system efficiency, equity, and healthy lives.

In 1970, life expectancy in the United States was one year above the OECD average but by 2016 it was almost two years below the average (Organization for Economic Cooperation and Development 2017). According to the Center for Disease Control and Prevention (CDC), in 2015, the average life expectancy at birth in the US was 78.6 years. For the first time in 50 years, life expectancy in the US had fallen two years in a row. In 25 other developed countries, life expectancy in 2015 averaged 81.8 years. Life expectancy at age 65 in the US ranked 26th among the 37 members of the OCED (Blumenthal 2018). The opioid epidemic has played a major role in the increased death rate for Americans aged 15 to 64 years. With 4 percent of the world's population, the US accounts for 27 percent of the world's overdose deaths. The European Union, with a population of 507 million, reported 6,800 overdose deaths in 2014, while in the US overdose death rate reported was 47,055 (Blumenthal 2018).

The United States also lags behind peer countries on child health outcomes. The US has ranked the worst in childhood deaths since the 1990s. A child born in the United States has a 70-percent greater chance of dying before adulthood than children born in other wealthy, democratic countries. Teenagers in the US are 82 times more likely to die from gun homicides and are twice as likely to die in car accidents as their peers in other countries (Thakrar et al. 2018).

The United States has the highest prevalence of obesity among the OECD countries—38 percent of adults compared to the OECD average of 19.4 percent. Obesity rates in the US have grown by 65 percent since the 1990s. On the positive side, daily smoking rates are lower in the US (11.4 percent) compared to an OCED average of 18.4 percent (Organization for Economic Cooperation and Development 2017).

What accounts for the fact that the United States spends more money on healthcare than any other country in the world but underperforms on a variety of health system performance indicators like access, equity, and health outcomes? Many experts point to factors such as lack of universal healthcare, cost of healthcare, lifestyle choices, profit-driven insurers, drug companies and hospitals, and a fragmented health system, among others. In recent years, increased attention has focused on the relationship between social services and health. A new argument that has been advanced is that the ratio of a country's social-service spending to healthcare spending is highly correlated with health outcomes. In the public health field, this has come to be called "social determinants" of health. We discuss this in the section on "the role of government in public health" later in this chapter and in Chapter 7.

In this chapter, we examine the historical development of healthcare policies in the United States. The major emphasis is placed on the evolution of federal government's role in the field of healthcare from the colonial times to the present. The chapter ends with a discussion of the role of different levels of government in the field of public health.

HEALTHCARE IN COLONIAL TIMES

Upon arrival in the new world, the new settlers soon discovered a world full of diseases such as malaria, typhoid, and yellow fever. Settlers also brought several diseases with them to America. Colonies were often swept by deadly epidemics such as smallpox, measles, scarlet fever, plagues, typhus, and diphtheria. During this period, colonists viewed diseases as an expression of divine providence. Diseases such as plagues were viewed as a divine force acting directly on the "Promised Land." Health, sickness, recovery, and death were considered acts of God that served a divine purpose. For example, the 1721 smallpox epidemic that struck New England was believed to be God's punishment to colonists for breaking their covenant with him. There was a strong link between medicine and theology and it was fused into the religious life of the Puritan community (Patel 2014). Thus, it is not surprising that health guides and brochures urged readers to avoid behaviors and emotions that could lead to disease. Strong emotions such as anger, fear, grief, and envy were seen as associated with illness by colonists (Patel and Rushefsky 2005a).

The progress of medicine, or the "healing arts," was very slow in the 1700s. Prior to 1800, medicine in the United States was very much considered a "family matter." A doctor was summoned only in case of serious illness. Medical practice by doctors essentially consisted of the use of home remedies and herbal medicine. Doctors did not possess the credentials required today and they traveled extensively to practice their medicine. Western medicine was based on the ancient Greek principle of the four humors—yellow bile, black bile, blood, and phlegm—and it was believed that balance among the humors was the key to health. Illness was caused by an imbalance among the four humors and treatment required a balancing of humors. Consequently, purging, puking, sweating, and bleeding were common medical treatments. There were very few European-trained doctors in the early settlements. Colonists trained their own doctors by a system of apprenticeship or by sending young men of promise to Europe for proper medical training. Physicians with medical degrees and scientific training started to appear in America during the late colonial period. In 1765, the University of Pennsylvania opened the first medical college. The Massachusetts Medical Society sought to license physicians (Tannenbaum 2012).

The Revolutionary War caused a significant disruption of civic life and crowded army camps became ideal grounds for the spread of diseases. The smallpox epidemic accompanied the American Revolution between 1775 and 1782. The use of inoculation ultimately brought smallpox under control. The aftermath of the Revolutionary War witnessed the emergence of government's role in the field of public health (see the section on "the role of government in public health" in the latter part of this chapter).

HEALTHCARE IN THE NINETEENTH CENTURY

Neither healthcare nor the biosciences received a great deal of popular support in the United States in the early 1800s. By the 1830s, vaccination had become an established practice for the prevention of epidemic and spread of diseases. From around 1800 to the 1830s there were limited advances in local governments' functions and responsibilities, including things such as garbage collection and street cleaning. The period of the 1830s to the start of the Civil War saw the emergence of vital statistics as an important public health tool. The American Medical Association (AMA) was formed in 1847. During the latter part of the nineteenth century, physicians and pharmacists were the sole dispensers of professionally recognized health services. Most physicians were trained through apprenticeships with practicing physicians. Physicians also established "diploma mills" to train several students at a time. Later, private and public schools set up medical schools to train physicians. Physicians made their living treating patients for fees and received very little money from the government. The same was true of pharmacists, who later developed drugstores to supplement their income from prescriptions. Thus, private practice and fees for services were firmly established in the early US healthcare system (Anderson 1985).

The biological sciences were not very popular with the general public. During the 1840s, a proposal for the establishment of a National Institute of Science, funded by the federal government, was rejected repeatedly by Congress. Finally, during the Civil War, the National Academy of Sciences was established in 1863 on the grounds of its usefulness to the Union armies (Hill 1976). During the Civil War, the state of American medicine was very poor. The use of ether and chloroform was crude and it was often unavailable. Many surgical procedures were performed on the battlefield or in a field hospital without anesthesia (Rutkow 2005).

The last quarter of the nineteenth century saw a steady advance in medical science (Stevens 2007; Stevens, Rosenberg, and Burns 2006; Warner and Tighe 2001). Antiseptic surgery was highly developed by 1875. In 1876, the discovery of the germ theory of disease by Louis Pasteur helped establish the empirical causal link between germs and diseases. The science of microbiology was introduced, and techniques of vaccination were developed.

General hospitals, as we know them today, did not exist. Poorhouses and almshouses provided care for destitute persons. The origin of a hospital system in the United States is associated with the establishment of the first marine hospital in 1799 (Raffel 1980). Both the US Army and the US Navy had their own requirements for treating sickness, and they differed from those of the US Marine Service. Between 1830 and 1860, marine hospitals proliferated. During the Civil War, the Marine Hospital Service was very much neglected and the number of hospitals decreased. In 1869, Congress reviewed the Marine Hospital Service and passed the first Reorganization Act in 1870. Under this law, the Marine Hospital Service was federalized and formally organized as a national agency with a central headquarters (US Health Resources Administration 1976). The building of mental hospitals also preceded the development of personal health services. Mental hospitals were and continue to be largely publicly owned and operated.

The advent of anesthesia and antisepsis made general hospitals a relatively safe place for surgery. Early general hospitals were established mostly by voluntary community boards and churches. The growing economy made it possible for hospitals to obtain capital funds from philanthropists and operating funds from paying patients. Voluntary hospitals, because of their charitable and non-profit charters, were obligated to provide care for the poor. Physicians began to admit patients to hospitals for surgeries. Patients paid for hospital charges and physicians' fees. In return, hospitals provided physicians with their facilities to give free care to the poor. In 1875 there were very few general hospitals in the country. The number of hospitals grew tremendously in the nineteenth century. By the end of 2003, there were a total of 5,764 registered hospitals in the United States (American Hospital Association 2005).

THE TRANSFORMATION OF US MEDICINE: 1900–1935

The rise of bacteriology and advances in pathology, physiology, and chemistry helped enhance the understanding of the causes of various diseases. The bacteriological revolution combined with other developments in medicine strengthened the position of the medical profession and physicians. The American Medical Association played a major role in this development (Patel and Rushefsky 2005a).

During the first decade of the twentieth century, the process of consolidation of medical education and the transformation of American medicine began to take shape. For a number of years, the AMA had been trying to force inferior medical schools to close in order to reduce the numbers of institutions competing for philanthropic support (Fox 1986). Reform of medical schools was the top priority of the AMA. The Council on Medical Education, established by the AMA in 1904, elevated and standardized requirements for medical education for physicians. In addition, in order to identify and pressure weaker institutions, the council began to grade medical schools and later extended its evaluation to include curriculum, facilities, faculty, and requirements for admissions (Starr 1982).

Philanthropic foundations often had power and influence, but they lacked authority. Their financial power was limited by their fear that legislatures that chartered them would restrict their power or tax them out of existence. Nevertheless, placing medical education on a more scientific basis had also become their top priority. Several foundations began to finance studies that recommended reorganization of medical education and medical care. The AMA Council invited an outside group, the Carnegie Foundation for the Advancement of Teaching, to investigate medical schools. Abraham Flexner, as a representative of the Carnegie Foundation, visited each of the medical schools in the country during 1909 and 1910. He saw a great discrepancy between medical science and medical education. His report, known as the Flexner Report, was published in 1910 and recommended adoption of the German model of medicine with scientifically based training, the strengthening of first-class medical schools, and the elimination of a great majority of inferior schools.

Following the Flexner Report, the process of consolidation of medical education proceeded at a rapid pace. By 1915, the number of medical schools had decreased from 131 to 95. Similarly, the number of graduates from medical schools dropped from 5,440 to 3,536. Mergers between class A and class B schools became common. The AMA Council became a national accrediting agency for medical schools, and many states came to accept its judgments regarding those schools. The new system increased the homogeneity and cohesiveness of the medical profession (Starr 1982). By the 1940s the AMA had become a powerful political force and a major player in shaping US healthcare policy (Campion 1984).

Another significant development during this period was the rise of the third-party payment system in US medicine. Prior to the 1930s, medical insurance programs were nonexistent. During the Great Depression of the 1930s, the incomes of hospitals and physicians declined. Many people could not afford to pay hospitals or physicians for their medical services. Realizing that they could operate better with a steady income, hospitals began to sponsor prepayment plans, which came to be known as the Blue Cross plans. Similarly, prepayment plans for physicians' services in the hospital, especially surgery, also began to appear. Sponsored by state medical societies, they became known as Blue Shield plans. Both the Blue Cross and the Blue Shield plans were very successful. During the 1940s, the federal government encouraged the development of private, voluntary insurance plans. For example, Congress gave voluntary plans a financial boost by legislating that health insurance and pensions were fringe benefits and exempt from a wartime freeze on wages. Thus, employers could offer their workers healthcare fringe benefits by paying for part or all of the cost of their insurance premiums. A ruling by the Internal Revenue Service in 1951 that employers' costs for premiums were a tax-deductible expense made the large-scale development of private health insurance viable.

The rise of third-party payment led to increases in visits to physicians and admissions to hospitals. The third-party payment system replaced the financing system based on one-on-one financial transactions between patient and physician. Third-party payers insulated healthcare consumers from the realities of healthcare costs, leading to overconsumption, a problem called "moral hazard" by economists. Physicians and hospitals prospered. Since insurance companies reimbursed hospitals for the charges and/or costs of hospital services received by the patient, third-party payments made hospitals financially secure and independent because they could count on a steady income. Physicians prospered because they were paid by voluntary health insurance according to generous fee schedules negotiated by the Blue Shield plans.

THE ROLE OF THE FEDERAL GOVERNMENT IN HEALTHCARE

During much of the nineteenth century, the role of the federal government was almost non-existent. In 1798, President John Adams signed a law that provided for the relief of sick and disabled seamen. This ultimately led to the development of Marine hospitals during the nineteenth century. Following the Civil War, Congress in 1878 passed a National Quarantine Act for the purpose of preventing entry into the country of persons with communicable diseases. The period of 1870 to 1910 saw the development of public health services by local and state governments.

Limited Federal Role: 1900s–1930s

During the late nineteenth and early part of the twentieth century, countries in Europe were establishing compulsory sickness insurance programs. Germany established the first national system of compulsory sickness insurance in 1883. Similar systems were established in Austria in 1888, Hungary in 1891, Norway in 1910, the UK in 1911, Russia in 1912, and the Netherlands in 1913. France and Italy required sickness insurance in only a few industries. Countries such as Sweden, Denmark, and Switzerland gave extensive state aid to voluntary funds and provided incentives for membership (Starr 1982).

The federal government in the United States, in contrast to happenings in Europe, took no action to subsidize voluntary funds or to make sickness insurance mandatory. This partly reflected existing political conditions and institutions in the United States, where, as a result of the influence of the public philosophy of classical liberalism, the government was highly decentralized and played a very small role in the regulation of the economy or in promoting social welfare.

Health insurance became a political issue in the United States on the eve of World War I. The progress of a workman's compensation (now referred to as worker's compensation) law between 1910 and 1913 encouraged reformers to believe that adoption of compulsory insurance against industrial accidents would lead to the adoption of compulsory sickness insurance. But the progressive reformers' hopes of strengthening government and adopting compulsory sickness insurance were soon dashed. Opposition from physicians and pharmaceutical and insurance companies defeated their reform proposals. In addition, both labor unions and business, fearing competition from the government in social welfare programs, failed to support the reformers. By 1920, the movement for compulsory sickness insurance had faded from the political agenda.

Under pressure from the labor movement and children's advocates, Congress passed the Sheppard-Towner Act in 1921. It established the first federal grant-in-aid program for local child health clinics. But many local health departments refused to accept these grants because the AMA and local medical societies strongly opposed the program. Congress allowed the program to terminate in 1928 (Roemer 1984). Thus, the federal government's role in healthcare remained very limited during the nineteenth and early twentieth centuries.

Expanded Federal Role: 1930s–1960s

Major Developments in Healthcare Field: 1930s

A number of significant developments took place in the healthcare field during the 1930s that brought about significant changes in the field of healthcare.

One major development, as mentioned earlier, was the start of a third-party payment system with the establishment of the Blue Cross and Blue Shield insurance plans. This revolutionized healthcare financing and led to employer-based health insurance programs.

A second development concerned advances in medical technology and the discovery of antibiotics. Antibiotics changed the focus of medical care from prevention of disease through inoculation and hygiene to cure of illnesses (Bernstein and Bernstein 1988). For the first time, sulfa drugs and penicillin gave physicians their true power to cure (Easterbrook 1987).

The third development was the increased emphasis on biomedical research by the federal government. In 1937, Congress passed the National Cancer Act. It established the National Cancer Institute (NCI) and set a national pattern for the federal support of biomedical research. The law authorized the NCI to conduct research in its own laboratories and to award grants to nongovernment scientists and institutions for training scientists and clinicians. The establishment of the National Cancer Institute in 1937, with a broad mandate for ascertaining the cause, prevention, and cure of disease, reflected the increased role of the federal government in healthcare in general and in public health services in particular. Later it paved the way for public funding of biomedical research through the National Institutes of Health (NIH) and later through the National Science Foundation (NSF). The fourth development was the shift from local control of health and welfare issues to state and especially federal government control. Workman's compensation, pensions, unemployment insurance, and certain medical services came to be perceived by the people as the responsibility of the federal government (Greifinger and Sidel 1978). This was because of the Great Depression and the economic problems of state and local governments. The problems facing the country were too large for any but federal solutions. In 1934, the Federal Emergency Relief Administration gave the first federal grants to local governments for public assistance to the poor, including financial support for medical care.

The fifth development was the creation of federal programs designed to provide general social benefits to the people. During the depression, there was an increased demand for social insurance as differentiated from insurance against specific risks. Most Western countries had placed a higher priority on establishing health insurance programs as a natural outgrowth of insurance against industrial accidents. Old-age pensions and unemployment insurance programs received a lower priority in these countries. In the United States, with millions of people out of work as a result of the Depression, unemployment insurance and old-age pensions received a higher priority. Thus, the United States, rather than move in the direction of providing free medical care or reimbursement for its costs, as many Western European countries had done, attempted to supply more general social security benefits.

The Social Security Act of 1935 provided for unemployment compensation, old-age pensions, and other benefits. The Social Security Act also extended the role of the federal government in healthcare by including provisions designed to strengthen public health services. These provisions called for federal matching grants-in-aid to states for maternal and infant care and diagnosis and treatment of crippled children. Federal grants were also made available for general public health purposes under the administration of the US Public Health Service (USPHS), which had evolved in 1912 from the Marine Hospital Service.

The sixth development was a failed effort to create a federal national health insurance program. The early planning of the legislation had initially included health insurance as part of the package. However, the Roosevelt administration did not want to jeopardize the enactment of the entire law because of strong opposition to health insurance by the medical profession. Therefore, national health insurance (NHI) was omitted from the final legislative proposal. During 1935–1936, the United States Public Health Service (USPHS) conducted a national health survey that revealed many untreated diseases in the population, especially in low-income groups. This led Senator Robert Wagner (D-NY), sponsor of the Social Security Act, to introduce an amendment to the Act that would have provided federal grants to the states for the organization of health insurance plans covering workers and their dependents. The onset of World War II postponed any serious consideration of such a plan (Roemer 1986). Similar attempts to establish a health insurance program under the Truman administration were defeated during the 1940s. The medical profession had succeeded in defeating proposals for establishing any national health insurance system.

Expansion of Health Facilities and Services: 1940s

After the war, the Truman administration called for the expansion of hospitals, more support for public health, maternal, and child health services, and federal aid for medical research and education. The administration's aim was to expand the country's medical resources and facilities, reduce the financial burden for their use, and in the process expand access to medical care (Starr 1982). One major problem was that no new hospital construction had taken place during the Depression or World War II, a period of some 16 years.

In 1946, Congress passed the National Hospital Survey and Construction Act, also known as the Hill-Burton Act. This program provided federal funds to subsidize construction of hospitals in areas of bed shortages, mainly in rural counties. State public health agencies were made responsible for surveying the hospital-bed supply in each state and for developing a master plan for the construction of new hospitals. They were also assigned the task of inspecting and licensing all hospitals and related facilities.

Physicians welcomed Hill-Burton funds and actively sought them for construction of new hospitals for reasons of prestige, convenience, and service. Many physicians did not have privileges to treat their patients in the limited number of hospitals that were in existence. These physicians, faced with a limited supply of hospitals and beds and restricted access to them, supported the construction of new hospitals in the hope that they would enjoy the privilege of treating their patients in newly constructed hospitals. In addition, local pressure favoring nearby facilities, tax-favored bonds, and assured income from insurance companies and later from Medicare contributed to the proliferation of hospitals (Bernstein and Bernstein 1988).

As the number of hospitals increased, a nongovernmental Joint Commission on Accreditation of Hospitals was established in 1952. Between 1947 and 1966, the number of voluntary, not-for-profit hospitals increased from 2,584 to 3,426. During the same period, state and local government general hospitals increased from 785 to 1,453. The total number of hospitals (for-profit, state and local government, and voluntary not-for-profit) increased from 4,445 to 5,736. The rate of hospital admissions per 1,000 population increased from 54 in 1935 to 129 in 1960 (Stevens 1989).

Congress, in 1946, also passed the National Mental Health Act. This law provided federal grants to states for the research, prevention, diagnosis, and treatment of mental disorders. During the 1950s, there was also further expansion of public health services at the federal level. The NIH greatly expanded support of biomedical research. By the end of the 1950s, the role of the federal government in healthcare had increased significantly compared to its role in the early 1900s. There was a corresponding increase in the role of state and local governments in the field of public health services.

Increasing Access to Healthcare: 1950s–1960s

From the 1920s to the 1950s, efforts to establish a national system of healthcare or health insurance for the entire population had failed because of charges from the medical profession and others that such plans would constitute "socialized medicine." The concept of socialized medicine went against the general public philosophy of classical liberalism, which advocates a limited role for government, and the specific philosophy of interest-group liberalism, wherein different interest groups exercise countervailing veto power over government policy decisions.

Faced with opposition to comprehensive change, advocates of a national system of healthcare or insurance changed their strategy and objectives and turned to an incremental strategy. They began to advocate increasing access to healthcare for the needy. Rather than push for universal coverage, under which the federal government would provide health insurance to all on a compulsory basis, they began to push for a limited system of health insurance for specific needy groups such as the elderly. The elderly were considered a perfect target group for providing help because of their greater medical need, inadequate financial resources, and loss of employment-based group medical insurance upon retirement. Additionally, the elderly were also deemed worthy and were not stigmatized as a failed group, as were welfare recipients (Schneider and Ingram 2004). The healthcare problems of the elderly would be faced by most of us; almost everyone grows old, after all. This new approach also accommodated the federal structure of government by emphasizing that such programs would be administered by state governments with the federal government providing financial aid to states.

The result was the passage of the Kerr-Mills Act (also known as the Medical Assistance Act) by Congress in 1960. The law provided federal matching payments to states for vendor (provider) payments and allowed states to include the medically needy (i.e., elderly, blind, and disabled persons with low income who were not on public assistance). The act also suggested the scope of services to be covered, such as hospitals, nursing homes, physicians, and other health services. It also required each state to plan for institutional and noninstitutional care as a condition of federal cost-sharing. State participation in the program was optional, and states were left free to determine eligibility and the extent of services provided. Most important, the act established the concept of "medical indigency."

The Kerr-Mills program proved to be neither effective nor adequate (Bernstein and Bernstein 1988). It failed to provide significant relief for a substantial portion of the elderly population. An investigation by the Senate Subcommittee on the Health of the Elderly in 1963 revealed that only 1 percent of the nation's elderly received help under the program. The report also highlighted several other problems such as stringent eligibility rules and high administrative costs of state governments (US Health Resources Administration 1976). Clearly, the issue of financing healthcare for the elderly had not been resolved and remained on the political agenda.

The Kennedy administration, on assuming office in 1961, was committed to increasing access to healthcare for millions of Americans. Having won a narrow victory in the 1960 presidential election, however, President Kennedy was not in a position to push for a universal insurance program. He faced a Congress that was not very amenable to his legislative proposals. He hoped that the 1962 congressional elections would produce a more receptive Congress. But he was able to keep the issue of healthcare needs of the elderly alive and on the political agenda (Fein 1986). On February 21, 1963, Kennedy delivered his "Special Message on Aiding Our Senior Citizens." The message contained 39 legislative recommendations. The key proposal was Medicare to meet the medical needs of the elderly. It had two objectives. One was protection against the cost of serious illness. The other was to serve as a base of insurance protection on which supplementary private programs could be added (David 1985). The assassination of Kennedy in November 1963 left the task of carrying on the battle for Medicare to his successor, Lyndon Johnson.

Lyndon Johnson adopted most of Kennedy's unfinished legislative proposals and incorporated them into the Great Society's War on Poverty program. After Civil Rights, Medicare was second in the administration's priorities. Johnson saw Medicare as an essential part of his War on Poverty (David 1985). Johnson won a landslide victory in the 1964 presidential election, which allowed him to claim a public mandate for his programs. Equally important was the fact that Democrats also won major victories in congressional elections. The administration now had enough votes in the House and the Senate for the passage of its healthcare proposals.

Health insurance was at the top of the legislative agenda in 1965. The Johnson administration proposed compulsory hospital insurance for the elderly, financed through payroll taxes. Republicans offered a proposal for subsidized, voluntary insurance for the aged, including coverage for physicians' services financed through general revenues. The AMA opposed both plans and advocated expansion of the Kerr-Mills program of matching grants to the states for vendor payments for the needy. Both opponents and proponents used traditional concepts, symbols, and clichés in the debate. Opponents, especially the AMA and insurance companies, opposed the Johnson administration's proposal on the grounds that it was compulsory, it represented socialized medicine, it would reduce the quality of care, and it was "un-American." The proponents defended the plan as designed to help the needy by providing them with access to medical care and thus compatible with American ideals of equity and equality (Skidmore 1970).

In 1965, Congress passed the Medicare program for the elderly and the Medicaid program for the poor as amendments to the Social Security Act of 1935. This final product was a classic compromise between three competing proposals. It included a compulsory health insurance program for the elderly, financed through payroll taxes (Medicare Part A, the Johnson administration proposal), a voluntary insurance program for physicians' services subsidized through general revenues (Medicare Part B, the Republican proposal), and an expanded means-tested program administered by the states (Medicaid, the AMA proposal).

In addition to Medicare and Medicaid, a number of other health programs, such as Maternal and Infant Care (MIC), the Children Supplemental Feeding Program, and community health centers, were created during the 1960s as part of Johnson's War on Poverty.

The principal objective of the Medicare and Medicaid programs was to provide equal access to healthcare for the elderly and the poor. Both programs dramatically increased access to healthcare (Darling 1986). Medicare helped alleviate substantial financially related barriers to healthcare access that existed before the program's enactment (Long and Settle 1984). It greatly expanded financial access to acute care for the elderly and disabled (Aaron 1991).

In recent years, concerns over rising healthcare costs and efforts at cost containment have led to tradeoffs between cost containment and access to healthcare. This situation has created new problems and gaps in access to healthcare. The next section provides a brief overview of the federal government's efforts to contain healthcare costs. Chapter 8 provides a more detailed examination and evaluation of major policy initiatives undertaken by federal and state governments, as well as the private sector, to contain these costs.

Efforts at Healthcare Cost Containment: 1970s–1980s

The 1970s represented a decade of transition in the US healthcare system. Prior to this time, federal healthcare policy was shaped by a number of assumptions. A major one was that the healthcare system suffered from too few healthcare facilities and services. The healthcare system needed more hospitals, physicians, technology, and biomedical research. Biomedical research was encouraged through federal funds for the National Institutes of Health, while new hospital construction was encouraged with federal funds provided through the Hill-Burton program. The second assumption was that one of the serious problems with the healthcare system was limited financial access to healthcare among disadvantaged citizens. The establishment of Medicare and Medicaid by the federal government was an effort to increase access to healthcare for the needy. The third assumption was that competitive markets and regulatory strategies do not work in the healthcare field (Brown 1986).

By the 1970s, these assumptions had come under increased scrutiny. As we discussed earlier in the chapter, the Hill-Burton program led to a significant expansion in the number of voluntary, not-for-profit, and state and local government hospitals. Policymakers came to recognize that the healthcare system was too large. This was in sharp contrast to the assumption before the 1960s that the healthcare system was too small. By the 1970s there was an increasing concern about the nation's sizable surplus of hospital beds and physicians. There was a realization that one of the reasons for increased healthcare costs was unconstrained diffusion of biomedical technology and an excess supply of hospitals and physicians, which encouraged excessive tests and treatments. Similarly, while Medicare and Medicaid had increased financial access to healthcare for the elderly and the needy, increased access had also led to increases in healthcare costs. From the beginning, outlays for Medicare and Medicaid greatly exceeded initial projections. When Medicare was established, the federal government had deliberately chosen to reimburse physicians in a generous manner to win their political support.

By the 1970s healthcare costs had risen dramatically. Total national healthcare expenditure had increased from $27.1 billion in 1960 to $74.3 billion in 1970. During this same period, federal healthcare expenditures increased from $2.9 billion to $17.8 billion, while state and local governments' healthcare expenditures increased from $3.7 billion to $9.9 billion. Similar increases were evident in hospital care and physician services (Levit et al. 1994). From 1966 to 1970, Medicare expenditures increased from $1.6 billion to $7.1 billion, while Medicaid expenditures increased from $1.3 billion to $5.3 billion. Increases in medical care inflation outstripped overall inflation (Levit et al. 1994).

Consequently, policymakers' concerns began to shift from providing access and quality healthcare to containing rising healthcare costs. During the 1970s and 1980s, the federal government and the states undertook a number of regulatory and market-oriented policy initiatives in an effort to contain costs (Brown 1987; Field 2007). They are briefly described below. These policy initiatives and their results are examined in more detail in Chapter 8, dealing with healthcare expenditures and cost containment.

During his first two years in office (1968–1970), President Nixon signed into law various acts designed to extend community mental health centers, migrant health centers, and programs designed to support training of healthcare personnel, among others. In 1971, Senator Edward Kennedy (D-MA) introduced the Health Security Act in Congress, which called for a comprehensive program of free medical care and would have replaced all public and private health plans with a single federally operated health insurance system. Since Nixon was seeking reelection in 1972, he felt compelled to respond to Kennedy's political challenge by proposing the National Health Insurance Partnership Act, which consisted of two parts. The first part, the Family Health Insurance Plan, was a federally financed plan to provide health insurance for all low-income families. The second part, the National Health Insurance Standards Act, would be financed by private funds, would set standards for employer health insurance programs, and would require coverage of employees through an employer mandate. However, this plan failed to win the necessary support in Congress for passage (Norris 1984).

Beginning in 1971, the Nixon administration sought to curtail healthcare costs. In his health message to Congress on February 18, 1971, Nixon argued that costs had skyrocketed and while we were investing more of the nation's resources in the health of people we were not getting a full return on our investment (Nixon 1971). Nixon sought curtailment in federal categorical health grant programs, vetoed legislation designed to renew and expand these programs, and impounded funds already appropriated. A struggle between the executive branch headed by a Republican president and a Congress controlled by Democrats ensued. The Democratic Congress was able to override some of Nixon's vetoes, and the battle over impoundment of funds ended up in the federal courts. It also ultimately led Congress in 1974 to enact the Congressional Budget and Impoundment Control Act, which Nixon signed into law a few days before he resigned from the presidency in the aftermath of the Watergate scandal. Despite Nixon's conflicts with Congress, a number of cost-containment initiatives were begun during this time.

PSROs and HMOs

One of the factors often cited as responsible for increased healthcare costs is the overutilization of healthcare resources. The rising costs of Medicare and Medicaid created concern in Congress about the cost as well as the quality of care provided in these programs. Congress created the Professional Standards Review Organizations (PSROs) through the Social Security Amendments Act of 1972. This was a regulatory mechanism to encourage efficient and economical delivery of healthcare in the two public programs—Medicare and Medicaid. More than 200 local PSROs were created and staffed by local physicians to review and monitor the care provided to Medicare and Medicaid patients by hospitals, skilled nursing homes, and extended-care facilities. The PSROs were given the authority to deny approval of payment to physicians who provided unnecessary or poor-quality services to Medicare and Medicaid patients.

In addition, the Nixon administration wanted a plan to control healthcare costs that would look uniquely Republican. Nixon hoped to promote market-oriented reforms designed to encourage competition in the healthcare market as a way of controlling costs. He was interested in developing a health strategy that would create a more efficient healthcare system, balance the supply of healthcare resources and demands, and at the same time ensure equal access to healthcare.

The Nixon administration's key proposal was to provide federal funds for the development of health maintenance organizations (HMOs). In 1973, nearly three years after Nixon first sent his proposal to Congress, the Health Maintenance Organization Act was passed. It was a much more modest plan than originally conceived and reflected the necessity of bargaining and compromises between the president and Congress. For example, the first Senate bill had authorized $5.2 billion over three years for start-up costs. The version signed into law authorized $375 million over three years for projects more limited in scope (Falkson 1980; Norris 1984). HMOs are a system in which enrollees pay a fixed fee (capitation) in advance, and in return, they receive a comprehensive set of health services. The Nixon administration believed that HMOs would promote competition with traditional healthcare delivery systems by creating incentives for shifting health services utilization from costlier inpatient services such as hospitals and skilled nursing facilities to less-costly outpatient services such as visits to doctors' offices.

Controlling Costs by Planning

During the late 1960s and the 1970s, the federal government also emphasized health planning to contain rising healthcare costs. The rationale for planning was based on the argument that there was an abundance of healthcare facilities and services—too many hospitals, too many hospital beds, and too much medical equipment. Unnecessary expansion and duplication led to overutilization of healthcare resources. The Comprehensive Health Planning Act of 1966 was an attempt at healthcare-facilities planning through the states. Comprehensive health-planning agencies were to be established in every state and in local areas. Their principal focus was hospital planning. In 1974, Congress passed the National Health Planning and Resource Development Act, which replaced the Comprehensive Health Planning Act and other health planning programs such as the regional medical and Hill-Burton programs. The law required all states to adopt certificate-of-need (CON) laws by 1980. CON laws require hospitals to document community need to obtain approval for major capital expenditures for expansion of facilities and services. The law also established a network of health system agencies at state and local levels to administer the CON laws.

Jimmy Carter, as a Democratic candidate for president in the 1976 election, had pledged his support for a comprehensive national health insurance program. Nevertheless, after assuming office in January 1977, Carter was hampered by budget constraints and was less anxious to push for a national health insurance program (Iglehart 1978). From 1971 to 1974, under the Nixon-imposed Economic Stabilization Program, economy-wide wage and price controls were in effect. Hospital prices were subject to control under this program; however, this had a limited impact on controlling hospital costs. In 1977, the Carter administration proposed a series of all-payer revenue controls on hospitals, known as the hospital cost-containment proposal. The Carter administration argued that controlling hospital costs was necessary because traditional market forces would not keep those costs down. The proposal was strongly opposed by the medical community in general and hospitals in particular. It also did not receive enthusiastic support in Congress. After three years of legislative battles, the proposal was defeated in favor of a promised voluntary effort by hospitals to contain costs. In a June 1979 message to Congress, President Carter proposed National Health Plan legislation to expand health insurance coverage and to protect Americans from the cost of catastrophic illness. Under the plan, Medicare and Medicaid would have been consolidated in a single administrative structure. It would have also included an employer mandate. The plan advocated increased competition through the development of HMOs and other alternative delivery-and-reimbursement systems (Carter 1979).

THE POLITICAL TRANSFORMATION OF THE US HEALTHCARE SYSTEM: 1981–2018

From about 1981 to 2008, the US healthcare system underwent a significant transformation. It took place largely through the political and legislative process under the ascendency of a conservative political ideology. The period of the 1930s through the 1960s had witnessed a significant increase in the federal government's role in healthcare. Federal health policies encouraged expansion of federal health grants to states, expansion of biomedical research, and expansion of hospitals and healthcare facilities, along with greater access to healthcare through Medicare and Medicaid programs.

The election of Richard Nixon in the 1968 election signaled an end to the liberal mandate and the rise of a conservative mandate. However, faced with a Democratic-controlled Congress, Nixon was forced to compromise his conservative agenda. The election of Ronald Reagan to the presidency elevated the conservative agenda. Under the conservatives, the period of 1981–2008 witnessed the initiation and implementation of several policy initiatives utilizing "managed competition" and "managed care" strategies to reduce the federal role in healthcare and expand the private-sector role. The "managed" part of "competition" and "care" recognized some role for the government in managing competition and care. Major elements of this competitive approach to healthcare were to provide consumers with an increased choice when they purchased insurance, the reduction and elimination of many regulatory approaches to cost containment, and new forms of prepaid healthcare delivery organizations to help contain costs (Ginsberg 1987).

The market approach to cost containment was designed to overcome perceived failures of the traditional system of health financing and services. These included: (1) the lack of motivation on the part of consumers to forgo consumption of health services since they shared little or no cost of each service; (2) the traditional fee-for-service mechanism that rewarded health professionals for providing more, not fewer, medical tests and treatment; (3) a lack of consumer knowledge about medical care, creating a dependence on healthcare providers that allowed them to control both demand and supply of services and thus the cost; and (4) that payments to hospitals and providers were based on the cost of care rather than on competitive prices (Oliver 1991). The goals of the market approach were to force consumers to share more of the cost of each medical procedure and health service and to emphasize competition between traditional fee-for-service organizations and alternative health delivery organizations (Oliver 1991).

As discussed in the previous section, the seeds of the market strategy were planted during the Nixon administration with the federal government encouraging the development of HMOs as an alternative healthcare delivery organization, but they developed deep roots during the period of 1980–2008. Health came to be treated more as a commodity than as a public good. Healthcare providers began to operate more like other businesses, relying on marketing strategies to attract new customers instead of outreach programs designed to bring needed health services to the community. The growing reliance on a market mechanism to address problems of the American healthcare system also led to the establishment of a medical-industrial complex consisting of a growing number of private for-profit hospitals, nursing homes, medical care organizations, and other businesses related to medical goods and services (Wallace and Estes 1989).

The Reagan Administration: 1981–1989

After campaigning on a platform of antiregulation and less government, Ronald Reagan became president in January 1981. Reagan sought to reduce expenditures for social programs, including healthcare. In this area, the Reagan administration reduced federal funding for preventive services, health professions education, community health centers, and Medicaid. The administration also shifted decision-making in health programs by consolidating health services and preventive programs into block grant programs and, as a part of deregulation, eliminated health planning and PSRO programs, giving state and local governments more responsibility and discretionary authority. In addition, the administration promoted competitive strategies in the healthcare market (Davis 1981; Robbins 1983; Wing 1984). All resulted in the reexamination of the role of federal government in financing and administration of health services and a significant change in the healthcare sector.

During the first three years of the Reagan administration, funding for health planning and health maintenance organizations was eventually eliminated. The PSRO program was renamed Peer Review Organizations (PROs), and its funding was reduced from $58 million in 1980 to $15 million in 1983, effectively ending the program. The Reagan administration also succeeded in combining 21 categorical grant programs in the areas of prevention, mental health, maternal and child healthcare, and primary care into four block grants. Funding for Medicare and Medicaid was also reduced (Etheredge 1983; Ginsberg 1987).

Medicaid Waivers

Two types of waivers are available under the Medicaid program. Section 1115 of the Social Security Act gives the executive branch authority to experiment with alternative state approaches to program delivery. These are called demonstration waivers. The second type of waiver, called program waivers, was established under Section 1915 of the Omnibus Budget Reconciliation Act of 1981 (Thompson and Burke 2008). This type of waiver gives the federal executive branch authority to allow states more freedom in their Medicaid programs in two areas. It gave states the opportunity to restrict the "freedom of choice" that beneficiaries had to select among Medicaid providers and adopt payment approaches other than fee-for-service. Using 1915(b) waivers, many states pursued various forms of managed care options for beneficiaries. The 1915(c) waivers, known as Home and Community-Based Services (HCBS) waivers, allow states to circumvent key requirements of the Medicaid law by providing alternatives to nursing home care in permitting states to offer home health benefits, such as personal assistance with daily living in a home or community setting, to the frail elderly, or to young persons with disabilities. The administrations of both President Reagan and President George H. W. Bush made frequent use of such waivers. Between 1981 and 1991, the number of HCBS waivers in operation grew from 6 to 113 (Thompson and Burke 2008). The Reagan administration saw this as an important mechanism for returning program decision-making authority to states and giving state governments more flexibility.

Prospective Payment System for Medicare

The biggest innovation of the Reagan administration was the introduction in 1983 of the Prospective Payment System (PPS), mandated by the Deficit Reduction Act of 1982, for reimbursement to hospitals under the Medicare program in the hope of reducing Medicare costs and making hospitals more efficient. As discussed earlier, when Medicare was created, it provided for a generous reimbursement to hospitals on a retrospective, reasonable-cost basis for services provided to Medicare patients. Under the new system, illnesses are classified into one of 468 diagnosis-related groups (DRGs). Each category is assigned a treatment rate, and hospitals are reimbursed according to these rates. If hospitals spend more money on treatment, they have to absorb the additional costs. If they spend less money than the established rates, they can keep the overpayment as profit. The new system was phased in over a period of time and went into full effect in 1987.

Medicare Catastrophic Coverage

By the mid-1980s, it was also becoming clear that the Medicare program was unable to meet all the health expenses of its beneficiaries. Their out-of-pocket expenses for services covered by Medicare were on the rise. In addition, the Medicare program did not provide coverage for certain basic services such as outpatient prescription drugs, custodial care, and most of the cost of nursing home care. The Reagan administration tried to address this problem of "Medigap." In his 1986 State of the Union message, President Reagan unveiled his proposal for an expansion of Medicare. Congress passed his proposal in 1988 as the Medicare Catastrophic Coverage Act.

The law modified both program benefits and financing, with changes to be phased in over a period of several years beginning in 1989. The Act provided for coverage of outpatient prescription drugs such as home-administered intravenous antibiotics and other FDA-approved drugs, as well as mammography screening for disabled beneficiaries. The act also expanded coverage of inpatient hospital days from 90 to an unlimited number of days per year. Similarly, the Act increased the number of days of coverage for skilled nursing facilities, home healthcare, and hospice care. The Act also reduced the amount of deductibles and coinsurance for certain services. The new benefits were to be financed entirely by the beneficiaries themselves through supplemental premiums. The Act increased monthly premiums for Part B of Medicare and increased the tax liability of higher-income beneficiaries.

The Medicare Catastrophic Coverage Act was very unpopular, particularly among the affluent elderly. One reason for their opposition was that they would shoulder most of the burden of financing the proposed changes through increases in their taxes. A second reason for the opposition was that many of the elderly were satisfied with the supplemental private insurance coverage they had purchased to cover the gaps in the Medicare program. Another major criticism of the Act was that while it made modest changes in Medicare nursing home benefits, it did not extend Medicare coverage to long-term nursing home care (Rice, Desmond, and Gable 1990). Long-term care is the type of care most likely to financially devastate the elderly (Rice and Gable 1986).

A plethora of bills based on competitive and market strategies were proposed during the Reagan administration. Many of them did not make it out of the Democratic Party-controlled Congress, although several of the initiatives, such as a reduced federal role in and reduced federal spending for healthcare, reduced regulations, giving state and local government more discretionary authority, and a prospective payment system for Medicare patients were successful.

The George H. W. Bush Administration: 1989–1993

George H. W. Bush was sworn in as president in January 1989. In November 1989 Congress repealed the Medicare Catastrophic Coverage Act due to significant protests against it. This defeat made Congress less enthusiastic about reforms in Medicare or undertaking any new initiatives with respect to long-term care (Rice, Desmond, and Gable 1990). Furthermore, the administration was too preoccupied with the Persian Gulf War (1990–1991) to undertake any major new initiatives in the area of healthcare. However, the Bush I administration did continue the practice started under the Reagan administration of granting Medicaid waivers to states.

Healthcare Reform

Polls in the early 1990s indicated that a majority of Americans had a negative view of the US healthcare system and were in favor of reforming it. Healthcare reform emerged on the national policy agenda with the approaching presidential elections in November 1992. President Bush announced new healthcare initiatives in February 1992. He proposed a series of reforms, including tax credits of up to $3,750 per year for families with incomes of up to $70,000 and a voucher for the same amount for poor families. The estimated cost, about $100 billion, was to be paid for by placing limits on Medicare and Medicaid programs. Under the plan, the self-employed would receive a tax deduction equal to the size of the premiums. Small businesses would receive tax inducements. There was also a proposal for mild insurance reform (Barnes 1991; Bocchino and Wakefield 1992; Dentzer 1992; Kinsley 1992; Wines 1992).

The Bush I initiative was clearly in response to the coming presidential election and to the promise of Bill Clinton, Arkansas governor and the Democratic candidate, that he would offer a plan for comprehensive reform of the US healthcare system. By October 1992, both President Bush and Democratic presidential nominee Clinton had endorsed managed care as the centerpiece of their healthcare plans. Comprehensive reform of the US healthcare system became one of the major campaign issues in the 1992 presidential election. Bill Clinton promised that, if elected, he would deliver a comprehensive reform of the US healthcare system that would provide universal coverage to all Americans. Clinton won the presidency, but he had managed to garner only 43 percent of the popular vote in a three-candidate race.

The Clinton Administration: 1993–2001

President Clinton was a "post-conservative" leader in the sense that he led a left-of-center Democratic Party to victory after an extensive period of conservative rule. As a candidate for president, Clinton had run as a new kind of Democrat by disassociating himself from more traditional liberal rhetoric and policy preferences. Under pressure to reduce government spending, to reduce or eliminate the federal deficit, and to push citizens who received public assistance toward more self-reliance and personal responsibility, in many areas the Clinton administration followed a moderate to right-of-center path, including antifederal interventionist leanings (Bashevkin 2000). This was evident in the Clinton administration's preference for and use of Medicaid waivers and support for welfare reform.

Medicaid Waivers

The arrival of the Clinton administration in 1993 created a more receptive environment for both Medicaid demonstrations (Section 1115) and program waivers (1915). During the Clinton years, the number of HCBS waivers increased by almost 50 percent from 155 to 231, and the number of Medicaid enrollees covered by waivers increased by 225 percent from 236,000 to 768,000. The hallmark of the Clinton years with respect to Medicaid waivers was the approval of 17 comprehensive waivers that moved a large number of Medicaid enrollees into managed care. Of the 89 proposals, including renewals, submitted during the Clinton years, 57 percent were approved (Thompson and Burke 2007). It is important to note that the granting of program waivers to states by the federal authority has become an important policy tool in the American federal system (Thompson and Burke 2008).

Healthcare Reform

President Clinton had promised, if elected, to propose a plan for comprehensive healthcare reform. His plan to overhaul the American healthcare system was presented to the nation in a speech before the joint session of Congress in September 1993, and a bill was sent to Congress in October. The six general principles underlying the reform were: security, simplicity, savings, choice, quality, and responsibility (Skocpol 1994). The proposal, entitled the Health Security Act, was very comprehensive; it proposed a fundamental restructuring of the US healthcare system. The bill provided universal coverage through an employer mandate. It also provided subsidies for poor persons and workers without insurance. The plan would provide a minimum benefits package covering a variety of services such as hospital, emergency, clinical preventive, mental health, substance abuse, family planning, pregnancy-related, hospice, home healthcare, extended care, outpatient laboratory, vision, hearing, and dental, among others (White House Domestic Policy Council 1993). "The healthcare plan that is always there" became the slogan for the Clinton plan (Clymer 1993). The plan was very much based on the concept of managed competition (Hanson 1994). Skocpol (1997, 41) described it as an ambitious plan for "inclusive managed competition."

The initial reaction to the Clinton plan was positive. Deliberation over healthcare reform in Congress did not begin until 1994, an election year. Several competing plans emerged in Congress on both sides of the aisle. The competing plans ranged from a more radical proposal of a single-payer system to proposals for only minor changes to the system, designed to deal with specific concerns. As the debate over these competing plans intensified, none of the plans managed to attract majority support. The initial positive reaction to the Clinton plan turned more negative as the plan was criticized and attacked by a variety of interest groups and Republicans in Congress. Republican leaders had made a strategic decision not to support the Clinton plan and to make the Clinton administration's failure to reform the healthcare system a campaign issue in the 1994 congressional elections. It was classic election-year politics. Public support for the Clinton plan as well as support for fundamental reform of the US healthcare system also declined as the debate continued. Opponents of comprehensive reforms argued that the US healthcare system was not facing a crisis requiring major changes and that the problems of the healthcare system could be addressed through incremental reforms.

Ultimately, this was the view that prevailed, and by late summer of 1994 President Clinton's Health Security Act was declared dead and buried. Some of the important reasons for this failure included the Clinton administration's miscalculation and mismanagement of the issue, attacks from interest groups opposed to the plan, partisan politics, election-year politics, a decline in President Clinton's popularity, and declining public support for comprehensive reform (Fallows 1995; Morin 1994; Patel 2003; Patel and Rushefsky 1998; Starr 1995). Another window of opportunity for reform of the US healthcare system had opened and closed without any comprehensive changes (Brady and Buckley 1995; Brodie and Blendon 1995; Canaham-Clyne 1995; Jacobs and Shapiro 1995; Navarro 1995; Patel and Rushefsky 1998; Steinmo and Watts 1995; Thomas 1995).

Republicans used a three-pronged approach in the 1994 election campaign: develop a positive governing agenda, derail Clinton's agenda, and amass a large campaign war chest (Balz and Brownstein 1996). The Republican Party also came up with the Contract with America, a ten-point platform that included a balanced-budget amendment, a line-item veto for the president, a crime bill, welfare reform, a family tax-cut plan, and parental rights in education. In addition, the Republican strategy of not cooperating with the president on the issue of comprehensive healthcare reform and then blaming President Clinton for its failure (on the basis that it was a bureaucratic, big-brother, big-government reform plan) paid handsome dividends in the 1994 congressional elections. The voters delivered the worst midterm repudiation that any president had received since Harry Truman in 1946. Republicans gained control of both the House and the Senate, establishing a divided government. The Republican victories extended to gubernatorial and state legislative races as well. A post-election survey conducted by President Clinton's pollster Stanley Greenberg identified the healthcare plan as the single item that directly linked Clinton with big government (Balz and Brownstein 1996). According to a survey conducted on election day, voters were strongly opposed to the comprehensive healthcare reform and instead favored an incremental solution to the nation's healthcare problems (Iglehart 1995).

Government Shutdown over Republican Proposal to Cut Spending for Medicaid and Medicare

The Republicans came up with a budget plan and Congress adopted a budget resolution for fiscal year (FY) 1996. It promised to balance the budget within seven years. It called for a $245-billion tax cut. It advocated reducing projected spending (growth rate) on Medicare by $270 billion and on Medicaid spending by $182 billion over the next seven years. The Medicaid program was to be changed into a block grant and turned over to the states. The Democrats went on the offensive and portrayed themselves as the saviors of the elderly (Medicare) and the poor (Medicaid) and argued that Republicans were willing to cut these programs to provide a tax cut for the wealthy. President Clinton refused to accept the Republican plan and was determined not to cave into Republican demands. The stalemate between the president and the Republican Congress led to the partial shutdown of the government twice. This confrontation backfired on the Republicans, as they saw public support for the Contract with America decline sharply. No action was taken on the proposed reduction in spending for Medicare and Medicaid.

In the 1996 legislation on the FY 1997 budget, the Republican leadership proposed block grants to replace the Medicaid and AFDC programs. President Clinton indicated that he strongly opposed turning Medicaid into a block-grant program, and twice he vetoed legislation that tried to transform both Medicaid and the AFDC program into block grants. Finally, the Republicans dropped their proposal to make Medicaid a block grant.

Welfare Reform

Republicans also wanted welfare reform, and President Clinton had indicated that he supported reforms. A welfare reform bill, after considerable bargaining between the president and congressional Republicans, did pass Congress, and President Clinton signed into law the bill known as the Personal Responsibility and Work Opportunity Reconciliation Act (PRWORA) of 1996. The new law included changes in welfare, supplemental security income, child support enforcement, and food stamps and social services. The main feature of the law is the Temporary Assistance to Needy Families (TANF) program, under which states are given a block grant to design their own welfare program. The Medicaid program was left virtually intact, but the linkage between Medicaid and welfare was broken.

Health Insurance Reform

Despite the partisan acrimony that dominated the 104th Congress in 1995 and 1996 over the issue of a balanced-budget amendment, Congress did succeed in passing some incremental healthcare reforms. One of the crowning achievements of the 104th Congress was the passage of the Health Insurance Portability and Accountability Act (HIPAA) of 1996, which President Clinton signed into law in August. Two of the major provisions of the bill include placing limits on insurance companies' authority to deny coverage or to impose preexisting condition exclusions and guaranteeing portability of insurance coverage when a person leaves their job voluntarily or involuntarily ("Kassebaum-Kennedy Health Insurance Bill Clears Congress" 1996).

Children's Health Insurance Program

President Clinton won an impressive reelection in 1996. The Republicans were able to retain their majorities in the House and the Senate with narrower margins. President Clinton and the Republican-controlled Congress managed to address another issue that had become an area of concern, the increased number of children who lacked health insurance coverage. The Balanced Budget Act of 1997 provided funds to expand health insurance coverage for children by creating the State Children's Health Insurance Program (SCHIP) as part of title XXI of the Social Security Act. State governments have taken advantage of this program and expanded health insurance coverage to uninsured children in their states (Congressional Budget Office 1998). When the program was reauthorized in 2009, it was renamed the Children's Health Insurance Program (CHIP).

When the SCHIP was passed, it was touted as enjoying broad bipartisan success. This bipartisan approach was symbolized by two of the cosponsors—Senator Edward Kennedy (D-MA) and Senator Orrin Hatch (R-UT). However, when the program came up for reauthorization in Congress in the summer and fall of 2007, bipartisanship was replaced by a bitter partisan and ideological divide and debate over the intended purpose of the program. The Republicans argued that the SCHIP should be a narrowly targeted means-tested program for poor, uninsured children. The Democrats argued that the SCHIP should be expanded further to guarantee that all children and some adults have some type of healthcare coverage. The administration of George W. Bush vetoed reauthorization and issued federal guidance restricting state flexibility around eligibility expansion (Gorin and Moniz 2007; Grogan and Rigby 2008). The SCHIP program is discussed in greater detail in Chapter 4 on Medicaid. The 1997 legislation also made significant changes to the Medicare program (see Chapter 5).

Patient's Bill of Rights

The expansion of managed competition in the healthcare marketplace as a way to cut costs led to a dramatic increase in the enrollment of millions of Americans in health maintenance organizations and preferred-provider organizations (PPOs). This, in turn, raised concerns about managed-care plans that deny or limit provision of healthcare services to their members in order to cut costs. Some legislators and consumer advocates pushed for the passage of a patient's bill of rights to protect patients against unfair, arbitrary, and capricious decisions by managed-care plans. President Clinton proposed such a bill, which would have allowed patients to sue their managed-care plans and/or managed-care organizations such as HMOs and PPOs. Republicans in Congress proposed their own version of a patient's bill of rights, which did not allow patients to sue their healthcare plans or provider organizations. Under the George W. Bush administration, Congress failed to enact a patient's bill of rights. However, a great deal of patients' rights have been incorporated into the Affordable Care Act (ACA) passed by Congress and signed into law by President Obama in 2010.

The George W. Bush Administration: 2001–2009

George W. Bush won the presidency in the election of 2000 by receiving 271 votes (270 needed to win) in the Electoral College, even though his opponent, Democratic Party candidate Al Gore, received more than half-a-million more popular votes. Bush had articulated a conservative political agenda during his presidential campaign of 2000. One of the very first health issues he had to confront was federal funding for stem cell research.

Stem Cell Policy and Politics

Embryonic stem cell research has generated a significant amount of controversy and heated discussion among its supporters and opponents, especially over the question of whether the federal government should fund such research. Supporters of stem cell research have argued that it could lead to the discovery of cures for diseases including Parkinson's, Alzheimer's, and diabetes. Such research, including therapeutic cloning, can help address problems of organ shortages and donor organ rejection. Supporters of stem cell research argue that such research is ethical because it promises to reduce human suffering and because thousands of frozen embryos are often discarded or destroyed at fertility clinics anyway. Opponents of stem cell research argue that this research is unethical and immoral because embryos are human and deserve the same full rights as humans, embryos should not be used to serve an instrumental value, taking life to prevent the suffering of others is unjustified, and research with embryonic stem cells so far is not very promising (Patel and Rushefsky 2005b).

Federal funding for embryonic stem cell research became a major issue in the 2000 presidential campaign. During the campaign, in order to attract the votes of Catholics and conservative evangelical Christians, George Bush indicated that he opposed federal funding for research that requires embryos to be destroyed or discarded. Upon assuming the presidency, Bush was confronted with the task of formulating a policy on the question of federal funding for stem cell research.

In August 2001, President Bush, in his first televised address to the nation, announced his policy decision. He argued that as a result of private research, more than 60 genetically diverse stem cell lines already in existence were created from embryos that were already destroyed. He further argued that these stem cell lines had the ability to regenerate themselves indefinitely, creating more opportunity for research. Thus, he argued that he would allow federal funds to be used for research only on these existing stem cell lines where the life-or-death decision had already been made.

President Bush's policy decision was essentially a political one designed to satisfy competing political interests and ethical values and was not based on any sound ethical principles, even though he tried to portray his decision as highly ethical (Patel and Rushefsky 2005b). The decision failed to satisfy completely either supporters or opponents of stem cell research. As Eric Cohen has pointed out, President Bush's decision is analogous to the Missouri Compromise, which permitted Missouri to enter the Union as a slave state and Maine as a free state. It sought to find a political compromise between competing interests and viewpoints (Cohen 2002). Furthermore, instead of more than 60 stem cell lines, in reality, there were only about 17 viable existing lines for researchers to work with because many of the other stem cell lines were damaged or lacked genetic diversity.

Given the fact that federal funding is limited to existing stem cells, embryonic stem cell research turned into a state-by-state battle between proponents and opponents. Some states moved ahead with stem cell research using only state funding. For example, California voters in November 2004 approved a ballot initiative to spend $3 billion on stem cell research (Kasindorf 2004). State laws vary considerably on the topic of stem cell research. States such as California, Connecticut, Illinois, Iowa, Maryland, Massachusetts, New Jersey, and New York encourage embryonic stem cell research, while some states strictly prohibit stem cell research regardless of the source. Even states that permit such research have established guidelines for scientists to follow with respect to things such as consent requirements, an approval and review process for research projects, the source of embryos for research, and cloning. Many states prohibit the sale of embryos or fetuses, while others prohibit research on live embryos; some states prohibit research on cloned embryos, while others prohibit human cloning only for the purpose of initiating a pregnancy, or reproductive cloning, but allow cloning for research. Some states limit the use of state funds for cloning or stem cell research. For example, Missouri law forbids the use of state funds for reproductive cloning but not for cloning research ("Stem Cell Research: Updated January 2008" n.d.).

The federal government exercises control only over stem cell research that it funds. There are no restrictions on stem cell research carried on in the private sector. Citing lack of leadership by the federal government, the National Academy of Sciences has proposed ethical guidelines to govern research with human embryonic stem cells. Major guidelines include: (1) laboratories doing such research should run proposed studies past a review board made up of community members and scientists; (2) women who donate eggs for embryonic stem cell research should not be paid; (3) no human embryo should be grown in a lab for more than 14 days; and (4) human embryonic stem cells may not be transplanted into an early human embryo. However, experiments in which human embryonic stem cells are transplanted into animals to study development and treatment of diseases is permitted with tight regulations ("Stem-Cell Guidelines: Ethics of a New Science" 2005; Wade 2005).

In 2005, the Republican-controlled House of Representatives passed a bill designed to expand federal funding for stem cell research beyond what President Bush's order allows. Bush had vowed to veto any measure that would expand federal financing of stem cell research (Stolberg 2005; Tumulty 2005). The Senate failed to act on the bill. President Obama in 2009 signed an executive order that allows federal tax dollars to be used for significantly broader research on embryonic stem cells ("Obama Ends Stem Cell Research Ban" 2009).

Medicaid Waivers

George W. Bush, like the Clinton administration, proved very receptive to HCBS waivers. In 2001, the administration announced the New Freedom Initiative, which called for the Centers for Medicare and Medicaid (CMS) to identify existing barriers to elderly and young people with disabilities in the community receiving health services. This initiative led to changes in some of the 1915(c) waiver practices. In 2002, the Bush administration started the Independence Plus initiative, under which waivers could be used for a cash payment and counseling. The number of 1915(c) waivers grew over 10 percent from the last year of the Clinton administration (Thompson and Burke 2008). The approval rate for Medicaid waivers increased considerably during the Bush administration. By August 2006, the administration had approved 72 percent of all waiver proposals and 44 states and the District of Columbia had obtained approval for 149 waivers (Thompson and Burke 2007). Virtually every aspect of the Medicaid program has been affected by the waivers. While broad and comprehensive reform of the Medicaid program has eluded national policymakers, waivers have allowed states to adopt smaller, incremental changes to the Medicaid program (Coughlin and Zuckerman 2008).

The Effort to Turn Medicaid into Block Grant

In 2003, President George Bush proposed converting Medicaid from an entitlement to a block-grant program. The proposal largely incorporated elements of similar but failed proposals by the Reagan administration in 1981 and congressional Republicans in 1995. Compared to categorical grants, block grants appeal to conservatives and Republicans since they are less restrictive, give states more flexibility, and eliminate the uncontrollable aspects of entitlement programs (Lambrew 2005). The proposal again failed to pass Congress.

Medical Liability Reform

President Bush also championed the cause of medical malpractice reform. Starting in 2003, in six consecutive State of the Union addresses, he urged Congress to pass medical liability reform. The proposed reform urged the capping of pain-and-suffering awards at $250,000. He justified this proposal as a way to control rising healthcare costs. The reform campaign was conducted against the backdrop of rising insurance premiums for US doctors ("U.S. Grapples with Solution to Preventable Medical Errors" 2009). Congress failed to pass such a reform.

Politics of Science and Reproductive Health

The term "reproductive health" is generally used to describe policies concerning abstinence, contraception, abortion, and assisted reproductive technologies. The topic of assisted reproductive technology and the court's role in dealing with ethical and legal issues raised by such technology are discussed in Chapter 9. The Bush administration played a major role in leading these policies in a more conservative direction.

Federal support for abstinence-only education flourished during the Bush administration, which launched a new abstinence program—Community Based Abstinence Education (CARE)—with more rigid guidelines. Under the program, grantees, often religious organizations, are required to teach that abstinence from sexual activity is the only way to avoid out-of-wedlock pregnancy and sexually transmitted diseases, and funded sex education curricula must accept the perspective that sexual activity outside marriage is likely to have harmful psychological and physical effects (McFarlane 2006). Under the Bush administration, annual funding for abstinence-only programs tripled from $60 million in 1998 to $176 million in 2006. The administration also altered performance measures to make the abstinence-only education program appear more successful. For example, outcome measures tracking pregnancy or sexual activity were replaced by measures of teenagers' attendance and attitudes. Abstinence-only programs also undermined more comprehensive sex education programs. The abstinence education movement was a key aspect of the Bush administration's attempt to promote a conservative moral framework and sexual ethics (Kulczycki 2007). Critics of the administration have argued that abstinence-only curricula blur religion and science, create stereotypes about boys and girls, and treat such stereotypes as scientific fact. For example, the curriculum teaches that women need financial support while men may need admiration and that women gauge their happiness/success by their relationships while men gauge their happiness/success by their accomplishments (Waxman 2006).

Given the Bush administration's commitment to abstinence, it also showed a great deal of ambivalence about the use of male condoms. Social conservatives have opposed efforts to support birth control by claiming that condoms are not very effective in protecting against sexually transmitted diseases. Administration officials, congressional lawmakers, and leaders of the religious right launched a series of campaigns that used the partial or misleading information to cast doubt on the effectiveness of condoms (Kulczycki 2007). In 2002, the Centers for Disease Control and Prevention (CDC) replaced a comprehensive online fact sheet about condoms, which included sections on their proper use and the effectiveness of different types of condoms, with one lacking crucial information on condom use and effectiveness. As a result, critics accused the Bush administration of suppressing and/or distorting scientific evidence (Waxman 2006). The administration also pushed for more parental involvement in minors' contraceptive decisions (McFarlane 2006). The Bush administration also pressured the Food and Drug Administration (FDA) to first deny and then to postpone repeatedly its decision on the over-the-counter availability of Plan B, which is a brand name for the most common form of emergency contraception. Opponents of Plan B tried to deny all women access to it over the counter. The agency in 2006 issued a compromise ruling that permitted over-the-counter status to Plan B, but only for women aged 18 and older (Kulczycki 2007; McFarlane 2006).

The Bush administration also tried to restrict access to abortion. During the first term, the domestic abortion-related issue that received the most attention was partial-birth abortion, which is not a medical term but a political one. President Bush signed the Partial Birth Abortion Ban Act into law on November 5, 2003. The law outlaws a specific abortion procedure medically called intact dilation and extraction (D&X). The law was challenged by opponents in courts and six federal courts ruled against the law on the grounds that it provided no exception for the protection of women's health, and for its imprecise language. The Bush administration pursued the ban to the US Supreme Court, which included two new Bush appointees. In April 2007 the Supreme Court upheld the law.

Consistent with its efforts to restrict domestic abortion, Bush also made two major changes to international abortion and family planning policy. He reinstated the "Mexico City policy" from the George H.W. Bush and Reagan era. Under the policy, the United States refuses to fund any foreign organization that provides abortion services (McFarlane 2006; Waxman 2006). Bush also signed a directive reviving the Global Gag Rule. This rule precludes awarding US government money earmarked for international population assistance and funded by the US Agency for International Development (USAID) to nongovernmental organizations in other countries that perform, counsel, or advocate for abortion services even in cases involving rape or incest (Kulczycki 2007).

Consumer-Driven Healthcare

Post the managed-care era, the Bush administration encouraged the idea of consumer-driven healthcare. Under this vision, patients are no longer just patients but take on the role of sophisticated consumers who use information and the Internet to comparison-shop and make informed choices about their own healthcare and tailor their own custom-made health benefit packages. The major instruments of consumer-driven healthcare are high-deductible health insurance plans (HDHP) and health savings accounts (HSAs) used to pay for routine healthcare expenditures until deductibles are met, at which point the HDHP's catastrophic coverage kicks in. The concept behind consumer-driven healthcare is that it would make consumers more cost-conscious, work against overinsurance and overutilization of health services, and lead to cost savings in healthcare (Oberlander 2006). The topics of managed competition, managed care, and consumer-driven healthcare are discussed in more detail in Chapter 8, which deals with healthcare cost containment.

Medicare Modernization Act of 2003 and Prescription Drug Benefit

By early 2000, rapidly rising prescription drug costs and growing concern about the affordability of needed drugs had helped elevate this issue on to the national policy agenda. According to a comprehensive report issued by the federal government on the nation's health, during 2001–2004, 46.7 percent of Americans reported taking at least one prescription drug. During the same period, 20.2 percent of Americans reported taking at least three prescription drugs (National Center for Health Statistics 2012). The number of Americans taking prescription drugs has continued to increase in the United States.

Americans spend a considerable amount of money on prescription drugs; for example, in 2000 they spent $120.9 billion on these drugs (National Center for Health Statistics 2012). In 2002, prescription drugs constituted about 10.4 percent of total national healthcare spending. Three factors have contributed to the increases in prescription drug expenditures. The first is increased use—from 2 billion prescriptions in 1993 to 3.4 billion in 2003, an increase of 70 percent. A second factor is the proliferation of different kinds of drugs, with newer and higher-priced drugs replacing older ones. The FDA, on average, approves about 30 new drugs annually. The third factor is the almost 25-percent increase in manufacturers' prices for existing drugs. Retail prescription prices increased an average of 7.4 percent a year from 1993 to 2003, double the average inflation rate of 2.5 percent (Kaiser Family Foundation 2004).

The problem of the high cost of prescription drugs is most acute for many seniors, especially those with low incomes and/or with multiple health problems. They often must make a difficult choice between healthcare and other consumption needs. The problem is dire for seniors on Medicare with low fixed incomes. The original Medicare program did not provide coverage for prescription drugs. Seniors with very low income qualify for Medicaid. Many seniors purchase additional insurance to cover expenses that Medicare does not cover. Yet, about one-third of Medicare beneficiaries in 2003 did not have coverage for prescription drugs, and it was also becoming increasingly more expensive to obtain (Fan, Sharpe, and Hong 2003).

The Bush administration saw a political opening. Democrats had for years talked about providing drug benefits to Medicare recipients but had failed to deliver. With the presidential election only a year away, Republicans saw an opportunity to take the issue of Medicare away from the Democrats by proposing and passing the Medicare Modernization Act (MMA) in 2003 (Nather 2003). The law added Part D, often referred to as the prescription drug benefit plan, to Medicare, which went into effect on January 1, 2006. Individuals are eligible for prescription drug coverage under a Part D plan if they are entitled to benefits under Medicare Part A and/or enrolled in Part B. Beneficiaries can obtain the Part D drug benefit either by joining a private prescription drug plan for drug coverage only, or under Medicare Part C by joining a Medicare Advantage plan that covers both medical services and prescription drugs. Chapter 5 provides a more detailed discussion of the politics surrounding the passage of the Medicare Modernization Act and the drug benefits provided under Part D.

The Barack Obama Administration: 2009–2017

Because the Patient Protection and Affordable Care Act of 2010 is the subject of the next chapter, we provide an abbreviated discussion of events related to the ACA in this section and the one on the Trump administration.

Reauthorization of the SCHIP

As discussed earlier, partisan differences regarding the goal of the SCHIP had delayed authorization of the program. The election of 2008 ushered in two years of unified government with the Democratic Party controlling both houses of Congress. One of the first actions undertaken by President Obama upon assuming office was to sign the Children's Health Insurance Program Reauthorization Act of 2009 (CHIPRA) on February 4, 2009. This legislation provides states with significant new funding, new program options, and a range of new incentives for covering children through Medicaid and the Children's Health Insurance Program (CHIP). The CHIPRA also provides flexibility to states to expand healthcare coverage to children who need it. Under the law, the secretary of Health and Human Services (HHS) is tasked with developing standards by which states can measure the quality of the care that children receive.

Healthcare Reform: The Affordable Care Act

By 2008, since the collapse of President Clinton's healthcare reform effort almost 15 years earlier, a consensus was emerging that a solution for the US healthcare system problems was overdue. The number of uninsured Americans had increased from 39.8 million in 2001 to 46.3 million in 2008 (Qazi 2009). There also appeared to be consensus across party lines that the American healthcare system served too few, cost too much, harmed too many and was too inefficient. However, the Democratic and Republican parties had different ideas about how to address these problems.

During the 2008 general election, Barack Obama, the Democratic nominee, and Senator John McCain, the Republican, were in agreement on a few points. Both candidates advocated conversion to electronic medical records, greater transparency, and consumer information, providing subsidies to low-to-moderate-income families for purchasing insurance, and more private insurance options. However, their agreements ended there. McCain's reform plan was more conservative. It opposed an individual mandate and advocated reforming the tax code to eliminate the bias toward employer-sponsored health insurance and to expand coverage through tax credits to families and individuals. To make insurance more affordable, McCain advocated expanding competition and expansion of Health Savings Accounts (Flint 2008).

Barack Obama's victory in the presidential election of 2008 set the stage for yet another major effort to reform the US healthcare system. According to Skocpol (2011), the political terrain had shifted with the election of Obama, and there were many reasons to believe that his election had opened a door for more than just incremental reform. One reason was that Barack Obama had won the presidency handily by garnering 53 percent of the popular vote and 365 electoral votes compared to 47 percent of the popular vote and 173 electoral votes for McCain. Second, congressional Democrats had also strengthened their majority in both houses of Congress. Third, the 2008 election was marked by the mobilization of a new bloc of voters, resulting in increased participation and enhanced support for the Democratic Party. Fourth, Obama assumed the presidency at a time when most Americans had become very disillusioned by his predecessor. Finally, during the campaign, Obama had clearly articulated his desire to change the direction of federal social and fiscal policies from years of conservative dominance (Skocpol 2011).

The Republican Party, just as it had done with the Clinton reform, decided to mount a strong opposition to Obama's reform plan. After more than a year of very partisan and divisive national and congressional debate, Congress passed and the president signed into law on March 23, 2010 the Affordable Care Act (ACA). The law aims to provide universal health insurance coverage through a combination of individual mandates, tax credits, insurance exchanges, expansion of Medicaid program, and several insurance market reforms. President Obama had finally broken a century-long logjam on healthcare reform.

However, the partisan battle over ACA was not over with the passage of the ACA. Opponents of the ACA launched an attack on two fronts—legal and political. The legal challenge included challenging the constitutionality of the different provisions of the ACA. On the political front, Republicans in Congress made many attempts to either defund, repeal, or repeal and replace the ACA. These are discussed in detail in Chapter 3.

One Supreme Court case (*NFIB v. Sebelius* 2012) ruled that states did not have to expand Medicaid, as called for by the ACA. As a result, Medicaid expansion became voluntary. In a second court case (*Burwell v. Hobby Lobby* 2014), the Court ruled that closely held for-profit corporations did not have to provide contraceptive coverage for their employees. A third case (*King v. Sebelius* 2015) unsuccessfully challenged federal tax subsidies on exchanges run by the federal government, as opposed to exchanges run by the states. A fourth case (*Zubik v. Burwell* 2016) challenged the contraceptive coverage mandate for religious-affiliated organizations (churches were already exempt). In this case, the Court was divided 4-4 after the death of Associate Supreme Court Justice Antonin Scalia. A fifth case (*Texas v. Azar* 2018) challenged the constitutionality of the ACA because Congress repealed the tax penalty in December 2017.

The ACA also faced electoral challenges. On the political front, in 2011, Republicans gained control of the House of Representatives, ushering in a period of divided government. Between 2011 and 2012 (112th Congress), Republicans had made 33 attempts at the partial or whole repeal of the ACA even though President Obama had stated that he would veto any bill passed by Congress designed to repeal the ACA ("House Obamacare Repeal: Thirty-Third Time's the Charm" 2012). During the 113th Congress, Republicans attempted to defund the implementation of ACA and in October 2013, the House Republicans refused to fund the federal government unless the implementation of the ACA was delayed, resulting in a partial government shutdown for two weeks (Montgomery and Kane 2013; Ornstein 2013). The efforts to repeal and replace the ACA continued throughout the Obama presidency and were renewed during the first year of the Trump presidency.

Despite various court challenges and repeal-and-replace efforts, the major provisions of the ACA have survived intact and thrived. As of April 2018, 32 states and the District of Columbia had expanded their Medicaid programs to cover more people while only 18 states had failed to expand their Medicaid program ("Status of State Action on the Medicaid Expansion Decision" 2018). Studies show that states that expanded their Medicaid program under the ACA significantly increased the number of individuals covered by Medicaid and reduced the number of uninsured in their states. Medicaid expansion has also had a positive effect on access to care, utilization of services, the affordability of care, and financial security among low-income individuals (Antonisse et al. 2018). The Affordable Care Act is discussed in more detail in Chapter 3 and Medicaid expansion under the ACA is discussed in more detail in Chapter 4.

The ACA has also succeeded in making health insurance more affordable to millions of Americans. In 2018, 11.7 million people had signed up for health insurance coverage on the ACA individual marketplaces ("National ACA Marketplace Signups Dipped a Modest 3.7 Percent this Year" 2018). Under the ACA the number of uninsured non-elderly Americans decreased from 44 million in 2013 (when the major provisions of the ACA went into effect) to less than 28 million at the end of 2016 and the uninsured rate dropped from 20.5 percent in 2013 to 12.2 percent in 2016 ("Key Facts About the Uninsured Population" 2017). Chapter 3 provides a comprehensive account of the political and legislative history of the ACA, the goals and major provisions of the law, and Republican efforts to repeal and replace the ACA.

The Trump Administration: 2017–

The Republican nominee Donald Trump won the presidency, defeating the Democratic Party nominee Hillary Clinton, in the November 2016 presidential elections. Since the Republican Party already had a majority in the

House and the Senate, the election of Donald Trump ushered in a unified government, giving Republicans hope for dismantling much of the Obama administration's policy agenda, especially healthcare initiatives and programs. However, while the Republican Party enjoyed a comfortable majority in the house, its majority was very slim in the Senate. The Trump administration moved quickly to implement some of its health policy agenda to satisfy its conservative base, which had played a major role in Trump's victory.

As with the previous section on the Obama administration, we briefly describe events related to the Affordable Care Act in this section; further and more detailed discussion appears in the next chapter.

Addressing the Affordable Care Act

The 2017–2018 period proved very challenging for those who supported the ACA. Legislatively, Republicans made a number of attempts to repeal and replace the ACA; ultimately all failed. The most successful proposal was the American Health Care Act, which passed the House of Representatives in 2017. In a mirror image of the passage of the ACA in 2010, no Democrats voted for the legislation.

The problem for the Republicans was in the Senate. Republicans had a very small majority, two votes, and were unable to get all Republicans behind the American Health Care Act or other repeal-and-replace legislation. The one legislative victory came in December 2017. Congress passed the Tax Cuts and Jobs Act, which cut taxes. But an amendment to the Act, a rider, repealed the tax penalty for failing to have health insurance.

Republicans were more successful at the administrative level. The Trump administration permitted and encouraged the purchase of what are called association plans, which would operate outside the ACA, as well as so-called "skinny" health insurance plans that people could purchase. These plans were temporary plans that did not have to meet the requirements of the ACA, such as mandatory benefits and bans on not covering people with pre-existing conditions. The administration also refused to pay insurance companies for keeping their premiums down, as called for by the ACA.

The Trump administration also tried to make it more difficult for people to sign-up for the exchanges. This effort included not paying for navigators to help people enroll on the web and shutting down the exchange website on Sundays during the enrollment period. The result for the 2019 period was a slight decrease in the number of people signing up for insurance on the exchanges.

The Trump administration also worked with states on the Medicaid expansion. Using waivers, the administration allowed states to add work requirements to Medicaid. Arkansas was the first of such states. States such as Arkansas agreed to expand Medicaid if the work requirements were approved. We discuss this more in Chapters 3 and 4.

The administration also sought ways to limit the contraception mandate in the Affordable Care Act. Under rules issued by the Obama administration, free coverage of contraceptives was part of the required essential benefits to be included in health insurance plans. The *Hobby Lobby* case allowed certain types of corporations to deny contraceptive coverage to their employees. The Obama administration sought to find ways around the ruling, which we discuss in Chapter 3.

In October 2017, the Trump administration issued new rules that opened doors for many companies or nonprofit organizations with religious or moral objections to stop offering contraceptive coverage if they had religious or moral objections offering such coverage (Andrews 2017; Facher 2017). In fact, it creates a new exception. Any employer that objects to contraceptive coverage on grounds of religious beliefs or moral convictions can opt out of providing contraceptive coverage. Under these new rules, an exception to contraceptive coverage would be available to various types of employers, including publicly traded companies (Rovner 2017). The administration's actions have been challenged and likely will be resolved by the judicial system.

From a judicial standpoint, the important case came in 2018. After Congress had repealed the tax penalty mentioned above, the Texas Attorney General filed suit in federal court, arguing that the ACA was now unconstitutional because the mandate was effectively removed. In December 2018, a federal district court judge ruled, in *Texas v. Azar*, that the ACA was unconstitutional. He later ruled that the ACA could continue as the case worked its way up to the US Supreme Court. It is likely that the Court will hear this case in its 2019–2020 session.

The failure of the Republican efforts to repeal and replace the ACA demonstrates several things about the policymaking environment we discussed in Chapter 1. One, even during a period of unified government there is no guarantee that the president and the majority party in Congress will always succeed in pushing its policy agenda if the majority party in either the House or the Senate enjoys a very slim and tenuous majority and fails to achieve almost a unanimity among its members. Second, the partisan and ideological polarization in the

American electorate and in the Congress makes consensus-building through bargaining and compromise very difficult. Third, major, fundamental policy changes and/or healthcare reforms are difficult to achieve. Fourth, public opinion often plays a very limited role (if any) in policymaking compared to partisan and ideological policy agenda designed to appeal to the party's base.

Mexico City Policy

On January 23, 2016, three days after being sworn into office, President Trump took executive action to reinstate the Mexico City Policy, which prohibits international non-governmental organizations (NGOs) from receiving US funding if they perform or promote abortions. During the Obama administration, US law banned direct funding of abortion services. The difference was that during the Obama administration, the NGOs that performed abortion procedures were allowed to receive funding for non-abortion services they provided such as access to contraceptives and post-abortion care. Under the new policy, NGOs that offer or promote abortion as part of family planning are prohibited from receiving any assistance from the US Agency for International Development. According to Marie Stopes International, a charity organization, the loss of its services could result in 6.5 million unwanted pregnancies, leading to unsafe abortions, in developing countries as well as the loss of general and gynecological checkups. The Trump administration reinstatement of the Mexico City Policy was condemned by many liberal Democrats and abortion rights activists, while it was applauded by many conservative Republicans and anti-abortion activists (Koran and Masters 2017).

The Trump Administration and the Opioid Crisis

More than 64,00 people died of drug overdose in 2016. In fact, between 2000 and 2014, the number of opioid overdose deaths soared 200 percent. The opioid epidemic had come to be viewed as a national emergency by most public health experts. In response, in October 2017, the Trump administration declared the US opioid epidemic as a public health emergency and directed the relevant executive agencies to use appropriate authority to fight the crisis. The declaration allows the quick hiring of personnel to deal with the issue, to allow remote prescribing of medicine and flexibility in the use of federal grant money to fight the problem. However, many in the healthcare field were disappointed that President Trump did not designate the crisis as a national emergency under the Stafford Act. The designation of the opioid crisis as a national emergency would have allowed the use of money from the federal Disaster Relief Fund from the Office of Emergency Management to deal with the crisis (Valverde 2017). The topic of the opioid crisis is discussed in more detail Chapter 10 of the book.

THE EVOLUTION OF PUBLIC HEALTH IN THE UNITED STATES

The Seventeenth Century

The New England colonies recognized public responsibility for the prevention of disease and taking care of those who became ill. Attempts to protect public health included quarantine of all ships arriving from ports afflicted with the disease. Based on the assumption that certain illnesses were contagious, quarantine legislation had become the most common practice. In addition, anyone afflicted with plague, smallpox, and malignant fever was isolated into a separate house, restricting their freedom. After initial resistance, the idea of inoculating people who had never contracted disease also became popular. Regulations were created to provide free inoculation and to isolate individuals who were inoculated in pest houses or in their homes during the course of their outbreak. By the middle of the seventeenth century, the concepts of keeping streets free of live or dead animals as well as regulating slaughterhouses were starting to take root (Parmet 1993).

The Eighteenth Century

State and local governments' involvement in public health can be traced back to the epidemics of the late eighteenth and early nineteenth century. The Revolutionary War caused major disruption of civil life and led to widespread disease. Overcrowded army camps became breeding grounds for the spread of diseases. As the war moved south, troops from the North suffered a lot from malaria. The smallpox epidemic was very common during the American Revolution between 1775 and 1782. Ultimately, the general use of inoculation brought the epidemic of smallpox under control. After the Revolutionary War, the basic pattern of sanitary regulations established during the colonial times continued with few modifications. There was an increase in public health regulations and renewed public attention to problems of health and sanitation. Quarantine laws became common and more stringent medical licensing laws were also enacted. In 1790, the New York City Dispensary was established with public and private monies to provide free medical care for the poor. The city also enacted comprehensive health legislation, which created the New York City Health Office, giving the city authority to enact sanitary ordinances (Parmet 1993). However, the situation changed dramatically when Philadelphia was struck with the yellow fever epidemic in 1793 and other epidemics such as cholera and smallpox became common during the next 50 years. Yellow fever also attacked many other cities such as Baltimore, New Haven, and New York in 1794 and 1795. Baltimore became the first city to establish a health department in 1798 (Altman and Morgan 1983).

The main causes of these epidemics were largely social and economic such as a growing and mobile population and urbanization of the eastern seaboard, resulting in overcrowding, bad housing, polluted water supplies, poor sanitary facilities, and contaminated food. The expansion into the West produced the same kind of conditions in Western towns and communities (Altman and Morgan 1983). Given the lack of scientific understanding of the diseases, quarantine became the main policy choice to deal with such epidemics. Cities and states also undertook some other activities such as providing medical care for the poor and sanitation measures such as cleaning filthy streets (Parmet 2007). However, what is clear is that during this period response to diseases was ad hoc, and no formal, standing bureaucracy existed to deal with public health crises either at state or local levels of government.

The origins of the federal government's involvement in public health can be traced to 1798 when President John Adams signed into law an Act that provided for the relief of sick and disabled seamen, and finance the construction and operation of the first public hospital for the medical care of merchant seamen. This was the first time that federal, state, or local government had established a health program for a specific group of people rather than a general health program for all people. This established the Marine Hospital Service and it ultimately led to the development of Marine hospitals during the nineteenth century. It was in 1912 that the Marine Hospital Service was renamed to what we know today as the Public Health Service (PHS) (Patel and Rushefsky 2005a).

The Nineteenth Century

The first third of the nineteenth century witnessed only limited advances in the functions and responsibilities of local governments. Such functions were largely confined to the emergence of garbage collection, street cleaning, temporary health boards, quarantine regulations, and nuisance ordinances. The period from about 1830 to the start of the Civil War witnessed the emergence of vital statistics as an important public health tool, which was helped by the establishment of the American Medical Association (AMA) in 1847. Consequently, medical societies also came to play an important role.

Public health as we know it today began to evolve around the latter half of the nineteenth century. Armed with new scientific discoveries and knowledge, health authorities began to apply this new knowledge to environmental sanitation techniques. One of the major developments was the publication of the Shattuck Report by the Massachusetts Sanitary Commission in 1950, heralded as the Magna Carta of public health. The report recommended the establishment of state health departments and local health boards in each town. Nineteen years later Massachusetts, in 1869, became the first state to establish a state board of health, followed by the state of California a year later (Altman and Morgan 1983). Also, between 1867 and 1860, several national sanitary conventions were held that called for sanitary and hygiene reforms.

The outbreak of Civil War in the Spring of 1861 delayed further developments in the field of public health. During the Civil War, sickness killed twice as many people as did battle wounds. Crowded army camps produced outbreaks of diseases such as mumps, measles, scarlet fever, and smallpox, and soldiers suffered from other disorders such as diarrhea, dysentery, and typhoid. President Lincoln in 1861 gave approval to the creation of the United States Sanitary Commission, which provided direct assistance to soldiers and helped reform the Army Medical Corps (Patel and Rushefsky 2005a). The end of the Civil War helped usher in the sanitation revolution in the United States (Duffy 1990). During the 1860s and 1870s, many major cities had established local health boards—New York in 1866, Chicago in 1867, Louisville in 1870, Indianapolis in 1872, and Boston in 1873 (Altman and Morgan 1983). The next 30 years saw the emergence of state health boards and the rapid expansion of local health departments.

The American Public Health Association was established in 1872, which ultimately led to the professionalization of public health. In 1876 the discovery of the germ theory of disease by Louis Pasteur established an empirical causal link between germs and diseases. In 1887, the first research facility, the Hygiene Laboratory established at the Staten Island Marine Hospital in 1891, was moved to Washington, DC. By the 1870s, public health reformers began to push for the creation of a national health board. In 1879, the United States Congress created the National Health Board with the power to enforce interstate quarantine laws.

During much of the nineteenth century, there was a great deal of overlap between public health and private medicine. Often, they acted as allies. In fact, many physicians were involved in the sanitation and public health reform movement. A majority of the members of the American Public Health Association were physicians. There was a humanitarian tradition in private medicine (Link 1992). This was a period of collaboration and accommodation. However, by the beginning of the twentieth century, a friction had begun to emerge between public health and private medicine; by the middle of the twentieth century it came to be characterized as an open hostility.

The Twentieth Century

The rise of bacteriology combined with advances in pathology, physiology, chemistry, and other fields had begun to advance scientific understanding of the causes of various diseases, helping identify many pathogenic organisms. Local public health departments became responsible for maintaining public health laboratories. Laboratory testing of water, milk, and other foods became an important function of local health departments. Between 1900 and the 1940s, state health boards transformed into strong state departments led by public health professionals. The bacterial revolution and other developments in medicine also strengthened the position of the medical professions.

By the beginning of the twentieth century, the interest and objectives of private medicine and public health had begun to diverge. Private medicine developed biologically grounded disciplines and began to explore the functioning of the human body and to diagnose and treat various illnesses and diseases. Private medicine started to focus on the individual and public health focused its attention on the health of the community as a whole. Two competitive models of healthcare emerged in the United States—the curative model and the preventive model. The curative model of healthcare represents the practice of private medicine focusing on the individual and diagnosing and curing the disease/illness after it emerges, while the preventive model of healthcare is represented by the practice of public health, which, rather than focusing on the individual, focuses on prevention and the spread of disease in the community as a whole. Since the second half of the twentieth century, the curative model has dominated the American healthcare system.

After World War I, public health and private medicine continued on their own separate ways. Each developed a separate system of financial, social, educational, and professional support. The American Medical Association played a crucial role in the professionalization of medical education following the Flexner report, helping to establish medical schools to train and ultimately license physicians. By 1915, there were 92 medical schools in the country. By 1932, most medical schools and state medical boards required a standard educational curriculum. The Welch-Rose Report of 1915 led to the establishment of separate institutionalized public health education, i.e., the establishment of schools of public health. The Johns Hopkins School of Hygiene and Public Health was established in 1916 and by 1922, schools of public health were established at Columbia, Harvard, and Yale Universities. Foundations such as the Rockefeller Foundation and the Carnegie Foundation played a major influential role in American medicine between 1910 and the 1930s (Patel and Rushefsky 2005a).

One of the major factors responsible for the separation of private medicine from public health was the divergence of economic interests between the two. In the late nineteenth and early twentieth century, the AMA and physicians welcomed government intervention and supported efforts to expand the regulatory powers of health departments. During the progressive era (1890s 1920s), the AMA not only supported but pushed for the establishment of a cabinet-level health department and also supported the idea of compulsory national health insurance. However, as the role of the national government began to expand, the AMA began to perceive such an expansion as harmful to the economic interests of physicians and started to oppose the expanded federal role in healthcare.

At the federal level, the national government started to become more active. In 1902, a permanent Census Bureau was created by the federal government to collect vital statistics. The Food and Drug Act was passed by Congress in 1906 to supplement state control and regulation of food. The hygiene laboratory established in 1887 became the National Institute of Health (NIH) in 1909. In 1912, the name of the United Marine Hospital was changed to the United States Public Health Service (USPHS). In 1921, Congress passed the Sheppard-Towner Act to provide federal grant-in-aid to states for maternal and child health programs to reduce maternal and infant mortality. The AMA opposed the law. As discussed in the previous sections, the federal government's role in healthcare expanded dramatically from the 1930s to the 1960s through the establishment of the Social Security system in 1935 and the Medicare and Medicaid programs in 1965.

By 1935, public health had become professionalized. Most states had established state health boards. Most cities had established public health departments and public laboratories. During World War II public health played a major role in American health because PHS was responsible for medical and sanitary support for the different branches of the armed forces. PHS also instituted a training program for nurses through the Cade Nurses Corps (Willever 1994). Medical research and science became the hallmark of healthcare and medicine after World War II. Changed societal conditions following World War II also necessitated a new definition and role for public health professionals. Public Law 78–184 in 1943 turned PHS service into a tightly knit bureaucracy managed by public health professionals. The Public Health Service Act passed in 1944 codified all PHS's responsibilities and strengthened the hands of the surgeon general (Snyder 1994a, 1994b). In 1946, the Communicable Disease Center (CC) was established. In 1948, the National Institute of Health (NIH) was established.

The second half of the twentieth century saw a dramatic expansion of the federal government's role in healthcare with the creation of several major new programs, such as Medicare and Medicaid and the War on Poverty programs in the 1960s. However, most of these programs bypassed existing public health structures at state and local levels. The Center for Medicare and Medicaid was put in charge of administering the Medicare and Medicaid programs and many War on Poverty programs were placed under existing or newly created federal agencies. In 1970, Congress created a new national agency, the Environmental Protection Agency (EPA), to deal with environmental concerns. Many federal programs focused on expanding healthcare facilities and access to care while medical areas most closely connected to public health such as infectious disease, family practice, pediatrics, medical social work, and such lost prestige and status compared to medical specialties connected to hospitals such as oncology, surgery, cardiology, and others, which gained money, status, and prestige (Garrett 2000). The AIDS epidemic of the 1980s and the slow response of public health to the crisis pointed to the weakness of the public health system. In fact, a report by the Institute of Medicine (1988), *The Future of Public Health*, provided a comprehensive examination of the weaknesses of the public health system. By the 1990s, the American public health system had come under a significant amount of criticism. One of the primary criticisms was that instead of being a coherent system, American public health was essentially made up of a hodgepodge of programs and agencies. Once the envy of the world, American public health was a shambles by the end of the twentieth century (Garrett 2000).

One positive development during the 1990s was the fact the animosity and apprehension that had developed between public health and private medicine since the 1950s was giving way toward cooperation and collaboration. In 1993, the AMA and APHA launched a joint initiative project to encourage cooperation between the two fields. The Robert Wood Johnson Foundation, along with other foundations, started providing grant money for collaborative initiatives and programs between the two fields. One of the outcomes of the private medicine and public health initiative was the creation of the Cooperative Action for Health Programs (CAHP) (Phillips 2000).

The Twenty-First Century

Stung by such criticisms, the American Public Health Association became more active in promoting laws aimed at improving public health. In response, Congress passed several laws to benefit public health activities. The Minority Health and Health Disparities Research and Education Act of 2000, also known as the Health Care Fairness Act, established a new center for research on minority health and health disparities. The Children's Health Act of 2000 expanded research and treatment on childhood concerns related to diabetes, asthma, and autism, among others. The Public Health Improvement Act of 2000 contained a comprehensive package of public health laws. The Public Health Threats and the Emergencies Relief Act strengthened the country's ability to detect and respond to serious public health threats such as a bioterrorist attack. Under the Twenty-First Century Research Laboratories Act of 2000, the NIH provided grants to improve the infrastructure of biomedical and behavioral research facilities throughout the country (Patel and Rushefsky 2005a). Following the terrorist attack of September 11, 2001 on the Twin Towers of the World Trade Center in New York and on the Pentagon, federal funding to state and local governments for bioterrorism-related programs and related activities increased dramatically. Today, all major cities and/or counties have an emergency management office or agency to plan and prepare for public health emergencies.

Two major reports issued by the Institute of Medicine (2000a, 2000b) called for an overhaul of the American public health system including public health education. Three of the major criticisms of the public health laws are: one, a great deal of public health laws are antiquated because they were formulated in the late nineteenth and early twentieth century. Second, public health laws in most states consist of successive layers of statutes and amendment built up over 100 years designed to deal with specific issues or problems. Disease-specific laws are ill-equipped to deal with today's emerging public health threats. Third, public health laws are highly fragmented, not only within states but also among states (Gostin 2001, 2002). In response to such criticism, a public health law reform movement has pushed for modernization of state public health laws. In 2000, with support from the CDC, the Center for Law and Public Health was established at Georgetown and Johns Hopkins Universities. In 2001, the Georgetown/Johns Hopkins Program on Law and Public Health drafted and proposed two model legislations. The Model State Public Health Privacy Act was designed to preserve states' and local health departments' ability to act to protect public health and at the same time provide strong privacy safeguards for public health data. The Model State Emergency Health Powers Act proposes to give significant emergency powers to state governors and public health agencies at state and local levels to deal with public health emergencies. The CDC has urged states to adopt both of the model legislations. However, both model legislations have been very controversial and have been criticized by both liberals and libertarians over concerns about potential abuse of power and restriction of civil liberties. Despite the controversy surrounding the Model State Emergency Health Powers Act, by August of 2011 most states had adopted at least a provision, a section, or some language of the model law into their state laws ("The Model State Emergency Health Powers Act: Summary Matrix" 2012).

Organization and Functions of Public Health

The mission of public health is to ensure healthy communities by maintaining and improving the health of the community as a whole through promotion of physical and mental health and healthy behavior/lifestyle, prevention of the spread of disease, injury, and disability, protection against environmental hazards, assurance of quality, equality, and access to healthcare, and response to public health emergencies and disasters such as hurricanes and other natural disasters, terrorist attacks, and epidemics, as well as aiding communities recover (Centers for Disease Control and Prevention 2013).

Since 1900, American life expectancy at birth has increased from 45 to 75 years and most of it is credited to public health actions such as improvements in living conditions through better sanitation, clean drinking water, safe foods, and elimination of environmental and occupational and worksite hazards. This is often accomplished by cooperative efforts between different levels of government, often forging partnerships between government and private organizations ("The Role of Public Health in Ensuring Healthy Communities" 1995).

The government public health system is made up of public health agencies from the federal government, 50 state governments, the District of Columbia, local governments (cities and counties), and federally recognized tribal agencies.

Federal Government

Federal government's responsibilities in public health include ensure that all levels of government have the capacity to provide essential public health services, to respond to public health threats when they involve more than one state or when solutions may be beyond the jurisdiction of one state, to help the states when they lack expertise or resources to deal with public health threats, and to help formulate public health goals in collaboration with state and local governments ("Trust for America's Health" 2006). The federal government is also responsible for working with local health leaders to ensure availability and coordination of essential public health services in insular areas such as the five US territories of Puerto Rico, Guam, the US Virgin Islands, American Samoa, and the Commonwealth of the Northern Mariana Islands (Centers for Disease Control and Prevention 2013).

A variety of federal agencies and offices are engaged, either directly or indirectly, in public health activities. Here, we discuss some of the most important ones and the functions they perform. Many of these agencies are located within the HHS (visit www.hhs.gov).

Within the HHS, under the Assistant Secretary of Health, a number of public health offices perform a variety of public health activities. For example, the National Vaccine Program Office (NVPO) coordinates vaccine and immunization activities of different federal agencies. The Office of Minority Health (OMH) deals with issues related to health status and quality of life for the minority population, while the Office on Women's Health (OWH) promotes improvement in women's health. For a comprehensive list of public health offices and their activities, visit www.hhs.gov/ash/public-health-offices/index.html.

Another important office housed under the Assistant Secretary of Health in the HHS is the Office of the Surgeon General (visit www.surgeongeneral.gov/). This office publishes the *Public Health Reports*, a key resource for those working in the public health field. The Surgeon General oversees the US Public Health Service Commissioned Corps (USPHS), made up of more than 6,700 uniformed public health professionals working throughout the federal government. Their mission is to protect, promote, and advance the health of our nation. The Surgeon General also provides Americans with the best scientific information on how to improve health and reduce the risk of illness and injury.

Some of the other important agencies within the HHS involved in public health activities include the Centers for Disease Control and Prevention, the Food and Drug Administration, the National Institutes of Health, the Substance Abuse and Mental Health Services Administration, the Agency for Healthcare Research and Quality, and the Indian Health Service.

The Centers for Disease Control and Prevention's (CDC) primary mission is to protect public health by providing leadership and direction in prevention and control of diseases, and to respond to public health emergencies. To perform this mission, the CDC engages in research and data collection about various diseases, promoting healthy living and environmental health, conducting vaccine and immunization campaigns, and preparing to deal with national emergencies involving natural disasters, pandemics, bioterrorism, and chemical and radiation emergencies (visit www.cdc.gov/).

The Food and Drug Administration (FDA) is responsible for ensuring the safety of the nation's food, animal and human drugs, biological products, and medical devices. The agency fulfills its mission by regulating the introduction of new drugs into the marketplace, fast-tracking the approval of important drugs, inspection of meat processing facilities, testing of products via clinical trials, and issuing alerts to warn consumers of potential problems in food supplies and often recalling products that are deeded to be unsafe and harmful (visit www.fda.gov/default.htm).

The National Institutes of Health (NIH) include many institutes and centers such as the National Cancer Institute, the National Eye Institute, the National Heart, Lung, and Blood Institute, the National Institute of Allergies and Infectious Disease, and the National Institute on Alcohol Abuse and Alcoholism, among others. These institutes and centers support biomedical and behavioral research, conduct research in their own laboratories, perform clinical trials, and promote the collection and sharing of medical knowledge. They also provide research grants. In fact, the NIH is the largest source of funding for medical in research in the world (visit www.nih.gov/).

The Substance Abuse and Mental Health Services Administration (SAMHSA) works to improve access and barriers to high-quality programs and services to individuals who suffer from or are at risk of addictive and mental disorders (visit www.samhsa.gov/).

The mission of the Agency for Healthcare Research and Quality (AHRQ) is to conduct research to make healthcare safer, to improve healthcare quality, and to make healthcare more accessible, equitable, and affordable (visit www.ahrq.gov/).

The Indian Health Service provides health services to American Indians and Alaska Natives (visit www.ihs.gov/). The tribal governments have a unique sovereignty and right to self-determination based on treaties made with the federal government. Part of the federal government's treaty obligation is to provide tribes with certain services, including health-related services. The IHS plays a major role in providing such services. Healthcare for American Indians and Alaska Natives is examined in more detail in Chapter 6.

To summarize, federal government functions and activities as they relate to population health include six areas: policymaking, the protection of public health, research, collection and dissemination of information about US health and the healthcare delivery system, capacity-building, and the direct management of certain services (Institute of Medicine 2003).

State Governments

A study by the Commonwealth Fund (2018) ranked all 50 states and the District of Columbia on their overall health system performance based on more than 40 measures of health access, quality of care, efficiency in the delivery of care, health outcomes, and income-based healthcare disparities. The top five-ranked states in health system performance were, in order, Hawaii, Massachusetts, Minnesota, Vermont, and Utah. The bottom five performers were Mississippi, Louisiana, Arkansas, West Virginia, and Kentucky. On the specific dimension of disease prevention and treatment, the top five performers were Massachusetts, Minnesota, Wisconsin, Iowa, and Maine, while the bottom five performers were Louisiana, Alaska, Florida, Mississippi, and Nevada.

While the administration of public health activities originally began in the cities, constitutional responsibility and authority for public health activities rest with the state governments. However, the organization and infrastructure vary considerably from state to state because state governments have significant latitude in defining public health authority through statutes and determining the breadth and depth of public health services to be provided and the manner in which they are organized, financed, and delivered (Salinsky 2010). The result is a very fragmented public health infrastructure throughout the country. Similarly, the relationship between state and local public health agencies also varies from one state to the other. In some states, public health infrastructure is highly centralized, whereby the state agency has direct control and authority for the supervision of local public health agencies. Some other states have a highly decentralized infrastructure in which local public health agencies have developed independently of the state agency and are run as counties or townships, reporting directly to local health boards or health commissions. Some states operate under a hybrid model, especially in large metropolitan areas in which local jurisdictions operate local public health agencies while state agencies assume responsibility for certain public health activities in local jurisdictions that do not have a health department or board. Two states—Hawaii and Rhode Island—do not have local public health agencies and all public health services are provided by state health agencies (Institute of Medicine 2003; Salinsky 2010).

The most common element among all 50 states is that every state has an agency that is responsible for public health activities. In the majority of states, the state health department is freestanding or independent. Some of them focus exclusively on public health while others have healthcare-related functions such as administration of the Medicaid program. In other states, the health department is one unit within a larger umbrella agency and includes a number of different functions such as providing services in areas such as mental health, public assistance, long-term care, and other human services. A majority of state public health departments are governed by a board or council of health that promulgates rules, advises elected public health officials on public health policies and concerns, develops state public health policies, and develops public health legislative agenda. Members are often appointed by the governor and generally include health professionals, citizens, consumer advocates, business people, and educators (Public Health Law Center 2015). In other states, the health department is led by a director who is appointed by the governor, often with confirmation by the state Senate.

The broad primary functions of the state health departments include the development of public policies that protect, promote, and improve public health, ensuring adequate resources are available to perform essential public health functions, ensuring laws are complied with, building community partnerships with relevant stockholders, monitoring, evaluating, and setting measurable outcomes for improving community health, and performing general oversight of all public health activities (Public Health Law Center 2015). Some of the more specific functions performed by state health agencies include the following: one, disease surveillance, epidemiology, and data collection. This includes collection, maintenance, and analysis of vital statistics records such as births and deaths and health-related information to identify trends in diseases and potential public health threats; two, provide laboratory services. This includes testing, such as testing newborns for rare genetic abnormalities and exposure to lead, bioterrorism, or emerging infectious agents like anthrax, West Nile virus, food-borne illnesses, screening individuals for exposure to toxins, and taking environmental samples for toxin contamination evaluation. Three, planning for public health emergencies. Four, the regulation of healthcare providers through inspection of healthcare facilities and licensing of healthcare professionals. Five, the administration of federal public health programs like Medicaid and the CHIP, as well as management of federal block grants (Salinsky 2010).

Local Governments

Local governments derive their authority from state governments. Thus, the scope and responsibilities of local public health authorities depend largely on a state's constitution and laws. Just like state governments, local health departments are structured in many different ways and vary from state-centralized, to local-centralized, to some mixed or hybrid pattern. All states typically have two levels of local governments: counties and municipalities. Municipalities can include cities, townships, towns, boroughs, villages, and hamlets. Metropolitan areas tend to have large local health departments that provide a wide range of services while in smaller geographic areas local health departments tend to be smaller and provide a narrow range of services. Local health departments/boards can also be structured as a locally governed health department, as part of a state health department, or as a state-centered district or region. Some local health departments serve a multi-county area (Public Health Law Center 2015). There are over 2,500 local health departments (Centers for Disease Control and Prevention 2013).

The responsibilities of the local health departments/boards include proposing, reviewing, and revising public health regulations as necessary, making sure community health assessment is conducted on a regular basis, collaborating with state health departments to recommend and establish public health priorities, and developing a strategic plan (Centers for Disease Control and Prevention 2013).

The most common services provided by local health departments are related to public health activities. An overwhelming majority of local health departments provide services such as adult and child immunization, communicable/infectious disease surveillance and epidemiology, restaurant inspections for health code violations, tuberculosis testing, food safety education, and population-based nutrition services. Some local health departments also provide services for maternal and child health; prenatal home visitation through maternal and child health services are typically restricted to high-risk populations (Centers for Disease Control and Prevention 2013; Institute of Medicine 2003).

Public Health Spending and Financing

As we have mentioned before, the United States spends more money on healthcare than any other country in the world. Yet, compared to the total amount of money spent annually on healthcare, the US spend very little money on public health activities. For example, in 2014, public health's share of total national health expenditure amounted to 2.6 percent. The percentage of public health expenditure of total health spending has fluctuated over the years but has remained less than 3 percent. Public health expenditure accounted for about 1.36 percent of the total in 1960 and had increased to 3.15 percent by 2002. However, it had dropped to 2.65 percent in 2014, a decline of 17 percent (Himmelstein and Woolhandler 2016). The growth in public health spending between 1960 and 2001 can largely be attributed to increased public health spending by state and local governments.

The federal government's funding for public health has remained relatively flat for many years. In 2011, federal public health spending through CDC averaged only about $20.28 per person. The amount of federal spending for disease prevention and improving community health ranged from a low of $14.20 per person in Ohio to $51.98 per person in Alaska (Trust for America's Health 2011). By 2015, per-capita CDC spending ranged from a high of $53.06 in Alaska to a low of $15.99 in Indiana (Trust for America's Future 2016).

In 2016, the total national health expenditure was $3.3 trillion, of which only $82.2 billion was spent on public health activities, 2.46 percent of the total (Hartman, Martin, Espinosa, and Catlin 2018). Of the $82.2 billion total spent on public health, the federal share was about $12 billion (14.6 percent) while the state and local government share was $70 billion (85.4 percent) (Center for Medicare and Medicaid Services n.d.). The proposed White House budget for FY 2018 aims to slash CDC funding by $1.2 billion. Since three-quarters of the CDC budget supports state and local public health programs, it will negatively impact state-local spending on public health activities. The budget also proposes to allocate some of the state public health funding on a pay-for-performance basis, requiring states to compete for available dollars. The proposed budget does include $500 million in new funding for a new block grant program administered through CDC for improving nutrition and physical activity for children and teens (Clary 2017).

State and local governments account for 80 to 90 percent of total public health spending in recent decades (Himmelstein and Woolhandler 2016). However, for the fiscal year 2014–2015, 16 states decreased their public health budget from the previous year. The median state funding for public health was $35.77 per person. The per-capita spending ranged from a low of $4.10 in Nevada to a high of $158.30 in Hawaii. Needless to say, some of the variations in states' public health spending is accounted for by wide variations among states in disease rates and other health statistics. Part of the variation is also accounted for by availability or lack of financial resources as well as states' level of commitment to public health (Trust for America's Future 2016).

Where does the funding for state and local health agencies come from? State governments rely heavily on federal funding to support their state agencies and programs. On average, almost 45 percent of their funding comes from federal funds (often through federal grants programs), around 23 percent comes from state general funds, another 16 percent from other state funds, 7 percent from state fees and fines, 4 percent from Medicare and Medicaid and the other 5 percent comes from other sources (Centers for Disease Control and Prevention 2013). The percentage of state health agency funding coming from the federal government varies widely between states due to differences in range and scope of services provided, level of resources committed by state health departments to public health activities, and distribution of federal grant dollars (Salinsky 2010).

The local health departments' funding tends to come from local government (26 percent), directly from the state (21 percent), federal grant money passed through state governments to their local governments (14 percent), Medicaid (13 percent), local fees (7 percent), direct money from the federal government (6 percent), Medicare (3 percent), with the remainder coming from other sources (Centers for Disease Control and Prevention 2013).

Public Health Accomplishments and Challenges

As noted earlier, much of the success in the expansion of average life expectancy at birth in the United States can be attributed directly to many of the public health activities and interventions. Some of the major accomplishments of public health in the twentieth century include vaccination, safer workplaces, safer and healthier food, improvements in motor vehicle safety, control of infectious disease, decline in death rate from coronary heart disease and stroke, family planning, recognition of tobacco's health hazards leading to a reduction in smoking, fluoridation of water, and healthier mothers and babies (Centers for Disease Control and Prevention 2013).

However, public health in the United States also faces many challenges. Despite a decline in smoking and deaths from coronary heart disease and strokes, heart disease, stroke, cancer, diabetes, accidents, Alzheimer's, and kidney disease still rank among the top leading causes of death in the United States. Addressing the dramatic increase in the rate of obesity and deaths resulting from opioid addiction and overdose remain major public health challenges.

In recent years, empirical research findings have demonstrated that the ratio of a country's social service spending to healthcare spending is highly correlated with health outcomes. In other words, increased spending on the "social determinants of health"—a set of home and community-based factors such as housing, electricity/heat, hunger, food assistance, education, environmental cleanup, and better urban design, i.e., built-in environment, among others—can produce positive health outcomes and reduced healthcare spending in the long run (Freedman 2018; Onie, Peria, and Lee 2016). One of the biggest challenges confronting public health professionals is how to persuade policymakers that investment in social determinants of health is a worthwhile endeavor. Success in addressing the challenges confronting public health would require a significant increase in funding for public health at all three levels of government. This ultimately may be the biggest challenge facing public health in the United States.

CONCLUSION

Healthcare policy in the United States results from a combination of decisions made and initiatives undertaken by various levels of government and the private sector. Though the role of federal, state, and local governments in healthcare policy has expanded significantly in the twentieth century, US healthcare remains a mostly private system. Policymakers in the United States have mainly followed a middle road between a totally private healthcare system and a publicly financed national healthcare system.

The federal government's health policy initiatives have focused on concerns about values of access (equality), quality of care, and cost efficiency. The federal role in healthcare has gone through four distinct stages. The first stage was characterized by policies designed to increase access through expansion of healthcare facilities, services, and resources; the second stage by policies specifically designed to provide equal access and quality care to needy groups such as the elderly and the poor; the third stage by policies designed to contain rising healthcare costs; and the fourth stage by the political transformation of the American healthcare system through managed care, managed completion, and consumer-driven healthcare.

The federal government in the past had always followed an incremental approach to creating specific policies such as Medicare, Medicaid, and numerous categorical grant programs targeted at narrowly defined groups or problems (Darling 1986). How the ACA changes the landscape of the American healthcare system remains to be seen.

Medicare, Medicaid, the CHIP, Medicare prescription drug benefit programs, and other federal grant-in-aid programs have increased access to healthcare by removing some of the financial obstacles facing needy groups. However, problems remain, and recent evidence suggests the emergence of new difficulties. The demise of the Medicare Catastrophic Coverage Act left many poor elderly with significant gaps in their Medicare coverage because they cannot afford to buy supplemental private insurance. This problem is likely to grow as the number of elderly in the population increases. One of the biggest problems is Medicare's failure to provide coverage for long-term care. Similarly, a significant number of poor people are not covered under Medicaid. More and more people are falling through the cracks in the healthcare safety net, as reflected in the increased number of uninsured Americans and the decline in employer-based health insurance. Moreover, hospitals in many major cities are facing a crisis situation (Beck et al. 1991; King 1990; Specter 1990).

Because government intervention in US politics takes place within the context of the public philosophy of interest-group liberalism and cynicism about government regulation, governmental input has tended to occur at the margins rather than at the core of the problem (Mechanic 1981). Powerful interest groups have been able to exercise veto power over proposed policies. For example, since the 1920s, numerous attempts by the federal government to establish some form of national health insurance that would guarantee healthcare access to everyone have been defeated by powerful interests such as the AMA and insurance companies. Such groups have successfully defended and protected their narrow interests, even if they have done so in the name of protecting the public interest by appealing to the value of freedom to choose one's doctor and by raising the specter of "socialized medicine," which they argue would lower the quality of healthcare. In recent years, the issue of national health insurance has been pushed back on the legislative agenda because of an economic environment characterized by huge federal budget deficits and a protracted recession. In light of this past history, the passage of the ACA was a major historical achievement for the Obama administration.

Both liberals and conservatives have had difficulty in carrying out an ideologically faithful healthcare policy. For example, while the Nixon administration advocated a competitive market strategy and successfully pushed for federal support for the development of HMOs, it also had to accept increased federal government regulations in the form of peer-review organizations. Similarly, the important innovation of the PPS for Medicare reimbursement under the Reagan administration relied on regulatory price-control mechanisms to encourage efficiency in the healthcare market. President George W. Bush, despite his strong conservative leanings, created the largest expansion of the Medicare program with prescription drug benefits. President Clinton's efforts to overhaul the US healthcare system through a national health insurance system failed to pass Congress.

Liberals and conservatives have also had to contend with powerful interest groups. For example, insurance companies, hospitals, and the medical profession have welcomed some regulatory relief, but they have not shown a great deal of enthusiasm for the conservative program of increased competition in the healthcare market (Starr 1982). Liberal efforts at major reforms to increase healthcare access were successfully thwarted by the same interest groups. Part of the reason for the success of the ACA was that the Obama administration from the very beginning courted and succeeded in winning over the support of some powerful interest groups through bargaining and achieving compromises. Also, it is important to remember that while Obama healthcare reform is a major accomplishment, the reform itself is modest. It did not create a single-payer universal healthcare system. Since undocumented individuals are not covered under the law, we can expect the number of individuals covered by health insurance to increase, but it will not achieve the goal of universal health insurance coverage. The law does not provide for a public option, and thus the American healthcare system will continue to remain a mostly private system despite opponents' charge that the law creates a "government-controlled" and/or "government-run" healthcare system.

The constitutional structure of separation of powers and checks and balances combined with the increased frequency of divided government has necessitated constant bargaining and compromises between the two houses of Congress and between the president and Congress. However, the increased partisanship and ideological divide between the two political parties have made bargaining and compromises more difficult. It is important to keep in mind that the ACA was passed largely on a party-line vote. Not a single Republican in the House voted for the law, while in the Senate only one Republican and two independents voted in line with the Democrats. The federal structure of government will continue to produce debate about the proper distribution of authority and responsibility between the different levels of government in health policy.

The election of Donald Trump to the presidency in 2016 established a unified government with the Republic Party in control of the presidency and both houses of Congress. This revived Republicans' hopes of repealing and replacing the ACA. However, efforts to repeal and replace the ACA failed given the slim Republican majority in the Senate and lack of consensus among conservative and moderate Republicans regarding the alternative proposals to replace it. Nonetheless, the Trump administration proceeded to weaken the ACA through the elimination of the Act's individual mandate in the tax reform legislation, expansion of the contraceptive mandate exemption on religious and moral grounds, and through a series of executive orders and administrative rules designed to reduce the length of the signup period for the ACA, reducing funding for healthcare navigators who helped individuals sign up for the ACA and the like. The long-term impact of these measures on the ACA remains to be seen.

Beginning in 1900, private medicine and public health parted ways and began to establish separate and distinct identities with private medicine focusing on the curative model of healthcare while public health focused on the preventive model of healthcare. By the 1950s, the curative model had become the dominant model of healthcare in the United States, despite the fact that public health was largely responsible for almost 30 years of expansion in life expectancy at birth in the United States. Despite many accomplishments of public health, the United States spends a minuscule amount of money on public health activities in comparison to the total national health expenditure. The history of the relationship between private medicine and public health is reflected in one Greek myth. According to this myth, Aesculapius, the Greek father of medicine, had two quarrelsome daughters, both of whom started life as equal. One daughter, Hygeia, the goddess of health, was known for preventing illness while the second daughter, Panacea, was known for treating illness. Over time, demand for Panacea's services grew so large that it exceeded her capacity to heal everyone and the price of her services became so high that many people could no longer afford her services anymore (Smith 1994).

STUDY QUESTIONS

1. Discuss how healthcare evolved in the United States in the eighteenth and nineteenth centuries.
2. Discuss the most important factors/developments that helped transform American medicine between 1900 and 1935.
3. What factors contributed to the separation and the schism that developed between public health and private medicine in early-twentieth-century America?
4. Discuss the evolution of the role of the federal government in healthcare from 1900 to the 1960s. What was the single most important goal/purpose of federal government healthcare policies during this time period?
5. Why and how did the political transformation of the American healthcare system come about between 1970 and 2008? What factors contributed to this transformation?
6. The failure of the Clinton administration's (1993–1994) attempt to overhaul the US healthcare system did lead to the passage of some important incremental healthcare reforms during the Clinton years. What were they?
7. Write an essay in which you discuss the major conservative health policy initiatives of the administration of George W. Bush (2001–2009).
8. Discuss the Trump administration's health policy initiatives with special focus on the administration's efforts to repeal and replace and to weaken the ACA.
9. Discuss the evolution of public health in the United States.
10. What are the major accomplishments and important challenges confronting public health in the United States?
11. Discuss the role and responsibilities of the federal, state, and local governments in public health in the United States.
12. How does the American healthcare system compare to healthcare systems of the other OCED countries?

REFERENCES

Aaron, Henry J. 1991. *Serious and Unstable Condition: Financing America's Health Care.* Washington, DC: Brookings Institution.
Abramson, John. 2004. *Overdosed America: The Broken Promise of American Medicine.* New York: HarperCollins.
Altman, Drew E. and Douglas H. Morgan. 1983. "The Role of the State and Local Government in Health." *Health Affairs*, 2, no. 4 (Winter): 7–31.
American Hospital Association. 2005. *AHA Hospital Statistics.* Chicago, IL: Health Forum Publishing.
Anders, George. 1997. *Health against Wealth: HMOs and the Breakdown of Medical Trust.* Thorndike, ME: G.K. Hall.
Anderson, Odin W. 1985. *Health Services in the United States: A Growth Enterprise since 1875.* Ann Arbor, MI: Health Administration Press.
Andrews, Michelle. 2017. "Want an IUD? Take Note of Trump's New Birth Control Policy." *Kaiser Health News.* Online at https://khn.org/.
Antonisse, Larisa, Rachel Garfield, Robin Rudowitz, and Samantha Artiga. 2018. "The Effects of Medicaid Expansion under the ACA: Updated Findings from a Literature Review." Issue Brief. March. Online at www.kff.org/.
Balz, Dan and Ronald J. Brownstein. 1996. *Storming the Gates: Protest Politics and the Republican Revival.* Boston, MA: Little, Brown.
Bartlett, Donald L. and James B. Steele. 2006. *Critical Condition: How Health Care in America Became Big Business and Bad Medicine.* New York: Broadway Books.
Barnes, Fred. 1991. "Rude Health." *New Republic*, 205, no. 23 (December): 9–10.
Bashevkin, Sylvia. 2000. "Rethinking Retrenchment: North American Social Policy during the Early Clinton and Cheretien Years." *Canadian Journal of Political Science*, 33, no. 1 (March): 7–36.
Beck, Melinda, Daniel Glick, Nadine Joseph, and Peter Katel. 1991. "State of Emergency." *Newsweek*, October 14.
Bernstein, Merton C. and Joan Broadshaug Bernstein. 1988. *Social Security: The System That Works.* New York: Basic Books.
Blumenthal, David. 2018. "Drop in U.S. Life Expectancy Is an 'Indictment' of the American Health Care System." *Stat.* Online at www.statnews.com/.
Bocchino, Carmella A. and Mary K. Wakefield. 1992. "Capitol Commentary: The Health Care Reform Debate: Competition Vs. Government Control." *Nursing Economics*, 10, no. 5 (September–October): 360–361.
Brady, David and Kara M. Buckley. 1995. "Health Care Reform in the 103d Congress: A Predictable Failure." *Journal of Health Politics, Policy and Law*, 20, no. 2 (Summer): 447–454.
Brill, Steven. 2015. *America's Bitter Pill: Money, Politics, Backroom Deals, and the Fight to Fix Our Broken Healthcare System.* New York: Random House.

Brodie, Mollyann and Robert J. Blendon. 1995. "The Public's Contribution to Congressional Gridlock on Health Care Reform." *Journal of Health Politics, Policy and Law*, 20, no. 2 (Summer): 403–410.

Brooks, Janet. "U.S. Grapples with Solution to Preventable Medical Errors." 2009. *Canadian Medical Association Journal*, 180, no. 7 (March 31): E4–E5.

Brown, Lawrence D. 1986. "Introduction to a Decade of Transition." *Journal of Health Politics, Policy and Law*, 11, no. 4: 569–583.

Brown, Lawrence D. 1987. *Health Policy in Transition: A Decade of Health Politics, Policy, and Law*. Durham, NC: Duke University Press.

Brownlee, Shannon. 2007. *Overtreated: Why Too Much Medicine Is Making Us Sicker and Poorer*. New York: Bloomsbury.

Budrys, Grace. 2011. *Our Unsystematic Health Care System*, 3rd edn. Lanham, MD: Rowman & Littlefield.

Campion, Frank D. 1984. *The AMA and U.S. Health Policy since 1940*. Chicago, IL: Chicago Review Press.

Canaham-Clyne, John P. 1995. "Clinton's Folly–The Health Care Debacle." *New Politics*, 5, no. 2 (Winter): 27.

Carter, Jimmy. 1979. "National Health Plan Legislation." *Challenge*, 22, no. 3 (July–August): 11–16.

Center for Medicare and Medicaid Services. n.d. "National Health Expenditures by the Type of Service and Sources of Funds: Calendar Years 1960–2016." Office of the Actuary, National Health Statistics Group. Online at www.cms.gov/.

Centers for Disease Control and Prevention. 2013. "United States Public Health 101." Atlanta, GA: Centers for Disease Control and Prevention. Office of State, Tribal, Local, and Territorial Support. Online at www.cdc.gov/stltpublichealth.

Clark, Cal and Rene McEldowney, eds. 2001. *The Health Care Financial Crisis: Strategies for Overcoming an "Unholy Trinity"*. Huntington, NY: Nova Science.

Clary, Amy. 2017. "Three Ways Proposed White House Budget Could Affect Public Health in States." Washington, DC: National Academy for State Health Policy. Online at https://nashp.org/.

Clymer, Adam. 1993. "Clinton Asks Backing for Sweeping Change in the Health System." *The New York Times*, September 23.

Cohen, Eric. 2002. "Bush's Stem Cell Ruling: A Missouri Compromise." In *The Future Is Now: America Confronts the New Genetics*, eds William Kristol and Eric Cohen, 316–318. Lanham, MD: Rowman & Littlefield.

Cohn, Jonathan. 2008. *Sick: The Untold Story of America's Health Care Crisis–And the People Who Pay the Price*. New York: HarperCollins.

Commonwealth Fund. 2014. "Mirror, Mirror On the Wall, 2014 Update: How the U.S. Health Care System Compares Internationally." New York: The Commonwealth Fund. Online at www.commonwealthfund.org/publications/fund-reports/2014/jun/mirror-mirror-wall-2014-update-how-us-health-care-system.

Commonwealth Fund. 2018. *2018 Scorecard on State Health System Performance*. New York: The Commonwealth Fund. Online at www.commonwealthfund.org/.

Congressional Budget Office. 1998. "Expanding Health Insurance Coverage for Children under Title XXI of the Social Security Act." February and August. Congressional Budget Office. Online at www.cbo.gov/.

Cortese, Denis A. 2006. "Healing America's Health Care System." *Mayo Clinic Proceedings*, 81, no. 4 (April): 492–496.

Coughlin, Teresa A. and Stephen Zuckerman. 2008. "State Responses to New Flexibility in Medicaid." *Milbank Quarterly*, 86, no. 2 (June): 209–240.

Darling, Helen. 1986. "The Role of the Federal Government in Assuring Access to Health Care." *Inquiry*, 23, no. 1 (Fall): 286–295.

Daschle, Thomas, Scott S. Greenberger, and Jeanne M. Lambrew. 2008. *Critical: What We Can Do about the Health Care Crisis*. New York: Thomas Dunne.

David, Sheri I. 1985. *With Dignity: The Search for Medicare and Medicaid*. Westport, CT: Greenwood Press.

Davidson, Stephen M. 2010. *Still Broken: understanding the U.S. Health Care System*. Stanford, CA: Stanford University Press.

Davis, Karen. 1981. "Reagan Administration Health Policy." *Journal of Public Health Policy*, 2, no. 4 (December): 312–332.

Dentzer, Susan. 1990. "America's Scandalous Health Care." *U.S. News and World Report*, March 12.

Dentzer, Susan. 1992. "Work-Care." *New Republic*, 206, no. 22 (June): 18–21.

Downing, Raymond. 2006. *Suffering and Healing in America: An American Doctor's View from Outside*. Seattle, WA: Radcliffe.

Duffy, John. 1990. *The Sanitarians: A History of American Public Health*. Chicago, IL: University of Illinois Press.

Easterbrook, Gregg. 1987. "The Revolution in Medicine." *Newsweek*, January 26.

Ehrenreich, Barbara. 1990. "Our Health-Care Disgrace." *Time*, December 10.

Elhauge, Einer, ed. 2010. *The Fragmentation of U.S. Health Care: Causes and Solutions*. New York: Oxford University Press.

Emanuel, Ezekiel J. 2014. *Reinventing America's Health Care*. New York: Public Affairs.

Etheredge, Lynn. 1983. "Reagan, Congress and Health Spending." *Health Affairs*, 2, no. 1 (Spring): 14–24.

Facher, Lev. 2017. "Trump Administration Rescinds Obamacare Birth Control Mandate." *Scientific American*. Online at www.scientificamerican.com/.

Falkson, Joseph L. 1980. *HMOs and the Politics of Health Service Reform*. Chicago, IL: American Hospital Association.

Fallows, James. 1995. "A Triumph of Misinformation." *Atlantic Monthly*, 275, no. 1 (January): 26–37.

Fan, Jessie X., Deanna L. Sharpe, and Goog-Soog Hong. 2003. "Health Care and Prescription Drug Spending by Seniors." *Monthly Labor Review Online*, 126, no. 3 (March): 16–26.

Fein, Rashi. 1986. *Medical Care, Medical Costs: The Search for a Health Insurance Policy*. Cambridge, MA: Harvard University Press.

Field, Robert E. 2007. *Health Care Regulations in America: Complexity, Confrontation, and Compromise*. New York: Oxford University Press.

Flint, Samuel S. 2008. "Health Care Reform in the 2008 Presidential Primaries." *Health & Social Work*, 33, no. 2 (May): 93–96.

Fox, Daniel M. 1986. *Health Policies, Health Politics: The British and American Experience: 1911-1965*. Princeton, NJ: Princeton University Press.

Freedman, David H. 2018. *"Health Care's 'Upstream' Conundrum."* Politico. Online at www.politico.com/.
Garrett, Lauri. 2000. *Betrayal of Trust: The Collapse of Global Public Health.* New York: Hyperion.
Geyman, John P. 2002. *Health Care in America: Can Our Ailing System Be Healed?* Boston, MA: Butterworth-Heinemann.
Geyman, John P. 2005. *Falling through the Safety Net: Americans without Health Insurance.* Monroe, ME: Common Courage Press.
Geyman, John P. 2010. *Hijacked: the Road to Single Payer in the Aftermath of Stolen Health Care Reform.* Monroe, ME: Common Courage Books.
Gibson, Rosemary. 2003. *Wall of Silence: The Untold Story of the Medical Mistakes that Kill and Injure Millions of Americans.* Washington, DC: LifeLine Press.
Ginsberg, David L. 1987. "Health Care Policy in the Reagan Administration: Rhetoric and Reality." *Public Administration Quarterly*, 11, no. 1 (Spring): 59–70.
Gorin, Stephen H. and Cynthia Moniz. 2007. "Why Does President Bush Oppose the Expansion of SCHIP?" *Health and Social Work*, 32, no. 4 (November): 243–246.
Gostin, Lawrence O. 2001. Public Health Law Reform." *American Journal of Public Health*, 91, no. 9 (September): 1365–1368.
Gostin, Lawrence O. 2002. "Public Health Law: A Renaissance." *Journal of Law, Medicine and Ethics*, 30, no. 2 (Summer): 136–140.
Gottfried, Dennis. 2009. *Too Much Medicine: A Doctor's Prescription for Better and More Affordable Health Care.* St. Paul, MN: Paragon House.
Greifinger, Robert B. and Victor William Sidel. 1978. "Three Centuries of Medical Care." In *Medical Care in the United States*, ed. Eric F. Oatman, 12–26. New York: H.W. Wilson.
Grogan, Colleen M. and Elizabeth Rigby. 2008. "Federalism, Partisan Politics, and Shifting Support for State Flexibility: The Case of the U.S. State Children's Health Insurance Program." *Publius*, 39, no. 1 (December): 47–69.
Hacker, Jacob S. 2002. *The Divided Welfare State: The Battle over Public and Private Social Benefits in the United States.* Cambridge, MA: Cambridge University Press.
Hadler, Nortin M. 2008. *Worried Sick: A Prescription for Health in an Overtreated America.* Chapel Hill, NC: University of North Carolina Press.
Hanson, Russell L. 1994. "Health Care Reform, Managed Competition and Subnational Politics." *Publius*, 23 no. 3 (Summer): 49–68.
Hartman, Micah, Anne B. Martin, Nathan Espinosa, and Aaron Catlin. 2018. "National Health Care Spending in 2016: Spending and Enrollment Growth Slow After Initial Coverage Expansion." *Health Affairs*, 37, no. 1 (December): 150–160.
Herzlinger, Regina. 2007. *Who Killed Health Care? America's $2 Trillion Medical Problem–And the Consumer-Driven Care.* New York: McGraw Hill.
Hill, Lister. 1976. "Health in America: A Personal Perspective." In *Health in America: 1776–1976*, ed. US Department of Health, Education, and Welfare, 3–15. Washington, DC: Government Printing Office.
Himmelstein, David U. and Steffie Woolhandler. 2016. "Public Health's Falling Share of US Health Spending." *American Journal of Public Health*, 106, no. 1 (January): 56–57.
"House Obamacare Repeal: Thirty-Third Time's the Charm." 2012. ABC News, July 11. Online at ABCNews.com.
Iglehart, John K. 1978. "The Carter Administration's Health Budget: Charting New Priorities with Limited Dollars." *Milbank Memorial Fund Quarterly*, 56, no. 1 (Winter): 51–77.
Iglehart, John K. 1995. "Health Policy Report: Republicans and the New Politics of Health Care." *New England Journal of Medicine*, 332, no. 14 (April 6): 972–975.
Institute of Medicine. 1988. *The Future of Public Health.* Washington, DC: National Academy Press.
Institute of Medicine. 2000a. *The Future of Public Health in the 21st Century.* Washington, DC: National Academies Press.
Institute of Medicine. 2000b. *Who Will Keep the Public Healthy? Educating Public Health Professionals for the 21st Century.* Washington, DC: National Academies Press.
Institute of Medicine. 2003. *The Future of Public's Health in the 21st Century.* Washington, DC: National Academies Press.
Jacobs, Lawrence R. and Robert Y. Shapiro. 1995. "Don't Blame the Public for Failed Health Care Reform." *Journal of Health Politics, Policy and Law*, 20, no. 2 (Summer): 411–423.
Kaiser Family Foundation. 2004. "Prescription Drug Trends." Fact-Sheet #3057-03. Kaiser Family Foundation. Online at www.kff.org.
Kasindorf, Martin. 2004. "States Play Catch-Up on Stem Cells." *USA Today*, December 17.
"Kassebaum-Kennedy Health Insurance Bill Clears Congress." 1996. Washington, DC: Families USA, August. Online at www.epn.org/families/Kafeka.html.
"Key Facts about the Uninsured Population." 2017. Kaiser Family Foundation. Online at www.kff.org/.
King, Peter. 1990. "The City as a Patient." *Newsweek*, February 19.
Kinsley, Michael. 1992. "Quack." *New Republic*, 206, no. 9 (March): 4.
Kleinke, J. D. 2001. *Oxymorons: The Myth of a U.S. Health Care System.* San Francisco, CA: Jossey-Bass.
Koran, Laura and James Masters. 2017. "Trump Reverses Abortion Policy for Aid to NGOs." CNN. Online at https://cnn.com/.
Kulczycki, Andrzej. 2007. "Ethics, Ideology, and Reproductive Health Policy in the United States." *Studies in Family Planning*, 38, no. 4 (December): 333–351.
Lambrew, Jeanne M. 2005. "Making Medicaid a Block Grant Program: An Analysis of the Implications of Past Proposals." *Milbank Quarterly*, 83, no. 1: 41–64.
Levine, Robert A. 2009. *Shock Therapy for the American Health Care System: Why Comprehensive Reform Is Needed.* Santa Barbara, CA: ABC-CLIO, LLC.
Levit, Katherine R. et al. 1994. "National Health Expenditures, 1993." *Health Care Financing Review*, 16, no. 1 (Fall): 247–294.

Lewis, Anthony. 1991. "A Sick System." *The New York Times*, June 3.
Link, Eugene P. 1992. *The Social Ideas of American Physicians (1776-1976): Studies of the Humanitarian Tradition in Medicine*. London: Associated University Press.
Long, Stephen H. and Russell F. Settle. 1984. "Medicare and the Disadvantaged Elderly: Objectives and Outcomes." *Milbank Memorial Fund Quarterly/Health and Society*, 62, no. 4 (Fall): 609–656.
Lynn, Joanne. 2004. *Sick to Death and Not Going to Take It Anymore! Reforming Health Care for the Last Years of Life*. Berkeley, CA: University of California Press.
Makover, Michael E. 1998. *Mismanaged Care: How Corporate Medicine Jeopardizes Your Health*. Amherst, NY: Prometheus Books.
McCarthy, Michael. 2001. "Fragmented U.S. Health-Care System Needs Major Reform." *Lancet*, 357, no. 9258 (March 10): 782.
McFarlane, Deborah R. 2006. "Reproductive Health Policy in President Bush's Second Term: Old Battles and New Fronts in the United States and Internationally." *Journal of Public Health Policy*, 27, no. 4: 405–426.
Mechanic, David. 1981. "Some Dilemmas in Health Care Policy." *Milbank Memorial Fund Quarterly/Health and Society*, 59, no. 1 (Winter): 1–14.
Mechanic, David. 2004. "The Rise and Fall of Managed Care." *Journal of Health and Social Behavior*, 45, no. Supplement 1 (December): 76–81.
Mechanic, David. 2008. *The Truth about Health Care: Why Reform Is Not Working in America*. New Brunswick, NJ: Rutgers University Press.
Montgomery, Lori and Paul Kane. 2013. "Shutdown Begins: Stalemate Forces First U.S. Government Closure in 17 Years." *The Washington Post*, October 1.
Moore, Thomas J. 1995. *Deadly Medicine: Why Tens of Thousands of Heart Patients Died in America's Worst Drug Disaster*. New York: Simon & Schuster.
Morin, Richard. 1994. "A Health Care Reform Post-Mortem." *The Washington Post National Weekly Edition*, September 12–18.
Nather, David. 2003. "GOP Hones 'Can Do' Pitch to Party Base, Swing Voters." *Congressional Quarterly Weekly*, 61, no. 48 (December 13): 3062–3064.
"National ACA Marketplace Signups Dipped a Modest 3.7 Percent This Year." 2018. Kaiser Family Foundation. Online at www.kff.org/.
National Center for Health Statistics. 2012. *Health United States, 2011: With Special Features on Socioeconomic Status and Health*. Hyattsville, MD: US Department of Health and Human Services.
Navarro, Vicente. 1995. "Why Congress Did Not Enact Health Care Reform." *Journal of Health Politics, Policy and Law*, 20, no. 2 (Summer): 455–462.
Nixon, Richard M. 1971. "Message to Congress." *Weekly Compilation of Presidential Documents*. Washington, DC: Office of the Federal Register, February 18.
Norris, Jonas. 1984. *Searching for a Cure: National Health Policy Considered*. New York: PICA Press.
"Obama Ends Stem Cell Research Ban." 2009. CBS News, June 18. Online at www.cbsnews.com/2100-503767_162-4853385.html.
Oberlander, Jonathan. 2006. "The Political Economy of Unfairness in U.S. Health Policy." *Law and Contemporary Problems*, 69, no. 4 (Autumn): 245–264.
Oliver, Thomas R. 1991. "Health Care Market Reform in Congress: The Uncertain Path from Proposal to Policy." *Political Science Quarterly*, 106, no. 3: 453–478.
Onie, Rebecca D, Rocco J. Peria, and Thomas H. Lee. 2016. "Population Health: The Ghost Aim." *NEJM Catalyst*. Online at https://catalyst.nejm.org/.
Organization for Economic Cooperation and Development. 2017. *Health at a Glance: OECD Indicators*. Paris, France: OECD. Online at www.oecd.org/.
Ornstein, Norm. 2013. "The Unprecedented and Contemptible Attempts to Sabotage Obamacare." *National Journal*, July 24.
Parmet, Wendy E. 1993. "Health Care and the Constitution: Public Health and the Role of the State in the Framing Era." *Hastings Constitutional Law Quarterly*, 20, no. 2: 267–335.
Parmet, Wendy E. 2007. "Public Health and Constitutional Law" Recognizing the Relationship." *Journal of Health Care Law and Policy*, 10, no. 1: 13–25.
Patel, Kant. 2003. "Presidential Rhetoric and the Strategy of Going Public: President Clinton and the Health Care Reform." *Journal of Health and Social Policy*, 18, no. 2: 21–42.
Patel, Kant. 2014. "Origins and Development of Government's Role in Health Care Policy (Colonial Era to Present)." In *Guide to U.S. Health and Health Care Policy*, ed. Thomas Oliver, 1–22. Thousand Oaks, CA: CQ Press.
Patel, Kant and Mark Rushefsky. 1998. "Health Policy Community and Health Care Reform in the United States." *Health: An Interdisciplinary Journal for the Social Study of Health, Illness and Medicine*, 2, no. 4 (October): 459–484.
Patel, Kant and Mark Rushefsky. 2005a. *The Politics of Public Health in the United States*. Armonk, NY: M.E. Sharpe.
Patel, Kant and Mark Rushefsky. 2005b. "President Bush and Stem Cell Policy: the Politics of Policy Making." *White House Studies Journal*, 5, no.1 (Special issue): 37–52.
Phillips, Donald F. 2000. "Medicine-Public Health Collaborative Tested." *Journal of American Medical Association*, 283, no.4 (January 26): 465.
Potter, Wendell. 2010. *Deadly Spin: An Insurance Company Insider Speaks Out on How Corporate PR Is Killing Health Care and Deceiving Americans*. New York: Bloomsbury Press.
Powell, Laurie. 2017. "Why are Healthcare Costs so High in the USA versus Other Countries?" Focus For Health. Online at https://focusforhealth.org/.

Public Health Law Center. 2015. "State and Local Public Health: An Overview of Regulatory Authority." St. Paul, MN: William Mitchell College of Law. Public Health Law Center. Online at www.publichealthlawcenter.org/.

Qazi, Khalid J. 2009. "Healthcare Reform in the United States: Fact, Fiction and Drama." *British Journal of Medical Practitioners*, 2, no. 4: 5–7.

Quadagno, Jill. 2005. *One Nation, Uninsured: Why the U.S. Has No National Health Insurance*. New York: Oxford University Press.

Raffel, Marshall W. 1980. *The U.S. Health System: Origins and Functions*. New York: Wiley.

Rangel, Charles B. 2009. "Fixing America's Health Care System." *New York Amsterdam News*, 100, no. 34 (August 20): 12.

Reagan, Michael D. 1999. *The Accidental System: Health Care Policy in America*. Boulder, CO: Westview Press.

Reid, T. R. 2010. *The Healing of America: A Global Quest for Better, Cheaper, and Fairer Health Care*. Reprint Edition. New York: Penguin Books.

Rice, Thomas, Katherine Desmond, and Jon Gable. 1990. "The Medicare Catastrophic Coverage Act: A Post-Mortem." *Health Affairs*, 9, no. 3 (Fall): 75–87.

Rice, Thomas and Jon Gable. 1986. "Protecting the Elderly against High Health Care Costs." *Health Affairs*, 5, no. 3 (Fall): 5–21.

Richmond, Julius B. 2005. *The Health Care Mess: How We Got into It and What It Will Take to Get Out*. Cambridge, MA: Cambridge University Press.

Robbins, Anthony. 1983. "Can Reagan Be Indicted for Betraying Public Health?" *American Journal of Public Health*, 73, no. 1 (January): 12–13.

Roemer, Milton I. 1984. "The Politics of Public Health in the United States." In *Health Politics and Policy*, eds Theodore J. Litman and Leonard S. Robins, 261–273. New York: Wiley.

Roemer, Milton I. 1986. *An Introduction to the U.S. Health Care System*, 2nd edn. New York: Springer.

Ropes, Linda B. 1991. *Health Care Crisis in America: A Reference Handbook*. Santa Barbara, CA: ABC-CLIO.

Rosenthal, Elisabeth. 2017. *An American Sickness: How Healthcare Became Big Business and How You Can Take It Back*. Reprint Edition. New York: Penguin Books.

Rovner, Julie. 2017. "Stunner on Birth Control: Trump's Moral Exception Is Geared toward Just 2 Groups." Kaiser Health News. Online at https://khn.org/.

Rutkow, Ira M. 2005. *Bleeding Blue and Gray: Civil War Surgery and the Evolution of American Medicine*. New York: Random House.

Salinsky, Eileen. 2010. "Governmental Public Health: An Overview of State and Local Public Health Agencies." National Health Policy Forum, Background paper no. 77. Washington, DC: George Washington University.

Sawyer, Bradley and Cynthia Cox. 2018. "How Does Health Spending in the U.S. Compare to other Countries?" Peterson-Kaiser Health System Tracker. Online at www.healthsystemtracker.org/.

Schneider, Ann L. and Helen M. Ingram. 2004. *Deserving and Entitled: Social Constructions and Public Policy*. New York: State University of New York Press.

Singer, Merrill and Hans Baer, eds. 2009. *Killer Commodities: Public Health and the Corporate Production of Harm*. Lanham, MD: AltaMira Press.

Skidmore, Max J. 1970. *Medicare and the American Rhetoric of Reconciliation*. University, AL: University of Alabama Press.

Skocpol, Theda. 1994. "From Social Security to Health Security? Opinion and Rhetoric in U.S. Social Policy Making." *PS: Political Science and Politics*, 27, no. 1 (December): 21–25.

Skocpol, Theda. 1997. *Health Care Reform and the Turn against Government*. New York: W.W. Norton.

Skocpol, Theda. 2011. "Obama and the Transformation of U.S. Public Policy: The Struggle to Reform Health Care." *Arizona State Law Journal*, 42, no. 4 (Winter): 1203–1232.

Smerd, Jeremy. 2006. "Stuck in the Waiting Room–Part 1 and 2." *Workforce Management*, 85, no. 18 (September 25): 25–28.

Smith, David R. 1994. "Porches, Politics, and Public Health." *American Journal of Public Health*, 84, no. 5 (May); 725–726.

Snyder, Lynne P. 1994a. "A New Mandate for Public Health." *Public Health Reports*, 109, no. 4 (July–August): 469–471.

Snyder, Lynne P. 1994b. "Passage and Significance of the 1944 Public Health Service Act." *Public Health Reports*, 109, no. 6 (November–December): 721–724,

Sparrow, Malcolm K. 2000. *License to Steal: Why Fraud Plagues America's Health Care System*. Boulder, CO: Westview Press.

Specter, Michael. 1990. "Putting Michigan Hospitals on the Critical List." *The Washington Post National Weekly Edition*, June 4–10

Starr, Paul. 1982. *The Social Transformation of American Medicine*. New York: Basic Books.

Starr, Paul. 1995. "What Happened to Health Care Reform?" *American Prospect*, no. 20 (Winter): 20–31.

Starr, Paul. 2011. *Remedy and Reaction: The Peculiar American Struggle over Health Care Reform*. New Haven, CT: Yale University Press.

"Status of State Action on the Medicaid Expansion Decision." 2018. Online at www.kff.org/.

Steinmo, Sven and Jon Watts. 1995. "It's the Institutions, Stupid! Why Comprehensive National Health Insurance Always Fails in America." *Journal of Health Politics, Policy and Law*, 20, no. 2 (Summer): 329–372.

"Stem Cell Research: Updated January 2008." n.d. National Conference of State Legislatures, Washington, DC. Online at www.ncsl.org/.

"Stem-Cell Guidelines: Ethics of a New Science." 2005. *Time*, May 9.

Stevens, Rosemary A. 1989. *In Sickness and in Wealth: American Hospitals in the Twentieth Century*. New York: Basic Books.

Stevens, Rosemary A. 2007. *The Public-Private Health Care State: Essays on the History of American Health Care Policy*. New Brunswick, NJ: Transaction Publishers.

Stevens, Rosemary A., Charles E. Rosenberg, and Lawton R. Burns. 2006. *History and Health Policy in the United States*. New Brunswick, NJ: Rutgers University Press.

Stolberg, Sheryl G. 2005. "In Rare Threat, Bush Vows Veto of Stem Cell Bill." *The New York Times*, May 21. Online at www.nytimes.com/.

Tannenbaum, Barbara J. 2012. *Health and Wellness in Colonia America*. Santa Barbara, CA: Greenwood Press.

Taurel, Sidney. 2005. "Critical Condition: The Ills of America's Health Care System and How We Can Heal Them." *Executive Speeches*, 19, no. 6 (June–July): 106.

"Tauzin to Head Pharmaceutical Lobbying Group." 2004. *The Washington Post*, December 15. Online at www.washingtonpost.com.

Taylor, Humphrey. 1990 "U.S. Health Care: Built for Waste." *The New York Times*, April 17.

Terris, Milton. 1990. "A Wasteful System That Doesn't Work." *Progressive*, 54, no. 10 (October): 14–16.

Thakrar, Ashish P., Alexandra D. Forrest, Mitchell G. Maltenfort, and Christopher B. Forrest. 2018. "Child Mortality in the US and 19 Other OECD Comparator Nations: A 50-Year Time-Trend Analysis." *Health Affairs*, 37, no. 1: 140–149.

"The Health Care System Is Broken and Here Is How to Fix It." 1991. *The New York Times*, July 22.

"The Model State Emergency Health Powers Act: Summary Matrix." 2012. The Network for Public Health Law. Online at www.networkforphl.org/_asset/80p3y7/MSEHPA-States-Table-022812.pdf.

"The Role of Public Health in Ensuring Healthy Communities." 1995. Policy no. 9521 (January 1): Washington, DC: American Public Health Association. Online at www.apha.org.

Thomas, W. John. 1995. "Clinton Health Care Reform Plan: A Failed Dramatic Presentation." *Stanford Law and Policy Review*, 7, no. 1: 83–104.

Thompson, Frank J. and Courtney Burke. 2007. "Executive Federalism and Medicaid Demonstration Waivers: Implications for Policy and Democratic Process." *Journal of Health Politics, Policy and Law*, 32, no. 6 (December): 971–1004.

Thompson, Frank J. and Courtney Burke. 2008. "Federalism by Waiver: Medicaid and the Transformation of Long-Term Care." *Publius*, 39, no. 1: 22–48.

Trust for America's Future. 2016. *Investing in America's Health: A State-by-State Look at Public Health Funding and Key Health Facts*. Washington, DC: Trust for America's Health. Online at http://healthyamericans.org/.

Trust for America's Health. 2011. *Investing in America's Health: A State-by-State Look at Public Health Funding and Key Health Facts*. Washington, DC: Trust for America's Health. Online at http://healthyamericans.org/.

Tumulty, Karen. 2005. "Stem Cells: Why Bush's Ban Could Be Reversed." *Time*, May 23, 26–30.

US Health Resources Administration. 1976. *Health in America: 1776-1976*. Rockville, MD: US Department of Health, Education, and Welfare.

Valverde, Miriam. 2017. "Donald Trump Declares Public Health Emergency over Opioid Crisis. Here Is What that Means." PolitiFact. Online at www.politifact.com/.

Veatch, Robert M. 2009. *Patient, Heal Thyself: How the New Medicine Puts the Patient in Charge*. New York: Oxford University Press.

Wade, Nicholas. 2005. "Group of Scientists Draft Rules on Ethics for Stem Cell Research." *The New York Times*, April 27. Online at www.nytimes.com/2005/04/27/health/27stem.html.

Wallace, Steven P. and Carroll L. Estes. 1989. "Health Policy for the Elderly." *Society*, 26, no. 6 (September–October): 66–75.

Warner, John H. and Janet A. Tighe. 2001. *Major Problems in the History of American Medicine and Public Health: Documents and Essays*. Boston, MA: Houghton Mifflin.

Waxman, Henry A. 2006. "Politics and Science: Reproductive Health." *Health Matrix: Journal of Law-Medicine*, 16, no. 1 (Winter): 5–25.

Welch, Gilbert H., Lisa Swartz, and Steve Woloshin. 2011. *Overdiagnosed: Making People Sick in the Pursuit of Health*. Boston, MA: Beacon Press.

White House Domestic Policy Council. 1993. *The President's Health Security Act: The Clinton Blueprint*. New York: Times Books.

Willever, Heather. 1994. "The Cadet Nurse Corps, 1943-1948." *Public Health Reports*, 109, no. 3: (May–June): 455–457.

Wines, Michael. 1992. "Bush Announces Health Plan, Filling Gap in Re-Election Bid." *The New York Times*, September 23.

Wing, Kenneth R. 1984. "Recent Amendments to the Medicaid Program: Political Implications." *American Journal of Public Health*, 74, no.1 (January): 83–84.

Section II
GOVERNMENT HEALTH PROGRAMS

3

THE AFFORDABLE CARE ACT

Stumbling Toward Universal Health Insurance?

I am not the first president to take up this cause, but I am determined to be the last. It has now been nearly a century since Theodore Roosevelt first called for healthcare reform. And ever since, nearly every president and Congress, whether Democrat or Republican, has attempted to meet this challenge in some way. A bill for comprehensive health reform was first introduced by John Dingell, Sr. in 1943. Sixty-five years later, his son continues to introduce that same bill at the beginning of each session.

Our collective failure to meet this challenge—year after year, decade after decade—has led us to a breaking point.
(—Barack Obama 2009)

The conditions in 2010 created a window for reform, but it was not a big one. To squeeze legislation through that window, Democrats had to work around the many constraints that might otherwise have doomed chances for passing a bill. And working around those constraints helped to shape the central choices they made, including the choices that left the law vulnerable to counterattack.
(—Paul Starr 2013, 16–17)

"What's past is prologue," William Shakespeare wrote—and it seems that's especially true when it comes to healthcare. The history of health reform in American spans a century of false starts, near misses, and historic advances that culminated when President Obama signed the Patient Protection and Affordable Care Act into law on March 23, 2010. It was a day that a lot of people thought would never come and a moment that almost didn't happen—and the story of how we got there is one of the most important stories in modern politics and public policymaking.
(—John Kerry 2010, 7)

As the above quotes suggest, getting comprehensive healthcare reform enacted was exceptionally difficult and contentious. The process of passage through Congress was treacherous, with land mines placed all over the place. It took some "unorthodox," though hardly unknown, maneuverings (Sinclair 2012) to finally achieve passage. The law relied heavily on past Republican initiatives, yet it garnered no Republican support. It sought to reform a highly fragmented system, yet left much of it in place. It was less than liberals had hoped for and more than conservatives wanted. And after enactment, it was the subject of challenges in Congress, the courts, and the White House.

This chapter focuses on healthcare reform that was enacted in 2010. We first look at the years preceding passage of the Affordable Care Act (ACA), 2006–2008. We follow that up with describing the process of passing the legislation and the controversies surrounding that passage. This is followed by an examination of threats to the Act, such as court challenges, elections, repeal attempts, White House opposition beginning in 2017, and implementation of the Act. We then look at Republican alternatives to health reform and conclude the chapter with some judgments about the legislation and its implementation and the future of healthcare reform.

THE ROAD TO THE AFFORDABLE CARE ACT (2006–2008)

Kingdon's Multiple Streams Model

One way of understanding the series of events leading up to the passage of the *Patient Protection and Affordable Care Act* (PPACA), informally known as the *Affordable Care Act* (ACA), is to make use of a model of agenda-building known as the *multiple streams model* (Kingdon 2010).

The model starts with three streams. The *problems stream* focuses on the problem-identification stage of the policy process (see Rushefsky 2017). In this stream, there is debate over whether a problem exists and, if so, what is the nature of the problem. Additionally, there is debate over whether a government response is necessary to address that problem. Different people and groups will have various perceptions about the nature of the problem and what to do about it. Further, there are often ideological differences that play a role in these perceptions. These ideological differences also play a strong role in perceptions about the Affordable Care Act.

The second stream is the *policies stream*. Here policy advocates or entrepreneurs push favored public policies and seek opportunities to get those policies adopted. As Kingdon (2010, 116) notes, policy solutions may stew in a "primeval soup," sometimes for decades, with some solutions emerging and others being cast aside.

The third stream is the *politics stream*. Here changes such as the results of elections or interest group activity provide an opportunity to seek innovative public policies.

An important aspect of this model is that these streams do not necessarily flow together. Problems can fester for years, or decades in the case of healthcare. Policy entrepreneurs may have spent years finding the right time for their proposed solutions. Political change is independent of the other two streams.

But there are certain times when the three streams come together, with the political stream being the most important. When all three streams are in sync, there is what is called a *window of opportunity*. Some big policy issues, such as healthcare reform, will assume a prominent place on the government agenda, and there is a real opportunity, though a brief one, for action (Kingdon 2010).

The Problems Stream

Cost

We have spent much of this book addressing the problems facing the American healthcare system. One problem that underlies all the rest is the cost of healthcare (see Chapter 8). We spend considerably more money on healthcare than any other industrialized nation. Healthcare costs increase faster than inflation and faster than the growth of the economy, so that more and more of our economic activity is taken up in paying for healthcare. The two large government programs, Medicaid (Chapter 4) and Medicare (Chapter 5), have seen continual increases in costs and pressure put on state and federal budgets. Employers face ongoing increases in the cost of healthcare for their employees and have begun placing more of those costs on them. As Kingdon (2010) points out, this puts American companies, especially manufacturers, at a disadvantage with much of their foreign competition. In other Western industrialized countries, the government pays for healthcare rather than the companies and, thus, the products of companies such as Toyota and Honda cost less than if they had to pay for their workers' health insurance costs. According to some estimates, health insurance premiums account for as much as $2,000 of the cost of a domestically produced car (Johnson 2012). Insurance premiums continue their dramatic rise. Individuals have problems paying for the cost of their healthcare, especially if they lack insurance or adequate coverage. Healthcare costs are an important cause of individual bankruptcy (National Patient Advocate Foundation 2012).

Even individuals with health insurance face problems. Some insurance policies have lifetime caps on how much they will pay out, and catastrophic healthcare could exceed those limits. Insurance companies, especially in the small business and individual markets, engaged in practices that left subscribers exposed to the full cost of their medical expenses (see Potter 2010). Companies would deny coverage for a claim because of an alleged pre-existing condition, a practice known as rescission (Potter 2010). These practices became so contentious that it led, in the late 1990s and early 2000s, to consideration of what was called "patient's bill of rights" legislation at both the state and federal level. While Congress did not enact such legislation (until 2010), many states did (Patel and Rushefsky 2006).

Access

The second major problem is one of access (Chapter 7). An estimated 47–50 million people lacked health insurance in 2008 (though some have disputed the numbers). There are ethnic/racial dimensions to the access issue. Minorities, such as Hispanics and African-Americans, are less likely to have health insurance than whites. Higher-income individuals and families are more likely to be covered than lower-income individuals and families. Lack of access to healthcare can also be a function of geography. People in rural areas and inner cities tend to have less access than people in suburbs. Employment-based insurance, the prime mechanism for insurance coverage in the United States, decreased throughout the twenty-first century. Lack of access to the healthcare system has health consequences (see Chapter 7; Patel and Rushefsky 2008).

These problems, cost and access, were captured on film, in books, and in articles. Three examples stand out. The first was Michael Moore's 2007 documentary *Sicko*. The documentary began by stating that it was not going to explore the problem of the uninsured, but rather the problems that affect those with inadequate insurance (the underinsured). For example, one of his cases focused on a man who damaged two of his fingers in an accident. His insurance company said it would pay to fix only one of his fingers, so he had to choose which finger to keep. After looking at these kinds of cases and the American healthcare system, Moore examined other healthcare systems and noted that the problems he describes would be taken care of by other healthcare systems at little or no cost.

Jonathan Cohn's (2007) similarly titled *Sick* also critically examined the American healthcare system. He provided case studies of people struggling with the healthcare system and argued that the system is unraveling.

Wendell Potter (2010) worked in the health insurance industry for a quarter of a century. His book, *Deadly Spin*, uncovered practices such as rescissions that are undercutting the country's healthcare system.

Of course, these critiques came from the left. The right also saw problems with the healthcare system, but rather than seeking a national health insurance policy, they have sought market reforms. For example, Herzlinger (2007, 1) casts her net widely in search of villains: "the health insurers, hospitals, government and doctors." Her solution is to have consumers take charge of their own healthcare through solutions like high-deductible health plans and health savings accounts (see below and Chapter 11).

The Policies Stream

Types of healthcare systems

There is no dearth of policy alternatives or solutions for the healthcare system's problems. One source is the healthcare systems of other Western industrialized countries. Reid (2010) provides a useful typology of different healthcare systems as well as indicating a major problem with the US healthcare system.

Reid (2010) distinguishes among four types of healthcare system. The first and oldest is the Bismarck model, developed in the late nineteenth century under Prussian and then German chancellor Otto von Bismarck. This model keeps much of the healthcare system private but utilizes a series of health insurance plans financed by workers and their employers. The plans are non-profit, and costs and services are tightly regulated.

The second type is the Beveridge model, adopted in the United Kingdom after World War II. This model approximates what has been called in the United States socialized medicine. The government owns the facilities (such as hospitals), and the workers are government employees, though doctors can take private paying patients.

The third type is the national health insurance model, typified by the Canadian system. The facilities and workers are private, but there is a single payer, the government, which collects taxes (premiums) and pays the providers.

The final type is what Reid (2010) calls the out-of-pocket model, which has virtually no public system and patients pay for their own healthcare if they can afford to.

So, we have these four models that can be drawn upon. One of Reid's (2010) most critical points is that there are elements of all four models in the United States. Employer-based health insurance represents the Bismarck model. Veterans and military personnel are in a Beveridge-type system (such as the VHA hospitals that we discuss in Chapter 6). Those on Medicare are in a national health insurance model. And those without health insurance are in the out-of-pocket model.

Looking at healthcare in the United States this way provides an insight as to why it has been and is so difficult to reform the system: we have these different sets of systems. American healthcare is highly fragmented. The politics of healthcare in America suggests that we are very unlikely to adopt any of these systems as *the* one system. But looking at other healthcare systems does give us a picture of possibilities. Other countries have faced many of the same problems that the United States has, but went in different directions. Despite the models of what other countries have done, the United States chose none of the above.

Policy Proposals

Policy proposals have been floating in Kingdon's (2010) primeval soup for decades. In general, liberals/Democrats have favored some type of national health insurance plan or public-sector program. At a minimum, they have advocated expansion of current programs, such as the Children's Health Insurance Program (CHIP) and Medicaid. Conservatives/Republicans have, in general, opposed the comprehensive plans and resisted expansion of current programs, though this is not entirely the case; Richard Nixon proposed the Comprehensive Health Insurance Plan (CHIP), and President Bush proposed, and Congress enacted, an expansion of Medicare to cover prescription drugs.

Another way of thinking about policy proposals is to focus on the role of government. Liberals/Democrats tend to favor programs that expand the role of government, whereas conservatives/Republicans tend to pursue plans that rely more on the private sector (see, for example, Capretta and Dayaratna 2013; Goodman 2012). Republican and conservative proposals focused on cost control and market mechanisms. Democratic/liberal proposals tended to focus more on access issues and public-sector solutions. Libertarians were mostly interested in government doing less. We can see these divides in healthcare reform proposals discussed in Chapter 11.

We begin with Democratic proposals.

Democratic Reform Proposals

One popular proposal was offered by Hacker (2007). Entitled "Health Care for America," it would retain employer-sponsored insurance, with an employer mandate: either employers would provide health insurance for their workers or pay 6 percent of their payroll into a pool that would be used to finance another feature of the plan. In health insurance policy language, this is known as "play-or-pay." A second part would keep Medicare for those currently eligible for it. The third part would be a new program, the Health Care for America plan (a Medicare-style plan) that would enroll those who had neither Medicare nor employer-sponsored insurance. Employers, Hacker wrote, could enroll their employees in Health Care for America and save administrative costs.

A fourth part would be an individual mandate. Those who were uninsured would be required to enroll in Health Care for America or purchase a private plan. Those enrolled in Medicaid or the CHIP would be moved to either Health Care for America or an employer-sponsored program. Thus, Medicaid would be eliminated under Hacker's proposal. There would be subsidies, depending on income, for low-income individuals and family.

Hacker wrote that under his plan there would be substantial cost savings. First, Medicare has lower administrative costs than private insurance, 2 percent versus 14 percent for private insurance (Hacker 2007; see discussion of the point in Chapter 8). Second, Health Care for America would be covering so many people—about half of the US population according to Hacker—that there would be administrative efficiencies. Third, both Medicare and Health Care of America would have leverage to bargain with providers of services and equipment. Cost savings would also occur at both the federal and state levels with the termination of Medicaid and the CHIP.

Hacker also described what changes would not take place. Here the contrast with conservative/Republican plans is set out very markedly:

> Equally important is what Health Care for America would not do. It would not eliminate private employment-based insurance. It would not allow employers to retreat from the financing of a reasonable share of the cost of health insurance. It would not leave Americans coping with ever-higher private insurance premiums with an inadequate voucher, or pressure them to enroll in HMOs that do not cover care from the doctors they know and trust. It would not break up the large insurance groups in the public and private sectors that are best capable of pooling risks today. And it certainly would not encourage individualized Health Savings Accounts that threaten to further fragment the insurance market and leave Americans even less protected against medical costs.
>
> (Hacker 2007, 2)

Davis and Schoen (2008) proposed keeping much of the public programs (Medicare, Medicaid, and the CHIP) and employer-based insurance. They suggested a series of reforms for the individual insurance market and the creation of what was called at that time an "insurance connector" (Davis and Schoen 2008, 3), what is now known as health exchanges, for individuals and small businesses. They envisioned the connector as a single national system. The exchanges would include a "public option," a plan similar to Medicare that would compete with private insurance plans. The insurance reforms focused on the kinds of problems mentioned above, such as rescissions.

The liberal think tank Institute for America's Future advocated a public option as part of healthcare reform (Clemente 2009). Its plan was based, in part, on work by Hacker (2009). The Institute argued that Medicare was a good model for such a plan, because it had controlled costs better than private insurance and, further, had taken action to cut back on what it called "excess growth" in health spending (Clemente 2009, 5). Another point for the public plan option was to provide competition to the private sector, which had become less competitive. Lower administrative costs and strong bargaining power were two other advantages of a public plan.

In 2008, Hillary Clinton, then a Democratic senator from New York and a candidate for the 2008 Democratic presidential nomination, offered the American Health Choices Plan (Hillary for President 2008). Her plan would first allow those who have health insurance and want to continue with that coverage to keep it. The plan promised those currently insured that their premiums would be lowered, and it would reduce cost-shifting. Those who want to change, which includes employers, employees, and individuals, would have a choice of plans. The plan called for enrolling these groups and people in the Federal Employees Health Benefit Program, which does have a large array of choices. Interestingly, the plan points out that this is the same program that members of Congress are enrolled in. The Clinton plan would include a public option as one of the choices. The plan noted that neither the public option nor the health choices menu would require additional bureaucracy, because the implementing agencies were already in place.

The Clinton plan also called for insurance reform, such as guaranteed issue (prohibiting insurance companies from turning down someone because of a preexisting condition), restraints on premium increases, and requirements that health insurance companies spend most of their money on paying for services (an issue known as the medical-loss ratio). The plan also called for an individual mandate and subsidies. It was, in fact, fairly close to what was included in the ACA.

The Clinton plan was important for two reasons. First, it was a specific plan proposed by a Democratic senator and a presidential aspirant. Second was Clinton's history of concern about health reform and her role in the deliberations over President Clinton's health reform proposal in 1993. Opponents of President Clinton's proposed Health Security Act referred to the bill as Hillarycare, a phrase later adapted to the ACA (Obamacare).

Liberal/Democratic proposals in the 2006–2009 period went in various directions. They were offered by think tanks such as the Economic Policy Institute, the Center for American Programs, and Families USA. Some wanted to expand employer-based health insurance. Others focused on expanding Medicare and Medicaid. A few would have preferred a single-payer system, but, in the American political system, this was not possible.

Conservative/Republican Reform Proposals

Republican plans, such as those included in the 2012 Republican Party platform, focused on the two large public-sector programs, Medicare and Medicaid. Medicare would be converted into a premium support or voucher program, a defined-benefits program (see Chapter 5). Medicaid would be turned into a block grant program, similar to what happened with welfare reform in 1996 (see Chapter 4; Kliff 2012). Both proposals would have the same effect of limiting the federal government's exposure to increases in healthcare costs. The size of the voucher and the block grant can be manipulated or remain the same in future years. Under current law, both are entitlements determined by the size of the recipient pool and their medical expenses.

Another set of health reform proposals came from, among other sources, Senator John McCain's (R-AZ) 2008 campaign. The McCain plan would end the decades-long tax treatment of employer-based insurance. Without the tax deduction, employers would likely end this benefit to workers. One of the interesting questions is whether, if such a proposal were enacted, employers would take the funds used to pay for their employees' insurance and add that to their salary or keep some or all to themselves. McCain's and similar plans would substitute an individual tax credit that could be used to purchase a healthcare plan. All three proposals would shift costs to consumers, and consumers/patients would have the responsibility for and choice of plans (Hacker 2006; Kliff 2012). Such proposals would rely more on private markets than is currently the case.

A related set of ideas would rely on consumer-driven or consumer-directed healthcare plans (CDHCP) and health savings accounts (see, for example, Capretta and Dayaratna 2013; Goodman 2012; Grassley 2009). Such healthcare plans, which are becoming more common, would have a much higher deductible than current employer-sponsored health insurance plans (an important feature to remember when Republicans criticized the Affordable Care Act; see below). The employee would establish a health savings account, similar to an individual retirement account, in which she would deposit money, tax-free, that could be used to pay for healthcare. Such plans were virtually unknown prior to 2006. By 2017, 28 percent of all employer-sponsored health plans were the high-deductible type (Claxton et al. 2017).

In 2009, four Republican senators proposed "The Patients' Choice Act." The act provided for a refundable tax credit that would be invested in a health savings account and could also be used to purchase insurance. The tax credit would be $5,700 per family and $2,300 per individual. A supplement up to $5,000 would be available for those at the lower end of the income scale (Turner and Antos 2009). Employers could still provide health insurance and receive a tax deduction. Under the proposal, states would set up health exchanges (virtual markets) from which consumers would choose a health insurance plan.

Other Republican ideas included converting the health insurance market from individual state markets to a national market. Under current laws, states have the prime responsibility for regulating health insurance plans. Each plan has to, effectively, be registered in any state in which it wishes to do business. The idea behind such proposals is that a national market would create more competition for consumers and thus produce lower health insurance costs or at least restrain them.

Health Insurance Industry Reform Proposals

The interest group representing insurance companies, America's Health Insurance Plans (AHIP), also took part in the debate. Long an opponent of national health insurance (Starr 1982, 2013), the insurance industry made a major effort to kill the Clinton healthcare plan. This included running a series of television spots, known as the "Harry and Louise" ads, which attacked various parts of the Clinton plan. But by the late 2008s, the healthcare problems had worsened, and AHIP could read the writing on the wall. Healthcare reform might very well succeed this time, and the industry wanted a seat at the table.

The AHIP proposals focused on access to health insurance and relying on the states more than the federal government. The plan, published in 2006, had five principles. First, the federal government should provide states with incentives to cover adults and children. Second, states should be encouraged by the federal government to expand Medicaid coverage to 100 percent of the federal poverty line (FPL) and 200 percent for those in the CHIP program. Third, the federal government should provide subsidies for low-income adults and families up to 400 percent of the federal poverty line. Interestingly, this principle states that those in the individual or small business market should purchase insurance using "existing market mechanisms" (America's Health Insurance Plans 2006, 4). The fourth principle was to provide a tax deduction for those with incomes over 400 percent of the federal poverty line to encourage them to purchase insurance. Finally, employers should be "encouraged" (America's Health Insurance Plans 2006, 4) to provide insurance for their employees. Further, the plan stated that the current business tax deductions for health insurance should be maintained.

In 2007, AHIP developed a follow-up plan, called the "Guaranteed Access Plan" (America's Health Insurance Plans 2007). This plan would essentially be a high-risk pool plan. High-risk pools are people with preexisting conditions or a history of high medical costs. If such a person applied for an individual policy (group plans, such as employer-sponsored plans, generally allow all members or employees to be a member of the plan) and were turned down, then she or he would have access to this state-based plan. Eligibility would be based on how much a person's healthcare costs would be. The criteria would be twice the average of claims in a particular state. If the person could not get into a guaranteed-access plan, then private health insurance would be the insurer of last resort. In both cases, the premiums charged would be limited to 150 percent of market rates.

The Massachusetts Model

Attempts at healthcare reform in the 1993–1994 period at the national level prompted some states, such as Massachusetts, to attempt its own reforms. The Massachusetts effort ultimately failed, but a later attempt in that state had a profound impact on the healthcare reform debates that began in 2008.

In 2006, the Massachusetts state legislature passed, and Republican governor Mitt Romney signed, an ambitious healthcare plan that was similar in many ways to the Affordable Care Act. The program contained the following elements (Long 2008): an individual mandate (all residents had to have health insurance), expansion of Medicaid, an employer mandate (play-or-pay), subsidies to pay for health insurance for low-income individuals and families, reform of the insurance market, and a virtual online health insurance market, known as the connector. In the ACA, the connector became the state health exchanges.

The Political Stream

The third stream in the Kingdon (2010) model is the politics stream. Here we can see the impact of elections, changes of administration and/or control of Congress, interest group activity, and public opinion. We begin with elections.

The unpopularity of the Iraq war and the general decline in public opinion approval of the George W. Bush administration led to several key Democratic victories. The first came in 2006 when Democrats regained control of both houses of Congress for the first time since the 1994 elections. Democrats began anticipating successful elections at the congressional and presidential levels and started preparing to jump-start healthcare reform. The anticipation was fulfilled in 2008. Democrats won bigger majorities in both the House and the Senate, and Illinois Democratic Senator Barack Obama defeated Republican Senator John McCain (AZ). By the time Obama took office in January 2009, the chair of the Senate Finance Committee, Max Baucus (D-MT), offered a plan that was almost identical to what eventually passed Congress.

The 2008 Presidential Elections

The 2008 presidential campaign itself lent momentum to healthcare reform. All three Democratic candidates—Barack Obama, New York Senator Hillary Clinton, and former North Carolina senator and 2004 Democratic vice-presidential candidate John Edwards—offered plans. They were fairly similar; for example, all had some type of health insurance exchange. The major difference between the two major candidates, Clinton and Obama, was that Clinton supported an individual mandate for all, whereas Obama supported it only for children (Jacobs and Skocpol 2010; Starr 2013). Of course, the Obama administration made healthcare reform a major priority for his first term.

Interest Groups

Interest group activity had certainly changed since the events of 1993–1994. Healthcare industry groups opposed the Clinton plan, though there were some exceptions, such as Physicians for a National Health Program. But 2009 was different. In May 2009, six healthcare industry associations indicated that they supported healthcare reform. The six were the Advanced Medical Technology Association (AdvaMed), the American Hospital Association (AHA), Pharmaceutical Researchers and Manufacturers of America (PhRMA), the American Medical Association (AMA), America's Health Insurance Plans (AHIP), and the Service Employees International Union (SEIU) (Jacobs and Skocpol 2010, 12). Not all of the support was wholehearted. While AHIP, for example, overtly supported healthcare reform, it also worked covertly to change or defeat it (Starr 2013).

Public Opinion

Where was the public on all this? The number-one issue on the public's mind in the months before the election was the economy, which at that time was in the midst of the worst recession since the Great Depression (Rushefsky 2017). Even so, 62 percent of respondents in a Kaiser Health Tracking Poll in October 2008 thought this was the right time to take on healthcare reform. The primary healthcare issue, according to the respondents, was costs. Overall support for healthcare reform was around the 50-percent mark (a percentage that remained fairly constant) with Democratic respondents much more supportive of change and Republican respondents much more supportive of keeping the system that currently existed (Kaiser Family Foundation 2008). This partisan divide would remain a key characteristic of debates over the Affordable Care Act before, during, and after enactment (see, for example, Weisman and Pear 2013).

An intriguing analysis of public opinion data in 2009 found that comparing it with 1993 was like watching the movie Groundhog Day, in which the day keeps repeating itself. Rivlin and Rivlin (2009) found that in 2008 about 82 percent of the public favored fundamental change compared to 92 percent in 1993. In 1993, 63 percent of the public supported reform versus 55 percent in 2008. Public support for reform was greater, at least initially, for the new Clinton administration than it would be for the new Obama administration.

THE LEGISLATIVE PROCESS: AN ORDEAL BY FIRE (2008–2010)

The Opening Moves

One of the lessons absorbed by the Obama administration from the failure of healthcare reform during the Clinton administration was not to make a specific policy proposal but to let Congress lead. President Obama would work for healthcare reform, often behind the scenes, sometimes very publicly. Late in the process the president would lobby members of his own party to support reform, offering deals when needed. But Congress would take the lead.

With Democrats anticipating a victory at the presidential level in 2008 as well as stronger legislative majorities, the party began to consider healthcare reform. This can be seen in the work of Senate Finance Chair Max Baucus (D-MT), who commenced meetings of Republicans and Democrats in the committee to garner support for healthcare reform and held numerous hearings (Starr 2013). In December 2008, Baucus issued a proposal that was very close to what the final legislation looked like. It called for national, rather than state, health insurance exchanges, allowing those aged 55 to 64 to enroll in Medicare, income-based subsidies to purchase health insurance, an individual mandate, reducing (over)payments to Medicare providers, free preventive services, and tax code reform (Baucus 2008).

In the meantime, interest groups were working to gather support for reform. Families USA, a consumer-oriented group, spent much of its time working for health insurance reform and attacking insurance companies. A group that sprang up in 2008 was Health Care for Americans Now (HCAN), "a coalition launched by progressive organizers ... bringing together labor unions, Moveon.org, Campaign for a New America, community organizations, and women's minority and faith-based groups" (Starr 2013, 191).

Industry interest groups played an important, positive role in the 2009–2010 events as compared to the 1993–1994 period. During the Clinton administration, industry interest groups opposed the plan. As we have seen, during the Obama administration, those interest groups decided that some type of reform would pass, and they wanted to help shape it. In turn, the Obama administration and Congress made deals with various segments of the industry.

One such group was the pharmaceutical industry. The industry received protection from the federal government's negotiating pharmaceutical prices, a deal also made as part of the Medicare Modernization Act (see Chapter 5). Additionally, the industry received protections against reimportation of cheaper drugs from foreign countries, such as Canada. In return, the industry promised to work to find $80 billion in savings, mostly related to closing the doughnut hole in the Medicare Modernization Act (see Chapter 5). However, the deal cost the head of the industry association, former congressman Billy Tauzin, his job (Altman and Shactman 2011).

The insurance industry was another major player. It was unalterably opposed to the Clinton Health Security Act proposal. Again, this time was different. The head of the industry interest group (AHIP), Karen Ignagni, publicly committed to support healthcare reform. AHIP agreed to discontinue industry practices that rejected applicants or refused to cover treatments, in return for the promise that everyone would have health insurance (the individual mandate), though it never made a deal with congressional committees (Starr 2013).

Much of the Affordable Care Act was insurance reform, and the for-profit health insurance companies remained wary of the proposed legislation. The Obama administration, for its part, saw the insurance industry as the cause of many of its problems and denounced the industry as part of a strategy for garnering support for the legislation. Covertly, the insurance industry began to oppose the legislation (Starr 2013).

In August 2009, AHIP sent a check for $86.2 million to the US Chamber of Commerce. The purpose was to fund a campaign against healthcare reform. The reason for doing it this way was that the opposition would be seen as coming from the Chamber and not AHIP. The Chamber was under no obligation to report the original source of funding. Further, AHIP was a middleman; the money was actually from the large for-profit insurance companies (Starr 2013). Thus, the insurance industry was both for and against health insurance reform.

The Legislative Process: Ideal versus Real

The legislative path to enactment itself was very complex. American government textbooks typically portray the legislative process as comprising a bill being sponsored by a congressional member; then being sent to a committee and subcommittee for hearings, discussions, and changes (known as markups); voted on and, if approved, sent to the floor of the legislative chamber; going through the Rules Committee in the House that places constraints on the length of debate and the number and type of amendments; and then debated and voted on in the floor of the chamber. The Senate, with its looser rules, allows more debate and amendments and procedures (such as the filibuster or the threat of a filibuster) that can slow down the process. If the legislation passes both houses of Congress, it would then go to a House-Senate conference committee to iron out differences in the two bills. The conference committee report then goes back to the House and the Senate for an up-or-down vote, again subject to the peculiarities of Senate procedures. If approved by both houses, the bill then goes to the president for either a signature or a veto. If it is vetoed, Congress could override the veto, though that is a very infrequent result. That is the way it is supposed to happen.

But in recent years, changes in partisanship, increases in polarization both inside and outside of Congress, have made this normal process much more difficult. The minority party, especially in the Senate, has acted more like an opposition party in a parliamentary system than a minority party that may oppose the majority on many occasions but also shows a willingness to compromise and get things done. Mann and Ornstein (2016), two very close and careful observers of Congress in particular and American politics in general, have noted how a parliamentary-oriented party system (the majority party controls the process and the minority party opposes) has been superimposed on the American constitutional system, leading to breakdowns. The failure of Congress, especially the Senate, to pass a budget resolution in recent years is one example of this (though the budget agreement reached after the October 2013 government shutdown is an exception to this; see below). The inability to pass the 12 appropriations bills every year and continual threats of government shutdowns because of the failure to resolve disagreements between the parties are two other examples. The partial federal shutdown at the end of 2018 over funding for a border wall is a good (or bad) example of this.

The number of clotures filed (motions to end debate) has dramatically increased. From 2001–2006, when Republicans controlled the Senate and the Democrats were in the minority for most of this period, there were a total of 65 cloture votes attempted. During the 2007–2012 period, when Democrats were the majority in the Senate and Republicans were a minority, there were 127 cloture votes attempted, more than double the previous period (Ornstein et al. 2013). During the 1979–2012 period, the average number of cloture votes when Republicans were in the minority was more than 30 percent higher (57.25) than when Democrats were in the minority (41.63) (Dews 2013). At the same time, the number of conference committees has dropped (Sinclair 2012).

Political Parties at War

Mann and Ornstein (2016) note that while both parties have played the obstructionist game, they attribute more of the problems to the growing conservatism within the Republican Party (see also Kaiser 2012; Ornstein et al. 2013; Poole et al. 2012). The polarization is thus, in Poole et al.'s (2012) phrase, asymmetric.

One can see this polarization via three measures: party unity, ideology, and what can be called the "outrage industry" (Berry and Sobieraj 2014). Party unity is the extent to which members of a particular party vote with that party. Looking at the 2009–2012 period, on average, 88.5 percent of House Democrats voted with their party compared to 89 percent of Republicans. The figures for the Senate were 91.5 percent (Democrats) and 84.3 percent (Republicans) (Ornstein et al. 2013). There was not much overlap in voting between the two parties.

The second measure is ideology. The Poole-Rosenthal ideological scale (Poole et al. 2012) measures ideology based on voting records in Congress. Looking at four years (1981, 1991, 2001, and 2011), we can see the changes in ideological makeup (see Table 3.1). Over this period of time, Democrats became more liberal and Republicans became more conservative. Not much of a surprise there. The important point, however, is that Republicans became much more conservative than Democrats became liberal. Indeed, the scores for Democrats in both the House and the Senate remained pretty close to each other (same scores for Senate Democrats) in 2001 and 2011, while Republicans became more conservative. This is consistent with Mann's and Ornstein's (Mann and Ornstein 2016) observation.

As Roarty (2013) notes in the *National Journal*'s annual rating of Congress, there is much less ideological overlap among the two parties than there was ten or 20 years ago. Both parties seem more like enemy camps in a military conflict. Compromise becomes difficult, though not impossible. This enhanced partisanship also affects any attempts to improve the ACA (see below). These are some of the political issues that we discussed in Chapter 1.

The third set of measures focuses on the "outrage industry." Berry and Sobieraj (2014) look at different types of media, such as cable news networks (Fox, CNN, MSNBC), talk radio, newspaper columns, and the blogosphere (Facebook, Twitter, Instagram, etc.). The outrage industry employs some combination of 13 modes of outrage: insulting language, name calling, emotional display, emotional language, verbal fighting/sparring, character assassination, misrepresentative exaggeration, mockery/sarcasm, conflagration, ideologically extremizing language, slippery slope, belittling, and obscene language (Berry and Sobieraj 2014, 40). They find that conservatives engage in more outrage activities than liberals, consistent with voting records and ideology. One can see this in the rise of the Tea Party movement within the Republican Party. Berry and Sobieraj (2014) observe, as did Roarty (2013), that the outrage industry has an impact on political discourse, elections, and congressional policymaking. To the last point, they note that it becomes more difficult for the parties to collaborate and compromise in this atmosphere.

Table 3.1

Ideological Change in Congress, Selected Years

House	Entire Chamber	Democrats	Republicans
1981	-0.044	-0.289	0.265
1991	-0.058	-0.317	0.359
2001	0.101	-0.374	0.542
2011	0.193	-0.394	0.675
Senate	Entire Chamber	Democrats	Republicans
1981	0.022	-0.286	0.275
1991	-0.049	-0.328	0.311
2001	0.013	-0.357	0.382
2011	0.038	-0.357	0.488

Note: A score of 0.0 would indicate a centrist ideology, a negative score indicates a more liberal ideology, and a positive score a more conservative ideology

Source: Ornstein et al. (2013, Tables 8–9 and 8–10).

Summers (2013) argues that gridlock can be a good thing. He notes that there are not sufficient checks and balances in the system, referencing the Vietnam and Iraq wars. He also argues that even in periods of gridlock, where it seems that Congress cannot do anything, things can get done:

> The great mistake of the gridlock theorists is to suppose that progress comes from legislation, and that more legislation consistently represents more progress. While people think the nation is gripped by gridlock, consider what has happened in the past five years: Washington moved faster to contain a systemic financial crisis than any country facing such an episode has done in the past generation. Through all the fractiousness, enough change has taken place that, without further policy action, the ratio of debt to gross domestic product is expected to decline for the next five years. Beyond that, the outlook depends largely on healthcare costs, but their growth has slowed to the rate of GDP growth for three years now, the first such slowdown in nearly half a century. At last, universal healthcare has been passed and is being implemented. Within a decade, it is likely that the United States no longer will be a net importer of fossil fuels. Financial regulation is not in a fully satisfactory place but has received its most substantial overhaul in 75 years. For the first time, most schools and teachers are being evaluated on objective metrics of performance. Same-sex marriage has become widely accepted.

While acknowledging Summers' point, all of the trends described above played out as the ACA wended its way through the House and, especially, the Senate.

Ornstein and Mann (2013) took objection to Summers' dismissal of the problems of gridlock. They noted that the ACA passed in spite of Republican opposition. But there was a price to pay for it. The legislation, Ornstein and Mann (2013) argued, was not as good as it could have been. Further, the lack of bipartisanship meant that about half the country would be opposed to the legislation and that opponents (Republicans) would continue efforts to hinder its implementation, repeal it, and delegitimize it.

Moving Through Congress

Healthcare reform bills were sent to two committees in the Senate (Finance; and Health, Education, Labor, and Pensions or HELP) and three committees in the House (Energy and Commerce; Ways and Means; and Education and Labor). The two Senate committees coordinated much of their work. But it would be up to the leadership in the House and the Senate to cobble together a single bill from the multitude of committee actions.

One potential barrier to the passage of healthcare reform was the need to get 60 senators to allow movement of the bill on the Senate. Republicans, it was clear, were going to oppose any effort at healthcare reform. Only

Olympia Snowe (R-ME) would vote for healthcare reform in the Senate Finance Committee; even then she voted against it on the floor of the Senate. One of the most important tools of a minority in the Senate is the filibuster. It takes 60 votes to end debate (invoking cloture), and the Senate has adopted the "rule of 60." If there are not 60 votes to end debate, then the bill will not come to the floor of the Senate. The threat of a filibuster is perhaps more important than the actual filibuster itself.

The 2008 elections gave Democrats a larger majority in the Senate, but not a filibuster-proof one. However, Bernie Sanders (I-VT) caucused with the Democrats, giving them 59 votes. The sixtieth vote came when Arlen Specter (R-PA), who was originally a Democrat and then switched to the Republican side, switched back to the Democrats. He felt that he would not be able to win the primary campaign for his seat in 2010 as a Republican because of challenges from the more conservative Tea Party wing of the party. (As it turned out, while Specter's defection to the Democrats helped move the passage of the Affordable Care Act, it did not help keep his Senate seat—he lost it in the November 2010 elections.)

The Democrats had their 60 votes. But it was a tenuous hold. Not a single one could be lost. In the summer of 2009, Senator Ted Kennedy (D-MA), the Senate's foremost advocate of comprehensive healthcare reform, died. Massachusetts governor Duval Patrick appointed Paul Kirk to fill Kennedy's seat until a special election in January 2010. In that election, Republican Scott Brown defeated Martha Coakley. The Democrats had lost their sixtieth vote, and it would influence the process in 2010.

Making Sausage

But that was only part of the Democrats' problems. The Democratic Party contains a wide range of views on politics, and the more conservative members (informally known as Blue Dog Democrats) raised objections and asked for deals. It is an old saw that there are two things one should never watch being made: one is sausage, the other is legislation. The ACA fit this well. Most of the negotiations over the bill among congressional members came within the Democratic Party. While the Democratic Party in the House was sufficiently large (and does not have the procedural barriers that exist in the Senate) that the loss of a few Blue Dog Democrats would not threaten health reform, that was clearly not the case in the Senate. Two examples illustrate this problem.

Senator Ben Nelson (D-NE) was an opponent of abortion (see below) and wanted additional restrictions on abortion within the legislation. He agreed to a provision that would separate government and personal funds paying for abortions in policies obtained through the state health exchanges. He also got a concession that allowed states to prohibit abortions being paid for by state health exchange policies. In return for agreeing to this, he asked for and received a promise that Nebraska would receive full federal funding for Medicaid expansion. Under the ACA, the federal government would pay 100 percent of the costs of Medicaid expansion for three years, and 90 percent thereafter. Nelson's price for compromise was that the federal government would permanently pay the full costs. This was known as the "Cornhusker Kickback" (Altman and Shactman 2011). The deal made quite a stir, though in the end the bill that accompanied the ACA eliminated it.

The second example is Senator Mary Landrieu (D-LA). Landrieu was opposed to the public option, a part of the House bill. But she had other concerns. In 2005, Hurricane Katrina had devastated Louisiana and other Gulf Coast states. Her price for not supporting a filibuster was additional money for her home state. Senate Majority Leader Harry Reid (D-NV) inserted an amendment in his manager's bill (the bill that combined the two Senate committee versions) that would provide additional Medicaid money to "certain states recovering from a major disaster" (Altman and Shactman 2011, 296). This was known, more colorfully than the deal Nelson got, as the "Louisiana Purchase." Deals such as these characterized much of the deliberations over healthcare reform.

Abortion

There also were issues that were, in one sense, tangential to healthcare reform but impacted passage as well as implementation. The most important of these was abortion. Abortion has been a festering public policy issue since the 1973 *Roe v. Wade* US Supreme Court decision. *Roe* effectively legalized abortion (though abortion was legal in some states prior to the decision). Following *Roe*, actions by the courts, the legislature, the executive branch, and the states limited the availability of abortion. In subsequent decades, states have enacted restrictions on abortion that, for the most part, have been upheld by the Supreme Court. In addition, in 1976 and every year thereafter, the Hyde Amendment, named after its sponsor, Representative Henry Hyde (R-IL), forbade the use of federal Medicaid funds to pay for an abortion. It also allowed states to prohibit the use of its contributions to Medicaid to pay for an abortion. There were limited exceptions for the health of the mother or in cases of rape and incest.

Some Democrats in the House were concerned that policies issued through the state health exchanges might allow abortions. Private health insurance plans frequently contained a provision that would pay for abortions. In the case of the state health exchanges, the federal government would provide assistance to the states in setting them up. But if states refused to set up a health exchange (as a number of states did; see the section on implementation), then the federal government would set them up using federal funds. Further, given the nature of the customers in the health exchanges, those not receiving employer-sponsored insurance or in one of the government programs would receive federal subsidies for purchase of the policies, depending on their income. Thus, federal dollars were involved with the exchanges.

Pro-life groups, such as the US Conference of Catholic Bishops, oppose abortion under any circumstances and certainly oppose public funding for abortion. There was, however, a split within the Catholic Church. The Leadership Conference of Women Religious (LCWR), though not necessarily all Catholic sisters, supported healthcare reform in opposition to the bishops' stance, though agreeing with the bishops on their abortion stance (Landsberg 2010). For the LCWR leaders, unlike the bishops, opposition to abortion did not lead to opposition to the ACA ("LCWR Stance on Healthcare Reform Draws Praise and Criticism" 2010).

In the House, Bart Stupak (D-MI) led the charge against inclusion of abortion coverage in any manner in the Affordable Care Act. One solution was to separate out the funding. A person wishing to have abortion paid for by her insurance company, under this proposal, would have to pay for a separate policy out of her own pocket. The Senate eventually went along with this Stupak amendment. Further, President Obama agreed to issue an executive order restating that federal dollars would not fund abortions. But this did not satisfy pro-life groups, and they continued to argue that the health reform bill would allow more abortions.

Misinformation Campaigns

Another problem that the Affordable Care Act and its sponsors faced was a misinformation campaign on the part of some its opponents. As an example, consider the charge that the bill contained so-called "death panels."

The provision that was in the legislation would pay doctors to provide end-of-life counseling and present options to the patient and the family. A bill outside of the health reform legislation would have permitted Medicare to pay for such counseling. It was introduced in 2009 by a bipartisan group of members of the House of Representatives. It was later incorporated into the healthcare reform legislation (Altman and Shactman 2011).

The idea that such counseling was a death panel came first from Betsy McCaughey. On her radio show, in 2009, McCaughey said: "Congress would make it mandatory—absolutely required—that every five years people in Medicare have a required counseling session that will tell them how to end their life sooner" (quoted in Starr 2013, 212). Other conservative/Republican opponents quickly picked up this call (part of the "outrage industry"; see Berry and Sobieraj 2014). The phrase "death panels" originated with a Facebook posting by former Alaska governor and 2008 Republican vice-presidential candidate Sarah Palin, who wrote that Medicare recipients

> will have to stand in front of Obama's "death panel" so his bureaucrats can decide, based on a subjective judgment of their "level of productivity in society," whether they are worthy of healthcare.
> (quoted in Starr 2013, 213; see also Altman and Shactman 2011)

Similar comments were made about cost-effectiveness research (CER). The idea behind CER is to evaluate treatments and procedures based on biomedical research and then rely more on the more cost-effective ones. This was transformed by opponents of healthcare reform as a form of rationing and bureaucratic meddling. The argument was that some agency would determine which procedures could be used (Altman and Shactman 2011).

These kinds of misinformation campaigns were part of a strategy set forth by Frank Luntz to defeat healthcare reform (Luntz 2009; McDonough 2011; Starr 2013). Luntz, a GOP strategist, has spent much of his career looking at how to frame policy debates that would advantage his party. Such framing is not confined to Republicans. Westen (2007) has written about the importance of appealing to emotion to frame political and policy debates from a Democratic Party perspective, arguing that Republicans were much better at framing debates than Democrats.

Luntz is a communications specialist and pollster who has been involved in policy debates since the mid-1990s for the Republican Party. For example, in 1995, Luntz counseled Republicans on how they should talk about the cuts they wanted to make in Medicare (for a discussion of the politics around the proposed 1995 Medicare cuts, see Rushefsky and Patel 1998). For example, Luntz advised the party not to talk about "improving" Medicare, because that sounded to seniors as if it would mean additional benefits. Instead, Republicans should talk about "strengthening" Medicare (quoted in Boxer 1995).

In 2009, Luntz gave Republicans similar advice as to how to talk about healthcare reform. For example, here is Luntz's fourth talking point:

> The arguments against the Democrats' healthcare plan must center around "politicians," "bureaucrats," and "Washington" … not the free market, tax incentives, or competition. Stop talking economic theory and start personalizing the impact of a government takeover of healthcare. They don't want to hear that you're opposed to government healthcare because it's too expensive (any help from the government to lower costs will be embraced) or because it's anti-competitive (they don't know about or care about current limits to competition). But they are deathly afraid that a government takeover will lower their quality of care—so they are extremely receptive to the anti-Washington approach. It's not an economic issue. It's a bureaucratic issue.
>
> (Luntz 2009, 1, emphasis in original)

Similarly, the first political use of the phrase "Obamacare," recalling how Republicans labeled the Clinton Health Security Act proposal "Hillarycare," was by Mitt Romney (who would be the Republican presidential candidate in 2012) in 2007. Other Republicans picked up the phrase, and eventually even Democrats, including President Obama, started calling the ACA Obamacare (Baker 2012).

Healthcare Reform and Public Opinion

An important reason why such messaging works is the nature of public opinion. Researchers have found that the public is not well informed about public policy issues, especially the details. For example, following the 2010 elections, less than half of the country knew that the Republicans had gained control over only the House of Representatives. The same survey found much ignorance about the Troubled Assets Relief Program (TARP), part of the effort to help the housing industry recover from the recession (Rushefsky 2013). Only about 16 percent of those surveyed knew that more than half of the money lent had been repaid. Respondents in previous surveys tended to incorrectly identify the TARP program with the Obama administration rather than the Bush administration (Pew Research Center 2010).

A further important finding about public opinion is what might be called "policy ambivalence." The public is concerned about the size of government and high taxes and supports private markets and individual autonomy. At the same time, it likes much of what government does, but does not want to pay for it (Cantril and Cantril 1999).

These dynamics can be seen in the 1993–1994 and the 2009–2010 debates over healthcare reform. As we know, the Clinton Health Security proposal was defeated in Congress. What was interesting was an article appearing in the March 10, 1994 issue of the *The Wall Street Journal* (Stout 1994). It found that a sizable majority liked the plan when presented with its features. That support diminished greatly when the participants were told that it was the Clinton plan. A similar dynamic was at work with the ACA. A majority of the public liked many of the provisions of the Act but disapproved of Obamacare (Kaiser Family Foundation 2011). Democrats and Independents tended to view the legislation much more favorably than Republicans, though Republicans liked some of the provisions, such as guaranteed issue (prohibiting insurance companies from rejecting applications) and the closing of the Medicare doughnut hole. The Obama administration drew the lesson that Congress, rather than the president, should be out in front on healthcare reform. Thus, proposals emanated from the legislature. The administration proposed only a general set of principles and only offered a program in 2010. Even then, it mirrored the consensus among congressional Democrats.

Another reason the Obama administration hesitated to submit its own proposal was the effect of presidential leadership on conflicts within Congress. Lee (2009) found that when presidents take the lead on an issue, even a relatively noncontroversial one, it tends to exacerbate whatever partisanship exists in the US Senate. It thus was good politics for the Obama administration not to be in the forefront. A 2013 public opinion poll (Rayfield 2013) found that when the law is referred to as Obamacare, supporters become even more supportive and opponents become even more opposed. In a time of hyper-partisanship, tying controversial legislation with a much-disliked president, as Republicans disliked Obama, can be politically effective.

One of the more interesting public opinion findings is that exposure to contradictory information does not necessarily change people's minds and may even reinforce their views. Paradoxically, those who are most informed about issues tend to hold on to their positions despite the contradictory information (Sunstein 2013). This suggests that disinformation campaigns are very powerful and hard to counter. It also shows the importance of the "outrage industry" (Berry and Sobieraj 2014). Advocates of health reform faced this problem during the legislative and implementation stage.

Town Hall Meetings

Another important series of events that surrounded passage of the ACA began in August 2009. While neither house of Congress had yet passed a bill, committees had, and the general outlines of what the legislation would look like was readily apparent. Congress normally takes a monthlong recess in August, which gives members a chance to get away from Washington, to refresh, to do some politicking back home, and to meet with constituents. An important means of doing this is with town hall meetings.

Senators and representatives, especially on the Democratic side, were taken by surprise at the town hall meetings that year. The meetings were packed with opponents of healthcare reform, especially against the requirement that everyone have health insurance—the individual mandate. In addition, the economy was in the midst of the Great Recession, and the federal government was spending billions of dollars bailing out financial institutions (begun under the Bush administration) and trying to stimulate/restart the economy (begun under the Obama administration). In the meantime, unemployment was rising, and home owners were losing their homes.

In this context came the phenomenon known as the Tea Party, self-named after the Boston Tea Party protesting British taxes in the colonial period. While there were legitimate concerns raised by those at the town halls, the Tea Party was not a spontaneous eruption against an aggressive, overreaching federal government. At least three groups planned the protests at the town hall meetings (Starr 2013). While supporters of healthcare reform mobilized to counteract the opposition, the Tea Party wing of the Republican Party and the town hall demonstrations were perfect opportunities for media coverage. The town hall protests provided visuals that made the conventional news media and also the newer Internet social media such as YouTube (Starr 2013).

Starr (2013) notes that the protests and media coverage had two important effects. First, the opponents of healthcare reform had a bigger impact in the media than the supporters. This was especially true of those who watched or listened to conservative-oriented media outlets, such as Fox News (Berry and Sobieraj 2014). Starr (2013, 217) writes: "an NBC poll at the time found that 45 percent of the public—and 75 percent of Fox News viewers—believed the legislation would give the government power to cut off care for the elderly."

The other point was that the protests and media coverage galvanized the supporters. Beleaguered Democrats asked Health Care for Americans Now (HCAN) for help. The protests also tended to move congressional Democrats more to the left on healthcare reform (Starr 2013).

A More Favorable Climate for Reform

Two articles suggested that despite the problems of gridlock and increased partisanship, the political situation was actually favorable to Obama and congressional Democrats. Beaussier (2012) argued that two factors enabled passage of the ACA. One was centralization of control by the leadership of both political parties, especially the Democrats. They were thus able to overcome the massive resistance of Republicans by making use of unorthodox or unusual legislative mechanisms that Sinclair (2012) wrote about (see below). A second factor was that the Democrats, normally a messy, undisciplined political party, were able to hold together (with the help of deals) to provide all the votes the ACA would need. Beaussier (2012) makes the intriguing observation that increased political polarization made it less likely that the parties would negotiate and therefore there was little need for bipartisan negotiation and support (which would not be forthcoming anyway). All the negotiations occurred within the Democratic Party.

Peterson (2011), focusing on the problems and political streams (Kingdon 2010), compared the Obama period to earlier efforts to pass national health insurance. He found that the various problems (such as costs and

Table 3.2

Affordable Care Act (ACA) Timeline

2006

(November)	Democrats regain control of both houses of Congress
	Massachusetts adopts healthcare reform that is a model for the Affordable Care Act
2007	Interest groups begin thinking about working toward reform
2008	Democratic presidential primaries: all three major candidates support reform; Democratic congressional staffers begin looking at reform proposals; Barack Obama defeats John McCain; Democrats win larger majorities in both houses of Congress; Senate Finance Committee chair Max Baucus (D-MT) issues "white paper" on reform containing most of the elements of what would be contained in the Affordable Care Act
2009	President Obama in State of the Union message calls for comprehensive healthcare reform; White House holds "summit" meeting with industry groups
July 15	Senate HELP Committee passes health reform bill
July 31	House Energy and Commerce Committee passes health reform bill
August	Town hall meetings demonstrate opposition to legislation
August 26	Senator Edward M. Kennedy dies
October 13	Senate Finance Committee passes health reform bill
November 7	House passes health reform bill by five votes
December 24	Senate passes health reform bill
2010	
January 19	Scott Brown wins special election to fill remainder of Kennedy's term; Democrats lose their filibuster-proof majority
February 25	Obama holds cost-containment summit
March 21	House passes Senate version of the Affordable Care Act
March 23	Obama signs executive order banning federal funds from being used to pay for abortions; Obama signs the Affordable Care Act
March 25	Congress passes the Health Care and Education Reconciliation Act
March 30	Obama signs the Health Care and Reconciliation Act
November	Republicans make gains in Senate and regain control of House
2012	
March 26–28	US Supreme Court hears oral argument in case challenging the Affordable Care Act
June 28	US Supreme Court rules on *NFIB v. Sebelius*, affirming part of the Affordable Care Act but rejecting other parts
November	President Obama reelected; Democrats gain seats in House and Senate, but Republicans retain control of House
2013	Health exchanges open for enrollment

insurance coverage) were worse than in any of the previous periods. Further, what he calls "contextual factors" (Kaiser Family Foundation 2011, 431–433) also were more favorable under Obama than in any previous administration. The public was more supportive of reform than in previous administrations, and interest groups were also more supportive, though not completely so. In other words, this time was different, more favorable, than past efforts.

The Affordable Care Act Clears the Obstacles

Table 3.2 presents a timeline of major events in the passage of the Affordable Care Act. The House of Representatives passed its version of healthcare reform on November 7, 2009. The Senate passed its version on December 24, 2009. Senate Majority Leader Harry Reid (D-NV) wanted the Senate to pass a bill before the Christmas break while they still had their filibuster-proof majority, so he kept the Senate in session until the bill was passed on Christmas Eve. By January 15, 2010, congressional leaders of both houses were pretty close to an agreement that would enable a conference report. Four days later, however, Republican Scott Brown won the special election in Massachusetts to replace Ted Kennedy. Senate Democrats no longer had a filibuster-proof majority.

This then led to the use of an unorthodox technique, reconciliation (Sinclair 2012), one that also played an important role in attempts to repeal/replace the ACA in 2017 (see below). Reconciliation is a process first put into place by the 1974 Congressional Budget and Impoundment Act. The original purpose of reconciliation was to order budget cuts felt necessary to stay within the congressional budget resolution (for a discussion of the federal budget process, see Mikesell 2013; Rubin 2009). One feature of reconciliation made it an ideal vehicle for those seeking to get legislation passed: by Senate rules, it was not subject to a filibuster. Thus, only a simple majority would be necessary to pass it. The reconciliation process has been used before. For example, the welfare reform legislation passed in 1996 made use of the process. The Bush-era tax cuts in 2001 and 2003 also employed the reconciliation path. The catch was that reconciliation legislation had to be related to the federal budget in some way, what is known as the "Byrd Rule," named after the late West Virginia Democratic senator Robert Byrd. The Senate parliamentarian would have to rule that the reconciliation bill was germane, related to the budget.

Because a conference committee was now out of the question, the House and the Senate resorted to a form of ping-pong, another example of unorthodox lawmaking (Sinclair 2012). President Obama and the House leadership worked to convince the more liberal House Democrats to accept the Senate bill, which had features that liberals did not like. For example, the House bill contained a public option for the state health exchanges, but the Senate bill did not. On March 21, 2010, the House voted to accept the Senate bill. Four days later, March 25, the Senate passed the Health Care and Education Reconciliation Act of 2010. Later that day, the House passed it as well. Healthcare reform had finally come to the United States.

THE PATIENT PROTECTION AND AFFORDABLE CARE ACT

Goals and Purposes

The Affordable Care Act is a complex piece of legislation superimposed on a complex healthcare system. A summary of the ACA by the Congressional Research Service was itself 55 pages (The Staff of the Washington Post 2010). In this section we describe the basic elements of the legislation, noting that some changes have occurred because of a 2012 US Supreme Court decision (see below), implementation issues, and efforts to undermine it (see below). The basic elements include expanded access, cost-sharing and subsidies, changes to the tax code, health insurance exchanges, benefit design, private insurance, Medicaid expansion, cost containment, improving quality and performance, prevention and wellness, long-term care, and Medicare. Implementation would take place over a period of time (see Figure 3.1).

Major Provisions

Mandates

The most important goal of the ACA was to increase access to the healthcare system by increasing health insurance coverage. A key part of this, as noted above, is the individual mandate. Because insurance companies agreed to accept all applicants regardless of pre-existing conditions (guaranteed issue), the only way an insurance system would work under these conditions was if everyone had insurance. If only sick people bought health insurance, then the premiums would have to be so high as to be unaffordable. Failure to have insurance would result in a penalty. Some exemptions were made, for example, for people who had religious objections and for those with very low incomes (Kaiser Family Foundation 2010). The individual mandate became the most unpopular provision of the ACA, pouring fire on the growing opposition to the legislation. As we shall see below, that part of the Act has been repealed.

A second, related feature is a modified employer mandate. Employers with 50 employees or more would either have to provide health insurance or pay a fee into a pool that would help pay for the legislation (what is known as "play or pay"). As in the case of the Massachusetts plan, the fee was considerably less than the cost of providing health insurance (Bernasek 2013). In addition, employers who have at least one employee receiving a tax credit to help pay for premiums would pay a fee.

Figure 3.1 **Healthcare Reform Implementation Timeline**

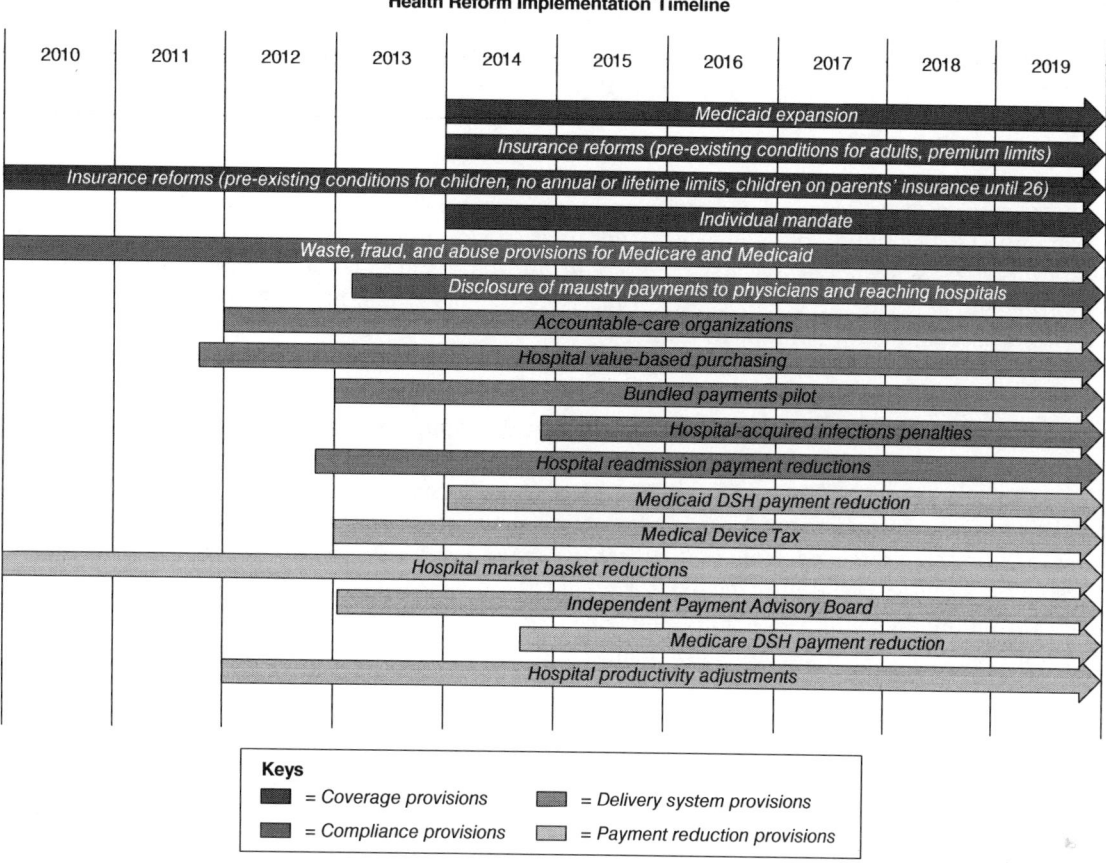

Source: Kaiser Family Foundation (2010). "Healthcare Reform Implementation Timeline." Menlo Park, CA: Henry J. Kaiser Family Foundation.

Medicaid Expansion

A third element is Medicaid. As we note in Chapter 4, eligibility for Medicaid varies dramatically depending on the state and the category someone falls into. Eligibility for children is easier than for adults. Childless adults have effectively no chance of getting on Medicaid. In some states, such as the authors' home state of Missouri, the income cut-off line for childless adults is 20 percent of the federal poverty line. The federal poverty level per year for a single adult in 2013 was $11,490; 20 percent of that is $2,298 annual income.

The Affordable Care Act required that states expand Medicaid eligibility for all persons up to 133 percent (or 138 percent of the federal poverty line, depending on how one reads the legislation). This would result in a significant increase in Medicaid enrollment. To ease the burden on states, the federal government would pay 100 percent of the costs of the expansion from 2014 through 2016; thereafter, the payments would be slightly reduced to 90 percent of the costs by 2020 and thereafter. Failure of states to expand as required would have meant the loss of a considerable portion of their Medicaid funds from the federal government. This last part was struck down by the US Supreme Court (see below).

Health Insurance Exchanges

One of the major ways that the ACA provides for increased insurance coverage is through the creation of health insurance exchanges. An exchange may be defined as:

a structured marketplace for the sale and purchase of health insurance. "Customers" can include individuals and businesses. The insurance companies ("issuers") that choose to sell their products through an exchange may be required to comply with consumer protections, such as offering insurance to every qualified applicant. Exchanges, however, are not issuers; rather, exchanges contract with issuers who will make insurance products available for purchase through exchanges. Essentially, exchanges are designed to bring together buyers and sellers of insurance, with the goal of increasing access to coverage.

(Fernandez and Mach 2013, 7)

The legislation calls on the states to create health exchanges, essentially a virtual marketplace, for those seeking nongroup insurance. The legislation notes that if a state fails to set up a health insurance exchange, the federal government will do so. In some cases, the federal government and a state may jointly run an exchange, what is known as a partnership exchange (Fernandez and Mach 2013). This is another area that has undergone some modification (see the section below on implementation).

The exchanges, whether state or federal, have numerous tasks to carry out. These include determining eligibility for the exchanges, helping people find the best exchange, helping determine eligibility for subsidies (both for premiums and for co-pays), and so forth. The exchanges also determine whether an individual might be eligible for a public program, such as Medicaid, and then help the individual enroll in that program (Fernandez and Mach 2013). Exchanges also certify plans as qualified. Exchanges assist individuals in picking plans and determining what their financial responsibility is. Examples of consumer assistance include toll-free telephone hotlines, a website, a calculator to help compare plans, outreach programs, and a Navigator program to help consumers and businesses find their way around the exchanges. Exchanges are also to oversee the finances of plans, including collecting and distributing premiums (Fernandez and Mach 2013).

The legislation creates different categories of plans, also known as benefit tiers, which would be available in the exchanges. The four tiers, from most costly and generous to least costly and less generous, are platinum, gold, silver, and bronze. All plans would have the same benefits, known as essential benefits, to be defined by regulations (see section on implementation below). The major difference is what percentage of the costs the plan would pay. Platinum plans would pay 90 percent of the benefits, versus the bronze plans, which would pay 60 percent. This would give consumers a range of choices when deciding which health plan to pick. The more generous the plan (such as platinum), the higher the premiums. All plans would limit out-of-pocket costs, which are set at whatever the out-of-pocket limit is for health savings accounts. The limit for out- of-pocket costs as of 2010 was $5,950 for individuals and $11,900 for families. For those who have incomes below 400 percent of the federal poverty line, the out-of-pocket spending limits would be reduced (Kaiser Family Foundation 2010).

There are also different types of exchanges (Fernandez and Mach 2013). One type is the SHOP (small business health options program) exchange for small businesses (99 or fewer employees) that qualify. Another type is multistate plans. Businesses and consumers could enroll in these plans regardless of plan location. Companies that participate in the exchange have to offer a child-only plan. Some plans may be non-profit, run by consumers; these are CO-OP (consumer-operated and oriented-plan) plans. Insurance plans can also offer catastrophic plans. Such plans have limited coverage, lower premiums, and higher cost-sharing. Another type of plan would provide only dental benefits (Fernandez and Mach 2013). The different types of plans and the requirements for the plans indicate the complexity of the ACA.

Subsidies

The writers of the Affordable Care Act recognized that some individuals and families would have difficulty paying for health insurance premiums in the exchanges. As a result, the legislation put into place a series of tax credits to pay for premiums. The premiums are refundable, paid in advance of normal tax refunds and are based on a sliding income scale. The subsidies would be available for those with incomes up to and including 400 percent of the federal poverty line. To illustrate, the federal poverty line for a family of four in 2013 was $23,550. Therefore, families of that size with incomes up to $94,200 would be eligible for some subsidy. Subsidies would also be available to small businesses that provide health insurance for their employees (Kaiser Family Foundation 2010). Lesser subsidies are also available to help pay for the cost-sharing features of a plan. As mentioned above, subsidies were also available to help pay for deductibles and co-pays, for those with incomes up to 250 percent of the federal poverty line.

Reforming Private Insurance Markets

An important series of provisions were directed at the private insurance market. Two features stand out. First, the states have traditionally had the major responsibility for regulating insurance sold within the states. The ACA is, effectively, a partial preemption of this state responsibility on the part of the federal government. Second, this section of the law, the patient protection part, is effectively a patient's bill of rights, the subject of state and federal activity in the late 1990s and early 2000s (see Patel and Rushefsky 2006).

The law requires that insurance companies spend 80–85 percent of premiums collected on healthcare. This is known as the medical loss ratio, an interesting phrase and indicative of some of the issues with insurance companies. Payments made for claims are considered a loss to the insurer. From the standpoint of investors, the lower the medical loss ratio (paying out smaller percentage in claims), the better the company was doing (on the problems with insurance companies, see Potter 2010). The legislation also addresses increases in insurance plan premiums. It requires that plans submit their premium increases to the federal government with the rationales for the increases.

The law modifies health insurance practices. It eliminates lifetime ceilings on benefits. Prior to the law, plans might limit lifetime coverage to, for example, $1 million. While that may seem like a great deal of money, the reality is that catastrophic illnesses such as cancer or chronic illnesses can result in costs that exceed the ceiling.

Pre-existing condition exclusions for children are prohibited. Further, children up to the age of 26 can stay on their parents' health insurance plan even if they are not living at home and are working. Beginning in 2014 insurance companies were prohibited from turning down anyone for a pre-existing condition (see Figure 3.1). The pre-existing conditions part of the legislation proved to be the most popular and helped block repeal-and-replace efforts (see below).

The legislation also affects differences in pricing of insurance policies. As we explain in Chapter 7, insurance companies have increasingly sold policies on the small group and individual market that are experience rated. That is, the price of policies would depend on risk factors of the subscriber, such as age or pre-existing condition or gender. This was one of the practices insurance companies engaged in that led to increased numbers of the uninsured. Under the ACA, insurance plans are limited to differential or experience pricing based on such factors as age, size of family, whether the subscriber is in a group or individual/small market plan, and whether the subscriber uses tobacco.

High-Risk Pools

As we shall discuss below, the ACA was designed to be implemented over a period of about ten years. Many of the insurance reforms/patient protections did not take place until 2014. Those in the individual market with pre-existing conditions faced alternatives—either they could purchase expensive policies that did not cover their pre-existing conditions, or they could not get any insurance. The first state to address the issue of the uninsurables and therefore create a high-risk pool was Minnesota in 1976. By 2013, nearly a quarter-of-a-million people were enrolled in state high-risk pools run by 34 states (Smith-Dewey 2013). That is a very small number compared to the size of the uninsured population.

ACA sought to address this transitional problem in a program called the pre-existing condition insurance plan (PCIP). In 18 states, the federal government ran the programs and lowered costs. In the District of Columbia and 23 states, the federal government lowered the standards for eligibility (Anderson 2013). The costs of the program were extremely high.

Because of the larger-than-expected enrollment and the high costs, the Obama administration ceased enrolling people into the pools in early 2013. The problem with high-risk pools is the same problem that led to the individual mandate. If the only people enrolled in a health insurance plan are sick people, premiums paid by enrollees will be very high and the costs of the program will be very high. These are not the characteristics of a sustainable program (Hall and Moore 2012; Lubell 2013).

Medicare

The Affordable Care Act also addresses Medicare. Two of the most important provisions affect Parts C and D (see Chapter 5 for a discussion of Medicare). Part C is the Medicare Advantage (MA) portion. It allows Medicare recipients to enroll in alternative delivery plans, such as a health maintenance organization or a preferred provider organization. These plans would then provide all Medicare-covered services, and many would provide additional services.

As we discuss in Chapter 5, the 2003 Medicare Modernization Act provided that the MA plans be paid at 115 percent of the average per-capita spending on Medicare recipients. This was to provide an incentive for plans to include Medicare recipients and for recipients to enroll in them. The political party division on this issue was pretty clear. Republicans wanted to transform Medicare into something else, and Democrats liked Medicare as it was and thought the plans were being overpaid. Democrats won on this issue. Over a period of time, payments to plans were slated to be lowered to the Medicare average per-capita payment.

The other important change to Medicare concerned prescription drugs (Part D). A prescription drug benefit was the major portion of the Medicare Modernization Act. But it contains an oddity known as the doughnut hole. At the point at which $2,970 is spent on covered pharmaceuticals (combining patient out-of-pocket expenses and Medicare coverage), the recipient would have to pay 100 percent of the cost of pharmaceuticals until the out-of-pocket costs reached $4,750 per year. The ACA gradually eliminates the doughnut hole.

The ACA also established an Independent Payment Advisory Board that would submit recommendations to Congress for changes if Medicare spending on a per-capita basis exceeds the growth of inflation plus 1 percent. This is one of those areas that was subject to misinformation (see, for example, the critique of comments by the 2012 Republican vice-presidential candidate and chair of the House Budget Committee, Paul Ryan [R-WI], in PolitiFact Florida 2012). The summary of the bill by the Kaiser Family Foundation (2010, 8) states:

> The Board is prohibited from submitting proposals that would ration care, increase revenues or change benefits, eligibility or Medicare beneficiary cost sharing (including Parts A and B premiums), or would result in a change in the beneficiary premium percentage or low- income subsidies under Part D.

The law also called for the reduction of disproportionate-share payments to hospitals. Medicare pays additional money to hospitals that have a large number of uncompensated claims and Medicaid patients (with their low reimbursement; see Chapter 4), thus a disproportionate share. But if much more of the population will be covered, there should be fewer uncompensated claims. This feature was dramatically affected by a 2012 US Supreme Court decision (see below). Congress never permitted the reductions to take place.

The ACA eliminates patient cost-sharing for a number of preventive services and treatments. The law also increases payments to primary care services under Medicaid. This is one way to increase the likelihood that primary care physicians will be willing to take on Medicaid patients (see Chapter 4).

Controlling Costs

The legislation also sought ways to reduce costs. One way the ACA attempts to do this is through the exchanges (Zuckerman and Holahan 2012). As with similar programs, such as Medicare Advantage, Part D of Medicare, the Federal Employees Health Benefits Program, and CalPERS (California Public Employee Retirement System), the exchanges are a form of managed competition. Consumers are faced with an array of plans and have to pay a portion of the premiums for the plan (with help from subsidies, depending on income). This should provide consumers with an incentive to purchase the type of plan they want, and the competition for subscribers should keep prices low. That, at least, is the theory of managed competition.

Medicare is the focus of several cost-constraining provisions. The ACA calls for cuts in provider reimbursements and cuts in DSH (disproportionate share hospital) payments, because if pretty much everyone has health insurance coverage, hospitals do not have to absorb losses from unreimbursed treatment (Zuckerman and Holahan 2012).

The legislation also includes some reforms in payment and reimbursement. For example, those hospitals treating Medicare patients with above-average hospital readmissions might find their Medicare payments reduced. A related provision calls for studies of "bundled" payments for those treating Medicare recipients. Under a fee-for-service system, providers are paid for each service rendered. Under a bundled system, similar in some ways to diagnostic-related groups (DRGs; see Chapter 5), the providers are given a single amount to cover all services (Zuckerman and Holahan 2012).

Another method for constraining costs is to tax so-called "Cadillac plans" (Orszag and Emanuel 2010). These are plans with very high premiums that cover almost all healthcare service expenses. The point of this is to reverse or limit the incentives currently in the system that lead to excessive use of healthcare services (Zuckerman and Holahan 2012).

Other parts of the law include funding cost-effectiveness research on medical treatments. Such research would help those involved in the system, such as patients, providers, and payers, to use the treatments or procedures most likely to prove beneficial (Zuckerman and Holahan 2012).

Another provision is coverage of preventive services. The idea behind this provision is that covering the cost of these services (such as mammograms) will encourage more people to get the services and, hopefully, catch health problems at an early stage.

The Independent Payment Advisory Board's task is to recommend changes if Medicare expenses exceed certain criteria. The law also seeks to reduce waste and fraud and create a somewhat less bureaucratic healthcare system (Orszag and Emanuel 2010).

Finally, the law promotes organizational changes. The Affordable Care Act encourages the creation of accountable care organizations that would better coordinate patient care and take responsibility for the full range of patient care. This is an attempt to create more efficiencies and decrease the fragmentation that characterizes the American healthcare system.

In short, there are a number of features of the ACA directed at cost control. But cost control is not the strongest component of the ACA. Critics of the ACA argue that these kinds of controls will not work (see, for example, Suderman 2012). Even those favorably disposed to the legislation have expressed some skepticism about the efficacy of the ACA's cost-control features (see, for example, Zuckerman and Holahan 2012). But spending increases have grown smaller in recent years, and perhaps the ACA has contributed at least a little to that slowdown (see Chapter 8). Nevertheless, the access features are much stronger than the cost-control features.

CHALLENGING THE AFFORDABLE CARE ACT

... the Affordable Care Act was both politically controversial and technically innovative, inviting constitutional challenge.

(Whittington 2013, 275)

The Affordable Care Act, passed by very small margins in the House and the Senate and with no Republican support, was challenged almost immediately after its passage. The challenges were judicial, administrative, electoral, and legislative. We begin with the judicial challenges.

The Affordable Care Act on Trial

National Federal of Independent Business v. Sebelius

Almost immediately after President Obama signed the Affordable Care Act, it faced a myriad of legal challenges, which came mostly from state attorneys general in Republican states. The challenges were twofold. First were challenges to the constitutionality of the ACA, particularly the individual mandate. The second challenge was based on the Medicaid expansion required under the ACA and what it would do to state budgets. In total, 27 states challenged the law (Stewart 2011). One private plaintiff was Liberty University in Virginia.

The cases started at federal district courts and then moved on to federal appellate courts. For the most part, the decisions were associated with political party. Those judges who had been appointed by Democratic presidents voted to uphold the law; those appointed by Republican presidents, with two exceptions, voted to deem the law unconstitutional. In a couple of instances, the judges ruled that if the individual mandate were unconstitutional, then the whole law was unconstitutional. This is the severability issue: would the ACA law hold up if a part of it (such as the individual mandate) was declared unconstitutional? This is an issue that was raised again in 2018 (see below).

Because of the variety of issues and decisions, the US Supreme Court combined the cases into one, *National Federation of Independent Business (NFIB) v. Sebelius* (2012). Generally speaking, oral argument before the Court takes 60 minutes: 30 minutes for the supporters and 30 minutes for the opposition. In this case, the Court broke the issues into three parts and heard oral argument over three days.

The first issue had to do with standing. Because the penalty or tax would not take place until 2014, under the Anti-Injunction Act challenges could not be made until imposed. The Court ruled that the payment for not having health insurance was not a tax but a penalty, and therefore standing was not an issue.

The two other issues were the important ones. We start with the individual mandate. Recall that the purpose of the individual mandate, part of the concept of shared responsibility, was that if no one could be turned down for health insurance coverage regardless of their health situation, then everyone had to have health insurance. Otherwise, premiums would skyrocket because only the sick would take insurance. This was the experience with high-risk pools as well as the guaranteed issue reform in New York State (prohibiting insurers from turning down applications because of pre-existing conditions [Parente and Bragdon 2009]). The individual mandate was an important part of the Massachusetts plan, the model for the Affordable Care Act.

The arguments against the individual mandate were, first, that it infringed on personal liberty and, second, that it went beyond congressional authority. The constitutional basis for the individual mandate was Congress's power to regulate commerce between the states.

Opponents of the ACA and the individual mandate argued that if the federal government could compel this activity (purchasing health insurance), then it could compel pretty much anything. Some, including US Supreme Court Associate Justice Antonin Scalia, used the "broccoli" argument: if Congress could compel purchase of insurance then it could compel eating of broccoli (Fried 2013). This was both a constitutional argument and a health policy argument (Hall 2013).

The third issue the Court faced was the extension of Medicaid. Under provisions of the ACA, failure of a state to extend coverage to people up to 133 (or 138) percent of the federal poverty line could result in the state's losing all its federal Medicaid funding. The question was whether this was too coercive (Kaiser Family Foundation 2012).

In recent years, highly charged court cases have produced a series of 5–4 decisions from the Court. The array of justices is political, with the four more conservative judges on one side and the four more liberal justices on the other side (see Toobin 2008, 2012). The swing justice has been Anthony Kennedy (who retired in 2018). The fate of the ACA was thus likely up to Justice Kennedy.

The big surprise was not that the ACA survived the court challenge but who the swing vote was: Chief Justice John Roberts. The first decision, over standing, was easily dismissed. All sides agreed that the Court should rule on the constitutionality of the Affordable Care Act. The Court ruled that for purposes of the Anti-Injunction Act, the fee to be paid by those who refused to purchase health insurance was not a tax but a penalty.

The second issue, on the constitutionality of the individual mandate, was a bit of a reach. A majority of the Court ruled that basing the mandate on the commerce clause was not valid. The majority distinguished between regulating an activity and regulating an inactivity (failure to purchase health insurance). The conservative majority (including Justice Kennedy) also thought that the ACA was stretching the commerce clause beyond acceptable limits, though a number of scholars disagreed with this interpretation (see Fried 2013).

That ruling would seem to have doomed the Affordable Care Act. Indeed, CNN reported, based on reading only the beginning of the summary of the case, that the Court had ruled the legislation as unconstitutional (Fried 2013). But for whatever reason, Chief Justice Roberts then went in a different direction (Toobin 2012).

Roberts, now siding with the liberals, wrote the majority opinion that the fee charged for not purchasing a health insurance policy was not a penalty but a tax. This would be acceptable under Congress's authority to tax and spend. Thus, the individual mandate and the constitutionality of the Affordable Care Act was upheld (Fried 2013; Mashaw 2013).

The Court's rulings on the first two issues were a perfect example of what Stone (2012) calls a policy paradox. A paradox is when something can be two different things at the same time. For purposes of the Anti-Injunction Act, the individual mandate was a penalty rather than a tax. For purposes of the constitutionality of the mandate, it was a tax rather than a penalty (Fried 2013).

The third issue was Medicaid expansion. The challenge from the states was that the penalty for noncompliance was too severe (Kaiser Family Foundation 2012). By a 7–2 majority, with two liberals joining the conservative justices, the Court ruled that the penalty was, indeed, too severe. There is no question that the federal government can attach conditions to grants it gives to state governments. But to the majority, the federal government had overreached.

In sum, the Affordable Care Act survived the court challenges, though lawsuits continued in 2013 and 2014. At the same time, the Court made it more difficult to meet the coverage expansion of the legislation. The Congressional Budget Office (CBO) predicted, after the Supreme Court decision, that

> in 2022, about six million fewer people will be covered by Medicaid as a result of some states deciding against expansion. The forecast estimates that roughly half of those individuals (three million) will instead receive subsidies through the exchanges, while the other half will remain uninsured.
>
> (Barnes et al. 2012, 4)

Burwell v. Hobby Lobby Stores, Inc.

The *Hobby Lobby* case (2014), the second of three major Supreme Court decisions regarding the Affordable Care Act, invoked values issues, including freedom of religion and women's access to contraceptives. Recall that the Affordable Care Act requires that insurance plans covered under the law contain ten essential benefits. The tenth benefit is preventive services, such as screening and payments for contraceptives for women. Contraceptives can be expensive, depending on the method and the income of the person. For example, looking at 2012 figures, the pill can cost between $160 and $600 a year. The initial cost of a diaphragm is between $15 and $75 plus the cost of a doctor's visit. An IUD (intrauterine device) has an upfront cost of $500 to $1,000. Female sterilization can cost between $1,500 and $6,000 (Palmer 2012).

Hobby Lobby argued that because of religious objections, it did not want to include contraceptives in its health insurance package for its employees. The corporation's lawyers argued that some of the contraceptives that would be covered are essentially abortion devices or abortifacients. While there is disagreement over that claim (Liptak 2014), the case, and a companion case, went to the US Supreme Court.

By a 5–4 decision, typical of splits in the Supreme Court, the Court held that a corporation such as Hobby Lobby, a privately held corporation, did have religious freedom rights and that under the Religious Freedom Restoration Act (1993), it did not have to comply with the ACA mandate on birth control. This is one of a number of decisions, such as the *Citizens United* decision in 2010 (allowing corporations to use their funds for electoral campaign purposes, though not direct contributions to candidates), where the Court has given corporations civil liberties found in the Bill of Rights. The majority was careful to limit its decision to privately held corporations, whose stock is not traded on public stock exchanges.

The Obama administration sought ways to both accommodate the religious objections while still providing insurance coverage for contraception. Subsequent to the decision, the administration offered a plan where an entity objecting to the benefit, including religious-based universities, would state in print its objection. At that point, the federal government would pay for the contraception devices. The various institutions subject to this process objected, stating that it would be, in effect, providing the benefit or complicit in providing the benefit (Radnofsky 2014).

As a follow-up, the Little Sisters of the Poor argued that the accommodation still violated their religious beliefs. In 2016, in *Zubik v. Burwick*, the Court ordered the parties to the case to work out an accommodation. In 2017, the Trump-administration Department of Health and Human Services issued a rule that provided "a broad exemption for non-profits like Little Sisters to prevent them from having to make available services in their healthcare plans that would violate their faith, like the week-after pill" (Martin 2017).

King v. Burwell

The next significant ACA Supreme Court case was *King v. Burwell* (2015). It is an interesting case, touching upon many aspects surrounding the Affordable Care Act, such as federalism, opposition, and statutory interpretation. The case begins with the new congressional process discussed above. Recall that once Senator Kennedy died in 2009 and the January 2010 special election to fill his seat was won by a Republican, Scott Brown, the Democrats were now one seat short of being able to end a filibuster and thus would have difficulty moving their legislation. The ACA had already passed in the Senate and the House had also passed its version. Instead of going to a conference committee, the House accepted the Senate version and then, through the reconciliation process, the Health Care and Education Reconciliation Act of 2010 was passed. But in going through all these twists and turns, the ACA was, perhaps, sloppier-written than it might otherwise have been.

The offending passage came in Section 1401 of the Affordable Care Act. The specific language was "through an exchange established by the state" (quoted in Carlson 2014). The problem these words, especially the last four, posed was that they referred to the refundable tax credits that were available to eligible persons to purchase insurance on the exchanges. As we shall see below, a sizable number of states chose not to set up their own exchanges, leaving it to the federal government to run exchanges in those states. The question raised was whether the tax credits or subsidies would be available in those states where the federal government ran the exchanges (Pear 2015).

Pear (2015) looks at the issue of how this phrase was put in to the law:

> How those words became the most contentious part of President Obama's signature domestic accomplishment has been a mystery. Who wrote them, and why? Were they really intended, as the plaintiffs in *King*

v. Burwell claim, to make the tax subsidies in the law available only in states that established their own health insurance marketplaces, and not in the three dozen states with federal exchanges?

The answer, from interviews with more than two dozen Democrats and Republicans involved in writing the law, is that the words were a product of shifting politics and a sloppy merging of different versions. Some described the words as "inadvertent," "inartful" or "a drafting error."

Opponents of the legislation, such as Michael Cannon, searched through the nearly-1,000-page legislation looking for a weakness. The four words were the one they found. Cannon argued, first, that the wording was a mistake and then argued then it was deliberate as a way to force the states to set up the exchanges. Cannon convinced Oklahoma Attorney General Scott Pruitt, later director of the Environmental Protection Agency in the Trump administration, to file the suit (see Kliff 2015 for a thorough discussion of the origins of the case).

If the suit were to win, then millions of people would no longer be eligible for subsidies to help them purchase insurance on the exchanges. The case ultimately depended upon statutory interpretation, a fancy expression for how we understand a law or a part of a law. The position that opponents of the law favored was a plain-text interpretation. In this case, one would look at the exact phrasing of the passage in dispute and follow that meaning. With this interpretation, and sticking to just this passage, the ACA seems to be saying that only those using state exchanges would be eligible for subsidies. The other position, the one taken by the ACA's supporters, was that if one looked at the entire legislation, it was clear that the writers of the law meant for the subsidies to be available for those on the federal exchanges as well. This was the position of the Internal Revenue Service under the Obama administration.

In June of 2015, the Court, by a 6–3 majority, decided that federal exchanges were eligible for the refundable tax credits.

House of Representatives v. Price

One of the deals made to obtain support for the passage of the Affordable Care Act was with the insurance industry. The industry promised to cut about $80 billion as a means of making insurance premiums more affordable. In return, the federal government would give the industry what were called cost-sharing reduction (or CSR) payments. In 2014, the House of Representatives, now led by Republicans, sued the Obama administration arguing that Congress had never appropriated the funds for it. If the CSR payments were not made, the insurance industry would still have to provide the discounts. Without the payments, premiums on the exchanges would rise and that would lead to fewer people enrolling on the exchanges (Kodjak 2017). The administration made several arguments against the House position, the major one being that the ACA implied the appropriations for the funds.

In 2016, a federal district court ruled that the House complaint had merit and that the CSR payments were unconstitutional. The administration could continue to make the payments, pending appeal. In December 2016, the House asked the DC Circuit Court of Appeal to delay any hearing because a new administration was coming in to office [the name of the case was changes to *House of Representatives v. Price*). With a Republican administration, the House leaders felt that a deal could be made. In February 2017, a deal was made between the House and the Justice Department that would allow the payments to be made but require quarterly reports. At present, the case remains on hold. Periodically, President Trump has threatened to withhold the payments (Kodjak 2017) but the administration has, so far, made all the payments.

Texas v. United States

The latest piece of litigation stems from congressional action in 2017 and the state of Texas (Goodnough and Hoffman 2018; Porter 2018). In December 2017, Congress passed the Tax Cut and Jobs Act. A rider, an amendment to the Act, repealed the penalty (tax) that lay under the individual mandate. In February, the State of Texas filed suit in federal court asking the court to declare the Affordable Care Act unconstitutional. In the first case discussed, *National Federation of Independent Business v. Sebelius*, there was some discussion about what was called severability. Recall that one of the issues was the constitutionality of the individual mandate. The question asked then was if the mandate was unconstitutional, would the entire law be unconstitutional? The question was not answered because the Supreme Court, as we have seen, upheld the individual mandate.

The Texas case, joined by some 19 other states led by Republicans, directly addresses the question. Unlike the situation in 2012, the Trump administration does not support the ACA and did not provide a defense of it.

Liberal states moved to oppose the Texas initiative. In September 2018, Maryland filed suit to force the Trump administration to enforce the ACA (Porter 2018).

In December 2018, a federal district court judge ruled that because the penalty for the individual mandate no longer existed, the entire law was unconstitutional. Those who opposed the Affordable Care Act cheered the decision. Those who supported the ACA argued that the judge's ruling was an overreach and wrongly decided. One basis for this side of the argument was that if Congress had wanted to repeal the entire ACA it would have; but it only repealed the tax penalty (see, for example, Ellement 2018). Other arguments included that there were major portions of the ACA that did not rely on the individual mandate or the tax penalty.

In any event, the ACA remained the law and the case awaited further deliberation in the federal court system.

Electoral Challenges

A second major challenge to the Affordable Care Act came via elections. If Republicans regained control of Congress and the presidency, they could repeal all or part of the legislation. And, as we shall below, such attempts were made.

The 2010 off-year elections produced mixed results. Republicans won (and Democrats lost) 63 seats in the House and thus did regain control. In the Senate, Republicans won (and Democrats lost) three seats, cutting into the Democratic majority. While the Republican House could set up roadblocks for implementation of the Affordable Care Act, a Democratic Senate and president ensured that the Act would survive.

In the 2012 elections, the presidency was at stake as well as Congress. While the economy was no longer in a recession, recovery was slow. The country was bitterly divided by party. The Republican presidential candidate was former Massachusetts governor Mitt Romney. Romney had worked with the Democratic-controlled Massachusetts legislature and Senator Kennedy to pass a health reform bill in 2006 that was a model for the Affordable Care Act. However, Romney insisted that while the 2006 legislation was good for the state, a similar piece of legislation was not good for the country as a whole. It was a difficult position to hold.

Obama won his reelection, and Democrats picked up seats in both the Senate and the House. Republicans retained control of the House and used that control to continually try to repeal all or parts of the ACA or to eliminate funding for implementation of it.

The 2014 mid-term elections produced significant gains for the Republicans. Republicans regained control of the Senate, with a 54–46 majority. Republicans increased their control in the House of Representatives, with a 247–188 majority. Republicans did not have a veto-proof majority, which requires a two-thirds vote in both houses. Nor did they have enough votes in the Senate to end a filibuster and deal with the rule of 60. But they controlled the legislative agenda and could, in a negative if not a proactive manner, undermine the Affordable Care Act. Republicans also did very well in state governorships and control of state legislatures. Republican hostility toward the Affordable Care Act meant that Medicaid expansion and establishment of state exchanges would be opposed (see below).

The 2016 election produced what appeared to be Republican victories, though the results were more mixed than most realized. The Republican candidate, Donald Trump, ran an insurgent campaign, which included promising to repeal the ACA. Going further, as president, Trump sought to undo much of the Obama agenda, in healthcare or elsewhere. Trump became president by winning a majority in the Electoral College, though his Democratic opponent, Hillary Clinton, won a majority of the popular vote by nearly 3 million people. Republicans maintained their majorities in the House and the Senate, but those majorities were smaller. In the Senate, the majority was a very narrow 52–48. In the House, the Republican majority shrunk slightly to 241–194, enough to control the agenda.

As a result of the 2016 election, Republicans controlled the presidency and Congress and the Affordable Care Act faced its greatest challenge.

Public Opinion

One problem that faced the Affordable Care Act was that the public, for a long time, did not support it. In 2010, 51.4 percent of the public opposed the Act, while only 39.9 percent supported it. Public opposition was reflected in Republican victories beginning with the 2010 elections ("Public Approval of Health Care Law" 2018).

The numbers stayed in that range until February 2017 when, for the first time, the percentage opposed and supportive was about the same. From that point on, supporters had the advantage ("Public Approval of Health

Care Law" 2018). The threat that the ACA might actually be repealed, including some of its more popular provisions, such as the ban on excluding coverage for pre-existing conditions, led to the increased public support and helped support efforts to maintain the legislation.

Public opinion was largely divided along partisan or party lines. Large majorities of Democrats supported the ACA, while large majorities of Republicans opposed it. Independents were somewhere in the middle. Sometimes, a majority of independents supported the ACA, sometimes a majority opposed (see, for example, Kaiser Family Foundation 2018).

IMPLEMENTING THE AFFORDABLE CARE ACT

The Affordable Care Act is a complex piece of legislation. It seeks to extend health insurance coverage and at the same time tries to control costs. Implementation of any policy is difficult, and, in the early years after passage, troublesome for the new legislation. One should view the ACA as being superimposed on top of an already-fragmented healthcare system.

The first point to make is that, as designed, full implementation of the ACA would take place over over a six-year period (see Figure 3.1). Some parts took effect immediately, such as allowing children up to the age of 26 to remain covered under their parents' insurance policy. Also, in 2010, insurance companies were prohibited from refusing coverage to children. The individual mandate took effect in 2014, as did establishment of the health exchanges.

A related point is that the legislation is complex and implementation of parts of the legislation (the exchanges) was rough, a problem acknowledged by the Obama administration (see, for example, "Obama Acknowledges" 2013). One scenario for the course of implementation is that it starts off bumpy or poorly and then gradually improves as learning takes place (Sabatier and Mazmanian 1980). This appears to have been the case, as the exchanges, both state and federal, in later years operated more smoothly.

The complexity of the problems (including political problems) can also be seen in three sets of rules issued by the Department of Health and Human Services (DHHS).

In March 2011, Health and Human Services issued a proposed rule on ACOs, defining what they are, how they have to operate, and how they have to be structured. The complexity of the rule is indicated by the number of federal agencies involved in crafting it: the Centers for Medicare and Medicaid Services (CMS), the Department of Health and Human Services Office of Inspector General (OIG), the Department of Justice (DOJ), the Federal Trade Commission (FTC), and the Internal Revenue Service (Hastings 2011). Later in October 2011, HHS issued its final rule. Interest groups were able to change or water down some of the provisions of the rule. Timetables were moved back, and the number of quality measures for evaluating ACOs was reduced. Community health centers could not participate in ACOs (Galewitz and Gold 2011).

Another example of complexity and politics mixing together is essential health benefits (ESBs). Insurance companies offering plans in the exchanges are supposed to have the same essential benefits, including free preventive care. Inclusion of the following ten categories of items is required:

> ambulatory patient services; emergency services; hospitalization; maternity and newborn care; mental health and substance use disorder services, including behavioral health treatment; prescription drugs; rehabilitative and habilitative services and devices; laboratory services; preventive and wellness services and chronic disease management; and pediatric services, including oral and vision care.
> (Office of the Assistant Secretary for Planning and Evaluation 2011)

One issue that arose over essential benefits was contraceptives as a covered preventive service. In July 2011, the Institute of Medicine, part of the National Academy of Sciences, recommended that contraceptive devices be included in the free provision of preventive services. In August of that year, the Department of Health and Human Services included them as part of the essential benefits (Pear 2011a, 2011b). Pro-life groups, such as Catholic bishops and Catholic institutions including universities and charities, immediately opposed including them (Pear 2011b) and urged the Obama administration to remove the benefit. Congressional Democrats opposed the change.

By early 2013, the Obama administration had made three compromises to try to appease religious organizations as well as Democrats. The administration exempted some businesses and organizations where there were religious objections to contraception. Instead the organizations would have a separate insurance policy that would cover contraceptives paid by insurance companies and beneficiaries. The compromise satisfied nobody

(Pear 2013a). Indeed, Liberty University in Virginia, founded by Jerry Falwell, filed suit in federal court in 2013 challenging the new rule, arguing that it violated the university's religious freedoms (requiring the provision of contraceptives that the university's counsel argued were essentially abortion drugs) and challenging the employer mandate as unconstitutional and beyond Congress's commerce clause powers (Haberkorn 2013). While the Liberty University suit was dismissed by the Court ("High Court Ends Liberty University Lawsuit over ObamaCare" 2013), the *Hobby Lobby* case discussed above exempted certain types of corporations from the requirement.

There were/are concerns about insurance company participation in the cases. Because of the difficulties of enrolling participants and hurdles set up by congressional Republicans, insurance companies found that they would have to either raise premiums substantially or pull out of markets. One reason for this problem was that more sick people enrolled in the early years than expected. Khazan (2017) points out that there would be fewer sick people on the exchanges if more states had expanded Medicaid (see below). Specifically, we are talking about people whose income was between 100 percent of the federal poverty level and 138 percent of that mark. In expansion states, they would have been eligible for Medicaid. In non-expansion states, they were not eligible for Medicaid, but were eligible for subsidies for purchase of insurance through the exchange. As a result, this group made up nearly 40 percent of those in the exchanges in non-expansion states, but only 6 percent in expansion states. Thus, insurers in non-expansion states were faced with a sicker population. As we shall see in Chapter 7, poorer people tend to be sicker. One can see the impact of this on the number of insurers for the exchange in a county. In 2016, 64 percent of counties had three or more insurers, 29 percent had two insurers, and 7 percent of counties had one insurer. The respective numbers for 2017 were 38 percent (3 or more), 31 percent (two insurers), and 31 percent (one insurer) (Khazan 2017). While there was concern that some counties would not have any insurers for the exchange, in 2018 (at least), all counties had at least one insurer (Soffen and Uhrmacher 2017).

The problem here is that the small number of insurers would mean limited competition and possibly higher prices for the plans. Insurers were concerned that those likely to use the healthcare system (such as those with pre-existing conditions) will enroll, while those less likely to use the healthcare system might hesitate to enroll (Johnson 2012). This is the adverse selection problem in health insurance and undermines the whole point of having an individual mandate. While insurers were facing high costs and, therefore, charging higher premiums, by 2018, the insurance market for the exchanges had stabilized and insurance companies were doing better from a financial standpoint (Fehr, Cox, and Levitt 2018). Indeed, for the first time, premiums on the exchanges decreased for 2019 (Galewitz and Appleby 2018).

A third example of the complexity of implementation issues is determining eligibility for the exchanges and the subsidies. In March 2013, the Department of Health and Human Services unveiled its application form—21 pages that could take up to three-quarters-of-an-hour to complete. It led to numerous complaints, and the next month DHHS issued a shorter form. There was still a bit of confusion about the form, because all the pages needed to be completed, and the time necessary to complete them was pretty short for single people. Families, however, had to fill out more of the form, depending on their size (see Gold 2013). Beyond filling out the eligibility forms is the complexity of choices given differences in premiums, subsidies (which depend on income), and cost-sharing. Loewenstein and Bhargava (2016) describe the difficulties facing those purchasing plans on the exchanges:

> While few financial decisions are as consequential as those related to the choice of health insurance, such decisions can be complicated, and even overwhelming, for consumers. When consumers choose among plans offered by their employer, the Affordable Care Act (ACA), or Medicare, they must evaluate options that differ not only in cost-sharing but also in non-financial dimensions, such as which doctors or hospitals are included "in-network" and the insurer's reputation for reliably processing claims. Furthermore, communication of critical plan details is frequently inconsistent across health plans, making it difficult for consumers to easily compare options.

The fourth example is employers' trying to avoid some of the coverage requirements of the ACA. Under the law, employers with over 50 employees must offer health insurance to those employees working more than 30 hours a week. Smaller businesses tried to get Congress to raise the number of hours that trigger the requirement. Some businesses began to reduce workers' hours to avoid either providing health insurance or paying penalties. Even states and non-profits considered this means of avoiding the mandate (Radnofsky 2013).

One part of the Affordable Care Act that died during the implementation stage was the CLASS Act (Glickman 2011). Long-term care, such as nursing homes and assisted living, is a problem that generally has not been well addressed in the United States (see Chapter 5). Long-term care is expensive, and while private long-term care insurance is available, a small percentage of the population has purchased such coverage, and the coverage itself is limited. The ACA attempted to remedy that problem. The CLASS (Community Living Assistance and Services and Supports) Act (part of ACA) sought to create a public insurance program that workers would purchase for later years. But in September 2011, the Senate Appropriations Committee deleted funding for the program, and the next month the administration abandoned the program completely. Questions were raised about the sustainability of the program, particularly since enrollment was voluntary. The ability of the Senate, with its Democratic majority, to form a conference committee with the House was limited by the lack of a filibuster-proof majority. The result was that while fixes were proposed by the Obama administration, the political support sufficient for passage and for an adequate program was never there (Glickman 2011).

The major and most publicized problems began in October 2013, though the origins of the problems precede that date. October 1, 2013 was the day when those eligible for insurance on the exchanges could begin to enroll in them. Under the ACA, enrollees had until December 23, 2013 to enroll and get insurance coverage by the beginning of 2014. The exchanges are virtual markets. People had to sign up online. The first few days saw a tremendous number of people trying to enroll, almost all of whom failed in the attempt. Part of the problem was that the large number of people who attempted to enroll was beyond the capacity of the computer systems to handle.

The major problems were with the computer systems. The systems were not completely pretested and the likelihood that they would work well at first was very small. Prospective enrollees would have to wait hours after initially attempting to enroll, or they would be knocked off the system, or they would receive incorrect information. They could not see the available plans and the costs associated with them before they were signed up, and insurance companies were sent incorrect information. The problems went on and on and were fodder for Jon Stewart and *The Daily Show* and, especially, for those opposed to the ACA. The problems were more severe for federally run exchanges, but some state exchanges also saw problems.

President Obama and the Department of Health and Human Services issued several delays and promised that the federal website, healthcare.gov, would be running more smoothly by the end of November 2013. By the end of December 2013, the federal website was handling about 40,000 people a day and nearly 1 million people had been enrolled. Better, but not nearly as many as originally predicted (about 7 million people) (Korte and Locker 2013). By 2015, the exchanges were running much more smoothly.

FEDERALISM AND THE AFFORDABLE CARE ACT

A critical feature of the Affordable Care Act is that it heavily involves the concept of federalism. States have an important role to play in the success or failure of healthcare reform in three areas: exchanges, Medicaid expansion, and insurance regulation (Beland, Rocco, and Waddan 2016). The exchanges and Medicaid expansion were designed to increase the number of insured people. Insurance or regulatory reform was designed to deal with things like premium increases (rate reviews), patient protections, and administrative costs of insurance companies. States are demonstrating varying perspectives on whether to cooperate, almost as if they were two different political systems, Republican or Democratic (Brownstein and Czekalinski 2013; Shaw 2017). The battle over healthcare reform is continuing at the state level. Beland, Rocco, and Waddan (2016) make the case that opposition to the ACA depended not only on partisanship but also which of the three issues are being considered. The most controversial was the exchanges, followed by Medicaid expansion, and regulatory reform.

Health Insurance Exchanges

Under the ACA, states were to set up state health exchanges, similar to the Health Connector established in Massachusetts in 2006, Part D under the 2003 Medicare Modernization Act and the market for Medicare supplementary insurance (medigap) policies. The purpose of the exchanges is to provide a virtual market by which individuals and those in small business could purchase insurance at a reasonable cost. The ACA stated that if the states did not set up health exchanges, the federal government would. Presumably, states would prefer to set up the exchanges under their own rather than federal control.

However, many of the opponents of the ACA, including states that challenged the constitutionality of the legislation, refused to set up the exchanges. This reaction should be considered a continuation of the legislative and judicial battles, with Democrats supporting the law and Republicans opposing it (Shaw 2017). There are three possibilities for states. One is to set up their own exchange. As of 2018, 11 states plus the District of Columbia had set up their own state-run exchanges. A second choice is for the state to set up an exchange but use the federal platform to run it. As of 2018, five states had chosen this option. The third option was for the state to not get involved in the exchanges and leave it up to the federal government. As of 2018, 34 states had chosen this path (National Academy of State Health Policy 2018). Setting up the exchanges in the recalcitrant states becomes a task for the Department of Health and Human Services. Further, when the federal government has the responsibility for setting up the exchanges, it still will have to work with state agencies. As we saw above, the rollout of the exchanges in the fall of 2013 was a disaster.

To complicate things even more, Republicans in Congress tried to stop federal funding of the exchanges. Because blocking legislation, such as appropriations bills, is easier than passing legislation, this was potentially a very real threat to the success of the ACA (Pettypiece and Salant 2013). And, as we saw above, the defunding effort led to a government shutdown just as the exchanges were rolled out. DHHS secretary Kathleen Sebelius then went to industry group executives seeking funds for implementation, which Republicans challenged (Kliff 2013b).

Then there is the problem of getting the word out about the exchanges so that people will enroll. A poll released in April 2013 indicated some of the problems. According to the poll (Kliff 2013a), 42 percent of the public were unclear as to whether the law was still on the books; another 7 percent thought that the Supreme Court had declared the law unconstitutional; and another 12 percent thought that Congress had repealed it. One of the administration's tasks was to inform the public about the exchanges. In 2013, the Obama administration began a campaign to inform the public about the law and to prepare people for enrolling in the health exchanges and choosing the appropriate insurance policy (Shapiro 2013). Even that was challenged by Republicans ("House GOP Expands Investigation" 2013). One strategy was to ask help from the National Football League and other sports enterprises to get the word out about the ACA and the exchanges (Galewitz 2013).

A related point has to do with navigators. Because of the complexity of the exchanges, navigators are employed to help people make their choices on the virtual marketplaces. States that oppose the Affordable Care Act and refuse to operate their own exchanges also make it difficult for navigators. These can be labeled "navigator suppression measures" (Health Care for America Now 2013, 3). These measures include stringent course requirements and training, residency requirements, high fees, background checks, and bans on providing advice (Health Care for America Now 2013). These are measures designed to make it more difficult for people to enroll. As we shall see below, the successor Trump administration continued this trend of undermining the ACA.

Supportive states engaged in considerable marketing to encourage eligible people to enroll in the marketplaces. The techniques utilized include informational videos, television commercials in English and Spanish, personal stories, and music and radio commercials (Stephens, Artiga, and Gates 2013).

For example, in Vermont a television commercial shows residents doing a variety of activities and then points to the marketplace (Vermont Health Connect) with the slogan "For Vermonters by Vermonters" (online at www.youtube.com/watch?v=yulTgIUERo4). An example of a personal story is "Ajay's Story," about a young woman with asthma who will now get coverage under Covered California (online at www.youtube.com/watch?v=Y7qQriEOu24).

Beland, Rocco, and Waddan (2016) argue that of the three major issues, the exchanges were the most controversial. Apart from the partisanship differences, states had little experience with the markets, compared to the other two issues. That lack of experience, or "lack of legacy," to use their words, reinforced opposition among those states, controlled by Republicans, whose leadership were already opposed to the new law. The result, as we have seen, was that fewer states ran their own exchanges than expanded Medicaid.

Most interesting was Kentucky. Kentucky had established a state exchange (KyNect) that was one of the more successful operations of state exchanges. In 2016, Republican governor Matt Bevin, a staunch opponent of the Affordable Care Act, asked the federal government for a waiver (i.e., permission) to close down its state exchange. In October 2016, the Obama administration granted the waiver and Kentucky residents had to enroll in the federal exchange (Gillespie 2016).

Medicaid Expansion and the States

The Medicaid issue was the result of the 2012 Supreme Court decision. Recall that the Court ruled that the penalty imposed on states for not extending Medicaid coverage was too coercive. It would be up to each state whether to comply with the Affordable Care Act.

As with the issue of health exchanges, the state reactions were split along party lines, though there was some division within the Republican Party on this. One factor was simply opposition, partisan and ideological, to the ACA. Another factor had to do with costs and federal payments.

The ACA called for states to extend Medicaid coverage to 133 percent (effectively 138 percent) of the federal poverty line. Eligibility for Medicaid varied by state and category of applicant. Coverage for children was greater than for parents and virtually zero for nonparental adults. Who would pay for the extension?

As we saw above, the ACA calls for the federal government to pay for 100 percent of the additional costs from 2014 to 2016. After that, the federal government would pay for 90 percent of the additional costs. States that hesitated or refused to expand had two concerns. One was whether the federal government would actually keep its part of the bargain, especially given the federal budget deficits and attempts to reduce them. The second concern was the cost of that 10 percent that states would have to cover after 2016. While that might seem like a small price, the impact on states, given their tight budgets, was not insignificant.

The calculations of the impacts of Medicaid expansion and the ACA on the state budgets (see Holohan et al. 2012) are complicated. States would gain from the ACA because fewer people would be uninsured even if the state does not extend Medicaid. Holohan et al. (2012) estimated that states would save about $10 billion through 2022 even without the extension.

The debate over Medicaid expansion has sometimes pitted Republicans against Republicans. Florida is a good example. The *Tampa Bay Times* noted that "Medicaid expansion is supported by the Florida Chamber of Commerce, Associated Industries, the healthcare industry and the majority of state voters" ("The Legislature's $51 Billion Failure" 2013; see also Campo-Flores 2013). Republican governor Rick Scott supported expansion in 2013, as did the Republican-controlled Florida Senate. But the Republican-controlled Florida House of Representatives did not, and the expansion bill died. Turning down the expansion meant giving up $51 billion in federal dollars and leaving about 1 million residents without insurance ("The Legislature's $51 Billion Failure" 2013).

As of October 2018, 20 states plus the nation's capital had agreed to the expansion. Another eight states expanded Medicaid through the 1115 waiver program. That is, these states agreed to expand Medicaid if they could make changes to the program. Such changes might include charging premiums and or work requirements (National Conference of State Legislators 2017). Seventeen states declined to expand Medicaid ("Status of Medicaid Expansion" 2018). Failure to expand Medicaid has consequences for states and businesses and residents in those states (Alonso-Zaldivar 2013). Obviously, it would leave millions of people uninsured. Pear (2013b) notes that 50 percent of those lacking health insurance live in the states that have refused to expand Medicaid. They are among the poorest in the country.

Another interesting, related quirk has to do with legal immigrants. Under the 1996 Personal Responsibility and Work Opportunities Reconciliation Act (welfare reform), legal immigrants were prohibited from enrolling in Medicaid for five years. Thus, poor legal immigrants cannot enroll in Medicaid, but under the ACA, they could enroll in the health exchanges, creating a situation where legal immigrants get health insurance, but citizens do not (Alonso-Zaldivar 2013). Illegal immigrants cannot get coverage under the ACA. About half of the illegal or undocumented immigrants have obtained insurance largely through their employers (Norris 2017). About one in five of the uninsured population is made up of undocumented immigrants (Norris 2017).

A third issue that Alonso-Zaldivar (2013) points to is the fairness issue. In states that reject Medicaid expansion, people with incomes just over the federal poverty line will be eligible for insurance and subsidies through the exchanges. Those with incomes just under the federal poverty line will not be covered.

One state that opposed Medicaid expansion, Arkansas, developed an intriguing proposal that might provide a way out of this political stalemate. Arkansas proposed that people who enroll under the expansion be allowed to participate in the state health exchanges, rather than in traditional Medicaid (Hancock 2013). This could meet Republican preferences by providing a private option rather than an expanded government program. This is similar reasoning to the prescription drug benefit (Part D) that was added to Medicare in 2003 (see Chapter 5). The advantages of the plan, apart from garnering Republican support, include access to a wider group of plans and providers. Physicians do not have to accept Medicaid recipients as patients. Providers would be paid at higher rates than Medicaid pays, and that would expand access. As Hancock (2013) notes, having assured access means that treatments that would otherwise be delayed can start earlier, thus producing a healthier and less costly population (see also Davidson 2010; Patel and Rushefsky 2008).

There are some disadvantages to the Arkansas plan. The major one is cost. Insurance on the exchanges will be costlier than Medicaid, perhaps as much as 50 percent more, according to a Congressional Budget Office report (Hancock 2013). On the other hand, supporters of relying more on private markets argue that competition among plans will restrain and perhaps even lower costs (Hancock 2013). Another issue is synchronizing the health exchange with Medicaid. Policies purchased under the health exchanges will come with substantial cost-sharing provisions. But cost-sharing is limited under Medicaid. The Arkansas plan seems to be one alternative that reluctant states might consider.

Some states that have been reluctant to expand Medicaid have agreed to do so if they could also impose work requirements on Medicaid recipients. Arkansas is a good example of this. Chapter 4 focuses on Medicaid and work requirements.

States' refusal to expand Medicaid means that fewer people will be covered than if all the states expanded Medicaid. As of 2018, an estimated 2.2 million adults did not have insurance because states did not expand Medicaid (Garfield, Damico, and Orgera 2018). These are generally people whose income is too low, ironically, to be eligible for subsidies on the exchange. Perhaps not surprisingly, the overwhelming majority of these people, often people of color, live in the South (Garfield, Damico, and Orgera 2018). There is clearly a partisan tinge to the decision (Shaw 2017). Republican-led states are more likely not to have expanded Medicaid than Democratic-led states. Interestingly, the states that are not expanding Medicaid already have very low eligibility standards, lower than those who are expanding (Rudowitz and Stephens 2013).

Additionally, these states will also not receive billions of dollars of assistance that would come with expansion. States not expanding will forego an estimated $346 billion over a ten-year period (2013–2022) (Rudowitz and Stephens 2013). Of course, one could argue that this will produce savings for the federal budget.

LEGISLATIVE CHALLENGES

Republicans, conservatives, and libertarians remain unalterably opposed to the ACA. Like much of the controversy surrounding the legislation, there is disagreement over how many times congressional Republicans attempted to repeal the ACA. A report by the Congressional Research Service, or CRS (Stephen and Kinzer 2017, ii), lists the types of actions taken in the House of Representatives:

> The House-passed legislation included stand-alone bills as well as provisions in broader, often unrelated measures that would have (1) repealed the ACA in its entirety and, in some cases, replaced it with new law; 2) repealed, or by amendment restricted or otherwise limited, specific provisions in the ACA; (3) eliminated appropriations provided by the ACA and rescinded all unobligated funds; (4) replaced the ACA's mandatory appropriations with authorizations of (discretionary) appropriations, and rescinded all unobligated funds; or (5) blocked or otherwise delayed implementation of specific ACA provisions.

York (2014) argues that in the 2013–2014 period, the House only voted six times to completely repeal the Affordable Care Act. The other 54 votes were delays or defunding, as mentioned in the previous paragraph. York also noted that some of the votes were on measures asked for by the Obama administration, such as delaying the employer mandate for a year or repealing the CLASS Act. Nevertheless, Republicans seemed to be busy trying to undo the law. This included five pieces of legislation offered in 2017 that would have repealed some though not all of the ACA.

Following the 2010 mid-term elections and by the 2014 elections, Republicans gained control of both houses of Congress. One problem for the Republicans was that Obama was president through 2016. The other problem was that when Donald Trump became president in 2017, Republicans did not have sufficient control of the Senate to repeal or replace the ACA. Here we focus on action or inaction in 2017.

The Republican difficulties were mostly in the Senate, with its rules that allow the minority party (in this case, the Democrats) to stall or delay or hinder passage of legislation. The main roadblock, not available in the House, is the filibuster, a problem that Democrats faced in 2010. A recent example of the use of a filibuster came in September 2013, when Senator Ted Cruz (R-TX), a member of what was then the minority party, gave a 21-hour-long speech on the floor of the Senate trying to delay action on the federal budget and calling for the defunding of Obamacare. Among other things, Senator Cruz read the Dr. Seuss story *Green Eggs and Ham*.

As we saw above, the reconciliation process played out both in the passage of a related bill to the ACA in 2010 and in attempts to repeal and replace the ACA in 2017. In the case of the Affordable Care Act, the Democrats controlled both houses of Congress and the presidency in 2009 and 2010. The Democrats were able to cobble together a 60-vote majority in 2009.

That brings us to 2017. As noted above, Donald Trump won the presidency in the 2016 elections and the Republicans maintained control of both houses of Congress and could strongly influence the makeup of the federal judiciary through new appointments. One would think that, given complete control over the federal government, the Republicans would be able to achieve one of their main goals, the repeal (and perhaps replacement) of the Affordable Care Act. Trump campaigned, partly, in 2016 on a promise to repeal the legislation. But the legislative path proved more difficult for the reasons mentioned above.

The first, and perhaps most important, problem for the Republicans was that they actually lost seats in both the Senate and the House. Again, because of unique rules of that chamber, we focus on the Senate. Republicans lost two seats in the Senate, leaving it with a narrow 52–48 majority. That margin became smaller after a special election in Alabama in December 2017 for an open seat. Jeff Sessions (R-AL) resigned his seat to become the Attorney General of the United States. In a surprise reminiscent of the 2010 special election to fill Ted Kennedy's seat, the Democrat Doug Jones beat the Republican Roy Moore. The Republican margin was now 51–49. The small Republican majority would have to use the reconciliation process to pass repeal-and-replace legislation. If two Republicans voted against any of the repeal-and-replace proposals, they would be defeated. That proved to be the case.

In 2017, Congress considered, in one house or the other, 12 pieces of legislation to repeal and replace the Affordable Care Act. These included the following: the Health Care Freedom Act, the Better Care Reconciliation Act of 2017, the Obamacare Repeal Reconciliation Act of 2017, the American Health Care Act, and the Cassidy-Graham-Heller-Johnson Amendment (Kaiser Family Foundation 2017). To get some idea of the various bills, we will look at the last one, the Cassidy-Graham bill.

The Cassidy-Graham bill retains some features of the ACA and changes others ("Summary of Cassidy-Graham-Heller-Johnson Amendment" 2017). Cassidy-Graham would repeal the individual mandate and the subsidies for those using the exchanges. Cassidy-Graham replaces the subsidies with block grants to the states. It repeals the Medicaid expansion and replaces Medicaid funding with per-capita block grants (see Chapter 4). It retains the provision that forbids exclusion for pre-existing conditions. It maintains the requirement for some coverage of maternity care. The essential benefits provisions are modified for Medicaid and limits on out-of-pocket payments under Medicaid are repealed. It enhances health savings accounts. The legislation effectively eliminates the exchanges. It maintains coverage of children on their parents' health plan up to the age of 26. It allows states to add a work requirement to their Medicaid programs. Cassidy-Graham repeals the tax revenue portions of the Affordable Care Act.

As with all the repeal-and-replace legislation (indeed all legislation), the Congressional Budget Office (CBO) "scores" or evaluates proposed legislation. In the case of Cassidy-Graham, the proposal was put together so swiftly that the evaluation, published in September of 2017, was preliminary. The two major points of evaluation, true for Cassidy-Graham as well as for other repeal-and-replace legislation, were the impacts on the federal budget and how many more people would be insured if the proposal were enacted. The CBO report (Congressional Budget Office 2017b) on this proposal was similar to its evaluation of other proposals.

On the first point, the impact on the federal budget, the CBO estimated at least a $133 billion savings over a ten-year period (the typical period for scoring). As to the second point, the CBO report did not provide a specific numerical source. Others did, however. Fielder and Adler (2017) estimated that 21 million more people might be uninsured than if the ACA remained in effect. This is in line with evaluations of the other repeal-and-replace legislation. For example, the CBO estimated that an additional 22 million people would be uninsured under the Better Care Reconciliation Act (Congressional Budget Office 2017a). The CBO report (Congressional Budget Office 2017b) said that reductions would be due to termination of the Medicaid expansion, termination of subsidies for purchase on exchanges, and repeal of the individual mandate. The report also noted that the block grants that replace the subsidies could, depending on how they are implemented by the various states, decrease the number of uninsured (see Fielder and Adler 2017). Finally, the protections for those with pre-existing conditions seem to be weaker than in the ACA.

Two other notes. First, none of the repeal bills went through the regular legislative process, with bills going to committee and then to the floor. In the case of the Affordable Care Act, consideration began, as we saw above, in 2008 and then proposals went to three committees in the House and two in the Senate. This was not true for the repeal legislation.

Second, none of the repeal-and-replace legislation passed Congress. In one case, three Republican Senators, John McCain of Arizona, Susan Collins of Maine, and Lisa Murkowski of Alaska, voted against the Republican bill. For Collins and Murkowski, it was concern about defunding Planned Parenthood, among other things. For all three, there was concern about the short-cutted process.

Republicans were able to achieve one of their goals. In December 2017, Congress passed and President Trump signed the Tax Cut and Jobs Act of 2017. A portion of that legislation eliminated the tax penalties for not having health insurance. The requirement that all people have health insurance remains in the Affordable Care Act. When the legislation passed, both opponents and supporters of the ACA thought the mandate was eliminated. However, it was only the enforcement mechanism that was eliminated, beginning in 2019 (Jost 2017). In effect, though not in law, the individual mandate has been repealed.

Opponents argued that this was the beginning of the end for the Affordable Care Act. The people most likely not to purchase insurance are younger, healthier adults. Here there is some combination of being a healthier part of the population and also facing the expense of health insurance even with subsidies that were available. One result of the repeal is that those on the exchanges are likely to be less healthy, use more services, and, thus, premiums would rise more than they otherwise would (Jost 2017). That, after all, was one of the major reasons for including everyone: to keep premiums from rising too much.

There are other potential effects of the repeal. First, the Congressional Budget Office estimated that by 2017 as many as 13 million more people would be uninsured than if the mandate were still in place.

Second, the legislation had an impact on court cases. Recall that in the first ACA court case, *NFIB v. Sebelius* (2012), the Supreme Court ruled that the individual mandate was constitutional because the penalty for not having insurance was a tax. Now that penalty is gone. But part of the argument in this case was that if the individual mandate were to be declared unconstitutional then the entire Act would also be unconstitutional. This is the severability issue. But it was not addressed in 2012. However, in the most recent case, again discussed above, *Texas v. Azar*, the argument was made, again, that the entire legislation is unconstitutional because of the absence of the mandate. The federal district court judge, as we discussed above, accepted that argument. With two new conservative Supreme Court justices, Neil Gorsuch and Brett Kavanaugh, on the bench it is not clear what direction the Court will take on this issue.

ADMINISTRATIVE CHALLENGES

While Barack Obama was president, the Affordable Care Act had a friend in the White House. With the Trump administration, the ACA has an avowed enemy.

During the 2016 presidential campaign, the Republican candidate promised to repeal the Affordable Care Act. He did not suggest an alternative policy to replace the ACA, but the emphasis was clearly on repeal (Saltzman and Eibner 2016). Where Congress had difficulty repealing and replacing the Affordable Care Act, the Trump administration could take actions on its own to undermine the legislation.

One simple example is the case just mentioned above. The Trump administration (the Justice Department) filed a brief in June 2018 stating that it would not defend the Act in *Texas v. Azar* (Keith 2018). Those supporting the ACA included unions, patient groups, and insurance companies, among others. Some Republican politicians, such as Lamar Alexander, Governor of Tennessee, and Senator Mitch McConnell of Kentucky, the Senate Majority Leader, also showed some support for the ACA. In the case of the Republican politicians, the concern was over the protections for those with pre-existing conditions (Keith 2018). This concern then became a key issue in the 2018 mid-term elections, as Democrats, such as Claire McCaskill of Missouri running for re-election, pounded Republicans, arguing that they wanted to take away protections for people with pre-existing conditions.

The administration made other efforts to undermine the ACA (Luhby 2018). One way was to place limits on enrollment for the exchanges. An example of this was stopping advertisement about enrollment. A related effort was to reduce the enrollment period from three months to six weeks. A third effort was, on several occasions, to stop or threaten to stop payment of subsidies to health insurance companies to allow for reductions in the cost-sharing provisions. The administration also shut down the exchange websites on Sundays during the six-week enrollment period.

A fourth effort focused on Medicaid (see Chapter 4). The administration has begun allowing states to impose work requirements on Medicaid recipients, similar to those used in the cash-welfare program Temporary Assistance to Needy Families (TANF). In addition, there are waiver provisions in both Medicaid and the ACA that the administration has taken advantage of. "States are requesting permission to charge recipients premiums, limit the time they can receive benefits, test them for drugs and lock them out if they fail to keep up with payments or paperwork" Luhby 2018).

A fifth effort was to loosen rules on health plans (Luhby 2018). The first such rule focused on *association health plans*. With such plans, small businesses and those who were self-employed could band together to form their own healthcare plans. While such plans have been available for years, the Obama administration insisted that they meet the requirements of the ACA. The Trump administration worked to loosen the requirements so that such plans would not have to meet all the essential benefits, nor would they be required to cover pre-existing conditions (Arensmeyer 2018). The rules issued by the Department of Labor in July 2017, however, made it less attractive to small business that had been hoped. The rules required substantial financial investment on the part of the firms. Two organizations that, in general, favor association health plans, the National Federation of Independent Businesses (NFIB) and the National Association of Realtors, both said that, given the new rule, they would not offer such plans to their members. Regardless of the rule, the intent was to provide an incentive for more people and groups to leave the exchanges, which would likely drive up premiums and the cost-sharing subsidies (Arensmeyer 2018).

A related attempt to undermine the Affordable Care Act was to encourage more healthy people to buy short-term health insurance policies outside the exchanges. Such plans, which are purchased for a limited time, originally about six months, do not have to meet many of the requirements of the ACA. For example, they do not have to cover essential benefits (such as maternal or contraceptive care), they can exclude people with pre-existing conditions, and they may not cover many hospital expenses. Nor would such plans have to meet the ACA requirement that they spend 80–85 percent of the premiums they collect on their subscribers. But they are cheap. These kinds of plans are sometimes referred to as "skinny plans." The administration issued a rule in 2018 allowing people to purchase these policies for as long as three years (Kodjak 2018). This would be attractive, again, to young, healthy people and thus narrow the types of people who purchase on insurance on the exchanges, i.e., sicker people, again resulting in higher premiums and cost-sharing subsidies.

The administration has also made it more difficult for people to sign up for insurance outside the designated enrollment period (end of fall/beginning of winter) (Luhby 2018). People might want to sign up for health insurance outside the enrollment period because of changes in their life circumstances. This might occur because of a divorce, the death of a spouse, or the loss of a job. Insurance companies, understandably, have a concern that people might want to "game" the system. Such gaming might occur if someone were anticipating a major health event, such as knee surgery or coronary bypass surgery. The prospective patient might not have insurance or have one of the temporary plans and then try to get on to the exchange, where such procedures would be covered. Following the procedure and rehabilitation, the person might then drop the exchange insurance and purchase the cheaper short-term plan. Relatedly, the Trump administration no longer looks to see whether insurance plans on the exchanges have a sufficient number of providers to meet the needs of their subscribers.

There is another way that the Trump administration is trying to undermine the Affordable Care Act. This method is the use of Section 1332 waivers (Pear 2018a; Scott 2018). Section 1332 is, in effect, a kind of backdoor for states built into the Affordable Care Act. It allowed states to refashion the Affordable Care Act beginning in 2017. States could modify the law to meet their own needs and desires, as long as the newly designed plan met the goals of the ACA. As of October 2018, 35 states were in some stage of seeking waivers, with some waivers having been granted (Cauchi 2018).

In October 2018, the Trump administration (Department of Health and Human Services) issued a rule that gave greater flexibility to the states (Cauchi 2018; Pear 2018a; Scott 2018). Scott (2018) lists the major points of the new rule.

- CMS wants states to prioritize private health insurance over public programs—remember, one possible use of a 1332 would be a state-level single-payer program.
- CMS is relaxing the requirement that state 1332 waivers provide as comprehensive benefits as Obamacare currently does.
- Instead, comprehensive coverage must be made available to anyone who wants it, but skimpier short-term plans will also count as coverage.
- In fact, CMS would *allow* Obamacare subsidies to be used to pay for short-term insurance—which, again, is not required to meet the ACA's preexisting conditions rules.

Such a rule would allow the purchase of cheaper, skinnier healthcare plans.

To summarize: while Congress has failed to repeal the Affordable Care Act, an argument can be made that legislative and executive branch actions have transformed legislation in Republican directions (Suderman 2018):

> Although the hastily written replacement bills that made their way through Congress were often vague and uneven, they tended to push the law in predictable directions: more federalism and individual choice, fewer mandates and more state flexibility, cheaper plans with less comprehensive coverage. They aimed to reduce some subsidies associated with the law while also, in some cases, providing funds to help states shore up Obamacare's unstable marketplaces. They pared back the law's Medicaid expansion and consistently took aim at its individual mandate.
> None of those plans or quasi-plans passed. But roughly speaking, this is the form that the Affordable Care Act is now starting to take, thanks to a series of changes that Republicans have ushered into place since the failure of repeal.

Republicans, having failed to repeal Obamacare, have stumbled, almost accidentally, into replacing it. For better and for worse, and with little coherent vision at work, they are making Obamacare their own. And over time, they are likely to embrace it.

(Suderman 2018)

EVALUATING THE AFFORDABLE CARE ACT

How well has the Affordable Care performed? Unfortunately, answering such a question often provokes a partisan divide. Democrats/liberals tend to believe it has had successes and Republicans/conservatives tend to believe it has been an out-and-out failure. Our reading of the literature suggests a more mixed, nuanced view.

Let us begin by thinking about the purposes of the Act. The name itself, the Patient Protection and Affordable Care Act, gives us a clue. The first part, patient protection, suggests three aspects. One is covering more people. The second is to provide patient protections such as coverage for pre-existing conditions and for certain procedures, such as maternity care. The third part suggests that implementation of the Act would create a situation where costs will be restrained, and the cost of insurance would be within reach of the population. A look at the evidence suggests a mixed picture, especially regarding costs.

Insurance Coverage

The biggest success of the ACA is extending health insurance coverage to a larger portion of the population. Figure 3.2 presents the data. As can be seen, with a few exceptions, the uninsured rate during the 1972–2010 period was in the 16–18 percent range. At the time of passage of the ACA, 2010, the uninsured rate was 18.2 percent of the population. We then saw a dramatic decline in the uninsured rate beginning in 2014. By the beginning of 2018, the uninsured rate was 10.3 percent.

Was this all due to the implementation of the Affordable Care Act? Probably not. The US experienced its worst recession since the Great Depression from 2007 to 2009. The economy was in a recovery mode by 2010. More people were finding work, and this generally leads to more people getting health insurance. But the slow recovery suggests that the ACA was largely responsible, through Medicaid expansion and the exchanges, for the dramatic decrease in the uninsured rate.

Looking at 2016, of the 76.1 million enrolled in Medicaid, 15.1 million were in the expansion group. Of those, almost 12 million were newly eligible enrollees. That is, they fell into the 100–138 percent of the federal poverty line created by the ACA ("Medicaid Expansion Enrollment" 2016). Buettgens (2018) estimates that if all states expanded Medicaid, as called for under the ACA, an additional 7.4 million people would be enrolled in Medicaid and about 2 million of those would be newly eligible. The uninsured rate would drop by about 16 percent in the expansion states and by over 25 percent in previously nonexpansion states (Buettgens 2018).

Now we look at the exchanges. Using 2018 data, about 11.8 million people signed up for the ACA exchanges in 2017. Nearly 74 percent of those enrolling were enrolled in the federal exchange (healthcare.gov) and the remaining in the state exchanges. Of those enrolling in 2017, 27 percent were new enrollees (Livingston 2018). The enrollment figures were good, but a bit down from the previous year. On the other hand, given attempts at suppressing enrollment, the numbers were pretty good. For 2019, enrollment was down about 4 percent from the 2018 period. Given the attempts by the Trump administration to undermine exchange enrollment, decline was fairly small (Pear 2018b).

If we compare the two expansion methods, Medicaid and the exchanges, we can see by the numbers that Medicaid expansion covered more people than in the exchanges. It is also cheaper to cover recipients of Medicaid than subscribers to the exchanges.

Glied, Stephanie and Borja (2017) find that Medicaid expansion and purchasing insurance on the exchanges increased access to healthcare (for a more detailed discussion of access issues, see Chapter 7), decreased the number of people who could not get care because of cost by 20–29 percent, and decreased the number of people without a usual source of care by about 47–86 percent (depending on the data source). Having insurance makes it more likely that people would be able to access the healthcare system.

The second part is the patient protections. This takes many forms. The most well-known is the ban on excluding people with pre-existing conditions from having insurance and from covering those pre-existing conditions. Chavez (2017) lists 36 conditions, a partial list that might not be covered under the American Health Care Act, one of the repeal-and-replace proposals briefly considered by Congress in 2017. One estimate is that about 27 percent of the under-65 population has a pre-existing condition (Chavez 2017; Claxton et al. 2016; Kliff 2017). This

Figure 3.2   **Uninsured Rate Among the Nonelderly Population, 1972–2018**

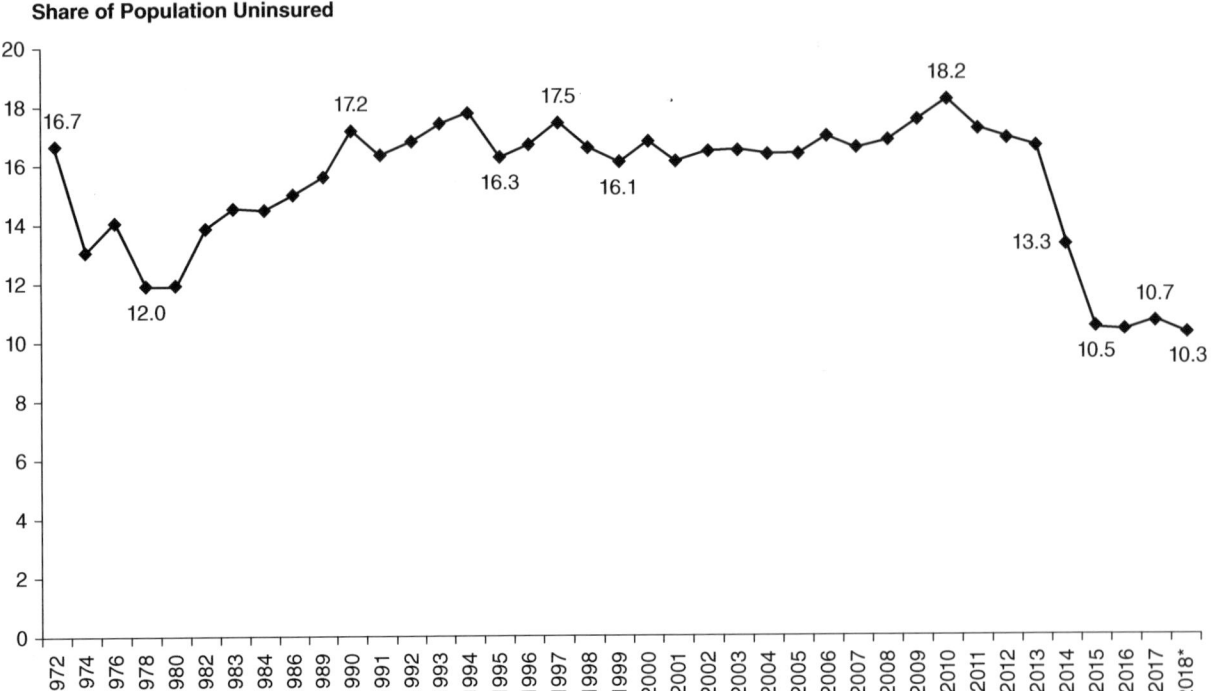

Source: Kaiser Family Foundation (2018).

amounts to an estimated 52 million people (Claxton et al. 2016). This is not to say that the pre-existing conditions would not be covered under a repeal-and-replace plan. Another possibility is that there may be limits placed on covering them and premiums might be higher for those with pre-existing conditions (Claxton et al. 2016).

Another, related, element focuses on women. It turns out that prior to the ACA, being a woman was a pre-existing condition. Health insurance companies engaged in "gender rating" (Grady 2010). Health insurance policies might not include coverage for maternity care, they might not cover women who had experienced domestic abuse, or who had Caesarean operations (Grady 2010). Women who did not smoke were charged more than men who did smoke. One reason health insurance companies charged women more was because women use the healthcare system more than men. Another problem is that there are small businesses, such as home healthcare, where women are major employees. Such businesses faced very high premiums for their workers and, therefore, did not offer health insurance as a premium (Grady 2010). The ACA changed all this.

Other patient protections included allowing children up to the age of 26 to remain on their parents' insurance and the ban on lifetime limits on how much a health insurance policy will pay out. All three are popular and the pre-existing conditions ban became one of the key issues in the 2018 mid-term elections, at least for Democrats.

The ACA has also made it easier for older people, aged 55–64, to afford insurance by limiting the age premium to three times that of younger people. Prior to the ACA, insurance companies could charge up to ten times as much as for younger people.

The problem here is that there has been very little evidence or research, apart from anecdotal evidence, as to how well these protections have worked. We can assume that more people got coverage because of this, but the evidence is limited.

Having said all that, we also know that the Affordable Care Act, even if it had been implemented without any glitches (an unlikely scenario) and without roadblocks set up by Republicans, would not have covered the entire population, despite statements by President Obama that it would (Robertson 2014). Robertson (2014) cites a Congressional Budget Office estimate that the ACA (and this was prior to the roadblocks) would leave an estimated 31 million people uninsured, leading to an uninsured rate of about 8 percent. The legislation contained provisions exempting people from the individual mandate (Robertson 2014):

> Some may choose to pay the tax penalty rather than buy insurance. Others may get an exemption from the requirement to have coverage. Those who make too little to file a tax return can be exempt, for instance, and the same is true for those who can't find affordable coverage—meaning if insurance would cost more than 8 percent of their household income. "Hardship" exemptions could be granted for several reasons, including bankruptcy, being a victim of domestic violence, a death in the family, unpaid medical bills, and having an individual market plan canceled and not finding "affordable" coverage among marketplace plans.

Also excluded from coverage under the ACA are undocumented immigrants. Whatever one thinks about the ACA, it does not and never was going to cover the entire population.

There is another aspect, related to the exchanges, that needs to be discussed. One of the advantages of the exchanges is that they are supposed to provide competition, which would then lead to constraints on costs (see the next section on healthcare costs and the ACA). Choosing among different plans, with different levels of premiums and cost-sharing, should lead, according to economic theory, to subscribers/consumers seeking out the lowest-cost plans that meet their needs. To do that, there actually needs to be competition, that is, several insurance companies offering plans. This is the idea behind the Massachusetts plan (the model for the ACA), Medicare Part D, and Medicare Advantage (see Chapter 5). But the instability and uncertainty in the market has led insurance companies to withdraw from many exchanges.

As a result, insurance companies were faced originally with more people needing healthcare than anticipated, which led to premium increases. More importantly, the instability and uncertainty led insurance companies to withdraw from the exchanges. Khazan (2017) and others (Corlette et al. 2018) point out that a significant number of counties, 31 percent, had only one insurer in the exchange, and 19 percent of enrollees lived in those counties. Another 31 percent of counties had two insurers, with 19 percent of enrollees. This is 2017 data. The 2016 data show much fewer counties with just one insurer (7 percent) and much fewer enrollees in those counties (2 percent). Data for 2018 again show a number of counties with just one insurer, with 2.9 million people living in such counties (Soffen and Uhrmacher 2017).

Khazan (2017) attributes the change to decisions by states about whether to expand Medicaid. Recall that the ACA expanded Medicaid coverage, subject to state determination, to up to 138 percent of the federal poverty level. In states that expanded Medicaid, those in the 100–138 percent of the federal poverty level were not eligible for subsides on the exchanges. But in those states that chose not to expand, this group was eligible for the exchange subsidies. This group made up about 40 percent of exchange enrollees in non-expansion states. For the expansion states, this group comprised only about 6 percent.

Khazan (2017) also notes that poorer people tend to be sicker than wealthier people. Therefore, their needs are more, causing more spending on the exchanges. It should also be pointed out that Medicaid spends less on its recipients than the subsidies that people get on the exchanges.

Finally, Khazan (2017) points out that many states allowed insurance plans to be sold that did not meet the demands of the Affordable Care Act. As a result, these plans were cheaper, though they were less likely to cover sick people. If someone on the plans got sick, they could go on the exchanges (during the enrollment period), thus, again, leaving the exchanges to cover a sicker population.

Affordable Care

The other major part of the ACA is costs. Here we get to the second part of the title of the legislation, Affordable Care. Affordable care has two parts. First, what has been the impact of the ACA on overall costs? Second, are people able to afford the premiums and cost-sharing that is part of health insurance? Note that here we are talking mainly about policies on the exchanges.

We know, as Chapter 8 discusses, that healthcare costs are high in the United States. They have taken up an increasing portion of our economy, as measured by gross domestic product (GDP). Healthcare costs have increased faster than the growth rate of the economy and the growth rate of wages.

As discussed in Chapter 8, yearly increases in healthcare expenditures have slowed. To what extent did the ACA contribute to that slowdown? We should note that we would expect healthcare expenditures to increase as insurance coverage increased as a result of the implementation of the ACA. That did happen in the first couple of years. But more recently the growth increases have slowed down. The ACA's impact on total expenditure increases seem to have been minimal (Hartman et al. 2018). Similarly, ten-year projections estimate that the ACA, if it should survive, would have little impact on increases in healthcare expenditures in the 2017–2026 period. Cuckler et al. (2018) argue that future healthcare expenditures will be affected by the "fundamentals": including increases in income, increases in prices, and the aging of the population.

The ACA contains some parts that address prices and overall expenditures, such as bundled payments and accountable care organizations. Both elements are experimental, mostly applying to Medicare, and, as discussed in Chapter 8, have had limited impact so far.

The other cost element is focused on the cost of insurance. Here the picture is mixed. The newness of the program, the instability of implementation, and the lower-than-expected number of healthy people enrolling led to significant increases in premiums on the exchanges (Medicaid has at most limited cost-sharing features; see Chapter 4). Increases were in the double digits, sometimes 30 percent or more. Most of the subscribers on the exchange saw little impact from the insurance premium increases because of the subsidies. As premiums rose, so did the subsidies. But it certainly meant higher expenses for the federal government, for the premium, cost-sharing, and reinsurance costs to insurance companies. It is clear that for some people, the cost of insurance on the exchanges was more than they could handle. This is especially true of those at the higher income levels not eligible for subsidies.

Looking at 2016 figures, average premiums for the bronze (lowest premium) plans on the federal exchanges increased an average of 16 percent over the previous year. The highest increase was in Arkansas, at 46 percent. For the popular silver plans, the average increase was 13 percent, with the highest increase in Oklahoma, at 44 percent (Pearson 2015). Significant price increases continued into 2018 (Mangan 2017b). The average price of the silver plan rose by 34 percent. The highest increase was in Iowa, with a 69-percent increase. The monthly premium for the Iowa silver plan was just over $1,000 (Mangan 2017b). Again, most people on the exchanges saw small increases because of the subsidies. Those who purchased plans on the exchanges without the subsidies (about 20 percent) were faced with paying the full costs. The two major factors leading to high exchange premium increases were uncertainties in the market and the decision by the Trump administration to end the reinsurance payments to insurance companies to provide cheaper policies (Mangan 2017b).

Given the previous very high increases and Trump's efforts to undermine the exchanges discussed above, it was very surprising that the increases for 2019 were exceptionally modest (Sloan, Carpenter, and Brooker 2018). Average premiums were projected to rise by only 3.1 percent and in some cases premiums declined. The reason was more stability in the market.

Criticisms of the Affordable Care Act

Early complaints about the ACA focused on the awkward implementation of the federal exchanges, a problem that has largely, though not entirely, been resolved. A second complaint revolved around some of the claims that President Obama made in 2009. One was that if you liked your health insurance policy, you could keep it. A similar one was that if you liked your doctor, you could keep him or her (Gore 2017). Both were promises or claims that the president probably should not have made. Many health insurance plans did not meet the requirements of the new legislation. Employers would change plans to get better deals. Health plans created narrow networks of providers to control costs and a patient's favorite physician might not be in the new list of providers for the patient's plan (Gore 2017).

Another criticism of the ACA was that for some the available health insurance plans were too expensive. This would include both premiums and cost-sharing. People with these complaints either did not buy insurance on the exchanges (and thus were not eligible for the subsidies) or their incomes were too high (above 400 percent of the federal poverty line) to qualify for assistance. One analysis suggests that there were over 17 million people purchasing individual insurance, both on and off the exchanges. Of those, 5.4 million purchased insurance outside of the exchange and nearly 2 million bought health insurance on the exchange. The total of these was about 43 percent of those purchasing non-group plans (Mangan 2017a; Rovner 2017).

Rovner (2017) provides a couple of examples of two couples with problems paying for insurance. The first couple paid a $15,000 a year in premiums and had deductibles for both partners of $6,550. Thus, this couple paid about $30,000 before their health insurance company would pay anything. A second couple faced premiums of almost $20,000 a year plus $7,500 deductible for each partner. This second couple decided to go without health insurance.

Most of the critiques of the Affordable Care Act, not surprisingly, came from the conservative side of the ideological spectrum. Goodman (2015) is a good example of this. He discusses six major problems with the ACA.

The first has to do with costs. Goodman writes that the ACA did not create the cost problem, but it is unable to alleviate it. Indeed, he argues, the ACA will make it worse. The ACA does this in two ways. First, it makes it difficult to pick a less costly health insurance package that would have fewer benefits and more cost-sharing. The second way, he notes, is that the ACA limits spending growth of Medicare, Medicaid, and the tax subsidies. That means that if healthcare costs continue in their upward path, the federal government will not be able to help as much.

Goodman's second complaint is that the subsidies are unfair. He gives us two examples of families making about the same amount of money. In the first case, the family might be eligible for Medicaid (he assumes the family makes just under 138 percent of the federal poverty level). If they make a bit more, they could buy insurance on the exchange and get tax subsidies for premiums and cost-sharing. His second example is a hotel employee who has to buy an expensive plan offered by her employer and does not get help from the federal government. But Goodman goes further. He argues that the subsidies hurt small businesses. For example, they would not have to provide health insurance to part-time employees and, therefore, have an incentive to hire such employees, or perhaps utilize contract workers.

The third problem is what Goodman (2015) labels as "perverse incentives for insurers." Here Goodman refers to the requirement not to charge more for people with pre-existing conditions. Everyone has to pay the same amount for insurance. The incentive, then, is to seek the healthy and try to avoid the sick. To make the plans attractive (less costly), insurers create narrow networks of providers and, often, do not include the best providers. There are incentives for buyers/purchasers of insurance to search for plans that have the best providers in the event they become sick.

The fourth problem, which given the tax legislation enacted in December 2017 mentioned above no longer applies, is that the mandate is weak. The tax is small relative to the cost of insurance, and hard to collect.

The fifth problem is lack of access. The ACA, Goodman (2015) asserts, increases the demand for healthcare, because much of the cost is covered by the plan and subsidies. Given the shortage of doctors, this would hurt access to care and certainly increase waiting times. Goodman (2015) notes that with the implementation of the ACA (Medicaid expansion and exchanges), there has not been a concomitant increase in doctor visits (sort of contradicting the point made just above). What there has been was an increase in visits to emergency rooms and urgent care centers for those newly on Medicaid (Goodman 2015). This is likely for two reasons. First, many of those newly on Medicaid did not have an established relationship with a family practitioner or a usual source of care. There is also a shortage of physicians and getting in to see a doctor and establish that relationship may take time. Second, going to the emergency room is a faster to way be seen and one that many of those newly on Medicaid are used to and comfortable with. Goodman (2015) correctly points out that the expansion is likely to put additional stress on already overcrowded (and expensive) emergency rooms.

The final criticism of the ACA by Goodman (2015) is that much of the savings in the ACA will come from cuts in Medicare spending. This would include cuts to providers and to Medicare Advantage plans (see Chapter 5 for a discussion of these plans). Provider reimbursement in Medicare is lower than what private insurance pays (and what individuals without insurance are charged), but higher than Medicaid. If provider reimbursements are cut, Goodman (2015) argues, then providers will be reluctant to take on Medicare patients, just as there is reluctance to take on any, or take on too many, Medicaid patients.

Turner et al. (2011, 24), arguing many of the same points as Goodman, provide a list of the portions of the ACA that they do not like:

1. federal mandates on individuals
2. federal mandates on employers
3. expanding federal entitlements
4. squeezing funds out of Medicare and choking off private plan choices
5. new federal taxes
6. health insurance exchanges
7. federal government-sponsored health plans
8. federal control over private insurance

What becomes clear is that their main criticism of the ACA is the expansion of federal government power over the healthcare system. Some of the features mentioned, such as federal taxes and employer mandates, have been subsequently reduced or repealed. And there are other elements of the ACA that they do not mention but are subsumed in the last point above: patient protections. This is, as we have seen, a very important part of the Affordable Care Act, perhaps the most popular.

Silver and Hyman (2018) provide one of the more interesting critiques of the ACA. First, they critique the US healthcare system. The write that the ACA should have addressed the following problems:

> Open-ended reimbursement for patented pharmaceuticals, regardless of price. Excessive use of medical treatments. Providers' conflicts of interest. The routine delivery of ineffective and unproven treatments. Games that providers play to maximize their revenues. Charges that bear no relation to costs. Surprise bills and other out-of-network rip-offs. Widespread quality problems tied to dysfunctional business models. Political corruption. And an ocean of fraud.
>
> (Silver and Hyman 2018, 272)

From their perspective, the major accomplishment of the ACA was to expand coverage, but in a way that increased spending. But for Silver and Hyman (2018), the Affordable Care Act failed to deal with the major problems of the American healthcare system. The major difficulty of that system, according to Silver and Hyman (2018), is that insurance covers so much of the expenses that no one really cares about the costs and the incentives in the system are cost-increasing. For example, the ACA does not address the cost of prescription medications. As we discussed earlier in this chapter, the ACA was better at expanding access to insurance than to controlling cost. That is Silver's and Hyman's main point.

CONCLUSION

> It was big—the most ambitious effort in recent decades to reorganize a major institution on a basis that agrees more closely with principles of justice and efficiency. Yet it was also comparatively limited—compared, that is, with the healthcare systems of other democracies or to the ideal remedies that many reluctant supporters of the legislation would have preferred.
> This is the puzzle of the Affordable Care Act. It calls for major changes, but it is also notable for what it leaves unchanged. After four decades of rising inequality and insecurity, it provides a major boost to the living standards of low-wage workers and their families and increases economic protection for the middle class. The central thrust of the law is to change how health insurance works and to make it affordable, though it also includes measures to improve the quality of medical care and control its costs. But the law does not substantially alter how medical care is organized, and it may not change the long-term trajectory of health spending. Most Americans with secure, employment-based insurance will see little different in their own coverage or healthcare.
>
> (Starr 2013, 239)

The attempt at comprehensive healthcare reform was seemingly like the Hundred Years' War (1337–1453) between England and France. Presidents and members of Congress spent decades trying to rationalize the American healthcare system, making it more efficient, controlling costs, and covering more people. While we made a series of incremental steps (such as the development of private health insurance, the passage of Medicare, Medicaid, and the CHIP), the development of the healthcare system made it difficult to make substantial changes without invoking opposition from various groups. This is the path-dependency argument. Once we took a particular direction, it was very hard to move in a different direction. This is the argument, using slightly different language, that Starr (2013) makes, referring to the policy trap of incremental healthcare policymaking.

What are we to make of the Affordable Care Act? There are many perspectives from which to view the ACA. Earlier in this chapter, we briefly examined the four major types of healthcare systems, following Reid (2010): Bismarck, Beveridge, national health insurance, and out-of-pocket models. The authors of the ACA chose to pick none of the above and stay with our hybrid, fragmented system. The focus of the ACA was on limiting the out-of-pocket model. The legislation is mostly insurance reform, providing additional access to people who did not have health insurance and patient protections (patient's bill of rights) for the entire population.

A second perspective is public opinion. For most of the period since the passage of the Affordable Care Act, a majority of the public was opposed to it (Kaiser Family Foudnation 2018). By April 2017, a plurality of the public favored the ACA. This was due to attempts to repeal and replace it on the part of congressional Republicans. As indicated throughout this chapter, there is a considerable partisan divide in thinking about the ACA; 73 percent of Democrats approved of the ACA, while the same percentage of Republicans had an unfavorable view of the legislation (these are October 2018 data) (Kaiser Family Foundation 2018). There is also a difference in approval ratings by race and ethnicity. For whites, 50 percent disapproved the act, while 43 percent approved. For blacks, 70 percent approved; for Hispanics, 55 percent approved (Kaiser Family Foundation 2018).

A third perspective, just mentioned above, is the partisanship one, and it combines with an institutional perspective. Other major legislative achievements, such as Medicare, Medicaid, Social Security, welfare reform, and the Bush-era tax cuts, had some support from both Republicans and Democrats. The ACA was not so fortunate.

Recall that in 1993–1994, Republicans, who were in the minority in both houses of Congress, opposed any kind of healthcare reform that could be attributable to the Democrats and the Clinton administration. This played out again in 2009 and 2010, and in the aftermath of enactment. Republicans, as Mann and Ornstein (2016) observed, acted pretty much in unison against healthcare reform. There were attempts on the part of Senate Democrats and the Obama administration to work with Republicans. Some of the changes to the legislation were the result of these attempts. Max Baucus (D-MT), the chair of the Senate Finance Committee, convened the gang of six (three Democrats including Baucus and three Republicans) to negotiate a compromise. In the end, not unexpectedly, the negotiations failed. But they did serve one purpose: they delayed action in the Senate. Had Senate Democrats, seeing that there would be no support from Republicans, moved ahead with their filibuster-proof majority, Congress would likely have passed a bill in 2009 rather than go through the convoluted process it went through in 2010. We should also note that none of the attempts to repeal and replace the ACA had any Democratic support. Clearly, partisanship was the perspective through which many viewed the legislation (Shaw 2017). As Shaw (2017) put it, the partisanship surrounding the ACA was dysfunctional.

It should also be noted that much of the Affordable Care Act relies on ideas that originated with Republicans—these include the individual mandate and the exchanges. An analysis of the legislation found that in the Senate "More than one-fourth of the linked ideas are found in bills sponsored by Republicans" (Wilkerson, Smith, and Stramp 2013, 25; Krugman 2011). The notion that Republicans had no input into the Affordable Care Act is not accurate. Shaw (2017) tells us that over a period of time, Republicans rejected ideas that they once championed.

The fourth perspective is the related institutional factor. In 1993, two political scientists, Sven Steinmo and Jon Watts, presented a paper, later published in 1995 (Steinmo and Watts 1995), predicting the failure of the Clinton administration effort. The title of the paper was "It's the Institutions, Stupid!" (a play on the internal Clinton 1992 campaign motto to focus on the economy, "It's the economy, stupid!"). Their argument was that the institutional barriers, particularly in the Senate, would prove insurmountable. Despite majorities in both houses of Congress in 1993–1994, Democrats could barely move the legislation. While Republican resistance was certainly responsible for the policy failure during the Clinton administration, the Democrats also share some blame. There was disagreement within the party about the Clinton plan or any other plan. Thus, there was no majority that supported healthcare reform.

Though comprehensive healthcare reform did pass in 2010, those institutional barriers remained difficult, though not impossible, to hurdle. In both 1993–1994 and 2009–2010, Republicans sought any means possible to thwart healthcare reform legislation. Part of the difficulty of getting anything passed was that in 2009–2010, as in the earlier period, most of the difficult negotiations occurred within the Democratic Party. Combine that with the need to get 60 votes in favor of reform, and the results were deals (Cornhusker Kickback, Louisiana Purchase) and unorthodox lawmaking (Sinclair 2012), such as the use of the reconciliation procedure, the absence of conference committees, and one house accepting what the other did (ping-pong).

The result of all this was legislation that pleased no one completely. Starr (2013) and Altman and Shactman (2011) assert that the Affordable Care Act was about as good as could be gotten from Congress. This sentiment is most picturesquely captured by Jacob Hacker. In 1997, Hacker published a book entitled *The Road to Nowhere* on the effort of the Clinton administration to pass the Health Security Act. During the subsequent debates beginning in 2007, Hacker advocated a more public role in the healthcare system, suggesting, first, that we use Medicare as the model, and then pushing for the public option in the exchanges. After the ACA was passed, he published an article (Hacker 2010) exploring why comprehensive healthcare reform passed this time but expressing some unhappiness with the outcome. The article was entitled "The Road to Somewhere." And these were supporters of the law.

The institutional and political problems that made passage of the Affordable Care Act so difficult also impeded any efforts to improve it. House Republicans have spent a considerable amount of time trying to repeal it. By May 2013, the House attempted to repeal the ACA 37 times (Mahar 2013). Most complex pieces of legislation have required subsequent changes to fix problems or make needed changes. As Weisman and Pear write:

> But as they prowl Capitol Hill, business lobbyists like Mr. DeFife, healthcare providers and others seeking changes are finding, to their dismay, that in a polarized Congress, accomplishing them has become all but impossible.
> Republicans simply want to see the entire law go away and will not take part in adjusting it. Democrats are petrified of reopening a politically charged law that threatens to derail careers as the Republicans once again seize on it before an election year.
> As a result, a landmark law that almost everyone agrees has flaws is likely to take effect unchanged.
> (Weisman and Pear 2013)

Klein (2013c) argues that the kind of gridlock described above effectively means that Congress defaults policymaking to other elements of government, such as an agency or a court or the president. Those other bodies may not be as accountable as Congress. Klein writes, "Gridlock doesn't mean nothing moves. It means that American policy ends up taking some very unusual detours" (2013c). As we saw, the Trump administration made a number of moves to undermine the ACA.

The fifth perspective is elections. The 2018 mid-term elections could have proved fatal to the Affordable Care Act. If the Republicans had retained control of the House and increased their majority in the Senate, further attempts to legislatively repeal the ACA would have taken place. To some extent, the 2018 mid-term elections were a referendum on the ACA. They could also be seen as a referendum on the Trump administration.

The results of the mid-terms were mixed. The turnout was exceptional for a mid-term election, with perhaps double the turnout from the previous mid-term (2014) and comparable to presidential elections, in some places over 60 percent of eligible voters. The concern that Republican repeal-and-replace plans would leave those with pre-existing conditions uncovered was considered an important issue, at least for Democrats. The 2018 elections showed that it was an impact, but not a decisive one, particularly in the Senate races (Rovner 2018).

The results of the 2018 election were that Republicans retained control of the Senate, gaining three seats, Democrats regained control of the House, picking up nearly 40 seats, and Democrats picked up seven governorships. We should note that, as in 2016, more people voted for Democratic House candidates than voted for Republican House candidates, a difference of nearly 9 million votes, greater than the difference in vote between Donald Trump and Hillary Clinton in 2016 (about 3 million in favor of Clinton). But the distribution of voters, as in 2016, favored Republicans. The importance of these results, from an ACA standpoint, is that attempts to legislatively replace and repeal the ACA will not pass the new Democratically controlled House. It is also possible, though not very likely, that the two parties will cooperate to make improvements/changes in the ACA. The elections also saw voter approval in several states for expanding Medicaid. Democratic gubernatorial victories might also mean Medicaid expansion in states, such as Kansas, that had refused to expand the program (Rovner 2018).

The Affordable Care Act still faces some threats. One is from the Trump administration. It has sought various ways to undermine the ACA, with some success. Another threat stems from the 2017 tax legislation, which repealed the individual mandate, the most unpopular part of the ACA. There is a question of how the repeal will affect enrollment in the exchanges. More importantly, the repeal immediately led to a court suits by state attorneys general that the ACA, without the individual mandate, is unconstitutional. *Texas v. Azar* (2018) will work its way up through the federal court system, likely appearing on the Supreme Court docket for the 2019–2020 term. It should be noted that President Trump nominated, and the Senate confirmed, two new US Supreme Court justices, Neil Garland and Brett Kavanaugh. It is not clear how they will vote, but it is clear that the Court, with those two additions, has become more conservative.

The final threat is the 2020 elections. A Republican wave, a second term for Donald Trump, would mean a renewed assault on the ACA.

Republicans remain opposed to the Affordable Care Act. This is pictured in a May 14, 2013 editorial cartoon by Steve Sacks for the *Minneapolis Star Tribune*. It shows an angry elephant (the symbol of the Republican Party) in the shower washing its head. The shampoo is "Repeal Obamacare Shampoo" and the directions read: "1) Work yourself into lather. 2) Rinse. 3) Repeat. And repeat. And repeat …" The caption of the cartoon is "Gonna Wash that Law Right Out of My Hair?" The October 2013 partial government shutdown was at least to some extent due to attempts to defund/repeal the ACA. The continuing attacks and the incremental nature of policymaking were nicely captured by Secretary of State George Schultz in 1986:

Nothing ever gets settled in this town. It's not like running a company or a university. It's a seething debating society in which the debate never stops, in which people never give up, including me, and that's the atmosphere in which you administer.

(quoted in Apple 1986)

Republicans, for the most part, prefer smaller government, lower taxes, and less regulation. Their opposition to the ACA is to the expansion of the federal role, what they call a "government takeover." This was on top of the financial bailout and large federal deficits that were the result of the Great Depression (Rushefsky 2013).

One interesting question that can and has been raised is what Trump supporters want to see in a healthcare plan. In late 2016 (Altman 2017), the Kaiser Family Foundation brought together six focus groups from the industrial Midwest, members of whom were all unhappy with the Affordable Care Act. The members of the groups complained about the ACA and also were skeptical of some Republican plans, including those with health savings accounts, tax credits, and high deductibles (see Chapter 11). There were elements of a healthcare plan that they wanted (Altman 2017).

If these Trump voters could write a health plan, it would, many said, focus on keeping their out-of-pocket costs low, control drug prices and improve access to cheaper drugs. It would also address consumer issues many had complained about loudly, including eliminating surprise medical bills for out-of-network care, assuring the adequacy of provider networks and making their insurance much more understandable.

To the extent that Republicans have a healthcare policy, it would include the following elements (Klein 2013a).

1. They want to end the tax bias in favor of employer-sponsored health insurance to create full portability (either through a tax credit, deductibility, or another method).
2. They want to reform medical malpractice laws (likely through carrot incentives to the states).
3. They want to allow for insurance purchases across state lines.
4. They want to support state-level pre-existing-condition pools.
5. They want to fully block-grant Medicaid.
6. They want to shift Medicare to premium support.
7. They want to speed up the FDA device and drug approval process.
8. They want to maximize the health savings account model, one of the few avenues proved to lower healthcare spending, making these high deductible and HSA plans more attractive where Obamacare hamstrung them.

Questions can be raised as to whether the plan would cover much of the population and whether it would control costs, but it does represent an alternative vision to the Affordable Care Act. Whether it meets the desires of Trump supporters is an interesting question.

Another way to judge the Affordable Care Act is the extent to which it "bends the cost curve." If healthcare costs and insurance premiums continue to rise at a rapid rate, then the ACA will be labeled a failure. As we shall see in Chapter 8, in recent years cost increases have diminished. Some of that is due to the severe recession and the slow recovery. But at least some may be due to the ACA. Klein (2013b) suggests that the ACA will result in a reduction in cost increases.

We argue that there are two major problems with the Affordable Care Act, apart from arguments by those who oppose the legislation or any kind of healthcare reform or larger government role. First, the legislation leaves in place a very fragmented system. While there are provisions in the Act that seek systemic changes, those changes are modest at best. It leaves in place much of what Michael Reagan (1999) calls "The Accidental System." The four types of healthcare systems that Reid (2010) discusses pretty much remain unexplored in the US. We understand that the ACA was a product of a difficult political process. Even supporters recognize that it was not what they wanted, and there are weaknesses that may be addressed in subsequent years.

The other, related, problem, discussed in some detail in this chapter, is the federal nature of the Affordable Care Act (Beland, Rocco, and Waddan 2016). It is not just that it requires states to do much of the heavy lifting in implementing the program (state health exchanges and Medicaid expansion, among others), but there is both opposition in many of the states to implementation and, equally as important, states will differ in how they shape their policies even when cooperating. Thus, it will continue to be the case that there really is no such thing as an

American healthcare system, but a set of systems, differing by geography and category (employer-insured, Medicare, Medicaid, etc.). A national system would have been easier to implement and simpler. But American exceptionalism suggests that we work within the time-honored constitutional principle of federalism.

The Affordable Care Act has already changed or evolved. Some of the changes came about because they simply could not work. Some have come about as a result of actions by Republicans. The question remains as to the future of the legislation: fix, repeal, replace. It may take the aftermath of the 2020 elections before we will know for sure.

STUDY QUESTIONS

1. There is an old saying that there are two things that one should never watch being made—one is sausage and the other is legislation. In what ways does the passage of the Affordable Care Act look like sausage making? Why were unorthodox congressional procedures utilized in getting the ACA passed?
2. The failed attempt at comprehensive reform during the Clinton administration provided lessons learned by the Obama administration and congressional Democrats in 2009 and 2010. What were those lessons?
3. What do you see as the strengths of the Affordable Care Act? What do you see as its weaknesses? Explain your answer. To what extent are answers to these questions influenced by ideology?
4. The most controversial part of the Affordable Care Act is the mandate that everyone purchase insurance. Why was this included in the legislation? Why was it so controversial? Do you agree with the mandate? Why or why not?
5. Since the passage of the Affordable Care Act, Republicans have continually tried to either repeal it in full or defund it. Why do they continually do this?
6. A number of states have refused to expand Medicaid and/or set up their own health exchanges. Why is that the case? What are the impacts of the refusal to participate?
7. The chapter notes that other countries have adopted national health insurance systems and have controlled costs better than the United States. Yet none of the policies adopted by these countries were adopted here or even seriously considered. Why not?
8. Why did the Obama administration succeed in passing comprehensive health reform when all previous efforts had failed?
9. In what ways did increased partisanship shape the Affordable Care Act?
10. In what ways does increased partisanship affect the ability to improve the Affordable Care Act?

REFERENCES

Alonso-Zaldivar, Ricardo. 2013. "Fallout for States Rejecting Medicaid Expansion." Associated Press, April 22. Online at http://bigstory.ap.org/article/fallout-states-rejecting-medicaid-expansion.
Altman, Drew. 2017. "Can We Learn from ACA Implementation and Improve the Law?" Menlo Park, CA: Kaiser Family Foundation. Online at http://kff.org/health-reform/perspective/can-we-learn-from-aca-implementation-and-improve-the-law/.
Altman, Stuart and David Shactman. 2011. *Power, Politics, and Universal Health Care: The inside Story of a Century-Long Battle*. Amherst, NY: Prometheus.
America's Health Insurance Plans. 2006. *We Believe Every American Should Have Access to Affordable Health Care Coverage: A Vision for Reform*. Washington, DC: America's Health Insurance Plans.
America's Health Insurance Plans. 2007. *Guaranteed Access to Coverage for All Americans*. Washington, DC: America's Health Insurance Plans.
Anderson, Steve. 2013. "Federal Reform: High-Risk Insurance Pools." Healthinsurance.org. Online at www.healthinsurance.org.
Apple, R. W., Jr. 1986. "A Lesson from Shultz." *The New York Times*, December 9.
Arensmeyer, John. 2018. "Buyer Beware of Association Health Plans." *The Hill*, July 25.
Baker, Peter. 2012. "Democrats Embrace Once Pejorative 'Obamacare' Tag." *The New York Times*, August 3.
Barnes, Julie et al. 2012. *Primer: Understanding the Effect of the Supreme Court Ruling on the Patient Protection and Affordable Care Act*. Washington, DC: Bipartisan Policy Center.
Baucus, Max. 2008. *Call to Action: Health Reform 2009*. Washington, DC: US Senate Finance Committee.
Beaussier, Anne-Laure. 2012. "The Patient Protection and Affordable Care Act: The Victory of Unorthodox Lawmaking." *Journal of Health Politics, Policy and Law*, 37, no. 5 (October): 741–778.
Beland, Daniel, Philip Rocco, and Alex Waddan. 2016. *Obamacare Wars: Federalism, State Politics, and the Affordable Care Act*. Lawrence, KS: University of Kansas Press.
Bernasek, Anna. 2013. "Why a Health Insurance Penalty May Look Tempting." *The New York Times*, June 22.

Berry, Jeffrey M. and Sarah Sobieraj. 2014. *The Outrage Industry: Political Opinion Media and the New Incivility.* New York: Oxford University Press.

Boxer, Sarah. 1995. "Word for Word/Sweetening the Bitter Pill; How a Republican Should Break Bad News to Grandma." *The New York Times*, September 17.

Brownstein, Ronald and Stephanie Czekalinski 2013. "Altered States." *National Journal*, 45, no. 15 (April 13): 12–21.

Buettgens, Matthew. 2018. *The Implications of Medicaid Expansion in the Remaining States: 2018 Update.* Washington, DC: Urban Institute.

Campo-Flores, Arian. 2013. "GOP Clashes Stymie Medicaid Expansion." *The Wall Street Journal*, May 2.

Cantril, Albert H. and Susan Davis Cantril. 1999. *Reading Mixed Signals: Ambivalence in American Public Opinion about Government.* Washington, DC: Woodrow Wilson Center Press.

Capretta, James C. and Kevin D. Dayaratna. 2013. "Compelling Evidence Makes the Case for a Market-Driven Health Care System." *Heritage Foundation Backgrounder*, no. 2867 (December 20).

Carlson, Joe. 2014. "Obamacare Legal Battle Threatens Subsidies for Millions." *Modern Healthcare*, June 14.

Cauchi, Richard. 2018. "State Roles Using 1332 Health Waivers." Washington, DC: National Conference of State Legislators, October 22. Online at www.ncsl.org.

Chavez, Nicole. 2017. "Here's a (Partial) List of All the Pre-Existing Conditions the GOP Bill May Not Cover." CNN, May 6.

Claxton, Gary et al. 2012. *Employer Health Benefits 2012 Annual Survey.* Menlo Park, CA: Henry J. Kaiser Family Foundation, and Chicago, IL: Health Research and Educational Trust.

Claxton, Gary et al. 2016. *Pre-Existing Conditions and Medical Underwriting in the Individual Insurance Market Prior to the ACA.* Menlo Park, CA: Kaiser Family Foundation.

Claxton, Gary et al. 2017. *Employer Health Benefits 2017 Annual Survey.* Menlo Park, CA and Chicago, IL: Henry J. Kaiser Family Foundation, and Health Research and Education Trust.

Clemente, Frank. 2009. *A Public Health Insurance Plan: Reducing Costs and Improving Quality.* Washington, DC: Institute for American's Future.

Cohn, Jonathan. 2007. *Sick: The Untold Story of America's Health Care Crisis–And the People Who Pay the Price.* New York: Harper Collins.

Congressional Budget Office. 2017a. *Cost Estimate: H.R. 1628: Better Care Reconciliation Act of 2017.* Washington, DC: Congressional Budget Office.

Congressional Budget Office. 2017b. *Preliminary Analysis of Legislation that Would Replace Subsidies for Health Care for Block Grants.* Washington, DC: Congressional Budget Office.

Corlette, Sabrina et al. 2018. *Insurers Remaining in Affordable Care Markets Prepare for Continued Uncertainty in 2018, 2019.* Washington, DC: Urban Institute.

Cuckler, Gigi A. et al. 2018. "National Health Care Expenditure Projections, 2017–26: Despite Uncertainty, Fundamentals Primarily Drive Spending Growth." *Health Affairs*, 37, no. 3 (March): 482–492.

Davidson, Stephen M. 2010. *Still Broken: Understanding the U.S. Health Care System.* Stanford, CA: Stanford Business Books.

Davis, Karen and Cathy Schoen. 2008. "Using What Works: Medicare, Medicaid, and the State Children's Health Insurance Program as a Base for Health Care Reform." Invited testimony before the House Committee on Energy and Commerce, Subcommittee on Health Hearing on "America's Need for Health Reform." September 18. Washington, DC: Commonwealth Fund.

Dews, Fred. 2013. "Chart: A Recent History of Senate Cloture Votes Taken to End Filibusters." Washington, DC: The Brookings Institution. Online at www.brookings.edu/blogs/brookings-now/posts/2013/11/chart-recent-history-of-senate-cloture-votes-to-end-filibusters#.

Ellement, John. 2018. "Here's Why Experts Say the Judge in the ACA Case Went Too Far." *Boston Globe*, December 18.

Fehr, Rachel, Cynthia Cox, and Larry Levitt. 2018. *Individual Insurance Market Performance in Mid-2018.* Menlo Park, CA: Kaiser Family Foundation.

Fernandez, Bernadette and Annie L. Mach. 2013. *Health Insurance Exchanges under the Patient Protection and Affordable Care Act (ACA).* Washington, DC: Congressional Research Service.

Fielder, Matthew and Loren Adler. 2017. *How Will the Graham-Cassidy Proposal Affect the Number of People with Health Insurance Coverage.* Washington, DC: The Brookings Institution.

Fried, Charles. 2013. "The June Surprises: Balls, Strikes, and the Fog of War." *Journal of Health Politics, Policy and Law*, 38, no. 2 (April): 225–241.

Galewitz, Phil. 2013. "NFL's Help Sought on Promoting Obamacare Insurance Plans." *Kaiser Health News*, June 24.

Galewitz, Phil and Julie Appleby. 2018. "Obamacare Premiums Dip for First Time. Some Call It a Correction." *Kaiser Health News*, October 11.

Galewitz, Phil and Jenny Gold. 2011. "HHS Releases Final Regulations for ACOs." *Kaiser Health News*, October 20.

Garfield, Rachel, Anthony Damico, and Kendal Orgera. 2018. *The Coverage Gap: Uninsured Poor Adults in States that Do Not Expand Medicaid.* Menlo Park, CA: Kaiser Family Foundation.

Gillespie, Lisa. 2016. "Kynect No More: Bevin's Move to Federal Exchange Approved." Online at www.wpfl.org.

Glickman, Howard. 2011. "Requiem for the CLASS Act." *Health Affairs*, 30, no. 12 (December): 2231–2234.

Glied, Sherry, Ma Stephanie, and Anaïs A. Borja. 2017. *Effect of the Affordable Care Act on Health Care Access.* New York: The Commonwealth Fund.

Gold, Jenny. 2013. "A Shorter Exchange Application, But Is It Simpler?" *Kaiser Health News*, April 30.

Goodman, John. 2015. "Six Problems with the ACA that Aren't Going Away." *Health Affairs*, June 25.

Goodman, John C. 2012. *Priceless: Curing the Healthcare Crisis.* Oakland, CA: The Independent Institute.

Goodnough, Abby and Jan Hoffman. 2018. "A New Lawsuit Threatens Obamacare. Here's What's at Stake and What to Expect in Oral Arguments." *The New York Times*, September 4.

Gore, D'Angelo. 2017. "Keeping Your Health Plan." *FactCheck.org*, November 11.

Grady, Denise. 2010. "Overhaul Will Lower the Costs of Being a Woman." *The New York Times*, March 29.

Grassley, Chuck. 2009. "Health Reform–A Republican View." *Health Affairs*, 361, no. 25 (December 17): 2397–2399.

Haberkorn, Jennifer. 2013. "Liberty University Pivots in Health Law Challenge." Politico, May 17. Online at www.politico.com.

Hacker, Jacob S. 2006. *The Great Risk Shift: The Assault on American Jobs, Families, Health Care, and Retirement and How You Can Fight Back*. New York: Oxford University Press.

Hacker, Jacob S. 2007. *Health Care for America: A Proposal for Guaranteed, Affordable Health Care for All Americans: Building on Medicare and Employment-Based Insurance*. Washington, DC: Economic Policy Institute, January 11.

Hacker, Jacob S. 2009. *The Case for Public Plan Choice in National Health Reform*. Washington, DC: Institute for America's Future.

Hacker, Jacob S. 2010. "The Road to Somewhere: Why Health Reform Happened." *Perspectives on Politics*, 8, no. 3 (September): 861–876.

Hall, Jean P. and Janice M. Moore. 2012. *Realizing Health Reform's Potential*. Washington, DC: Commonwealth Fund.

Hall, Mark A. 2013. "Health Care Law Versus Constitutional Law." *Journal of Health Politics, Policy and Law*, 38, no. 2 (April): 267–272.

Hancock, Jay. 2013. "The Arkansas Medicaid Model: What You Need to Know about the 'Private Option.'" *Kaiser Health News*, May 1.

Hartman, Micah et al. 2018. "National Health Care Spending in 2016: Spending and Enrollment Growth Slow after Initial Coverage Expansions." *Health Affairs*, 37, no. 1 (January): 150–160.

Hastings, Douglas. 2011. "The Medicare ACO Proposed Rule: Legal Structure, Governance, and Regulatory Sections." *HealthAffairs Blog*, April 5. Online at http://healthaffairs.org/blog/2011/04/05/the-medicare-aco-proposed-rule-legal-structure-governance-and-regulatory-sections/.

Health Care for Americans Now. 2013. *Anti-Obamacare States Try to Throw Navigators Off-Course*. Washington, DC: Health Care for Americans Now.

Herzlinger, Regina. 2007. *Who Killed Health Care? America's $2 Trillion Medical Problem–And the Consumer-Driven Cure*. New York: McGraw-Hill.

Hess, Jeffrey. 2013. "Political Fight Jeopardizes Mississippi's Entire Medicaid Program." *Kaiser Health News*, June 22.

"High Court Ends Liberty University Lawsuit over ObamaCare." Fox News, December 2. Online at www.foxnews.com/politics/2013/12/02/high-court-ends-liberty-u-lawsuit-over-health-law/.

Hillary for President. 2008. "The American Health Choices Plan." Hillary for President. Online at www.hillaryclinton.com.

Holohan, John et al. 2012. *The Cost and Coverage Implications of the ACA Medicaid Expansion: National and State-by-State Analysis*. Washington, DC: Kaiser Commission on Medicaid and the Uninsured.

"House GOP Expands Investigation of Sebelius' ACA Donation Requests." 2013. *California Healthline*, May 28. Online at www.californiahealthline.org.

Jacobs, Lawrence R. and Theda Skocpol. 2010. *Health Care Reform and American Politics: What Everyone Needs to Know*. New York: Oxford University Press.

Johnson, Toni. 2012. *Healthcare Costs and U.S. Competitiveness: Backgrounder*. Washington, DC: Council on Foreign Relations, March 26.

Jost, Timothy. 2017. "The Tax Bill and the Individual Mandate: What Happened, and What Does It Mean?" *Health Affairs*, December 20.

Kaiser Family Foundation. 2008. *Kaiser Health Tracking Poll: Election 2008*. Menlo Park, CA: Henry J. Kaiser Family Foundation.

Kaiser Family Foundation. 2010. *Summary of the Affordable Care Act*. Menlo Park, CA: Henry J. Kaiser Foundation.

Kaiser Family Foundation. 2011. *Kaiser Health Tracking Poll: Public Opinion on Health Care Issues*." Menlo Park, CA: Henry J. Kaiser Family Foundation, November.

Kaiser Family Foundation. 2012. *A Guide to the Supreme Court's Decision on the ACA's Medicaid Expansion*. Menlo Park, CA: Henry J. Kaiser Family Foundation, August.

Kaiser Family Foundation. 2017. *Proposals to Replace the Affordable Care Act*. Menlo Park, CA: Kaiser Family Foundation.

Kaiser Family Foundation. 2018. *Kaiser Health Tracking Poll: The Public's View of the ACA*. Menlo Park, CA: Kaiser Family Foundation, October 18.

Kaiser, Robert G. 2012. "'It's Worse than It Looks: How the American Constitutional System Collided with the New Politics of Extremism' by Thomas E. Mann and Norman J. Ornstein." *The Washington Post*, April 30.

Keith, Katie. 2018. "The Latest in Texas V. United States." *Health Affairs*, June 22.

Kerry, John. 2010. "Foreword." In *Power, Politics, and Universal Health Care: The inside Story of a Century-Long Battle*, ed. Stuart Altman and David Shactman, 7–9 Amherst, NY: Prometheus.

Khazan, Olga. 2017. "Why So Many Insurers Are Leaving Obamacare." *The Atlantic*, May 11.

Kingdon, John. 2010. *Agendas, Alternatives, and Public Policies*, updated 2nd edn. Glenview, IL: Longman.

Klein, Ezra. 2013a. "The Republican Plan for Replacing Obamacare Doesn't Replace Obamacare." *The Washington Post*, April 3.

Klein, Ezra. 2013b. "One Way Obamacare May Already Be Working." *Bloomberg*, May 29. Online at www.Bloomberg.com.

Klein, Ezra. 2013c. "Congress, Today Is Your Fault." *The Washington Post*, June 25.

Kliff, Sarah. 2012. "The Republican Plan to Overhaul Health Care." *The Washington Post*, August 27.

Kliff, Sarah. 2013a. "Poll: 42 Percent of Americans Unsure if Obamacare Is Still Law." *The Washington Post*, April 30.

Kliff, Sarah. 2013b. "Budget Request Denied, Sebelius Turns to Health Executives to Finance Obamacare." *The Washington Post*, May 10.
Kliff, Sarah. 2015. "The Accidental Case Against Obamacare." *Vox*, May 26.
Kliff, Sarah. 2017. "15 Charts that Show How Obamacare Works Now—How Republicans Would Overhaul It." *Vox*, January 4.
Kodjak, Alison. 2017. "Halt in Subsidies for Health Insurers Expected to Drive up Costs for the Middle Class." *National Public Radio*, October 13.
Kodjak, Alison. 2018. "Under New Rules, Cheaper 'Short-Term' Health Care Plans Now Last up to Three Years." *National Public Radio*, August 1.
Korte, Gregory and Ray Locker. 2013. "Insurance Sign-Ups Surpasses 1 Million." *USA Today*, December 30.
Krugman, Paul. 2011. "Conservative Origins of Obamacare." *The New York Times*, July 27.
Landsberg, Mitchell. 2010. "Nuns in U.S. Back Healthcare Bill despite Catholic Bishops' Opposition." *Los Angeles Times*, March 18.
"LCWR Stance on Healthcare Reform Draws Praise and Criticism." 2010. *Update: A Publication of the Leadership Conference of Women Religious*, April. Online at cwr.org/sites/default/files/publications/filesZLCWRnewsletter4-10.pdf.
Lee, Frances E. 2009. *Beyond Ideology: Politics, Principles, and Partisanship in the U.S. Senate*. Chicago, IL: University of Chicago Press.
"The Legislature's $51 Billion Failure." 2013. *Tampa Bay Times*, May 3.
Liptak, Adam. 2014. "Supreme Court Rejects Contraceptives Mandate for Some Corporations." *The New York Times*, June 30.
Livingston, Shelby. 2018. "Final 2018 Exchange Enrollment Comes up Slightly Short of 2017." *Modern Healthcare*, April 3.
Loewenstein, George and Saurabh Bhargava. 2016. "The Simple Case Against Health Insurance Complexity." NEJM Catalyst, August 23. Online at www.catalyst.nejm.org.
Long, Sharon K. 2008. "On the Road to Universal Coverage: Impacts of Reform in Massachusetts at One Year." *Health Affairs*, June 3: w270–w284.
Lubell, Jennifer. 2013. "ACA High-Risk Pool Failings Offered as Cautionary Tale." *American Medical News*, April 15. Online at www.amednews.com/article/20130415/government/130419966/7.
Luhby, Tami. 2018. "8 Ways Trump Hurt Obamacare in His First Year." CNN, January 20. Online at money.cnn.com.
Luntz, Frank. 2009. "The Language of Healthcare 2009." Campaign for America's Future. Online at http://thinkprogress.org/wp-content/uploads/2009/05/frank-luntz-the-language-of-healthcare-20091.pdf.
Mahar, Maggie. 2013. "The 37th Vote to Repeal Health Care Reform: Why?" May 21. Healthinsurance.org. Online at www.healthinsurance.org.
Mangan, Dan. 2017a. "Obamacare's Crushing Cost to Some Families: 49 Percent since 2014, Premiums of $14,300." *CNBC*, May 11.
Mangan, Dan. 2017b. "Most Popular Obamacare Plans Cost Average of 34 Percent More for 2018." *CNBC*, October 25.
Mann, Thomas E. and Norman J. Ornstein. 2016. *It's Worse than It Looks: How the American Constitutional System Collided with the New Politics of Extremism*. New York: Basic Books.
Martin, Mark. 2017. "Supreme Court Win Not Enough? Little Sisters of the Poor Back in Court." CBNNews, November 22.
Mashaw, Jerry L. 2013. "Legal, Imagined, and Real Worlds: Reflections on *National Federation of Independent Business V. Sebelius*." *Journal of Health Politics, Policy and Law*, 38, no. 2 (April): 257–266.
McDonough, John E. 2011. *Inside National Health Reform*. Berkeley, CA: University of California Press.
"Medicaid Expansion Enrollment." 2016. Menlo Park, CA: Kaiser Family Foundation. Online at www.kff.org.
Mikesell, John. 2013. *Fiscal Administration*, 9th edn. Farmington Hills, MI: Cengage.
National Academy of State Health Policy. 2018. "State Health Insurance Market Plan Enrollment." Washington, DC: National Academy of State Health Policy. Online at www.nashp.org.
National Conference of State Legislatures. 2017. *Section 1115 Waivers: A Primer for State Legislators*. Denver, CO: National Conference of State Legislators.
National Patient Advocate Foundation. 2012. *Issue Brief: Medical Debt, Medical Bankruptcy and the Impact on Patients*. Washington, DC: National Patient Advocate Foundation.
Norris, Louise. 2017. "How Immigrants Are Getting Health Coverage." January 18. Healthinsurance.org. Online at healthinsurance.org.
"Obama Acknowledges Possible 'Glitches' in ACA Implementation." 2013. *California Healthline*, May 1.
Obama, Barack. 2009. "Obama's Health Care Speech to Congress." 2013. *The New York Times*, September 9.
Office of the Assistant Secretary for Planning and Evaluation. 2011. *Essential Health Benefits: Individual Market Coverage*. Washington, DC: US Department of Health and Human Services.
Ornstein, Norman J. et al. 2013. *Vital Statistics on Congress*. Washington, DC: American Enterprise Institute, the Campaign Finance Institute, and the Brookings Institution.
Ornstein, Norman J. and Thomas E. Mann. 2013. "Gridlock Is No Way to Govern." *The Washington Post*, April 18.
Orszag, Peter R. and Ezekiel J. Emanuel. 2010. "Health Care Reform and Cost Control." *New England Journal of Medicine*, 363, (August 12): 601–603.
Palmer, Kimberly. 2012. "The Real Cost of Birth Control." *U.S. News & World Report*, March 5.
Parente, Stephen T. and Tarren Bragdon. 2009. "Why Health Care Is So Expensive in New York." *The Wall Street Journal*, October 16.
Patel, Kant and Mark E. Rushefsky. 2006. *Health Care Politics and Policy in America*, 3rd edn. Armonk, NY: M.E. Sharpe.
Patel, Kant and Mark E. Rushefsky. 2008. *Health Care in America: Separate and Unequal*. Armonk, NY: M.E. Sharpe.
Pear, Robert. 2011a. "Panel Recommends Coverage for Contraception." *The New York Times*, July 19.

Pear, Robert. 2011b. "Democrats Urge Obama to Protect Contraceptive Coverage in Health Plans." *The New York Times*, November 19.
Pear, Robert. 2013a. "Birth Control Rule Altered to Allay Religious Objections." *The New York Times*, February 1.
Pear, Robert. 2013b. "States' Policies on Health Care Exclude Some of the Poorest." *The New York Times*, May 24.
Pear, Robert. 2015. "Four Words that Imperil Health Care Law Were All a Mistake, Writers Say." *The New York Times*, May 25.
Pear, Robert. 2018a. "Trump Officials Make It Easier for States to Skirt Health Law's Protections." *The New York Times*, October 22.
Pear, Robert. 2018b. "Despite Challenges, Health Exchange Enrollment Falls Only Slightly." *The New York Times*, December 19.
Pearson, Caroline. 2015. "Avalere Analysis: 2016 Exchange Premiums." Washington, DC: Avalere Health. Online at www.avalere.com.
Peterson, Mark A. 2011. "It Was a Different Time: Obama and the Unique Opportunity for Health Care Reform." *Journal of Health Politics, Policy and Law*, 36, no. 3 (June): 429–436.
Pettypiece, Shannon and Jonathan D. Salant. 2013. "Health Law Critics Seek to Gut Program by Undermining Exchanges." *Bloomberg Businessweek*, May 28. Online at www.bloomberg.com.
Pew Research Center. 2010. "Public Knows Basic Facts about Politics, Economics, but Struggles with Specifics." Washington, DC: Pew Research Center, November 18. Online at www.pewresearch.org/2010/11/18/public-knows-basic-facts-about-politics-economics-but-struggles-with-specifics/.
PolitiFact Florida. 2012. "Paul Ryan Said '15 Unelected, Unaccountable Bureaucrats' Could 'Lead to Denied Care for Current Seniors'." *Tampa Bay Times*, August 18. Online at www.politifact.com/florida/statements/2012/aug/23/paul-ryan/paul-ryan-said-15-unelected-unaccountable-bureaucr/.
Poole, Keith T. et al. 2012. "Polarization Is Real (And Asymmetric)." Voteview Blog, May 16. Online at http://voteview.com/blog/?p=494.
Porter, Steven. 2018. "Maryland Sues to Head off Texas-Lead ACA Challenge." HealthLeaders Media. Online at www.healthleadersmedia.com.
Potter, Wendell. 2010. *Deadly Spin: An Insurance Company Insider Speaks Out on How Corporate PR Is Killing Health Care and Deceiving Americans*. New York: Bloomsbury.
"Public Approval of Health Care Law." 2018 RealClearPolitics. Online at www.realclearpolitics.com.
Radnofsky, Louise. 2013. "Employers Push Back on Health Law's Insurance Trigger." *The Wall Street Journal*, May 3.
Radnofsky, Louise. 2014. "Administration Offers Contraception Compromise for Religious Employers." *The Wall Street Journal*, August 22.
Rayfield, Jillian. 2013. "Poll: Dems like 'Obamacare' More than They like 'Health Care Law.'" *The Wall Street Journal*, June 19.
Reagan, Michael. 1999. *The Accidental System: Health Care Policy in America*. Boulder, CO: Westview.
Reid, T. R. 2010. *The Healing of America: A Global Quest for Better, Cheaper, and Fairer Health Care*. New York: Penguin.
Rivlin, Sheri and Allan Rivlin. 2009. "Public Opinion on Healthcare Reform 2009 and 1993—Is This a New Day or 'Groundhog Day'?" *Huffington Post*, March 24.
Roarty, Alec. 2013. "Can This Congress Be Saved?" *National Journal*, February 21. Online at nationaljournal.com.
Robertson, Lori. 2014. "Not 'Everybody' Is Covered Under ACA." FactCheck.org, April 2. Online at www.factcheck.org.
Rovner, Julie. 2017. "Steep Premiums Challenge People Who Buy Health Insurance without Subsidies." *NPR*, October 7.
Rovner, Julie. 2018. "Midterm Results Show Health Is Important to Voters but No Magic Bullet." *Kaiser Health News*, November 7.
Rubin, Irene S. 2009. *The Politics of Public Budgeting: Getting and Spending, Borrowing and Balancing*, 6th edn. Washington, DC: Congressional Quarterly.
Rudowitz, Robin and Jessica Stephens. 2013. *Analyzing the Impact of State Medicaid Decisions*. Menlo Park, CA: The Kaiser Commission on Medicaid and the Uninsured.
Rushefsky, Mark E. 2013. *Public Policy in the United States*, 5th edn. New York: M.E. Sharpe.
Rushefsky, Mark E. 2017. *Public Policy in the United States*, 6th edn. New York: Routledge.
Rushefsky, Mark E. and Kant Patel. 1998. *Politics, Power & Policy Making: The Case of Health Care Reform in the 1990s*. Armonk, NY: M.E. Sharpe.
Sabatier, Paul and Daniel Mazmanian 1980. "The Implementation of Public Policy: A Framework of Analysis." *Policy Studies Journal*, 8, no. 4 (January): 538–560.
Saltzman, Evan and Christine Eibner. 2016. "Donald Trump's Health Care Reform Proposals: Anticipated Effects on Insurance Coverage, Out-of-Pocket Costs, and the Federal Deficit." New York: The Commonwealth Fund.
Scott, Dylan. 2018. "The Trump Admin Has Cooked up a New Plan to Bring Back Preexisting Conditions." *Vox*, October 22.
Shapiro, Ari. 2013. "Obama's Next Big Campaign: Selling Health Care to the Public." *Morning Edition*, *NPR*, May 28. Online at www.npr.org/2013/05/28/186496205/obamas-next-big-campaign-selling-health-care-to-the-public.
Shaw, Greg M. 2017. *The Dysfunctional Politics of the Affordable Care Act*. Santa Barbara, CA: Praeger.
Silver, Charles and David A. Hyman. 2018. *Overcharged: Why Americans Pay Too Much for Health Care*. Washington, DC: Cato Institute.
Sinclair, Barbara. 2012. *Unorthodox Lawmaking: New Legislative Process in the U.S. Congress*, 4th edn. Washington, DC: CQ Press.
Sloan, Chris, Elizabeth Carpenter, and Chad Brooker. 2018. "2019 Premium Increases Lowest on Average since 2015." New York: Avalere Health,, September 13. Online at sss.avalere.com.
Smith-Dewey, Chuck. 2013. "Traditional State Health Risk Pools." January 3. Healthinsurance.org. Online at www.healthinsurance.org.

Soffen, Kim and Kevin Uhrmacher. 2017. "Where the Obamacare Exchanges Lost Insurers for 2018." *The Washington Post*, October 10.

Starr, Paul. 1982. *The Social Transformation of American Medicine*. New York: Basic Books.

Starr, Paul. 2013. *Remedy and Reaction: The Peculiar American Struggle over Health Care Reform*, rev edn. New Haven, CT: Yale University Press.

"Status of Medicaid Expansion." 2018. Washington, DC: Commonwealth Fund.

Steinmo, Sven and Jon Watts 1995. "It's the Institutions, Stupid! Why Comprehensive National Health Insurance Always Fails in America." *Journal of Health Politics, Policy and Law*, 20, no. 2 (Summer): 329–372.

Stephen, Redhead C. and Jane Kinzer. 2017. *Legislative Actions in the 112th, 113th, and 114th Congresses to Repeal, Defund, and Delay the Affordable Care Act*. Washington, DC: Congressional Research Service.

Stephens, Jessica, Samantha Artiga, and Alexandra Gates. 2013. *Getting into Gear for 2014: An Early Look at Branding and Marketing of New Health Insurance Marketplaces*. Menlo Park, CA: Kaiser Family Foundation.

Stewart, Brandon. 2011. "List of 27 States Suing over Obamacare." *The Foundry*, January 17. Online at http://blog.heritage.org/2011/01/17/list-of-states-suing-over-obamacare/.

Stone, Deborah. 2012. *Policy Paradox: The Art of Political Decision Making*, 3rd edn. New York: Norton.

Stout, Hilary. 1994. "Many Don't Realize It's the Clinton Plan They Like." *The Wall Street Journal*, March 10.

Suderman, Peter. 2012. "Why Obamacare's Health Care Cost Controls Won't Work." Reason.com, December 13. Online at http://reason.com/archives/2012/12/13/why-obamacares-health-care-cost-controls.

Suderman, Peter. 2018. "Republicans Didn't Repeal Obamacare, But They Did Replacce It." Reason.com, March 12. Online at https://reason.com/2018/03/12/republicans-didnt-repeal-obamacarebut-th/.

"Summary of Cassidy-Graham-Heller-Johnson Amendment." 2017. Menlo Park, CA: Kaiser Family Foundation.

Summers, Lawrence. 2013. "When Gridlock Is Good." *The Washington Post*, April 14.

Sunstein, Cass R. 2013. "Why Well-Informed People Are Also Close-Minded." Bloomberg View, April 15. Online at www.bloombergview.org.

The Staff of the Washington Post. 2010. *Landmark: The inside Story of America's New Health-Care Law and What It Means for Us All*. New York: Public Affairs.

Toobin, Jeffrey. 2008. *The Nine: Inside the Secret World of the Supreme Court*. New York: Knopf Doubleday.

Toobin, Jeffrey. 2012. *The Oath: The Obama White House and the Supreme Court*. New York: Knopf Doubleday.

Turner, Grace-Marie et al. 2011. *Why Obamacare Is Wrong for America*. New York: Broadside.

Turner, Grace-Marie and Joseph R. Antos. 2009. "The GOP's Health Alternative." *The Wall Street Journal*, May 20.

Weisman, Jonathan and Robert Pear. 2013. "Partisan Gridlock Thwarts Effort to Alter Health Law." *The New York Times*, May 26.

Westen, Drew. 2007. *The Political Brain: The Role of Emotion in Deciding the Fate of the Nation*. New York: Public Affairs.

Whittington, Keith E. 2013. "'Our Own Limited Role in Policing Those Boundaries': Taking Small Steps on Health Care." *Journal of Health Politics, Policy and Law*, 38, no. 2 (April): 272–282.

Wilkerson, John, David Smith, and Nick Stramp. 2013. "Tracing the Flow of Policy Idea in Legislatures: A Text Reuse Approach." September 17: 1–34. Ken Benoit. Online at www.kenbenoit.net/pdfs/NDATAD2013/PolicyIdeas2013TextasData.pdf.

York, Byron. 2014. "No, House Republicans Haven't Voted 50 Times to Repeal Obamacare." *Washington Examiner*, March 15.

Zuckerman, Stephen and John Holahan. 2012. "Despite Criticism, the Affordable Care Act Does Much to Contain Health Care Costs." Washington, DC: Urban Policy Center, Urban Institute.

4

MEDICAID AND THE CHILDREN'S HEALTH INSURANCE PROGRAM

Healthcare for the Poor and the Disabled

The establishment of Medicare and Medicaid in 1965 was the result of a lengthy debate during the early part of the twentieth century over the role of the federal government in financing healthcare. The debate among policymakers focused on two competing models. Under the universal coverage model, the federal government would provide health insurance to all people on a compulsory basis, financed by taxes on earnings. The second model envisioned a more limited role for the federal government, providing assistance only to needy groups in society. Throughout the twentieth century, all federal healthcare laws followed the second model (Ginsburg 1988). The political environment, institutional structures, and legislative processes made such an incremental approach feasible.

In the 1930s, President Herbert Hoover established the Committee on the Costs of Medical Care (CCMC). This committee's assessment of US healthcare specifically focused on challenges facing low-income Americans in obtaining care. Prior to the passage of Medicaid in 1965, a hodgepodge of poorly funded federal programs existed for meeting the healthcare needs of the poor (Goldfield 2003). The 1950 amendments to the Social Security Act authorized matching grants to the states for direct vendor (provider) payments for treatment of individuals on public assistance. During the late 1950s, the debate focused on the problem of hospital costs faced by the aged, which had doubled over the decade. Support increased for addressing this problem because the aged were presumed to be both needy and deserving (Starr 1982). In 1960, Congress passed the Kerr-Mills Act, creating the Medical Assistance for the Aged (MAA) program. This Act expanded federal matching funds to the states for vendor payments, and, more importantly, it allowed states to include the "medically needy"—that is, elderly, blind, and disabled persons with low incomes who were not on public assistance. However, many states moved very slowly or failed to move at all to take advantage of the Kerr-Mills Act.

The Democratic Party's sweep of the 1964 elections guaranteed further action with respect to the role of the federal government in healthcare. Lyndon Johnson was elected to the presidency with an overwhelming popular vote. The Democrats gained a two-to-one majority in the House of Representatives. This made it possible for Congress in 1965 to create the Medicare and Medicaid programs. Both were at the forefront of Lyndon Johnson's Great Society programs designed to help the poor and the disadvantaged (Davis and Reynolds 1977). Medicare was established as a program for the elderly, Medicaid as a program for the poor. The final shape of both programs represented compromises among competing models and approaches. The Democratic plan for a compulsory hospital insurance program, financed through payroll taxes under Social Security, became Part A of Medicare. The Republican-supported plan of a government-subsidized, voluntary insurance program financed through general revenues to cover physicians' bills became Part B of Medicare. The AMA opposed both plans and pushed a plan of its own to expand the Kerr-Mills program to the needy. An expanded means-tested program for the poor administered by the states became the Medicaid program.

The generally accepted political explanation for the creation of Medicaid is that the program was created almost as an afterthought to Medicare (Grannemann and Pauly 1983). Medicaid was intended to "pick up the pieces" left over by Medicare. It was designed to cover deductibles and coinsurance for indigent Medicare patients. The program was intended to pay for services not covered, or covered only inadequately, by Medicare (i.e., outpatient and nursing home care), and to pay the cost of medical care of indigent persons other than the elderly (Brown 1984).

It is important not to confuse the Medicaid and Medicare programs. Although Medicare and Medicaid were adopted at the same time, there are fundamental differences between the two. First, the Medicare program has enjoyed public popularity and legitimacy because it is tied to Social Security, a program that is contributory in nature (i.e., through Social Security taxes paid by workers). In contrast, from the beginning, Medicaid was burdened by the stigma of being associated with public assistance (i.e., welfare) programs since eligibility for Medicaid was often tied to the cash assistance provided through programs such as Aid to Families with Dependent Children (AFDC) or Supplemental Social Security Income (SSI). However, such is not the case today. As the Medicaid program has expanded over the years to cover more children, women, and poor adults it has also become disassociated from the welfare programs. In recent years, the Medicaid program has enjoyed considerable popular support. Second, Medicare is financed and administered solely by the federal government, while Medicaid is financed by both the federal and state governments on a matching basis. Third, Medicare is administered by the federal government, while Medicaid is administered by the state governments. Fourth, Medicare has uniform national standards for eligibility and benefits. In sharp contrast, Medicaid, to a large extent, lets states decide on eligibility standards and benefits within the framework of meeting minimum federal requirements. Fifth, physician reimbursement under Medicaid is lower than under Medicare or private insurance; consequently, fewer physicians participate in the Medicaid program (Starr 1982).

IMPORTANT FACTS ABOUT THE CURRENT MEDICAID PROGRAM

To understand today's Medicaid program, it is important to understand the following key facts about the Medicaid program as it exists today, because these facts contradict some of the negative stereotypes a number of Americans have about the program and its beneficiaries (Gunja and Collins 2016; *Kaiser Health News* 2017; Park 2015; Rudowitz and Garfield 2018; Waldron 2017).

First, Medicaid is the country's health insurance program for low-income individuals.

Second, the program has evolved over time to expand coverage to more low-income individuals and to meet their changing needs.

Third, the program is structured as a partnership between the federal and state governments.

Fourth, the program is jointly financed by the federal and state governments. The federal government matches state spending on Medicaid based on a formula under which the poorest states receive more federal funding.

Fifth, the program primarily covers single parents, children, people with disabilities, low-income seniors, pregnant women, and other low-income adults. Children make up the largest group of beneficiaries, amounting to 41 percent of all recipients.

Sixth, the program provides a wide range of services to meet the diverse group of eligible beneficiaries, ranging from neonatal care for pregnant women, immunization and early screening for children, mental health and physician services for people with disabilities to long-term care for the elderly.

Seventh, the program provides assistance to around 76 million people—one in every five low-income Americans.

Eighth, about 60 percent of non-disabled program enrollees have a job.

Ninth, 41 percent of the program enrollees have a university degree or some college education, 33 percent have a high school diploma or GED, and about 26 percent have less than a high school degree.

Tenth, a large majority of the program enrollees receive their healthcare services through private managed care plans.

Eleventh, the program has a positive impact on access to healthcare and health outcomes. A growing body of research has demonstrated that the program's coverage of pregnant women has contributed to the decline in infant and child mortality. Similarly, access to Medicaid in early childhood has led to a reduction in teen mortality, and lower rates of hospitalization and emergency-department visits later in life.

Twelfth, on a per-enrollee basis, Medicaid is a low-cost program compared to private insurance. For example, Medicaid costs 27 percent less for children and 20 percent less for adults than private insurance (Park 2015). However, it is important to note that this is largely due to the low reimbursement rates paid by the Medicaid program to health providers. This is also the reason why many physicians do not accept Medicaid patients.

Thirteenth, the participation rate in the Medicaid program is very high. About 65.6 percent of low-income adults and children who are eligible are enrolled in the program (Park 2015).

Fourteenth, most low-income adults with Medicaid coverage express satisfaction with the program and rate it very highly (Gunja and Collins 2016).

Fifteenth, recent public polling data suggests that the program has broad public support. In a poll, 65 percent of respondents opposed cutting funding for Medicaid (Waldron 2017). In another poll, 74 percent said that they had a very favorable to a somewhat favorable opinion of the program (Rudowitz and Garfield 2018).

In the remainder of the chapter, we examine in more detail some of the key facts about the Medicaid program outlined above.

PROGRAM OBJECTIVE AND STRUCTURE

The primary objective of Medicaid when it was created in 1965 was to provide a limited number of poor individuals with financial assistance to meet their medical needs. The Medicaid program incorporated the Elizabethan notion of "deserving" or "worthy" poor from the times of colonial America. The state governments, in order to receive federal funding, had to operate within a set of minimum federal requirement and guidelines. State governments were given the primary responsibility for establishing program requirements with respect to eligibility and benefits. States were also given the option of making the administration of the program a local rather than state responsibility. Thus, initially the purpose and objective of the program were to provide financial help to a limited number of poor, aged, blind, disabled, and children to meet their healthcare needs. The program was perceived by many as "medical welfare" since it was also closely tied to some of the welfare programs. The original Medicaid program was a safety net program with many holes in it that left a large number of poor without health insurance coverage. "Able-bodied" poor adults were not eligible to receive coverage under the program (Huberfeld and Roberts 2015). Over the years, the objective of the program has expanded and today it provides health insurance coverage to a broad range of Americans who meet expanded eligibility requirements.

The Medicaid program was created as a partnership between federal and state governments to improve access and quality of healthcare for the poor. The national government establishes broad program guidelines, promotes and monitors program development, and provides federal funds through matching grants. State governments are given significant control over important aspects of the scope and structure of the program. For example, state governments enjoy discretionary authority for establishing eligibility standards, the nature and scope of benefits provided, and mechanisms used to reimburse healthcare providers.

The Centers for Medicare and Medicaid Services (CMS) issues program guidelines in the form of letters to state Medicaid directors and state health officials. The CMS also issues regulations to codify policies based on legislative provisions. It does this through issuing notices of proposed rulemaking, seeking inputs on proposed rules, and issuing interim and final rules. The Center for Medicaid and CHIP Services (CMCS), created in 2000, also uses informational bulletins to communicate with state officials and other stakeholders in the Medicaid program ("Medicaid and CHIP Program Information" n.d.).

Medicaid is an excellent example of how the federal structure of government shapes the dynamics of policymaking and implementation. On the one hand, the federal structure, with its multiple governments, shared authority, political autonomy, and constitutional ambiguities, has allowed states to act as laboratories for innovation and experimentation in the Medicaid program. On the other hand, the same federal structure of government produces overlapping jurisdictions and duplications, encourages the promotion of narrow and parochial interests, and creates inefficiencies and inequities. Instead of a "unified system of healthcare" for low-income individuals as originally envisioned, the Medicaid program varies a great deal from state to state with respect to eligibility, services, and benefits creating many inequities in the program. It allows one level of government to pass the buck or to blame another level of government by playing the federalism game.

MEDICAID ELIGIBILITY AND COVERAGE, SERVICES AND BENEFITS

Eligibility and Coverage

As mentioned previously, the Medicaid program has evolved considerably from the time of its creation in 1965 to the present day. Over the years, the federal government has expanded eligibility and coverage requirements to include a large number and category of poor individuals. For example, the Social Security Act Amendments of 1967 and 1972 required states to provide comprehensive medical coverage to children and expanded coverage of the aged, blind, and disabled to meet the federal government's Supplemental Security Income (SSI). During the 1980s, federal mandates required states to expand eligibility for pregnant women and children. The Children's Health Insurance Program (CHIP) gave state governments the option to expand health insurance coverage to children as part of an existing Medicaid program, a standalone separate program, or a combination of both. The Medicare Prescription Drug and Modernization Act of 2003 provided prescription drug coverage to individuals enrolled in both Medicaid and the Medicare Program. (See Chapter 5 for more discussion.) The Affordable Care Act (ACA) of 2010 required states to expand the Medicaid program to cover everyone under the age of 65 earning up to 133 percent of the Federal Poverty level (FPL). The ACA also expanded Medicaid to non-elderly adults earning up to 138 percent of the FPL and significantly increased federal matching funds for the expansion. The ACA changes effectively eliminated "categorical" eligibility and allowed adults without children to be covered. However, the US Supreme Court in *NFIB v. Sebelius* in 2012 ruled that the federal government cannot force states to expand Medicaid under the threat of withdrawal of federal matching funds, making Medicaid expansion by state governments optional at their discretion (Huberfeld and Roberts 2015; Rudowitz and Garfield 2018).

Mandatory Eligibility Groups

In order to participate in Medicaid, the federal government requires states to cover certain population groups called "mandatory eligibility groups." The "mandatory eligibility groups" include:

- pregnant women with income below 138 percent of the Federal Poverty Level (FPL);
- children through age 18 in families with income below 138 percent of FPL;
- parents whose incomes fall within the state's eligibility limit for cash assistance that was in place prior to welfare reforms enacted in 1996; and
- most elderly and persons with disabilities who receive cash assistance through the Supplemental Security Income (SSI) program (Center for Budget and Policy Priorities 2016).

Optional Eligibility Groups

States can also receive federal matching funds to cover "optional population." Thus, states have the option to cover other populations beyond the mandatory eligibility groups under their Medicaid programs. They are called the "optional eligibility groups." These include pregnant women, children, parents with income above the "mandatory" coverage income limits, seniors and persons with disabilities with income below the poverty line, as well as "Medically needy" individuals whose income exceeds the state's regular eligibility limits but who have high medical expenses, such as nursing-home care. Medically needy individuals can also become eligible by "spending down" the amount of their income that is above a particular's state's medically needy income standards.

Due to the fact that (1) many state governments have expanded while other states have opted not to expand their Medicaid program under the ACA, and (2) states have broad flexibility to decide which of the "optional" groups to cover and at what income level, Medicaid eligibility varies significantly from state to state (Center for Budget and Policy Priorities 2016).

Dual Eligibility

Some seniors are enrolled in both the Medicaid and Medicare program because they qualify for both programs by criteria of low income (Medicaid) and age (Medicare); such individuals are referred to as "dual eligible."

Financial Eligibility

The ACA established a new methodology for determining income eligibility for Medicaid. It is based on what is called modified adjusted gross income (MAGI). MAGI is used to determine income eligibility for Medicaid and the CHIP, as well as for premium tax credits and cost-sharing reductions available through the health insurance marketplace under the ACA. The MAGI methodology relies on taxable income and tax filing relationships to determine financial eligibility for the Medicaid program. By using one set of income counting rules and a single application, the ACA has made it easier for people to apply and enroll in the appropriate program.

Some individuals—for example, individuals whose eligibility for Medicaid is based on blindness, disability or age (65-plus)—are exempt from MAGI-based income counting rules. Their eligibility is determined using a different methodology, used by the SSI program administered by the Social Security Administration. Certain other eligibility groups do not require a determination of income because their eligibility is based on enrollment in another program, such as SSI or the breast and cervical cancer treatment program (Centers for Medicare and Medicaid Services n.d.).

Non-Financial Eligibility

Finally, to be eligible for the Medicaid program individuals also must meet some non-financial eligibility criteria, such as the fact that Medicaid beneficiaries must generally reside in the state in which they are receiving

Table 4.1

Medicaid Benefits

Mandatory Benefits	Optional Benefits
• Inpatient hospital services	• Prescription drugs
• Outpatient hospital services	• Clinic services
• Early and periodic screening, diagnostic and treatment (EPSDT) services	• Physical therapy
	• Occupational therapy
	• Speech, hearing, and language disorder services
• Nursing facility services	• Respiratory care services
• Home health services	• Other diagnostic, screening, preventive, and rehabilitative services
• Physician services	• Podiatry services
• Rural health clinic services	• Optometry services
• Federally qualified health center services	• Dental services
	• Dentures
• Laboratory and X-ray services	• Prosthetics
• Family planning services	• Eyeglasses
• Nurse-midwife services	• Chiropractic services
• Certified pediatric and family nurse practitioner services	• Other practitioner services
	• Private-duty nursing services
• Freestanding birth center services (when licensed or otherwise recognized by the state)	• Personal care
	• Hospice
	• Case management
• Transportation to medical care	• Services for individuals age 65 or older in an institution for mental disease (IMD)
• Tobacco cessation counseling for pregnant women	• Services in an intermediate care facility for individuals with intellectual disability

- State-planned Home and Community Based Services—1915(i)
- Self-Directed Personal Assistance Services—1915(j)
- Community First Choice Option—1915(k)
- TB-related services
- Home health for enrollees with chronic conditions
- Inpatient psychiatric services for individuals under the age of 21
- Other services approved by the secretary[1]

[1] These includes services furnished in a religious non-medical healthcare institution, emergency hospital services by a non-Medicare-certified hospital, and critical-access hospitals (CAH).

Source: Centers for Medicare and Medicaid Services, Baltimore, MD. 201. Online at www.medicaid.gov/medicaid/benefits/list-of-benefits/index.html.

Medicaid. They must be a citizen or legal permanent resident of the United States (Centers for Medicare and Medicaid Services n.d.).

Finally, while Medicaid eligibility has expanded considerably since 1965, it is important to note that not all low-income Americans are eligible for Medicaid. Childless adults who are not disabled, pregnant, or elderly are generally not eligible for Medicaid in states that have opted not to expand their Medicaid program under the ACA. Also, with the exception of some states, legal immigrants are prohibited from participation in the Medicaid program for the first five years in the country, even if they meet all of the program's eligibility requirements (Center for Budget and Policy Priorities 2016).

Benefits and Services

States are required to cover certain "mandatory benefits" in their Medicaid programs. These benefits include inpatient and outpatient hospital services; physician services; nursing facility services; rural health clinic services; prenatal care; vaccines for children; family planning services and supplies; and laboratory and X-ray services, among others. States can also receive federal matching funds if they elect to provide other "optional benefits" such as diagnostic and clinic services, intermediate care facilities for those suffering from intellectual disability, prescribed drugs and prosthetic devices, optometrist services and eyeglasses, transportation services, rehabilitation and physical therapy services, and home and community-based care for certain persons with chronic impairment (see Table 4.1 for a list of mandatory and optional benefits).

Medicaid also provides coverage for a host of long-term care services to beneficiaries in a variety of settings. For example, Medicaid pays for most of the cost of nursing home care once a person living in a nursing home has exhausted all of his/her own financial resources/assets to pay for such care. Nursing home care is very expensive, ranging from $5,000 to $8,000 a month or more, and can easily deplete the lifelong savings of an elderly couple if one of them has to live in a nursing home. In 1988, Congress enacted provisions called "spousal impoverishment," to prevent a spouse living at home in the community with little or no income or resources. Under the provision, a certain amount of the couple's combined resources is protected for the spouse living at home in the community. The topic of long-term care is discussed in more detail later in the chapter.

MEDICAID FINANCING

Federal Financing

The Medicaid program is jointly financed by the federal and state governments. The federal government pays a specified percentage of each state's Medicaid program expenditures. The Federal Medical Assistance Percentages (FMAPs) are used in determining the amount of federal matching money paid to the states. The FMAPs vary from state to state because they are based on a formula that takes into consideration factors such as per-capita income in the state. Thus, the FMAPs vary from a minimum match rate of 50 percent to a maximum of 75 percent. Consequently, the poorer states receive a larger percentage of federal matching funds. The Secretary of Health and Human Services (HHS) is required to calculate and publish the FMAPs each year (Centers for Medicare and Medicaid Services n.d.; Federal Register 2015).

The Enhanced Federal Medical Assistance Percentages (EFMAPs) are for the Children's Health Insurance Program (CHIP). Title XXI of the Social Security Act, Section 2105(b) specifies the formula to be used in calculating this. Beginning in 2015 the ACC increased the EFMAPs by 23 percentage points.

State Financing

State Financing Sources

A state's share of Medicaid expenditures comes from state legislative appropriations, intergovernmental transfers of funds (IGTs), certified public expenditures (CPEs), and permissible taxes and provider donations. States are permitted to restrict the amount of services per beneficiary. For example, a state may limit the number of days in hospital or the number of visits to a physician per year that it would cover.

Cost-Sharing

State governments have the option to charge a limited amount of premiums and enrollment fees to Medicaid enrollees. They can also require enrollees to pay out-of-pocket expenses such as co-payments, coinsurance, and deductibles. States can impose higher charges for certain targeted groups, such as enrollees with a higher income. On the other hand, certain vulnerable groups such as children and pregnant women are exempted from most out-of-pocket expenses. States can also use out-of-pocket charges to promote the most cost-effective use of prescription drugs. To encourage enrollees to use low-cost drugs, states can also establish different co-payments for generic drugs or drugs listed on a preferred-drug list compared to name-brand drugs. States can also impose high co-payments when enrollees visit a hospital emergency department for non-emergency services. However, states cannot impose out-of-pocket costs for certain services such as family planning, pregnancy-related services, or preventive care for children. In general, cost sharing for most services is limited to nominal or minimum amounts (Centers for Medicare and Medicaid Services n.d.).

Provider Taxes

State governments have increasingly come to rely on provider taxes as a way of increasing their share of Medicaid matching funds. A provider tax, sometimes also referred to as a fee or assessment, is a state law that authorizes the collecting of revenue from certain targeted groups of providers, such as hospitals. In most instances, states use this as a tool to generate new in-state funds for the Medicaid program and match them with a federal fund to receive additional federal Medicaid dollars. In the majority of cases, the cost of the tax is paid back to providers through an increase in reimbursement for the treatment and services provided to Medicaid patients. However, under federal laws and regulations, revenues generated through such provider taxes cannot exceed 25 percent of the state's (non-federal) share of Medicaid expenditures. Nor can a state guarantee a health provider that the taxes will be returned to them. According to the National Conference of State Legislatures in 2018, 49 states plus the District of Columbia had some type of Medicaid-related provider or insurance taxes or fees. Such taxes generate millions of dollars in revenue for the state's Medicaid program (National Conference of State Legislatures 2017).

Provider taxes allow states to produce revenues that go into the state treasury, and then that revenue is directly appropriated to the state Medicaid agency. Provider taxes give states two advantages. One, as states are faced with the ever-increasing costs of the Medicaid program and tight budgets, provider taxes generate added revenue to pay for their share of the program costs. Second, by coming up with more money for Medicaid, states receive more federal matching funds (Miller 2010).

Disproportionate-Share Hospital Payments

Federal law requires state Medicaid programs to make Disproportionate-Share Hospital (DSH) payments to qualifying hospitals that serve a large number of Medicaid and uninsured persons. The federal government annually allocates DSH payments to the states. The allocations for each state are established by law. In order to receive such payments, states must submit an independent certified audit and annual report to the secretary of the Department of Health and Human Services (HHS) explaining the DSH payments made to each of their DSH hospitals.

Medicaid DSH payments are the largest source of federal funding for uncompensated hospital care provided to Medicaid beneficiaries and uninsured individuals. States are required to make supplemental payments or adjustments to the DSH payment rates. The federal government distributes the DSH allocation to states based on a formula and states, in turn, use this money to cover the costs of hospital care they are required to provide to low-income individuals and that are not covered by other payers such as Medicaid, Medicare, and the CHIP. Providers participating in Medicaid must accept Medicaid rates as payment in full. Payment rates are often updated based on factors such as an economic index or an inflation index. The DSH payments vary considerably from state to state. The Affordable Care Act requires annual percentage reduction in DHS, and it will be eliminated by 2020. As a result, hospitals in states that do not expand the Medicaid program under the ACA could face much higher uncompensated care costs (Haeder and Weimer 2015).

State Medicaid Reimbursement to Providers

States enjoy significant discretion with respect to the method and rate of payment to healthcare providers. Medicaid operates as a vendor payment program. States can establish their own Medicaid provider payment rates within federal guidelines. Consequently, every Medicaid program differs based on state laws and regulations. Most Medicaid reimbursement models use fee-for-service, managed care, or a combination of both to pay providers. The fee-for-service reimbursement model pays providers by the volume of services provided to the Medicaid beneficiaries. Most Medicaid fee-for-service models set rates by a charge for services or maximum allowable price—whichever is lesser. Thirty-eight out of 50 states use this method. Medicaid fee-for-service rates tend to be significantly lower than Medicare reimbursement rates, which explains the lower rate of physician participation in the Medicaid program and the difficulty Medicaid beneficiaries face in getting physician services.

Medicaid managed-care models fall into three types. First, some states use a comprehensive risk-based managed-care model in which a plan receives a capitated rate for Medicaid covered services. The plan is paid a fixed amount per member, per month and aims to cover a specific set of services for the beneficiary. However, the plans assume the financial risk if care exceeds the capitated amount. In the second model, the limited-benefit managed-care plan, states partner with limited-benefit plans to provide services for the specific patient population. The third model is a primary-care case management model in which primary-care providers receive a monthly case management fee ("The Difference Between Medicare and Medicaid Reimbursement" n.d.). In recent years there has been a shift from fee-for-service to alternative models for Medicaid reimbursements.

THE CHILDREN'S HEALTH INSURANCE PROGRAM (CHIP)

The Origins and Evolution of the CHIP

The failed attempt at comprehensive reform of the US healthcare system under the Clinton administration in 1993–1994 led advocates of reforms to push for incremental changes. The result was the passage of the Health Insurance Portability and Accounting Act (HIPAA) of 1996, which provided some protection to uninsured adult Americans by placing limits on insurance companies' ability to deny coverage for pre-existing conditions and by allowing portability of insurance from one job to the next.

In the past, Medicare and Medicaid programs had targeted specific groups of Americans for protection. Following this model, the advocates of reforms argued that the next logical group that needed government protection was a large number of children who lacked any health insurance (Flint 1997). From the mid- to late 1980s Congress passed several mandates requiring states to expand their Medicaid program to cover more poor children (Cunningham and Kirby 2004). As a result, the uninsured rate among the very poor children declined for those living in families whose income was up to 100 percent of the federal poverty level. However, the uninsurance rate continued to increase for low-income children whose family incomes were between 100 and 200 percent of the federal poverty level and thus not low enough for Medicaid eligibility.

The issue of health insurance coverage for children has been an important topic for policymakers, as children are uniquely vulnerable because of their dependent status; that is, their health insurance status often generally depends on the economic status of their parents. Since the US legal system gives parents the authority and legal responsibility to make decisions about their children's healthcare with some constraints, the government was generally not seen as having a positive obligation to promote and support children's health programs (Huntington and Scott 2015). Research evidence points to the fact that poverty affects health and often begins quite early in life (Kindig 2015). Even though government spending on children's health has increased over time, the United States has lagged behind other industrialized nations in various measures of children's health. The federal government has taken the lead in supporting healthcare needs of the elderly and the poor via Medicare, SSI, and Medicaid programs while state governments have generally taken the lead in children and families through education and social programs. Federal government spending on the welderly easily surpassed total overall spending by states on children (Rosenbaum and Blum 2015).

After the failed healthcare reform effort under the Clinton administration in 1993–1994, a consensus was beginning to emerge among policymakers that federal government's investment in children's health was a good idea and uninsured children were the next logical group that needed the support of the federal government. Proponents of expanding health insurance coverage to a larger pool of children had argued that, first, allowing 10 million-plus children to go without health insurance was scandalous; second, insuring children was smart public policy because it was an investment in the country's future workforce and its citizens; and third, child health coverage was a relatively low-cost method of reducing the growing number of uninsured in the country (Flint 2014a). Consequently, a bipartisan consensus emerged in support of the expansion of children's health insurance programs. Congress created the State Children's Health Insurance Program (SCHIP) in 1997 as part of Title XXI of the Social Security Act under the 1997 Balanced Budget Act (Cunningham and Kirby 2004).

Initially, states were given three options to expand health insurance coverage to children: expanding their Medicaid program to cover more children by raising their Medicaid income-eligibility standards; developing new or expanding existing insurance programs for children; or using a combination of the two options (Congressional Budget Office 1997). Under the first option, states build on existing Medicaid program institutional structures to implement the CHIP with few program modifications. Many advocates favored this approach because Medicaid already provides a comprehensive benefits package for children. However, opponents argued that some low-income families may not apply for coverage because of the perceived stigma associated with the Medicaid program. Under the second option, states could create an alternative new insurance program, separate from Medicaid, with the SCHIP funds. Such an approach was attractive to states that already had such a program in place funded by state and local governments. This option also gave such states the advantage of not having to satisfy all the federal requirements of the Medicaid program, such as the mandatory benefits and limits on cost-sharing. Since such a program is not an individual entitlement, program outlays can be capped. Under the third option, states could use a combination of the first two approaches. Within three years of its establishment, all states had implemented the SCHIP (Rosenbaum and Budetti 2003).

The Struggle over the Renewal of the CHIP

When the SCHIP was created in 1997 it was touted as enjoying broad bipartisan success. The fact that legislation was cosponsored in the Senate by a liberal Democrat and a conservative Republican—Senator Edward Kennedy (D-MA) and Senator Orrin Hatch (R-UT)—was viewed as a symbol of its bipartisanship. It was this bipartisanship and incrementalism that had helped stitched the Children's Health Insurance Program together (Flint 2014a).

However, as Grogan and Rigby (2009) have pointed out, not only partisan cleavages existed when the SCHIP was enacted in 1997 because Republicans wanted a block-grant approach and the Democrats preferred Medicaid expansion. A mirage of partisanship was created by Congress giving its blessings to both approaches. Also, state implementation of the SCHIP had become increasingly partisan over the years. In addition, as states experimented with the program over the ten-year period, by the time the program came up for renewal in 2007, the Democratic and Republican positions on sate flexibility had completely reversed, with Democrats favoring giving states more flexibility while the Republicans favored a more nationally standardized program.

Thus, when the program came up for reauthorization in Congress in the summer and fall of 2007, a bitter partisan debate emerged over the program's intended purpose. Republicans argued that the SCHIP should be a narrowly targeted means-tested program for poor, uninsured children. The Democrats argued that the SCHIP should be expanded further to guarantee that all children and some adults could have some type of healthcare coverage (Grogan and Rigby 2009). Congress passed a reauthorization bill that would have expanded the SCHIP; however, in October of 2007, President George W. Bush vetoed the reauthorization bill on the grounds that it would federalize healthcare and expand the SCHIP program beyond its original intent. Instead, the Bush administration issued new federal guidelines restricting state flexibility around eligibility expansion (Gorin and Moniz 2007; Grogan and Rigby 2009). Ultimately, Congress passed a law extending SCHIP funding until March 2009, which President Bush signed into law. President Obama's victory and increased Democratic majorities in both houses ultimately paved the way for breaking the political stalemate, and in February 2009 President Obama signed the Children's Health Insurance Program Reauthorization Act (CHIPRA), extending the program through October 2015. The name of the program was changed from the State Children's Health Insurance Program (SCHIP) to the Children's Health Insurance Program (CHIP). Hence, we refer to it as the Children's Health Insurance Program (CHIP) throughout the book, except for when the use of "SCHIP" is appropriate in the context of the discussion.

The Act provided states with more flexibility, significant new funding, programmatic options, and new incentives for covering children, and it helped states develop strategies to identify, enroll, and retain children who were eligible for Medicaid or the CHIP but were not yet enrolled/covered. Several states received millions of dollars in bonuses from the federal government between 2009 and 2011 ("Children's Health Insurance Program Reauthorization Act" n.d.).

By 2015, the CHIP had extended health insurance coverage to nearly 9 million children nationwide and the nation's percentage of uninsured children had declined from almost 14 percent when the program started to about 4.5 percent (Resnick 2017a). In 2015, the CHIP was reauthorized under the Obama administration for another two years (until 2017).

The election of Republican Donald Trump to the presidency ushered in a period of a unified government, with the Republican Party controlling the presidency and both houses of Congress. The reauthorization of the CHIP got entangled in the political environment of increased partisanship and ideological polarization in Congress surrounding Republican efforts to repeal and replace the ACA and passing the tax reform legislation. The deadline to pass a reauthorization of the CHIP passed on September 20, 2017, creating a crisis in many states as they faced the prospect of CHIP funding running out and thousands of children losing health insurance coverage. A bipartisan group of governors in December sent a letter to Congress urging reauthorization of the program (Ingold 2017). Almost three months after the reauthorization deadline for the CHIP came and went, Congress voted in December 2017 to provide an additional $2.85 billion for the CHIP as a means of propping up the program until March of 2018 (Resnick 2017b). By end of January 2017, ten states were expected to run out of money for the CHIP. Three days into the federal government shutdown over the budget impasse, Congress finally reached a deal to reopen the government and reauthorize and fund the CHIP for six more years (Quinn 2018a). President Trump signed it into law on January 22, 2018. On February 9, 2018, as part of the Bipartisan Budget Act of 2018, Congress voted to extend the CHIP for four more years on top of the six-year extension authorized in January. President Trump signed the Budget Act into law, extending the CHIP through 2027.

CHIP Eligibility, Benefits, Financing, and Cost-Sharing

Today, all states participate in the CHIP program. Eight states, five territories, and the District of Columbia have expanded their Medicaid program to implement the CHIP. Eleven states have created their own stand-alone CHIP separate from the Medicaid program. Twenty-nine states use a combination of Medicaid expansion and a separate CHIP ("Children's Health Insurance Program: Plan Activity as of May 1, 2015" 2015).

Eligibility

The ACA created a national minimum Medicaid eligibility level at 133 percent of the FPL. The CHIP provides health insurance coverage to children up to the age of 19 in families with income too high to qualify them for Medicaid. The Medicaid and CHIP upper-income eligibility level varies by state. Forty-six states and the District of Columbia cover children up to or above 200 percent of the FPL. Of these states, 24 offer coverage to children in families with an income of 250 percent of the FPL. States that offer coverage up to 300 percent of the FPL receive an enhanced federal match rate that is higher than the Medicaid federal matching fund rate ("Children's Health Insurance Program" n.d.).

Most states have eliminated or shortened the waiting periods. Many states have also, under the CHIPRA, opted to restore Medicaid and/or CHIP coverage to children and pregnant women who are lawfully residing in the United States. The CHIPRA also created an explicit category of pregnant women to receive coverage through the CHIP under certain circumstances. The ACA provides states the option to extend CHIP eligibility to the children of state employees ("Children's Health Insurance Program" n.d.).

Benefits

Each state is free to decide on the benefits provided under the CHIP within federal guidelines. Thus, the benefits provided in the CHIP vary by state. However, all states cover health services such as routine checkups, immunizations, hospital care, dental care, and laboratory and X-ray services. Children get free preventive care, but low premiums and other cost-sharing may be required for other services.

States that expanded their Medicaid programs to cover additional children (Medicaid Expansion CHIP) provide the standard Medicaid benefit package, including early and periodic screening, diagnostic and treatment services, which include all medically necessary services like mental health and dental ("Children's Health Insurance Program" n.d.).

States that created separate CHIPs have the option to provide benchmark coverage, benchmark-equivalent coverage, or HHS Secretary-approved coverage ("Children's Health Insurance Program" n.d.). Benchmark coverage must be based on one of the following: (1) the standard Blue Cross/Blue Shield preferred-provider organization service benefit plan offered to federal employees; (2) a state employees' coverage plan; or (3) the HMO plan that has the largest commercial, non-Medicaid enrollment within the state. Benchmark-equivalent coverage must be actuarially equivalent and include inpatient and outpatient hospital services, physician's services, surgical and medical services, laboratory and X-ray services, and well-baby and well-child care, including immunizations.

Secretary-approved coverage can include any other health coverage deemed appropriate and acceptable by the secretary of the US Department of Health and Human Services ("Children's Health Insurance Program" n.d.).

Financing

Just as in the Medicaid program, state governments are responsible for administering the CHIP, but it is funded jointly by the federal and state governments through a formula based on the Medicaid Federal Medical Assistance Percentage (FMAP). To encourage states to expand coverage to children, Congress created an "enhanced" federal matching rate for the CHIP that is generally 15 percentage points higher than the Medicaid rate. Thus, the overall average federal matching rate is about 71 percent; that is, the federal government funds about 71 percent of the total program costs. Each fiscal year CMS determines the federal share of the program funding and allocates funds to states. Under the ACA the federal matching rate can be increased by almost 23 percent. Thus, the average federal match rate now for the CHIP is 93 percent and will continue until September 2019 ("Children's Health Insurance Program" n.d.).

Cost Sharing

States have discretionary authority to impose limited enrollments fees, premiums, deductibles, coinsurance, and co-payments for children and women enrolled in the CHIP. Cost-sharing is generally limited to 5 percent of a family's annual income and is prohibited for services such as well-baby and well-child visits ("Children's Health Insurance Program" n.d.).

THE AFFORDABLE CARE ACT OF 2010 AND MEDICAID EXPANSION

The Affordable Care Act (ACA) passed in 2010 will impact many aspects of the Medicaid program in a variety of ways (Guterman et al. 2010; Landers and Leeman 2011). We have discussed some of these throughout this chapter. A more detailed analysis of the ACA and all its provisions is provided in Chapter 3.

One of the major goals of the ACA is to reduce the number of uninsured persons in the country by making affordable health insurance available to everyone. This is to be accomplished by following two strategies: (1) requiring virtually all Americans to have basic health insurance coverage or pay a penalty in the form of a tax beginning in 2014; and (2) by expanding the Medicaid program to cover a large number of uninsured low-income individuals who are currently not eligible for Medicaid. Our discussion here focuses on this second strategy.

The law in effect creates a national eligibility standard for Medicaid instead of each state establishing its own eligibility standards constrained only by the minimum federal guidelines, as currently is the case. Under the law, effective January 2014, all states would have been required to cover all adults (under age 65) with income below 133 percent of the FPL with a 5-percentage-point offset. Thus, in practice, at a minimum, states have to cover all non-elderly persons making up to 138 percent of the FPL (Ku 2010). In 2018, 138 percent of the FPL amounts to $16,573 for an individual and $34,638 for a family of four (Paying for Senior Care 2018). Because Medicaid imposes certain categorical restrictions at present, it covers only about two out of five "poor" Americans, as defined by the federal poverty standards. The ACA established a new mandatory eligibility group and ended Medicaid's exclusion of individuals from coverage based on family status (Landers and Leeman 2011). States are free to expand coverage beyond the mandatory minimum threshold of 138 percent of the FLP by covering individuals making up to 200 or 300 percent of the FPL.

To encourage states to expand the Medicaid program under the ACA the federal government used the carrot-and-stick approach. The law provided for the federal government to pay 100 percent of the cost of covering the newly eligible Medicaid population under the Medicaid expansion from 2014 to 2016, followed by a 95-percent federal share in 2017, a 94-percent federal share in 2018, a 93-percent federal share in 2019 and a 90-percent federal share starting in 2020 and going forward (Flint 2014b). However, the law also threatened that if states refused to participate in the expansion, they could lose not only the federal funding relating to the expansion but also all of their federal Medicaid dollars, including their federal matching funding under the original Medicaid program (Pear and Cooper 2012).

A great deal of political controversy surrounded the enactment of the ACA in general and Medicaid expansion in particular. The law itself was passed largely along party lines, with almost all Republicans voting against the law and a majority of Democrats voting for it. The partisan and ideological divide was also clear in the debate over the

Medicaid expansion in Congress, with most Republicans and conservatives opposing it. Several lawsuits were filed challenging the constitutionality of the whole law itself, as well as the individual mandate, and the Medicaid expansion. One of the lawsuits, which included a Florida district court, included attorney generals of 26 states, two private citizens, and the National Federation of Independent Businesses, ultimately reached the US Supreme Court. After hearing oral arguments, the Supreme Court in the case of *NFIB v. Sebelius*, in June of 2012, by a 5–4 majority, upheld the constitutionality of the law and the individual mandate under Congress's power to tax. However, by a 7–2 majority, the court ruled that requiring states to expand their Medicaid program was unconstitutional and that the states are free to voluntarily join or to opt out of the expansion without fear of losing federal matching funds for the original Medicaid program. Thus, Medicaid expansion under the ACA was not mandatory but optional.

The Implementation of Medicaid Expansion under the ACA

The original Medicaid program as well as the expansion of the program under the ACA is a joint federal-state program and is viewed as a partnership between the federal and state governments. The history of American federalism shows that almost all joint federal-state programs share some of the same characteristics: implementation is often slow and uneven across states; program features often vary widely across states; federal government is generally accommodating to the states; partisan and political ideological conflicts permeate enactment and early implementation; federal grants/matching funds create financial incentives for states to respond to them; finally, not all eligible individuals are going to participate in the joint program (Haeder and Weimer 2015). Such has been the case with Medicaid expansion under the ACA.

Since almost all joint federal-state programs emphasize shared governance between the two levels of government, the federal government has to rely heavily on states to implement many such programs. This leads to intergovernmental negotiating and bargaining and both levels of governments use the leverage at their disposal to achieve their own goals. Often the goal of the federal government is to get states to participate in the program and help it achieve its policy objectives. The goal of the state governments is to achieve as much flexibility as they can from federal control in the implementation of the program within their respective states. The ACA was no exception. In fact, the Supreme Court ruling making state Medicaid expansion optional gave state governments even more leverage in bargaining with the federal government.

When it came to Medicaid expansion and implementation, the reactions of state officials can be classified into three groups. One group of officials immediately committed to participate and expand their Medicaid programs and viewed the expansion as financially beneficial to their states. This group included many Democratic officials and eventually included some Republican governors. The second group of officials included many Republican governors and a vast majority of Republican state legislatures who opposed expansion because of added cost to the state coffers in the out years after 2020 in light of the fact that state Medicaid costs were often the largest or the second-largest item in state budgets and also often the fastest-growing item. The third group of officials were those who were ambivalent and in general inclined to oppose expansion but would not completely rule out participating in the program at some point in the future. These officials were under pressure from hospitals to expand because of their fear of taking a big financial hit due to cuts and ultimate phasing out of the DSH payments for uncompensated care (Dinan 2014).

The federal government was eager to get as many states as possible to participate in the expansion of the Medicaid program under the ACA as a way to reduce the number of uninsured individuals in the country as well as to increase access to healthcare by reducing overall healthcare costs and insurance premiums. The biggest leverage the federal government had to encourage states to participate was the financial incentive. Under the law, the federal government picked up 100 percent of the cost of covering the newly eligible Medicaid population for three years, after which the federal government would continue to pick up 90 percent of the cost beginning in 2020. On their part, the state governments used the leverage of the threat of refusal to expand the program to win several concessions from the federal government. Some of the concessions states won from federal officials included announcement by the federal government that states could opt in or opt out of the expansion at any time, signing off on state waiver requests by granting states more flexibility in operating and experimenting in their Medicaid program—including agreeing to allow some states (e.g., Arkansas) to use federal Medicaid funds to purchase private insurance policies for newly eligible beneficiaries through the exchanges—and backing away from the threat of reducing federal Medicaid funding and passing off more cost to the states (Dinan 2014).

What Factors Explain States' Decisions to Expand or Not to Expand?

Income eligibility under Medicaid and the CHIP varies widely across states and by groups. As of January 2018, 32 states cover parents and other adults with income up to 138 percent of the FPL under the ACA Medicaid expansion to low-income adults. Most states extend coverage to pregnant women beyond the minimum of 138 percent of the FPL through Medicaid and the CHIP. Almost all states cover children with income up to at least 200 percent of the FPL, while some states cover children up to 300 percent of the FPL through Medicaid and the CHIP ("Where are States Today" 2018).

Since 2014 a steady stream of states have expanded their Medicaid programs to extend the coverage. In fact, many states have expanded their coverage in the Medicaid and the CHIP for different groups beyond the minimum threshold of 138 percent of the FPL established by the ACA. Initially, in 2012 only three states—Nevada, New York, and Vermont—expanded Medicaid. As can been seen from Table 4.2, most expansion occurred in 2013, when 21 states expanded their Medicaid programs. By 2014, a total of 27 states and the District of Columbia had expanded their Medicaid programs. That number had reached 31 states and DC by July of 2016. As of June 7, 2018, 33 states and DC had expanded their Medicaid programs, three were considering expansion and 14 states had no plans to expand ("Status of Action on Medicaid Expansion Decision" 2018).

As a result of the November 2018 elections, three more states will expand their Medicaid programs. In three states—Utah, Nebraska, and Idaho—voters approved ballot measures that require states to expand Medicaid coverage under the ACA beginning in 2019. This brings the total number of states with Medicaid expansion under the ACA to 36, plus the District of Columbia. However, it should be noted that Montana voters rejected a measure in the November ballot that would have extended Medicaid expansion beyond June 30, 2019, when it is set to sunset unless the state legislature acts to expand it ("Status of Action on Medicaid Expansion Decision" 2018).

Why did some states decide to expand their Medicaid programs under the ACA, while some others have not expanded their Medicaid programs despite the tremendous financial incentive provided by the federal government? What factors help explain states' decisions to expand or not to expand? Researchers have explored these questions and have identified several factors that help explain states' decisions.

Barrilleaux and Rainey (2014) have argued that states' decisions to expand or not to expand Medicaid under the ACA are driven entirely by partisan politics and to a much lesser extent by public opinion. The economic conditions or the financial needs of the states have had very little effect on the expansion decision.

Olson (2015) has also argued that partisanship and ideology have played a major role in states' expansion decisions. She points to the fact that of the 26 state attorney generals who opposed the ACA's individual mandate and Medicaid expansion and launched a court challenge, all but one were Republicans. Even after the Supreme Court made Medicaid expansion under the ACA optional, a vast majority of Republican governors and Republican-controlled state legislatures initially balked and refused to expand. According to Olson, two competing partisan narratives emerged around the issue of expansion. The Democrats supported expansion because it fit into their neoliberal ideology, which envisioned a robust role for the national government combined with private-sector market approaches as a way to reach near-universal health insurance coverage for the working poor. The Republican narrative at the national (Congressional) level was to repeal the ACA and/or dismantle it piece by piece. At the state level, Republicans have argued that Medicaid is an expensive and inefficient program and it fosters federal government encroachment into the private sector and state rights and authority. Olson points to the fact that around three-quarters of 29 Republican governors initially opposed expansion, while 20 Democratic governors (14 of them backed by Democratic-controlled state legislatures) and one independent governor supported it. Thus, Olson argues that the decision to adopt Medicaid expansion or not has largely been a partisan one.

Research suggests that while partisanship has played a significant role in the expansion decision, it is not the only factor. There are other factors besides partisanship that have also played a role in state governments' decisions. Callaghan and Jacobs (2014) found that the presence of a Republican legislature had a negative influence on the expansion decision, while the presence of a Republican governor had a more nuanced effect. Conversely, the stronger the Democratic Party control over state government, the more likely a state was to implement Medicaid expansion. After controlling for party domination, they found that the trajectory of established policy for the vulnerable population and state learning about the process of intergovernmental bargaining were other factors that also exercised influence on the expansion decision. States with well-established and generous social programs for low-income individuals create self-reinforcing and positive feedback (path dependency), making such states more willing to expand their Medicaid program. Similarly, states with experience in negotiating and

Table 4.2

State Action on Medicaid Expansion under the ACA, December 2018

Year Expanded	Expanded	Has Not Expanded
	36 States and DC	14 States
2010	Washington (state) Washington DC	Alabama
2012	Nevada	Florida
	New York	Georgia
	Vermont	Kansas
2013	Arizona	Mississippi
	Arkansas	Missouri
	California	North Carolina
	Colorado	Oklahoma
	Connecticut	South Carolina
	Delaware	South Dakota
	Hawaii	Tennessee
	Illinois	Texas
	Iowa	Wisconsin
	Maryland	Wyoming
	Massachusetts	
	Michigan	
	Minnesota	
	New Jersey	
	North Dakota	
	New Mexico	
	Ohio	
	Oregon	
	Rhode Island	
	Washington	
	West Virginia	
2014	Kentucky	
	New Hampshire	
	Pennsylvania	
2015	Alaska	
	Indiana	
	Montana	
2016	Louisiana	
2017	Maine	
2018	Virginia	
2019[a]	Idaho	
	Nebraska	
	Utah	

[a] Voters in these three states approved ballot measures to expand Medicaid in 2019.

Sources: "Where the States Stand on Medicaid Expansion." http://advisory.com/Daily-Briefing/Resources/Primers/Medicaid Map; "Status of State Action on the Medicaid Erxpansion Decision." www.kff.org/.

Table 4.3

Expenditures for Medicaid and CHIP Programs, Selected Calendar Years

Expenditure Amount (Millions)	1966	1997	1998	2000	2005	2010	2011	2012	2013	2014	2015	2016
Total National Health Expenditures	46,081	1,135,224	1,201,451	1,369,125	2,023,744	2,598,823	2,689,349	2,797,260	2,879,008	3,026,157	3,200,815	33,37,248
Medicaid (Title XIX) (Total $)	1,304	160,849	169,011	200,345	309,275	397,226	406,744	422,688	445,361	496,645	544,073	5,65,550
Federal $	632	94,954	98,648	116,821	177,461	266,360	247,125	243,251	256,907	305,106	343,123	358,095
Federal %	48%	59%	58%	58%	57%	67%	61%	58%	58%	61%	63%	63%
State and Local $	672	65,896	70,363	83,524	131,814	130,865	159,619	179,438	188,454	191,540	200,951	207,454
State and Local %	52%	41%	42%	42%	43%	33%	39%	42%	42%	39%	37%	37%
CHIP (Title XIX and Title XXI) Total $			399	3,012	7,566	11,540	11,990	12,629	13,509	13,215	14,853	16,883
Federal $			276	2,097	5,254	8,052	8,377	8,780	9,362	9,217	11,106	15,309
Federal %			69%	70%	69%	70%	70%	70%	69%	70%	75%	91%
State and Local $			123	915	2,313	3,489	3,613	3,848	4,146	3,998	3,747	1,573
State and Local %			31%	30%	31%	30%	30%	30%	31%	30%	25%	9%

Source: Centers for Medicare & Medicaid Services, Office of the Actuary, National Health Statistics Group. Online at www.cms.gov/Research-Statistics-Data-and-Systems/Statistics-Trends-and-Reports/NationalHealthExpendData/index.htm.

working with CMS and HHS over Medicaid changes are more likely to decide to expand their Medicaid program, having learned the skills to effectively bargain with the federal government. Finally, they also find that affluence/economic conditions of the state and state institutional and administrative capacity have also played some role in expansion decisions.

Callaghan and Jacobs (2016) found that state party control has a positive and statistically significant effect on Medicaid expansion, but it is not a sufficient explanation for Medicaid expansion since several states like Arizona, Iowa, New Mexico, Ohio, and North Dakota, in which Republicans wield power, also expanded their Medicaid programs. They found that interest-group dynamics in the state also played a role, with business and professional interest groups having a negative influence and public advocacy interest groups having a positive influence on the decision to expand Medicaid. The influence of state affluence and economic circumstances on the expansion decision was not statistically significant. How does one explain the fact that some states where Republicans wield power have gone against the general national Republican narrative and implemented Medicaid expansion? Jacobs and Callaghan (2013) have suggested that the explanation may lie in the fact that such states were under cross-pressure, whereby political party orientation tilted them against expansion, but other state dynamics, such as level of state affluence, past policy trajectory and institutional and administrative capacity, have pushed them to adopt the expansion.

In summary, research suggests that the most significant factor in the decision to expand or not to expand the Medicaid program under the ACA is partisanship (state party control). However, factors such as the trajectory of the already-established program, experience and learning from intergovernmental bargaining, dynamics of interest-group interplay in the state, state affluence and the state's institutional and administrative capacity also play a role—but a lesser role—in influencing states' Medicaid expansion decisions.

Justifications for Expansion and Consequences

The fact that thus far 33 states and the District of Columbia have expanded their Medicaid programs under the ACA suggests that they must have seen some advantages in doing so. Why expand Medicaid under the ACA? The reasons often cited for expansion include the following. First, Medicaid expansion is a good policy for both uninsured patients and healthcare providers. The expansion provides health insurance protection to low-income individuals and providers benefit because it would help reduce the cost of uncompensated care. Second, extending health insurance coverage under Medicaid expansion is good for both the physical and mental health of the uninsured and it offers financial protection to a population that is more vulnerable to the cost of healthcare. Third, the federal financial incentive is too good to pass up. Given the high federal match rate, a state's spending for the expansion (added cost to the state) as a proportion of its economy would be very small. Fourth, since under the expansion states would receive hundreds of millions of dollars in federal matching funds, expansion would help stimulate a state's economy by promoting job and income growth. It would generate a larger tax base for the state, and lower unemployment due to new jobs created by federal spending. Fifth, many social work services funded entirely by states and local governments would be underwritten with federal matching dollars, saving money (Flint 2014b; Frakt and Carroll 2013).

Research suggests that states that have expanded their Medicaid programs have experienced many positive benefits as a result of expansion. The benefits include the following.

- States that have expanded Medicaid have experienced significant health insurance coverage gains without diverting coverage from traditional groups and reduction in uninsured rates (Antonisse et al. 2018; McCarter 2015; McMorrow et al. 2016; Rudowitz and Antonisse 2018). Since the passage of the ACA, it is estimated that 20 million Americans have gained health insurance coverage, lowering the rate of uninsured to around 10 percent nationwide. Most of this gain has been due to Medicaid expansion (Bloomberg and Holahan 2016; Mattoon 2016).
- Studies have also demonstrated that Medicaid expansion has increased access to healthcare and increased utilization of healthcare services (Antonisse et al. 2018; Choi et al. 2017; Rudowitz and Antonisse 2018). Increased Medicaid eligibility is associated with a higher probability of having a general doctor visit and improved mental health status among the low-income population (McMorrow et al. 2016).
- Medicaid expansion has improved the affordability of care and financial security among low-income individuals (Antonisse et al. 2018; Rudowitz and Antonisse 2018). Expanding Medicaid eligibility has reduced the unmet needs of low-income individuals due to cost consideration (McMorrow et al. 2016).

- The expansion of Medicaid eligibility under the ACA has protected low-income Americans not only from out-of-pocket medical costs but has also improved their overall financial health. Expansion has significantly reduced the number of unpaid medical bills (Drum 2016; "Medicaid Expansion Under Obamacare has Improved Financial Health of Low-Income Americans" 2016).
- The healthcare disparity with whites narrowed more for both blacks and Hispanics on three access indicators among expansion states compared to non-expansion states—the percentage of uninsured working-age adults, the percentage who skipped care because of costs and the percentage who lacked a regular care provider (Hayes et al. 2017).
- Medicaid expansion under the ACA has had positive economic effects largely tied to the infusion of federal dollars and has resulted in a reduction in uninsured visits and uncompensated care costs for hospitals, clinics and other providers (Antonisse et al. 2018).
- Medicaid expansion has had either some positive or neutral effects on employment and the labor market (Rudowitz and Antonisse 2018).

Justifications for Non-Expansion and Consequences

As of June 2018, 14 states have not expanded their Medicaid programs, while three (Nebraska, Utah, and Idaho) are considering expansion. Republicans are in control (Republican governors and/or Republican-controlled state legislatures) in all 14 states that have not expanded Medicaid. This again indicates that partisanship is one of the important factors in Medicaid expansion decisions. However, the decision not to expand is never couched in partisan terms. Rather, the justifications cited for not expanding Medicaid include the following. First, opponents of expansion claim that Medicaid is an inefficient program that is riddled with waste, fraud, and abuse, despite research evidence that contradicts such claims (Grant 2014). Second, even though the federal government would pay 90 percent of the cost of the expansion, it would cause additional cost to the state Medicaid budget, which states cannot afford. Third, the federal government cannot be trusted to keep its promise of funding 90 percent of the cost of expansion in the future. Fourth, Medicaid expansion would lead to more federal control and authority. Fifth, the Medicaid expansion would largely benefit Democratic constituents and not Republican constituents (Frakt and Carroll 2013). It is important to remember, as noted earlier, that there are several Republican-controlled states that have expanded Medicaid and have decided to keep expansion under the Trump administration.

What are the consequences of states' decisions not to expand Medicaid under the ACA? Research has demonstrated several negative consequences of a decision not to expand.

- Non-expanding states will forgo or lose millions of dollars of federal funds coming into the states. For example, according to one estimate, Texas will forgo about $9.58 billion, Florida $5 billion, and Georgia $4.9 billion in federal funding in 2022 (Glied and Ma 2013).
- The Urban Institute estimated that non-expansion states caused 6 million people to remain uninsured in 2016, with Texas, Florida, and Georgia accounting for half of the total (Barofsky 2015).
- A higher proportion of low-income individuals in non-expanding states do not have a usual source of care and have lower rates of dental checks, routine physical checks, blood-pressure checks, and flu vaccinations (Han et al. 2015).
- Compared to Medicaid expansion states, low-income individuals in non-expansion states are more likely to be black and reside in rural areas and are less likely to have a regular source of care. In addition, the racial and ethnic composition of the population that falls into the coverage gap disproportionately affects people of color, particularly black Americans. This could lead to increased disparity between two sets of states among disadvantaged groups (Garfield, Damico, and Orgera 2018; Han et al. 2015).
- Poor uninsured adults who fall into a coverage gap because of a decision not to expand are likely to face barriers to needed health services and may face serious financial consequences if they need medical care (Garfield, Damico, and Orgera 2018).
- It is estimated that if all states that have not expanded Medicaid did so, hundreds of thousands of low-income poor would have a usual source of care, preventive care and regular checkups, and fewer people would face catastrophic out-of-pocket medical costs and trouble paying medical bills (Buettgens 2018; Council of Economic Advisors 2014).

CHANGES IN MEDICAID ENROLLEES, ENROLLMENT, AND EXPENDITURES

Characteristics of Program Enrollees

Today, Medicaid and the CHIP provide health insurance coverage to low-income children, pregnant women, people with disabilities, adults, and elderly who meet the eligibility qualification. In 2016, of all Medicaid enrollees, 54 percent were women and 46 percent were men; 47 percent were under the age of 21, 7 percent were between the age of 21 and 26, 35 percent were between the age of 27 and 64, while 11 percent were elderly ("Who Enrolls in Medicaid and CHIP?" 2017). The number of men and adults enrolled in the Medicaid program has increased since the implementation of the ACA. In 2013, prior to Medicaid expansion under the ACA, 58 percent of enrollees were women, while 42 percent were men and 31 percent were adults between the ages of 27 and 64 ("Medicaid Enrollment by Gender and Age" 2013).

Medicaid Enrollment and Expenditures

Enrollment and expenditures of the Medicaid program can fluctuate and are influenced by two major factors, one of whch is the economy. During the economic downturn and recession, individuals lose jobs, incomes decline and consequently more people become eligible and enroll in the Medicaid program. Higher enrollment in the program also leads to higher expenditures for the program. In addition, economic downturn also negatively impacts state revenues, which places additional pressure on Medicaid state budgets, and demands for other forms of assistance such as food stamps and unemployment compensation also increase. When the economy improves or is doing well, lower unemployment and rising income can lead to a decline in enrollment and expenditures for the program. The second factor that can influence enrollment and expenditures is the introduction of major policy changes in the program, such as the creation of the CHIP in 1997 and the ACA in 2010.

For example, after the economic recession started in 2008, the unemployment rate in the country had reached 10 percent by 2009. State governments not only experienced high unemployment rates but their revenue also declined. Medicaid enrollment jumped from a 3.1-percent increase in 2008 to a 7.6-percent increase in 2009. Correspondingly Medicaid spending jumped from a 5.8-percent increase in 2008 to a 7.8-percent increase in 2009. As the economy began to recover from the recession, the enrollment growth had slowed to 2.3 percent and the total spending was -4.0 percent in 2012 ("Medicaid Enrollment and Spending Growth: FY 2015 & 2016" 2015).

Similarly, the passage of the ACA in 2010 and the implementation of Medicaid expansion in the following years significantly impacted total Medicaid enrollment. The Medicaid annual enrollment growth rate increased by 1.5 percent in 2013, 5.3 percent in 2014, and 13.2 percent in 2015. By 2016, the annual enrollment growth rate declined to 3.9 percent ("Medicaid Enrollment and Spending Growth: FY 2016 & 2017" 2016). The annual enrollment growth rate slowed even further in 2017, to 2.7 percent ("Medicaid Enrollment and Spending Growth: FY 2017 & 2018" 2017).

In April of 2018, 67.3 million were enrolled in Medicaid and 6.4 million were enrolled in the CHIP. The number of children enrolled in the CHIP and Medicaid stood at 35.6 million, making up about 50 percent of the total enrollment in the programs ("Medicaid and CHIP Enrollment Data Highlights: April 2018 Report" 2018).

One way to examine the impact of the ACA on total Medicaid enrollment is to examine Medicaid enrollment in 2013 prior to the start of the first open enrollment period under marketplace exchanges and before Medicaid expansion was in full swing. From July to September 2013, the total Medicaid enrollment (including in the CHIP) stood at 56.5 million, of which 37.9 million enrollees lived in expansion states and 18.6 million lived in non-expansion states. According to the preliminary data, by April of 2018, the total number of Medicaid enrollees stood at 73.7 million, of which 52.9 million were in expansion states while 20.9 million were in non-expansion states. As the data indicate, the number of Medicaid enrollees increased 39 percent in expansion states, compared to 12 percent in non-expansion states ("Medicaid and CHIP Enrollment Data Highlights: April 2018 Report" 2018). Clearly, Medicaid expansion under the ACA played a major role in expanding health insurance coverage to millions of low-income individuals.

Needless to say, with a significant increase in the number of enrollees, the expenditures for Medicaid also increased considerably after Medicaid expansion. Medicaid spending grew 11.5 percent in 2014 and 9.5 percent in 2015. The high growth in spending in 2014 and 2015 is largely attributed to the initial impact of Medicaid expansion in 2013 and 2014 and the resulting growth in total Medicaid enrollment. As the Medicaid expansion tapered off, so did the expenditures. Medicaid spending increases slowed to 3.9 percent in 2016 and 2.9 percent in 2017 ("National Health Expenditure 2016 Highlights" n.d.; "National Health Expenditure Projections 2017–2026" n.d.).

However, Medicaid spending growth is projected to average 6.1 percent over 2021–2026 largely because of higher per-enrollee spending; the proportion of aged and disabled enrollees is expected to grow, and they require more expensive care ("National Health Expenditure 2016 Highlights" n.d.; "National Health Expenditure Projections 2017–2026" n.d.).

The total Medicaid spending for financial year 2016 was $553 billion, with the federal government contributing, on average, 63 percent of the total cost and the state governments contributing 37 percent. When we examine the spending pattern in Medicaid by different groups enrolled in the program, some interesting facts emerge. An analysis of breakdown in Medicaid spending by enrollment groups revealed that while children constituted almost 43 percent of the total enrollees in 2014, they accounted for only 19 percent of the total Medicaid spending. Thus, providing health insurance coverage to low-income children is cost-effective and a good long-term investment. In contrast, disabled individuals constituted only 14 percent of the total enrollees but they accounted for 40 percent of the total Medicaid spending. Similarly, the aged constituted 9 percent of the total enrollment, but accounted for 21 percent of the total spending. Elderly and disabled enrollees combined account for almost 50 percent of the Medicaid spending. These two groups face more health problems and need more expensive and longer-term care ("Medicaid Enrollees by Enrollment Groups" 2015; "Medicaid Spending Per Enrollees" 2015).

MEDICAID WAIVERS

What are Medicaid Waivers?

The Medicaid program varies among states for two reasons. First, the federal government only sets minimum standards related to eligibility and benefits and states enjoy discretionary authority to make decisions about program eligibility and benefit options. Thus, a waiver is not always needed to implement certain changes by the states. Second, states can apply for a waiver from certain federal requirements, giving them additional flexibility to experiment and reform the Medicaid program within their state to meet their unique needs and circumstances.

Types of Medicaid Waivers

Medicaid waivers can be divided into three major categories.

Section 1115 Research and Demonstration Project Waivers

Section 1115 of the Social Security Act gives states permission to experiment with innovative ways to design and deliver Medicaid services to enrollees. This type of waiver allows states to experiment with new or existing approaches to financing and delivering health services under Medicaid and the CHIP. For example, states can provide coverage to otherwise-ineligible populations, provide services typically not covered by Medicaid, experiment with cost-sharing and other payment reforms, and implement changes to the service delivery system. States must demonstrate in their application for a waiver that federal Medicaid expenditures will not exceed what would have occurred without the demonstration. In addition, states must demonstrate that if granted, a waiver would increase and strengthen the overall coverage of the low-income population in the state, would improve health outcomes for Medicaid and other low-income populations in the state, would increase access to providers and strengthen provider networks, and would increase efficiency and quality of care for low-income individuals by transforming the service delivery network in an innovative way. Finally, states are required to provide matching funds through a variety of sources such as general funds, intergovernmental transfers or state-funded health programs ("Medicaid Waivers in the States: Seven FAQS" 2018).

Section 1915 Waiver Programs

Under the Social Security Act's Section 1915 waiver program, individual enrollees are required to meet criteria set by the state based on their level of needs. There are different types of waivers states can apply for under Section 1915 waiver programs.

Under a Section 1915(a) waiver, states can implement a voluntary managed-care program by executing a contract with companies via competitive bidding to procure Medicaid managed-care services. A Section 1915(b) waiver allows states to provide Medicaid services through managed-care delivery systems or to limit beneficiaries' choice of providers. Section 1915(c) waivers allow states to provide long-term care services in home and community settings rather than institutional settings such as nursing homes. Under Section 1915(i), states can offer a wide range of services under a State Plan Home and Community-Based Services benefit. Under Section 1915(j), states can offer self-directed personal assistance services. Finally, Section 1915(k) established under the ACA the Community First Choice Option allowing states to provide home and community-based attendant services ("1915 Wavier Processing Tools for States" n.d.).

Under concurrent Section 1915(b) and 1915(c) waivers, states can simultaneously implement both types of waivers to provide a continuum of services to the elderly and people with disabilities as long as all federal program requirements are met ("Medicaid Waivers in the States: Seven FAQS" 2018; The Commonwealth Fund 2018).

Section 1332 Innovation Waivers under the Affordable Care Act

Section 1332 of the ACA allows states to waive some portions of the Act, such as requirements-related qualified health plans, health benefit exchanges, and cost-sharing, within limits, as long as they retain the basic protections guaranteed under the ACA. The states can establish an alternate health reform network within the limits of the law. States can apply for waivers from Medicaid, the CHIP, Medicare and any federal law related to the provision of healthcare items or services. Such a waiver is often called an "innovation waiver" because it allows states to experiment with new and innovative methods for providing health coverage and service delivery (McDonough 2014).

Title 1 in Section 1332 allows states to seek waivers from the requirement of establishing qualified health plans, including minimum essential benefits, specified standards, and coinsurance limits; the creation of government or non-profit Health Benefit Exchanges; reduced cost-sharing for low-income individuals and families enrolled in qualified health plans; and IRS regulations related to refundable tax credits for premiums. States applying for such waivers have to demonstrate how an innovation waiver will meet the ACA's goal of coverage expansion, affordability, and comprehensiveness, implementation timeline, economic analysis and actuarial certification, as well as how the waiver might impact provisions of the ACA that are not waived, like access to health services and the deterrence of fraud, abuse and waste, and specific plans for filing periodic reports (McDonough 2014). Typically, waivers granted under Section 1332 are limited to five years and must be renewed.

States can coordinate 1332 and 1115 waivers to achieve better alignment across insurance programs related to premiums, cost-sharing, purchasing, eligibility, and enrollment. States can seek multiple waivers to obtain permission to change the Medicaid program under Section 1115 of the Social Security Act and their marketplace coverage under the Section 1332 waiver of the ACA. To obtain a Section 1332 waiver, state legislatures must pass authorizing legislation to implement Medicaid reform under such a waiver. As of January 2017, states are allowed to implement approved waivers ("Medicaid Waivers in the States: Seven FAQS" 2018).

Medicaid Waivers and State Medicaid Reforms, 1980s–2010s

Since the establishment of the Medicaid program in 1965, states have been granted waivers. Such waivers tended to be small in scope and number. However, beginning in the 1980s and accelerating in the 1990s, states began to use waivers for a wide range of purposes. Many administrations going back to 1980s began to view waivers as an important tool to decentralize federal authority and give state governments more flexibility to experiment with the Medicaid program. The administrations of both President Reagan (1981–1989) and President George H. W. Bush (1989–1993) made frequent use of Medicaid waivers (Thompson and Burke 2009). President Clinton (1993–2001) pursued his own vision of Medicaid devolution (Thompson 1998). The Clinton administration allowed states more flexibility on Medicaid funds and supported states' efforts at innovation and experimentation. The Clinton administration created a more receptive environment for both Medicaid demonstrations (Section 1115) and program waivers (Section 1915). The hallmark of the Clinton years with respect to Medicaid waivers was the approval of 17 Section 1915(b) comprehensive waivers that moved a large number of Medicaid enrollees into managed care (Thompson and Burke 2007).

During the 1980 and 1990s, many of the state Medicaid reforms carried out through the use of Medicaid waivers involved the following.

- *Cutbacks in eligibility, benefits and coverage*: in efforts to cut Medicaid expenditures, states engaged in narrowing eligibility and cutting benefits and services (Altman 1983; Altman and Morgan 1983; Bovbjerg and Holahan 1982; Johnson 1983).
- *Increased use of co-payment*: several states started to make use of co-payment in the hope of making Medicaid beneficiaries more cost-conscious (Johnson 1983).

- *Use of competitive bidding and contractual and prudent buyer arrangements*: this was done in the hope of reducing Medicaid expenditures by introducing competition in the marketplace. For example, in 1982 the state of Arizona implemented the Arizona Health Care Cost Containment System (AHCCCS), which relied on providers bidding for the delivery of healthcare to the indigent (Vogel 1984). Starting in 1983, California's Medicaid Program—Medi-Cal—began to rely on negotiated fixed-price arrangements by establishing selective contracting with hospitals in 1983 (Johnson 1983).
- *Healthcare rationing*: in 1994, Oregon implemented the Oregon Health Plan, under which the state agreed to cover all poor people in the state but not to cover all medical services (Kosterlitz 1990).
- *Replacing traditional Medicaid with a state plan*: in the mid-1990s, Tennessee made history when it replaced its traditional Medicaid program by implementing TennCare. Under this program, the state extended coverage to uninsured and uninsurable adults and children and provided a wide range of medical services.
- *Managed-care plans*: many states made increased use of managed-care plans to address the problems of cost and access through the use of Medicaid research and demonstration projects, especially for the most costly Medicaid beneficiaries—the elderly and the disabled (Iglehart 2011). Under both the Oregon Health Plan and TennCare, all beneficiaries were to be serviced by capitated managed-care organizations that were known as Health Maintenance Organizations (HMOs) (Bonnyman 1996; Larson and Williams 2003; Schwartz and Aaron 1985).
- *Privatization of Medicaid*: some states moved in the direction of "privatization" of their Medicaid programs. Under such arrangements, states and the federal government continue to fund the program jointly, but the day-to-day control of health plans for the poor is turned over to managed-care organizations or private insurers. Many states required Medicaid recipients to enroll in some form of Medical Care Organizations (MCOs).
- *New approaches to reimbursing providers*: state governments, through the use of waivers, implemented new approaches to reimbursing providers, such as paying physicians a set fee or capitation payment rather than the traditional fee-for-service, limits or ceilings on physician payments or the use of fee schedules.
- *New Medicaid hospital payment models*: finally, many states also implemented new Medicaid hospital payment models. Many states have adopted some form of hospital rate review or a prospective reimbursement system. Rate-setting programs fall into three broad strategies to control Medicaid costs: multiple-payer rate setting, Medicaid-only prospective payment, and selective contracting (Holahan 1988). State rate-setting programs have produced mixed results.

The Current State of Medicaid Waivers and Reforms

It is important to note that the landscape of Medicaid waivers is constantly changing. It is impossible to discuss all different waivers and Medicaid reforms undertaken by each of the 50 states. Thus, we first provide a brief overview of approved and pending waivers at present and then we focus our discussion on some of the more important state Medicaid reforms/experiments and trends.

Broad Overview of Approved and Pending Waivers

Section 1115 Medicaid Demonstration Waivers

As of July 2018, under Section 1115, 45 Medicaid demonstration waivers were approved across 38 states, while 22 waivers are pending approval across 22 states. Many states have multiple waivers approved or pending and they fall into different categories. Of the approved waivers, 7 involve implementing Medicaid expansion through alternative models that differ from federal law; 7 involve implementing certain eligibility and enrollment restrictions; 6 involve implementing health behavior incentives tied to premium or cost-sharing reductions and charging co-payments in excess of the federal maximum for non-emergency use of the emergency room; 21 involve the use of federal funds to pay for certain behavioral health issues, such as in-patient substance use and/or mental health services for non-elderly adults in institutions for mental disease, and fund other behavioral health or supportive services; 16 waivers involve states using federal Medicaid funds to reform or experiment with delivery of healthcare services for Medicaid patients; 12 involve authorizing delivery of Medicaid long-term services and supports (MLTSS) through capitated managed care; 16 involve providing services such as acute care services or community-based services to certain "targeted groups" such as persons with HIV/AIDS, seniors and persons with disabilities; and 3 involve work requirements. Of the 23 pending Medicaid waivers,

7 involve eligibility enrollment restrictions; 7 involve work requirements; 6 involve benefit restriction and co-payments; 15 involve dealing with behavioral health; 4 involve MLTSS; and 2 involve targeted population waivers ("Medicaid Waiver Tracker: Which States Have Approved or Pending Section 1115 Medicaid Waivers" 2018).

Section 1332 Innovation Waivers under the ACA

It should be noted that Section 1332 innovation waivers under the ACA are very broad; a state can seek a waiver from various requirements of the ACA as it pertains to Medicare, the CHIP, and Medicaid. Thus, a waiver under Section 1332 is not limited only to the Medicaid program. States can also submit innovation waivers under Section 1332 of the ACA in conjunction with a Medicaid waiver under Section 1115 of the Social Security Act. However, innovation waivers cannot be used to change Medicaid program requirements (Tolbert and Pollitz 2017). Initially one of the purposes of Section 1332 of the ACA was to encourage reluctant states such as Arkansas, Iowa, and Michigan to expand their Medicaid programs (McDonough 2014).

Since the implementation of innovation waivers approved under Section 1332 began only in January of 2017, as of May 2018, only four states—Alaska, Hawaii, Minnesota, and Oregon—had implemented innovation waivers. The innovation waivers for Alaska, Minnesota, and Oregon essentially allow federal pass-through funding to partially finance reimbursement to insurers. The Hawaii waiver requires employers to provide more generous coverage than is required under the ACA. Waiver applications from two states, Maine, and Wisconsin, are awaiting approval. Six states—Massachusetts, Ohio, Vermont, California, Iowa, and Oklahoma—having initially applied for waivers, have withdrawn their applications for the time being because they were deemed incomplete by the CMS ("Tracking Section 1332 State Innovation Waivers" 2018; "Section 1332: State Innovation Waivers" n.d.).

Section 1915 Medicaid Waivers

Today, a large majority of Medicaid enrollees are in managed-care programs under Section 1915(b) waivers. Similarly, today, all states implement at least one home and community-based services (HCBS) as an alternative to institutional care, leading to a shift away from care provided in an institutional setting such as a nursing home. More states have also adopted capitated payment systems instead of the traditional fee-for-service method for Medicaid managed long-term services and supports (MLTSS) under Section 1115 Medicaid demonstration waivers to streamline program administration, improve care coordination and increase beneficiary access to community-based services. In 2016, 11 states were using Section 1115 waivers to provide capitated MLTSS with 900,000 beneficiaries enrolled. Almost all such waivers were approved since 2012 (Watts, Musumeci, and Ubri 2017).

Trends in Medicaid Reforms and Experiments: Private-Sector Approaches

Managed Care

Under a managed-care delivery system, providers deliver health benefits and services to Medicaid enrollees through contracted arrangements between state Medicaid agencies and managed-care organizations (MCOs) that accept a set per-member, per-month payment for those services, i.e., a capitated payment system. The primary goals of the use of a managed-care delivery system are to improve the performance of health plans, health quality and health outcomes. Since the early 1990s state Medicaid agencies began to utilize managed care in efforts to contain costs and improve healthcare delivery. By the end of the 1990s, more than half of Medicaid beneficiaries were enrolled in a managed-care plans (Smith, Arose, and Coustasse 2014).

Today, states are implementing a wide range of initiatives to coordinate and integrate the delivery of care beyond traditional managed care. Some of these initiatives include improving care for Medicaid enrollees with chronic and complex medical conditions, aligning payment incentives with performance goals and creating accountability for high-quality care.

Federal managed-care regulations recognize four types of managed-care entities: managed-care organizations (MCOs), primary-care case management (PCCM), pre-paid inpatient health plans (PIHP), and pre-paid ambulatory health plans (PAHP),

The dominant model is the comprehensive managed-care MCOs, in which the managed-care organization provides comprehensive acute care, and, in some cases, long-term services and support. MCOs can be grouped into to Medicaid-only (100 percent of plan enrollment consists of Medicaid enrollees), Medicaid-dominant (Medicaid enrollees count for 75 to 99 percent of total plan enrollment), or Medicaid-focused (Medicaid enrollees account for less than 75 percent of total enrollment).

A PCCM provider physician or group practice physician contracts directly with the state Medicaid agency to locate, coordinate and monitor primary care. PIHP is a pre-paid in-patient health plan providing less-than-comprehensive services that arranges, provides and is responsible for any in-patient hospital and institutional services. PAHP is a pre-paid ambulatory health plan that provides less-than-comprehensive services on an at-risk or other-than-state-reimbursement basis and does not typically provide or coordinate in-patient hospital or institutional services ("Medicaid Managed Care Enrollment and Program Characteristics 2016" 2018).

In April of 2016, the CMS issued final regulations that revised and significantly strengthened existing Medicaid managed-care rules. The major goals of these new rules were to align Medicaid and CHIP managed-care requirements, enhance and protect beneficiaries' care, to promote quality of care and to strengthen actuarial soundness or payment provisions and program integrity (Paradise and Musumeci 2016).

Comprehensive Medicaid managed-care plans serve a wide range of population including pregnant women, children, non-disabled adults and ACA adults in states that expanded Medicaid programs. In addition, such plans also serve special-needs populations such as people with disabilities or HIV/AIDS, dual-eligible individuals, children with special healthcare needs, and children in foster care. Some plans are specifically designed as "specialty plans" designed to serve targeted populations (Garfield et al. 2018a).

Over the years, the number of the Medicaid population enrolled in managed-care plans has grown substantially; in 2002, the total Medicaid population was 40 million, of which 23 million (57 percent) were enrolled in managed-care plans ("Medicaid Management Care Enrollment Report: Summary Statistics as of July 1, 2011" 2011). On July 1, 2016, the total number of Medicaid enrollees nationwide was 80.2 million, of which 65 million (81 percent) were enrolled in managed-care plans. Of the 80.2 million enrollees, 55.6 million (68 percent) were enrolled in comprehensive Medicaid managed plans with the remainder enrolled in other types of plans. Medicaid enrollment in comprehensive managed-care plans increased by 7.2 percent from 2015 to 2016. More than 12 million low-income adults covered under the ACA Medicaid expansion were enrolled in comprehensive managed-care plans ("Medicaid Managed Care Enrollment and Program Characteristics 2016" 2018).

While it is clear that a large majority of Medicaid beneficiaries are enrolled in some type of managed-care plan, the plans do face several challenges. In a 2017 survey of Medicaid managed-care plans carried out by the Kaiser Family Foundation, respondents listed some of the following challenges they faced in ensuring access to care. The top two challenges listed were provider supply shortages in certain specialties (65 percent) and certain geographic areas (62 percent). Others listed were capitation rate paid by states being too low (48 percent), lack of continuous eligibility for Medicaid members (46 percent), and lack of member education about how to access care (Garfield et al. 2018a).

Consumer-Directed Healthcare

Consumer-directed healthcare plans emerged in the 1990s in a response to the backlash against managed care and to address the problem of rising health expenditures. They were intended to reduce healthcare spending by exposing consumers to the financial implications of their treatment decisions by giving them more control over decisions affecting their own health and treatment (Goodell and Bundorf 2012). The underlying assumption of consumer-directed healthcare plans is that consumers would make more informed choices and forego unnecessary medical care if they had to use more of their own money to pay for it. This would help avoid the problem of moral hazard in health insurance, which posits that if the consumer does not have to pay for any of the cost of their health insurance, they are more likely to engage in risky and wasteful health behavior (Yi 2010). Consumer-directed health plans generally are low-premium, high-deductible insurance plans and generally involve some form of health savings accounts. Many employers have begun to offer such plans to their employees.

State governments and the federal government also became interested in the concept of consumer-directed healthcare to address the problem of rising Medicaid expenditures and their impact on state budgets. In the early 1990s, several states enacted laws authorizing Medical Savings Accounts (MSAs) and in 1996 the federal government authorized the establishment of MSAs under the Health Insurance Portability and Accountability Act (HIPAA). Workers/employees could set aside pre-tax dollars through MSAs to pay for their healthcare. In 2002, the Treasury Department authorized tax-favored Health Reimbursement Arrangements (HRAs), which allowed employers to structure a portion of their benefits package as a durable fund that employees can use to pay for covered services or accumulate for future healthcare needs. With the Medicare Modernization Act of 2003, Congress authorized the creation of Health Savings Accounts (HSAs) to give consumers even more control of their own healthcare choices. HSAs allow eligible persons and their employers to make a tax-free contribution to the HSA account. However, the HSAs are held exclusively by the individual and not the employer. There are no income limits on who can participate and withdrawals are not taxed if they are used to pay for qualified medical services such as deductibles, coinsurance, co-payments, and uncovered medical expenses—and the HAS can grow from year to year (American College of Physicians 2005).

State governments saw consumer-driven healthcare as a way to control utilization costs and unnecessary services and to encourage the use of low-cost preventive services. The CMS encouraged states to submit innovation proposals under the Deficit Reduction Act of 2005. States such as Florida, South Carolina, West Virginia, Kentucky, and Idaho, under approved Section 1115 demonstration waivers, experimented with things such as insurance premiums, defined contribution, and options to opt out of private employer-sponsored insurance, and allowed individuals to choose from state-approved managed-care plans, personal health accounts, and pre-paid plans such as Managed Care Organizations (MCOs), Preferred Provider Organizations (PPOs), and Medical Home Networks (MHNs). Many states included healthy behavior incentives for things such as smoking cessation and nutrition education (Folkemer 2006).

The Obama administration granted Section 1115 demonstration waivers as a way to encourage reluctant states to experiment with and expand their programs under the ACA. These states have used their political leverage to negotiate and bargain for more flexibility to experiment with private-sector approaches in their Medicaid programs in return for expansion.

Of the 33 states and the District of Columbia that have thus far expanded Medicaid under the ACA, 25 states and DC did a straightforward expansion by building on the traditional Medicaid program. In contrast, seven states used the Section 1115 Medicaid innovation waiver under the ACA as a major element in expanding their Medicaid program and to implement private-sector approaches. While each state's plan is unique and is known by a different name, the states also share certain common elements in the types of changes they made. These states include Arkansas, Indiana, Michigan, Iowa, Pennsylvania, Montana, and New Hampshire. Two states—Tennessee and Utah—attempted but failed to pass expansion under Section 1115 innovation waivers.

Many of these states were controlled by conservative Republican legislatures and/or governors who were opposed to expanding the Medicaid program by simply building on traditional Medicaid, since it was viewed as faulty and dysfunctional. These states were persuaded by proponents of expansion on the ground that they could expand their Medicaid program under a Section 1115 innovation waiver by introducing more private-sector and conservative elements such as charging premiums and imposing cost-sharing on beneficiaries, and creating economic incentives to modify beneficiaries' lifestyle choices (Grogan, Singer, and Jones 2017).

Arkansas, Iowa, and Michigan were the first three states to expand Medicaid under Section 1115 of the ACA in 2013; Pennsylvania did it in 2015, while Indiana, New Hampshire, and Montana did it in 2015. The private-sector elements that all these states share in the Medicaid expansion plan include enrollment in private managed-care plans and cost-sharing requirements for enrollees; five states require enrollees to pay premiums, four states include healthy behavior incentives, while three states include providing premium assistance to purchase Qualified Health Plans (QHP) on insurance exchanges, voluntary work incentives, and health savings accounts (Grogan, Singer, and Jones 2017). The rhetoric surrounding Medicaid expansion in all of the seven states included conservative themes of personal responsibility, deservingness of Medicaid enrollees (limiting the program to the "truly needy"), discouraging dependency and private (non-governmental) options (Grogan, Singer, and Jones 2017; McKenzie 2015).

Most of the 17 states (three states are considering it) that have thus far not expanded their Medicaid programs are politically conservative states. The Section 1115 Medicaid innovation waiver may provide a pathway for future expansion in these states.

The election of Donald Trump to the presidency in 2016, combined with Republican control of both houses of Congress (unified government), the trend toward consumer-directed healthcare is likely to accelerate. The Trump administration has demonstrated a willingness to grant states more flexibility with respect to their Medicaid programs (Singer, Nelson, and Tipimeni 2017).

It is too early to draw any conclusions about the success of the implementation of private-sector-driven consumer-directed healthcare approaches in the Medicaid program, since most of them have been in effect only a few years. One early study provides some insights. Conducted in 2017, the study was based on a telephone survey of low-income, non-elderly adults in three states—Ohio, which used traditional Medicaid expansion, Indiana, which expanded its program through a Section 1115 Medicaid demonstration waiver and uses a private-sector approach, including a health savings account called the "Power Account," and Kansas, which has not expanded its

Medicaid program. The study found that cost-related barriers were more common in Ohio than Indiana. Additionally, among eligible Medicaid beneficiaries in Indiana, 39 percent had not heard of Indiana's health savings account—the "Power Account"—and 36 percent reported making their required payments. In other words, two-thirds potentially stood to lose their benefits or coverage. Thus, some of the Medicaid innovation may lead to some unintended consequences (Sommers et al. 2018).

Work Requirements

Several politically conservative states had asked the Obama administration to allow them to impose work requirements on able-bodied Medicaid recipients. This has been a long-sought goal of conservatives. The Obama administration had rejected such requests on the ground that such a policy went against the very purpose of the program, which was to give more low-income individuals access to health insurance. However, the Trump administration in 2017 signaled its willingness to approve states' waiver requests to impose work requirements. The head of the CMS, Seema Verma, in a speech to the directors of the state Medicaid program, stated that the CMS will approve proposals that promote employment or volunteer work (Galewitz 2017). The CMS issued new guidelines for states seeking Section 1115 demonstration waivers to impose a work requirement on "able-bodied" individuals. The new guidelines exempt children, individuals with disabilities and people in treatment for substance-abuse disorders, pregnant women and the elderly from the work requirements. The CMS also indicated that states must comply with federal disabilities and civil rights laws to accommodate disabled people and the medically frail from being denied coverage. The new guidelines define work to include job training, volunteering, or caring for relatives. This is a major policy shift that could affect millions of low-income individuals (Quinn 2018b).

For conservative states, this policy change represents a politically acceptable way for them to accept billions of federal funds to expand health insurance coverage to more low-income individuals under the ACA. Not surprisingly, in Republican-dominated states, either the governor or state legislature were the first to rush to seek waivers to add a work requirement as part of Medicaid expansion under the ACA. As of July 2018, 11 states have sought Section 1115 Medicaid waivers to add work requirements for Medicaid recipients. Of the 11 states, four states—Kentucky, Arkansas, Indiana, and New Hampshire—have had their waiver application approved. Waiver applications from seven states—Maine, Wisconsin, Ohio, Mississippi, Kansas, Utah, and Arizona—are currently pending a decision by the CMS ("Medicaid Waiver Tracker: Which States Have Approved and Pending Section 1115 Medicaid Waivers?" 2018).

Kentucky became the first state to adopt new Medicaid work requirements. Kentucky's work requirement policy, which went into effect in July 2018, requires Medicaid beneficiaries between the age of 19 and 64 who do not meet exemption qualifications to complete at least 80 hours per month of community engagement, which could include work, school, job skill training, or community service. Failure to meet the requirement would result in suspension of Medicaid eligibility (Abramson 2018; Goodnough 2018). In Indiana, required work hours will be phased in over 18 months and would eventually reach 20 hours per week (Goldstein 2018). In Arkansas, Medicaid enrollees who did not work or volunteer at least 80 hours a month were scheduled to lose their health insurance coverage as early as September of 2018 (Galewitz 2018a). However, the implementation of such work requirements in Kentucky and Arkansas has been blocked by lower courts, pending appeals.

Kentucky's Section 1115 waiver includes not only a work requirement but also monthly premiums and coverage lockout among other requirements. Sixteen Medicaid enrollees filed a lawsuit challenging the waiver. On June 29, 2018, the DC federal district court issued a decision in the case of *Stewart v. Azar*. The court ruled that the plaintiffs had the ability to file a lawsuit since they were actually injured by the waiver; the court had the ability to review the waiver approval; and the waiver approval violated the Administrative Procedure Act because the secretary of the HHS did not adequately consider how the waiver would promote health insurance coverage. The court vacated Kentucky's waiver and remanded the HHS secretary to correct the error and to make a decision supported by the administrative records. Perhaps even more importantly the court's decision affirmed Medicaid's status as a health insurance program and the program's equal treatment of all groups covered by the law (Musumeci 2018). This court decision is not likely to be the last word on such a waiver given the potential for appeal in this case as well as similar court challenges that are likely to occur in other states. For the time being, the court decision has caused some states like Arizona, Utah, and Ohio to put a pause on their waiver requests to see how the CMS responds to the court's ruling before proceeding, while other states such as Arkansas, Indiana, and New Hampshire, whose waiver requests have already been granted, plan to proceed with the implementation of the work requirement (Galewitz 2018b; Quinn 2018c).

According to two analyses by the Kaiser Family Foundation, nationwide, 62 percent of Medicaid enrollees who can work are already working, with 43 percent working full-time and 19 percent working part-time. Of the remaining 38 percent who are not working, 15 percent do not work because of disability or fair/poor health, 6 percent do not work because they are attending schools, 11 percent are not working because they are caregivers, and 6 percent are not working for other reasons. Still, millions of individuals face the prospect of disenrollment from the Medicaid program because of the added work requirement. Furthermore, these individuals are likely to face barriers in complying with the reporting requirements. Also, part-time work and low wages often are not sufficient to overcome poverty. Even when working, adults with Medicaid face financial insecurity because they are still living in or near poverty (Garfield, Rudowitz, and Musumeci 2018; Garfield et al. 2018b). Finally, the work requirement by itself does not necessarily help people find jobs, and the red tape associated with work requirements can cause people to lose access to important supports (Hahn 2018).

Encouraged by the Trump administration's willingness to grant states waivers to impose work requirements on Medicaid recipients, several states are requesting work requirements to include things such as drug testing and placing limits on the length of Medicaid coverage. For example, both Arizona and Maine have requested a five-year time limit on someone being able to stay on Medicaid while Wisconsin wants to impose drug tests on job applicants (Quinn 2018b). The Trump administration seems receptive to the idea of placing a limit on how long a person can stay on Medicaid (Baird 2018). In fact, the work requirement is moving beyond just the Medicaid program. Some state lawmakers are proposing not only a work requirement for Medicaid recipients but also for people receiving food stamps under the Supplemental-Subsidized Nutrition Assistance Program, known as SNAP, making it difficult to receive and keep welfare benefits (Fifield 2018).

LONG-TERM CARE: TRANSITION FROM INSTITUTIONAL TO COMMUNITY-BASED/HOME CARE

Over time, institutional long-term care for the frail elderly has shifted from local government funding and administration to state-level oversight to a shared federal-state concern. Long-term care has often been referred to as Medicaid's 800-pound gorilla because of the costs of institutional care and its impact on state budgets (Olson 2010).

Long-term care policy in the United States has undergone several phases. During the seventeenth century, colonial statutes assigned the responsibility for taking care of the impoverished frail elderly and disabled to local governments funded by the local poor tax. From the late 1800s to the early 1900s, public almshouses became the primary residence for the elderly and were funded by the public, and state governments played a primary role in providing long-term care. Following the Great Depression, the federal government's role in long-term care began to grow as the federal intergovernmental grant system expanded and the federal government became more involved in financing services for the elderly. With the passage of the Social Security Act, several states moved to close their almshouses. The 1954 amendments to the Hill-Burton Act allowed federal grants to public and non-profit entities for nursing homes and rehabilitation services. The 1965 Medicaid law mandates certain basic medical services that include "skilled nursing home" care. The law also includes a provision for long-term care for those receiving any kind of cash welfare benefits from federal programs. This provision provided a backdoor entryway for the elderly into nursing home care. Most states quickly moved to access this new source of funding (Ogden and Adams 2009). Consequently, the nursing home population and costs started to rise.

The Omnibus Budget Reconciliation Act of 1980 included the Boren Amendment, which linked Medicaid's nursing home payment policy with minimum federal and state quality-of-care standards and required that Medicaid nursing home rates be "reasonable and adequate." During the 1980s and 1990s, Medicaid had become the major financier for all US nursing home patient days (Grogan and Patashnik 2003). The Balanced Budget Act of 1997 repealed the Boren Amendment and gave states more flexibility to set costs for nursing home care.

In response to the increased financial burden of long-term care and specifically the burden of nursing home care costs on Medicaid, Section 2176 of the Omnibus Budget Reconciliation Act of 1981 allowed states to seek Medicaid 1915(c) waivers from the Department of Health and Human Services for a variety of home and community-based services (HCBS) provided to certain individuals—the elderly, the physically disabled, the developmentally disabled, and the mentally ill—who would otherwise require nursing home care. States that have approval from the HHS can receive matching funds. The objective of Section 2176 was to encourage a move away from the use of the more expensive treatment in nursing homes and other long-term care facilities and toward less-expensive HCBS when appropriate. Such waiver programs became popular with many states and grew rapidly. During the Reagan administration, between 1981 and 1991, the number of 1915(c) HCBS waivers in operation grew from 6 to 113. During the Clinton years, the number of HCBS waivers increased from 155 to 231

(Thompson and Burke 2009). Today, all states implement at least one home and community-based service program (HCBS). By 1997, every state was participating in the 1915(c) waiver program. During the 1990s, there was a 285-percent increase in waiver participants (Kitchener et al. 2005).

As a result of the 1915(c) waivers and the repeal of the Boren Amendment in 1997, there has been a major shift in Medicaid's long-term care policy, away from an acute-care program for the disabled, poor adults and children toward a long-term care program for the elderly and chronically ill. Today, more states are shifting Medicaid long-term care spending from institutional care to non-institutional HCBS. This is often referred to as rebalancing (Kaye 2012; Robison et al. 2012).

Several factors have contributed to states' increased reliance on HCBS and less reliance on nursing facilities for long-term care services in their Medicaid programs. First, many older persons prefer the HCBS alternative because it gives them more privacy and control over their own lives. Second, the US Supreme Court in its 1999 *Olmstead v. L.C.* ruling supported seniors' preference for HCBS by prodding states to reduce their reliance on nursing facilities' institutionalization and to their integration of seniors in the community. Third, HCBS alternatives are generally less expensive per resident in the long run (Lockhart, Giles-Sims, and Klopfenstein 2009). Fourth, HCBS options have broad-based ideological appeal. Conservative states like HCBS waivers as a relatively inexpensive way to provide services to a narrowly defined group of recipients. Liberal states like waivers, especially for the very expensive special-needs population, because they view such waivers as part of their policy toolkit to expand services (Thompson and Burke 2009).

The long-term landscape is changing as a result of the shift from institutional/nursing facility care to more focus on home and community-based long-term services. A great deal of long-term care services are provided informally by unpaid family caregivers. Most formal long-term care services are paid by government sources (Ng, Harrington, and Kitchener 2010). For example, a large majority of older Americans with cognitive or physical disabilities live at home and are taken care of by their spouses or adult children (Olson 2010). Some of the new consumer-directed service delivery approaches adopted by states have given individuals with disabilities and their families greater choice and control over publicly funded long-term care services (Doty, Mahoney, and Sciegaj 2010).

The emphasis on "rebalancing" as a policy priority indeed has led to considerable growth in HCBS programs as well as the number of participants. The rebalancing has been successful to the extent that in 1990, 87 percent of state Medicaid spending on long-term care went to institutional care, i.e., nursing homes. By 2012, almost 50 percent went to HCBS (Konetzka 2014). However, long-term care in the United States still faces several challenges. One of the major challenges is the recruitment and retention of a well-trained and stable workforce. This has been made difficult by poor public perception, perceived lack of respect and value, the demanding nature of the job, insufficient training, lack of autonomy, and limited opportunities for career advancement. The second challenge is the problem of insufficient quality of care. The third challenge is the financing and the cost of long-term care. The fourth challenge is coordination of chronic care and the dual eligible (Miller 2012).

The Affordable Care Act attempts to address some of these challenges through its various provisions. One of the major provisions in the ACA related to long-term care was the Community Living Assistance Services and Supports Act (CLASS Act). It would have resulted in the creation of a government-run long-term care insurance program. However, the CLASS Act was abandoned by the Obama administration. But the ACA provided added incentives and options to states to expand HCBS programs. One, it provided enhanced federal matching payments from 2011 to 2015 for states increasing the proportion of spending HCBS. Second, financial incentives (an enhanced 6-percent federal medical assistance matching rate) to states to establish what is known as the Community First Choice Option to provide community and home-based attendant support and services to individuals with disabilities. Third, grants for demonstration projects to enhanced training for professional and paraprofessional workers. Fourth, authorizing research and demonstration projects for improving chronic care coordination. Fifth, the ACA extends the mandatory spousal impoverishment protection to community-based spouses of the person receiving HCBS (Harrington et al. 2012; Miller 2012). Finally, to coordinate care for Medicaid beneficiaries who suffer from chronic conditions the ACA created an optional Medicaid state plan benefit for states to establish Health Homes. Services provided by Health Homes include comprehensive care management, coordination, transitional care, health promotion, patient/family support, and referral to community and social support services ("Medicaid—Long Term, Home, and Community Based Services" 2016).

The end result is that today, state governments are perusing three common strategies to expand and improve long-term services and support (LTSS) for adults with disabilities and functionally impaired adult individuals—expanding non-institutional care, integrating payment and care delivery, and realigning incentives through market-based reforms (Naylor et al. 2015).

According to Statista, Inc. (2018), in 2018, 46 states were participating in HCBS waiver programs and all 50 states were participating in HCBS expansion. In addition, 95 percent of Americans age 40 and older who received long-term care got it through HCBS; 5 percent received it in an institutional setting, with 2 percent in nursing homes. Medicaid is the largest payer of long-term care services and support (LTSS). In financial year 2016, the total Medicaid LTSS expenditures were $167 billion, accounting for approximately 30 percent of total Medicaid expenditures. In 1981, institutional care accounted for 99 percent and HBS for 1 percent of the Medicaid spending on LTSS. In 2016, institutional care accounted for 43 percent while HCBS accounted for 57 percent of the Medicaid spending on LTSS. The most dramatic growth in HCBS expenditures happened in the 1980s and 1990s (Eiken et al. 2018). The data clearly indicate the significant rebalancing of expenditures that has happened between institutional care and HBCS. It has taken states over 35 years to shift from institutional care to HCBS programs.

The federal government is pushing states to keep more of their low-income out of nursing homes and to enroll them in HCBS programs due to increased demand for long-term care and because of the high cost of institutional care. About half of all people turning 65 today will need daily help as they age, either at home or in nursing homes (Gorman and Ostrov 2016). People are also living longer. By 2050, the number of people over the age of 85 is expected to triple and reach 18 million (Cancino 2016). Thus, demand for long-term care will continue to rise. Long-term care costs continue to surge upward and private insurance and Medicare offer only limited help. Most seniors do not have long-term care insurance because of the high cost. Medicaid ends up bearing the heaviest financial burden for nursing home care. According to a survey by the Genworth Group (2017), the median cost for a private room in a nursing home room can cost as much as $97,000 annually, imposing a significant financial burden on individuals or families. While less costly, for homemaker services the annual median cost is about $47,934, and for home aid services about $49,192.

Konetzka (2014) has argued that while the policy goal of shifting funding from intuitional care to HBCS—i.e., rebalancing—has been achieved through the expanded provisions of HCBS services under the Medicaid state option plan and the use of Medicaid Section 1915(c) waivers, there might be some hidden costs associated with rebalancing. The intended and unintended consequences of rebalancing are often complicated to measure for three reasons. First, even when using a common matrix, a comparison of state Medicaid dollars spent on institutional care versus HCBS often is meaningless because at the state level states with older and sicker populations have greater need for nursing home/institutional care and at individual level residents of nursing homes are substantially in worse health on average compared to enrollees in HCBS. Second, even though most residents of long-term care express a strong preference to remain at home, the reality is that such preferences depend on one's health status and as persons get older and cognitive impairment sets in, preference for institutional care becomes stronger. Third, there is surprisingly very little known about the health outcomes of HCBS compared to other alternatives.

MEDICAID PAY-FOR-PERFORMANCE

Pay-for-Performance (P4P) originally began in the private sector. There are some 115 P4P programs in the US, which can take a variety of forms ("Medicaid Pay-for-Performance: Ongoing Challenges, New Opportunities" n.d.). The programs' main targets are hospitals, medical groups and physicians, who are provided with financial incentives to achieve assigned quality goals. The most common financial incentives are bonuses or add-on per-diem rates. Most such programs are sponsored by private health insurance plans and employer purchasing cooperatives,

The P4P movement quickly spread to the public sector. The CMS defines P4P as "the use of Payment Methods and other incentives to encourage quality improvement and patient-focused high-quality care" ("Medicaid Pay-for-Performance: Ongoing Challenges, New Opportunities" n.d.). The CMS launched its first P4P pilot program in 2003 and since that time has participated in many demonstration projects that have tested different types of P4P methods (Baird 2016).

Since the state of Wisconsin began using P4P in its Medicaid program beginning in 1991 to incentivize health plans with which it contracts to improve their performance, P4P has spread to many other states. As states struggle to cope with rising healthcare costs, more are implementing Medicaid P4P incentive programs. State governments are providing incentives directly to providers such as physicians and hospitals. They are also using P4P incentives in Medicaid managed-care plans. Some states are considering providing P4P incentives to nursing homes and other institutional settings to also address the problem of racial and ethnic disparities in care. Almost half of the state Medicaid programs operate one or more P4P programs ("Medicaid Pay-for-Performance: Ongoing Challenges, New Opportunities" n.d.).

However, there are several challenges confronting the use of P4P programs in the Medicaid system. Congress in 2015 imposed the use of P4P in the Medicaid program. According to recent research, the prospect of P4P achieving significant success is doubtful. Research has found that Medicare P4P programs did not improve quality, nor did they reduce costs. They made matters worse by penalizing doctors for caring for the poorest and sickest patients because their "quality scores" suffered. In fact, in 2018, the Medicare Payment Advisory Commission recommended that Congress repeal the Medicare P4P program because it was costly and ineffective (Sullivan and Soumerai 2018).

CONCLUSION

Medicaid is the biggest government health insurance program, providing coverage to almost 80 million low-income people in the United States. While Medicare serves only people over the age of 65, Medicaid serves a wide variety of low-income individuals, including children, pregnant women, adults with income below 138 percent of the federal poverty level, persons with disabilities, and seniors who are eligible for both Medicaid and Medicare programs, i.e., dual-eligible. Medicaid has improved access to healthcare, providing financial support to millions of low-income beneficiaries. Medicaid has also helped reduce the number of uninsured Americans. Since the Medicaid expansion and new marketplace insurance exchanges in 2014 under the ACA the number of uninsured Americans has dropped from 43 million to 26 million. A greater reduction in the uninsured rate has occurred among adults in expansion states compared to non-expansion states. Medicare is also cost-effective. Medicaid costs 27 percent less for children and 20 percent less for adults than private insurance (Park 2016, 2015). Most adults with Medicaid coverage express satisfaction with the program and rate it very highly; Medicaid helps people get needed care and improves their health (Gunja and Collins 2016; Katch 2017). The Medicaid program has been described as the "workhorse" of the US healthcare system because whenever policymakers want to provide health insurance to new population groups, they turn to Medicaid (Weil 2003).

Yet, Medicaid often receives mixed reviews. Some have described Medicaid as the "Pac-Man" of the state budgets because it eats up costs and crowds out state spending on other programs (McDonough 2003). Others have argued the Medicaid program is not the bogeyman that it is made out to be (Miller 2003). Still others have argued that Medicaid gets very little respect because, like Cinderella, the program has ended up in the wrong household—state government. While state governments may not be the "evil stepmother," the reality is that the financial condition of state governments is linked to that of the US economy, and health sector spending tends to be countercyclical. This means that health sector spending rises fastest when the economy experiences a downturn. Such was the case during recessions of the mid-1970s, the early 1990s, the late 1980s/early 1990s, and the early 2000s (McDonough 2003).

Republicans and Democrats have pursued very different strategies with different political agendas. Republicans, since the early 1980s, have followed a long-term strategy aimed at dramatically changing entitlement programs in a more conservative direction. Republicans' efforts to turn Medicaid into a block-grant program, to reduce eligibility and benefits and to experiment with private-sector approaches under Medicaid waivers reflect this strategy. Democrats, on the other hand, have always attempted to broaden Medicaid to expand healthcare coverage to additional groups. President Clinton, in the 1990s, for example, suggested that Medicaid was not just a safety-net program designed to protect the poor but also a broad-based entitlement that protected all Americans. Significant expansion in the Medicaid program came about as a result of the passage of the ACA during the Obama administration.

The origin and the evolution of the Medicaid policy is a byproduct of a variety of constitutional, institutional, and political factors discussed in Chapter 1 of this book. Factors such as unified/divided governments, federalism, partisanship and political ideology have played a major role in shaping the Medicaid program and policy. The Supreme Court has undoubtedly influenced the shape and the direction of the Medicaid expansion. Finally, factors in the economic environment such as the state of the economy and budgetary constraints have also impacted Medicaid policy.

Medicaid policy reflects the dictum that the more things change, the more they stay the same. The Medicaid policy process is driven to a significant extent by the incremental approach to policymaking that often produces policies geared toward short-term, patchwork answers, rather than long-term solutions. All the new state experiments and innovations have failed to produce any consensus on how best to contain costs. These experiments have yielded different models of cost containment but none that is satisfactory to all parties, nor have they resulted in significant overall cost-containment in the program. The Medicaid program, in many ways, represents the best and the worst of American politics. It reflects the best of the American tradition of helping the poor and disadvantaged groups who cannot help themselves. It also reflects the worst of American politics and policy-making—that of an incremental, patchwork approach to policymaking—influenced by the vagaries of electoral and economic cycles and partisan and ideological battles that often produce irrational and incomprehensible public policy.

STUDY QUESTIONS

1. What factors contributed to the successful passage of Medicare and Medicaid in 1965? What are some of the fundamental differences between the two programs?
2. Compare and contrast the role of the federal versus state governments with respect to administration, financing, cost-sharing, and setting eligibility requirements and benefit standards in the Medicaid program.
3. Write an essay in which you discuss the objective, structure/organization, and financing of Medicaid. How has the federal-state financing arrangement changed for Medicaid expansion under the ACA?
4. Describe the basic eligibility requirements for Medicaid under the ACA and the mandatory and optional benefits and services provided by Medicaid.
5. Describe the nature of Medicaid reforms/experiments adopted by state governments during the 1980s and 1990s.
6. What is a Medicaid waiver? What are the different types of Medicaid waivers available to states?
7. What factors help explain states' decisions to expand or not to expand the Medicaid program under the ACA?
8. In the American federal system, state governments are often heralded as laboratories of experiments. Write an essay in which you discuss how state governments have experimented with the Medicaid program, with a special focus on private-sector approaches used by state governments.
9. Discuss long-term care policy in the United States. How has it changed over the years? What are some of the major challenges confronting long-term care in the United States?
10. What role has the Children's Health Insurance Program (CHIP) played in addressing the problem of uninsured children? Describe options available to states with respect to the implementation of the CHIP, and eligibility and benefits provided under it.
11. Is investing in a health insurance program like Medicaid for a low-income population a good public policy? Why or why not? Be sure to cite specific examples and research findings.
12. Write an essay in which you describe how constitutional, institutional, political, and economic factors have shaped Medicaid policy.

REFERENCES

"1915 Wavier Processing Tools for States." n.d. Online at www.medicaid.gov/.
Abramson, Alana. 2018. "It Will Be Transformational: Kentucky Becomes First State to Adopt New Medicaid Work Requirement." *Time*, January 13. Online at http://time.com/5102167/kentucky-medicaid-work-requirement/.
Altman, Drew E. 1983. "Health Care for the Poor." *Annals of the American Academy of Political and Social Sciences*, no. 468 (July): 103–121.
Altman, Drew E, and Douglas A. Morgan. 1983. "The Role of State and Local Government in Health." *Health Affairs*, 2, no. 4 (January): 7–31.
American College of Physicians. 2005. *Consumer-Directed Health Care and Health Savings Accounts*. Philadelphia, PA: American College of Physicians.
Antonisse, Larisa, Rachel Garfield, Robin Rudowitz, and Samantha Artiga. 2018. "The Effects of Medicaid Expansion under the ACA: Updated Findings from a Literature Review." Kaiser Family Foundation. Online at www.kff.org/medicaid/.
Baird, Addy. 2018. "Trump Administration to Allow Lifetime Limits on Medicaid Coverage for Thousands at Risk." ThinkProgress.org. Online at https://thinkprogress.org/.
Baird, Courtney. 2016. "Top Healthcare Stories for 2016: Pay-For-Performance." Committee for Economic Development. Online at www.ced.org/.
Barofsky, Jeremy. 2015. "What are the Effects of Not Expanding Medicaid?" Brookings. Online at www.brookings.edu/.
Barrilleaux, Charles and Carlisle Rainey. 2014. "The Politics of Need: Examining Governors' Decision to Oppose the 'Obamacare' Medicaid Expansion." *State Politics and Policy Quarterly*, 14, no. 4 (December): 437–460.
Bloomberg, Linda J. and John Holahan. 2016. "Early Experience with the ACA: Coverage Gains, Pooling of Risks, and Medicaid Expansion." *Journal of Law, Medicine, & Ethics* 44, no. 4 (December): 538–543.

Bonnyman, G. Gordon, Jr. 1996. "Stealth Reform: Market-Based Medicaid in Tennessee." *Health Affairs* 15, no. 2 (Summer): 306–314.

Bovbjerg, Randall R. and John Holahan. 1982. *Medicaid in the Reagan Era: Federal Policy and State Choices*. Washington, DC: Urban Institute.

Brown, Richard E. 1984. "Medicare and Medicaid: Band-Aids for the Old and Poor." In *Reforming Medicine: Lessons of the Last Quarter Century*, eds Victor W. Sidel and Ruth Sidel, 50–76. New York: Pantheon.

Buettgens, Matthew. 2018. "The Implication of Medicaid Expansion in the Remaining States: 2018 Update." Urban Institute. Online at www.urban.org/.

Callaghan, Timothy and Lawrence R. Jacobs. 2014. "Process Learning and the Implementation of Medicaid Reform." *Journal of Federalism* 44, no. 4: 541–563.

Callaghan, Timothy and Lawrence R. Jacobs. 2016. "Interest Group Conflict over Medicaid Expansion: The Surprising Impact of Public Advocates." *American Journal of Public Health*, 106, no. 2 (February): 308–313.

Cancino, Alejandra. 2016. "New Push to Keep Seniors in Home, Community-Based Programs." MedicalXpress. Online at https://medicalxpress.com/news/2016-04-seniors-home-community-based.html.

Center for Budget and Policy Priorities. 2016. "Introduction to Medicaid." Center for Budget and Policy Priorities. Online at www.cbpp.org/.

Centers for Medicare and Medicaid Services. n.d. Baltimore, MD: Centers for Medicare and Medicaid Services. Online at www.medicaid.gov/.

"Children's Health Insurance Program." n.d. Baltimore, MD: Centers for Medicare and Medicaid Services. Online at www.medicaid.gov/chip/index.html.

"Children's Health Insurance Program Reauthorization Act." n.d. Maryland: Centers for Medicare and Medicaid Services. Online at http://medicaid.gov/Medicaid-CHIP-Program-Information/.

"Children's Health Insurance Program: Plan Activity as of May 1, 2015." 2015. Baltimore, MD: Centers for Medicare and Medicaid Services. Online at www.medicaid.gov/chip/.

Choi, Sunha, Sungkyu Lee, and Jason Matejkowski. 2017. "The Effects of State Medicaid Expansion on Low-Income Individuals' Access to Health Care: Multilevel Modeling." *Population Health Management*, 21, no. 3 (September): 235–244.

Congressional Budget Office. 1997. *Expanding Health Insurance Coverage for Children under Title XXI of the Social Security Act*. Washington, DC: Congressional Budget Office.

Council of Economic Advisors. 2014. "Missed Opportunities: The Consequences of State Decisions Not to Expand Medicaid." Council of Economic Advisors. Online at https://obamawhitehouse.archives.gov/.

Cunningham, Peter and James Kirby. 2004. "Children's Health Coverage: A Quarter-Century of Change." *Health Affairs*, 23, no. 5 (September/October): 27–38.

Davis, Karen and Roger Reynolds. 1977. *The Impact of Medicare and Medicaid on Access to Medical Care*. Washington, DC: Brookings Institution.

Dinan, John. 2014. "Implementing Health Reform: Intergovernmental Bargaining and the Afforcable Care Act." *Publius* 44, no. 3 (June): 399–425.

Doty, Pamela, Kevin J. Mahoney, and Mark Sciegaj. 2010. "New State Strategies to Meet Long-Term Care Needs." *Health Affairs*, 29, no. 1 (January): 49–56.

Drum, Kevin. 2016. "Unsurprisingly, Medicaid Expansion Helps Poor People Get More Medical Care." *Mother Jones Magazine*. Online at www.motherjones.com/.

Eiken, Steve, Kate Sredl, Brian Burwell, and Angie Amos. 2018. "Medicaid Expenditures for Lon-Term Services and Support in FY 2016." Baltimore, MD: Centers for Medicare and Medicaid Services. Online at www.medicaid.gov/.

Federal Register. 2015. 80, no. 227 (November 25): 73779–73782.

Fifield, Jen. 2018. "Where the Work-for-Welfare Movement Is Heading." Pew Research Center. Online at www.pewtrusts.org/.

Flint, Samuel S. 1997. "Insuring Children: The Next Steps." *Health Affairs*, 16, no. 4 (July/August): 79–81.

Flint, Samuel S.2014a. "How Bipartisanship and Incrementalism Stitched the Children's Health Insurance Safety Net (1982–1997)." *Health & Social Work*, 39, no. 2 (May): 109–116.

Flint, Samuel S. 2014b. "Who Loses When a State Declines the Medicaid Expansion?" *Health & Social Work*, 39, no. 2 (May): 69–72.

Folkemer, John G. 2006. *Consumer Directed Health Care: Medicaid Style*. Falls Church, VA: The Lewin Group.

Frakt, Austin B. and Aaron E. Carroll. 2013. "Sound Policy Trumps Politics: States Should Expand Medicaid." *Journal of Health Politics, Policy and Law*, 38, no. 1 (February): 165–178.

Galewitz, Phil. 2017. "Medicaid Chief Says Feds are Willing to Approve Work Requirements." *Kaiser Health News*. Online at https://khn.org/news/.

Galewitz, Phil. 2018a. "Feds Issue Split Decision on Arkansas Medicaid Waiver." Online at www.governing.com/.

Galewitz, Phil. 2018b. "Despite U.S. Court's Ruling, Medicaid Work Requirements Advance in Other States." *Kaiser Health News*. Online at https://khn.org/news/.

Garfield, Rachel, Anthony Damico, and Kendal Orgera. 2018. "The Coverage Gap: Uninsured Poor Adults in States that Do Not Expand Medicaid." Kaiser Family Foundation. Online at www.kff.org/medicaid/.

Garfield, Rachel, Elizabeth Hinton, Elizabeth Cornachione, and Cornelia Hall. 2018a. *Medicaid Managed Care Plans and Access to Care*. Washington, DC: Kaiser Family Foundation.

Garfield, Rachel, Ronin Rudowitz, and MaryBeth Musumeci. 2018. "Implications of a Medicaid Work Requirements: National Estimates of Potential Coverage Losses." Kaiser Family Foundation. Online at www.kff.org/.

Garfield, Rachel, Ronin Rudowitz, MaryBeth Musumeci, and Anthony Damico. 2018b. "Implications of Work Requirement in Medicaid: What Does the Data Say?" Kaiser Family Foundation. Online at http://files.kff.org/.

Genworth Group. 2017. "2017 Cost of Care Survey." Genworth Group. Online at www.genworth.com/dam/.

Ginsburg, Paul B. 1988. "Public Insurance Programs: Medicare and Medicaid." In *Health Care in America: The Political Economy of Hospitals and Health Insurance*, ed. H.E. Frech III, 179–215. San Francisco, CA: Pacific Research Institute for Public Policy.

Glied, Sherry and Stephanie Ma. 2013. "How States Tend to Gain or Lose Federal Funds by Opting in or Out of the Medicaid Expansion." The Commonwealth Fund. Online at www.commonwealthfund.org/.

Goldfield, Norbert. 2003. "The Crisis Confronting Medicaid." *Journal of Ambulatory Care Management*, 26, no. 4 (October–December): 277–284.

Goldstein, Amy. 2018. "Indiana Wins Federal Permission to Adopt Medicaid Work Requirements." *The Washington Post*. Online at www.washingtonpost.com/.

Goodell, Sarah and Kate Bundorf. 2012. "Consumer Directed Health Plans: Do They Deliver?" Robert Wood Johnson Foundation. Online at www.rwjf.org/.

Goodnough, Abby. 2018. "Kentucky Rushes to Remake Medicaid as Other States Prepare to Follow." *Time*. Online at http://time.com/5102167/kentucky-medicaid-work-requirement/.

Gorin, Stephen H. and Cynthia Moniz. 2007. "Why Does President Bush Oppose the Expansion of SCHIP?" *Health and Social Work*, 32, no. 4 (November): 243–246.

Gorman, Anna and Barbara F. Ostrov. 2016. "Long-Term Care Is an Immediate Problem – For the Government." *Kaiser Health News*. Online at https://khn.org/news/.

Grannemann, Thomas W. and Mark V. Pauly. 1983. *Controlling Medicaid Costs: Federalism, Competition, and Choice*. Washington, DC: American Enterprise Institute for Public Policy Research.

Grant, Roy. 2014. "The Triumph of Politics over Public Health: States Opting Out of Medicaid Expansion." *American Journal of Public Health*, 104, no. 2 (February): 203–205.

Grogan, Colleen M. and Eric M. Patashnik. 2003. "Universalism within Targeting: Nursing Home Care, the Middle Class, and the Politics of the Medicaid Program." *Social Service Review*, 71, no. 1 (March): 51–71.

Grogan, Colleen M. and Elizabeth Rigby. 2009. "Federalism, Partisan Politics, and Shifting Support for State Flexibility: The Case of the U.S. State Children's Health Insurance Program." *Publius*, 39, no. 1 (December): 47–69.

Grogan, Colleen M., Phillip M. Singer, and David K. Jones. 2017. "Rhetoric and Reform in Waiver States." *Journal of Health Politics, Policy and Law*, 42, no. 2 (April): 247–284.

Gunja, Munira and Sara R. Collins. 2016. "Five Facts About Medicaid." The Commonwealth Fund. Online at www.commonwealthfund.org/.

Guterman, Stuart, Karen Davis, Kristof Stremikis, and Heather Drake. 2010. "Innovation in Medicare and Medicaid Will Be Central to Health Reform's Success." *Health Affairs*, 29, no. 6 (June): 1188–1193.

Haeder, Simon F. and David L. Weimer. 2015. "You Can't Make Me Do It, But I Could Be Persuaded: A Federalism Perspective on the Affordable Care Act." *Journal of Health Politics, Policy, and Law*, 40, no. 2 (April): 281–323.

Hahn, Heather. 2018. "Work Requirements in Safety Net Programs: Lessons for Medicaid from TANF and SNAP." Urban Institute. Online at www.urban.org/.

Han, Xuesong, Binh T. Nguyen, Jeffrey Drope, and Ahmedin Jemal. 2015. "Health-Related Outcomes among Poor: Medicaid Expansion V. Non-Expansion States." *PLoS One*, 10, no. 12 (December): 1–11.

Harrington, Charlene, Terence Ng, Mitchell LaPlante, and Stephen H. Kaye. 2012. "Medicaid Home-And Community-Based Services: Impact of the Affordable Care Act." *Journal of Aging and Social Policy*, 24, no. 2 (April/June): 169–187.

Hayes, Susan L., Pamela Riley, David Radley, and Douglas McCarthy. 2017. "Reducing Racial and Ethnic Disparities in Access to Care: Has the Affordable Care Act Made a Difference?" The Commonwealth Fund. Online at www.commonwealthfund.org/.

Huberfeld, Nicole and Jessica L. Roberts. 2015. "An Empirical Perspective on Medicaid as Social Insurance." *University of Toledo Law Review*, 46, no. 3 (Spring): 545–558.

Huntington, Clare and Elizabeth Scott. 2015. "Children's Health in a Legal Framework." *Future of Children*, 25, no. 1 (Spring): 177–197.

Iglehart, John K. 2011. "Desperately Seeking Savings: States Shift More Medicaid Enrollees to Managed Care." *Health Affairs*, 30, no. 9 (September): 1627–1629.

Ingold, John. 2017. "In Letter to Congress, Hickenlooper and Other Governors Say CHIP Should Be "One Thing We Can All Agree On." December 12. Online at www.denverpost.com/.

Jacobs, Larry and Timothy Callaghan. 2013. "Why States Expand Medicaid? Party, Resources, and History." *Journal of Health Politics, Policy and Law*, 38, no. 5 (October): 1023–1050.

Johnson, Kathryn. 1983. "Major Surgery for Ailing Medicaid Program." *U.S. News and World Report*, October 17.

Kaiser Health News. 2017. "10 Ways Medicaid Affects Us All." Kaiser Health News. Online at https://khn.org/news/.

Katch, Hannah. 2017. "Medicaid Works, in 5 Charts." Center on Budget and Policy Priorities. Online at www.cbpp.org/.

Kaye, Stephen H. 2012. "Gradual Rebalancing of Medicaid Long-Term Services and Support Saves Money and Serves More People, Statistical Model Shows." *Health Affairs*, 31, no. 6 (June): 1195–1204.

Kindig, David A. 2015. "Improving Our Children's Health Is an Investment Priority." *Milbank Quarterly*, 93, no. 2 (June): 255–258.

Kitchener, Martin, Terence Ng, Nancy Miller, and Charlene Harrington. 2005. "Medicaid Home and Community-Based Services: National Program Trends." *Health Affairs*, 24, no. 1 (January–February): 206–212.

Konetzka, Tamara R. 2014. "The Hidden Cost of Rebalancing Long-Term Care." *Health Service Research*, 49, no. 3 (June): 771–777.

Kosterlitz, Julie. 1990. "Rationing Health Care." *National Journal*, 22, no. 26 (June 30): 1590–1595.

Ku, Leighton. 2010. "Ready, Set, Plan, Implement: Executing the Expansion of Medicaid." *Health Affairs*, 29, no. 6 (June): 1173–1177.

Landers, Renee M. and Patrick A. Leeman. 2011. "Medicaid Expansion under the 2010 Health Care Reform Legislation: The Continuing Evolution of Medicaid's Central Role in American Health Care." *National Academy of Elder Law Attorneys Journal*, 7, no. 1 (March): 143–164.

Larson, Celia and Jannie Williams. 2003. "Sociological Context of TennCare: A Public Health Perspective." *Journal of Ambulatory Care Manager*, 26, no. 4 (October–December): 315–321.

Lockhart, Charles, Jean Giles-Sims, and Kristin Klopfenstein. 2009. "Comparing States' Medicaid Nursing Facilities and Home and Community-Based Services Long-Term Care Programs: Quality and Fit Inclination, Capacity, and Need." *Journal of Aging and Social Policy*, 21, no. 1 (January/March): 52–74.

Mattoon, Richard H. 2016. "Medicaid Expansion and the Affordable Care Act: A Fiscal Checkup." Federal Reserve Bank of Chicago. Online at www.chicagofed.org/.

McCarter, Joan. 2015. "Medicaid Expansion Reducing Uninsured Rate, Where Political Leadership Is Allowing It." October 10. *Daily Kos*. Online at www.dailykos.com/.

McDonough, John E. 2003. "The Clouded Future of Medicaid." *Journal of Ambulatory Care Management*, 26, no. 4 (October–December): 369–372.

McDonough, John E. 2014. "Wyden's Waiver: State Innovation on Steroids." *Journal of Health Politics, Policy, and Law*, 39, no. 5 (October): 1099–1111.

McKenzie, Anne. 2015. "Section 1115 Waivers, the Future of Medicaid Expansion." *Health Lawyer*, 27, no. 3 (February): 12–21.

McMorrow, Stacey, Genevieve M. Kenney, Sharon K. Long, and Dana E. Goin. 2016. "Medicaid Expansion from 1997 to 2009: Increased Coverage and Improved Access and Mental Health Outcomes for Low Income Parents." *Health Service Research*, 51, no. 4 (August): 1347–1367.

"Medicaid and CHIP Enrollment Data Highlights: April 2018 Report." 2018. Baltimore, MD: Centers for Medicare and Medicaid Services. Online at www.medicaid.gov/.

"Medicaid and CHIP Program Information." n.d. Baltimore, MD: Centers for Medicare & Medicaid Services. Online at www.medicaid.gov/Medicaid-CHIP-Program-Information/.

"Medicaid Enrollees by Enrollment Groups." 2015. Kaiser Family Foundation. Online at www.kff.org/.

"Medicaid Enrollment & Spending Growth: FY 2015 & 2016." 2015. Kaiser Family Foundation. Online at www.kff.org/medicaid/.

"Medicaid Enrollment and Spending Growth: FY 2016 & 2017." 2016. Kaiser Family Foundation. www.kff.org/medicaid/.

"Medicaid Enrollment and Spending Growth: FY 2017 & 2018." 2017. Kaiser Family Foundation. Online at www.kff.org/medicaid/.

"Medicaid Enrollment by Gender and Age." 2013. Kaiser Family Foundation. Online at www.kff.org/.

"Medicaid Expansion under Obamacare Has Improved Financial Health of Low-Income Americans." 2016. PBS. Online at www.pbs.org/newshour/.

"Medicaid Managed Care Enrollment and Program Characteristics 2016." 2018. Baltimore, MD: Centers for Medicare and Medicaid Services. Online at www.medicaid.gov/.

"Medicaid Management Care Enrollment Report: Summary Statistics as of July 1, 2011." 2011. Baltimore, MD: Centers for Medicare and Medicaid Services. Online at www.medicaid.gov/.

"Medicaid Pay-for-Performance: Ongoing Challenges, New Opportunities." n.d. The Commonwealth Fund. Online at www.commonwealthfund.org/.

"Medicaid Rates Have Not Kept up with Medicare's." 2009. *State Health Watch*, 16, no. 8 (August): 10–11.

"Medicaid Spending Per Enrollee." 2015. Kaiser Family Foundation. Online at www.kff.org/.

"Medicaid Waiver Tracker: Which States Have Approved or Pending Section 1115 Medicaid Waivers." 2018. Kaiser Family Foundation. Online at www.kff.org/medicaid/.

"Medicaid Waivers in the States: Seven FAQS." 2018. National Conference of State Legislatures. Online at www.ncsl.org/.

"Medicaid—Long Term, Home, and Community Based Services." 2016. Baltimore, MD: Centers for Medicare and Medicaid Services. Online at www.medicaid.gov/.

Miller, Andy. 2010. "States Weigh Taxes to Help Fund Medicaid—And Raise Federal Contributions." *Kaiser Health News*, March 17. Washington, DC: Kaiser Family Foundation. Online at www.kff.org/medicaid/upload/.pdf.

Miller, Edward A. 2012. "The Affordable Care Act and Long-Term Care: Comprehensive Reform or Just Tinkering around the Edges?" *Journal of Aging and Social Policy*, 24, no. 2: 101–117.

Miller, Michael. 2003. "The Policy and Political Context of Defending Medicaid." *Journal of Ambulatory Care Management*, 26, no. 4 (October–December): 307–314.

Musumeci, MaryBeth. 2018. "Explaining Stewart V. Azar: Implications of the Court's Decision on Kentucky's Medicaid Waiver." Kaiser Family Foundation. Online at http://files.kff.org/.

National Conference of State Legislatures. 2017. "Health Provider and Industry State Taxes and Fees." National Conference of State Legislatures. Online at www.ncsl.org/.

"National Health Expenditure Projections 2017–2026." n.d. Centers for Medicare and Medicaid Services. Online at www.cms.gov/.

"National Health Expenditures 2016 Highlights." n.d. Centers for Medicare and Medicaid Services. Online at www.cms.gov/.

Naylor, Mary D., Ellen T. Kurtzman, Edward A. Miller, and Peter Fitzgerald. 2015. "An Assessment of State-Led Reform of Long-Term Services and Supports." *Journal of Health Politics, Policy and Law*, 40, no. 3 (June): 531–564.

Ng, Terence, Charlene Harrington, and Martin Kitchener. 2010. "Medicare and Medicaid in Long-Term Care." *Health Affairs*, 29, no. 1 (January): 22–28.
Ogden, Lydia L. and Kathleen Adams. 2009. "Poorhouse to Warehouse: Institutional Long-Term Care in the United States." *Publius*, 39, no. 1 (Winter): 138–163.
Olson, Laura. 2015. "The Affordable Care Act and the Politics of the Medicaid Expansion." *New Political Science*, 37, no. 3: 295–320.
Olson, Laura. 2010. *The Politics of Medicaid*. New York: Columbia University Press.
Paradise, Julia and MaryBeth Musumeci. 2016. "CMS's Final Rule on Medicaid Managed Care: A Summary of Major Provisions." Kaiser Family Foundation. Online at www.kff.org/medicaid/.
Park, Edwin. 2015. "Medicaid at 50: Ten Key Facts." Center on Budget and Policy Priorities. Online at www.cbpp.org/.
Park, Edwin 2016. "Medicaid Works: 10 Key Facts." Center on Budget and Policy Priorities. Online at www.cbpp.org/.
Paying for Senior Care. 2018. "2018 Health and Human Services Poverty Guidelines—Federal Poverty Levels." Paying For Senior Care. Online at www.payingforseniorcare.com/.
Pear, Robert and Michael Cooper. 2012. "Reluctance in Some States over Medicaid Expansion." *The New York Times*, June 30. Online at www.nytimes.com/.
Quinn, Mattie. 2018a. "Shutdown and Children's Health Insurance Saga Comes to an End." *Governing*. Online at www.governing.com/.
Quinn, Mattie 2018b. "Work Requirement May Be Just the Beginning of Medicaid Changes under Trump." *Governing*. Online at www.governing.com/.
Quinn, Mattie 2018c. "After Medicaid Ruling, Most States Hit Pause but Some Proceed." *Governing*. Online at www.governing.com/.
Resnick, Gideon. 2017a. "Congress Created a Health-Care Crisis for Kids in Time for the Holidays." *The Daily Beast*. Online at www.thedailybeast.com/.
Resnick, Gideon. 2017b. "States to Congress: You've Still Left US a Children's Health Care Mess." *The Daily Beast*. Online at www.thedailybeast.com/.
Robison, Julie, Noreen Shugrue, Martha Porter, Richard H. Fortinsky, and Leslie A. Curry. 2012. "Transition from Home Care to Nursing Home: Unmet Needs in a Home- and Community-Based Program for Older Adults." *Journal of Aging and Social Policy*, 24, no. 3 (July/September): 251–270.
Rosenbaum, Sara H. and Robert Blum. 2015. "How Healthy are Our Children?" *Future of Children*, 25, no. 1 (Spring): 11–34.
Rosenbaum, Sara H. and Peter Budetti. 2003. "Low-Income Children and Health Insurance: Old News and New Realities." *Pediatrics*, 112, Supplement E1 (December): 551–553.
Rudowitz, Robin and Larisa Antonisse. 2018. "Implications of the ACA Medicaid Expansion: A Look at the Data and Evidence." Kaiser Family Foundation. Online at www.kff.org/medicaid/.
Rudowitz, Robin and Rachel Garfield. 2018. "10 Things about Medicaid: Setting the Facts Straight." Kaiser Family Foundation. Online at http://files.kff.org/.
Schwartz, William B. and Henry J. Aaron. 1985. *Health Care Costs: The Social Tradeoffs*. Washington, DC: Brookings Institution.
"Section 1332: State Innovation Waivers." n.d. Centers for Medicare and Medicaid Services. Online at www.cms.gov/.
Singer, Phillip M., Daniel B. Nelson, and Renuka Tipimeni. 2017. "Consumer-Directed Health Care for Medicaid Patients: Past and Future Reforms." *American Journal of Public Health*, 107, no. 10 (October): 1592–1594.
Smith, Rick, Nick Arose, and Alberto Coustasse. 2014. "The Impact of the Affordable Care Act in the Medicaid-Focused Managed Carte Plans." *Insights to a Changing World*, 2014, no. 3 (September): 15–29.
Sommers, Benjamin D., Carrie E. Fry, Robert J. Blendon, and Arnold M. Epstein 2018. "New Approaches in Medicaid: Work Requirements, Health Savings Accounts, and Health Care Access." *Health Affairs*, Online at https://dash.harvard.edu/.
Starr, Paul. 1982. *The Social Transformation of American Medicine*. New York: Basic Books.
Statista, Inc. 2018. New York. Online at www.statista.com/topics/2925/long-term-care/.
"Status of Action on Medicaid Expansion Decision." 2018. Kaiser Family Foundation. Online at www.kff.org/.
Sullivan, Kip and Stephen Soumerai. 2018. "Pay for Performance: A Dangerous Health Policy Fad that Won't Die." January 30. *Stat*. Online at www.statnews.com/.
The Commonwealth Fund. 2018. "1115 Medicaid Waivers: From Care Delivery Innovation to Work Requirements." The Commonwealth Fund. Online at www.commonwealthfund.org/.
Thompson, Frank J. 1998. "The Faces of Devolution." In *Medicaid and Devolution: A View from the States*, ed. Frank J. Thompson, 15–55. Washington, DC: Brookings Institution.
Thompson, Frank J. and Courtney Burke. 2007. "Executive Federalism and Medicaid Demonstration Waivers: Implications for Policy and Democratic Processes." *Journal of Health Politics, Policy and Law*, 32, no. 6 (December): 971–1004.
Thompson, Frank J. and Courtney Burke. 2009. "Federalism by Waiver: Medicaid and the Transformation of Long-Term Care." *Publius*, 39, no. 1 (Winter): 22–46.
Tolbert, Jennifer and Karen Pollitz. 2017. "Section 1332 Innovation Waivers: Current Status and Potential Changes." Kaiser Family Foundation. Online at www.kff.org/.
"The Difference between Medicare and Medicaid Reimbursement." Revenue Cycle Management and Healthcare. Online at https://revcycleintelligence.com/.
"Tracking Section 1332 State Innovation Waivers." 2018. Kaiser Family Foundation. Online at www.kff.org/.
Vogel, Ronald J. 1984. "An Analysis of Structural Incentives in the Arizona Health Care Cost-Containment System." *Health Care Financing Review*, 5, no. 4 (Summer): 13–32.
Waldron, Amanda. 2017. "8 Key Facts About Medicaid." *Brookings*. Online at www.brookings.edu/.

Watts, Molly O., MaryBeth Musumeci, and Petry Ubri. 2017. "Medicaid Section 1115 Managed Long-Term Services and Support Waivers: A Survey of Enrollment, Spending, and Program Policies." Kaiser Family Foundation. Online at www.kff.org/medicaid/report/.

Weil, Alan. 2003. "There Is Something About Medicaid." *Health Affairs*, 22, no. 1 (January–February): 13–30.

"Where are States Today." 2018. Kaiser Family Foundation. Online at www.kff.org/medicaid/.

"Who Enrolls in Medicaid and CHIP?" 2017. Baltimore, MD: Centers for Medicare and Medicaid Services Online at www.medicaid.gov/.

Yi, Song G. 2010. "Consumer-Driven Health Care: What Is It, and What Does It Mean for Employees and Employers?" Bureau of Labor Statistics. Online at www.bls.gov/.

5

MEDICARE

Healthcare for the Elderly

> Much of the current debate is about Medicare's future mistakes, what Medicare is, and what it is designed to achieve. Medicare isn't just a trust fund. Medicare isn't just a certain kind of health care system called fee for service. And Medicare is a lot more than just another number in the federal budget debate. Medicare is designed, at bottom, for two purposes. First, Medicare helps assure that older Americans and those with disabilities have access to the same standard of quality health care services as most Americans. Second, Medicare is an essential part of economic security. It is an insurance system that protects beneficiaries and their families from the high and unpredictable costs of health care services.
>
> —*John C. Rother (n.d.)*

Medicare is the largest public-sector healthcare program in the United States in terms of dollars and second (to Medicaid) in numbers of people covered. It began as an alternative to national health insurance and remains one of the most popular government programs. Despite its popularity, it continues to be a target for those seeking to curtail government spending and shrivel what government does. The 1990s and 2000s saw legislation that both expanded Medicare benefits and threatened the very nature of the program itself. Cost and coverage problems remain an issue, as does the lack of coverage for long-term care. The passage of the Patient Protection and Affordable Care Act, also known as the Affordable Care Act (ACA), in 2010 presented new changes and challenges to the program. The election of a new administration in 2016 calls into question the future of the program.

In this chapter, we closely examine Medicare. We begin by looking at its origin and structure. We then look at some of the changes and problems with the program and how those problems have been addressed. We next turn to the problem of long-term care and how that has been addressed in the United States. We conclude the chapter by considering the impact of the ACA on Medicare and proposals to reform it.

THE ORIGINS OF MEDICARE

As mentioned in Chapter 2, national health insurance (NHI) was first mentioned in the United States in the early twentieth century, during the presidential elections of 1912 (Starr 1982, 2013). But the onset of World War I, the linkage between NHI and Germany (which was the first to adopt NHI), and opposition to national health insurance on the part of the American Medical Association (AMA) killed the program. During the development of what eventually became the Social Security Act of 1935, policy formulators considered and rejected the idea of adding a national health insurance provision. They believed, based on responses to the mere mention of it, that including national health insurance would sink the entire Social Security bill (Marmor 2000; Oberlander 2003; Starr 1982, 2013). Beginning in 1939, bills for national health insurance were introduced in Congress (e.g., the Murray-Wagner-Dingell legislation). Marmor (2000, 7) points out that, though the Democrats had a numerical majority, they did not have a "programmatic majority" to enact the legislation. That is, there was insufficient unity within the majority Democratic Party in favor of an NHI program, a problem that was repeated in 1994 during the Clinton administration. The 1948 Democratic national platform called for national health insurance. Despite Truman's victory in that election, the Murray-Wagner-Dingell proposal died, never coming out of committee in Congress.

Advocates of national health insurance then tried an alternative strategy. The new strategy was incremental in nature, focusing on a group or groups that could garner sympathy but could not afford health insurance. The ideal group was the elderly. Marmor (2000, 15) describes the politics behind the new strategy:

The concentration on the burdens of the aged was a ploy for sympathy. The disavowal of aims to change fundamentally the American medical system was a sop to AMA fears, and the exclusion of physician services benefits was a response to past AMA hysteria. The focus on the financial burdens of receiving hospital care took as given the existing structure of the private medical care world and stressed the issue of spreading the costs of using available services within that world. The organization of healthcare, with its inefficiencies and resistance to cost-reduction, was a fundamental but politically sensitive problem which consensus-minded reformers wanted to avoid when they opted for 60 days of hospitalization insurance for the aged in 1951 as a promising "small" beginning.

The above quote contains several important points. It shows the attempt to accommodate potential opposition, primarily from the medical profession. It did this in several ways. This incremental strategy excluded coverage of physician services (though Medicare as enacted did include such coverage but treated it differently from hospital care). It limited the number of hospital days covered, the "small beginning," a feature that remains an integral part of Medicare. Finally, it left the structure of American medicine alone. That structure was the private practice of physicians and the fee-for-service system (Krause 1977). Some of these features would eventually be changed beginning in the 1980s, but they were at least partly responsible for some of the problems that Medicare has continued to face. The finance committees in Congress held hearings on Medicare from 1958 to 1965 (Marmor 2000).

In 1960, Congress passed the Kerr-Mills bill, which provided federal assistance (50–80 percent) to states to help with hospital care for the aged poor. In other words, Kerr-Mills was a welfare program, with all the accompanying problems and stigma of means-tested (income-based) programs. Few states made any effort to implement the program (Starr 1982).

John F. Kennedy's campaign platform in 1960 included health insurance for the aged. Attempts were made to push a narrow program for the elderly from the beginning of the Kennedy administration. The conservative coalition (Republicans and southern Democrats) that had long opposed liberal legislation was able to delay enactment of the program, but the great electoral victory of Lyndon Johnson in 1964, accompanied by a large liberal Democratic majority in Congress, allowed the passage of a number of programs, part of the Johnson administration's Great Society. For our purposes, the important bill was Medicare, passed in 1965.

The law (Title 18 [XVIII] amendments to the 1935 Social Security Act) was broader than envisioned under the incrementalist strategy following the defeat of national health insurance during the Truman administration. It included physician services and covered a large section of the aged population—not just those who were poor, but also those covered by Social Security. Thus, it embodied a social insurance concept whereby subscribers made contributions, rather than assistance to the poor, which required means testing, though means testing for premiums would eventually be incorporated into the program. Medicare would cover a large portion of the population, and virtually all would contribute and benefit. It was, effectively, national health insurance for the elderly and eligible disabled (Reid 2009).

PROGRAM OBJECTIVES AND STRUCTURE

Objectives

The original design or theory of the program has been aptly stated by Thompson: "If Washington paid mainstream rates to providers for delivering medical care to the elderly, they would receive increased amounts of needed care" (1981, 155).

The problem facing the elderly was that, for several reasons, they could not afford health insurance. First, health insurance was available to individuals and families largely through the workplace. As retirees, the elderly were in most cases no longer eligible to receive health insurance benefits. Second, because retirees were no longer part of a larger group through their jobs, they would not be able to gain the benefits of group insurance. Individual insurance rates are considerably higher than group rates. Finally, the elderly were (and remain) more at risk of needing medical care (more likely to experience periods of illness, especially extended illness) and more expensive care than those of working age. The combination of these three factors meant that few private health insurance companies would offer a policy to retirees, and those that were offered were prohibitively expensive. In 1963, only about 54 percent of the elderly (65 years and older) had hospital insurance (calculated from US Bureau of the Census 1966).

Medicare resolved many, but not all, of these problems. In 2009 (prior to the enactment of the Affordable Care Act), 98.7 percent of those 65 or older were covered by insurance. By comparison, nearly 15 percent of those under 18 had no health insurance (US Bureau of the Census 2012). Medicare had achieved its primary goal of providing health insurance for the elderly. Whether it was adequate is another story.

Structure

Medicare is open to those over 65 years of age, those disabled and receiving Social Security cash benefits, and those suffering from end-stage renal disease (ESRD, or kidney failure) or amyotrophic lateral sclerosis (ALS, also known as Lou Gehrig's disease) (Cubanski et al. 2015).

Medicare originally had two parts (A and B), with Part C added in 1997 (and modified in 2003), and Part D in 2003. The hospital insurance (HI, or Part A) program covers inpatient hospital expenses for specified periods. Recipients are covered for up to 90 days for a benefit period and have a lifetime reserve of 60 hospital days. Payment is made for room and board in semiprivate rooms and for such hospital services as nursing and pharmaceuticals. Part A also pays for hospice services, home healthcare, and limited skilled nursing care (Cubanski et al. 2015). Table 5.1 lists the services covered under Part A.

The second part of Medicare is the supplemental medical insurance (SMI), or Part B program. It is a voluntary program, though most Medicare recipients (nearly 93 percent, calculated from Cubanski et al. 2015) subscribe to it. SMI covers a wide range of physician and outpatient services, including diagnostic and surgical procedures and radiology. It also covers ambulance services, medical supplies, clinical services, and blood transfusions. Table 5.2 lists the services covered under Part B.

The third part of Medicare, Part C, focuses on alternative delivery systems. Under the Balanced Budget Act (BBA) of 1997, the new program was entitled "Medicare+Choice." Under the 2003 Medicare Prescription Drug, Improvement, and Modernization Act, also known as the Medicare Modernization Act or MMA, Part C was renamed "Medicare Advantage." It is through this program that Medicare recipients enroll in managed-care programs such as health maintenance organizations (HMOs) as an alternative to what is now called traditional Medicare (see below). By 2017, 33 percent or 19 million Medicare beneficiaries were enrolled in a Medicare Advantage plan (Jacobson et al., 2017). The final, and newest, part of Medicare is Part D. Under the MMA, Medicare recipients beginning in January 2006 were eligible for prescription drug coverage. We will discuss this program in more detail below.

Table 5.1

Medicare Part A: Hospital Insurance-Covered Services, 2019

Services	Benefit	Recipient Pays	Medicare Pays
Hospitalization: semiprivate room and board, general nursing, inpatient drugs, and other hospital services and supplies	First 60 days	$1,364 deductible for each benefit period	All but deductible
	Days 61–90	$341 coinsurance for each day	All but coinsurance
	Days 91 and beyond	$682 coinsurance of lifetime reserve days	All but coinsurance
	Beyond lifetime reserve days	All costs	
Skilled nursing facility: semiprivate room and board, meals, skilled nursing care, variety of services	Days 1–20		All costs
	Days 21–100	$170.50 coinsurance per day	All but coinsurance
	Days 101 and beyond		All costs
Home healthcare: part-time or intermittent skilled care, home health aide services, durable medical equipment and other supplies and services	Unlimited as long as recipient meets Medicare conditions	Nothing for services; 20 percent of approved amount for durable medical equipment	100 percent of approved amount; 80 percent of approved amount for durable medical equipment
Hospice care	For as long as doctor certifies need	$5 per prescription for outpatient drugs;	5 percent of approved amount for hospital respite care

Source: www.medicare.gov

Table 5.2

Medicare Part B: Medical Insurance-Covered Services, 2019

Premium	$135.50–$460.50 per month, depending on income		
Services	Benefit	Recipient Pays	Medicare Pays
Outpatient medical services including doctor and laboratory services	Unlimited if medically necessary	$185 deductible; 20-percent co-payment for approved services	80 percent of approved amount after deductible
Wide range of preventive services	Various screenings and shots	Free if medically necessary	100 percent depending on plan
Durable medical equipment	Medically necessary	20 percent of approved payment after deductible	80 percent after deductible
Hospital outpatient services	emergency of observational services, lab tests billed by hospital, radiological services, medical supplies, some drugs and pharmaceuticals	20 percent of approved payment after deductible, though may be higher depending on service and setting	80 percent after deductible
Home health care	Unlimited as long as recipient meets Medicare conditions	Nothing for services; 20 percent of approved amount for durable medical equipment	100 percent of approved amount; 80 percent of approved amount for durable medical equipment

Source: www.medicare.gov

As important as what is covered is what is not covered. In two major areas Medicare coverage is extremely limited: catastrophic coverage, that is, coverage of hospital stays that exceed the specified limits, and long-term care coverage. We will address these issues later in this chapter.

FINANCING MEDICARE

Medicare is financed through a combination of subscriber and tax payments. The hospital insurance and supplemental medical insurance programs are financed differently. We begin with the hospital program.

The bulk of revenue for the hospital insurance trust fund comes from the payroll tax (2.90 percent), a part of the Social Security tax that employees and employers pay (1.45 percent each) (Baicker and Chernew 2011; "Medicare Spending and Financing: Fact Sheet" 2011). In addition, there are deductibles (initial out-of-pocket costs before Medicare pays anything) and co-payments when Medicare recipients use hospital services. There is a one-time deductible (paid before Medicare starts paying) equal to the average cost of one day in the hospital. For 2018, that amount was $1,340 for each benefit period (Centers for Medicare and Medicaid Services 2018a). Medicare then pays for the entire cost of hospitalization for the next 59 days. If the hospitalization lasts longer than 60 days, there is a co-payment equal to one-quarter of a hospital day ($335 as of 2018) for days 61 through 90. Each Medicare recipient has a reserve equal to 60 hospital days, which can be used past day 90. Under Part A, Medicare also pays for hospice and home healthcare with very limited deductibles. Approved home healthcare services do not have a deductible, and there is a 20-percent co-payment for durable medical equipment, such as oxygen and wheelchairs. Those eligible for skilled nursing home services do not have to pay a deductible. For the next 80 days, the coinsurance (the percentage of remaining costs the patient has to pay) is $167.50 per day as of 2018. After the 100th day (an unlikely scenario in Medicare), the cost to the patient is zero (Centers for Medicare and Medicaid Services 2018a).

The supplemental insurance program, or Part B, is financed through a combination of general federal revenues and Medicare subscriber premiums. Premiums and tax contributions were approximately equal in 1971; since that time, tax contributions have dwarfed premiums. The federal government pays about 75 percent of the costs, and premiums cover the remaining 25 percent (Cubanski et al. 2015). That is why, even given the cost increases in Part B co-payments, SMI remains a bargain. Medicare beneficiaries with higher incomes face higher premiums ranging from 35 to 80 percent, depending on income (Cubanski et al. 2015).

As mentioned above, most Medicare recipients are enrolled in the supplemental insurance program (Part B). The 2018 premium (the amount paid each month) was $134, though it could rise to as much as $428 for those at the highest range of income (depending on income and whether the unit is an individual or a couple), and is deducted from Social Security checks (Centers for Medicare and Medicaid Services 2018a). There is also a $183 deductible as of 2018, and a 20-percent co-payment for Part B services (with the exception of some preventive services), with Medicare paying 80 percent of those services (Centers for Medicare and Medicaid Services 2018a). Physician charges are determined under the physician fee scale phased in from 1992. Physicians elect each year whether to accept full assignment, that is, whether to accept the Medicare fee schedule (participating). If the physician does accept the fee schedule, Medicare is billed by the physician and the recipient pays the balance. Physicians do not have to accept full assignment. They can charge up to 115 percent of the Medicare fee schedule.

An example may help explain the fee schedule. Assume that you are a Medicare recipient who needs to visit a doctor for a Medicare-approved service. Your doctor would normally charge $200, given the services provided. According to the Medicare physician fee schedule, the visit is worth $142. Medicare then will pay 80 percent of the $142, or $113.60. Now it gets complicated. Consider these two cases: in case 1, the physician accepts full assignment, or the $142. He or she then sends the paperwork in to Medicare and receives a reimbursement of $113.60. You, the Medicare patient, pay the balance, or $28.40, to the doctor. Now take case 2: the physician does not accept full assignment. He or she can charge up to 115 percent of the $142, or $163.30. The physician bills the patient for the entire amount. The patient pays the doctor and files for reimbursement from Medicare. The Medicare recipient receives $113.60 from Medicare and has to pay the physician $49.70. From the standpoint of the recipient, using a physician who does not accept full assignment would cost an additional $21.30, an increase in the co-payment of 75 percent. It obviously pays the Medicare recipient to use physicians who accept assignment.

Over time, Medicare cost-sharing has become a significant proportion of the elderly's expenses. One definition of those who are underinsured, who have insurance but whose healthcare costs still total a significant portion their budget, is that 10 percent or more of a person's or family's expenses are spent on healthcare. By that definition, many Medicare beneficiaries are underinsured. On average, in 2016, Medicare beneficiaries spent 14 percent of their income on healthcare (Cubanski et al. 2018). For those whose income is at the lower end (relying primarily on Social Security), the burden is higher. Indeed, employing a definition of poverty that takes into account the cost of medical care, the poverty rate among the elderly increases from 9 percent (in 2010) under the more traditional measure to 15.9 percent (Komisar 2012).

SUPPLEMENTING MEDICARE

Because of the substantial and growing cost-sharing provisions (premiums, deductibles, and co-payments) and coverage gaps, many Medicare recipients have looked for ways to supplement their Medicare plans. As of 2010, 86 percent of the beneficiary population had some kind of health coverage in addition to traditional Medicare. Of these, 23 percent were covered through a current or former employer, 17 percent owned individual coverage (e.g., a medigap policy), 12 percent were also Medicaid beneficiaries (dual eligibles), and 33 percent participated in HMOs or other private plans, or Medicare Advantage plans. About 19 percent had no supplemental coverage ("An Overview of Medicare" 2017; Cubanski et al. 2015; Medicare Payment Advisory Commission 2017).

Medicaid Buy-In

For Medicare beneficiaries who are also eligible for Medicaid (i.e., low-income individuals), known as dual eligibles, there is state buy-in coverage. States pay Part B premiums and any cost-sharing. What is covered under Medicare is paid for by Medicare, and what is covered under Medicaid (such as long-term care) is paid for by Medicaid. A sizable proportion of the dual eligibles are disabled and under 65 years of age. Dual eligibles tend to be sicker than the overall Medicare population, and many of them are in long-term care institutions; 73 percent of the dual eligibles have incomes less than 125 percent of the federal poverty line (Jacobson, Neuman, and Damico 2012; Medicare Payment Advisory Commission 2012; Young et al. 2013). Dual eligibles are disproportionately female and minority (Hispanic and African-American). They are also more likely to be in poorer health. Spending on them is much higher than for nondual Medicare and Medicaid recipients (Jacobson, Neuman, and Damico 2012; Musumeci 2017; Young et al. 2013).

There are three groups of Medicare beneficiaries who qualify for the Medicaid buy-in. One group consists of those who are either categorically (eligible for programs such as Supplemental Security Income) or medically needy. Additionally, there are two low-income groups that also qualify for the buy-in: those whose income is below the poverty line with limited assets (qualified Medicare beneficiaries, or QMBs) and those whose income is just over the poverty line (120 percent of poverty) with limited assets (specified low-income Medicare beneficiaries, or SLMBs). QMBs are limited to help with paying for Part B premiums and cost-sharing, while SLMBs are limited to help with Part B premiums (Young et al. 2013).

The state buy-ins changed somewhat beginning in 2006, when the Medicare Modernization Act's prescription drug benefit took effect. The law requires that states pay for their Medicaid/Medicare beneficiaries (see below).

Medigap

Another alternative is private supplemental medical insurance, so-called medigap policies. Such policies are provided by insurance companies or group organizations such as the American Association of Retired Persons (AARP). In 2013, 23 percent of Medicare recipients purchased such policies ("An Overview of Medicare" 2017). Medigap policies raise the average cost of healthcare because policyholders pay the full cost of that insurance, which includes administrative and advertising costs plus profits for insurance (Moon 1996). Such policies, as might be expected, are expensive. There are ten standardized medigap policies, labeled A through N, with different policies and benefits. The monthly premiums vary depending on the plan chosen and can range from about $72 (for a plan with a high deductible) to $414 a month (as of 2016) (Health Markets 2017).

Employment Retiree Benefits

A third way that beneficiaries can supplement Medicare coverage is through their former employers. A number of those companies that insure their workers also insure their retirees. As of 2010, some 28 percent of Medicare enrollees were in employer retirement plans (Cubanski et al. 2012).

However, there has been a major drop in such coverage. Large employers, the ones most likely to cover workers and retirees, significantly decreased their coverage of retirees, from 66 percent in 1988 to just 36 percent five years later (Cubanski et al. 2012). This is part of a larger trend of reducing employer coverage, primarily due to the cost problems.

TRANSFORMING MEDICARE

Parts A and B compose what is now called traditional Medicare, as it was designed in the 1965 legislation. But Congress has tinkered with the program since then, with some of the changes being fairly significant. This illustrates the incrementalist nature of American public policymaking. It is rare that a piece of legislation is the final say. We continually visit and revisit programs. Indeed, since 1997, Medicare has been affected by ten pieces of legislation, including the Patient Protection and Affordable Act of 2010, the Medicare Modernization Act of 2003, and the Deficit Control Act of 2011 (Cubanski et al. 2012).

In this section, we focus on the two newest parts of Medicare, Parts C and D, and changes from 1995 to 2012. The changes are profound and have transformed Medicare into something quite different from its original design. We might label this process as "Ending Medicare as We Know It" (Rushefsky 2004; see also Oberlander 2003; Oliver, Lee, and Lipton 2004).

In the 1980s, Medicare began enrolling recipients in managed-care organizations (MCOs), such as HMOs, as a means of restraining cost increases while maintaining quality of care for recipients. In addition, it was hoped that Medicare recipients would gain access to the same range of services as other patients (Brown et al. 1993). The plans often offered important additional services that Medicare did not at that time, such as prescription drugs. The plans also did not originally charge for their services and allowed Medicare beneficiaries to avoid the high costs of medigap policies (Freudenheim 1997).

A major move toward Medicare managed care and greater choice came in 1997 (see Marmor 2000; Oberlander 2003; Palazzolo 1999; Rushefsky and Patel 1998). To understand what happened, we need to go back to 1995. The Republicans gained control of Congress following the 1994 off-year elections. Their policy agenda, most of which was stated in the "Contract with America," was to balance the federal budget and to cut taxes. Doing so required significant budget cuts. Medicare and Medicaid were important targets because of their size. The fiscal year (FY) 1996 budget that Congress passed called for $270 billion in savings over a seven-year period (Marmor 2000; Rushefsky and Patel 1998).

Here we have an interesting play of semantics and politics. The Republican proposal called for cuts in projected spending increases. It did not call for actual reductions in Medicare spending, at least on the surface.

Managed-care organizations and HMOs would be one way to reduce spending increases, by making the system more efficient—at least, so claimed the Republicans (Rushefsky and Patel 1998).

Democrats, especially President Clinton, saw the proposed cuts as real, not just as a slower increase in spending. The reasoning here was twofold. First, as the population ages, Medicare enrollment will increase. By definition, then, Medicare spending will have to increase, even if spending per beneficiary is kept constant or decreases. And Medicare spending per beneficiary was, in fact, decreasing.

In politics, sometimes things can get topsy-turvy. One of the provisions of the Affordable Care Act calls for savings from Medicare spending—again, a decrease in the increase rather than an actual decrease in spending. But now the political roles were reversed. Republicans, who unanimously opposed ACA, argued that it cut spending, while Democrats, who mostly supported it, argued that it only cut the increases and focused on waste (Kessler 2011).

From our perspective, the most important part was the creation of Part C and its focus on managed care. Enrollment in these alternative plans was slow. One reason might have been that there was insufficient choice among types of plans. Prior to the BBA of 1997, the choice was between traditional Medicare and HMOs. The BBA of 1997 expanded choice through the *Medicare+Choice Program*.

Under the BBA, Medicare recipients had a choice of seven different types of plan. Recipients would now be able to have a selection of plans that would rival that of private employer-based plans. The Medicare+Choice program (Part C) undermined traditional or regular Medicare. It attempted to fragment the Medicare community. The idea that everybody had the same plan—an idea that underlay the consensus about Medicare (Oberlander 2003)—was eliminated. The proponents of choice hoped to wean beneficiaries away from Medicare, modernize Medicare, and move Medicare to more efficient healthcare plans. The plans were to be competitive, based on price and quality (Newman and Langwell 1999).

As subsequent data showed, the program did not work as planned. For one thing, enrollment in managed-care plans declined in 2000 and 2001. HMOs withdrew from some areas, leaving recipients without any similar health plan. In 2001, nearly 1 million recipients lost their healthcare plan (Gold 2001). Further, plans that remained became less generous to their beneficiaries. More of them were requiring premiums and fewer were covering prescription drugs (Gold 2001; see also Biles, Dallek, and Nicholas 2004).

One of the more interesting aspects of the debate over Medicare+Choice and the withdrawal of plans—one that also affected the 2003 and 2010 legislation—had to do with payments to plans by Medicare. The Health Care Financing Administration (HCFA, now the Centers for Medicare and Medicaid Services, or CMS) reasoned that HMOs would be able to save money serving their clientele. Because of this reasoning, the reimbursement rate for HMOs was set at 95 percent of the average spending on Medicare beneficiaries (adjusted average per-capita cost, or AAPCC). Paradoxically, both HCFA and HMOs claimed that they were losing money on the deal. The HCFA's claim was based on HMOs' enrolling healthier segments of the Medicare population, whose costs would be less than average. The HMOs' claim was based on recipients making more use, particularly of the prescription drug benefit, than anticipated.

The next stage came in 2003.

The Medicare Prescription Drug, Improvement, and Modernization Act of 2003

Medicare, when it was adopted and throughout most of its existence, had some important gaps. A major one was in prescription medications. Medicare pays for such medications while the recipient is in a hospital or a skilled-nursing home. It did not, traditionally, pay for outpatient prescription drugs. The 1988 Medicare Catastrophic Coverage Act provided for the addition of such a benefit. But because of the politics surrounding it (Marmor 2000; Oberlander 2003), the law was repealed the next year. In 2003 a new law, the Medicare Prescription, Drug, Improvement, and Modernization Act of 2003 (MPDIMA), more popularly known as the *Medicare Modernization Act* (MMA), was enacted, which provided a prescription drug benefit plus much more. The politics surrounding that new law and the policy implications of what that law has done represent the greatest change in Medicare since the 1997 Balanced Budget Act and possibly since the origin of Medicare itself (Oliver, Lee, and Lipton 2004; Rushefsky 2004).

The Need for Prescription Drug Coverage

Before we look at the history of drug coverage proposals and the 2003 proposals in particular, we should examine why such an addition to Medicare was necessary. Much of the biomedical revolution in the late twentieth and early twenty-first centuries was in the area of pharmaceuticals. One measure of the revolution in the use of pharmaceuticals can be seen in national health expenditure data. Overall spending on prescription medications rose fairly rapidly, especially in the 1999–2003 period. For 2002, spending on prescription medications accounted for 11 percent of all national healthcare expenditures, but also represented 16 percent of the *increase* in expenditures in 2002 (Levit et al. 2004). Further, one set of projections suggested that spending on prescription medications would increase from $162.4 billion in 2002 to $483.2 billion in 2021 (Keehan et al. 2012).

One reason this is important is that the elderly population (65 plus) makes higher use of prescription medications than younger people because they are more likely to have chronic conditions that require such use. Xu's (2003) analysis finds that the non-elderly are more likely to rate their health as good or excellent than the elderly. The elderly are also more likely than the non-elderly to have chronic conditions such as cancer, asthma, and arthritis (HIV/AIDS is the one area where the younger group has a higher incidence of chronic conditions). Of course, spending on prescription medications is not uniformly distributed among the elderly; average spending is misleading. Those with fewer or no chronic conditions will spend considerably less than those who have chronic or more serious conditions (Steinberg et al. 2000). We can see this pattern in what is known as *concentration of healthcare spending*. Looking at 2014 data, we find that 6 percent of enrollees accounted for 46 percent of spending on prescription medications outside the hospital, 11 percent accounted for 57 percent of such spending, and the top 27 percent accounted for 81 percent of prescription drug spending (Part D) (Medicare Payment Advisory Commission 2017). The impact of Part D on overall prescription drug spending can be easily demonstrated. In 2006, when Part D went into effect, Medicare spending on prescription medications accounted for 18 percent of total prescription spending; by 2015, the number had increased to 29 percent, even as overall prescription spending increased as well ("10 Facts about Medicare and Prescription Spending" 2017). There are three reasons for increases (projected and actual) in prescription medication spending: increasing prices of medications (Medicare Payment Advisory Commission 2017), the increasing size of the beneficiary population, and the Part D coverage of outpatient prescriptions. Seniors who lack prescription drug coverage tend to be less likely to use needed prescriptions.

Of course, most seniors now have prescription drug coverage (see Table 5.3), largely because of the 2003 legislation. A couple of points need to be made about Table 5.3. First, the percentage of retirees who have employer- or union-sponsored plans has declined. In 2003, the year the MMA was passed, but three years before it was fully implemented, 34 percent of Medicare beneficiaries had such drug coverage. By 2014, that was down to 10 percent (Cubanski et al. 2015). Second, in 2003, 10 percent of beneficiaries had medigap policies with prescription drug benefits. The MMA eliminated that benefit, so now no beneficiaries have such policies. Similarly, the MMA eliminated drug coverage by Medicaid for dual eligibles.

What is in the Law: The New Drug Benefit (Part D)

The Medicare Prescription Drug, Improvement, and Modernization Act of 2003 is a complex piece of legislation. The first portion of the new law was a transitional discount card program until the benefit became effective in January 2006.

The major part of the Medicare legislation is the drug benefit itself, the new Part D. The benefit is available to seniors on a "voluntary" basis. "Voluntary" is used advisedly, because those who do not meet the exceptions (for example, being part of an employee retirement program that offers a prescription drug benefit at least as good as Medicare's) and not enrolled by January 2006 face a 1-percent penalty for each month they do not enroll if they choose to do so later. It could be argued that Part D is effectively an individual mandate for Medicare beneficiaries, similar to that contained in the ACA.

Table 5.3

Sources of Prescription Drug Coverage for the Elderly, 2015

Type of Plan	Number of Medicare Beneficiaries (in Millions of Beneficiaries
Stand-alone	19.3
Medicare Advantage	13.4
Employer/union retiree	6.6

Source: Hoadley, Cubanski, and Neuman (2015)

Seniors have some choices to make even before they get to choose a plan. To receive the Part D benefits, they will either have to join a preferred-provider organization (PPO) or HMO (a Medicare Advantage plan) and get all their healthcare, including prescription drugs, from them (an MA-PD plan). Alternatively, seniors could stay with Medicare but enroll in a private insurance plan that only offers a prescription drug benefit. And some seniors will have coverage through an employer or union retiree plan—although, as we have seen, this benefit has declined. A fourth choice, for low-income seniors on Medicaid (dual eligible), is to have Medicaid provide the benefit.

Seniors pay a monthly premium and a deductible. The premiums depend on the type of plan chosen, the type and number of prescriptions the beneficiary has, the beneficiary's income, and the area in the country in which the beneficiary lives. Thus, it is not possible to look at what average costs are. But to provide some sense of costs, we present two scenarios. Both are based on available plans in Springfield, MO (where the authors live) for 2018. The numbers can be found at Medicare.gov.

In the first scenario, the beneficiary is in good health and takes only one type of medication, pravastatin, a medicine designed to reduce cholesterol. Pravastatin is one of the earliest of the statins and one of the least expensive. Given these parameters, there are 24 plans to choose from in Springfield, MO. In this case we are selecting an AARP MedicareRX Walgreens plan offered by UnitedHealthcare. The monthly premium is $26.80, with an annual deductible of $405 (some plans have no deductibles or smaller deductibles). The drug co-payment varies from $0 to $32 and the coinsurance varies from 25 to 32 percent. Again, shopping for a plan every year becomes important because plan payments vary, and the AARP plans tend to be expensive.

In the second scenario, the beneficiary has multiple sclerosis (MS). The average retail price for the medication (Aubagio [brand name]) is $8,304.97 a month. On a yearly basis, that would amount to over $99,000 a year, much more than most of the population can afford (data from goodrx.com). With a discount, the monthly cost at Walgreen's would be $6,922.79 (higher than other pharmacies). The yearly cost with the discount would be just a bit over $83,000—again, far beyond the capabilities of most Americans. For our Medicare beneficiary, we go back to Medicare.gov. There are 24 plans available in Springfield and we, as with the first scenario, chose the AARP MedicareRX Walgreens plan offered by UnitedHealthcare. Now the premium is $83.30 (high compared to other plans). There is no annual deductible, but between co-payments and coinsurance the beneficiary's total cost would be over $8,600 a year (authors' calculation from Medicare.gov.) That is substantially less than paying full retail or the discount mentioned above. It should be noted that because Medicare beneficiaries are not especially wealthy, that $8,600+ would still represent a substantial portion of the beneficiary's income.

For stand-alone plans, the monthly premium in 2018 was $43.48. In 2011, the monthly premium averaged $38.29. This represents a 13.6-percent increase since 2011 and almost a 68-percent increase since 2006. MA-PD plans are a bit more expensive. For those in the MA-PD (Medicare Advantage-Part D) plans, the premiums averaged $36 a month ("Medicare Advantage: Fact Sheet" 2017). In a complex architecture, particularly for those in private drug plans, benefits and co-payments rise and fall and rise again depending on the level of spending on the part of the individual.

For example, there are standard Part D plans (and comparable alternatives) and enhanced Part D plans (Cubanski et al. 2017a; "Medicare Part D: Types of Alternative Part D Plans" 2017). Enhanced plans have a premium (usually higher than standard plans) and a deductible. Additionally, such plans can add features such as drugs that might not normally be covered under Part D; some reduced cost-sharing, particularly for those recipients in the coverage gap (see below). A majority of Part D plans are enhanced plans (Cubanski et al. 2017a).

Plans have deductibles ($405 in 2018; Cubanski et al. 2017b) and there is tiered cost-sharing. The most common type of tiered cost-sharing "includes tiers for preferred generics, generics, preferred brands, non-preferred drugs (including a mix of brands and generics), and specialty drugs" (Cubanski et al. 2017b, 8). The more expensive the medication—for example, speciality drugs such as the MS drug mentioned above—the more the cost-sharing. For the most expensive medications, the cost-sharing often is coinsurance rather than co-payments. A co-payment is a specific amount paid after the deductible is paid. Coinsurance is a percentage of the remaining costs after the deductible. Coinsurance is costlier than co-payments. Co-payments are more common with preferred medications (Cubanski et al. 2017b).

Another element of the Part D plans is that some Medicare beneficiaries are eligible for low-income subsidies. Such plans waive the premiums for beneficiaries, though, depending on the plan, beneficiaries would have to pay a portion of the premium (Cubanski et al. 2018). This was put into place by the Affordable Care Act.

Then comes the famous "doughnut hole," or coverage gap. The reason for this complex structure was to keep the costs of the program within the $400-billion cap that President Bush insisted upon (even though the administration knew that it would cost much more than that). Subsidies are available for low-income seniors. In 2006, the coverage gap worked as follows. Every year, the recipient would pay a deductible of $250 and then a co-payment of 20 percent for the next $2,000 in drug costs, for a total of $2,250. Then the beneficiary would hit the donut hole. The beneficiary would have to pay all of the next $2,850 up to the catastrophic limit of $5,100. The beneficiary would have to pay 5 percent of all costs after that and the plan would pay 95 percent of the costs. The total out-of-pocket costs up to the catastrophic limit would be $3,600. Costs were projected to go up. One estimate is that in 2015, the total out-of-pocket costs up to the catastrophic limit would be $6,800 (National Committee to Preserve Social Security and Medicare 2006).

The Affordable Care Act made changes to the coverage gap. Most private plans make no provision for any coverage in the gap, though the percentage of plans offering some coverage has increased. Those that do offer additional coverage for the gap charge higher premiums—on average about 250 percent higher for plans with additional coverage. Cubanski et al. (2017a) argue that recipients are likely better off not having the additional coverage. Again, gap coverage is complex: how much required coverage there is depends on the drugs used. For 2018, 50 percent of the gap is required to be covered plus another 15 percent for name-brand drugs and 56 percent of generics (Cubanski et al. 2017a). The ACA requires that pharmaceutical manufacturers provide a 50-percent discount of brand-name drugs in the coverage gap (Cubanski et al. 2017b). The overall goal of the ACA was to reduce, by 2020, the co-payments in the doughnut hole from 100 percent to 25 percent ("Summary of Key Changes to Medicare in 2010 Health Reform Law" 2010).

One interesting part of the new drug benefit, because of the politics involved, concerns dual enrollees and the states. Under the new law, the states have to pay Medicare for the prescription drug costs of covering those enrolled in both Medicare and Medicaid. Some states have calculated that they will be paying for a federal service and will pay more than they spent on the benefit for their enrollees. As a result, some states have decided not to make the payments. For example, Texas Governor Rick Perry vetoed legislation in 2005 that would have appropriated money for that purpose (Pear 2005; see also Smith, Gifford, and Kramer 2005).

A major problem facing some Medicare recipients is that there is no cap on prescription drug spending. Recall, again, our recipient with MS. That person easily passes the catastrophic limit. Looking at 2015 data, about 2 percent or 1 million Medicare recipients had spending above the gap or catastrophic limit (Cubanski et al. 2017b). Those with spending outside the limit spent about six times as much as average spending and about 1100 percent more than those who did not reach the gap (our patient who uses Pravastatin) (authors' calculations from Cubanski et al. 2017b). Those in the top 1 percent of prescription drug spending spent nearly $9,484 in 2015 (Cubanski et al. 2017b). The low-income subsidies (LIS) help protect beneficiaries at the lower end of the income scale (Cubanski et al. 2017b). It should also be noted that Medicare beneficiaries, on the whole, are not especially wealthy, so such spending can comprise a large percentage of their income. Those with high-out-of-pocket costs tended to have chronic conditions, such as MS, HIV/AIDS, viral hepatitis and schizophrenia (Cubanski et al. 2017b). As we shall see in Chapter 8, a small percentage of people, whether in the overall healthcare system, Medicaid, or Medicare, account for a large percentage of spending. What we are seeing are more people with chronic conditions using more expensive medications.

Subsidies for the Favored

> Another part of the legislation involves subsidies and other favors. One set of favors concerns provider reimbursement. Historically, the federal government has tried restraining the costs of Medicare by reducing payments to providers ... Doctors and hospitals are on fee schedules that have been the subject of negotiations over the years [Laugesen 2016]. For example, the 1997 Balanced Budget Act significantly reduced payments to providers. This created the problem that physicians are becoming more reluctant to accept Medicare patients. The 2003 Medicare law included increases, rather than the proposed decreases, in payments to providers.
>
> (Altman 2004)

A second related feature is centered around health plans, such as PPOs and HMOs. Recall that in the late 1990s and early 2000s, some HMOs exited the Medicare field, claiming that they were losing money on Medicare recipients. The new legislation provided for additional payments to those plans—some $14 billion. As Oliver, Lee, and

Lipton (2004) pointed out, this means that these healthcare plans would be getting more per Medicare enrollee than Medicare on average would normally spend.

Third, employers who offer healthcare benefits for their retirees would also get subsidies. The subsidy amounted to about $81 billion and was intended to provide an incentive for employers to maintain their coverage. Interestingly, employers who reduced their coverage would still get the subsidy (Antos and Calfee 2004).

If there was an overall winner in the legislation, it was the pharmaceutical industry, which has historically opposed the addition of a drug benefit for fear that it would lead to price controls. The MMA alleviated all such fears. Under the law, Medicare cannot negotiate drug prices. The states do engage in such negotiation under Medicaid, as does the Department of Veterans Affairs, but Medicare cannot. It is up to the private drug plans to engage in the negotiations. Further, the legislation banned the reimportation of drugs from other countries. Under the law, the Food and Drug Administration will explore drug importation from Canada (Oliver, Lee, and Lipton 2004).

Medicare Advantage

The story of Part C is another thread in the transformation of Medicare. In 1982, Medicare enabled participation of health maintenance organizations (HMOs) in Medicare as an alternative to what is now called traditional Medicare. Private plans were also a way to make greater use of markets, according to advocates, and control costs. Growth of Medicare beneficiary enrollment in the private plans, however, was small. That brings us, again, to the Balanced Budget Act of 1997.

The BBA created Part C, Medicare+Choice. Medicare beneficiaries could choose among seven plans, including traditional Medicare and a medical savings account (a high-deductible plan with Medicare paying for catastrophic expenses).

HMOs were thought to be more efficient than traditional Medicare in the sense that they could deliver the same services for less cost. This was because such plans are generally paid on a per-capita (capitation) rather than fee-for-service basis. In a fee-for-service system, providers are paid for each service delivered. In a capitation system, the organization is paid a certain amount for each of its members. In that sense, private plans were effectively assuming the risk of enrollee illness. Congress took these ideas into consideration, and Medicare, as we saw above, paid HMOs 95 percent of what, on average, Medicare spends per beneficiary. Further, enrollees would not have to pay extra. Plans would cover Part A and Part B services and cost-sharing such as deductibles and copayments, plus some would offer additional services, including prescription drug coverage beginning in 2006.

The program did not work out as planned, which laid the groundwork for the 2003 legislation. A four-year evaluation found that risk plans (whereby the plan would not get more money from the Health Care Financing Administration if its costs increased) tended to enroll healthier-than-average Medicare recipients. Those enrolled in risk plans had 20-percent lower Medicare reimbursements than those not so enrolled. Further, beneficiaries enrolled in HMOs were less likely to be disabled or have chronic health problems than those not enrolled in risk plans. Such a pattern of enrollment, called favorable selection, has often been charged to HMOs. The evaluation study estimated that, given favorable selection, costs to Medicare were actually 5.7 percent higher than with the fee-for-service system (Brown et al. 1993; see also Biles, Dallek, and Nicholas 2004; Congressional Budget Office 1997; Oberlander 1997).

On the other hand, HMOs did tend to reduce the length of hospital stays compared to the fee-for-service system, though they did not reduce the number of admissions. For other services, HMOs tended to reduce the intensity of services (the number of services provided) by 10–20 percent (Congressional Budget Office 1997). The effects were greatest for those who were chronically ill (Oberlander 1997). Quality of care for HMO Medicare recipients was about equal to that of fee-for-service Medicare recipients (Brown et al. 1993).

One question that could be asked is how satisfied Medicare recipients are with managed care plans. A study by Nelson (1997) found that most Medicare HMO enrollees were satisfied with their access to care, such as being admitted to a hospital, seeing a specialist, making an appointment, or receiving desired home healthcare. Most were able to select their primary-care physician and had received enough information to obtain care. Those more likely to report access problems were from "vulnerable subgroups" (Nelson 1997, 151–152), such as the non-elderly disabled, those whose health was less than good, the oldest beneficiaries, and those with functional disabilities. African-Americans seemed less satisfied with their HMOs than whites. Even so, most of these groups said they would recommend the plan to others with health problems. Adequacy of home healthcare services appears more likely under Medicare fee-for-service than under managed care.

In the late 1990s and early 2000s, Medicare+Choice plans began to drop out of the market and avoid rural areas. By 2003 some 2.4 million HMO enrollees had been dropped by their plans (Peck 2003). This obviously caused disruptions for beneficiaries, as they had to find another plan or, more likely, enroll in traditional Medicare. Further, HMOs and PPOs limited the availability of physicians. Only those providers who were included in the plan or network were available to beneficiaries (going outside plans costs beneficiaries more money), a phenomenon that recurred in 2013 with the rollout of the ACA. Disenrollment—beneficiaries dropping plans—was also a problem. Disenrollees tended to be sicker, had more chronic conditions, and were older than those who stayed (Riley, Ingber, and Tudor 1997). One can see the impact of disenrollment and dropping beneficiaries. In 1999, 6.9 million Medicare recipients, 18 percent of all Medicare recipients, were in private plans. By 2003, that number had declined to 5.3 million people, 13 percent of Medicare recipients (Gold et al. 2012).

The 2003 Medicare Modernization Act sought to fix this problem. The legislation, including the new prescription drug benefit (Part D) discussed above and health savings accounts (HSAs), sought to move Medicare beneficiaries to private plans.

Medicare+Choice was renamed Medicare Advantage (MA) (employing the symbolic use of names to describe a program). More importantly, it changed Medicare payments to private plans from the 95-percent average per-capita Medicare spending as it was under the Balanced Budget Act to 113 percent. This was designed to encourage private plans to return or stay with Medicare. The extra money could be used to provide additional benefits, including prescription medications.

Beneficiaries began to move to MA plans. By 2017, 13.1 million or 33 percent of beneficiaries were enrolled in a Medicare Advantage plan ("Medicare Advantage: Fact Sheet" 2017). Most of them (63 percent) were in traditional health maintenance organizations, 26 percent were in local preferred-provider organizations, 7 percent in regional preferred-provider organizations, and 1 percent in private fee-for-service plans ("Medicare Advantage: Fact Sheet" 2017). There are also HMO Point of Service Plans, which pay a higher rate for out-of-network care than do traditional HMOs. Medical savings account plans represented another alternative. Under such plans, the federal government puts money into an account that can be used to pay for needed services ("Different Types of Medicare Advantage Plans" 2012).

Complaints on the part of those opposed to private plans cropped up almost immediately after the passage of the Medicare Modernization Act. A major objection was to the higher payments to the plans, with the result that Medicare is spending more than it otherwise might, an estimated $157 billion more from 2009 to 2019 (Jaffe 2009).

Additionally, according to the then-majority (Democratic) staff of the US House Committee on Energy and Commerce, administrative costs are much higher for private plans than for traditional Medicare. These costs include marketing, profits, and so on (Committee on Energy and Commerce 2009). Further, such plans paid out less for services than traditional Medicare. As an extreme case, one MA plan spent only 36 percent of what it received from Medicare on services (the medical loss ratio). Many of the companies had a medical loss ratio of nearly 85 percent, a figure contained in the Affordable Care Act. Further, MA plans tended to advertise for (tried to attract) health beneficiaries (see Cai et al. 2008).

The Affordable Care Act (2010), as it did with Part D, made some changes to Part C. The additional payments were supposed to be phased out through 2017, and the medical loss ratio will be mandated at 85 percent (Potetz, Cubanski, and Neuman 2011). Cuts were made through 2014, but the latter years, through 2018, have seen payment increases to MA plans (Norris 2018).

Lessons from the Medicare Modernization Act

One last consideration about the Medicare Modernization Act concerns its parallels with the ACA. One such parallel already mentioned is that the MMA is effectively an individual mandate for Medicare beneficiaries, similar to the individual mandate in the ACA (though the tax penalty for the individual mandate in the ACA was repealed in the 2017 tax legislation; see Chapter 3). Under the MMA, a Medicare beneficiary who is not enrolled in some type of drug benefit plan must, upon enrollment, pay a penalty equal to 1 percent of the premiums for each month the person was not enrolled. The ACA, likewise, contained a penalty (officially a tax) for not having health insurance (though, again, effectively repealed with the 2017 legislation).

Second, beneficiaries who received their drug benefit through private plans under the MMA purchased plans on virtual markets yearly during enrollment periods, the equivalent of the health exchanges contained in both the 2006 Massachusetts plan (see Chapter 11) and the ACA.

Third, implementation of the prescription drug benefit plan under the MMA was very bumpy. Beneficiaries were confused about the program and did not understand it well. Over the years, the confusion has diminished, and the program has worked better, though there are still some problems. One problem was that the helpline for the program did not always provide accurate information. Further, a large number of beneficiaries signed up for the program on the last day of 2005, and when they went to purchase their medications in early 2006, there was no record of them in the system (Kliff 2013).

Fourth, Medicare Part D was very unpopular when it passed and as it approached the 2006 implementation year. Indeed, it was even more unpopular in 2005 and 2006 than the ACA was in 2013 (Kliff 2013). Over the years, the program has become much more popular among Medicare beneficiaries. In a 2017 survey (the most recent of such surveys dating back to the start of the program), over 85 percent of seniors were satisfied with the program (*Medicare Today* 2017).

Of course, there are differences between the two programs. The ACA is more complex and covers much more of the population than Medicare. There was less political opposition to Part D than there has been for the ACA. Medicare, as a federal program, did not rely on the states for implementation as ACA does with the Medicaid expansion and the health exchanges. Nevertheless, there are lessons from Part D that can be applied to the implementation of the ACA (see Chapter 11).

CONTROLLING COSTS

From the beginning, a chief concern about the Medicare program was cost. Several dimensions of cost play a role. One discussed earlier is costs to the Medicare beneficiary. Here we can look at the co-payments and deductibles that recipients have to pay under Parts A and B and premiums under Part B (and the new Parts C and D). We have also looked, to a certain extent, at the problem of cost through HMOs and medigap policies.

A second major dimension of cost control is cost to the federal government. As Medicare became more expensive for a variety of reasons, federal administrators and policymakers sought ways to curb those costs. Some of this could be done by raising premiums and deductibles for Medicare recipients. By far the largest target of cost control was providers: physicians, hospitals, and so forth. From the beginning, the politics of Medicare revolved around the issue of provider payment, beginning with hospitals and then expanding to doctors (Feder 1977; Thompson 1981). In addition, the size of the Medicare program made it a tempting target for those seeking to cut government spending and/or reduce the budget deficit. Medicare played a key role in the 1995–1997 budget debates—debates that ultimately led to significant changes in the program. The enormous budget deficits that appeared beginning in 2007 renewed the debate over the role of Medicare in the federal budget. Table 5.4 presents data on Medicare expenditures for selected years.

Third, and related, are questions about the long-term viability of the program. The trust fund, which affects Part A, is predicted to be depleted by 2029 (Boards of Trustees 2017; Cubanski and Neuman 2017).

Consider, first, the increase in expenditures and enrollments in Medicare (see Tables 5.4 and 5.5). Medicare expenditures in 1970 were about $7.7 billion, almost 42 percent of federal health expenditures and 10.3 percent of total personal health expenditures. In 1995, Medicare expenditures were about $184.43 billion, representing just over 50 percent of federal personal healthcare expenditures and almost 18 percent of total personal healthcare expenditures. By 2016, Medicare expenditures were over $672 billion, representing almost 60 percent of federal health expenditures and over 21 percent of total personal health expenditures (calculated from Hartman et al. 2018). As fast as overall health expenditures were increasing, Medicare expenditures increased more rapidly in the 2010–2013 period and then at a slower rate (Hartman et al. 2018). Considering the concern about overall increases in healthcare, increases in Medicare could not help but raise alarms.

One of the reasons for the increase in program expenditures was the upsurge in the number of Medicare beneficiaries (see Table 5.5). When the program began operation in 1966, it had a little over 19 million enrollees. By 1970, that number had increased to over 20 million. The 1972 amendments to the Social Security Act added the disabled and those suffering from end-stage renal disease (kidney failure). By 1995, there were just over 37 million Medicare enrollees, 4.4 million of whom were disabled. That represents an increase of about 83 percent in total recipients. By 2017, there were more than 55 million beneficiaries, including almost 9 million disabled (Centers for Medicare and Medicaid Services 2018a). This represents an almost-50-percent increase in the total number of beneficiaries since 1995. The number of disability eligible Medicare beneficiaries doubled over the same period.

Another reason is the growing generosity of Medicare in the sense that cost-sharing on the part of Medicare recipients has become relatively smaller. In 1980, cost-sharing amounted to about 19.6 percent of total

Table 5.4

Medicare Expenditures, Selected Years, 1970–2016 (in $ billions)

1970	$7.67	1997	$210.37
1975	$16.34	1998	$209.21
1980	$37.39	2000	$224.34
1985	$71.83	2005	$338.77
1990	$110.18	2010	$519.8
1995	$184.39	2016	$672.1

Source: Centers for Medicare and Medicaid Services (2012b); Hartman et al. (2018).

Table 5.5

Medicare Beneficiaries, Selected Years, 1970–2017 (in millions)

	Total Enrollees	Aged	Disabled
1970	20.4	20.4	
1975	25.3	22.5	2.2
1980	28.1	25.1	3.0
1985	29.6	26.7	2.9
1990	33.7	30.5	3.3
1995	37.1	32.7	4.4
2000	39.2	33.8	5.4
2005	42.0	35.3	6.7
2010	46.9	39.0	7.9
2017	55.5	49.8	8.8

Source: Centers for Medicare and Medicaid Services (n.d.); Centers for Medicare and Medicaid Services (2018a).

expenditures. By 2010, the number had decreased to 17.6 percent (calculated from Centers for Medicare and Medicaid Services 2011). That percentage continued to decline, decreasing to 13 percent in 2013 (Medicare Payment Advisory Commission 2017). Even with these numbers, Medicare recipients still pay a sizable portion of their income on healthcare. Looking at 2012 data, Medicare recipients pay almost 14 percent of their income on healthcare, compared to 5.2 percent of the non-Medicare population (Cubanski et al. 2015). Other reasons for greater expenditures include general inflation, healthcare inflation over and above general inflation, increasing costs for prescription medications, and changes in the technology of healthcare.

When policymakers began to seriously consider imposing cost-control measures on Medicare, they focused first on hospitals. As is true for overall national healthcare expenditures, hospitals accounted for the largest single portion of Medicare expenditures. In 2015, Medicare hospital inpatient services cost about $140 billion, approximately 22 percent of total Medicare payments. By contrast, physician services accounted for about $70 billion, approximately 11 percent of total payments. These numbers apply to fee-for-service beneficiaries; 29 percent of Medicare spending went to Medicare Advantage plans in 2017 (Medicare Payment Advisory Commission 2018).

When Medicare began, it contained the usual compromise provision that "the federal insurance program would not interfere in the practice of medicine or the structure of the medical care industry" (Feder 1977, 1; Krause 1977). But it was inevitable that the federal government would have to take steps as the program became relatively more expensive. One way to understand that inevitability is to consider the theory of imbalanced political interests and its application to Medicare (Marmor, Wittman, and Heagy 1983).

At the beginning of the program, Medicare amounted to a relatively small percentage of federal expenditures. In FY 1970, five years after it was established, Medicare accounted for 3.7 percent of federal expenditures.

Hospitals and physicians were faced with concentrated benefits and costs of payment and regulatory policies. The program was too small in the early years for the federal government to give it much concern. By 1980, Medicare as a percentage of total federal spending had nearly doubled to 6.1 percent. By 2010, Medicare accounted for 15.2 percent of federal spending (calculated from Office of Management and Budget 2011). As Medicare spending continued to increase faster than overall spending, the federal government developed its own set of interests in cost containment that would counterbalance provider interests. Additionally, there was, and is, the continual concern that the hospital trust fund will eventually become insolvent. In the early 1980s, the federal government looked at hospital cost containment in Medicare. During the latter part of the decade, it turned to physician payments. Eventually, other providers, such as nursing homes and home healthcare agencies, were covered by prospective payment.

Prospective Payment System

With the enactment of Medicaid and Medicare in the mid-1960s, the federal government became a major purchaser of services in the healthcare market. Part of the increase in overall healthcare costs is attributed to dramatic increases in the cost of Medicaid and Medicare. By 1980, spending had reached about $61.2 billion, constituting about 27.8 percent of total national health spending—financing healthcare for about 50 million people (Levit et al. 1994). At the same time, hospital costs were also rising dramatically, from $28 billion in 1970 to $102.7 billion in 1980 (Levit et al. 1994). From 1977 to 1982, Medicare hospital expenditures grew at an average annual rate of 18 percent compared to a 14.6-percent increase in overall hospital spending (Gibson et al. 1984).

The burden on the federal health budget created the political environment for federal regulation of hospital costs (Marmor, Wittman, and Heagy 1983; Steinwald and Sloan 1981). Advocates of regulation argued that cost controls on hospitals would limit waste and inefficiency without sacrificing quality of care.

President Carter, in response to rising hospital costs, proposed hospital cost-containment legislation designed to constrain the rate of increase in hospital charges and to limit the rate of increase in hospital revenues. Not surprisingly, the hospital industry strongly opposed such a measure and proposed a voluntary plan to control costs on its own. The controversy surrounding both plans led to their demise in 1979.

As mentioned earlier, President Reagan came to office in 1981 with the express intent of eliminating federal regulatory healthcare programs in favor of a market-oriented, competitive strategy to contain healthcare costs. Federal funding was cut for health planning programs, and the Professional Standards Review Organizations (PSROs) program was renamed Peer Review Organizations (PROs) and given reduced funding. Budget cuts were made in Medicaid and Medicare, and new federal grants for health maintenance organization startups were eliminated.

Minor changes were made in Medicare by the Omnibus Budget Reconciliation Act of 1981. This included tightening Medicare reimbursement payments. The 1982 Tax Equity and Fiscal Responsibility Act (TEFRA) limited the increase in Medicare hospital payment rates, created an early basis for prospective payment based on a case-mix index, and called for incentive payments to hospitals defined as efficient. The TEFRA required that the Department of Health and Human Services (HHS) design a new plan for the Medicare program. That new system, implemented in 1983, was the Prospective Payment System (PPS) for Medicare reimbursement to hospitals. The PPS was based on the New Jersey diagnosis-related groups (DRGs) program. This is an example of the federal government embracing a program originally implemented at the state level. In the same manner, the Affordable Care Act was based on, or at least similar to, the plan adopted in Massachusetts in 2006.

Under the PPS, hospitals are paid according to a schedule of preestablished rates linked to over 500 DRGs, effectively a form of price regulation. The categories depend on the type of case or what is called case mix. Case mix includes such factors as the severity of the disease, the amount of resources needed to treat the patient, and the prognosis.

Each category is assigned a treatment rate. Hospitals are reimbursed according to these rates. There are economic incentives in the form of rewards and punishments built into the system. If a hospital spends more money than the preestablished rate for a particular diagnostic treatment, the hospital must absorb the additional cost. If the hospital spends less money than the preestablished rate, it is still paid the preestablished rate and can keep the overpayment as profit. The HCFA (now the CMS) within the HHS was assigned the responsibility of establishing the DRG payment schedule. To safeguard against reduction in quality of care as a result of the PPS, Congress assigned PROs the responsibility of monitoring the quality and appropriateness of care for Medicare patients. If a PRO finds inappropriate or substandard care, the hospital may be denied Medicare payment. If a pattern of inappropriate or substandard care is discovered, the hospital's Medicare provider agreement may be terminated.

The rationale behind replacing the retrospective (fee-for-service or FFS) payment system was that under that system, hospitals had no incentive to economize in their use of healthcare resources in treating Medicare patients. If anything, such a system tended to encourage overutilization of health resources, since hospitals were assured that they would be reimbursed for all reasonable costs incurred. The PPS was based on the assumption that, given built-in incentives, hospitals would be forced to consider cost factors in treatment and would be encouraged to be economically more efficient. Thus, inefficient hospitals would be forced to close. An economically more efficient hospital sector would help contain increases in hospital costs. The PPS was viewed as a method of influencing hospital activities, creating cost-containment constraints, and introducing incentives into hospital payments (Shaffer 1983). The cost-control incentive was the primary purpose in establishing the PPS (Quade 1989). Additional Medicare prospective payment mechanisms were imposed on physicians in 1989 and on nursing homes, home healthcare agencies, and hospice agencies in 1997 (the latter as a result of the 1997 Balanced Budget Act).

How well has the prospective payment system constrained hospital and other cost increases? Our analysis of national health expenditure data (available at cms.gov) shows significant declines in the rate of increase in Medicare hospital expenditures in the first seven years of the DRG system, declining from an annual almost-19-percent change to less than half that annual change (9.2 percent) over the next eight years. Additionally, increases in Medicare hospital expenditures prior to the implementation of the prospective payment system were higher than overall hospital expenditures, but lower afterward. Though there has been some variation from year to year, the general trend remains that such Medicare hospital expenditures are lower than overall hospital expenditures. In the later years, some of the difference might be at least partly a function of the move toward managed care (Medicare Advantage) plans within Medicare.

One way of looking at the impact of the PPS is to consider PPS margins, effectively a measure of profits and the balance of revenue and expenses. Data from 1999 to 2010 (Medicare Payment Advisory Commission 2012) show that the margins declined from 13.7 percent in 1999 to -0.3 percent in 2004. Since then, the margins have remained below zero (Medicare Payment Advisory Commission 2018). Hospitals still made money on Medicare patients (Medicare Payment Advisory Commission 2018).

Between 1984 and 1991, the PPS payment per caseload rose at an annual rate of 6.4 percent (2.5-percent faster than the CPI). Between 1991 and 1995, the PPS payment per case had decelerated to 4.2 percent per year. The PPS cost per case actually declined in 1994 and again in 1995 (Guterman 1998). Medicare payments per hospital discharge were flat from 1996 to 2000 and then began a steep rise in 2001 and 2002 (Medicare Payment Advisory Commission 2004). The most recent data indicate that over the past several years the hospital industry has managed to improve the balance of revenue and expenses in the face of strong pressure from private payers. Hospital inpatient margins were negative in 1991 (-2.4 percent), reached a peak in 1997 (16.7 percent), and declined significantly through 2002 (4.7 percent). The overall margin (including most institutional care) declined from 10.3 percent in 1996 (the first year for which such data were collected) to 1.7 percent in 2002 (Medicare Payment Advisory Commission 2004). From 2004 to 2011, hospital inpatient margins were consistently negative, reaching a low of -4.7 percent in 2008 (Medicare Payment Advisory Commission 2013). In 2016, the margin was -9.6 percent, lower than in the previous year (Medicare Payment Advisory Commission 2018). As a result, cost-shifting to outpatient care has occurred. The prospective payment system has had similar effects on physicians (after 1989) and nursing homes, home healthcare agencies, and hospices with the passage of the Balanced Budget Act in 1997.

There have been criticisms of the payment system. Some suggest that hospitals seek ways to limit the impact of the new hospital regulations (see, for example, Lave 1984). Because price regulation is a tax on hospital behavior, it affects not only price but also hospital output and quality and quantity of services. Hospitals respond by attempting to reduce the use of affected services or resources by modifying their practices and products (Cook et al. 1983). Hospitals modify the cost of regulation by seeking an area unaffected by the regulation, that is, the "unregulated margin." Organizations respond to regulation through institutional, managerial, and technical changes (Parsons 1956). Hospitals altered services, influenced practices, and changed the products offered to decrease the impact of regulation at the expense of Medicare patients. They also changed the mix of services offered in the inpatient Medicare market and expanded the surgical market because surgical DRGs are more profitable than medical DRGs. Often, services were cut (Gay et al. 1989).

Controlling Physician Costs

The Prospective Payment System focused on hospitals, but it also had an indirect effect on doctors. Hospitals are the structure or framework, but doctors decide medical or surgical treatment. The PPS, by creating a ceiling on hospital reimbursements, caused hospitals to pressure doctors so as to limit hospital expenditures. But physicians had independent effects on Medicare expenditures and government budgets.

General revenues make up a significant portion of Part B expenditures—73 percent in 2013. Beneficiaries pay 25 percent of Part B expenditures (Cubanski et al. 2015). With hospital expenses easing a bit, attention naturally turned to expenditures on the next-biggest item, physicians. By 1995, such expenses accounted for 21.7 percent of total Medicare spending (Levit, Lazenby, and Stewart 1996).

In some ways, though Medicare based payments on usual and customary fees, the process was administratively complex and created inequities in physician income and dissatisfaction among physicians. In 1984, Congress froze Medicare physician reimbursements and then limited balance billing (the amount doctors could charge above Medicare). Further, there were significant increases in Medicare beneficiary cost-sharing above increases in Social Security benefits. A final factor leading to change was the passage and implementation of the Prospective Payment System for hospitals. As Oliver points out, PPS "demonstrated that health cost containment was both technically feasible and politically feasible" (Oliver 1993, 120).

Although the Reagan administration did not consider a physician payment schedule program, Congress acted. It froze physician fees in Medicare and ordered the (now defunct) Office of Technology Assessment to evaluate different payment schemes. In 1985, Congress created the Physician Payment Review Commission (PPRC), through an omnibus budget reconciliation Act, and ordered it to make recommendations regarding a payment system. It simultaneously ordered the Department of Health and Human Services to develop a fee schedule, based on a resource-based relative-value scale (RBRVS). Such a scale was adopted in 1989, again through an omnibus budget reconciliation Act. HCFA began implementing the fee schedule in 1992, and it was fully implemented in 1996 (Moon 1996).

A relative-value scale (RVS) compares the complexity and time of services offered (Moon 1996). Thus, a simple office visit would have a lower RVS than a coronary bypass operation. The fee schedule also contains adjustments for geography, and there is a conversion factor that translates the results into dollar amounts. Additionally, volume standards help in establishing growth rates in physician payments (Moon 1996).

The impact of the fee schedule varied depending on the kind of service. Fees for office and hospital visits were generally increased; fees for surgery were significantly reduced. It is no wonder that physicians and their associations were unhappy with the fee schedules. Political pressure by interest groups, Congress, and the Bush administration led HCFA to liberalize the fee schedule (Oliver 1993). In 1998, HCFA began using a single conversion factor for all physician services, effectively raising the conversion factor for primary care and nonsurgical care and lowering it for surgical services ("Victory" 1997). The 1997 Balanced Budget Act called for changes in the fee schedule components to be fully implemented by 2002 (Physician Payment Review Commission 1997). By FY 2004, physician spending was down to 17.4 percent of total Medicare spending (Centers for Medicare and Medicaid Services 2004b). The fee schedules are developed with the assistance of various medical societies and those recommendations are generally adopted by CMS. In a sense, physicians get to determine their own fees (Laugesen 2016).

The figures through 2002 show the impact of cost controls, especially the Balanced Budget Act of 1997. Consider the 1998–2002 period. Overall health expenditures increased by about 35 percent, and federal health expenditures increased by about 37 percent. Medicare expenditures, on the other hand, grew by only about 27 percent during the same time period (Centers of Medicare and Medicaid Services 2004b).

The Balanced Budget Act of 1997 also focused on physician reimbursement and created a problem that festered until April 2015. The problem was something called the sustainable growth rate (SGR). The idea behind this was to put a leash on physician payments (Part B) as part of the reimbursement rates that CMS sets each year. SGR resulted in cutbacks in physician payments. The problem, apart from the impact on physicians, is that the cutbacks actually made each year were less than those targeted under the program. The differences become cumulative. By 2010, physician reimbursement should have been cut by 21 percent (American Medical Association 2009).

Each year Congress was faced with the decision of whether to allow the scheduled cuts to take place or to change the reimbursements. Naturally, physicians and their organizations, such as the American Medical Association, opposed the cuts. Physicians were unhappy with the Medicare program because of the relatively low reimbursement rates, which were higher than for Medicaid but lower than for privately insured patients. Congress responded by either not allowing the cuts to take place or, in some cases, increasing reimbursements to physicians (American Medical Association 2009). This yearly ritual was known as the "doc fix." But each year that Congress delayed action, the targeted cuts got bigger. Recall the 2010 cumulative figure. For 2013, the cumulative cuts would be 27 percent (Congressional Budget Office 2012). Actually allowing the SGR reimbursement cuts to take effect would reduce Medicare spending by over $200 billion (Steinbrook 2015; Walker 2011).

Finally, in 2015, Congress passed a law, supported by both Republicans and Democrats, to repeal the SGR. This was the *Medicare Access and CHIP Reauthorization Act of 2015*. The legislation created a new payment system, the *Merit-Based Incentive Payment System* (MIPS), that is supposed to begin in 2019. Steinbrook (2015) lists the four criteria by which payments will be determined: "quality, resource use, meaningful use of electronic health records, and clinical practice improvement activities." Veuger and Clemens (2015) observe that the point of the new payment system is to provide better quality and value, while not necessarily using more resources. They also note that Medicare payments to physicians strongly influence payments to physicians by the private sector. As has been true of Medicare payments since the program's inception, figuring out the fee schedule is administratively complex and highly political (Laugesen 2016).

Reorganizing Payment Mechanisms and Service Delivery

Another set of reforms reorganizes how services are delivered and how providers are paid. These reforms are administered by the *Center for Medicare and Medicaid Initiatives* (created by the ACA). One such reform is *Accountable Care Organizations* (ACO). Here, providers (physicians, hospitals, etc.) come together to provide services for their patients. ACOs have financial incentives to provide high-quality services in a timely fashion. The financial incentives are penalties or bonuses for providing the services. In a sense, ACOs take a risk treating their patients. If they perform well, then they receive bonuses; if they do not perform well, they are penalized. Often the penalty is not being reimbursed for services provided that were unnecessary or of low value (Kaiser Family Foundation n.d.). Studies have shown that ACOs have produced savings for Medicare while maintaining or improving the quality of services compared to traditional Medicare patients (Kaiser Family Foundation n.d.).

A second set of reforms is *bundled payments*. Under such a system, similar to DRGs but broader, when a patient experiences a health incident, such as a heart attack, Medicare would pay one amount for all the care by all the providers. This would end or trim fee-for-service. If the cost of providing the services is less than the Medicare payment, then the providers keep the difference; if the cost is more than the payment, the providers take the loss. As with ACOs, there are a variety of models of bundled payments (Kaiser Family Foundation, n.d.). Again, research has shown modest savings from using bundled payments and quality of care equal to that of traditional Medicare (Kaiser Family Foundation, n.d.).

The third reform was the *medical home* or *patient-centered medical home* (PCMH). Under this model, a Medicare patient would be part of a primary-care practice that would be responsible for much of the patient's medical needs and coordinate with other providers as necessary. Medicare would pay a management fee and, depending on the model, provide other resources. The medical home model was terminated in 2016 (Kaiser Family Foundation n.d.). Evaluations showed that they tended not to produce savings (Kaiser Family Foundation n.d.). Further, as with the other reforms, they were extremely complicated (see, for example, Sullivan 2015).

THE PROBLEM OF LONG-TERM CARE

Although the impetus behind the nation's quest for healthcare reform is public dissatisfaction over glaring deficiencies in America's acute-care health system—primarily excessive cost and the inability of millions of Americans to get health insurance—the way the nation provides for the financing and delivery of long-term care (LTC) may be even more badly in need of reform. Strong considerations, both public-policy and moral, argue for addressing healthcare for the uninsured first, before long-term care. Yet no other part of the healthcare system generates as much passionate discontent as does long-term care (Weiner and Illston 1994, 17).

With prescription medications now covered under Medicare, perhaps the most important gap in Medicare pertains to long-term care. We begin this section by looking at some of the data.

A first point is the increase in expenditures on nursing homes. Data on nursing homes and other continuing-care retirement communities show projected spending for 2018 was $174.6 billion, an increase of 18 percent since 2013 (Hartman et al. 2018; percentage increase calculated by authors). This growth rate was less than for overall national health expenditures. Additionally, using 2018 projections, nursing home and other continuing-care retirement communities made up about 4.6 percent of total spending (authors' calculations from Hartman et al. 2018).

Second, Medicare (and most private medical insurance) focuses on short-term or acute care. It provides limited coverage for skilled nursing care, and then only after a hospital episode on physician orders. The bulk of spending on nursing homes is from Medicaid and out-of-pocket expenditures. Of the $162.7 billion spent on nursing homes nationally in 2016, Medicare accounted for only about 23 percent, or $37.5 billion. By contrast, Medicaid accounted for almost 31 percent (almost $50 billion), out-of-pocket payments accounted for about 27 percent, and long-term care health insurance accounted for a little over 9 percent ($14.8 billion) (calculated from Centers for Medicare and Medicaid Services 2018b).

Having looked at expenditure data, we can look at the population likely to need long-term care. The number of elderly (those 65 and over) is growing rapidly, and the segment of the elderly population growing the fastest is the 85-and-older group. Thus, there are projections that the need for long-term care services, especially nursing homes, will double over the next 20 to 30 years. The aged, those 65 and older, accounted for an estimated 15.2 percent of the population in 2016—roughly 49.2 million people. By 2035 there will be a projected 78 million elderly people, and by 2060 a projected 94.7 million elderly, about 23.5 percent of the overall population (Mather, Jacobsen, and Pollard 2015; US Bureau of the Census 2017).

Not all elderly people will go to, or need to go to, a nursing home. In 2014, about 1.4 million or 2.9 percent the elderly population were in nursing homes. If we use the 2.9-percent rate, then we should expect that about 2.3 million elderly people will be in nursing homes in 2035 and 2.7 million in 2060.

Similar increases are projected for the use of home healthcare and hospice services. One reason is the growth in the number of the elderly population and their increased life span. Another reason is the surge in disabilities among the elderly. This includes the rising number of people with AIDS who survive the disease because of medications, the increasing prevalence of obesity and the chronic diseases that accompany it, and the increasing incidence of asthma within the population (Gittler 2009).

The nursing home industry was born of two actions by the federal government. One, in 1950, was an amendment to the Social Security Act prohibiting payments to residents living in institutional settings, such as boardinghouses, that did not provide healthcare. The other major development was the establishment of Medicaid. Though Medicaid does not pick up all nursing home costs, it does pay for the medically indigent in nursing homes. These two developments created a situation in which long-term care became synonymous with nursing homes.

Despite the relatively small number of the elderly in nursing homes, the threat of a nursing home stay is that it can wipe out lifetime savings. In 2018, the national median yearly cost for a semiprivate room in a nursing home was $89,297. Nor is home healthcare cheap. The national median yearly cost for homemaker services was $48,048; for a home health aide, $50,366. Adult day healthcare costs a median $18,720 a year. The median annual cost of living in an assisted-living facility is $48,000 (Genworth Financial 2018). The impact of these high costs should be compared to the income available to the elderly. While members of the Baby Boomer generation are relatively better prepared for retirement than previous (and perhaps future) generations, they are hardly wealthy. Just over half of elderly Social Security beneficiaries depend on the program for more than half of their income, especially minority groups (Caldera 2012). Social Security benefits are not overly generous. The average monthly benefit for a retired worker in 2018 was $1,413, with a maximum monthly benefit of $2,788 (Brandon 2018). To put this into perspective, compare the above numbers on the cost of long-term care with the yearly benefits from Social Security: its average cost is $16,956 and the maximum is $33,456, less than the cost of living in an assisted-living facility and much less than the cost of living in a nursing home. And those who receive the maximum are more likely to have other sources of income, such as retirement accounts and pensions, than those at the lower end.

Long-term care thus presents several problems at different levels. At the level of the individual, the problem is financial: being able to afford long-term care, or in some cases being able to arrange it. From the standpoint of government, the problem is long-term care's ever-increasing costs. From a societal standpoint, the problem is the increasing demand for long-term care in the twenty-first century.

Much care for the elderly is given in the home by relatives, that is, unpaid informal assistance. This includes meals, transportation, and home healthcare. Only a small minority of the elderly at any one time live in a nursing home. Relatives (mainly spouses and children) caring for the elderly need help and understanding as they deal with work and home conflicts (Tilly, Goldenson, and Kasten 2001). One way that these informal caregivers, the overwhelming majority of whom are women, can be assisted is by employers (both public and private) providing options for their employees that will help them assist their disabled relatives, such as stronger medical and family leave policies.

A 2015 study by the AARP Public Policy Institute estimated the value of such home caregiving at $470 billion (2013 data) (Reinhard 2015). The report identified a number of efforts/initiatives at the federal and state levels to address issues raised by family caregiving. At the state level, a number of states have mandated paid family leave and/or extended leave. Some have provided for family leave insurance (think of Aflac for families). Medicare, as of 2015, for example, allows for telehealth coverage for rural families, including counseling and mental health.

In 2018, Congress passed, and President Trump signed in to law, a bipartisan piece of legislation, the RAISE Family Caregivers Act (AARP 2018). The acronym RAISE stands for **R**ecognize, **A**ssist, **I**nclude, **S**upport, and **E**ngage. The purpose of the legislation is to bring together appropriate members of the public and private sectors in an advisory council that has 18 months to create a strategy to deal with the many issues raised by family caregivers. The advisory council should consider the following issues (AARP 2018):

- promoting greater adoption of person- and family-centered care in all health and LTSS settings, with the person and the family caregiver (as appropriate) at the center of care teams
- assessment and service planning (including care transitions and coordination) involving care recipients and family caregivers
- information, education, training supports, referral, and care coordination
- respite options
- financial security and workplace issues

An alternative to informal home care and nursing homes (institutionalization) is the use of home healthcare agencies. Under Parts A and B, Medicare will pay for services if the enrollee is "under the care of a physician, confined to home, and need[s] skilled nursing services on an intermittent basis" (Moon 1996, 79; see also Centers for Medicare and Medicaid Services 2004a, 27). Since 1989, after a Supreme Court decision, Medicare has relaxed eligibility requirements for home healthcare. Medicare will pay 100 percent of home healthcare visits and 80 percent of durable equipment costs (Centers for Medicare and Medicaid Services 2012a). The result has been a massive increase in use of services and increased costs. In 2004, total home healthcare expenditures were $43.8 billion, of which Medicare paid $15.5 billion, or 35.8 percent. By 2017, total home healthcare expenditures had increased to $97 billion, of which Medicare paid $38.8 billion, or 40 percent (calculated from Centers for Medicare and Medicaid Services 2018b).

The major change that occurred in regard to home healthcare agencies came in the Balanced Budget Act of 1997. It called for a prospective payment system, similar to what already existed for hospital and physician services, for nursing homes, home healthcare agencies, and hospice services.

Long-Term Care Insurance

One policy alternative for addressing the cost of long-term care is long-term care (LTC) insurance. LTC is an indemnity-type policy. It pays a certain amount per day that the recipient is in a facility, usually with some limits on how long the policyholder will be covered (Congressional Budget Office 2004). Insurance could be sold to the elderly, say, when they become 65 years old, or to younger people where they work so that a reserve fund could be established.

Long-term care insurance is not cheap, and its premiums depend on the age of the holder at the time the policy is purchased. A 55-year-old male, on average, would pay an annual premium of $1,870 (2018 numbers). A 55-year-old female would pay, on average, an annual premium of $2,965. The respective premiums for those at age 65 would be $2,460 and $4,720. The average benefit per day is $150 (American Association of Long-Term Care Insurance 2018). This compares to an average of $250 a day for a stay in a nursing home facility. The difference in costs by age is due to the greater likelihood that older people would need the benefit than younger people, and women are more likely to need it then men.

There are other issues with long-term care insurance. Those purchasing such insurance undergo risk evaluations and as many as 20 percent of applicants are denied coverage based on health risks. The policies are complex to understand and there is a long period between the time when one purchases the policy and when one needs to make use of it—as long as several decades (Tumlinson, Aguiar, and Watts 2009). Often the payments from the policy last for three years at most. The result of all this (along with the unwillingness on the part of many to think about the issue) is that only a small percentage (10 percent) of the senior population has such coverage (Andrews 2010).

The Affordable Care Act of 2010 contained a provision that addressed the long-term care insurance issue. The Community Living Assistance and Services and Supports (CLASS) Act would have created a voluntary program whereby workers would enroll in long-term care policies through the workplace (implying that people with serious disabilities would not be part of the program). Unlike private insurance, benefits would be for the lifetime of the purchaser, and there would be subsidies for low-income purchases ("CLASS Act Provision of Health Care Reform" 2011).

Several provisions of the law led the Obama administration to decide not to implement it. One was that participation in the program was voluntary, a problem that the ACA in general had to face (see Chapter 3). Those most likely to need the benefit are also those most likely to participate, an issue known in the insurance world as adverse selection. And the resulting premiums would be much less than for private LTC insurance, at between $235 and $391 a month. A third feature is the lifetime benefit versus the normal three-year benefit of private plans. Finally, the subsidies for low-income people would have been substantial.

POLICY OPTIONS: TRANSFORMING MEDICARE

Oberlander (2003) views the process leading to the Medicare Modernization Act as the end of the consensus about what Medicare was supposed to be. Indeed, the process that began with the 1997 Balanced Budget Act led to drastic changes in the nature of Medicare. As we discussed earlier, Medicare represents a significant portion of federal spending at a time when the federal deficit is large. The large Baby Boomer generation (those born between 1946 and 1964 or so) is entering its retirement stage, healthcare costs continue to increase, and Medicare benefits have improved (especially for outpatient prescription drugs and subsidies to private plans). Johnson and Kwak (2012; see also Wessel 2012) argue that healthcare costs in general are the major problem behind long-term deficits. Because Medicare is such a large part of the federal deficit, it is only natural that thought would be given as to how to rein in the future costs of the program—what is called "bending the curve."

Before we look at reform proposals, we should point out that the problems that Medicare faces are at least partly a function of how the American healthcare system is constructed. Because Medicare is specifically designed for the elderly, demographic changes loom large. The Baby Boomer generation is the largest generation in American history, some 75 million people. As that generation moves into the Medicare-eligible age, obviously, the number of Medicare recipients dramatically increases. It is a shock to the system. A national health system of some sort (see Reid 2009) would not experience this kind of shock because everyone is already enrolled. Even if Medicare is able to control costs per capita, there will be more per-capitas. That presents a major public policy problem for the program itself and for the federal government's budget.

Some of the reform proposals are fairly straightforward, amounting to incremental change or tinkering. Such policy tools would include some combination of reducing demand, increasing revenue, and reducing provider reimbursements. Others would fundamentally change the nature of Medicare. Having said that, none of the proposals for change is politically easy to do. Some would affect the beneficiaries. But seniors are a potent political force and would likely push back on policies that would adversely affect them. Others would affect providers, also obviously not a group to be taken lightly. And the future of Medicare became tied to the 2012 presidential race.

Incremental Policy Alternatives

The simplest way to control costs is to raise the age of eligibility for Medicare, currently at 65. Social Security, a program that in some ways resembles Medicare, has raised the full retirement age to 67. The argument for it is obvious. If people are on Medicare for a shorter period of time, say, two years less, Medicare will spend less money on them.

But simple, straightforward, and easy is not necessarily the same as a good or effective policy. There are several reasons why such a change might have little effect. One is that younger seniors, aged 65–67, are generally healthier than older seniors. One thing we know about Medicare, and healthcare spending in general, is that a small percentage (10 percent) of the senior population accounts for a large percentage (42 percent) of Medicare expenditures (Cubanski et al. 2012). Raising the eligibility age will not change this. Aaron (2011) points out that Medicare premiums are based on average costs. Taking out the lower-costing recipients would lead to higher premiums for the beneficiaries.

Further, there is concern over how those in the two additional years before eligibility will be covered. Many of them might spend those years without coverage, or perhaps be covered by Medicaid, raising that program's costs.

A second possibility is to raise premiums for Part B and Part D. To some extent this has already been done for higher-income beneficiaries, effectively income-related or means-tested premiums. But as Stuart Butler (AARP Public Policy Institute 2012) notes, premiums for the higher-income beneficiaries would need to be higher to pay the full costs of their benefits, and the income threshold for designating the higher-income should be lowered somewhat. A variation on this is to raise premiums on all beneficiaries. This is one example of cost-shifting, asking some (if not all) beneficiaries to pay more.

One question that can be raised is where the threshold should be. If the threshold is lowered, as Butler suggests, then more recipients will face the considerably higher premiums. If the threshold is frozen, then the incomes of more and more recipients will exceed the threshold in future years. Another concern is that higher-income beneficiaries might decide that Parts B and D are not worthwhile for them, and pay for that coverage themselves. This would, again, make premiums higher for the many remaining in the program.

Another possibility is to generate additional revenue by raising the payroll tax. The total Medicare payroll tax is 2.9 percent, split between employer and employee (or the full 2.9 percent for self-employed people). Unlike Social Security, there is no cap or limit on how much of earned income is subject to the Medicare payroll tax. An increase of the total tax to 3.9 percent would eliminate much of the Part A trust fund deficits (AARP Public Policy Institute 2012).

But raising taxes is difficult in the United States, even if by a relatively modest amount (see Wessel 2012). Congress and the Obama administration cut the Social Security payroll taxes in 2010 through 2012, going the other way in a program with a similar trust fund problem. Butler (AARP Public Policy Institute 2012) argues that increasing taxes would slow economic growth and the burden of taxation would be on younger people (because they would be in the workforce the longest). He also argues that raising taxes would eliminate any incentive on the part of Congress to make needed changes in the program.

Another possibility would be to increase cost-sharing, including deductibles (how much recipients have to pay before Medicare begins paying for a service) and co-payments (how much of the remaining part of the bill recipients would have to pay). Some have suggested that increased cost-sharing could be combined with limits on out-of-pocket expenses, which currently do not exist. Increased cost-sharing does tend to reduce the use of services. The combined impact of these effects would be sizable. A major problem with this proposal is that it would adversely affect lower-income beneficiaries who would reduce their use of necessary services (AARP Public Policy Institute 2012).

The most common approach to controlling Medicare costs has focused on provider reimbursements, as we discussed above. The two major examples of this focus are prospective payment systems (applied to hospitals, doctors, nursing homes, etc.) and the sustainable growth rate issue. CMS could certainly reduce provider payments. The problem is that as provider payments are reduced and begin to approach the levels of reimbursement that Medicaid pays, providers will be increasingly reluctant to take on Medicare patients. That is one reason why the SGR issue took so long to resolve (the other is the impact of eliminating the SGR on the federal budget).

Another possibility is to require Medicare beneficiaries to enroll in managed-care plans. As of 2017, about one-third of Medicare beneficiaries were in Medicare Advantage plans. It is not clear whether such plans produce savings or are more efficient than the current system.

One set of incremental plans comes from the National Commission on Fiscal Responsibility and Reform, better known as the Bowles-Simpson report, named after the chairs of the commission, former Wyoming Republican Senator Alan K. Simpson and Erskine Bowles, former chief of staff in the Clinton White House. The commission was formed by President Obama, with members nominated by Obama and Democratic and Republican leaders in both houses of Congress. The purpose of the commission was to develop a set of proposals to address the fiscal problems (slow recovery from the recession, large federal government debts and deficits). While the commission was unable to gain the supermajority needed to adopt the proposals, they did address Medicare. One reason for doing this is that Medicare and Medicaid represent growing slices of the federal budget. Resolving, or at least alleviating, the cost increases would go a long way toward facing those fiscal challenges.

The commission made seven recommendations to restrain cost increases in Medicare (National Commission on Fiscal Responsibility and Reform 2010). The first recommendation, one of the smaller in terms of monetary impact (an estimated $9 billion in savings through 2020), was to reduce fraud in the program by enhancing CMS oversight of Medicare and providing more resources to achieve these savings.

The second recommended change, with a much larger impact ($110 billion through 2020), focused on cost-sharing. The commission pointed out that cost-sharing provisions in Medicare are complicated and confusing. The recommendation would replace all the different types of cost- sharing with a simpler plan that would have a single $500 deductible for Parts A and B and a 20-percent coinsurance rate after that. The commission recommended a cap or limit on cost-sharing by lowering the coinsurance to 5 percent after $5,500 of out-of-pocket costs and no cost-sharing after expenses exceed $7,500. Cost-sharing for Part D (the prescription drug benefit) would not be changed (though it was reduced by the ACA).

The remainder of the recommendations collectively were smaller. The third recommendation would prohibit medigap (or supplementary policies) from paying for the first $500 of expenses and also require that such plans pay for no more than half of the next $5,000 of expenses, a high-deductible policy and similar to consumer-directed health plans (see Chapter 11). Recommendation number 4 would extend prescription drug rebates under Medicaid to those Medicare recipients eligible for both programs (dual eligibles). The fifth recommendation would reduce payments to hospitals that engage in medical education. The sixth recommendation, following the practice of private insurance companies, over a period of time would terminate payment to providers for bad debts. The final recommendation suggested accelerating home healthcare cost savings called for by the ACA. The savings from these seven recommendations total $298 billion through 2020.

Ultimately, both House Republicans and President Obama rejected Bowles-Simpson, though not necessarily because of the Medicare provisions. The Republicans, including 2012 Republican vice-presidential candidate Paul Ryan, rejected the report because it called for tax increases (though dwarfed by spending reductions). The president's concern was cuts to Social Security and a cap on federal spending (Pianin 2011).

Comprehensive Policy Alternatives

The most significant proposed change is to transform Medicare into a premium-support program. This was a policy favored by a majority of commissioners of the National Bipartisan Commission on the Future of Medicare. There is a distinctive political edge to such proposed reforms. For the most part, premium support proposals are supported by Republicans, particularly House Speaker Paul Ryan (R-WI). Ryan included premium support in his series of policy proposals in 2016 (Kliff 2016).

The idea behind premium support is that Medicare beneficiaries would choose from a number of plans and receive some portion of the plans' premiums as a subsidy from the federal government. There would be some regulation of the plans and, depending on the proposal, some minimum or common level of benefits. The federal government's contribution would be a fixed amount. Depending on the proposal, traditional Medicare (i.e., fee-for-service) would stay in some form or be replaced entirely (Fuchs and Potetz 2011; Kliff 2016).

From the standpoint of the Medicare beneficiary, she would be faced every year with a choice of plans. The beneficiary would choose the plan that would meet her needs as well as be affordable. Some plans will offer more benefits and less cost-sharing, while others will offer fewer benefits and more cost-sharing. Premiums for the former would be greater than premiums for the latter. The beneficiary would also want to know which doctors and other providers are included in the plan. Under premium support, the federal government would pay some percentage of the average premium of all plans, perhaps 80 percent. Plans would likely include some additional cost-sharing, such as deductibles and co-payments. Medicare Part D and the ACA exchanges are similar to premium support, though the financing mechanism is different.

Premium support proposals, according to their advocates, have several advantages over Medicare as it currently exists. One is that they would create conditions under which competitive markets could operate. In this case the competition is among plans rather than providers. Certainly, one of the problems of the healthcare system is that it operates much differently than other markets, such as those for automobiles or shoes (for the classic discussion of market failures in healthcare, see Arrow 1953). Creating those conditions would, hopefully, restrain costs, either through reducing use of services or reducing the price for services (Fuchs and Potetz 2011).

A second advantage of such plans is that they reduce the federal government's role in the healthcare sector. The federal government, through Medicare, Medicaid, employee health benefits (the Federal Employees Health Benefits Program [FEHBP]), and the Department of Veterans Affairs, is the single largest purchaser/provider of healthcare services. Especially with Medicare, the federal government is involved in rate setting, quality control, and so forth. Recall the discussion about DRGs and SGR. Under the more radical premium support plans, government's role would be very much constrained.

A third advantage of premium support plans may be even more significant than the other two. Under the current program, Medicare is largely an uncontrolled expense for the federal government. Expenditures depend on a combination of utilization and prices. As the Baby Boomer generation ages, utilization will increase, and expenditures will go up. That is a large part of the problem that Medicare causes the federal budget.

Under premium support, the uncontrollable becomes the controllable. One way of understanding this is to think about the difference between a defined-benefit plan and a defined-contribution plan (Aaron 2011). Medicare and most pension plans (private as well as public such as Social Security) are defined-benefit plans. Beneficiaries are guaranteed a certain set of benefits, and the plan pays for all or part of the cost of those services or benefits. If more services are used, then the plan pays more. That has been the experience with Medicare (of course, the cost of healthcare has risen, so that also plays a major role).

Under a defined-contribution plan, the plan is limited to paying a specific portion of, in this case, premiums. Utilization of services then becomes less important. The expense is controllable and knowable in advance because we know how many people will be on Medicare.

Further, premium support proposals allow the federal government to control future expenses. Let's say that premiums, on average, go up by 6 percent next year (a lower-than-normal amount for many plans) and the federal government's program pays 80 percent of the average premium for all plans. The federal government could decide to maintain its 80-percent rate, or it could decide to allow only a portion of the increase, so the effective premium support might be 77 percent.

The most prominent recent plan is Representative Paul Ryan's (R-WI) proposal, "The Path to Prosperity: Restoring America's Promise." Ryan was the chair of the House Budget Committee, so his proposal drew a great deal of attention ("Proposed Changes to Medicare in the "Path to Prosperity" 2011). The Ryan plan took center stage when, in August 2012, he was chosen to be the vice-presidential running mate by Mitt Romney; media attention on Medicare greatly increased after Ryan's selection. In 2016, now the Speaker of the House, Ryan offered a similar proposal (Ryan 2016; see Chapter 11).

Under Ryan's plan, the eligibility age would gradually rise to 67. In the 2011 version of the plan, new beneficiaries as of 2022 could only choose private plans, and the federal government would pay the support to the plans. Under the 2012 revision, new beneficiaries would have a choice between the premium support programs and traditional Medicare (House Budget Committee 2012). The 2016 plan would begin the new retirement age in 2020. Those currently in Medicare or entering it before 2022 could choose between private plans or traditional Medicare. Beneficiaries would go to virtual markets—private exchanges—to pick plans, similar to what is done with Part D plans, the California Public Employees' Retirement system (CalPERS), the Federal Employees Health Benefits Program (FEHBP), the Massachusetts plan, and the healthcare exchanges or marketplaces under the ACA. The Centers for Medicare and Medicaid Services would regulate the plans ("Comparison of Medicare Premium Support Proposals" 2012).

Premiums would be adjusted depending on age, income, and health of the recipient (Fuchs and Potetz 2011; "Proposed Changes to Medicare in the 'Path to Prosperity'" 2011). The premium support payment or voucher would be paid to the plans. Those whose income is below the federal poverty line would receive a medical savings account with $7,500 deposited in it. Those whose income is between 100 and 150 percent of the federal poverty line would receive 75 percent of that amount. The deposits would be indexed to the consumer price index ("Proposed Changes to Medicare in the 'Path to Prosperity'" 2011).

An important element of the plan is how the premiums would increase over time. The key to the plan is that competition, a "competitive bidding process" (House Budget Committee 2012, 53), would keep growth under control. Under the original Ryan plan, government's contribution would be based on increases in the consumer price index. Other proposals would be based on changes in gross domestic product (GDP). The modified Ryan plan would base increases, as a backup in case competitive bidding does not work, on GDP plus one-half of a percent. Because healthcare costs exceed either indicator, over time the relative value of the premium support would decrease ("Proposed Changes to Medicare" 2011).

Not surprisingly, there have been many critics of the premium support proposals. One of the more interesting critics is Henry Aaron, an economist with the Brookings Institution. In 1995, Aaron and another economist, Robert Reischauer, coined the phrase "premium support" (Aaron 2011). They wanted to distinguish premium support from the similar concept of vouchers. Voucher proposals would be based not on the cost of services but on government budget considerations. But Aaron thought three changes were necessary to make the proposal stronger and move from a voucher to premium support.

The first change would be to link increases in the value of the voucher (and medical savings account deposits) to increases in the cost of healthcare, rather than linking them to either changes in gross domestic product or overall price changes. The second change would be to create what are effectively regulated insurance markets, providing information so that consumers can make appropriate choices. Third, premiums should be adjusted for factors such as health risk and age. By these standards, Aaron continued, all such premium support proposals had some defects.

For example, Aaron (2011) notes that if the original Ryan plan had been in force over the last 20 years, recipient benefits would have been nearly 50 percent lower than they are now. But that, of course, is the point of such plans.

An analysis of the original Ryan plan by the Kaiser Family Foundation ("Proposed Changes to Medicare in the 'Path to Prosperity'" 2011) found that the plan would not, according to the Congressional Budget Office, reduce the cost of healthcare spending on the elderly. What it would do is constrain government spending on Medicare. Under the current system and projecting to 2022, healthcare spending for a 65-year-old would average $13,500; the federal government's share would be just over 59 percent, and the beneficiary's share would be about 41 percent. Under the original Ryan plan, healthcare spending for a 65-year-old that same year would average

$20,500; the federal government's share would drop to about 39 percent, and the beneficiary's share would rise to about 61 percent. It follows that under the Ryan plan, beneficiaries would be paying a larger amount of their income than under the current Medicare program. According to the Kaiser report, the typical 65-year-old in 2022 would have an average income of $25,000. Under the current plan, healthcare costs would amount to about 22 percent of her income. Under the original Ryan plan, it would amount to nearly 50 percent of her income ("Proposed Changes to Medicare" 2011). A Congressional Budget Office analysis of premium support proposals in 2013 (Congressional Budget Office 2013) found that total costs for beneficiaries, which included premiums, deductibles, and co-payments, would rise over time for beneficiaries as compared to the current program.

The next question then becomes: why would healthcare spending on the elderly increase by so much under the Path to Prosperity Plan? Aaron (2011) and the Kaiser study ("Proposed Changes to Medicare" 2011) provide the same answer. Private plans have substantially higher administrative costs than Medicare, including marketing and sales, and also pay providers at higher rates than Medicare.

While not true for all who propose premium support/voucher programs, Park et al.'s comment about an earlier proposal rings true for some:

> In short, while the idea of introducing more competition into Medicare through the expanded use of private plans has been promoted as a "reform" that can restrain rising Medicare costs, the reality is that the legislation *increases* Medicare costs by overpaying private plans in order to induce more beneficiaries to enroll in them. Examination of the details of the legislation indicates that the ideological goal of privatizing more of Medicare trumped the stated goal of using "competition" to restrain the rate of growth in Medicare costs.
>
> (Park et al. 2003, 5)

Alice Rivlin suggests a compromise. She notes the inconsistency of Republican and Democratic arguments. "Ironically, Democrats favor competiton among private plans in the ACA, but oppose it in Medicare, while Republicans push competition in Medicare but want to repeal the ACA. But who expects campaign politics to be logical?" (Rivlin 2012).

Paul Ryan teamed up with Democratic Senator Ron Wyden (Oregon) to propose the "Guaranteed Choices" plan (Wyden and Ryan 2011). The plan, which Rivlin endorsed—and indeed called for a similar measure—would be a hybrid, similar to Ryan's 2012 revision. New seniors in 2022 would have a choice of traditional Medicare (changes proposed by Democrats) and private plans. Should the program not restrain cost increases, a cap of GDP plus 1 percent would be put in place in 2023. If the cap is exceeded, reductions in payments to providers and pharmaceutical companies would be made, among other changes. It should be pointed out that this element of the plan gives it one year to succeed before taking these other measures, a goal that is nearly impossible. But Rivlin's point is an interesting one, and it falls into the tradition of compromise that can be seen back to the founding of the republic.

There are also some proposals that would expand Medicare. Some proposals would extend Medicare eligibility to those 55 to 64 years of age. Others, such as plans offered by Senator Bernie Sanders (I-VT), a candidate for the 2016 and 2020 presidential nominations, and the Center for American Progress would extend Medicare to everyone—"Medicare for all," effectively a single-payer plan. If the premium support plans were largely, though not entirely, supported by conservatives/Republicans, the Medicare extension plans were supported by liberals/Democrats. We consider these plans in detail in Chapter 11.

MEDICARE AND THE AFFORDABLE CARE ACT

In March 2010, Congress passed, and President Obama signed, the ACA. The legislation impacts much of the healthcare system, including Medicare. We discussed the ACA in detail in Chapter 3, as well as efforts to repeal and replace it; here, we briefly summarize the legislation's provisions concerning Medicare. Some of the changes provide additional benefits to Medicare recipients (and increase expenditures), and some seek to control costs.

One important change provided in the ACA is the shrinking of the "doughnut hole" that is part of Part D. Recall that after a certain point ($2,250), Medicare recipients would pay for their entire drug costs up to about $5,100. That "hole" began to shrink in 2010 with small rebates, and by 2020 recipients would have to pay only 25 percent of drug costs in the hole ("Summary of Key Changes to Medicare in 2010 Health Reform Law" 2010).

A second change is to eliminate cost-sharing for specified prevention benefits. A third set of changes is designed to either provide for more revenue for the program, or reform or cut provider payments. One change, mentioned above, is reduction of payments to Medicare Advantage plans. Payments to MA plans declined from 114 percent in 2009 to 100 percent of the average annual costs of benefits to beneficiaries in traditional Medicare (Guterman, Skopec, and Zuckerman 2018). Another change is in provider payments, with some reductions in payments to specialists but increases in payments to primary-care physicians. Income-related premiums will be instituted for the Part D benefit as will a higher payroll tax for the Part A trust fund targeted at high-income wage earners.

Other changes focus on payment structure and reorganization. These include bundled payments (discussed above) and accountable care organizations ("Summary of Key Changes to Medicare in 2010 Health Reform Law" 2010). As discussed above, there have been savings from these two changes, but the savings have been modest (Baseman et al. 2016).

CONCLUSION: THE POLITICS AND POLICY OF MEDICARE

> The challenges posed by rising costs today combined with the future burdens that will arise from an aging population will require that changes be made in Medicare. But we should not begin this process of reassessment under the mistaken claim that the program is a failure.
>
> (Moon n.d.)

Financial considerations have been an important part of the politics and policy deliberations surrounding Medicare since the program's inception. One such problem, already mentioned, is the sheer size of the program combined with its rapid growth and its impact on the federal budget. Another aspect is that the increase in the size of Medicare beneficiary population (especially as the massive Baby Boomer generation begins to retire) places increased pressure on Medicare. This is most clearly seen in estimates that the Hospital Insurance (Part A) Trust Fund is expected to be depleted sometime in the 2020s. The trust fund and budget impacts of Medicare came together in the politics of balanced budgets in the twenty-first century.

On the one hand, there have been enhancements of Medicare benefits. The Medicare Modernization Act, however controversial, represents a major, but not the only, example. Beginning January 1, 2005, there were new preventive benefits, such as physical exams and screening for diabetes, elevated blood pressure, and hearing and vision losses (Rainey 2004). On the other hand, there are continual warnings that the financial future of Medicare is bleak. Not all researchers are quite as alarmed as the authors of these reports. Haase (2004) points out that long-range projections are notoriously inaccurate (see also Johnson and Kwak 2012). He also notes that the aging of the population is only a small factor in increased medical costs. Increased utilization of services and medical price inflation are more important factors. These two factors affect all costs, not just Medicare (see Chapter 8).

Medicare remains a popular program among the population at large (Norton, DiJulio, and Brodie 2015). This can be seen in public opinion polls during the 2012 election. The selection of Paul Ryan as the Republican vice-presidential candidate placed his Medicare premium support proposal and Medicare in general front and center on the public agenda. An August 2012 poll found that majorities from both parties supported Medicare as it currently existed over the premium support plan. Further, Medicare was considered a more important issue than the ACA. Only the cost of healthcare exceeded Medicare as a concern ("Public Opinion on Health Care Issues" 2012; Viebeck 2012). And Medicare has done a better job of controlling costs than the healthcare system as a whole and private insurance in particular (Miller 2012; Van de Water 2016).

But problems remain in both the long and the short term. First, the cost of Medicare and the increases in those costs affect both recipients and the federal government. Second, as the Baby Boomer generation began retiring in 2010–2011, additional pressures were placed on the program. Additionally, Medicare has significant gaps in its coverage, particularly in long-term care. Even with the new prescription drug benefit, financial pressure on beneficiaries will remain. A 2017 estimate by Fidelity Investments suggests that a couple retiring that year would need about $275,000 to pay for their future healthcare costs (Fidelity Investments 2017).

The past four-plus decades have seen significant change in the structure of Medicare. The 1980s saw the imposition of fee schedules for hospitals and physicians and the beginning of Medicare managed care. The Balanced Budget Act of 1997 brought more potentially fundamental restructuring of Medicare. It extended fee schedules to other providers (e.g., home healthcare agencies) and instituted the Medicare+Choice program, which increased the types of plans beneficiaries could choose, even giving some (the wealthier ones) an opportunity to effectively drop out of the program. The 2003 Medicare Modernization Act created even more changes and challenges. It provided a prescription drug benefit, however limited it might be, and revamped the managed-care program (Medicare Advantage). At the same time, it increased the fiscal pressure through the new benefits and provisions that create new threats (the 45-percent cap on general revenue funding). The ACA also promises changes, including savings to the program.

The consensus that had existed from the beginning of the program about what Medicare would be has dissolved. Oberlander (1997, 2003) argues that the politics of Medicare up to 1994 led to a consensus, first that Medicare would be a public program, operated by the federal government. The other element of the consensus was that the politics of Medicare was bipartisan, supported by Republicans and Democrats. The politics of Medicare subsequent to the November 1994 elections saw the unraveling of the consensus. Medicare was depicted by some as a failure, a throwback to the 1960s Great Society programs, and a problem of intergenerational equity (younger people paying for older people). Medicare+Choice was the result, with its medical savings accounts and private fee-for-service provisions. This has been supplanted by the MMA.

One simple example will show the changing nature of Medicare. From its beginning until the mid-1990s, Medicare was the equivalent of a universal national health insurance program for the elderly (Reid 2009). All seniors were eligible, and all had the same benefits, regardless of residence (unlike Medicaid). The MMA changed this by making it more of (though not nearly entirely) a means- or income-tested program, more like Medicaid or welfare. This is done by giving subsidies and more generous benefits to low-income recipients and by having higher Part B premiums for higher-income seniors (Moon 2004; Pauly 2004).

The Balanced Budget Act of 1997 had, for a while, protected the fiscal future of Medicare. This was combined with a vibrant economy in the late 1990s and the brief reappearance of federal budget surpluses during the Clinton administration. But the new legislation and the reappearance of substantial budget deficits in the twenty-first century have placed Medicare in a more precarious financial position.

A variety of proposals have been suggested that would affect Medicare in the twenty-first century, from the incremental, tinkering type to dramatically changing the nature of the program. The debate over the future of Medicare is part of a larger debate, about not only government deficits and balanced budgets, but also the role of government in American society.

The twenty-first-century Medicare program is being built around the ideas found in the Balanced Budget Act of 1997, the Medicare Modernization Act of 2003, and the Affordable Care Act of 2010. We live in a brave and scary new world.

STUDY QUESTIONS

1. Medicare as it is currently configured is the product of accommodations made over the years, starting from the original 1965 legislation. What were those accommodations? Who was accommodated? Why were they accommodated? What has been the impact of those accommodations?
2. A number of researchers/experts have argued that Medicare (along with Medicaid) will have an important negative impact on federal budget deficits. Why might that be the case? Do you agree that Medicare will lead to increased federal budget deficits? Republicans and Democrats disagree on the potential impact of Medicare on federal budget deficits. What are their disagreements? Who do you agree with? Why?
3. Write an essay in which you discuss the objective, structure, eligibility/coverage requirements, and benefits and services provided by Medicare.
4. The chapter has the following statement: "Ending Medicare as we know it." What does this mean? What is the nature of the changes? Have they strengthened or improved Medicare?
5. In the chapter on the safety net (Chapter 7), we offer the following definition of the concept "underinsured": individuals and families who spend at least 10 percent of their income on healthcare (including premiums). By that definition, many Medicare beneficiaries are underinsured. Do you think this is a problem that should be addressed? Why? If so, what changes would you recommend?
6. A frequently suggested Republican proposal to reform Medicare is to transform it into a voucher or premium support program (defined contribution program). What are the advantages and disadvantages of this proposal? Why do you think Republicans rather than Democrats have proposed this? If it were adopted, how would it affect Medicare beneficiaries?

REFERENCES

Aaron, Henry J. 2011. *Medicare Reform: Rhetoric Versus Substance*. Washington, DC: Brookings Institution.
AARP. 2018. *RAISE Family Caregivers Act Now Law*. Washington, DC: AARP. Online at www.aarp.org/politics-society.
AARP Public Policy Institute. 2012. *Options for Reforming Medicare*. Washington, DC: AARP.

Altman, Drew E. 2004. "The New Medicare Prescription-Drug Legislation." *New England Journal of Medicine*, 350, no. 1 (January 1): 9–10.

American Association of Long-Term Care Insurance. 2018. *2018 National Long-Term Care Insurance Price Index*. Westlake Village, CA: American Association of Long-Term Care Insurance. Online at www.aaltc.org.

American Medical Association. 2009. *Medicare Physician Payment System: Permanently Reforming the Sustainable Growth Rate (SGR)*. Washington, DC: American Medical Association.

Andrews, Michelle. 2010. "Few Seniors Have Long-Term Care Insurance." Kaiser Health News.

Antos, Joseph and John E. Calfee 2004. *Of Sausage-Making and Medicare. Health Policy Outlook* (January–February). Washington, DC: American Enterprise Institute for Public Policy Research. Online at. www.aei.org.

Arrow, Kenneth J. 1953. "Uncertainty and the Welfare Economics of Medical Care." *American Economic Review*, 53, no. 5: 941–973.

Baicker, Katherine and Michael E. Chernew 2011. "The Economics of Financing Medicare." *New England Journal of Medicine*, 10, no. 1056 (July 28): e7(1)–e7(3).

Baseman, Susan et al. 2016. *Payment and Delivery System Reform in Medicare*. Menlo Park, CA: Kaiser Family Foundation.

Biles, Brian, Geraldine Dallek, and Lauren Hersch Nicholas. 2004. "Medicare Advantage: Deja Vu All Over Again?" *Health Affairs* (December 15): W4-586–W4-597. Online at www.healthaffairs.org.

Boards of Trustees, Federal Hospital Insurance and Federal Supplementary Medical Insurance Trust Funds. 2017. *2017 Annual Report of the Boards of Trustees, Federal Hospital Insurance and Federal Supplementary Medical Insurance Trust Funds*. Washington, DC: Government Printing Office.

Brandon, Emily. 2018. "How Much You Will Get from Social Security." *U.S. News & World Report*, August 20.

Brown, Randall S., Dolores G. Clement, Jerold W. Hill, Sheldon M. Retchin, and Jeanette W. Bergeron 1993. "Do Health Maintenance Organizations Work for Medicare?" *Health Care Financing Review*, 15, no. 1 (Fall): 7–23.

"The Bush Prescription Drug Plan." 2000. *The New York Times*, September 11.

Cai, Xiaomei et al. 2008. *Pitching Private Medicare Plans: An Analysis of Medicare Advantage and Prescription Drug Plan Advertising*. Menlo Park, CA: Kaiser Family Foundation.

Caldera, Selena. 2012. *Social Security: Who's Counting on It?* Washington, DC: AARP Public Policy Institute.

Center for American Progress. 2004a. *Your Medicare Benefits*. Washington, DC: Centers for Medicare and Medicaid Services.

Center for American Progress. 2004b. *2004 CMS Statistics*. Washington, DC: Centers for Medicare and Medicaid Services.

Center for American Progress. 2011. *Medicare and Medicaid Statistical Supplement, 2011*. Washington, DC: US Department of Health and Human Services.

Center for American Progress. 2012a. *Medicare and Home Health Care*. Washington, DC: US Department of Health and Human Services.

Center for American Progress. 2012b. *National Health Expenditures by Type of Service and Source of Funds: Calendar Years 1960 to 2010*. Washington, DC: Centers for Medicare and Medicaid Services.

Center for American Progress. 2018a. *Medicare 2018 Costs at a Glance*. Washington, DC: Centers for Medicare and Medicaid Services.

Center for American Progress. 2018b. *National Health Expenditures by Type of Service and Source of Funds: Calendar Years 1960 to 2017*. Washington, DC: Centers for Medicare and Medicaid Services.

Centers for Medicare and Medicaid Services. n.d. *Medicare Enrollees*. Washington, DC: Centers for Medicare and Medicaid Services.

"CLASS Act Provision of Health Care Reform Depicts a Practical but Disappointing Reality." 2011. News Medical Life Sciences. Online at www.news-medical.net/news/20111105/CLASS-Act-provision-of-health-care-reform-depicts-a-practical-but-disappointing-reality.aspx.

Committee on Energy and Commerce. 2009. *Profits, Marketing, and Corporate Expenses in the Medicare Advantage Market*. Washington, DC: US House of Representatives, Committee on Energy and Commerce, Majority Staff.

"Comparison of Medicare Premium Support Proposals." 2012. Menlo Park, CA: Kaiser Family Foundation.

Congressional Budget Office. 1997. *Predicting How Changes in Medicare's Payment Rates Would Affect Risk Sector Enrollment and Costs*. Washington, DC: Congressional Budget Office.

Congressional Budget Office. 2004. *Financing Long-Term Care for the Elderly*. Washington, DC: Congressional Budget Office.

Congressional Budget Office. 2012. *Medicare's Payments to Physicians: The Budgetary Impact of Alternative Policies Relative to CBO's March 2012 Baseline*. Washington, DC: Congressional Budget Office.

Congressional Budget Office. 2013. *A Premium Support System for Medicare: Analysis of Illustrative Options*. Washington, DC: Congressional Budget Office.

Cook, Karen et al. 1983. "A Theory of Organizational Response to Regulation: The Case of Hospitals." *Academy of Management Review*, 8, no. 2 (April): 193–205.

"Costs of Care." 2017. Washington, DC: US Department of Health and Human Services. Online at longtermcare.gov.

Cubanski, Juliette et al. 2012. *Health Care on a Budget*. Menlo Park, CA: Kaiser Family Foundation.

Cubanski, Juliette et al. 2015. *A Primer on Medicare*. Menlo Park, CA: Kaiser Family Foundation.

Cubanski, Juliette et al. 2017a. *Medicare Part D: A First Look at Prescription Drug Plans in 2018*. Menlo Park, CA: Kaiser Family Foundation. October.

Cubanski, Juliette et al. 2017b. *No Limit: Medicare Part D Enrollees Exposed to High Out-of-Pocket Costs without a Hard Cap on Spending*. Menlo Park, CA: Kaiser Family Foundation.

Cubanski, Juliette et al. 2018. *The Financial Burden of Health Care Spending: Larger for Medicare Households than for Non-Medicare Households*. Menlo Park, CA: Kaiser Family Foundation.

Cubanski, Juliette and Tricia Neuman 2017. *The Facts on Medicare Spending and Financing*. Menlo Park, CA: Kaiser Family Foundation.
"Different Types of Medicare Advantage Plans." 2012. Washington, DC: Centers for Medicare and Medicaid Services.
Feder, Judith M. 1977. *Medicare: The Politics of Federal Hospital Insurance*. Lexington, MA: DC Heath.
Fidelity Investments. 2017. "Health Care Costs for Retirees Rise to an Estimated $275,000 Fidelity Analysis Shows." Fidelity Analysis, August 24. Online at www.fidelity.com.
Freudenheim, Milt. 1997. "Medicare H.M.O.'s To Trim Benefits for the Elderly." *The New York Times*, December 2.
Fuchs, Beth and Lisa Potetz 2011. *The Nuts and Bolts of Medicare Premium Support Proposals*. Menlo Park, CA: Kaiser Family Foundation.
Gay, E. Greer et al. 1989. "An Appraisal of Organizational Response to Fiscally Constraining Regulation: The Case of Hospitals and DRGs." *Journal of Health and Social Behavior*, 30, no. 1 (March): 41–55.
Genworth Financial. 2018. *Cost of Care Survey 2018*. Richmond, VA: Genworth Financial.
Gibson, Robert M. et al. 1984. "National Health Expenditures, 1983." *Health Care Financing Review*, 6, no. 2 (Winter): 1–29.
Gittler, Josephine. 2009. "Government Regulation and Oversight of Nursing Homes: Improving Quality of Care for Nursing Home Residents and Protecting Residents from Abuse and Neglect." PowerPoint presentation delivered to the Geriatric Grand Rounds, Institute on Aging, Iowa Geriatric Education Center.
Gold, Marsha. 2001. "Medicare+Choice: An Interim Report Card." *Health Affairs*, 20, no. 4 (July/August): 120–138.
Gold, Marsha et al. 2012. *Medicare Advantage 2012 Data Spotlight: Enrollment Market Update*. Menlo Park, CA: Kaiser Family Foundation.
"GOP to Unveil Drug-Benefit Plan." 2002. Associated Press, May 1.
Guterman, Stuart. 1998. "The Balanced Budget Act of 1997: Will Hospitals Take a Hit on Their PPS Margins?" *Health Affairs*, 17, no. 1 (January/February): 159–188.
Guterman, Stuart, Laura Skopec, and Stephen Zuckerman 2018. *Do Medicare Advantage Plans Repond to Payment Changes? A Look at the Data from 2009 to 2014*. New York: The Commonwealth Fund.
Haase, Leif Wellington. 2004. *The Debate over Medicare Costs: A Primer*. New York: Century Foundation.
Hartman, Micah et al. 2018. "National Health Care Spending in 2016: Spending and Enrollment Growth Slow after Initial Coverage Expansion." *Health Affairs*, 37, no. 1 (January): 150–160.
Health Markets. 2017. "What Is the Cost of Supplemental Health Insurance for Seniors?" Health Markets, May 25. Online at www.healthmarkets.com/resources/medicare/cost-of-supplemental-health-insurance-for-seniors.
Hoadley, Jack, Juliette Cubanski, and Tricia Neuman. 2015. "Medicare Part D at Ten Years: The 2015 Marketplace and Key Trends, 2006-2015." Menlo Park, CA: Kaiser Family Foundation, October 5.
House Budget Committee. 2012. *The Path to Prosperity: A Blueprint for American Renewal: Fiscal Year 2012 Budget Resolution*. Washington, DC: US House of Representatives, House Budget Committee.
"House GOP Unveils Final Version of Medicare Package." 2002. Kaisernetwork.org, June 18.
"In 'Rare' Agreement, Republicans, Democrats Say Bush's Proposed Allocation for Medicare Drug Benefit Not Enough." 2002. Kaisernetwork.org, February 26.
Jacobson, Gretchen et al. 2017. *Medicare Advantage 2017 Spotlight: Enrollment Market Update*. Menlo Park, CA: Henry J. Kaiser Family Foundation.
Jacobson, Gretchen, Tricia Neuman, and Anthony Damico 2012. *Medicare's Role for Dual Eligible Beneficiaries*. Menlo Park, CA: Kaiser Commission on Medicaid and the Uninsured.
Jaffe, Susan. 2009. "Health Policy Brief: Medicare Advantage Plans." *Health Affairs*, April 29.
Johnson, Simon and James Kwak. 2012. *White House Burning: The Founding Fathers, Our National Debt, and Why It Matters to You*. New York: Pantheon Books.
Kaiser Family Foundation. n.d. *Medicare Delivery System Reform: The Evidence Link*. Menlo Park, CA: Kaiser Family Foundation.
Keehan, Sean P. et al. 2012. "National Health Expenditure Projections: Modest Annual Growth until Coverage Expands and Economic Growth Accelerates." *Health Affairs*, 31, no. 7 (June 12): 1600–1612.
Kessler, Glenn. 2011. "Fact Checking the GOP Debate: $500 Billion in Cuts to Medicare." *The Washington Post*, June 15.
Kliff, Sarah. 2013. "Part D Was Less Popular Than Obamacare When It Launched." *The Washington Post*, June 21.
Kliff, Sarah. 2016. "Republicans Have a Clear Plan to Cut Medicare—But They Might Not Go through with It." *Vox*, December 6. Online at vox.com.
Komisar, Harriet. 2012. *Key Issues in Understanding the Economic and Health Security of Current and Future Generations of Seniors*. Menlo Park, CA: Kaiser Family Foundation.
Krause, Elliott A. 1977. *Power and Illness: The Political Sociology of Health and Medical Care*. New York: Elsevier.
Laugesen, Miriam J. 2016. *Fixing Medical Prices: How Physicians Are Paid*. Cambridge, MA: Harvard University Press.
Lave, Judith R. 1984. "Hospital Reimbursement under Medicare." *Milbank Memorial Fund Quarterly/Health and Society*, 62, no. 2 (Spring): 251–278.
Levit, Katharine et al. 2004. "Health Spending Rebound Continues in 2002." *Health Affairs*, 23, no. 1 (January/February): 147–159.
Levit, Katharine R. et al. 1994. "National Health Spending Trends: 1960-1993." *Health Affairs*, 13, no. 5 (November): 14–31.
Levit, Katharine R., Helen C. Lazenby, and Madie W. Stewart 1996. "DataView: National Health Expenditures, 1995." *Health Care Financing Review*, 18, no. 1 (Fall): 175–214.
Marmor, Theodore. 2000. *The Politics of Medicare*, 2nd edn. Chicago: Aldine.
Marmor, Theodore R., Donald A. Wittman, and Thomas C. Heagy 1983. "The Politics of Medical Inflation." In *Political Analysis and American Medical Care*, ed. Theodore R. Marmor, 61–75. Cambridge: Cambridge University Press.

Mather, Mark, Linda A. Jacobsen, and Kevin M. Pollard 2015. "Aging in the United States." *Population Bulletin*, 70, no. 2 (December).

"Medicare Advantage: Fact Sheet." 2017. Menlo Park, CA: Kaiser Family Foundation, October 20.

"Medicare and Medicaid Statistical Supplement, 1997." 1998. Washington, DC: Health Care Financing Administration.

"Medicare Part D: Types of Alternative Type D Plans." 2017. Arlington, VA: National Center on Aging.

Medicare Payment Advisory Commission. 2004. *Healthcare Spending and the Medicare Program: A Data Book*. Washington, DC: Medicare Payment Advisory Commission.

Medicare Payment Advisory Commission. 2012. *Health Care Spending and the Medicare Program: A Data Book*. Washington, DC: Medicare Payment Advisory Commission.

Medicare Payment Advisory Commission. 2013. *Health Care Spending and the Medicare Program: A Data Book*. Washington, DC: *Medicare* Payment Advisory Commission.

Medicare Payment Advisory Commission. 2017. *Health Care Spending and the Medicare Program: A Data Book*. Washington, DC: *Medicare* Payment Advisory Commission.

Medicare Payment Advisory Commission. 2018. *Health Care Spending and the Medicare Program: A Data Book*. Washington, DC: Medicare Payment Advisory Commission.

"Medicare Spending and Financing: Fact Sheet." 2011. Menlo Park, CA: Kaiser Family Foundation, August.

Medicare Today. 2017. "New National Survey: Nearly 9 in 10 Seniors Satisfied with Medicare Part D." Online at http://medicaretoday.org/2017/07/new-national-survey-nearly-9-in-10-seniors-satisfied-with-medicare-part-d-2/.

Miller, Mark. 2012. "Top Six Myths About Medicare." Reuters. Online at Reuters.com.

Miller, Mark. 1996. *Medicare Now and in the Future*, 2nd edn. Washington, DC: Urban Affairs Press.

Miller, Mark. 2004. "Medicare Means-Testing: A Skeptical View." *Health Affairs* (December 8): W4-558–W4-560. Online at www.healthaffairs.org.

Moon, Marilyn. n.d. "Ensuring a Future for Medicare." AARP. Online at www.aarp.org/monthly/medicare3/viewmm.htm.

Musumeci, MaryBeth. 2017. *Medicaid's Role for Medicare Beneficiaries*. Menlo, CA: Kaiser Family Foundation.

National Commission on Fiscal Responsibility and Reform. 2010. *The Moment of Truth*. Washington, DC: National Commission on Fiscal Responsibility and Reform.

National Committee to Preserve Social Security and Medicare. 2006. *Medicare's Donut Hole: A Bitter Pill to Swallow*. Washington, DC: National Committee to Preserve Social Security and Medicare. Online at ncpssm.org.

Nelson, Lyle. 1997. "Access to Care in Medicare HMOs, 1996." *Health Affairs*, 16, no. 2 (March/April): 148–156.

Newman, Patricia and Kathryn M. Langwell 1999. "Medicare's Choice Explosion? Implications for Beneficiaries." *Health Affairs*, 18, no. 1 (January/February): 150–160.

Norris, Louise. 2018. *Medicare and Health Care Reform*. St. Louis Park, MN: HealthInsurance.org. Online at www.medicareresources.org.

Norton, Mira, Bianca DiJulio, and Mollyann Brodie. 2015. *Medicare and Medicaid at Fifty*. Menlo Park, CA: Kaiser Family Foundation.

Oberlander, Jonathan B. 1997. "Managed Care and Medicare Reform." *Journal of Health Care Politics, Policy and Law*, 22, no. 2 (April): 595–631.

Oberlander, Jonathan B. 2003.*The Political Life of Medicare*. Chicago, IL: University of Chicago Press.

Office of Management and Budget. 2011. *Historical Tables; Budget of the U.S. Government, Fiscal Year 2012*. Washington, DC: Executive Office of the President.

Oliver, Thomas R. 1993. "Analysis, Advice and Congressional Leadership: The Physician Payment Review Commission and the Politics of Medicare." *Journal of Health Politics, Policy and Law*, 18, no. 1 (Spring): 113–174.

Oliver, Thomas R., Philip R. Lee, and Helene L. Lipton 2004. "A Political History of Medicare and Prescription Drug Coverage." *The Milbank Quarterly*, 82, no. 2 (June): 283–354.

"An Overview of Medicare." 2017. Menlo Park, CA: Kaiser Family Foundation.

Palazzolo, Daniel J. 1999. *Done Deal? the Politics of the 1997 Budget Agreement*. New York: Chatham House.

Park, Edwin, Melanie Nathanson, Robert Greenstein, and John Springer 2003. *The Troubling Medicare Legislation*. Washington, DC: Center on Budget and Policy Priorities, December 8.

Parsons, Talcott E. 1956. "Suggestions for a Sociological Approach to a Theory of Organizations." *Administrative Science Quarterly*, 1, no. 1 (June): 63–85.

"Part B Costs." 2012. Washington, DC: Centers for Medicare and Medicaid Services.

Pauly, Mark V. 2004. "Means-Testing in Medicare." *Health Affairs* (December 8): W4-546–W4-557. Online at www.healthaffairs.org.

Pear, Robert. 2005. "States Rejecting Demand to Pay for Medicare Cost." *The New York Times*, July 4.

Peck, Benjamin. 2003. *Private Insurance Plans & Medicare: The Disappointing History*. Washington, DC: Public Citizen.

Physician Payment Review Commission. 1997. "A New Law Changes Practice Expense." *PPRC Update* no. 24 (August).

Pianin, Eric. 2011. "Super Flaw: If Only Obama Had Upheld Bowles-Simpson." *Fiscal Times*, November 22.

Potetz, Lisa, Juliette Cubanski, and Tricia Neuman 2011. *Medicare Spending and Financing: A Primer*. Menlo Park, CA: Kaiser Family Foundation.

"Proposed Changes to Medicare in the 'Path to Prosperity': Overview and Key Questions." 2011. Kaiser Family Foundation. Menlo Park, CA: Kaiser Family Foundation.

"Public Opinion on Health Care Issues." 2012. Menlo Park, CA: Kaiser Family Foundation.

Quade, E.S. 1989. *Analysis for Public Decisions*, 3rd edn. New York: Elsevier.

Rainey, Richard. 2004. "Medicare Adds Preventive Benefits." *Los Angeles Times*, November 10.

Reid, T.R. 2009. *The Healing of America: A Global Quest for Better, Cheaper, and Fairer Health Care*. Farmington Hills, MI: Gale Group.

Reinhard, Susan C. 2015. *Valuing the Invaluable: 2015 Update*. Washington, DC: AARP Public Policy Institute.

Riley, Gerald F., Melvin J. Ingber, and Cynthia G. Tudor 1997. "Disenrollment of Medicare Beneficiaries from HMOs." *Health Affairs*, 15, no. 5 (September/October): 117–124.

Rivlin, Alice M. 2012. "The Great Medicare Compromise." Brookings Institution. Online at brookings.edu.

Rother, John C. n.d. "A Medicare in the 21st Century." AARP. Online at www.aarp.org/monthly/medicare3/viewjr.htm.

Rushefsky, Mark E. 2004. "Ending Medicare as We Know It?" Paper presented at the annual meeting of the American Political Science Association, September 2–5, Chicago.

Rushefsky, Mark E. and Kant Patel 1998. *Power and Policy Making: The Case of Health Care Reform in the 1990s*. Armonk, NY: M.E. Sharpe.

Ryan, Paul. 2016. *A Better Way: Our Vision for A Confident America: Health Care*. Washington, DC: US House of Representatives, Speaker's Office. Online at abetterway.speaker.gov.

Shaffer, Franklin A. 1983. "DRGs: History and Overview." *Nursing and Health Care*, 4, no. 7 (September): 388–389.

Smith, Vernon, Kathleen Gifford, and Sandy Kramer. 2005. *Implications of the Medicare Modernization Act for States*. Menlo Park, CA: Henry J. Kaiser Foundation.

Starr, Paul. 1982. *The Social Transformation of American Medicine*. New York: Basic Books.

Starr, Paul. 2013. *Remedy and Reaction: The Peculiar American Struggle over Health Care Reform*. New Haven, CT: Yale University Press.

Steinberg, Earl P. et al. 2000. "Beyond Survey Data: A Claims-Based Analysis of Drug Use and Spending by the Elderly." *Health Affairs*, 19, no. 2 (March/April): 198–211.

Steinbrook, Robert. 2015. "The Repeal of Medicare's Sustainable Growth Rate for Physician Payment." *Jama*, 313, no. 20 (May 26): 2025–2026.

Steinwald, Bruce and Frank A. Sloan. 1981. "Regulatory Approaches to Hospital Cost Containment: A Synthesis of the Empirical Evidence." In *A New Approach to the Economics of Health Care*, ed. Mancur Olson, 273–308. Washington, DC: American Enterprise Institute for Public Policy.

Sullivan, Kip. 2015. *CMS' 'Medical Home' Experiment Is a Mess*. Chicago, IL: Physicians for a National Health Program, February 24. Online at pnhp.org/blog.

"Summary of Key Changes to Medicare in 2010 Health Reform Law." 2010. Menlo Park, CA: Kaiser Family Foundation.

"Ten Essential Facts about Medicare and Prescription Spending." 2017. Menlo Park, CA: Kaiser Family Foundation.

Thompson, Frank J. 1981. *Health Policy and the Bureaucracy: Politics and Implementation*. Cambridge, MA: MIT Press.

Tilly, Jane, Susan Goldenson, and Jessica Kasten. 2001. *Long-Term Care: Consumers, Providers, and Financing; A Chartbook*. Washington, DC: Urban Institute.

Tumlinson, Anne, Christine Aguiar, and Molly O'Malley Watts. 2009. *Closing the Long-Term Gap: The Challenge of Private Long-Term Care Insurance*. Menlo Park, CA: Kaiser Commission on Medicaid and the Uninsured.

US Bureau of the Census. 1966. *Statistical Abstract of the United States, 1966*. Washington, DC: US Government Printing Office.

US Bureau of the Census. 2012. *Statistical Abstract of the United States, 2012*. Washington, DC: US Department of Commerce.

US Bureau of the Census. 2017. *An Aging Nation: Projected Number of Children and Older Adults*. Washington, DC: US Department of Commerce. Online at www.census.gov/library/visualizations/2018/comm/historic-first.html.

Van de Water, Paul N. 2016. *Medicare Leads in Controlling Costs*. Washington, DC: Center on Budget and Policy Priorities.

Veuger, Stan and Jeffrey Clemens. 2015. *Repeal of the Medicare Sustainable Growth Rate: Direct and Indirect Consequences*. Washington, DC: American Enterprise Institute. Online at aei.org.

"Victory: Family Physicians Make Gains in Medicare Fee Schedule." 1997. *AAFD Directors' Newsletter*, November 13. Online at www.aafp.org/dn;/971113dl/2.html.

Viebeck, Elise. 2012. "New Poll Finds Medicare More Important to Voters than Healthcare Reform Law." The Hill. Online at thehill.com.

Walker, Emily 2011. "Medicare Commission Votes to Scrap SGR Pay Formula." *MedPage Today*, October 6. Online at www.medpagetoday.com/PublicHealthPolicy/Medicare/28919.

Weiner, Joshua M. and Laurel Hixon Illston. 1994. "How to Share the Burden: Long-Term Care Reform in the 1990s." *Brookings Review*, 12, no. 2 (Spring): 16–21.

Wessel, David. 2012. *Red Ink: Inside the High-Stakes Politics of the Federal Budget*. New York: Crown Business.

Wyden, Ron and Paul Ryan. 2011. "Guaranteed Choices to Strengthen Medicare and Health Security for All: Bipartisan Options for the Future." Washington, DC: US Congress. Online at www.budget.house.gov/bipartisanhealthoptions.

Xu, K. Tom. 2003. "Financial Disparities in Prescription Drug Use between Elderly and Nonelderly Americans." *Health Affairs*, 22, no. 5 (September/October): 210–221.

Young, Katherine et al. 2013. *Medicaid's Role for Dual Eligible Beneficiaries*. Menlo Park, CA: Kaiser Commission on Medicaid and the Uninsured.

6

HEALTHCARE FOR AMERICAN INDIANS, ALASKA NATIVES, AND VETERANS

AMERICAN INDIANS AND ALASKA NATIVES

Achieving an accurate count of the American Indian and Alaska Native (AI/AN) population has been a challenge for the US Census Bureau. Census data are very important because they are used to determine how billions of federal dollars are distributed among various social services, healthcare, and education programs. Since Indian land is held in trust by the federal government it is nontaxable and thus AIs/ANs were excluded from the first six censuses from 1790–1850. Starting in 1860, only those Indians who were considered assimilated in American society were officially counted, and noted as "civilized Indians" in the census documents. In the 1880 census, another issue that complicated the process of counting American Indians was the controversy over whether to count or not count Indian people of "mixed blood." The 1930s census was the first to include a thorough account of the American Indian population. In censuses from 1940 to 1970, the enumerator decided the race of the respondent. The 1980 census showed a 72-percent increase in the American Indian and Alaska Native population over the 1970 census. This was attributed largely to the fact that, starting with the 1980 census, respondents were allowed to self-identify their own race instead of the enumerator determining the race of the respondent. The 1990 census revealed a 38-percent increase in the American Indian and Alaska Native population over the 1980 census (Lujan 2014).

In the 2000 and 2010 censuses the American Indian and Alaska Native populations were combined into one category. More importantly, for the first time, respondents were given the option to self-identify with more than one race. American Indian and Alaska Native respondents who identified themselves with only one race are referred to as the "American Indians and Alaska Natives alone," while those who identified themselves with more than one race are referred to as "American Indians and Alaska Natives combination" (US Census Bureau 2012). The term "American Indians and Alaska Natives" refers to people having origins in any of the original people of North and South America (including Central America), and who maintain tribal affiliation or community attachment (US Census Bureau 2012).

Conceptualizing, operationalizing, and counting the American Indian and Alaska Native population continues to remain a challenge for the US Census Bureau. Ironically, despite the fact that several censuses have reported a significant increase in the number of American Indians and Alaska Natives, a great deal of research has demonstrated an underdocumentation and undercounting of the American Indian and Alaska Native population for several reasons. One reason is high mobility due to lower education and higher unemployment rates among this population. The second reason is the distrust of the federal government and thus resistance to the US Census. The third reason is the changes in census methodology, and the uncertain and inconsistent definition of "Indian," which often leads to misclassification of the American Indian and Alaska Native population. Finally, the US census is based on the concept of a nuclear family household, while American Indian and Alaska Native tribes are based on the concept of extended family (Lujan 2014).

Censuses over several decades have seen the American Indian and Alaska Native population increase substantially more than expected. However, this may be a result of changes in individuals' self-identified race responses. Research has demonstrated a considerable race response change, especially among multiple-race and/or Hispanic American Indians. In other words, some of the population increase recorded in censuses may be due to changes in how respondents report their race on the census form and race response changes do not necessarily mean identity changes (Liebler and Bhaskar 2016). Finally, among the American Indian and Alaska Native population, most aspects of ethnicity are associated with the person's tribal origins. In the 2000 census, almost 1 million American Indians failed to respond to the tribal affiliation part of the race question. Also, it is difficult to understand and interpret what people intend to communicate when they answer questions about race, i.e., are the respondents reporting how they see themselves or how others see them? (Liebler and Zacher 2013.)

Given the above discussion, a few words of caution are in order. First, because of the change from the enumerator identifying respondent's race to self-identification of the race by the respondents, the 2000 and 2010 census data on race are not directly compatible with the censuses of 1990 and earlier. Second, starting with the 2000 census, allowing respondents to self-identify with one race or multiple races and thus categorizing the American Indian and Alaska Native population into "American Indians and Alaska Natives alone," and "American Indians and Alaska Natives combination" makes it difficult to compare and analyze statistical data, including health data, on this population group between the pre-2000 census and post-2000 censuses. Third, while census reports published since the 2000 census identify data for American Indians and Alaska Natives alone, other published research does not specifically identify "alone" and "combination population groups" and uses the generic term "American Indians and Alaska Natives." Fourth, the accuracy and reliability of data, such as mortality rates and other indicators derived from sources such as death certificates, etc., can be problematic because of frequent misclassification of American Indians and Alaska Natives.

In light of the above discussion, it is necessary to mention that for our purposes, for the remained of this chapter, American Indians and Alaska Natives are referred to as AIs/ANs. When the data is identified as "AIs/ANs alone" or "AIs/ANs combination," we have utilized this identification. When such specific identification is missing, we have used the more generic term AIs/ANs.

Population Characteristics and Trends

In comparison to African-Americans and Hispanics, AIs/ANs constitute a very small minority in American society. In 2016, the total AI/AN population was 6.7 million, making up about 2 percent of the total population in the United States. Of the 6.7 million, 2.6 million residents (39 percent) identified themselves as "American Indians and Alaska Natives alone," while the remainder (61 percent) identified themselves with more than one race, i.e., "American Indians and Alaska Natives combination" ("American Indian and Alaska Native Heritage Month" 2017; "New Detailed Statistics on Race, Hispanic Origin, Ancestry, and Tribal Groups" 2017).

The term Alaska Natives refers to all indigenous groups who live in the state of Alaska. Alaska Natives include the three primary groups of Eskimo, Indian, and Aleut. The majority of rural residents in Alaska are Alaska Natives who live in small villages (Barnhardt 2001). An estimated 15.3 percent of Alaska residents identify themselves as American Indians and Alaska Natives alone ("Quick Facts: Alaska" 2017).

According to the 2010 census, 41 percent of AIs/ANs, alone or in combination, live in the West. The second-largest concentration of AIs/ANs is in the South, followed by the Midwest and the Northeast. The AI/AN-in-combination population is geographically more dispersed in the United States than the AI/AN-alone population (US Census Bureau 2012).

In 2016, 21 states had 100,000 or more AI/AN residents, alone or in combination. Alaska has the largest concentration of AIs/ANs. Almost 20 percent of Alaska's population identified themselves as AI/AN residents, alone or in combination. Alaska was followed by Oklahoma (13.7 percent), New Mexico (11.9 percent), South Dakota (10.4 percent), and Montana (8.4 percent) ("American Indian and Alaska Native Heritage Month" 2017).

The AI/AN-alone population as a group enjoy lower socioeconomic status in American society compared to the rest of the population. Socioeconomic status is generally determined by one's level of education, occupation, and income. For example, in 2016, 79.9 percent of the AI/AN-alone population aged 25 and over had at least a high school diploma, GED certificate, or alternative credentials, compared to 87.5 percent of the overall population. Similarly, 14.5 percent of the AI/AN-alone population had obtained a bachelor degree or higher, compared to 31.3 percent of the total population. Fifty-three percent of the AI/AN-alone population owned their own home, compared to 63 percent of the overall population. The median household income of the AI/AN-alone population was $39,719, compared to $57,617 for the nation as a whole. The percentage of the AI/AN-alone population who lived in poverty was 26.2, compared to a 14-percent poverty rate nationwide. Finally, 19.2 percent of the AI/AN-alone population lacked health insurance, compared to 8.2 percent for the country as a whole ("American Indian and Alaska Native Heritage Month" 2017).

There were 567 federally recognized AI/AN tribes and 326 federally recognized American Indian Reservations including federal reservations and off-reservation trust land in 2016. In addition, there are more than 265 state or non-federally recognized tribes. Contrary to popular myth, most AIs/ANs do not live on or near the reservation. In fact, over 70 percent of the AI/AN population lives in cities and urban areas ("American Indian and Alaska Native Heritage Month" 2017; "Health Coverage and Care for American Indians and Alaska Natives" 2013; "Myths and Realities" n.d.)

Federally recognized tribes are provided health and educational assistance through the Indian Health Service (IHS) within the US Department of Health and Human Services (DHHS). The majority of those who receive health and educational services from the IHS live on reservations and in rural communities. AIs/ANs living in urban areas receive health services through Urban Indian Health Organizations (UIHOs) funded by the IHS.

It is also important to remember that the Indian Health Service is not a government health insurance program like Medicaid or Medicare. The treaties signed by the federal government in exchange for Indian lands established a trust relationship and a government responsibility for providing healthcare services to the AI/AN people. The relationship between the federal government and the AI/AN population has been formed and defined by the US Constitution and subsequent case law. Thus, healthcare for AIs/ANs is delivered from a system that is separate from that of mainstream America. This system has evolved from the unique and complex history of interaction between the various AI/AN tribes and the United States government (Shelton 2004).

HISTORICAL BACKGROUND

The immigration from Europe that began in the sixteenth century impacted the historical sovereignty of American Indian tribes and healthcare for their people. The colonizing nations of Europe used the doctrine of discovery as a first step in obtaining the right to land from the local native population. Under this doctrine, the first discoverer had the right to control the land they discovered. The right of the local Indians was relegated to mere occupancy, that is, the right to be on the land without being found guilty of trespassing. Treaties of peace and treaties of war were used to eliminate the right of American Indians to own the land. In return, tribes were provided with some medical supplies and physician services (Shelton 2004). The doctrine of conquest was used to remove Indians who were not willing to move from their land. It claimed that when a nation defeats another nation in a war, it gains the right to the defeated nation's land and control of its people. The United States was born into this established legal tradition based on the doctrines of discovery and conquest (Shelton 2004).

Between 1778 and 1868, around 367 treaties with AI/AN tribes were ratified by the federal government. In the initial treaties of 1784, the federal government recognized certain responsibilities toward the indigenous people. Many such treaties included language that contained the promise of taking proper care of and providing protection for the indigenous people in exchange for tribal land and natural resources. The federal government's obligations toward the AIs/ANs were subsequently reconfirmed, formalized, and defined by US Supreme Court decisions, congressional laws, presidential executive orders, and other federal policies. The US Constitution also establishes that federally recognized tribes are sovereign nations with all inherent rights. This is what distinguishes AIs/ANs from all other ethnic groups in the United States ("The First Fifty Years of the Indian Health Service" n.d.; Warne and Frizzell 2014).

Prior to contact with the European immigrants, the North American Indians lived a very healthy lifestyle that included a good diet and natural exercise. The European colonizers introduced many infectious diseases among the native populations, such as measles, cholera, diphtheria, and smallpox. Epidemics of such diseases often wiped out whole tribes, leading to the ultimate subjugation of Native people (Pfefferbaum et al. 1995/1996).

Colonial powers used imperial medicine—European or Western—as an important tool in colonies established by conquest, occupation, and settlement for further colonial expansion. For example, as early as the 1780s, Catholic missionaries used the live smallpox virus to inoculate Native Americans in Guatemala and southern Mexico. The first recorded inoculation of an American Indian occurred in 1797 (Pearson 2004). Thomas Jefferson ordered Meriwether Lewis to use the smallpox vaccine as a diplomatic tool on the Lewis and Clark expedition. One of the major goals of the expedition was to use imperial medicine to advance colonization among the indigenous population by gaining diplomatic and political access to American Indians (Pearson 2004).

THE LEGAL AND CONSTITUTIONAL STATUS OF AMERICAN INDIANS AND ALASKA NATIVES

American Indians

Upon gaining independence, the United States assumed the role previously held by England with respect to American Indians. The commerce clause (Article I, Section 8, clause 3) and the treaty clause (Article II, Section 2, clause 2) of the US Constitution grant the federal government exclusive authority to regulate commerce and to make treaties with Indian tribes on behalf of the United States. The four most basic principles of federal Indian law established early in the United States were: (1) tribes retain all of their inherent sovereignty that the federal government has not encroached upon; (2) the federal government, and not states, is in charge of Indian affairs;

(3) the federal government deals only with tribes it has recognized; and (4) the United States has assumed trust responsibility toward the Indian nations (Shelton 2004).

As America's original people, AIs/ANs hold a distinct legal, cultural, and historical position in American society. Many AI/AN peoples are entitled to certain services of the federal government as a result of, first, their membership in sovereign Indian nations and negotiated treaties, agreements, legislative enactments, and compacts signed between the various tribes and the federal government and, second, as citizens of local, state, and federal government (Pfefferbaum et al. 1995/1996). The federal government's responsibility toward the AIs/ANs originates from a variety of sources, including specific treaties through which land and other resources were given up by Indians in exchange for promises of healthcare and other services such as education. However, the federal government's obligation is often not clearly defined with respect to specific rights and responsibilities and is influenced by the courts' interpretations and rulings. For example, courts have ruled that benefits provided to AIs/ANs by the government are provided voluntarily rather than in response to the federal government's trust responsibility for the Indian tribes; that is, the government's trust responsibility alone cannot constitute a basis for a claim against the government nor does it constitute a legal entitlement to benefits. On the other hand, Congress has passed laws that require the federal government to provide the best possible health status to Indians and to provide all resources necessary to the Indian Health Service (IHS) to make that possible (Pfefferbaum et al. 1995/1996, 1997).

Alaska Natives

The United States acquired Russia's rights to Alaska in 1867. The Treaty of Cession provided that Alaska Natives would be treated the same as aboriginal peoples in the rest of the United States (Shelton 2004). Between 1778 and 1871, almost 400 treaties were negotiated between the US government and Indian nations. Alaska Natives were not part of these treaties since Alaska did not become part of the United States until 1867. The US government never negotiated treaties with Alaska Natives, and few reservations were created in Alaska. The federal government did not initially deal with Alaska Natives as dependent Indian communities, and it was not until 1905 that a distinction was made between Native and non-Native residents of the territory for the purpose of education (Barnhardt 2001).

Initially, Congress placed responsibility for Alaska Natives under the Bureau of Education, the sole federal agency responsible for Alaska Native services. In 1931, responsibility for Alaska Natives was shifted to the Office of Indian Affairs (OIA) and later to the Bureau of Indian Affairs (BIA) (Huhndorf and Huhndorf 2011). The federal government, through the Bureau of Indian Affairs, pursued its relationship with Alaska Natives on a village-by-village basis. Since the 1930s Alaska Natives have generally been subject to the same policies and are eligible for the same programs as American Indians (Huhndorf and Huhndorf 2011).

It wasn't until the Alaska Native Claims Settlement Act of 1971 (ANCSA) that the land claims of Alaska Natives were addressed. Native corporations were created to hold settlement funds and lands. In general, regional Native non-profit corporations provide healthcare to Alaska Natives (Shelton 2004).

THE EVOLUTION OF HEALTH POLICY

The federal government's relationship with the AI/AN population has always reflected a great deal of ambivalence. As a result, the government's policy toward AIs/ANs has vacillated between aggression and paternalism, reflecting two images of the American Indians in the mind of white people: "noble savages" and "ignoble savages" (Pfefferbaum et al. 1995/1996). A vague sense of obligation has guided successive generations of policymakers and often has led to a great deal of fluctuation and inconsistent policies that have been described as "a great patchwork quilt pieced together with fragments of faded, long-abandoned programs and bright, new policies cut from shiny, new cloth" (Pfefferbaum et al. 1995/1996, 366).

The Nineteenth Century

At the beginning of the 1800s, primary administrative responsibility for Indian healthcare was assigned to the War Department (Pfefferbaum et al. 1997). The main efforts in the area of healthcare were designed to prevent the spread of infectious diseases such as smallpox. Army physicians undertook emergency measures to curb such infectious diseases among Indians living in the vicinity of military posts (Bergman et al. 1999; Pfefferbaum et al. 1995/1996). In 1824, the Bureau of Indian Affairs (BIA) was created within the War Department and charged with the overall responsibility for overseeing treaty negotiations, administering trade with the Indians, managing Indian schools, as well as handling all expenditures and correspondence concerning Indian affairs.

In 1832, Congress appropriated $12,000 to hire physicians and to provide vaccinations to American Indians (Pfefferbaum et al. 1995/1996). This was the first large-scale smallpox vaccination authorized by Congress, aimed more at protecting American soldiers than protecting American Indians (Bergman et al. 1999). Some health services were also provided through general educational appropriations made available to religious and philanthropic organizations engaged in the "civilization" of Indians (Shelton 2004). In 1849, the BIA was transferred to the newly created Department of the Interior, and thus Indian healthcare passed from military to civilian control (Kunitz 1996; Shelton 2004).

By the early 1830s, the US government's relationships with Indian tribes had changed and President Andrew Jackson had come to view the tribes as obstacles to American expansion. Consequently, the Indian Removal Act was signed into law by President Jackson in 1830, authorizing him to negotiate with the Indians in the southern United States for their removal to federal territories west of the Mississippi in exchange for their homeland. The BIA enthusiastically advocated the "civilization" of Indians through the creation of the reservations system by negotiating with the tribes for their settlement on the reservations. By 1840, despite opposition to the Act by some Christian missionaries, the BIA and the US military had removed and relocated about 40 Indian tribes to the west of the Mississippi. Thousands of American Indians, often by force, were made to emigrate to the West.

The Indian Removal Act (IRA) was strongly supported in the South, where states were eager to gain access to lands inhabited by the Five Civilized Tribes. This refers to five Native American nations—the Cherokee, Chickasaw, Choctaw, Creek, and Seminole—the first five tribes that Europeans considered "civilized." States such as Virginia, North Carolina, and South Carolina sought to make Indian land available to white farmers. During the antebellum period (pre-Civil War) the primary factors that contributed to the dispossession of southern Indians were greed, racism, and political posturing (Perdue 2012). One of the common strategies used in the Southern states was to categorize Indians as "colored," insisting that intermarriage with African-Americans had tainted native Indian people's blood, thus closing "white" facilities to them and refusing to record them as Indian on official documents (Perdue 2012). As a way of maintaining white power and authority as well as justifying slavery and the dispossession of Indian land, "race" was systematically categorized by rules governing identity, that is, the amount of blood required to be Indian or black. Individuals belonging to several of the Southeast's tribal nations were often reclassified and their collective identity disbanded (Gonzales, Kertesz, and Tayac 2007).

However, the Indian removal policy of the 1830s, designed to rid the South of Indian nations with communal land and sovereign powers, had fallen short. Following the Civil War, to deal with the federal government's "Indian problem," a policy of assimilation gained favor over the policy of eradication and removal. The main goal of the policy was to try to assimilate Indians into the mainstream of American society by encouraging them to abandon their way of life (Shelton 2004). Under the Indian Appropriation Act of 1871, making treaties with Indian tribes was discontinued. The major tool used for implementation of the assimilation policy was the General Allotment Act of 1887, under which the group title of a tribe to the land on its reservation was abolished in favor of providing individual land ownership. The law also provided US citizenship to allottees via the Fourteenth Amendment (Pfefferbaum et al. 1995/1996; Shelton 2004). By the end of the nineteenth century, the number of Indian tribes had decreased and they were geographically dispersed and isolated.

Toward the end of the nineteenth century, a more organized health service structure for AIs/ANs was established in the country. By 1880, the BIA was operating four hospitals and employed 77 physicians to serve the Indian population (Pfefferbaum et al. 1995/1996). However, westward expansion and removal of Indians to reservations also produced harmful health effects on them because of a shift away from a traditional diet. Many of the health problems faced by AIs/ANs today, such as diabetes, cancer, and heart disease, are related to this change. Many traditional healthcare activities were prohibited, and the detention of "medicine men" was authorized. The development of federal healthcare for AIs/ANs during the period of assimilation helped establish the early framework for the modern AI/AN healthcare system (Shelton 2004).

The Twentieth Century

Congress began formally appropriating funds for BIA healthcare services in 1910. In 1912 President Taft sent a special message to Congress summarizing the results of several surveys that described the deplorable conditions of health and sanitation on Indian reservations (Shelton 2004). Congressional appropriations for Indian health services increased from $200,000 in 1914 to $300,000 in 1915 and 1916, to $350,000 in 1917 (Pfefferbaum et al.

1995/1996). World War I delayed further advancement in AI/AN health policy, and it was not until the 1920s that Indian health needs again received serious public attention (Pfefferbaum et al. 1995/1996).

The Snyder Act passed by Congress in 1921 provided formal legislative authorization for Indian healthcare and provided for regular congressional appropriations (Pfefferbaum et al. 1997). Under the law, formal federal health services were established within the War Department (Bergman et al. 1999). This was Congress's first explicit legislative authorization for federal provision of healthcare services to members of all federally recognized American Indian tribes and for the conservation of the health of Indian communities (Roubideaux 2002).

The Merriam Report, published in 1928 by the nongovernmental Institute for Government at the request of the secretary of the interior, described the devastation caused by land allotment, the failure of Indian education, and the dreadful health status of American Indians. This set the stage for an era of reorganization of health services for AIs/ANs (Shelton 2004). The Johnson-O'Malley Act of 1934 authorized the secretary of the interior to contract with states and territories for the provision of services, which allowed the BIA to contract for the provision of Indian health services.

The Indian Reorganization Act of 1934 encouraged economic development and provided for Indian tribes' self-determination (Gonzales, Kertesz, and Tayac 2007; Shelton 2004). Yet, the health status of AIs/ANs remained poor during the period of 1920 to 1950. Many studies during this period documented high infant mortality and excessive deaths among AIs/ANs from infectious disease ("The First Fifty Years of the Indian Health Service" n.d.).

By the early 1950s, an assimilation policy reemerged. The prevailing political philosophy was that the interests of AIs/ANs would be served best by assimilating them into the larger American society (Bergman et al. 1999). The Hoover Commission's Task Force on Indian Policy had advocated this approach. Thus, assimilation became the formal federal Indian policy during the Eisenhower years of 1953–1961 (Kunitz 1996). However, assimilation was to be accomplished by terminating federal recognition of Indian tribes, eliminating their reservations, and encouraging the relocation of Indians from reservations to cities, and ultimately the weakening and dismantling of the BIA (Kunitz 1996). Thus, this policy has also been referred to as the policy of termination because congressional acts terminated the special federal–tribal trust relationship with 109 tribes and bands (Shelton 2004). This move was promoted as a way to "free" Indians from supervision and control by the BIA. The result was a marked increase in the Indian population in cities across the country.

In 1954, the Transfer Act moved responsibility for Indian health to the Public Health Service, which at that time was part of the Department of Health, Education, and Welfare (Shelton 2004). The Indian Health Service was established as an agency under the Public Health Service in 1955. The Indian Sanitation Facilities Act of 1959 authorizes the IHS to construct sanitation facilities for Indian communities and homes.

Today, the IHS within the Public Health Service is part of the US Department of Health and Human Services (DHHS). The IHS is the main federal agency with primary responsibility for fulfilling the United States' trust obligation to provide healthcare for AI/AN people (Shelton 2004). At the time of the transfer of responsibilities to IHS, Congress had identified four major functions for the IHS: advocacy for Indian health, providing comprehensive health services, providing training and technical assistance, and coordinating health resources between federal, state, and local programs for the benefit of AIs/ANs (Kunitz 1996; Pfefferbaum et al. 1995/1996).

The health policy during the 1950s and 1960s focused on assimilation and termination of federal trusteeship over AIs/ANs on the belief that if they were relocated from their reservations to urban areas they would assimilate into the general society more rapidly, move away from their traditional ways of living, and ultimately become part of the larger culture and society. During the termination period, Congress enacted laws that terminated the federal–tribal trust relationship with 109 tribes and bands ("The First Fifty Years of the Indian Health Service" n.d.).

The American Indian Movement of the 1960s and 1970s brought about a shift from a policy of assimilation/termination toward a policy of self-determination for American Indian tribes. President Nixon specifically rejected the "forced termination" policy of the Eisenhower years in a message to Congress on the grounds that: (1) federal responsibility was not simply an act of generosity toward a disadvantaged people but a solemn obligation; (2) the practical result of forced termination had been clearly harmful in instances where it has been tried; and (3) the fear of one extreme policy, forced termination, had produced the opposite extreme, excessive dependence on the federal government (Kunitz 1996). The Nixon administration's Indian policy was embodied in two major pieces of legislation passed by Congress: the Indian Self-Determination and Education Assistance Act (ISDEAA) of 1975 and the Indian Health Care Improvement Act (IHCIA) of 1976.

The Indian Self-Determination and Education Assistance Act of 1975 directed the Secretary of the Interior and the Secretary of Health and Human Services, upon the request of any Indian tribe, to enter into self-determination contracts or compacts with tribal organizations for planning, conducting, and/or administering programs that are provided by the federal government for the benefit of Indians.

The Indian Health Care Improvement Act of 1976 contained many provisions designed to increase the quantity and quality of Indian health services and to improve the participation of Indians in planning and providing these services, with the national goal of establishing the highest health conditions for Indians and providing existing Indian health services with all necessary resources to affect that policy. For the first time, the law authorized Medicare and Medicaid reimbursement for services performed at Indian health facilities. The primary goal of the Act was to improve the health status of AIs/ANs. It also authorized services for AIs/ANs living in urban areas, including the establishment of urban health centers (Pfefferbaum et al. 1995/1996). Charles Trimble, the executive director of the National Congress of American Indians from 1972 to 1978, called those years the golden era of Indian policies (Bergman et al. 1999).

In 1981, Everett R. Rhoads became the first American Indian Director of the IHS. Under his leadership (1981–1993), the 1980s witnessed increases in funding for Indian health programs. Major emphasis was placed on the construction of modern health facilities, professional excellence, and a movement toward tribal involvement. In 1988, the IHS was elevated to Agency-status within the United States Public Health Service (USPHS) from its status as a bureau within the Department of Health and Human Services ("The First Fifty Years of the Indian Health Service" n.d.).

The 1990s witnessed the evolution of the policy of self-determination to a policy of self-governance. The 1992 amendments to the IHCIA of 1976 (a) reauthorized the Indian Self-Determination Act, (b) provided for tribal self-governance demonstration projects through the IHS, and (c) authorized the Secretary of Health and Human Services to negotiate and implement a compact of Self-Governance and Annual Funding with tribes participating in demonstration projects (Pfefferbaum et al. 1995/1996).

President Clinton, in 1994, issued executive orders to facilitate tribal involvement in the administration of Indian programs. One of the initiatives undertaken by the Clinton administration was called "compacting." Compacting involves a looser arrangement than contracting and gives tribes more flexibility in their use of government funds. American Indian and Alaska Native corporations differ greatly in their use of contracting and compacting with the IHS. Some tribal corporations have participated a great deal in such arrangements, while others have not. The Navajo tribe, for example, has been reluctant to engage in contracting. However, the reality is that they are forced to undertake contracting and compacting in the fear that if they do not, a larger share of the limited funding available through the IHS budget will be absorbed by those willing to engage in such arrangements. Thus, even though contracting and compacting are supposed to be a matter of free choice for tribal governments, the reality is that if they do not engage, they risk losing IHS funding. The result is increased competition not only between tribes but also within tribes for limited federal resources (Kunitz 1996).

In 1994, Congress passed legislation to extend tribal self-governance on a demonstration basis to allow tribes to contract for programs, services, functions, and activities within the HHS and the BIA. The success of the demonstration period led to the creation of a permanent authority in 2000. Today, the IHS has come to be identified with three distinct sectors—services managed by the IHS, those managed by tribes, and those categorized as Urban Indian Health Programs ("The First Fifty Years of the Indian Health Service" n.d.).

The administration of George W. Bush continued the policy of tribal consultation (Shelton 2004), as did the Obama administration. Today, under the broad authorization of the 1921 Snyder Act, Congress every year appropriates funds to the IHS to fulfill the federal government's trust responsibility to provide health services to AI/AN people.

The Twenty-First Century

The Affordable Care Act and AIs/ANs

The 2010 ACA has several positive implications for the AI/AN community. The law included permanent reauthorization of the Health Care Improvement Act of 1976 and authorizes new programs and services within the IHS. The Act invests in prevention and wellness programs as well as increasing access to affordable healthcare to help address the problem of health disparities experienced by AIs/ANs.

The ACA also provides AIs/ANs with more choices in accessing healthcare depending on eligibility and coverage available in the state in which they reside. AIs/ANs can select between three options for health services. First, they can continue to use IHS, tribal, and/or urban Indian health programs. Second, they can enroll in a qualified health plan (QHP) through the health insurance marketplace exchanges. Third, they can access coverage to healthcare through Medicare, Medicaid, and the Children's Health insurance program if they meet the eligibility requirements ("Affordable Care Act" n.d.). These options provide enhance opportunities for uninsured AIs/ANs to access affordable healthcare. Nearly 30 percent of the AI/AN-combination population lack health insurance. They have limited access to employer-sponsored coverage because they have a high unemployment rate and tend to be employed in low-wage jobs that do not offer health insurance coverage ("Health Coverage and Care for American Indians and Alaska Natives" 2013).

The ACA provides additional healthcare benefits and protections to AIs/ANs beyond those provided to the general population. For example, the law exempts AIs/ANs in a federally recognized tribe from the "individuals shared responsibility" requirements to have adequate health insurance coverage. The law also provides cost-sharing subsidies for individuals enrolled in the federal or state health insurance marketplace and these subsidies cover all or some of the out-of-pocket healthcare costs to AIs/ANs (Erb and Speidel 2015). One in three (33 percent) of uninsured AIs/ANs have income in the range to qualify for the tax credit subsidies to purchase QHP through the new marketplace. Thus, the new marketplace and tax subsidies will provide other important affordable healthcare coverage options for AIs/ANs.

The Medicaid expansion under the ACA provides an additional opportunity for AIs/ANs to gain access to affordable healthcare coverage. Many AIs/ANs are eligible for Medicaid but often remain uninsured due to barriers in enrollment. AIs/ANs who meet state eligibility standards are entitled to Medicaid coverage in the state in which they live. Federal Medicaid funding is also available for covered services through the IHS or facilities operated by tribes under the urban Indian health programs. In fact, the federal government covers 100 percent of the cost of Medicaid services provided to AIs/ANs through any of these three facilities ("Health Coverage and Care for American Indians and Alaska Natives" 2013). Medicaid provides coverage to more than one in four non-elderly AIs/ANs and half of AI/AN children.

The Medicaid expansion under the ACA increases the number of health insurance coverage options for many uninsured AIs/ANs in states that have implemented it since it expanded Medicaid to low-income adults with income up to 138 percent of the federal poverty level. Due to this, AIs/ANs have experienced significant gains in coverage since the implementation of the Medicaid expansion in 2012 under the ACA. Between 2013 and 2015, the percentage of non-elderly uninsured AIs/ANs fell from 24 percent to 17 percent. Needless to say, AIs/ANs living in Medicaid expansion states have experienced much larger gains in coverage compared to those living in non-expansion states (Artiga, Ubri, and Foutz 2017).

THE INDIAN HEALTH SERVICE: ORGANIZATION AND STRUCTURE

The Indian Health Service has evolved from a very centralized and regionalized service at the time of its creation in 1955 to a highly decentralized service today involving contracting and compacting (Bergman et al. 1999). The IHS is a division of the Department of Health and Human Services. The division consists of local administrative units called service units. These units provide healthcare in their designated areas, generally centered on a reservation or on multiple small reservations. In Alaska, service units provide healthcare where there is a concentration of Alaska Natives. Service units are grouped into larger jurisdictions administered by area offices. Each area office is responsible for overseeing the operation of IHS programs within its jurisdiction. The heavy reliance on service units reflects the high degree of decentralization that exists in today's IHS (Pfefferbaum et al. 1997).

The IHS is headed by a director. Three of the major offices within the IHS include the Office of Tribal Self-Governance, the Office of Direct Services and Contracting Tribes, and the Office of the Urban Indian Health Programs. Health services are administered through 12 Area Offices (regions), with each office responsible for covering a certain geographic area in the country, and 170 IHS and tribally managed service units, which operate at a local level. Also, there are 34 urban programs operated by local nongovernmental and non-tribal organizations that provide clinical services to help urban Indians gain access to health services ("The First Fifty Years of the Indian Health Service" n.d.).

In addition, tribes have the option of exercising their right to self-determination and self-governance under the Indian Self-Determination and Education Assistance Act of 1975 and subsequent amendments. Today, over 60 percent of the IHS appropriation is administered by tribes through self-determination contracts or self-governance compacts ("IHS Profile" 2018).

Healthcare facilities under the IHS consist of 45 hospitals (26 IHS and 19 tribal), 343 health centers (59 IHS and 284 tribal), 111 health stations (32 IHS and 79 tribal), and 163 tribal-run Alaska village units. IHS employs 15,369 persons, including 2,648 nurses, 725 physicians, 698 pharmacists, 271 dentists, 115 physician assistants, and 110 sanitarians ("IHS Profile" 2018).

Organization and Delivery of Health Services

The federal government, in order to fulfill its responsibility for healthcare of AIs/ANs, has established a separate system of healthcare. AIs/ANs are entitled to certain health services as a result of treaty provisions and a long legislative history. There are also certain health services for which they qualify as US citizens and state residents (Pfefferbaum et al. 1997).

The IHS provides a comprehensive range of health services that includes traditional public health services along with inpatient and ambulatory clinical services. The IHS places great emphasis on community and preventive medicine. It administers a variety of programs ("Community Health" n.d.). For example, the IHS's Environmental Health Program provides services in the areas of injury prevention and institutional environmental health. The program helps identify environmental hazards and risk factors in tribal communities and proposes preventive measures. The Sanitation Facilities Construction Program is designed to provide safe drinking water and sewerage systems. The Environmental Health program strives to enhance the health and quality of life of AIs/ANs by focusing its priorities on creating a safer environment for children, providing safe drinking water and food, and preventing the spread of communicable diseases.

The Behavioral Health Program focuses on problems of alcohol and substance abuse, mental health disorders, suicide, violence, and behavior-related chronic diseases in AI/AN communities. The Injury Prevention Program promotes building the capacity of tribes through increased understanding of preventable injuries and finding effective solutions. The HIV/AIDS Program focuses primarily on the care of individuals and facilitating a preventive approach to reduce the impact of HIV/AIDS in AI/AN communities.

The Health Promotion and Disease Prevention Program focuses on preventive efforts at local, state, and regional levels. Its primary focus areas include diabetes, obesity, nutrition, physical activity and exercise, and tobacco cessation.

The IHS is primarily a rural healthcare delivery system. There are three major ways in which the IHS delivers health services. First, the IHS uses its own hospitals, outpatient health centers, and smaller health stations. Second, the IHS contracts with tribes under the Indian Self-Determination and Education Act to operate its hospitals, health centers, and health stations. Third, the IHS purchases services not available through its own facilities from non-tribal, private-sector hospitals and health practitioners. IHS services are provided free of charge to eligible AI/AN people (Forquera 2001). However, the IHS has a limited reach because eligibility for its services does not extend to all AIs/ANs for two reasons. First, IHS services are available only to members of federally recognized tribes. Thus, AIs/ANs who are not members of federally recognized tribes are ineligible to receive IHS services (Katz 2004). Second, IHS services are provided only to AIs/ANs living on or near reservations. By the year 2000, over 60 percent of AI/AN people were living in metropolitan areas ("American Indian/Alaska Native Profile" n.d.). These two factors combine to considerably limit the IHS service population (Forquera 2001).

Urban Indian Health Programs

Historically, most AI/AN individuals lived in remote rural areas on reservations or nearby. Only about 8 percent of the AI/AN population lived in cities according to the 1940 US census. During the 1950s and 1960s under the federal government's termination policy and Indian Relocation Program, thousands of AI/AN individuals and families were relocated to urban areas with promises of job training and placement, temporary housing, healthcare, and other types of assistance to help them adjust to living in an urban environment and to be assimilated into larger American society. By the 1970 census, 38 percent of AIs/ANs were living in urban centers and by the 2010 census the number of AIs/ANs living in urban areas had increased to 78 percent ("Office of Urban Indian Health Program Strategic Plan 2017–2021" n.d.). As a result, many Indians, including those who are members of federally recognized tribes, lost access to healthcare and other benefits granted to them when they lived on reservations.

As the urban Indian population increased, in part due to the government's relocation program, the need for health services for Indians living in urban areas also increased. Several cities, particularly those designated as relocation sites, independently developed health services for urban Indians. The Indian Health Care Improvement Act of 1976, in recognition of the plight of urban Indians who lacked access to health services, provided for the creation of an urban Indian health program (Bergman et al. 1999). This was a major departure for the IHS because previously it had not included Indians living outside IHS service areas. The purpose was to make outpatient health services available to urban Indians directly or by referrals. The IHS administers a program of grants and contracts to non-profit organizations, controlled by urban Indians often called Urban Indian

Organizations (UIOs). The UIOs vary in geographic area, size, and services offered. This program is referred to as the Urban Indian Health Program (UIHP).

Today, UIHP consists of 34 non-profit UIOs, which provide services such as comprehensive primary care, information, outreach and referrals, dental services, community health, substance abuse and behavioral health, immunization, health promotion, and disease prevention, among other services. The outpatient health services and referrals to urban Indians are on an income-based, sliding-scale fee schedule. Thus, this service is not free. The patients are asked to pay what they can afford. Most UIOs receive their income from patient fees, public and private insurers, tribal funds, and a mix of public and private grants, including funding from IHS contracts. More than half of the UIOs are certified as federally qualified health centers, making them eligible for additional federal funds (Renfrew 2006). The services at urban health centers are restricted to primary care, and referrals for inpatient hospital care, specialty services, diagnostics, and the like are at the patient's expense (Forquera 2001). It is important to note that UIHP operates separately from reservation-based IHS programs. The UIHP receives funding from IHS as well as non-IHS sources.

Urban Indians, like other American citizens, are also eligible for health coverage under Medicaid, Medicare, or the State Children's Health Insurance Program (SCHIP) if they meet the eligibility requirements. However, some Indians do not enroll in public programs because they believe the federal government is obligated by treaty and laws to pay for their healthcare and they should not have to enroll in healthcare programs for the general population. Despite this reluctance, many urban Indians are enrolled in public programs. Since UIOs are recognized by law as federally qualified health centers, they have an opportunity to enroll eligible urban Indians in Medicaid. In their benefits package, state Medicaid programs are required to cover the services provided by federally qualified health centers and such centers are entitled to payments for these services at a specified rate under the law (Forquera 2001).

One of the major changes made by the Indian Health Care Improvement Act of 1976 was a provision that allowed the IHS to bill Medicaid for services provided to Medicaid-eligible patients. This was not the case prior to 1976. Since Medicaid is a joint federal–state program funded on a matching basis, this would have increased costs to the state government. To limit state resistance to this provision, Congress provided a 100-percent federal medical assistance percentage (FMAP). This opened a new stream of federal funding for the IHS.

The Indian Health Service and Funding

The IHS receives its funding from three major sources. The largest source of funding is the annual discretionary appropriations by the Congress. The discretionary appropriations are divided into three separate accounts—Indian Health Services, Contract Support Costs, and Indian Health Facilities. The second major source of funding consists of funds received as payments for services provided to AIs/ANs from third-party payers such as Medicare, Medicaid, and the Children's Health Insurance program, the Department of Veterans Affairs, and private insurance. The third and smallest source of funding is a mandatory appropriation of $150 million annually to support the Special Diabetes Program for AIs/ANs. President Trump's budget request proposes shifting the FY 2019 appropriation under the discretionary funding category ("Indian Health Service (IHS) FY 2019 Budget Request and Funding History: A Fact Sheet" 2018.)

In 2017, the IHS collected $1.2 billion from third-party payers. Medicaid accounted for 68 percent, Medicare 21 percent, private insurance 9 percent, and the Department of Veterans Affairs 2 percent of all third-party collection in FY 2017. Medicaid is the largest source of the IHS's third-party payment collection ("Indian Health Service (IHS) FY 2019 Budget Request and Funding History: A Fact Sheet" 2018.)

Table 6.1 shows the total discretionary budget for the IHS fiscal years 2014 through 2019. As can be seen from the table, the IHS's annual discretionary budget increases have fluctuated between 3 and 5 percent, except for FY 2018. The FY 2018 discretionary budget showed a significant increase of 12 percent. This is due to the fact that FY 2018 appropriation included increases in a number of programs funded under the Indian Health Facilities account, which included money for the construction of new facilities as well maintenance and improvement of already-existing facilities. Also, the appropriation included increased funding for mental health and alcohol and substance abuse services. In addition, $50 million in appropriation was specifically targeted to go to tribes and tribal organizations to address the opioid crisis by increasing access to treatment- and recovery-related activities ("Indian Health Service (IHS) FY 2019 Budget Request and Funding History: A Fact Sheet" 2018; "President Trump Signs FY 2018 Omnibus" 2018).

It is important to note that President Trump's FY 2019 appropriation request represents a 2-percent decrease from FY 2018.

Table 6.1

Indian Health Service Funding History and Budget Request, 2014–2019 (in $ millions)

	FY 2014	FY 2015	FY 2016	FY 2017	FY 2018	FY 2019 Request
Indian Health Service account	4,714	4,820	4,909	5,035	5,295	5,290
Contract support costs account	587	663	718	718	718	822
IHS facilities account	460	469	532	554	876	515
Program-level total	5,761	5,951	6,160	6,307	6,889	6,627
Less funds from other sources	1,327	1,309	1,353	1,350	1,353	1,203
Total discretionary budget	4,435	4,642	4,808	4,957	5,536	5,424
% change from previous year		5	4	3	12	-2

Source: Congressional Research Service. 2018. "Indian Health Service FY 2019 Budget Request and Funding History." Online at www.everycrsreport.com/reports/R45201.html#Content.

HEALTH STATUS AND TRENDS

When Columbus arrived in the Western hemisphere, he found American Indians to be clean, fit, and without illness. Today, American Indians have higher occurrences of diseases than other racial/ethnic minorities (Ambler 2003). For example, American Indians have a higher prevalence of disease risk factors such as obesity, hypertension, high cholesterol, and tobacco smoking than other racial/ethnic minorities (Liao, Tucker, and Giles 2003). While the average life expectancy of AIs/ANs has increased by ten years since 1955, their life expectancy is five years shorter than the rest of the overall US population (Horwedel 2016; "The First Fifty Years of the Indian Health Service" n.d.). AIs/ANs make up a small percentage of the US population but suffer from disproportionate rates of diseases. For example, AIs/ANs have the highest rates of mortality for tuberculosis (450 percent higher), alcoholism (520 percent higher), diabetes mellitus (117 percent higher), unintentional injuries (141 percent higher), homicides (86 percent higher), pneumonia and influenza (37 percent higher), and suicide (60 percent higher) of any group in the United States (Donalee 2018).

AIs/ANs living in cities also continue to face a host of health problems. The infant mortality rate among urban AIs/ANs is 33 percent higher than that of the general population. The death rate due to accidents is 38 percent higher, diabetes is 54 percent higher, and chronic liver disease is 126 percent higher than the general population. The rate of alcohol-related deaths is 178 percent higher compared to the general population (Urban Indian Health Commission 2007).

There are several factors that impact health and contribute to poor health in Indian country. One of the major factors is poverty. AIs/ANs experience higher rates of poverty than the rest of the general US population. Unemployment is often closely related to poverty and both contribute to health problems because they can limit access to doctors and good nutrition, and affect the choices a person makes. The second factor that impacts AI/AN health is the cultural barriers, including access to care due to health providers' lack of knowledge about tribal language and culture. The third factor that impacts the health status of AIs/ANs is geographic location or residence. Many AIs/ANs lives in remote, rural areas and geographic distance often can make access to healthcare as well as healthy food such as fresh fruits, vegetables, and whole grain, etc., more difficult. The CDC calls such areas "food deserts," and research demonstrates their negative impact on health. The fifth factor, especially as it relates to AI/AN communities, is "historical trauma." The term refers to emotional and psychological wounds spanning across generations resulting from 500 years of mistreatment of AIs/ANs caused by forced removal and relocation, displacement of families, and lots of negative impact on racial and cultural identity (Horwedel 2016).

Table 6.2 provides data on some selective health status indicators for AIs/ANs in comparison to the general total US population. As can be observed, on almost all indicators, AIs/ANs rate poorer compared to the general total population. Over 16 percent of AIs/ANs rate their own health as fair to poor, compared to only 9.2 percent of the general population. Similarly, 20 percent of AIs/ANs report suffering from two to three chronic health conditions, compared to 18.8 percent of the general population.

Table 6.2

Comparison of Selective Health Status Indicators for American Indians/Alaska Natives and the General Population, 2014–2015

	General Population	AI/AN-Alone Population
Respondent-reported incidence of		
heart disease (18 years and older)	10.7%	13.4%
Cancer (18 years and older)	6.9%	5.3%
Stroke (18 years and older)	2.4%	*2.6%
Respondent-reported		
fair to poor health status	9.2%	16.6%
Suffering from two to three chronic conditions	18.8%	20.1%
Death rates per 100,000 population		
Firearm-related injuries	11.1%	14.4%
Homicide	5.7%	9.8%
Use of substances in the past month (age 12 years and older)		
Any illicit drug	12.1%	14.2%
Marijuana	8.3%	11.2%
Tobacco	23.9%	37.0%
Cigarettes	19.4%	29.5%
Alcohol	51.7%	37.9%
Binge alcohol use	24.9%	24.1%
Serious psychological distress in the past 30 days	3.3%	*11.8%

Notes * estimates may be unreliable due to high relative standard error of 20–30 percent.
Source: National Center for Health Statistics. 2018. *Health United States 2016*. Available online at www.cdc.gov/nchs/hus/contents2016.htm#American_Indian_or_Alaska_Native_Population.

Over 13 percent of AIs/ANs report suffering from heart disease and 2.6 percent report suffering from a stroke, compared to 10.7 percent and 2.4 percent, respectively, of the general population. In fact, stroke mortality rates among AIs/ANs are among the highest of all racial and ethnic groups in the United States. AIs/ANs with stroke often also suffer from hypertension, high cholesterol, or high rates of smoking—all of which are widely recognized for cerebrovascular risk factors (Harris et al. 2015). Only for cancer (18 years and older) do AIs/ANs report lower incidence rates, with 5.3 percent compared to 6.8 percent of the general population. However, it is important to note that a long time ago, cancer was a rare disease among AIs/ANs. The incidence of cancer and cancer deaths has increased among AIs/ANs over many years due to increased smoking, changes in diet, an aging population, and a sedentary lifestyle (Plescia et al. 2014).

The data in Table 6.2 also demonstrate a higher incidence of firearm-related injuries and homicide rates among AIs/ANs compared to the general population. The death rate per 100,000 population in 2014–2015 was 14.4 percent for AIs/ANs, compared to 11.1 percent in the general population. Similarly, the homicide rate per 100,000 population was 9.8 percent among AIs/ANs, compared to 5.7 percent in the general population.

Finally, Table 6.2 demonstrates a higher level of risky lifestyle and behavior that can negatively impact health among AIs/ANs than the general population. For example, the use of illicit drugs, marijuana, tobacco, and cigarettes is much higher among AIs/ANs compared to the general population. Even though the use of alcohol is lower among the AI/AN population than the general population, engaging in binge drinking is about the same in both groups. Binge drinking among young persons is a serious problem in the AI/AN population.

The high prevalence of risky behavior can lead to excessive deaths from chronic diseases, injuries, cancer, diabetes, obesity, and the like among AIs/ANs. For example, excessive drinking can lead to deaths from motor vehicle accidents in the short run and death from liver disease in the long run. High prevalence of tobacco use can contribute to heart disease and lung cancer. Changes in diet and nutrition, particularly from a reliance on vegetables, fruits, and meats from farming and hunting to a reliance on fast food and a mainstream American diet caused by movement from reservations to urban areas through a policy of removal, relocation, and assimilation have also contributed to increased risk factors for cancer, obesity, and diabetes (Cobb, Espey, and King 2014; Landen et al. 2014; Suryaprasad et al. 2014).

Table 6.3 shows data about the leading causes of death among AIs/ANs for 1980 and 2015. It demonstrates that some significant changes have taken place in the ranking of causes of death within the AI/AN community. For example, diabetes mellitus was the eighth-leading cause of death in 1980, but by 2015 it had become the fourth-leading cause. Two of the top ten leading causes of death in 1980—certain conditions originating in the prenatal period, and homicide—had dropped out of the top ten in 2015 and were replaced by chronic lower respiratory diseases (ranked sixth) and nephritis, nephrotic syndromes, and nephrosis (ranked ninth). Influenza and pneumonia ranked sixth in 2008 had dropped to tenth in 2015. Thus, in some areas, progress has been made because of better education, awareness, training, and vaccination.

Diseases of the heart were the number-one leading cause of death among AIs/ANs in 1980 and remain so in 2015. The largest percentage of deaths from heart disease is caused by diabetes. Another startling fact is that in recent years, type-2 diabetes has become a significant threat to Native American children. Type 2 diabetes in the past was largely confined to adults. The IHS has documented a 54-percent increase since 1996 in the prevalence of diagnosed diabetes among Native American youth of 15 to 19 years of age ("Diagnosed Diabetes" 2006; Fagot-Campagna, Pettitt, and Engelgau 2000; US Commission on Civil Rights 2004). Perhaps related to the high rate of diabetes in the AI/AN population is the fact that the AI/AN community also suffers from a higher prevalence of visual impairment and normal-tension glaucoma compared to other racial/ethnic groups (Mansberger et al. 2005). AIs/ANs also have the highest rate of premature death from heart diseases among all racial/ethnic groups (O'Connell et al. 2012).

Cardiovascular disease is another major health problem confronting AI/AN communities. In the past, heart disease and strokes were rare among AIs/ANs. Cardiovascular disease rates among AIs/ANs are twice that of the general population. The soaring rates of cardiovascular disease can be traced to the high rates of diabetes, high blood pressure, and the presence of other risk factors such as poor diet and a more sedentary lifestyle (US Commission on Civil Rights 2004).

Cancer is another growing concern among AIs/ANs. While AIs/ANs have lower cancer incidence and mortality rates than the general population (see Table 6.2), cancer has become the leading cause of death for Alaska Native and American Indian women. Also, the ratio of cancer deaths to new cancer cases is higher for AIs/ANs than the ratio for all other races (US Commission on Civil Rights 2004). AIs/ANs have the poorest cancer-survival rates among any racial group in American society. Furthermore, among AIs/ANs there has been a steady increase in cancer incidence and mortality.

Table 6.3

Leading Causes of Death for American Indians and Alaska Natives, 1980 and 2015

Rank	1980	2015
1	Diseases of the heart	Diseases of the heart
2	Unintentional injuries	Malignant neoplasms
3	Malignant neoplasms	Unintetional injuries
4	Chronic liver disease and cirrihosis	Diabetes mellitus
5	Cerebrovascular diseases	Chronic liver disease and cirrihosis
6	Pneumonia and influenza	Chronic lower respiratory diseases
7	Homocide	Cerebrovascular diseases
8	Diabetes mellitus	Suicide
9	Conditions originating in prenatal period	Nephritis, newphrotic syndromes and nephrosis
10	Suicide	Influenza and pneumonia

Source: National Center for Health Statistics. 2018. *Health United States, 2016*. Available online at www.cdc.gov/nchs/data/hus/2016/019.pdf.

The most common types of cancer among AIs/ANs are breast, colon, rectum, and lungs. In eight of the nine IHS areas, death caused by lung cancer is the most common, and 87 percent of all lung cancer deaths can be linked to tobacco smoking (UCLA Center for Health Policy Research 2004). AIs/ANs have a high rate of tobacco use, especially cigarette smoking, compared to the general population. Epidemiological data from a population-based, cross-sectional study of Southwestern and Northern Plains American Indians ages 15 to 54 found that 19 percent of Southwestern men, 10 percent of Southwestern women, 49 percent of Northern Plains men, and 51 percent of Northern Plains women smoked regularly (Henderson, Jacobsen, and Beals 2005). It is important to point out that racial misclassification and undercounting are often major obstacles to obtaining accurate and informative data on the AI/AN population (Swan et al. 2006). In reality, cancer rates among the AI/AN population are shown to be considerably higher when more accurate methods are used to estimate the incidence of cancer (Puukka, Stehr-Green, and Becker 2005).

Another area of concern is that unintentional injuries are another leading cause of death for AIs/ANs under the age of 44. In 1980, unintentional injuries ranked as the second-leading cause of death among AIs/ANs. In 2015, they were the third-leading cause of death among AIs/ANs. Three leading causes of unintentional injury mortality among AIs/ANs are motor vehicle traffic crashes, poisoning, and falls (Murphy et al. 2014). Alcohol abuse also contributes to mental health problems. Studies show that drinkers in the highest risk category for alcohol dependence are also more likely to report drug use disorders, mood/anxiety disorders, alcohol-related physical disorders, and a lower quality of life (Novins et al. 2006).

AIs/ANs have the highest prevalence of diabetes among all racial/ethnic groups in the United States, and their mortality attributable to diabetes is three to four times higher (O'Connell et al. 2012). Diabetes is one of the most serious health problems confronting AIs/ANs and is responsible for significant morbidity and mortality rates among the population. Most AIs/ANs with diabetes have type-2 diabetes, also known as adult-onset diabetes, which is characterized by high levels of blood glucose stemming from impaired insulin secretion and/or the body's resistance to the action of insulin. In fact, Native Americans have the highest prevalence of diabetes in the world.

Furthermore, the rate of diabetes among AIs/ANs has increased in almost epidemic proportions. For example, the number of AIs/ANs aged 35 or younger with diabetes diagnosed through the IHS more than doubled from 6001 in 1994 to 12,313 in 2004. While the rates of diabetes increased among both males and females, the prevalence of diabetes was greater among females than males in all age groups ("Diagnosed Diabetes" 2006). Diabetes is not only more prevalent among AIs/ANs, but they also develop diabetes at a younger age, making them more vulnerable to complications of diabetes. The good sign is that there is a decline in diabetes-related mortality among AIs/ANs because of better education and management of the disease (Cho et al. 2014).

Diabetes is related to obesity, and American Indians of all ages and both sexes have a high prevalence of obesity. AIs/ANs have a higher rate of obesity and being overweight than whites or Hispanics (Anderson, Spicer, and Peercy 2016). Obesity has become a major health problem among American Indians in the past one to two generations. Obesity is believed to be associated with the relative abundance of high-fat foods and the rapid changes in AI/AN lifestyle—from an active to a more sedentary lifestyle (Story et al. 1999; Welty 1991).

AIs/ANs have the highest rates of smoking by adults among all ethnic groups (US Department of Health and Humans Services 2000). As Table 6.2 indicates, 29.5 percent of the AI/AN population smoke cigarettes, compared to 19.4 percent of the general population. According to a national telephone survey conducted by the Centers for Disease Control and Prevention (CDC) (2000), 30.8 percent of AIs/ANs were smokers. Thus, the numbers have not changed much. Having more than one risk factor for heart disease is also more common among older AIs/ANs. A sizable percentage of AIs/AN suffered from specific risk factors such as high blood pressure (22 percent), high cholesterol (16 percent), and obesity (21.5 percent).

The most significant public health concerns in AI/AN communities are substance abuse, depression, anxiety, violence, and suicide. Up to 30 percent of AIs/ANs suffer from depression (Urban Indian Health Commission 2007). American Indians experience the highest rate of suicide of all racial/ethnic groups in the United States (Olson and Wahab 2006). It was the eighth-leading cause of death among AIs/ANs in 2015. Research also shows that many suicidal young people avoid asking for help. For example, in a study of a sample of 101 American Indians between the ages of 15 and 21 who had thought about or attempted suicide, 74 participants indicated that they had avoided seeking help because of largely internal factors, such as embarrassment, lack of problem recognition, or a belief that nobody could help. Participants rarely cited structural factors such as lack of money or service availability as reasons for not seeking help (Freedenthal and Stiffman 2007).

AIs/ANs are consistently overrepresented among the high-need population in mental health services. According to a report by the Surgeon General of the United States, this overrepresentation may be associated with high rates of homelessness, incarceration, alcohol and drug abuse, and stress and trauma (Satcher 2001). An examination of the prevalence of trauma in two large American Indian communities revealed that members of both tribes witnessed traumatic events, experienced trauma to loved ones, and were victims of physical attacks more often than in the overall US population (Manson et al. 2005).

A higher percentage of AI/AN veterans compared to veterans of all other races served in the military during the pre-9/11 and post-9/11 era ("Selected Research Highlights" 2015). Consequently, AI/AN veterans have experienced higher rates of trauma and posttraumatic stress disorder (PTSD). PTSD is associated with bodily pain, lung disorders, general health problems, substance abuse, and gambling (Bassett, Buchwald, and Manson 2014). A panic attack is another common mental health issue in the AI/AN community (Sawchuk et al. 2017). Mental disorders are among the top ten leading causes of HIS hospitalization and ambulatory care visits. AIs/ANs have equal or greater prevalence of psychiatric disorders compared to other US population groups (Brave Heart et al. 2016).

ACCOMPLISHMENTS OF THE IHS

Since the establishment of the IHS in 1955, there have been considerable improvements in the health status of AIs/ANs, and healthcare disparities between AIs/ANs and the general US population have narrowed somewhat. Mortality rates for AIs/ANs have declined and life expectancy has improved. There have also been major improvements in infant and child mortality and a decline in infectious diseases. In the first 25 years of the IHS, infant mortality rates dropped by 82 percent, maternal death rates declined by 89 percent, mortality rates from tuberculosis declined by 96 percent, and deaths from diarrhea and dehydration declined by 93 percent (Bergman et al. 1999).

Between 1940 and 1990, life expectancy at birth among AI/AN men increased by 17.8 years to 69.1 years. During the same time, life expectancy at birth for AI/AN women increased by 25.6 years to 77.5 years. The most significant decline in mortality has been for two infectious diseases—tuberculosis and gastroenteritis (Young 1997).

The IHS has been effective in reducing preventable and treatable conditions/diseases but has not had much impact on certain chronic conditions such as diabetes and certain types of cancers (Kunitz 1996). While the burden of mortality and morbidity has decreased since World War II, the relative contribution of various diseases and health conditions has changed, reflecting what might be called epidemiologic transition (Young 1997).

Among more recent accomplishments of the IHS include strengthened partnership with tribes to improve the health of the AI/AN community, reforming the IHS with an eye toward improving financial management, making business operations more efficient and effective, better management and monitoring of budgets, reducing pay disparities to help the recruitment of qualified health professionals, and improving the quality and access to healthcare through new programs such as the Special Diabetes Program for Indians (SDPI) and the methamphetamine and suicide prevention initiative. Finally, IHS Health Care Facilities Construction funding has increased 132 percent since FY 2008, allowing for the construction of new health facilities ("Fiscal Year 2011 Accomplishments" n.d.).

Despite some of the successes, it is clear that AIs/ANs still experience significant healthcare disparities when it comes to health status/outcome, access to healthcare, and quality of healthcare in comparison not only to whites but also to the general US population. In certain areas, AIs/ANs fare even worse than do African-Americans or Hispanics. The topic of healthcare disparities and AIs/ANs is discussed further in Chapter 7.

CHALLENGES CONFRONTING THE IHS AND HEALTHCARE POLICY FOR AIS/ANS

The health status of AIs/ANs is the result of a variety of health determinants such as exposure to risk factors, affordability, availability, and accessibility of health services, social factors, and individual behavioral factors. AIs/ANs have a high poverty rate, with nearly one-third of non-elderly living in families with income below the federal poverty level and nearly half living in families with income below 200 percent of the federal poverty level (James, Schwartz, and Berndt 2009). As a result, more than 25 percent of AIs/ANs are eligible for Medicaid, but only 17 percent report that they are covered by Medicaid or any other public program (Urban Indian Health Commission 2007). Part of the reason is that some AIs/ANs do not apply for Medicaid even when eligible, and the reach of the Medicaid program to childless adults is limited due to eligibility restrictions (James, Schwartz, and Berndt 2009). One in five AIs/ANs lives in families without a worker. Also, one in five AIs/ANs adults does not have a high school diploma. Among those under the age of 65, AIs/ANs have the lowest rate of private health insurance coverage of any racial/ethnic group, and one in three non-elderly AIs/ANs is uninsured or depends solely on services provided by the IHS (James, Schwartz, and Berndt 2009).

Increasing Funding for the IHS

The IHS's annual discretionary budget increases have fluctuated between the 3 and 5-percent rate, except for FY 2018. The FY year 2018 discretionary budget showed a significant increase of 12 percent. This is due to the fact that FY 2018 appropriation included new money for construction of new facilities as well maintenance and improvement of already-existing facilities. Also, the appropriation included increased funding for several new programs such as mental health and alcohol and substance abuse services and programs to address the opioid crisis by increasing access to treatment and recovery-related activities. It is important to note that President Trump's FY 2019 appropriation request represents a 2-percent decrease from FY 2018 ("Indian Health Service (IHS) FY 2019 Budget Request and Funding History: A Fact Sheet" 2018; "President Trump Signs FY 2018 Omnibus" 2018).

Critics have argued that one of the major shortcomings of the IHS in providing healthcare services is that it is critically underfunded (Lillie-Blanton 2005; Noren, Kindig, and Sprenger 1998; Warne 2007). In 2003, per-capita expenditure for AI/AN health services was only $1,914. In contrast, per-capita expenditure for Medicaid recipients was $3,879 in 2003, for Medicare recipients $5,815, for Veterans Administration beneficiaries $5,214, and for federal inmates, in the Bureau of Prisons, it was $3,803 (Warne 2007). In 2013, IHS spending on patient health services was $2,849 per person, compared to $7,717 for healthcare spending per person nationally (Friedman 2016).

One of the consequences of this low level of expenditures is that IHS hospitals provide a more limited range of diagnostic and therapeutic services than community hospitals do in general. Because of the underfunding of the IHS and tribal programs and the fact that a significant number of AIs/ANs are poor, the IHS and tribal programs have become heavily dependent on third-party revenue sources such as Medicaid (Warne 2007).

Underfunding also affects the ability to recruit and retain competent healthcare providers, which in turn has a direct bearing on the quality of care received by AIs/ANs. Overworked staff develop burnout, resulting in high turnover rates, which also negatively affects the quality of care provided. It has been well documented that, historically, the IHS has experienced shortages of doctors, dentists, pharmacists, and nurses. The IHS also faces problems in recruiting and retaining healthcare providers because of the remoteness of some of the health clinics. It is difficult to recruit and retain healthcare providers who are willing to live and work in remote tribal communities (US Commission on Civil Rights 2004). The problem is further compounded by factors such as a lack of parity in pay, insufficient or inadequate housing, lack of jobs for spouses, and insufficient opportunities for continuing education. It is clear that a shortage of healthcare providers negatively affects the quality of care for AIs/ANs (US Commission of Civil Rights 2004). Staffing and budget shortages put the IHS at high risk (Davidson 2017).

Another problem caused by high provider-turnover rates is that AI/AN patients do not receive consistent care from the same provider. This, combined with a lack of resources and the remoteness of healthcare facilities, often leads to misdiagnosis or late diagnosis of diseases, which can negatively affect health outcomes. For example, early detection of cancer can increase the patient's chance of survival, while late diagnosis decreases the chances. Unfortunately, in AI/AN communities, misdiagnosis of a disease is too common (US Commission on Civil Rights 2004).

Thus, the most important challenge is to increase funding for AI/AN healthcare services, since it affects access to care as well as the quality of care received. The IHS has been underfunded over the years, and increases in funding would go a long way toward improving the quality of health services provided to AIs/ANs.

Increasing Access to Healthcare Services

A second important policy challenge for AI/AN healthcare is increasing access to healthcare services and increasing funding for the IHS and tribal programs may help. Research has shown that a lack of health insurance negatively affects people's health because they are less likely to receive preventive care, are more likely to be hospitalized for avoidable health problems, and are more likely to be diagnosed in the late stages of the disease. AIs/ANs have the lowest rate of private health insurance coverage among all racial/ethnic groups in American society. Those who lack health insurance coverage are more financially vulnerable to the high cost of care and end up paying more out-of-pocket costs for care. In contrast, having health insurance improves overall health and could reduce the mortality rates of those currently uninsured by 10 to 15 percent (Kaiser Commission on Medicaid and the Uninsured 2006). Having health insurance coverage increases the chances of having a "medical home" and thus improves access to preventive screening, medical care for acute illness, and ongoing care for chronic medical conditions (Kaiser Commission of Medicaid and the Uninsured 2006).

Availability of medical providers, place of residence, travel time, and financial issues are some of the other major factors strongly associated with the use of healthcare services by AIs/ANs (Cunningham and Cornelius 1995). High rates of poverty, low rates of other health insurance coverage, and the lack of private providers in many areas inhabited by AIs/ANs also contribute to less access and utilization (Cunningham and Altman 1993).

The US Commission on Civil Rights (2004), in its report *Broken Promises: Evaluating the Native American Health Care System*, found that structural factors such as high staff turnover and loss of continuity of care, long distances to travel to receive even primary care, lengthy waiting lines upon arrival, and many outdated health facilities act as added barriers to healthcare access.

The US Government Accountability Office (2005) conducted a study of the availability of health services for AIs/ANs and whether they were accessible to AIs/ANs in the IHS facility area. The study found that the availability of primary care—medical, dental, and vision service—largely depended on the extent to which AIs/ANs were able to gain access to the services offered at the thirteen IHS-funded facilities. While IHS facilities generally offered primary-care services, access to these services was not assured because of factors such as waiting times between the call to make an appointment and the delivery of service, and long travel distances to facilities or lack of transportation. Waiting times often ranged from two to six months for certain types of appointments, and some Native Americans were required to travel over 90 miles one way to obtain care. The study further found that certain services were not always available to Native Americans. Gaps in services were found in diagnosis and treatment of nonurgent conditions such as arthritis, knee injuries, and chronic pain. Gaps were also found in specialty dental and behavioral healthcare.

Providing Culturally Competent Care

Racial/ethnic minorities often have cultural values that may differ from the mainstream cultural values and influence perceptions about health and illness, healing, and treatment, and can affect nutrition and lifestyle behaviors. This is also true in the case of AI/AN communities. The cultural values shared by AIs/ANs certainly influence their lifestyle and risk and health behaviors.

In contrast to AIs/ANs and African-Americans, many other ethnic groups voluntarily emigrated to the United States and assimilated into the majority American culture. In the case of American Indians, the majority culture forced its beliefs, values, and practices on them and removed them from their ancestral lands. In addition, many American Indians continue to reside on geographically remote reservations isolated from mainstream culture (Herman-Stahl, Spencer, and Duncan 2003). Perhaps more than any other ethnic group in American society, traditional AIs/ANs have consistently resisted acculturation into mainstream society. Many traditional American Indian cultural values such as sharing, cooperation, importance of the group, and harmony and balance with nature are in sharp contrast to the mainstream European-American values of domination over nature, competition and aggression, winning, individualism, the nuclear family, and a preference for scientific explanations of everything (Garrett and Garrett 1994).

Consequently, traditional AIs/ANs often encounter difficulties when dealing with Western medicine and practices and the mainstream healthcare system. For example, American Indians' emphasis on a nonverbal communication style, avoiding direct eye contact, respect for authority figures, speaking slowly and softly, and the like, may be misinterpreted by mainstream healthcare providers as slow, lazy, uncooperative, passive, withdrawn, and nonassertive. This creates communication barriers and room for misunderstanding between healthcare providers and patients (Garrett and Garrett 1994). AIs/ANs, in general, do perceive various barriers to obtaining social and health services based on a mutual misinterpretation of cultural norms and etiquette (Kramer 1992).

Research also suggests a high incidence of behavioral risk factors such as substance and alcohol abuse in the AI/AN communities (Herman-Stahl, Spencer, and Duncan 2003). Such behavioral risk factors are often found to be associated with the cultural values and belief system.

For centuries, many indigenous cultures in America have used nonpharmacologic methods such as sleep deprivation, drumming, pain, and fasting to achieve altered mind states. Prior to contact with the Europeans, mind-altered states were viewed as a social good in cultures of the Plains Indians, associated with a quest for enlightenment, powers of healing, and facilitation of war-making. In more contemporary times, it is common to see the use of alcohol in an Iroquois vision quest as well as the use of non-alcoholic psychotropic substances such as jimsonweed, peyote, and tobacco. The use of such substances and the states they induced occur under the umbrella of religious and social sanctions (Frank 2000).

Some scholars have also traced the roots of the epidemic of alcohol-related problems among AIs/ANs to a cultural response to the European arrival and the use of alcohol in frontier society. It has been suggested that Native Americans' responses to alcohol were heavily influenced by the example of white frontiersmen who drank a lot and engaged in unacceptable behavior while drunk. Whites also deliberately pressed alcohol upon the natives because it was a very profitable trade good. Alcohol was used as a tool of "diplomacy" in official dealings between authorities and natives. Alcohol was also used as a bargaining chip in the appropriation of traditional land holdings (Frank 2000).

Another area where cultural values play a role among AIs/ANs is in the use of healers such as herbalists, spiritual healers, and medicine men to deal with their health problems (Marbella et al. 1998). The US Commission on Civil Rights (2004) found that social and cultural factors such as a healthcare system that is insensitive to AI/AN peoples' unique culture, bias among healthcare workers, disproportionate poverty, and low levels of education among AIs/ANs acted as significant barriers to Native Americans' access to healthcare and contribute to healthcare disparities.

Thus, the third challenge is to increase the number of culturally competent healthcare providers. This would include providing necessary training to healthcare professionals currently serving AI/AN communities as well as increasing the number of AI/AN healthcare professionals. It would require a coordinated educational policy that encourages young AIs/ANs to enter healthcare profession education by providing more scholarships. Currently, there is a significant shortage of minority, especially AI/AN, health professionals, and researchers. African-Americans, Hispanics/Latinos, and AIs/ANs together make up more than 25 percent of the population, but they make up less than 9 percent of nurses, 6 percent of physicians, and 5 percent of dentists. If fewer and fewer minorities enter health professions, it is likely to negatively impact the availability and quality of healthcare services for minorities (Warne 2009). The long history of AI/AN nonparticipation in research processes and policy development has often created misunderstanding and mistrust about motivations of researchers and policymakers. It is important to include AIs/ANs in the research agenda for dealing with their health status, as well as in policy discussions and developments that arise out of research findings (Warne 2009).

Conclusion

In comparison to African-Americans and Hispanics, American Indians and Alaska Natives (AIs/ANs) constitute a very small minority in American society, but they experience some of the worst health status. Healthcare for members of American Indian tribes and Alaska Natives is delivered from a system that is separate from that of mainstream America. This separate healthcare delivery system has evolved from the unique and complex history of interaction between the various tribes and the US government. The Indian Health Service (IHS) is primarily responsible for delivering health services to the AI/AN population.

Since its establishment in 1955, the IHS has accomplished a lot and significant progress has been made in improving the health status of AIs/ANs in certain areas such as life expectancy, infant mortality, and reducing the incidence of certain preventable diseases. Yet, many challenges remain. The AI/AN community suffers some of the worst health indicators compared to other racial/ethnic groups in American society. Inconsistent and often conflicting policies pursued toward AIs/ANs, such as relocation, assimilation, eradication, and self-determination, combined with apprehension and ambiguities in dealings with AIs/ANs, have often produced negative health consequences. In the last several decades, policies to enhance self-determination and empowerment of AIs/ANs are steps in the right direction.

Critics have argued that one of the reasons for the healthcare disparity is that the IHS is critically underfunded. Consistent underfunding of health programs is negatively impacting healthcare access, quality of care, and health status of AI/AN communities and remains a threat, undermining any progress already made. The fact that AIs/ANs constitute a very small minority in American society, that they do not participate in large numbers in political processes, and that they have very little representation of their community in policymaking institutions of government speaks to their lack of political power, which makes them more invisible and vulnerable.

HEALTHCARE FOR VETERANS

Population Characteristics and Trends

In 2016, the total veteran population was about 19.7 million. Of the total veteran population, 91.4 percent were male and 8.6 percent were female. The racial makeup of the veterans consisted of about 77.6 percent white and 22.6 percent minorities. Of the 22.6 percent minorities, 10.9 percent were black, 6.1 percent were Hispanic, 1.5 percent were Asian, 0.9 percent were AI/AN and Native Hawaiian and other Pacific Islander, and the remaining 3 percent were other races, including those identifying with more than one race (www.statista.com). Overall, the total veteran population is projected to decline to 13.6 million by the year 2037. The overall minority veteran population is projected to increase to about 32.8 percent while the female veteran population is projected to increase to over 16 percent by the year 2037. As the share of minorities and females rises in the active-duty force, so will their share in the veteran population. Beginning in 2016, the Gulf-era veterans became the largest veteran cohort, followed by veteran cohorts made up of those who served in Vietnam, the Korean Conflict, and World War II. Fifty percent of veterans resides in ten states—California, Texas, Florida, Pennsylvania, New York, Ohio, North Carolina, Virginia, Georgia, and Illinois—with more veterans moving to the West and the South ("Veteran Population Projections 2017–2037" n.d.; "Projected Veteran Population 2013 to 2043" 2014; Parker, Cilluffo, and Stepler 2017). The United States is in the midst of a significant long-term change in both the size and profile of its veteran's population with respect to gender, race/ethnicity, and the era of service (Livingston 2016; Trimble 2017).

In 2016, the median age of male veterans was 65, compared to 50 for female veterans. Almost 65 percent of male veterans were married, compared to 49 percent of female veterans. Female veterans were more likely to have some college education, a bachelor's, or an advanced degree compared to male veterans. For example, 43 percent of female veterans had some college education, 22 percent had a bachelor, and 15 percent had an advanced college degree, compared to 28 percent of male veterans having some college education, 16 percent having a bachelor's degree, and 11 percent having an advanced college degree. Similarly, the percentage of female veterans working in management and professional occupation was about 15 percent higher than male veterans—50 percent compared to 35 percent. Another 27.6 percent of female veterans worked in sales/offices compared to 19.2 percent of male veterans. The fact that more female veterans were employed in management/professional and sales/office occupations compared to male veterans is not too surprising given the fact that female veterans are more likely to have had a higher level of educational attainment compared to their male counterparts. Yet, the median personal income of male veterans was higher than female veterans. For example, in 2016, the median personal income of male veterans who worked year-around and full-time was $37,991, compared to $30,493 for female veterans ("Profile of Veterans: 2016" 2018).

Both male and female veterans are more likely to have health insurance coverage and are less likely to be unemployed or live in poverty compared to the non-veteran US population. For example, in 2016, 2.8 percent of male veterans and 3.5 percent of female veterans did not have any health insurance coverage, compared to 13.3 percent of the male and 8.5 percent of the female non-veteran US population. Similarly, 6.4 percent of male veterans and 9.5 percent of female veterans lived in poverty, compared to 11.5 percent of the male and 14.3 percent of the female non-veteran US population ("Profile of Veterans: 2016" 2018).

Finally, another important trend in the veteran population is that while the total veteran population has been declining since 1986, the number of veterans with a service-connected disability has been on the rise. Since 1973 the lowest number of disabled veterans was recorded in the fiscal year 1990. However, since 1990 the number of veterans with a service-connected disability has increased 60 percent. The rate of increase in cash payment is outpacing the growth in the number of veterans with a service-connected disability ("Trends in Veterans with a Service-Connected Disability: 1985 to 2014" 2015).

HISTORICAL BACKGROUND: THE DEVELOPMENT OF VETERANS' BENEFITS

The United States has a very comprehensive veterans' benefits system. The origins of this system can be traced back to 1636, when pilgrims of the Plymouth Colony passed a law supporting disabled soldiers in the war with the Pequot Indians. In 1776, the Continental Congress passed the country's first pension law, in which it granted half-pay for life in case of loss of limb or other serious disability. However, the law left it up to the individual states to make pension payments. In 1789, after the ratification of the US Constitution, the first Congress passed the first federal pension law and assumed the responsibility of paying veterans' benefits ("VA History in Brief" n.d.).

In 1811, the federal government authorized the first domiciliary and medical facility for veterans. The establishment of the first Naval Home in Philadelphia in 1812 was the first national effort to provide for the medical care of disabled veterans. This was followed by the Soldiers Home in 1853 and St. Elizabeth's Hospital in Washington, DC. The Revolutionary War Pension Act of 1818 provided a fixed pension for life for those who had served in the War of Independence and needed assistance. The Commissioner of Pensions was established by Congress in 1833, administered from within the War Department until 1840, and from 1840 to 1849 under the Secretary of the Navy. The office was then renamed the Bureau of Pensions and was placed under the new Department of the Interior ("VA History in Brief" n.d.). In 1862, President Lincoln signed a law authorizing the creation of the National Cemeteries system for veterans, and in 1865 he signed another law creating the National Home for Volunteer Soldiers in Maine. Homes for disabled Civil War veterans were subsequently opened in several states (Kizer, Demakis, and Feussner 2000).

By the end of the Civil War in 1865, 1.9 million veterans had been added to the pension rolls. Initially, pension was limited to Union soldiers only. However, in 1958, Congress pardoned Confederate soldiers and extended pension benefits to one single remaining survivor ("VA History in Brief" n.d.). After the Civil War (1861–1865), two factors contributed to significant increases in veterans' benefits. One was the fact that their claims for increased benefits were legitimized by their patriotic service to the country. Second, veterans had become a large and well-organized interest group with political clout and were able to successfully lobby for increased benefits (Holcombe 1999). After the Civil War, veterans made up 5 percent of the total population, but due to the limited franchise (eligible voters) at the time, they made up a much larger fraction of the voting population. In 1865, the United States Soldiers' and Sailors' Protective Society was organized to help veterans. In 1866, the Grand Army of the Republic (GAR) was formed as a political group to lobby for veterans' benefits. Laws passed by Congress between 1865 and 1868 helped define federal benefits to Civil War veterans. Under these Acts, pension payments were made to disabled veterans and surviving widows and the children of those killed in the war. Veterans who survived the war uninjured were not entitled to a pension. Another Act by Congress in 1868 specified that to be eligible for a disability pension, the disability had to have occurred in the line of duty (Holcombe 1999). The Arrears Act of 1879 specified that veterans' benefits started from the time of discharge from the army or for dependents from the time of the death, and not at the time of application, as was the case prior to the Act. In 1890, veterans' benefits were broadened to provide benefits to disabled veterans and survivor benefits to widows of veterans, regardless of whether they were injured in the war and regardless of need. Under this policy, veterans who became physically or mentally disabled after the war were entitled to a pension, as were their widows (Holcombe 1999).

The Sherwood Act of 1912 awarded pensions to all veterans. When the United States entered World War I in 1917, Congress established a new system of veterans' benefits that included programs for disability compensation, insurance for service persons and veterans, and vocational rehabilitation for the disabled. The Vocational Rehabilitation Act of 1918 established an independent agency, the Federal Board for Vocational Education, and made honorably discharged disabled veterans of World War I eligible for vocational rehabilitation training. In 1919, the Public Health Service was assigned the responsibility of medical care for veterans and a number of military hospitals were transferred to its remit. In 1921, veterans' programs managed by three separate agencies were consolidated into a newly created Veterans Bureau. In 1930, President Hoover signed a law uniting three separate bureaus, the Veterans Bureau, the Bureau of Pensions, and the National Homes for Disabled Volunteer Soldiers, into an independent federal agency called the Veterans Administration (VA). The VA assumed responsibility for healthcare/medical services for war veterans, disability compensation and allowances for World War II veterans, and life insurance and other services. By 1941, the number of VA hospitals had increased to 91 from 64 in 1931 (Kizer, Demakis, and Feussner 2000; "VA History in Brief" n.d.).

The Servicemen's Readjustment Act of 1944, famously known as the "GI Bill of Rights," provided three major benefits: first, federally guaranteed low-interest loans for veterans to purchase homes, farms, or small businesses, without any down payment; second, financial assistance for up to four years of education or training; and third, unemployment compensation. The Veterans' Preference Act of 1944 gave veterans hiring preference in programs that spent federal funds. By 1950, the number of VA hospitals had increased to 151 from 91 in 1941. Following the Korean War, The Veterans' Readjustment Assistance Act of 1952, known as the Korean GI Bill, provided benefits similar to those offered to World War II veterans. Congress in 1966 passed the Veterans' Readjustment Benefits Act, known as the Vietnam GI Bill. The education program for Vietnam veterans was highly successful and 76 percent of those eligible participated, compared to 50.5 percent of World War II veterans and 43.4 percent of Korean conflict veterans. In the 1980s and 1990s, Congress also passed legislation providing disability compensation for disability resulting from exposure to herbicides used in Vietnam and veterans suffering from a disease associated with exposure to radiation ("VA History in Brief" n.d.).

In 1988, under the Reagan administration, the Veterans Administration was elevated to the new status of a cabinet-level department—the Department of Veterans Affairs (DVA). In response to an increase in the number of female veterans, the Veterans Health Benefit Act of 1992 provided authority for several gender-specific services and programs to care for women veterans. In 1997, the Women Veterans Health Program Office was established. On July 21, 2005, the VA celebrated its 75th Anniversary. The VA had grown from an operating budget of $786 million serving 4.6 million veterans in 1930 to its new title as the Department of Veterans Affairs, with a budget of $63.5 billion and serving close to 25 million veterans ("VA History in Brief" n.d.).

VETERANS' HEALTH POLICY DEVELOPMENT

A month before the end of the Civil War, in March 1865, President Lincoln authorized the first ever National Soldiers' and Sailors' Asylum to provide medical and convalescent care for discharged members of the Union Army and Navy volunteer forces. In 1873, it was renamed as the National Home for Disabled Volunteer Soldiers. Such National Homes, often called "soldiers' homes" or "military homes," housed thousands of veterans. The first National Home, opened in Augusta, Maine in 1966, is now the VA's oldest military hospital. By 1929, the National Homes had grown to 11 institutions spread across the country. World War I brought about the establishment of the second-largest system of veterans' hospitals. Two agencies in the Department of the Treasury, the Bureau of War Risk Insurance and the Public Health Service, were tasked with operating hospitals specifically for returning World War I veterans. They leased hundreds of private hospitals and hotels to treat returning injured war veterans and started a program of building new hospitals ("History—VA History" n.d.; "Our History: A Brief History of the Veterans Health Administration" n.d.).

In 1921, three World War I programs were combined and housed in the newly created Veterans Bureau. In 1924, veterans' benefits were liberalized to cover disabilities that were not service-related and in 1928 admission to Veterans Bureau hospitals and National Homes was extended to women, national guards, and militia veterans ("History—VA History" n.d.; "Our History: A Brief History of the Veterans Health Administration" n.d.). In January 1946, Congress passed, and President Truman signed into law, Public Law 293, formally creating the Veterans Health Administration (VHA) within the Veterans Administration (now the Department of Veterans Affairs). Also in 1946, the Department of Medicine and Surgery was established within the VA. Veterans Affairs hospitals immediately sought affiliation with university medical schools in order to improve the quality and number of physicians. This helped establish a very successful partnership between the VA and the country's medical schools, allowing the veterans' healthcare system to grow rapidly during the 1940s and 1950s. By 1948, 60 medical schools were affiliated with VA hospitals. VA hospitals were a training ground for America's medical, nursing, and allied health professionals. Around 60 percent of all medical residents received a portion of their training at VA hospitals. Over the years this collaboration between VA hospitals and university medical schools led to major advances in medicine, nursing, medical research, and prosthetics. The addition of more than 70 new hospitals, combined with the establishment of university medical school affiliations and teaching programs, dramatically expanded research activities as well as new avenues of care for the veterans. During this time period, most emphasis was placed on providing hospital inpatient care for veterans, with healthcare provided by medical specialists (Kizer and Dudley 2009; "Our History: A Brief History of the Veterans Health Administration" n.d.).

In 1956, the Dependents Medical Care Act provided the Department of Defense the authority to provide civilian healthcare to eligible dependents of military service members. The Civilian Health and Medical Program of Uniformed Services (CHAMPUS) was established in 1966 for family members of those on active duty and was later extended to retired service members and their dependents. This program provided supplemental care in addition to what was available in both the military and the Public Health Service (PHS), inpatient as well as outpatient care, and pharmacy benefits (Jackonis, Deyton, and Hess 2008).

As the veterans' healthcare system grew, it also became more complex and bureaucratic. During the 1970s and 1980s, the media reported several embarrassing incidents involving the poor quality of healthcare received by veterans in several VA hospitals. Also, the number of Vietnam War veterans needing healthcare increased significantly during this time. Many of these veterans became alienated by what they perceived as a lack of response from the VA to their healthcare needs. Several veterans' service organizations sought a higher status for veterans' programs. In response, President Reagan in March 1989 elevated Veterans Affairs to the cabinet-level Department of Veterans Affairs (Kizer and Dudley 2009). However, by the early 1990s, the veterans' healthcare system had come to be perceived as very dysfunctional, fragmented, disjointed, and insensitive to individual veterans' needs. This popular sentiment was often captured in movies such as *Article 99* and *Born on the Fourth of July* (Kizer and Dudley 2009).

In 1991, the Physicians' Pay bill substantially raised physicians' salaries and helped attract high-quality staff to the VHA (Oliver 2007). Under the authority of the CHAMPUS Reform Initiative of 1988, several reforms were introduced in the CHAMPUS program and implemented in 1993. The thrust of the reform initiatives was to bring the military healthcare system in line with the emerging concept of managed care. The revised program was named TRICARE, and it incorporated financial practice management, and established provider networks for managed care in most healthcare delivered directly at military treatment facilities.

By 1994, a consensus had emerged that the veterans' healthcare system needed a major overhaul. A plan to dramatically transform the veterans' healthcare system was developed during 1994–1995 under the VHA leadership of Kenneth Kizer, who was appointed undersecretary for health, the chief executive officer of the VHA. Kizer wrote two reports. In *Vision for Change* (Kizer 1995), he outlined his vision for reorganizing the VHA. In *Prescription for Change* (Kizer 1996), he outlined the underlying principles and strategic objectives for accomplishing the transformation of the VHA. Based on these two reports, Congress in 1996 passed the Veterans Eligibility Reform Act, which went into effect on October 1, 1998.

Under the Veterans Eligibility Reform Act, veterans' benefits were expanded. For example, it made the VHA more accessible for the nonindigent and for those without service-related disabilities, and it also offered access to pharmaceuticals in outpatient care. The VHA keeps the cost of prescription drugs low by using its bargaining powers with pharmaceutical companies. Ironically, the Centers for Medicare and Medicaid Services are explicitly prohibited by congressional law from bargaining with drug companies for lower prices for Medicare and Medicaid patients (Oliver 2007).

The Veterans Eligibility Reform Act dramatically changed the VHA. It relied on five major strategies to bring about the change. First, to create an accountable management structure and management control system within the VHA, the law established 22 Veterans Integrated Service Networks (VISN), implemented a new performance management system, and decentralized decision-making. Second, to integrate and coordinate services, the VHA created a number of primary-care projects and changed its focus from inpatient hospital care to outpatient care for veterans in any medically appropriate setting. Third, to improve the quality of care received by veterans, a performance-based management system was implemented and promoted the use of evidence-based clinical guidelines. Also, a Patient Safety Initiative was launched in 1997. Fourth, to align system finances to desired outcomes, a new global fee-based resource reallocation system called the Veterans Equitable Resource Allocation (VERA) was developed to allocate funds based on actual service needs to VISNs and not to individual hospitals or clinics. Fifth, to modernize its information system, the VHA upgraded its information technology infrastructure and implemented a nationwide Computerized Patient Record System (CPRS) platform in 1997. When the CPRS was combined with a new graphical interface, the VHA's new electronic health record (EHR) became known as the Veterans Health Information System and Technology Architecture or VistA. The CPRS/VistA was implemented in all VHA medical centers over the years (Kizer and Dudley 2009). All these changes transformed the VHA into a model integrated healthcare system. Research evidence points to the improved quality of care and clinical performance, higher levels of service satisfaction, greater operational efficiency, an improved information management system, and improved research and education programs (Kizer and Dudley 2009).

In October 2000, the National Institutes of Medicine issued a report linking exposure to Agent Orange (an herbicide used by the US military in Vietnam) to the onset of diabetes among Vietnam veterans. In response to this report, the VA defined diabetes as a service-connected disability for veterans who served in the Vietnam War beginning in 2001. The defining of diabetes as a service-connected disability does not apply to Vietnam-era veterans who did not serve in Vietnam. This policy change increased the number of Vietnam veterans enrolled in the veteran's disability compensation program (Duggan, Rosenheck, and Singleton 2010).

The Patient Protection and Affordable Care Act of 2010, also known as the Affordable Care Act (ACA) was created to expand access to healthcare, control costs, and improve the quality of care. The ACA does not impact VA healthcare benefits or veterans' out-of-pocket costs. Those who are enrolled in VA healthcare do not need to take any additional steps to meet the law's new coverage standards. Veterans not enrolled in VA healthcare can apply to enroll at any time. The VA is required by law to notify the IRS of veterans' enrollment status in the VA's healthcare system. Family members of veterans who are not enrolled in the VA healthcare program and who do not meet healthcare law coverage standards can use the insurance marketplace exchange to get coverage ("What is the Affordable Care Act?" n.d.).

In 2010, an estimated 1.5 million veterans had no health insurance, including VA coverage. Uninsured veterans are more likely to be young and poorer and they have less access to needed healthcare. Two provisions under the ACA can help uninsured veterans gain health coverage. First, veterans with income of less than 138 percent of the federal poverty level could be eligible for Medicaid coverage, and, second, veterans can gain private insurance coverage via the Health Insurance Marketplace. In addition, veterans with an income of between 128 and 400 percent of the federal poverty level may also be eligible to receive premium subsidies in the Health Insurance Marketplace. Thus, the ACA has the potential to decrease the number of uninsured veterans (Silva et al. 2016).

The initial data on the effect of the ACA on reducing the number of uninsured veterans are very encouraging. The number of new enrollees in the health insurance marketplace from the low-income priority group of veterans increased significantly during the open enrollment period between 2013 and 2014. Also, Medicaid expansion states experienced a somewhat higher increase in new VA enrollment than the non-expansion states. This may be due to the fact that in non-expansion states, low-income veterans could meet the ACA's mandate by enrolling in VA or obtaining insurance through the health insurance marketplace (Silva et al. 2016). Two years after the implementation of the ACA, nearly half-a-million veterans under the age of 65 gained health coverage. This represents a 40-percent drop in veterans without health insurance between 2013 and 2015. The Veterans with the lowest income saw the greatest increase in health insurance coverage. The uninsured rate among non-elderly veterans fell from 9.1 percent in 2013 to 5.8 percent in 2015 (Boddy 2015; Dworsky, Farmer, and Shen 2017).

In response to the long delays veterans faced in getting appointments at VA health facilities and to address the problem of access, Congress in 2014 passed the Veterans Access, Choice, and Accountability Act. The Act provided new funding, authorities, and other tools to support and reform the VA. The law established A "Veterans Choice Fund" to implement a Veterans Choice Program. The program was designed to operate for three years or until the fund is exhausted. Under the program, veterans who enrolled as of August 1, 2014 and who are unable to schedule an appointment within 30 days of their preferred date or a clinically appropriate date, or live more than 40 miles' driving distance from the nearest VA facility, can elect to receive care from eligible non-VA healthcare facilities or providers. The law allowed roughly 1.7 million veterans to receive care from private-sector providers. The eligible non-VA entities or providers must enter into an agreement with the VA to furnish care; they must maintain similar credentials and licenses as VA providers. This is a separate program from the VA's existing programs that provide veteran care outside of the VA system. The law also called for the establishment of an independent commission to undertake a comprehensive evaluation and assessment of access to healthcare at VA facilities (Sheetz and Shulkin 2018; "Veterans Access, Choice, and Accountability Act of 2014" n.d.).

Despite this new effort, the problem of waiting times and delays in getting access to needed healthcare continues, and calls for more private-sector competition to the VA remains (Lee and Bagley 2017; Sheetz and Shulkin 2018; Shulkin 2017). The 2016 Inspector General's report indicated that despite Congressional attention and funding provided for the Veterans Choice Fund, problems of long wait times and difficulty in accessing healthcare services by veterans remained a problem for two main reasons. First, since the VA was given only 90 days to set up the new private-sector choice system, the VA used private-sector providers that already had ongoing contracts with the VA, whether or not they were the best choice for the new work. The VA and the contractors each blamed the other for delays in providing required authorization and changing the requirement on short notice. Also, private-sector providers complained of the VA's delay in processing claims and making prompt payment, i.e., reimbursements. The second reason was the increased demand for services by veterans (Wilensky 2016).

The VA Mission Act of 2018 attempts to address some of these concerns. The law would combine the VA's seven community care programs into one and extend the Veterans Choice Program for one year while the VA implements the consolidated community care program. The law injected an additional 5.2 billion into the Veterans Choice Program, under which veterans can obtain healthcare from non-VA providers, including county-owned and supported healthcare facilities. The law also expanded the circumstances under which veterans can obtain care from non-VA healthcare providers. It also established a prompt payment standard system to make sure that non-VA providers are reimbursed promptly for services rendered to veterans. Finally, the law authorized the secretary of the VA to enter into consolidated and competitively bid contracts to establish provider networks to ensure sufficient access to healthcare services (Igleheart 2018; Waxman 2018).

THE VETERANS HEALTH ADMINISTRATION

Mission

The Veterans Health Administration (VHA) has a fivefold mission. Its primary mission is to provide medical care to eligible veterans, especially those with service-connected health conditions. Its second mission is to train healthcare professionals. The VHA's third mission is to conduct medical research in basic biomedical sciences, rehabilitation, health service delivery, and quality of care aimed at improving care for veterans. The fourth mission is to provide contingency support to the military healthcare system and to the Department of Homeland Security. The fifth mission of the VHA is to serve homeless veterans (Kizer, Demakis, and Feussner 2000; Kizer and Dudley 2009).

Organization and Structure

The Department of Veterans Affairs (DVA) includes three administrative offices—the Veterans Health Administration, the Veterans Benefits Administration, and the National Cemetery Administration. The deputy secretary of the DVA is the second in command and serves as the chief executive officer of the VHA. Various program offices within the VHA help carry out the mission of the agency. The Office of Academic Affiliations provides information for VA staff, clinical trainees, and other learning organizations about VHA higher education programs. The National Center for Ethics addresses complex problems pertaining to ethical issues that arise in patient care and research. The Office of Health Information supports the computer information needs of VHA clinical and administrative staff. The Office of the Medical Inspector examines healthcare issues raised by veterans and conducts surveys. The Office of Patient Care Services oversees the VHA's clinical programs. The National Center for Patient Safety deals with patient safety issues. The Office of Public Health protects the health of veterans through research and new initiatives. The Office of Policy and Planning coordinates various aspects of national health policy development and programs. The Office of Quality and Performance supports the VHA mission of providing high-quality care to veterans. The Office of Research and Development publishes research articles and reports. The Office of Research Oversight oversees safety and protection of human subjects in research activities. Finally, the financial staff deals with budget formulation and execution of VHA programs ("VHA Program Offices" n.d.).

The VHA is the United States' largest integrated healthcare system, providing comprehensive healthcare at 1,243 healthcare facilities to about 9 million enrolled veterans every year out of a total veteran population of around 20 million. The VHA's healthcare system consists of 172 medical centers (VA hospitals), about 1,062 community-based outpatient clinics, 300 VA Vet Centers, plus many community living centers and domiciliaries. There are 23 Veterans Integrated Service Networks (VISN) located throughout the country. Medical centers/VA hospitals provide traditional hospital-based services such as surgery, critical care, mental health, pharmacy, and radiology. Many medical centers offer additional medical and surgical specialty services such as audiology and speech pathology, dermatology, dental, geriatrics, neurology, oncology, podiatry, prosthetics, urology, and vision care ("About VHA" n.d.).

Community-based outpatient clinics provide common outpatient services such as health and wellness visits. Community living centers are essentially skilled nursing facilities. Vet Centers provide readjustment counseling and outreach services to veterans who served in combat zones. Domiciliaries provide medical, psychiatric, vocational, educational, and other services to veterans in a homelike setting. These facilities employ more than 53,000 independent licensed healthcare practitioners. The United States is divided into 22 Veterans Integrated Service Networks, that is, regional healthcare centers ("About VHA" n.d.).

In 1988, the Women Veterans Health Program was established to streamline services for women veterans. As part of the realignment of the Veterans Health Administration, effective March 27, 2011, Women's Health became part of the Office of Patient Care Services (PCS). The name of the program office was changed to Women's Health Services in August 2012. Women's Health Services addresses the healthcare needs of women veterans. It works to ensure that timely, equitable, high-quality, comprehensive healthcare services are provided to women veterans in a sensitive and safe environment at VA health facilities nationwide. At present, women veterans constitute about 8.6 percent of the total veteran population, and this number is on the rise ("About the Women Veterans Health Care Program" n.d.).

TRANSITIONING FROM TRICARE TO VA HEALTHCARE

TRICARE is the Department of Defense's government-managed health insurance available worldwide and is considered the gold standard for medical coverage. The programs' beneficiaries include (1) active-duty service members, National Guards, reserves, military retirees, and survivors of deceased service members, and (2) eligible family members, i.e., spouses and children registered in the Defense Eligibility Enrollment Reporting System (DEERS). TRICARE provides several health plan options and provides healthcare, dental, and pharmacy services. Some of the major TRICARE health plans include TRICARE Prime, TRICARE Select, TRICARE for Reserve and Guard. TRICARE Prime is a managed care option available in the prime service area and active-duty service members are required to enroll in this plan. This plan offers fewer out-of-pocket costs but less freedom of choice in providers. Those active-duty service members who do not live in the prime service area have the option to enroll in other prime options. TRICARE Select is a fee-for-service insurance plan that allows enrollees the freedom of choice in doctors. This plan is available to family members, veterans, and retirees and is available worldwide. TRICARE for Reserve and Guard provides some of the same benefits as those offered to active-duty members while other benefits are different. TRICARE Reserve Select is a premium-based health insurance program that is also available worldwide ("TRICARE" n.d.).

Since its creation, TRICARE has undergone several changes, including realignment of TRICARE contract regions for better coordination and delivery of services; base realignment and closure; the addition of TRICARE for Life benefits for Medicare-eligible individuals; and expansion of the program to military reservists (Jackonis, Deyton, and Hess 2008). In 2018, TRICARE Standard and TRICARE Extra plans were combined into a new TRICARE Select plan including some new regions and contractors ("Major Tricare Changes Kicked Off Jan. 1" 2017).

When service members leave active duty, they may be eligible for benefits offered by TRICARE as well as the VA. A retiring service member is eligible for TRICARE as a military retiree and may also be eligible for VA healthcare benefits. Service members who separate from the military due to service-connected disease or injury may be eligible for VA healthcare benefits as well as certain TRICARE benefits. Once active-duty service members have received their separation and/or retirement orders, they can transition from TRICARE by applying for enrollment in the VA healthcare system ("Active Duty Servicemembers: Transitioning from TRICARE to VA Health Care" n.d.).

THE VA HEALTHCARE SYSTEM

Eligibility and Enrollment

In principle, all veterans are eligible for lifetime VA medical treatment, but in reality, of the total veteran population of about 20 million, only about 9 million veterans (about 45 percent) are enrolled in the veterans' healthcare system. While the total veteran population has been declining since 1986, the number of veterans with a service-connected disability has increased from around 2.3 million to about 3.8 million by 2014, an increase of 60 percent ("Trends in Veterans with a Service-Connected Disability: 1985 to 2014" 2015).

It is also important to remember that many veterans constitute a dual-enrolled population, that is, they can be enrolled in a veterans' health benefits program and at the same time can be enrolled in a Medicaid program if they are poor and meet Medicaid's eligibility criteria. Similarly, since many veterans are older than 65 years of age, they can be enrolled in veterans' health benefits as well as Medicare. The Medicaid program plays a major role in covering veterans. Since 2015, Medicaid has covered one in ten veterans between the ages of 19 and 64. In 2015, among the 10 percent of veterans covered by Medicaid, 39 percent had Medicaid as their only source of coverage while 41 percent supplemented their Medicaid coverage with veterans' health coverage, 11 percent with Medicare coverage, and 9 percent with private coverage ("Medicaid's Role in Covering Veterans" 2017).

Basic eligibility for VA health benefits includes any individual who served in the active military, naval, or air service and who was discharged and released honorably. Active service means full-time service. Certain benefits require wartime service. Reservists and national guards may also qualify if they were called to active duty by a federal order and completed the full period for which they were called or ordered to active duty. Veterans who enlisted after September 7, 1980, and entered active duty after October 16, 1981, must have served 24 continuous months or the full period for which they were called to active duty in order to be eligible ("Federal Benefits for Veterans, Dependents and Survivors" 2017).

Applying for enrollment is the first step of entry into the VA health system for most veterans. Once enrolled, veterans can receive health services at any VA healthcare facility in the country. During enrollment, each veteran is assigned a priority group. This is done in order to balance demand with resources. The priority groups range from one to eight, with priority group one receiving the highest priority and priority group eight receiving the lowest priority for enrollment. Priority groups are based on factors such as severity of service-connected disability, household income, prisoner-of-war (POW) status, veterans awarded service-related medals, and certain health conditions related to service in combat. For example, priority group one consists of veterans with service-connected disabilities rated 50 percent or more and determined to be unemployable due to their disabilities, while priority group eight includes veterans with gross household income above the VA national income limit and the geographically adjusted income limit for their resident location and who agree to pay co-payments ("Federal Benefits for Veterans, Dependents and Survivors" 2017).

Four categories of veterans who are not required to enroll but are urged to enroll for better planning of healthcare resources include: (1) veterans with a service-connected disability of 50 percent or more; (2) veterans seeking care for a disability incurred or aggravated in the line of duty within 12 months of discharge but who have not been yet rated; (3) veterans seeking care for a service-connected disability only; and (4) veterans seeking care for registry examination for exposure to ionizing radiation or Agent Orange, depleted uranium, or who served in Gulf War/Operation Iraqi Freedom ("Federal Benefits for Veterans, Dependents and Survivors" 2017).

Benefits and Services

The VA provides a comprehensive health benefits package to all enrolled veterans. It includes a full range of preventive outpatient and inpatient health services within the VA healthcare system. Once enrolled, a veteran can seek health services at any VA facility in the country. All VA patients receive comprehensive care from a primary-care team. Throughout the country, VA healthcare facilities offer a broad range of medical, surgical, and rehabilitative care for acute and chronic health conditions. A variety of specialized care suited for individual needs of the patient is also offered, such as prosthetic devices, rehabilitative services for spinal cord injury, posttraumatic stress disorder, psychological counseling for war-related trauma, as well as rehabilitative services for veterans suffering from alcoholism, drug abuse, and homelessness (Vandenberg, Bergofsky, and Burris 2010).

Outpatient services covered by VA include medical, surgical, and mental health including substance abuse. VA inpatient care includes services such as medical, surgical, mental health, dialysis, acute care, and access to specialized care units such as intensive care, transplant services, traumatic brain injury, spinal cord injury centers, and polytrauma centers. In addition, other services covered by the VA include prescription drugs, bereavement counseling, medical equipment and prosthetic and orthotic devices, medically necessary reconstructive plastic surgery, and home healthcare, along with preventive care immunization, periodic medical exams, screening tests, and the like. A variety of other programs that veterans may be eligible for include blindness rehabilitation, posttraumatic stress, HIV/AIDs treatment, and radiation treatment, among others. Services typically excluded from the medical benefit package include abortion and abortion counseling, non-medically necessary cosmetic surgery, health club and spa membership, in-vitro fertilization, and drug, biological, and medical devices not approved by the Food and Drug Administration (FDA) ("Veterans Health Benefits" n.d.; "Veterans Medical Benefit Package" n.d.).

The VA also maintains several health registries, and certain veterans can participate in a VA health registry and receive free medical examinations that include laboratory and other diagnostic tests considered necessary by the examining health clinician. For example, the Gulf War Registry was established for veterans who served on active military duty in Southwest Asia during the Gulf War. It was established to identify possible diseases resulting from serving in that part of the world. Similarly, the Agent Orange Registry was established for veterans possibly exposed to dioxin and other toxic substances in herbicides used during the Vietnam War. Other health registries maintained by the VA include the Depleted Uranium Registry and the Ionizing Radiation Registry ("Health Benefits: Federal Benefits for Veterans, Dependents, and Survivors" n.d.).

For older veterans, the VA provides a wide range of institutional and non-institutional long-term care services. Institutional long-term care is provided through VA Community Living Centers, that is, nursing homes, community nursing homes, state veterans' homes, and domiciliaries (Vandenberg, Bergofsky, and Burris 2010). In 1998, an expert external review of VA management of older veterans concluded that the system was much too dependent on institutional long-term care and recommended that the VA should make non-institutional care alternatives to long-term care widely available (Shay and Yoshikawa 2010). Today, older veterans have a broad range of non-institutional home and community-based services available to them, including hospice and palliative care, respite care, geriatric evaluation and management care, community residential care, home-based primary care, adult day healthcare, and homemaker/home health aide services (Vandenberg, Bergofsky, and Burris 2010).

The VA's Women Health Services Office addresses the healthcare needs of women veterans and offers gender-specific comprehensive primary care such as cervical cancer screens, breast cancer screens, birth control counseling, and hormone replacement therapy at every VA facility. Specialty care provided includes management and screening of chronic conditions such as heart disease, diabetes, and sexually transmitted diseases, along with reproductive healthcare including maternity care and infertility evaluation ("About VA Women's Health" n.d.).

The VA also provides a comprehensive range of health services for blind and visually impaired veterans, mental health services, a suicide prevention lifeline for veterans experiencing emotional distress/crisis, and outpatient dental care. Finally, under the Civilian Health and Medical Program of the Department of Veterans Affairs (CHAMPVA), certain dependents and survivors can receive reimbursement for most medical expenses ("Health Benefits: Federal Benefits for Veterans, Dependents, and Survivors" n.d.).

Health Benefits for Family Members of Veterans

Family members of veterans are eligible for health benefits under certain circumstances. Some of the programs offered include the Civilian Health and Medical Program of the Department of Veterans Affairs (CHAMPVA), the Spina Bifida Health Care Program (SB), Children of Women Vietnam Veterans (CWVV), Foreign Medical Program (FMP), Camp Lejeune Family Member Program (CLFMP), and Caregiver.

The CHAMPVA program provides health benefits coverage to the spouse or widow and dependent children of veterans who are or were rated permanently and totally disabled due to a service-connected disability, died of a service-connected disability or died on active duty, and if dependents are not eligible for TRICARE benefits. VA shares the cost of the covered healthcare services for eligible beneficiaries. The Spina Bifida Health Care Program is a health benefit program for Vietnam and certain Korean veterans' birth children who have been diagnosed with spina bifida (except spina bifida occulta). The program provides reimbursement for medical services and supplies. The CWVV Health Care Program is another health benefits program for children with certain birth defects born to women Vietnam veterans. The CWVV program is a fee-for-service (indemnity plan) program, which provides reimbursement for medical care-related conditions associated with certain birth defects, except for spina bifida, which is covered under the Spina Bifida Health Care Program. Both of these programs are administered by the Department of Veterans Affairs ("Health Benefits: Family Members of Veterans" n.d.).

The CLFMP is for family members of veterans who were stationed at Camp Lejeune between August 1, 1953 and December 31, 1987, who were potentially exposed to drinking water contaminated with industrial solvents, benzene, and other chemicals. The program reimburses eligible Camp Lejeune family members for healthcare costs related to one or more of the 15 specified illnesses or medical conditions. Finally, under the Caregiver program, caregivers of veterans of the war in Afghanistan, Operation Enduring Freedom (OEF), and the war in Iraq, Operation Iraqi Freedom (OIF), may be eligible to receive a stipend and access to health coverage if they are not entitled to care or service under a health plan contract including Medicaid, Medicare, unemployment compensation, and the like ("Health Benefits: Family Members of Veterans" n.d.).

THE HEALTH STATUS OF VETERANS

In front of the Department of Veterans Affairs building is inscribed President Abraham Lincoln's charge to the nation he laid out in his Second Inaugural Address, "to care for him who shall have borne the battle and for his widow and his orphan." As it relates to veterans' healthcare, it is an expression of the country's covenant with those who serve and have served, and has been the VA's motto for a long time. However, the current Veterans Health Administration (VHA) system is not funded to meet the needs of the entire veteran population. In reality, a multiplicity of healthcare and health insurance programs exist side by side with the VHA, like Medicaid, Medicare, private insurance, and the like, in which active-duty service members, retirees, their family members, and veterans may participate (Jackonis, Deyton, and Hess 2008). Veterans' health and their physical as well as mental well-being can be affected negatively by the type, intensity, and duration of their service and the transition from full-time military service to civilian life. A variety of factors connected to military services such as intensive physical activity, physical and psychological trauma, exposure to toxic substances, long-term and sustained exposure to loud noises, and the like can contribute to the development of physical, mental, and social health problems. Similarly, the transition from military to civilian life itself can contribute to the development of health problems among veterans who feel disconnected from civilian life due to the significant differences between the two worlds

(Fullwood 2015; Oster et al. 2017). For example, in a *Washington Post*/Kaiser Family Foundation survey of Iraq and Afghanistan active-duty soldiers and veterans, 69 percent expressed the feeling that average Americans did not understand their experiences and 55 percent indicated that they felt disconnected from civilian life. Forty-three percent indicated that their physical health and 31 percent indicated that their mental and emotional health were worse after the war than before the war ("Visualizing Health Policy: *The Washington Post*/Kaiser Family Foundation Survey of Iraq and Afghanistan Active Duty Soldiers and Veterans" 2014). In this section, we focus on the health status and health problems encountered by veterans.

Some of the major health problems facing veterans include musculoskeletal injuries and pain in their back, neck, knees, or shoulders, physical injuries and symptoms such as fatigue, cognitive disturbances, memory and concentration problems, autoimmune disorders, and diseases that occur when the immune system attacks healthy tissues, infectious diseases, hearing loss caused by exposure to loud noises from gunfire, aircraft, heavy weapons, etc., lung problems caused by exposure to chemicals and toxins, urological injuries caused by penetrating injuries to the groin area, mental health problems including depression, violent behavior, anger control, substance and alcohol abuse, and posttraumatic stress disorder (PTSD), traumatic brain injury (TBI), and physical and/or psychological trauma. Homelessness, which is found in high incidence among veterans, can also lead to numerous health issues (Bains n.d.; "Critical Issues Facing Veterans and Military Families" 2017; Goldberg 2013; Salamon 2010; White 2017).

Veterans as a whole are more likely to be homeless and to lack health insurance coverage than the general population. Factors responsible for this include difficulty in transitioning from military to civilian employment, higher incidence of mental health and substance abuse problems, and the fact that single men are generally ineligible for Medicaid. Homeless veterans tend to be male, non-Hispanic white, between the ages of 31 and 50, and disabled ("Profile of Sheltered Homeless Veterans for Fiscal Years 2009 and 2010" 2012). Veterans report higher rates of substance use and mental health problems as the primary cause of homelessness compared to non-veterans (Dunne et al. 2015). Homeless veterans have many health problems that can be classified into four categories: addiction, psychosis, vascular disorders, and generalized medical and psychiatric illness. Factors most closely associated with homelessness appear to be sociodemographic factors such as age, ethnicity, and employment status. Psychosis, especially schizophrenia and substance abuse, typically seem to precede the onset of homelessness. However, the stereotype that all homeless veterans suffer from PTSD or alcohol or drug abuse is not true. Some homeless veterans have a significant medical illness without accompanying the psychiatric disorder. Some have major substance abuse problems, while others have some form of mental illness. The health status of homeless veterans is a complex problem that defies a single explanation (Goldstein et al. 2010).

In 2010, veterans were overrepresented among the homeless population in the country. They accounted for 10 percent of the total population but composed about 13 percent of the sheltered homeless adults and 16 percent of the total homeless adult population ("Profile of Sheltered Homeless Veterans for Fiscal Years 2009 and 2010" 2012). In 2009, to address the problem of homeless veterans, the Veterans Administration announced an ambitious goal of ending homelessness among veterans. In 2010 the first comprehensive strategic plan to end homelessness, called "Opening Doors: Federal Strategic Plan to Prevent and End Homelessness," was presented to Congress, and was amended in 2012 and 2015 (United States Interagency Council on Homelessness 2015).

In 2018, the plan was updated and called, "Home, Together: The Federal Strategic Plan to Prevent and End Homelessness" (United States Interagency Council on Homelessness 2018). According to a report by the US Department of Housing and Urban Development (2017), the number of homeless veterans dropped from 74,087 in 2020 to 40,056 in 2017, a 45-percent drop. However, the number of homeless veterans increased by 585 between 2016 and 2017, and 40,056 veterans were experiencing homelessness in a single night. Ninety-one percent of the homeless veterans were men, and 57 percent were white. Veterans experiencing homelessness were twice as likely to be Hispanic. Between 2016 and 2017, the number of homeless veterans who were women increased by 7 percent compared to 1 percent for men, while the number of Hispanic veterans who were homeless increased by 9 percent. Thus, while considerable progress has been made in addressing the problem of homelessness among veterans, the problem still persists.

One of the consequences of war is the physical injuries suffered by soldiers in combat. The "war on terror" launched by the United States following the September 11, 2001 terrorist attack on the US has resulted in continuous combat that has lasted over a decade. Between 2011 and 2018, the US military conflicts/wars involving Operation Iraqi Freedom (OIF), Operation New Dawn (OND), Operation Enduring Freedom (OEF), Operation Inherent Resolve (OIR), and Operation Freedom's Sentinel (OFS) have resulted in 6941 military casualties and 52,682 have been wounded in action ("Department of Defense Casualties Report" 2018). Blast injuries resulting from the use of improvised explosive devices (IEDs) by the enemy have included loss of limbs, traumatic brain injuries, and severe burns suffered by soldiers. The number of soldiers suffering from a service-related disability has also increased dramatically along with the cost of the disability compensation program. The proportion of veterans with service-connected disabilities who used VA healthcare services increased from 58.9 percent in 2007 to 69.6 percent in 2016 ("VA Utilization Profile: FY 2016" 2017).

Among the many consequences of war are the psychological stress and toll that soldiers suffer. One of the unique features of the Global War on Terror (GWOT) includes multiple, longer, and indeterminate deployment resulting in greater risk of developing mental health problems. According to a study, more than one-third of the US Army and Marine troops have consulted mental health professionals after returning from Iraq, and 19 percent screened positive for mental health concerns (Hoge, Auchterlonie, and Milliken 2006). Forty-nine percent of National Guard service members, 38 percent of the Army, and 31 percent of the Marines reported suffering from psychological symptoms within 120 days of returning from combat. According to a task force appointed by the Pentagon, as many as one-half of active-duty and reserve troops deployed to combat zones reported various mental health symptoms, including possible posttraumatic stress disorder (PTSD) and traumatic brain injury (TBI) ("An Achievable Vision" 2007).

One of the often-invisible wounds of combat is PTSD, which is an anxiety disorder resulting from an overwhelming or dangerous event. PTSD is associated with flashbacks, emotional numbness, depression, insomnia, and angry outbursts. According to the VHA, 286,134 veterans of the wars in Iraq and Afghanistan had been seen for possible PTSD at the end of 2012. This number does not include those diagnosed and treated outside of the VA health system. A study of about 290,000 veterans of the GWOT treated at the VA health system between 2002 and 2008 found that 37 percent had been diagnosed with mental health problems such as PTSD and depression (Baker 2014).

Another serious and invisible potential result of the GWOT is a traumatic brain injury (TBI), an injury that may not show up on physical examination but can be found during surgical exploration or through imaging scans that can result in significant disability. TBI can be anything from a major head injury to a mild concussion. However, even mild TBI can lead to cumulative health problems. The symptoms associated with TBI can include headaches, confusion, problems with concentration, and attention deficits, among others. Since the year 2000, nearly 300,000 TBIs have been diagnosed in US service members worldwide. About 89 percent of these can be classified as mild in severity. Veterans of OEF and OIF are more susceptible to such injuries due to exposure to blasts from mines, roadside bombs, and improvised explosive devices (Amara et al. 2014). Based on self-reported data, around 15 percent of the troops engaged in active combat in Iraq and Afghanistan could have suffered TBI. Thirty-three present of combat-related injuries and 60 percent of blast-related injuries seen at Walter Reed Army National Medical Center had sustained TBI (Baker 2014). The Department of Defense has documented almost 250,000 cases of TBI since the year 2000 and more than 60 TBI programs have been created at military medical treatment facilities at US bases to address the problem (Rizzo 2012). The societal cost of TBI has been estimated at around $590 to $910 million across all levels of severity. The one-year cost associated with the treatment of TBI has been estimated at around $32,000 (Kulas and Rosenheck 2018).

Some of the consequences of veterans suffering from PTSD or TBI are that they often have difficulty completing school, holding jobs, keeping the family together, and are often more likely to become homeless. They are also more likely to engage in risky behavior such as substance abuse, fighting, drunk-driving, and smoking. For example, the rates of substance abuse among veterans diagnosed with PTSD range from 21 to 35 percent (Baker 2014).

Studies also indicate that TBI may increase the risk of suicide because of depression (Gradus et al. 2015). According to the VHA, there are 18 suicides per day among the entire veteran population and 1000 suicide attempts per month among all veterans seen at VHA medical facilities (Baker 2014). Sixteen percent of veterans reported unmet mental healthcare needs and 18 percent reported having thoughts of suicide (Becerra et al. 2016). The rate of suicide among those serving in the military has been on the rise. A mental health diagnosis is a very strong suicide risk factor (Hyman et al. 2012). In 2008, the DVA implemented a suicide event reporting system designed to collect standardized information on all suicide attempts reported to VA clinicians. Since then, the VA has collected information on about 46,000 suicide attempts ("Surveillance of Suicide and Suicide Attempts Among Veterans" 2012). Preventing suicide has become a high-priority issue for the military and specifically the VHA, given the fact that the rate of suicide among active-duty soldiers has doubled since 2005 ("Preventing Suicide by Preventing Lethal Injury" 2012). Furthermore, a new pattern emerged in 2012 when there were more suicides among veteran soldiers than among younger GIs (Zoroya 2012).

A study that examined the mental and physical health of veterans within one year of returning from war zone deployment found that their mental health functioning was significantly worse compared with the general population. Almost 14 percent screened positive for probable posttraumatic stress disorder, 39 percent for probable alcohol abuse, and 3 percent for probable drug abuse. Men reported more alcohol and drug abuse than women (Eisen et al. 2012).

In 2016, women veterans comprised about 8.6 percent of the total veteran population, a number that is projected to increase to over 16 percent by the year 2037. Thus, the health status of female veterans and their health service needs have become an important topic in the veterans' healthcare system. Women have been involved in many military conflicts in a variety of roles, and they have suffered deaths and injuries just like their male counterparts. Overall, most women veterans report good to excellent health. However, evidence suggests that for female veterans, military service is associated with increased risks of suffering from a variety of physical conditions and illnesses.

Military sexual trauma (MST) is the term the DVA uses to refer to sexual assault or repeated threatening sexual harassment that occurs during military service. This includes any sexual activity against one's will, being pressured into sexual activity, and events where an individual may have been unable to consent to sexual activity or may have been physically forced into sexual activity ("VA Services for Military Sexual Trauma: Help, Hope, Healing" n.d.). For women veterans, in-service sexual assaults and sexual harassment have long-term health implications. Research shows that psychosocial health complications of sexual assault include increased risk of suicide, depression, alcohol and drug abuse, sexual dysfunction, and PTSD. Similarly, in-service sexual harassment is also demonstrated to be related to adverse psychiatric outcomes such as depression, anxiety, and PTSD. Women veteran VA patients also suffer as heavy a burden of physical and mental illness as do men in the VA system (Frayne et al. 2006; Murdoch et al. 2006). Sexual harassment is also associated with many later mental health symptoms including PTSD and anxiety (Carlson, Stromwall, and Lietz 2013).

According to the latest estimate, MST is a significant health issue faced by today's younger female veterans returning from Iraq and Afghanistan, with about one in five women being traumatized while serving in the military. National data from the VA's National Screening Program, in which every veteran who is seen for healthcare is asked whether he or she experienced MST, reveal that one in four women and 1 in 100 men reported that they had experienced MST ("Military Sexual Trauma" 2015). Women veterans who experienced MST are not only at higher risk for gynecological issues but have a 60-percent greater risk of developing mental health issues (Cramer n.d.). MST is also associated with chronic pain conditions among female veterans (Cichowski, Rogers, and Clark 2017). Also, in the nationally sourced sample of 4544 female veterans, 25.5 percent reported medically diagnosed depression conditions varying from mild to severe (Sairsingh et al. 2018; Thomas et al. 2016). Military sexual harassment is also found to be significantly associated with emotional problems during pregnancy and postpartum (Miller and Ghadiali 2018).

FUNDING AND EXPENDITURES OF THE VA AND VHA

The VA is financed through the regular annual congressional appropriations process. The VA's total budget can be divided into three parts. The mandatory budget consists of funding for benefits mandated by law. This includes things such as disability compensation, pensions, educational benefits, vocational rehabilitation, and employment benefits. These mandatory benefits are administered by the Veterans Benefit Administration (VBA). The discretionary budget consists of things such as medical care programs, information technology, discretionary benefit programs, construction of VA facilities, and administration. Programs funded under the discretionary budget are primarily administered by the Veterans Health Administration (VHA) and medical care/health benefits make up the largest part of the discretionary budget. The third (and a relatively minor) part of the VA's total budget is made up of what is called the Medical Care Collection Fund (MCCF). The MCCF was established under the Balanced Budget Act of 1997 and it authorizes the VA to bill reasonable charges for health services provided to veterans by private healthcare providers. The MCCF supplements congressional appropriations to help finance the cost of providing medical care to veterans ("Audit of the Medical Care Collection Fund Program" 2002; Auerbach, Weeks, and Brantley 2013).

The 2014–2015 overall annual average healthcare expenditure per veteran was $9,338 for all veterans, $12,411 for VA users, and $7,525 for non-VA users. Thus, the average medical expenditure per veteran was 65-percent higher for VA users than non-VA users. Among VA service users, of the total medical expenditures, 36 percent went for hospital inpatient stays, 24.2 percent went for office-based provider visits, 16.7 percent went for prescription medicine, 9.7 percent went for outpatient hospital visits, and the remaining 13.4 percent went for other services (Machlin and Muhuri n.d.).

Table 6.4 provides some data on the budget for the VA and VHA, and where most of the expenditures of the VA and VHA are concentrated. The VA's total budget has grown from $163 billion in 2015 to $186 billion in 2018. In 2018, the VHA's medical care budget of $72.3 billion accounted for 39 percent of the total VA budget.

Table 6.4

The VA's Budget, FY 2015–2019 (in $ billions)

	2015	2016	2017[a]	2018[b]	2019[c]
Mandatory	95.1	92.5	104.3	104.3	109.7
Discretionary	65.1	70.9	74.3	78.8	85.5
MCCF[d]	3.2	3.5	3.5	3.3	3.4
Total	163.4	166.9	182.1	186.4	198.6
% Increase from previous year		2.1	8.3	2.3	6.1
VHA medical care budget			68.0	72.3	76.5
% of VA budget			37	39	39
Compensation/pension budget			86.1	90.1	97.2
% of VA budget			47	48	49
% Total medical care/compensation/pension			84	87	88

Notes: a = actual; b = estimate; c = requested; d = Medical Care Collection Fund.
Sources: "Department of Veterans Affairs—Budget in Brief 2019." Congressional Submission. Online at www.va.gov/budget/docs/summary/fy2019VAbudgetInBrief.pdf.

Also, in 2018, of the VA's discretionary budget of $78.8 billion, spending for medical care accounted for $72.3 billion. In other words, 92 percent of the VA's discretionary budget goes toward spending for medical care. Similarly, of the VA's mandatory budget of $104.3 billion in 2018, $90.1 billion (48 percent) was payment for disability compensation and pensions. Finally, it is also worth noting that in 2018, spending for veterans' medical care and disability compensation/pensions combined accounted for 87 percent of the total VA budget.

The 2019 VA budget request represents a 6.1-percent increase from the 2018 budget. The increase is designed to enable the VA to deliver healthcare to 9.3 million veterans enrolled in the VA's healthcare system. In addition, the increase in the budget request is also to modernize the VA's electronic health record system to improve the quality of care, expand mental health services, strengthen the VA's infrastructure, and to meet the anticipated increase in the number of patient visits/treatment and outpatient visits. For example, the 2019 budget requests $8.6 billion for veterans' mental health services, an increase of 5.8 percent over the 2018 estimate, of which $190 million would go toward suicide prevention outreach ("Department of Veterans Affairs—Budget in Brief 2019" n.d.).

VETERANS' USE OF BENEFITS AND SERVICES

Not all veterans are automatically eligible for VA healthcare. Of those who are eligible, not all use VA services. Some rely primarily on the VA to meet their healthcare needs, while others rely on multiple public and private sources for health coverage. Some veterans remain uninsured and without any health coverage.

Under current VA policy, around 60 percent of veterans are eligible for VA care based on the length of their service, service-connected injuries and/or disability, service in designated combat areas, and income. Fewer than half of eligible veterans use VA health benefits and a majority of those who use VA care also have other sources of care, such as Medicare, Medicaid, or private health insurance (Farmer, Hosek, and Adamson 2016).

In 2010, about 5 million US veterans did not have any health insurance coverage, including VA coverage. The Affordable Care Act helped extend health coverage to uninsured veterans. This is demonstrated in two ways. First, the number of enrollees from low-income priority groups increased markedly during the open enrollment period between 2013 and 2014, and, second, Medicaid non-expansion states experienced slightly higher percentage increases in the new enrollment of veterans than Medicaid expansion states. This can be explained by the fact that low-income veterans in non-expansion states could meet the ACA's individual mandate by enrolling in VA or obtaining insurance in the marketplace exchanges. While the ACA helped extend coverage to many low-income veterans, one of the concerns it raises is the possibility that veterans' reliance on multiple sources of coverage can make coordination of health services more difficult and can lead to increased fragmentation of healthcare (Silva et al. 2016).

Table 6.5 provides a profile of veterans' utilization of VA benefits and services. In 2016, 9.7 million veterans (47.5 percent) used at least one VA benefit (not limited to health benefits) while 10.7 million (52.5 percent) did not use any VA benefits. Of all the program benefits offered by the VA, an overwhelming majority of veterans (7.5 percent) relied heavily on two benefits, healthcare and disability compensation/pension, while all other program benefits were used by only 24.5 percent. Among veterans with a service-connected disability, 69.7 percent enrolled in the VA health system and used health benefits, while 23.8 percent enrolled but did not use health benefits; another 6.6 percent did not enroll. Also, among veterans with a service-connected disability, blacks/African-Americans, American Indians and Alaska Natives, Native Hawaiians/Pacific Islanders, and Hispanics used healthcare benefits in higher numbers compared to whites, Asians, and other races.

Some other trends to note with respect to veterans and use of VA benefits are the following. First, as the number of women serving in the armed forces has increased, so has the number of female veterans and their use of VA benefits. For example, the presence of female veterans who used VA benefits increased from 35 percent in 2007 to 47 percent in 2016. Second, veterans between the ages of 25 and 34 and over the age of 65 are more

Table 6.5

Veterans Administration Utilization Profile, 2016

Number of Veterans Who Used/Did Not Use VA Benefits	Millions
Used at least one benefit	9.7
Did not use any benefits	10.7
Number of Veterans Using Benefit by Programs	Millions
Healthcare	6.0
Compensation/pensions	4.6
Loan guarantee	2.6
Life insurance	1.1
Education	0.7
Memorial benefits	0.3
Vocational rehab	0.1
Breakdown of Veterans' Use of Program Benefits	%
Healthcare or disability compensation	75.5
All other benefits	24.5
Service-Connected Diasabled Veterans	%
Enrolled and used healthcare	69.6
Enrolled but did not use healthcare	23.8
Not enrolled	6.6
Use of Health Care by Service-Connected Disabled Veterans by Race	%
White	68.1
Asian	64.1
Black/African-American	75.6
Native Hawaiian/Pacific Islander	74.4
American Indian/Alaska Native	74.3
Hispanic	72.1
Other	69.8

Source: "VA Untilization Profile: FY 2016" 2017. National Center for Veterans Analysis and Statistics. US Department of Veterans Affairs. Online at www.va.gov/vetdata/docs/Quickfacts/VA_Utilization_Profile.pdf.

likely to use VA benefits than veterans of other ages. Third, black/African-American and Hispanic veterans are more likely to use VA benefits than any other racial groups. Fourth, VA patients have a higher prevalence of serious health conditions compared to other veterans (non-VA) and non-veterans (general population). For example, 25 percent of VA patients suffer from mental health issues compared to 13 percent of non-VA veterans and 18 percent of non-veterans. Similarly, 19 percent of VA patients suffer from cancer compared to 11 percent of non-VA patients, and 5 percent of non-veterans. Fifth, despite a steady decline in the veteran population, the number of veterans who use VA healthcare has increased. For example, in 1995, the total veteran population was 27.9 million but only 2.5 million (9 percent) were VA patients. In 2014, the veteran population has declined to 21.6 million but the number of VA patients had increased to 5.9 million (27 percent). One of the reasons for this is the increase in the number of veterans with service-connected disabilities resulting from the Global War on Terror (Farmer, Hosek, and Adamson 2016; "VA Utilization Profile FY 2016" 2017).

Service-connected disability means that the disability was a result of disease or injury incurred or aggravated during active military service. The severity of a veteran's disability is evaluated by the Department of Veterans Affairs and disability ratings are graduated based on the degree of the veteran's disability on a scale of 0 to 100 percent in increments of 10 percent ("Trends in Veterans with a Service-Connected Disability: 1985 to 2014" 2015). With respect to service-connected disability and VA benefits, certain facts stand out. First, healthcare and disability compensation account for the largest share of VA utilization. Second, the number of service-connected disability veterans using VA healthcare increased from 59 percent in 2007 to 70 percent in 2016. In fact, over 90 percent of service-connected disabled veterans were enrolled in the VAH health system regardless of whether they used VA healthcare or not. Third, the likelihood of veterans with a service-connected disability seeking VA healthcare increases with a higher disability rating. Fourth, the likelihood of a disabled veteran seeking VA healthcare varies by race and ethnicity with blacks/African-Americans, American Indians and Alaska Natives, Native Hawaiians and Pacific Islander, and Hispanics more likely to seek treatment from VA facilities compared to whites and Asians ("VA Utilization Profile FY 2016" 2017). Fifth, while the veteran population has been declining since 1986, the number of veterans with a service-connected disability has been on the rise. Since 1990, there has been a 60-percent increase in the number of veterans with a service-connected disability. Sixth, the rate of increase in cash payment for disability compensation is outpacing the growth in the number of veterans with a service-connected disability. Seventh, the growth in the number of veterans with a service-connected disability is concentrated among those rated 50 percent or higher, i.e., more severe disability ("Trends in Veterans with a Service-Connected Disability: 1985 to 2014" 2015). This will place more strain on the VA budget.

A HISTORY OF SCANDALS AT THE VETERANS ADMINISTRATION

The Veterans Administration has many accomplishments to its credit, especially in the areas of research and development dealing with medical advances in prosthetics, new surgical and treatment techniques, and rehabilitation. Veterans' hospitals have also been an excellent training ground for America's future doctors ("Timeline of Accomplishments" n.d.). Yet, the VA's history has also been tainted by a variety of scandals spanning its history.

When the Veterans Bureau was created in 1921, its first director, Colonel Charles R. Forbes, was relieved of his job and later sent to prison for conspiracy to defraud the government on hospital contracts ("VA History in Brief" n.d.). In 1930 the Veterans Administration was established to replace the troubled Veterans Bureau. In 1932 federal troops were used to forcibly remove veterans of World War I and their families who had marched to Washington, DC to demand payment of promised war bonuses. In 1945, after a series of new reports dealing with shoddy care in VA hospitals were published, the VA administrator, Frank Hines, was forced to resign. Two government reform commissions in 1947 and 1955 found tremendous waste, duplication, and widespread instances of poor care of veterans in the VA system. In 1974, Ron Kovic, a Vietnam veteran and subject of a book and movie titled "Born on the Fourth of July," led a 19-day hunger strike to protest poor treatment of veterans in the VA hospitals (Pearson 2014).

In 1982, Robert Nimmo, director of the VA, was forced to resign under pressure from veterans' groups. He was accused of wasteful spending including expensive office redecoration and using a chauffeured car. In 1986, the VA's Inspector General's Office discovered that 93 physicians working for the agency had sanctions against their medical licenses, including suspension and revocation. In 1991, the *Chicago Tribune* reported that doctors at the VA's North Chicago Hospital sometime ignored test results, failed to treat patients in a timely manner, and performed unnecessary surgeries. A General Accounting Office (GAO) report in 2000 found significant problems with the VA's handling of research trials involving human subjects. In 2003, a commission appointed by President

George W. Bush reported that over 200,000 veterans had been waiting for six months or more for an initial or follow-up appointment (Pearson 2014).

In interviews conducted by the Department of Veterans Affairs in August 2004, seriously wounded recuperating soldiers at the Walter Reed Army Medical Center in Washington, DC expressed anger and a great deal of frustration in dealing with the hospital bureaucracy. They also reported substandard living conditions at the facility. In 2005, the Base Realignment and Closure Commission (BRCC) recommended closing down the hospital and moving its staff and services to the National Naval Medical Center (Blum and Fee 2008).

The Washington Post, in a series of articles published in February 2007, exposed the shortcomings and deficiencies at Walter Reed Army Medical Center involving substandard living conditions, inadequate management of outpatient care, insufficient resources, and poor leadership (Jackonis, Deyton, and Hess 2008). President George W. Bush appointed a bipartisan commission to investigate the matter. The commission recommended the creation of recovery coordinators, restructuring the disability and compensation system, and improving the prevention, diagnosis, and treatment of posttraumatic stress disorder and traumatic brain injury (United States President's Commission 2011). An independent review group appointed by the US Secretary of Defense, Robert Gates, submitted a report, *Rebuilding the Trust* (2007), concluding that a variety of factors such as the decision to close Walter Reed by BRCC, pressure to outsource traditional military service functions, military-to-civilian personnel conversions, inadequate facilities, inattentive leadership, combined with the increased number of soldiers returning from wars in Iraq and Afghanistan had contributed to the shortcomings and failures at Walter Reed. Finally, in 2011, under the order from the Department of Defense, Walter Reed Army Medical Center was merged and integrated with the National Naval Medical Center and renamed Walter Reed Bethesda. Today, Walter Reed Bethesda is the largest state-of-the-art military treatment facility in the Department of Defense, and it integrates Army, Navy, and Air Force medical expertise into one tertiary-care facility (Regan and Hobbs 2012).

In the 2012 presidential elections, then-candidate Barack Obama made taking care of veterans a pledge and priority. However, the Obama administration found it difficult to address the VA's backlog problem due to a surge in veterans' claims. For example, the VA received 1 million new claims during Obama's first year in office. The number of claims had reached 1.3 million by 2013. The rise in the number of claims and the backlog was the result of the VA having to deal with a sudden influx of Afghanistan and Iraq veterans as the US reduced its troop levels. Around 970,000 Iraqi and Afghanistan war veterans deployed since 9/11 had filed a disability claim (Carney and Kaper 2014).

CNN's ground-breaking coverage of veterans' issues—veterans dying while they waited for care, allegations of secret waiting lists for tests and treatment, and charges of cover-up—brought national attention to the VA's problems. Reports of mismanagement at VA hospitals had started to emerge across the country in 2012 (Gold 2014). News reports included allegations of VA employees cooking books to hide long waiting lines in Fort Collins, Colorado, workers at VA hospitals in Austin and San Antonio being instructed by superiors to list official wait times as close to zero as possible, employee bonuses at VA in Chicago being tied to manipulated wait-time data, the Texas VA being run like a crime syndicate, and many more (Roy 2014; Siegel 2014).

On May 16, 2014, VA Secretary Eric Shinseki accepted the resignation of Dr. Robert Petzel, the VA undersecretary for Health, amid a scandal involving allegations of deadly healthcare delays (Stewart and Alexander 2014). Critics called it a window dressing. A scathing report issued by the VA Inspector General's Office released May 28, 2014 confirmed allegations of excessive delay in care in Phoenix, Arizona, with an average 115-day wait for a first appointment for those on the waiting list—nearly five times longer than the Phoenix Hospital System had reported to the national VA administration (Skoloff and Daly 2014). Under increased pressure, the Secretary of the Department of Veterans Affairs, Eric Shinseki, resigned his position on May 30, 2014 and President Obama named Sloan Gibson as Acting Secretary (Dovere 2014; Felsenthal 2014). The acting secretary stated that retaliation against whistleblowers would not be tolerated and that the agency was putting out bids for "purchased care," allowing veterans to be treated at other hospitals at the VA's expense while it cut backlogs at VA facilities (Forsyth 2014; Lozano and Daly 2014). In June 2014, President Obama nominated Robert McDonald for the position of Secretary of the Department of Veterans Affairs and vowed to continue to push for reform at the VA (Epstein 2014). McDonald's nomination was confirmed by the US Senate by a vote of 97–0 and he was sworn in as VA secretary on July 30, 2014. In August of 2014, Congress passed, and President Obama signed into law, a $16.3-billion plan including $10 billion in new emergency spending to allow veterans to use private doctors at the VA's expense if they cannot get a VA appointment in fewer than 30 days ("Obama Signs $16.3 Billion Veterans Spending Bill" 2014).

Some of the explanation offered for the scandals and failures of the VA have included increased demand, the VA's ambiguous scheduling policies, a lack of federal oversight over the VA's local medical centers, and a lack of sufficient funding by Congress for the VA (Lopez 2014).

Who did Americans blame for the 2014 VA scandals? According to a CBS News telephone survey conducted in May 2014, Americans were divided about who to blame, with 33 percent placing the blame on Veterans Affairs Secretary Eric Shinseki, 28 percent on local VA hospitals, and 17 percent on President Obama. The survey also showed how the issue was viewed through partisan lenses, with 31 percent of Republican respondents placing the blame on the VA secretary and 30 percent placing the blame on President Obama, while fewer Democrats and independents placed the blame on President Obama ("Who do Americans Blame for the VA Scandal?" 2014).

Even a year after the outrage over about the long waiting list for healthcare, the Department of Veterans Affairs was facing a new crisis. The number of veterans who had been on the waiting list for one month or longer grew 50-percent higher than it was at the height of the problem in 2014. The department was also facing a $3-billion budget shortfall (Oppel 2015). As the Trump administration assumed office in January of 2018, the problems of the VA continued. During 2017 and early 2018, newspapers reported more scandals at the VA. In 2017, a USA Today investigation found that the VA for years had concealed mistakes and misdeeds by staff members. In a review of hundreds of confidential VA records, in at least 126 cases, the VA had initially found mistakes and misdeed by workers that were so serious they should have been fired. Instead, in three-quarters of settlements with such workers, the VA had agreed to purge the negative records from their personnel files or had agreed to give them neutral or positive references to prospective employers (Slack and Sallah 2017). At a veteran's hospital in Oregon, a push for better rating put patients at risk, while at a VA medical center in Bedford, Massachusetts, when it needed landscaping and snow removal, one employee contracted her own brother for $1 million of supplies, which were never delivered. The employee was allowed to keep her federal job and was demoted only one pay grade (Philipps 2018; Wax-Thibodeaux 2018). In March of 2018, President Trump fired Veterans Affairs Secretary David Shulkin and nominated his own personal White House doctor, Ronny Jackson, who had virtually no experience with the veterans' agency, to replace him. Trump's pick blindsided the VA staff and threw the agency into further disarray (Woellert, Johnson, and O'Brien 2018; Yen and Miller 2018). Prior to his Senate confirmation hearing, when a slew of misconduct charges came to light, Ronny Jackson withdrew his name from consideration to head the VA. In fact, independent investigations in 2012 and 2013 had found that Ronny Jackson had exhibited unprofessional behavior and recommended that the White House consider removing him from the White House Medical Staff (Slack 2018). In May of 2018, President Trump nominated Robert Wilkie, Jr., for the secretary position. He was confirmed by the Senate and assumed his position as secretary of the VA on July 30, 2018.

A report by the Office of the Inspector General of the VA released in August 2018 concluded that the Department of Veterans Affairs had improperly denied hundreds of military sexual trauma (MST) claims in recent years, leaving potentially thousands of veterans suffering from PTSD without benefits. The report found that in 2017, the VA had mishandled as many as 1300 of the 2700 MST-related claims, a 49-percent error rate. The report attributed the errors to claim reviewers' lack of specialization, lack of additional levels of review, and inadequate training (Veterans Benefits Administration 2018).

All the recent VA scandals have revived the debate among liberals and conservatives about government versus private-sector healthcare. Liberals argue that government healthcare is free of perverse incentives like the "profit motive," which drives up the cost of healthcare due to unnecessary tests, medical procedures, and greed. For example, In 2011, Paul Krugman, a liberal economist, hailed VA healthcare as a triumph of socialized medicine. However, conservatives argue that the egalitarians ignore the fact that a government healthcare system contains its own perverse incentives such as global budgets and a rationing that leads to treatment delays and preventable deaths, which government bureaucracy tries to cover up. In addition, the conservatives argue that free or low-cost healthcare creates an ever-increasing demand for more healthcare ("Government Health-Care Model" 2014).

While it is probably true of many government agencies, perhaps the VA best exemplifies the old adage, "the more things change, the more they stay the same."

CHALLENGES CONFRONTING THE VA HEALTHCARE SYSTEM

The veterans' healthcare system has undergone a major organizational and management transformation since the passage of the Veterans Eligibility Reform Act, which went into effect on October 1, 1998. It has led to improved patient safety and quality of care. However, scandals have continued to plague the agency. Both the VA and VHA continue to face many challenges.

One of the major challenges facing the VA is the instability produced by the vacuum of leadership at the top. Between 1998 and 2018, the Department of Veterans Affairs had 15 secretaries, including seven who served as acting secretaries. This instability of qualified senior leadership positions is both a short-term and long-term challenge. There is also a lack of rigorous job performance evaluation of senior leadership positions at the VA. Despite all the scandals and delays in processing veterans' compensation claims and delays in accessing care over the last four years, all of the 470 senior executives at the VA received an annual rating indicating that they were "fully successful" in their jobs. In 2013, nearly 80 percent of all senior executives were rated either "outstanding" or "fully successful in their job performance," with 65 percent of them receiving performance awards averaging about $9,000 (Oppel 2014). The problem of instability and the vacuum of leadership also translate to management problems with respect to the delivery of care and benefits to veterans, and issues in areas of financial management, procurement, and information management practices ("FY 2017 Agency Financial Report: Management Challenges" 2018).

The second challenge confronting the VA is the struggle to strike a balance between the call for more private-sector care and the call to invest more and innovate across the VA. As we have discussed, adequate and timely care has been a long issue at VA, which in turn has led to calls for more privatization of veterans' healthcare services by some. Others have pointed out that some of these problems are a result of increased demand for services and limited or inadequate funding and have called for more funding for the VA to meet the increasing demand.

The solution is not as simple as telling veterans to seek more private-sector care for their health needs. Many veterans face interrelated physical and mental health issues that require integrated care and not all private-sector providers are capable of providing such integrated care. Many such providers often lack the contextual understanding of veterans' healthcare needs compared to VA physicians. In fact, a study by the Rand Corporation found that a civilian care setting may not be prepared to serve the needs of veterans (Hendricks and Broadwell 2018). The debate about the public sector versus privatization is often colored by a partisan and ideological lens.

The demographics of the US Armed Forces and the veterans' population are changing rapidly. As the number of female and minorities serving in the US Armed Forces continues to rise, so will their numbers among the ranks of veterans (Bialik 2017).

The third challenge confronting the VA is addressing the unique healthcare needs of the increasing number of women veterans. Women are serving in forward positions in combat in larger numbers. Their increased involvement has resulted in increased physical and mental health risks (Resnick, Mallampalli, and Carter 2012). The VA needs to be prepared to deal with health issues faced by female veterans such as military sexual trauma and related problems of PTSD, mental health, depression and substance use, and homelessness. For example, female veterans are twice as likely to be homeless compared to the non-veteran population ("Six Challenges Facing Today's Women Veterans" n.d.). Conducting research on women veterans, identifying their unique healthcare needs, and meeting these needs is important given the fact that they are a rapidly growing segment of the total veteran population (Washington 2004).

The VA's healthcare system also needs to address the problem of perceived racial disparity. The perceived racial/ethnic discrimination is more prevalent among patients who use Veterans Affairs facilities than among those who do not (Hausmann et al. 2009). There continues to be a gap in clinical outcomes between African-American and white veterans (Trivedi et al. 2011). Racial/ethnic discrimination during military service is also strongly associated with lower physical health. Better mental health among minority veterans also seems to be related to satisfaction with healthcare providers' sensitivity toward the racial/ethnic background of patients (Sohn and Harada 2008). Part of the problem in studying racial-ethnic disparities with respect to veterans is that VHA databases used to study this problem do not necessarily capture all care received by VHA patients (Halanych et al. 2006).

CONCLUSION

Inscribed on the wall of the Department of Veterans Affairs headquarters in Washington, DC is a quotation from Abraham Lincoln, "To care for him who shall have borne the battle, and for his widow and his orphan" (quoted in Oliver 2007, 13). Unfortunately, that has not always been the priority. Benefits for veterans (including healthcare benefits) and their dependents have slowly and steadily expanded only after political struggles and political lobbying and pressure-group politics. But, even today, not all veterans or their dependents receive healthcare benefits through the veterans' healthcare system because enrollment is based on a priority rating system designed to balance resources with needs. Poor and minority veterans have come to rely exclusively on the veterans' healthcare system to meet all their healthcare needs. A significant number of veterans still lack health insurance coverage, and despite progress, homelessness continues to be a problem confronting many veterans. Many also suffer from psychological stress and mental health problems and are at higher risk for suicide and alcohol and substance abuse. Many have found the transition from military to civilian life difficult after returning from battlefields.

The Veterans Eligibility Reform Act, passed in 1996 and implemented in 1998, expanded veterans' health benefits and fundamentally and dramatically changed the veterans' healthcare system. Today, the veterans' healthcare system is the largest integrated healthcare system in the United States.

The wars in Iraq and Afghanistan have dramatically increased the number of veterans who are physically wounded, have lost their limbs, and suffer from service-related disabilities. While the total veteran population is in decline, the number of claims for disability compensation has increased dramatically. In fact, the number of disability compensation claims has outpaced the growth in the number of disabled veterans. This has put increased financial strain on the disability compensation program.

Since the establishment of the Veterans Health Administration in 1946, the veterans' healthcare system has had ups and downs. It showed improvement after the scandal-plagued days of the 1970s and 1980s and those involving Walter Reed Army Medical Center in the mid-2000s. However, scandals again plagued the VA during the 2010s.

The VA and its healthcare system continue to face many challenges in meeting the healthcare needs of veterans. Scandals have left the VA with a leadership vacuum and instability. Despite some of the reform and privatization efforts to reduce the long wait list, veterans continue to struggle to meet their healthcare needs in a timely manner. Significant demographic changes are happening in the veteran population and meeting the healthcare needs of the increased number of women and minority veterans continues to be an important challenge.

STUDY QUESTIONS

1. Discuss the legal and constitutional status of American Indians and Alaska Natives in the United States.
2. Discuss the evolution of US health policy for American Indians and Alaska Natives.
3. Discuss the role of the Indian Health Service (IHS) in providing healthcare for American Indians and Alaska Natives. Be sure to include in your discussion the IHS and its role in service delivery.
4. What are the major accomplishments of the IHS? What are the major challenges confronting the IHS?
5. Discuss the trends and health status of American Indians and Alaska Natives. What factors help explain their relatively poor health status compared to white Americans?
6. Discuss how US health policy for veterans has evolved over the years.
7. Discuss the mission and organization of the Department of Veterans Administration (DVA) and Veterans Health Administration (VHA) and the VHA's role in delivering health services to veterans.
8. Discuss the eligibility requirements for veterans to receive health services. What are some of the major trends in veterans' enrollment? What health services and benefits are they entitled to?
9. What are some of the major and unique health issues confronted by American veterans?
10. What are some of the major trends in the utilization of VA benefits, including health benefits among veterans in general and veterans with service-connected disability in particular?
11. Write an essay in which you describe the scandal-plagued history of the VA and the factors that have contributed to such scandals.
12. What are some of the problems and challenges facing the VA?

REFERENCES

"2010 National Survey of Veterans: Understanding and Knowledge of VA Benefits and Services." 2011. Washington, DC: National Center for Veterans Analysis and Statistics, US Department of Veterans Affairs. Online at www.va.gov/vetdata/docs/.

"About the Women Veterans Health Care Program." n.d. Washington, DC: US Department of Veterans Affairs. Online at www.womenshealth.va.gov/.

"About VHA." n.d. Washington, DC: US Department of Veterans Affairs. Online at www.va.gov/health/aboutVHA.asp.
"Active Duty Servicemembers: Transitioning from TRICARE to VA Health Care." n.d. Washington, DC: US Department of Veterans Affairs. Online at www.va.gov/.
"Affordable Care Act." n.d. Indian Health Service. Online at www.ihs.gov/aca.
Amara, Jomana, Terri K. Pogoda, Maxine Krengel, Kathrine M. Iverson, Errol Baker, and Ann Hendricks. 2014. "Determinants of Utilization and Cost of VHA Care by OEF/OIF Veterans Screened for Mild Traumatic Brain Injury." *Military Medicine*, 179, no. 9 (September): 964–972.
Ambler, Marjane. 2003. "Reclaiming Native Health." *Tribal College Journal*, 15, no. 2 (Winter): 8–9.
"American Indian and Alaska Native Heritage Month." 2017. United States Cencus Bureau. Online at https://census.gov/.
"American Indian/Alaska Native Profile." n.d. Rockville, MD: Office of Minority Health, US Department of Health and Human Services. Online at http://minorityhealth.hhs.gov/.
"An Achievable Vision: Report of the Department of Defense Task Force on Mental Health, June 2007." 2007. Falls Church, VA: Defense Health Board Task Force on Mental Health. Online at www.health.mil/dhb/mhtf/mhtf-report-final.pdf.
Anderson, G. Kermyt, Paul Spicer, and Michael T. Peercy. 2016. "Obesity, Diabetes, and Birth Outcomes among American Indians and Alaska Natives." *Maternal and Child Health Journal*, 20, no 12 (December): 2548–2556.
Artiga, Samantha, Petry Ubri, and Julia Foutz. 2017. "Medicaid and American Indians and Alaska Natives." Kaiser Family Foundation. Online at www.kff.org/.
"Audit of the Medical Care Collection Fund Program." 2002. Washington, DC: US Department of Veterans Affairs. Online at www.va.gov/.
Auerbach, David I., William B. Weeks, and Ian Brantley. 2013. *Health Care Spending and Efficiency in the U.S. Department of Veterans Affairs*. Santa Monica, CA: Rand Corporation.
Bains, Wesley. n.d. "Problems Facing Veterans: The Wounds of War are Both Visible and Invisible." Beliefnet. Online at www.beliefnet.com/wellness/8-health-problems-veterans-face.aspx?.
Baker, Michael. 2014. "Causalities of the Global War on Terror and Their Future Impact on Health Care and Society: A Looming Public Health Crisis." *Military Medicine*, 179, no. 4 (April): 348–355.
Barnhardt, Carol. 2001. "A History of Schooling for Alaska Native People." *Journal of American Indian Education*, 40, no. 1: 1–30.
Bassett, Deborah, Dedra Buchwald, and Spero Manson. 2014. "Posttraumatic Stress Disorder and Symptoms among American Indians and Alaska Natives: A Review of the Literature." *Social Psychiatry and Psychiatric Epidemiology*, 49, no. 3 (March): 417–433.
Becerra, Monideepa B., Benjamin J. Becerra, Christina M. Hassija, and Nasia Safdar. 2016. "Unmet Mental Healthcare Need and Suicidal Ideation among U.S. Veterans." *American Journal of Preventive Medicine*, 51, no. 1 (July): 90–94.
Bergman, Abraham B., David C. Rossman, Angela M. Erdrich, John G. Todd, and Ralph Forquera. 1999. "A Political History of Indian Health Service." *Milbank Quarterly*, 77, no. 4: 571–604.
Bialik, Kristen. 2017. "Changing Face of America's Veteran Population." Pew Research Center. Online at www.pewresearch.org/.
Blum, Nava and Elizabeth Fee. 2008. "Critical Shortcomings at Walter Reed Army Medical Center Create Doubt." *American Journal of Public Health*, 98, no. 12 (December): 2159–2160.
Boddy, Jessica. 2015. "Many Veterans Gain Health Care through the Affordable Care Act." *NPR*. Online at www.npr.org/.
Brave Heart, Maria Yellow Rose, Roberto Lewis-Fernandez, Janette Beals, Deborah S. Hasin, Luisa Sugaya, Shuai Wang, Bridget F. Grant, and Carlos Blanco. 2016. "Psychiatric Disorders and Mental Health Testament in American Indians and Alaska Natives." *Social Psychiatry and Psychiatric Epidemiology*, 51, no 7 (July): 1033–1046.
Carlson, Bonnie E., Layne K. Stromwall, and Cynthia A. Lietz. 2013. "Mental Health Issues in Recently Returning Women Veterans: Implications for Practice." *Social Work*, 58, no. 2 (April): 105–114.
Carney, Jordain and Stacy Kaper. 2014. "Obama Has Every Reason to Fix the VA. Why Hasn't He?" *NationalJournal*. Online at www.nationaljournal.com/s/57617.
Centers for Disease Control and Prevention. 2000. *Facts about Heart Disease and Stroke among American Indians and Alaska Natives*. Centers for Disease Control and Prevention. Online at www.cdc.gov.
Cho, Pyone, Linda S. Geiss, Nilka R. Borrows, Diana L. Roberts, Ann K. Bullock, and Michael E. Toedt. 2014. "Diabetes-Related Mortality among American Indians and Alaska Natives, 1990–2009." *American Journal of Public Health*, 104, no. 3 (Supplement): 496–502.
Cichowski, Sara B., Rebecca G. Rogers, and Elizabeth A. Clark. 2017. "Military Sexual Trauma in Female Veterans Is Associated with Chronic Pain Conditions." *Military Medicine*, 182, no. 9 (September): e1895–e1899.
Cobb, Nathaniel, David Espey, and Jessica King. 2014. "Health Behaviors and Risk Factors among American Indians and Alaska Natives, 2000–2010." *American Journal of Public Health*, 104, no. 3 (Supplement): 481–489.
"Community Health." n.d. Indian Health Service. Online at www.ihs.gov/communityhealth/.
Cramer, Tom. n.d. "Female Veterans of Today Facing Vastly Different Health Issues than Their Predecessors." US Department of Veterans Affairs. Online at www.va.gov/.
"Critical Issues Facing Veterans and Military Families." 2017. SAMHSA. Online at www.samhsa.gov/.
Cunningham, Peter J. and Barbara M. Altman. 1993. "The Use of Ambulatory Health Care Services by American Indians with Disabilities." *Medical Care*, 31, no. 7 (July): 600–616.
Cunningham, Peter J. and Llewellyn J. Cornelius. 1995. "Access to Ambulatory Care for American Indians and Alaska Natives: The Relative Importance of Personal and Community Resources." *Social Science & Medicine*, 40, no. 3 (February): 393–407.
Davidson, Joe. 2017. "Staffing, Budget Shortages Put Indian Health Service at 'High Risk'." *The Washington Post*. Online at www.washingtonpost.com/.

"Department of Defense Casualties Report." 2018. Washington, DC: US Department of Defense. Online at www.defense.gov/casualty.pdf.

"Department of Veterans Affairs – Budget in Brief 2019." n.d. Washington, DC: US Department of Veterans Affairs. Online at www.va.gov/.

"Department of Veterans Affairs Statistics at a Glance." 2012. Washington, DC: National Center for Veterans Analysis and Statistics, US Department of Veterans Affairs. Online at www.va.gov/vetdata/.

"Department of Veterans Affairs: Veteran Surveys and Studies." 2011. Washington, DC: National Center for Veterans Analysis and Statistics, US Department of Veterans Affairs. Online at www.va.gov/vetdata/.

Donalee, Unal. 2018. "Sovereignty and Social Justice: How the Concepts Affect Federal American Indian Policy and American Indian Health." *Social Work in Public Health*, 33, no. 4 (April): 5.

Dovere, Edward-Isaac. 2014. "Eric Shinseki Exit Marks a Course Shift for Obama." *Politico*. Online at www.politico.com/.

Duggan, Mark, Robert Rosenheck, and Perry Singleton. 2010. "Federal Policy and the Rise in Disability Enrollment: Evidence for the Veterans Affairs' Disability Compensation Program." *Journal of Law and Economics*, 53, no. 2 (May): 379–398.

Dunne, Eugene M., Larry E. Burrell II, Allyson D. Diggins, Nicole E. Whitehead, and William W. Latimer. 2015. "Increased Risk of Substance Use and Health-Related Problems among Homeless Veterans." *American Journal on Addictions*, 24, no. 7 (October): 676–680.

Dworsky, Michael, Carrie M. Farmer, and Mimi Shen. 2017. "Veterans' Health Insurance Coverage under the Affordable Care Act and Implications of Repeal for the Department of Veterans Affairs." Santa Monica, CA: Rand Corporation. Online at www.rand.org/.

Eisen, Susan, Mark R. Schultz, Dewne Vogt, Mark E. Glickman, Rani Elwy, Mari-Lynn Drainoni, Princess E. Osei-Bonsu, and James Martin. 2012. "Mental and Physical Health Status and Alcohol and Drug Use following Return from Deployment in Iraq or Afghanistan." *American Journal of Public Health*, 102, no. S1 (Supplement): S66–S73.

Epstein, Jennifer. 2014. "Barack Obama Announces VA Pick." *Politico*. Online at www.politico.com/.

Erb, Heather and Christine Speidel. 2015. "The ACA, the Service, and the Indian Health Care Delivery System." *Newsquarterly*, 34, no. 4 (Summer): 1–21.

Fagot-Campagna, Anne, David J. Pettitt, and Michael M. Engelgau. 2000. "Type 2 Diabetes among North American Children and Adolescents: An Epidemiologic Review and a Public Health Perspective." *Journal of Pediatrics*, 136, no. 5 (May): 664–672.

Farmer, Carrie M, Susan D. Hosek, and David M. Adamson. 2016. "Balancing Demand and Supply for Veterans Health Care." *Rand Health Quarterly*, 6, no. 1: 3–8.

"Federal Benefits for Veterans, Dependents and Survivors." 2017. Washington, DC: US Department of Veterans Affairs. Online at www.va.gov/.

Felsenthal, Mark. 2014. "Obama Taps Army Ranger as Interim Head of Troubled Veterans Agency." Yahoo. Online at www.yahoo.com/.

"First Fifty Years of the Indian Health Service: Caring and Curing." Washington, DC: HIS Gold Book – Parts 1–4. Indian Health Service, US Department of Health and Human Services. Online at www.ihs.gov/newsroom/factsheets/.

"Fiscal Year 2011 Accomplishments." n.d. Indian Health Service, Washington, DC: US Department of Health and Human Services. Online at www.ihs.gov/.

Forquera, Ralph. 2001. *Urban Indian Health*. Washington, DC: Henry J. Kaiser Family Foundation.

Forsyth, Jim. 2014. "New VA Secretary Plans More 'Purchased Care' to Relieve Backlogs." Yahoo. Online at www.yahoo.com/.

Frank, John W. 2000. "Historical and Cultural Roots of Drinking Problems among American Indians." *American Journal of Public Health*, 90, no. 3 (March): 344–351.

Frayne, Susan M., Victoria A. Parker, Cindy L. Christiansen, Susan Loveland, Margaret R. Seaver, Lewis E. Kazis, and Katherine M. Skinner. 2006. "Health Status Among 28,000 Women Veterans." *Journal of General Internal Medicine*, 21, no. 3 Supplement (March): S40–S46.

Freedenthal, Stacey and Arlene R. Stiffman. 2007. "They Might Think I Was Crazy: Young American Indians' Reasons for Not Seeking Help When Suicidal." *Journal of Adolescent Research*, 22, no. 1 (January): 58–77.

Friedman, Misha. 2016. "For Native Americans, Health Care Is a Long, Hard Road Away." *NPR*. Online at www.npr.org/.

Fullwood, Danielle. 2015. "Understanding and Managing the Health Needs of Veterans." *Nursing Standard*, 30, no. 10 (November): 37–43.

"FY 2017 Agency Financial Report: Section A: Management Challenges." 2018. Washington, DC: Office of Inspector General, US Department of Veterans Affairs. Online at www.va.gov/.

Garrett, J. T. and Michael W. Garrett. 1994. "The Path of Good Medicine: Understanding and Counseling Native American Indians." *Journal of Multicultural Counseling and Development* 22, no. 3 (July): 134–144.

Gold, Hadas. 2014. "Anatomy of a Veterans Affairs Scandal." *Politico*. Online at www.politico.com/.

Goldberg, Eleanor. 2013. "5 Growing Problems Iraq, Afghanistan Wars Veterans Face (And What Is Being Done)." *The Huffington Post*. Online at www.huffingtonpost.com/.

Goldstein, Gerald, James F. Luther, Gretchen Haas, Cathleen Appelt, and Adam Gordon. 2010. "Factor Structure and Risk Factors for the Health Status of Homeless Veterans." *Psychiatric Quarterly*, 81, no. 4 (December): 311–323.

Gonzales, Angela, Judy Kertesz, and Gabrielle Tayac. 2007. "Eugenics as Indian Removal: Sociohistorical Processes and the De(con)struction of American Indians in the Southeast." *Public Historian*, 29, no. 3 (Summer): 53–67.

"Government Health-Care Model." 2014. *The Wall Street Journal*. Online at www.wsj.com/.

Gradus, Jaimie L., Blair E. Wisco, Matthew T. Luciano, Katherine M. Iverson, Brian P. Marx, and Amy E. Street. 2015. "Traumatic Brain Injury and Suicidal Ideation among U.S. Operation Freedom and Operation Iraqi Freedom Veterans." *Journal of Traumatic Stress*, 28, no. 4 (July): 361–365.

Halanych, Jewell H., Fie Wang, Donald R. Miller, Leonard M. Pogach, Hai Lin, Dam R. Berlowitz, and Susan M. Frayne. 2006. "Racial/Ethnic Differences in Diabetes Care for Older Veterans: Accounting for Dual Health System Use Changes Conclusions." *Medical Care*, 44, no. 5 (May): 439–445.

Harris, Raymond, Lonnie A. Nelson, Clemma Muller, and Dedra Buchwald. 2015. "Stroke in American Indians and Alaska Natives: A Systematic Review." *American Journal of Public Health*, 105, no. 8 (August): 16–26.

Hausmann, Leslie R., Kwonho Jeong, James E. Bost, Nancy R. Kressin, and Said A. Ibrahim. 2009. "Perceived Racial Discrimination in Health Care: A Comparison of Veterans Affairs and Other Patients." *American Journal of Public Health*, 99, no. S3 (November): S718–S724.

"Health Benefits: Family Members of Veterans." n.d. Washington, DC: US Department of Veterans Affairs. Online at www.va.gov/.

"Health Benefits: Federal Benefits for Veterans, Dependents, and Survivors." n.d. Washington, DC: US Department of Veterans Affairs. Online at www.va.gov/.

"Health Coverage and Care for American Indians and Alaska Natives." 2013. Kaiser Family Foundation. Online at www.kff.org/.

"Health Insurance Coverage, Poverty, and Income of Veterans: 2000 to 2009." 2011. Washington, DC: National Center for Veterans Analysis and Statistics, US Department of Veterans Affairs. Online at www.va.gov/vetdata/.

Henderson, Patricia N., Clemma Jacobsen, and Janette Beals. 2005. "Correlates of Cigarette Smoking among Selected Southwest and Northern Plains Tribal Groups: The AL-SUPERRFP Sud." *American Journal of Public Health*, 95, no. 5 (May): 867–872.

Hendricks, Kate T. and Paula Broadwell. 2018. "Beyond the Leadership Vacuum: Challenges Facing Veterans Affairs." *The Hill*. Online at http://thehill.com/.

Herman-Stahl, Mindy, Donna L. Spencer, and Jessica E. Duncan. 2003. "The Implications of Cultural Orientation for Substance Use among American Indians." *American Indian & Alaska Native Mental Health Research*, 11, no. 1: 46–66.

Hoge, Charles W., Jennifer L. Auchterlonie, and Charles S. Milliken. 2006. "Mental Health Problems, Use of Mental Health Services, and Attrition from Military Service after Returning from Deployment to Iraq or Afghanistan." *Journal of the American Medical Association*, 295, no. 9 (March): 1023–1032.

Holcombe, Randall G. 1999. "Veterans Interest and the Transition to Government Growth: 1870–1915." *Public Choice*, 99, nos. 3–4: 311–326.

Horwedel, Dina. 2016. "It Is No Secret that American Indian Populations Experiences Significantly Higher Rates of Disease." *Tribal College Journal*, 27, no. 4 (May): 21–24.

Huhndorf, Roy M. and Shari M. Huhndorf. 2011. "Alaska Native Politics since the Alaska Claims Settlement Act." *South Atlantic Quarterly*, 110, no. 2 (Spring): 385–401.

Hyman, Jeffrey, Robert Ireland, Lucinda Frost, and Linda Cottrell. 2012. "Suicide Incidence and Risk Factors in an Active Duty U.S. Military Population." *American Journal of Public Health*, 102, no. S1 (Supplement): 38–46.

Igleheart, Austin. 2018. "Congress Passes VA Mission Act of 2018." National Association of Counties. Online at www.naco.org/.

"IHS Profile." 2018. Washington, DC: Indian Health Service. Online at www.ihs.gov/nrewroom/factsheets/.

"IHS Year 2012 Profile." n.d. Washington, DC: Indian Health Service, Department of Health and Human Services. Online at www.ihs.gov/.

Jackonis, Michael J., Lawrence Deyton, and William J. Hess. 2008. "War, Its Aftermath and U.S. Health Policy: Toward a Comprehensive Health Program for America's Military Personnel, Veterans and Their Families." *Journal of Law, Medicine, and Ethics*, 36, no. 4 (Winter): 677–689.

James, Cara, Karyn Schwartz, and Julia Berndt. 2009. *A Profile of American Indians and Alaska Natives and Their Health Coverage*. Washington, DC: Henry J. Kaiser Family Foundation.

Kaiser Commission on Medicaid and the Uninsured. 2006. *The Uninsured: A Primer. Key Facts about Americans without Health Insurance*. Washington, DC: Henry J. Kaiser Family Foundation.

Katz, Ruth J. 2004. "Addressing the Health Care Needs of American Indians and Alaska Natives." *American Journal of Public Health*, 94, no. 1 (January): 13–14.

Kizer, Kenneth W. 1995. *Vision for Change: A Plan to Restructure the Veterans Health Administration*. Washington, DC: US Department of Veterans Affairs.

Kemp, Janet, and Robert M. Bossarte. "Surveillance of Suicide and Suicide Attempts among Veterans: Addressing a National Imperative." 2012. American Journal of Public Health, 102, no. S1 (Supplement): e4–e5.

Kizer, Kenneth W. 1996. *Prescription for Change: The Guiding Principles and Strategic Objectives Underlying the Transformation of the Veterans Health Care System*. Washington, DC: US Department of Veterans Affairs.

Kizer, Kenneth W., John G. Demakis, and John R. Feussner. 2000. "Reinventing VA Health Care: Systematizing Quality Improvement and Quality Innovation." *Medicare Care, Supplement*, 38, no. 6 (June): I-7–I-16.

Kizer, Kenneth W. and Adams R. Dudley. 2009. "Extreme Makeover: Transformation of the Veterans Health Care System." *Annual Review of Public Health*, 30, no. 1: 313–339.

Kramer, Josea B. 1992. "Cross-Cultural Medicine: A Decade Later." *Western Journal of Medicine*, 157, no. 3: 281–285.

Kulas, Joseph F. and Robert A. Rosenheck. 2018. "A Comparison of Veterans with Post-Traumatic Stress Disorder, with Mild Traumatic Brain Injury and with Both Disorders: Understanding Multimorbidity." *Military Medicine*, 183, no. 3/4 (March/April): e114–e122.

Kunitz, Stephen J. 1996. "The History and Politics of U.S. Health Care Policy for American Indians and Alaskan Natives." *American Journal of Public Health*, 96, no. 10 (October): 1464–1473.

Landen, Michael, Jim Roeber, Tim Naimi, Larry Nielsen, and Mack Sewell. 2014. "Alcohol-Attributable Mortality among American Indians and Alaska Natives in the United States, 1999–2009." *American Journal of Public Health*, 104, no. 3 (Supplement): 343–349.

Lee, Doohee and Charles E. Bagley. 2017. "Delays in Seeking Health Care: Comparison of Veterans and General Population." *Public Health Management*, 23, no. 2 (March-April): 160–168.

Liao, Y., P. Tucker, and W. H. Giles. 2003. "Health Status of American Indians Compared with Other Racial/Ethnic Minority Population." *Morbidity & Mortality Weekly Report*, 52, no. 47: 1148–1152.

Liebler, Carolyn A. and Renuka Bhaskar. 2016. "Joining, Leaving, and Staying in American India/Alaska Native Race Category between 2000 and 2010." *Demography*, 53, no. 2 (April): 507–540.

Liebler, Carolyn A. and Meghan Zacher. 2013. "American Indians without Tribes in the Twenty-First Century." *Ethnic and Racial Studies*, 36, no. 11 (November): 1910–1934.

Lillie-Blanton, Marsha. 2005. "Understanding and Addressing the Health Care Needs of American Indians and Alaska Natives." *American Journal of Public Health*, 95, no. 5 (May): 759–761.

Livingston, Gretchen. 2016. "Profile of U.S. Veterans Is Changing Dramatically as Their Ranks Decline." Washington, DC: Pew Research Center. Online at www.pewresearch.org/.

Lopez, German. 2014. "The VA Scandal, Explained." *Vox*. Online at www.vox.com/.

Lozano, Juan A. and Matthew Daly. 2014. "VA Acting Chief: Retaliation Will Not Be Tolerated." *Savannah Morning News*. Online at www.savannahnow.com/.

Lujan, Carol C. 2014. "American Indian and Alaska Natives Count." *American Indian Quarterly*, 38, no. 3 (Summer): 320–341.

Machlin, Steven R. and Pradip Muhuri. n.d. "Statistical Brief # 508: Characteristics and Health Care Expenditures of VA Health System Users Vs. Other Veterans, 2014–2015." Medical Expenditure Panel Survey. Online at https://meps.ahrq.gov/.

"Major Tricare Changes Kicked Off Jan. 1." 2017. Military.com. Online at www.military.com/.

Mansberger, Steven L., Francine C. Romero, Nicole H. Smith, Chris A. Johnson, George A. Cioffi, Beth Edmunds, Choi Dongseok, and Thomas M. Becker. 2005. "Causes of Visual Impairment and Common Eye Problems in Northwest American Indian and Alaska Natives." *American Journal of Public Health*, 95, no. 5 (May): 881–886.

Manson, Spero M., Janette Beals, Suzell A. Klein, and Calvin D. Croy. 2005. "Social Epidemiology of Trauma among 2 American Indian Reservation Populations." *American Journal of Public Health*, 95, no. 5 (May): 851–859.

Marbella, Anne M., Mickey C. Harris, Sabina Diehr, Gerald Ignace, and Georginna Ignace. 1998. "Use of Native American Healers among Native American Patients in an Urban Native American Health Center." *Archives of Family Medicine*, 7, no. 2 (March–April): 182–185.

"Medicaid's Role in Covering Veterans." 2017. Kaiser Family Foundation. Online at www.kff.org/.

"Military Sexual Trauma." 2015. Washington, DC: US Department of Veterans Affairs. Online at www.mentalhealth.va.gov/.

Miller, Matthew. "Preventing Suicide by Preventing Lethal Injury: The Need to Act on What We Already Know." 2012. *American Journal of Public Health*, 102, no. S1 (Supplement): e1–e2.

Miller, Laura J. and Nafisa Y. Ghadiali. 2018. "Mental Health across the Reproductive Cycle in Women Veterans." *Military Medicine*, 183, no. 5/6 (May/June): e140–e146.

Murdoch, Maureen, Arlene Bradley, Susan H. Mother, Robert E. Kline, Carole L. Turner, and Elizabeth M. Yano. 2006. "Women at War." *Journal of General Internal Medicine*, 21, no. 3 Supplement (March): S5–S10.

Murphy, Tierney, Pallavi Pokhrel, Anne Worthington, Holly Billie, Mack Sewell, and Nancy Bill. 2014. "Unintentional Injury Mortality among American Indians and Alaska Natives in the United States, 1990–2009." *American Journal of Public Health*, 104, no. 3 (Supplement): 470–480.

"Myths and Realities." n.d. National Council of Urban Indian Health. Online at www.ncuih.org/about.

"New Detailed Statistics on Race, Hispanic Origin, Ancestry, and Tribal Groups." 2017. Washington, DC: United States Census Bureau. Online at www.census.gov/.

Noren, Jay, David Kindig, and Audrey Sprenger. 1998. "Challenges to Native American Health Care." *Public Health Reports*, 113, no. 1 (January/February): 22–33.

Novins, Douglas K., Janette Beals, Calvin Croy, Anna E. Baron, Paul Spicer, and Dedra Buchwald. 2006. "The Relationship between Patterns of Alcohol Abuse and Mental and Physical Health Disorders in Two American Indian Populations." *Addiction*, 101, no. 1 (January): 69–83.

"Obama Signs $16.3 Billion Veterans Spending Bill." 2014. Yahoo. Online at www.yahoo.com/.

O'Connell, Joan M., Charlton Wilson, Spero M. Manson, and Kelly J. Acton. 2012. "The Cost of Treating American Indian Adults with Diabetes within the Indian Health Service." *American Journal of Public Health*, 102, no. 2 (February): 301–308.

"Office of Urban Indian Health Program Strategic Plan 2017–2021." n.d. Indian Health Service. Online at www.ihs.gov/.

Oliver, Adam. 2007. "The Veterans Health Administration: An American Success Story?" *Milbank Quarterly*, 85, no. 1: 5–35.

Olson, Lenora M. and Stephanie Wahab. 2006. "American Indians and Suicide: A Neglected Area of Research." *Trauma, Violence & Abuse*, 7, no. 1 (January): 19–33.

Oppel, Richard A. 2014. "Every Senior V.A. Executive Was Rated 'Fully Successful' or Better over 4 Years." *The New York Times*. Online at www.nytimes.com/.

Oppel, Richard A. 2015. "Wait List Grows as Many More Veterans See Care and Funding Falls Short." *The New York Times*. Online at www.nytimes.com/.

Oster, Candice, Andrea Morello, Anthony Venning, and Sharon Lawn. 2017. "The Health and Wellbeing Needs of Veterans: A Rapid Review." *BMC Psychiatry*, 17, no. 1 (December): 1–14.

"Our History: A Brief History of the Veterans Health Administration." n.d. Washington, DC: US Deparment of Veterans Affairs. Online at www.washingtondc.va.gov/about/history.asp.

Parker, Kim, Anthony Cilluffo, and Renee Stepler. 2017. *6 Facts about U.S. Military and Its Demographics*. Washington, DC: Pew Research Center. Online at www.pewresearch.org/.

Pearson, Diane J. 2004. "Medical Diplomacy and the American Indian: Thomas Jefferson, the Lewis and Clark Expedition, and the Subsequent Effects on American Indian Health and Public Policy." *Wicaza Sa Review*, 19, no. 1: 105–130.

Pearson, Michael. 2014. "VA's Troubled History." *CNN*. Online at www.cnn.com/.

Perdue, Theda. 2012. "The Legacy of Indian Removal." *Journal of Southern History*, 78, no. 1: 3–36.

Pfefferbaum, Betty, Rennard Strickland, Everett R. Rhoades, and Rose L. Pfefferbaum. 1995/1996. "Learning How to Heal: An Analysis of the History, Policy, and Framework of Indian Health Care." *American Indian Law Review*, 20, no. 2: 365–397.

Pfefferbaum, Rose L., Betty Pfefferbaum, Everett R. Rhoades, and Rennard J. Strickland. 1997. "Providing for the Health Care Needs of Native Americans: Policy, Programs, Procedures, and Practices." *American Indian Law Review*, 21, no. 2: 211–258.

Philipps, Dave. 2018. "At VA Hospital in Oregon, A Push for Better Ratings Puts Patients at Risk, Doctors Say." *The New York Times*. Online at www.nytimes.com/.

Plescia, Marcus, Sarah J. Henley, Anne Pate, Michael Underwood, and Kris Rhoads. 2014. "Lung Cancer Deaths among American Indians and Alaska Natives: 1990–2009." *American Journal of Public Health*, 104, no. 53 (Supplement): s388–s394.

"President Trump Signs FY 2018 Omnibus." 2018. Southern Plains Tribal Health Board. Online at https://www.spthb.org/.

"Profile of Sheltered Homeless Veterans for Fiscal Years 2009 and 2010." 2012. Washington, DC: National Center for Veterans Analysis and Statistics, US Department of Veterans Affairs. Online at www.va.gov/vetdata/.

"Profile of Veterans: 2016." 2018. Washington, DC: National Center for Veterans Analysis and Statistics, US Department of Veterans Affairs. Online at www.va.gov/vetdata/.

"Projected Veteran Population 2013 to 2043." 2014. Washington, DC: US Department of Veterans Affairs. Online at www.va.gov/vetdata/docs/.

Puukka, Emily, Paul Stehr-Green, and Thomas M. Becker. 2005. "Measuring the Health Gap for American Indians/Alaska Natives: Getting Closer to the Truth." *American Journal of Public Health*, 95, no. 5 (May): 838–843.

"Quick Facts: Alaska." 2017. Washington, DC: United States Census Bureau. Online at www.census.gov/quickfacts/.

Rebuilding the Trust: Report on Rehabilitative Care and Administrative Processes at Walter Reed Army Medical Center and National Naval Medical Center. 2007. Arlington, VA: Independent Review Group on Rehabilitative Care and Administartive Processes.

Regan, Ann-Francis C., and Loretta M. Hobbs. 2012. "Walter Reed Bethesda—Much More than Changing Name." *OD Practitioner*, 44, no. 3 (Summer): 31–36.

Renfrew, Megan J. 2006. "The 100% Federal Medical Assistance Percentage: A Tool for Increasing Federal Funding for Health Care for American Indians and Alaska Natives." *Columbia Journal of Law and Social Problems*, 40, no. 2 (Winter): 173–224.

Resnick, Eileen M, Monica Mallampalli, and Christine L. Carter. 2012. "Current Challenges in Female Veterans' Health." *Journal of Women's Health*, 21, no. 9 (September): 895–900.

Rizzo, Jennifer. 2012. "The Medical Legacy of a Decade at War." *CNN*. Online at http://security.blogs.cnn.com/.

Roubideaux, Yvette. 2002. "Perspectives on American Indian Health." *American Journal of Public Health*, 92, no. 9 (September): 1401–1406.

Roy, Avik. 2014. "No, the VA Isn't A Preview of Obamacare – It's Much Worse." *Forbes*. Online at www.forbes.com/.

Sairsingh, Holly, Phyllis Solomon, Amy Helstrom, and Dan Tregilia. 2018. "Depression in Female Veterans Returning from Deployment: The Role of Social Factors." *Military Medicine*, 183, no. 3/4 (March/April): e133–e139.

Salamon, Maureen. 2010. "After the Battle: 7 Health Problems Facing Veterans." LiveScience. Online at www.livescience.com/.

Satcher, David. 2001. *Mental Health: Culture, Race, and Ethnicity—A Supplement to Mental Health: A Report of the Surgeon General*. Washington, DC: US Department of Health and Human Services.

Sawchuk, Craig N., Peter Roy-Byrne, Carolyn Noonan, Julia R. Craner, Jack Goldberg, Spero Manson, and Dedra Buchwald. 2017. "Panic Attacks and Panic Disorder in the American Indian Community." *Journal of Anxiety Disorder*, 48 (May): 6–12.

"Selected Research Highlights." 2015. Washington, DC: National Center for Veterans Analysis and Statistics, US Department of Veterans Affairs. Online at www.va.gov/vetdata/.

Shay, Kenneth and Thomas T. Yoshikawa. 2010. "Overview of VA Healthcare for Older Veterans: Lessons Learned and Policy Implications." *Journal of the American Society on Aging*, 34, no. 2 (Summer): 20–28.

Sheetz, Kyle and David J. Shulkin. 2018. "Why the VA Needs More Competition." *New England Journal of Medicine*, 378, no. 25 (June): 2356–2357.

Shelton, Brett L. 2004. *Legal and Historical Roots of Health Care for American Indians and Alaska Natives in the United States*. Washington, DC: Henry J. Kaiser Family Foundation.

Shulkin, David J. 2017. "Understanding Veteran Wait Time." *Annals of Internal Medicine*, 167, no.1 (July): 52–54.

Siegel, Jacob. 2014. "Texas VA Run like a 'Crime Syndicate'." *The Daily Beast*. Online at www.thedailybeast.com/.

Silva, Abigail, Elizabeth Tarlov, Dustin D. French, Zhiping Huo, Rachel N. Martinez, and Kevin T. Stroupe. 2016. "Veterans Affairs Health System Enrollment and Health Care Utilization after the Affordable Care Act: Initial Insights." *Military Medicine*, 181, no. 5 (May): 469–475.

"Six Challenges Facing Today's Women veterans." n.d. Veterans Assembled, November 15. Online at https://vaellc.com/advice/challenges-facing-todays-women veterans/.

Skoloff, Brian and Matthew Daly. 2014. "IG: Phoenix VA Hospital Missed Care for 1,700 Vets." *The Seattle Times*. Online at www.seattletimes.com/.

Slack, Donovan. 2018. "Ronny Jackson Staying on as White House Doctor despite Misconduct Charges." *USA Today*. Online at www.usatoday.com/.

Slack, Donovan and Michael Sallah. 2017. "VA Conceals Shoddy Care and Health Workers' Mistakes." *USA Today*. Online at www.usatoday.com/.

Sohn, Linda and Nancy D. Harada. 2008. "Effects of Racial/Ethnic Discrimination on the Health Status of Minority Veterans." *Military Medicine*, 173, no. 4 (April): 331–338.

Stewart, Phil and David Alexander. 2014. "Top U.S. Veterans' Healthcare Official Resigns Amid Scandal." Yahoo. Online at www.yahoo.com/news/.

Story, Mary, Marguerite Evans, Richard R. Fabsitz, Theresa E. Clay, Bonnie Holy Rock, and Brenda Broussard. 1999. "The Epidemic of Obesity in American Indian Communities and the Need for Childhood Obesity-Prevention Programs." *American Journal of Clinical Nutrition*, 69, no. 4 (April): 747–754.

Suryaprasad, Anil, Kathy K. Bird, John T. Redd, David G. Perdue, Michell Manos, and Brian McMahon. 2014. "Mortality Caused by Chronic Liver Disease among American Indians and Alaska Natives in the United States, 1999–2009." *American Journal of Public Health*, 104, no. 3 (Supplement): 350–357.

Swan, Judith, Nancy Breen, Linda Burhansstipanov, Delight E. Satter, William W. Davis, Timothy McNeel, and Matthew C. Snip. 2006. "Cancer Screening and Risk Factor Rates among American Indians." *American Journal of Public Health*, 96, no. 2 (February): 340–350.

Thomas, Kate H., M. M. Albright, Kaufman E. Shields, Plummer S. Michaud, and Hamner K. Taylor. 2016. "Predictors of Depression Diagnoses and Symptoms in United States Female Veterans: Results from a National Survey and Implications for Programming." *Journal of Military and Veterans Health*, 24, no. 3 (July): 6–16.

"Timeline of Accomplishments." n.d. Washington, DC: Office of Research and Development, Veterans Administration. Online at www.research.va.gov/about/history.cfm.

"Trends in Veterans with a Service-Connected Disability: 1985 to 2014." 2015. Washington, DC: National Center for Veterans Analysis and Statistics, US Department of Veterans Affairs. Online at www.va.gov/vetdata/docs/Quickfacts/SCD_trends_FINAL_2014.pdf.

"Tricare." n.d. Military.com. Online at www.military.com/benefits/tricare.

Trimble, Megan. 2017. "A Look at the Changing Future of American Veterans." *U.S. News & World Report*. Online at www.usnews.com/.

Trivedi, Amal N., Regina C. Grebla, Steven M. Wright, and Donna L. Washington. 2011. "Despite Improved Quality of Care in the Veterans Affairs Health System, Racial Disparity Persists or Important Clinical Outcomes." *Health Affairs*, 30, no. 4: 707–715.

UCLA Center for Health Policy Research. 2004. "American Indian and Alaska Native Cancer Fact Sheet." Los Angeles, CA: UCLA Center for Health Policy Research. Online www.healthpolicy.ucla.edu.

"Unemployment Rates of Veterans: 2000 to 2009." 2010. Washington, DC: National Center for Veterans Analysis and Statistics, US Department of Veterans Affairs. Online at www.va.gov/vetdata/.

United States Interagency Council on Homelessness. 2015. *Opening Doors: Federal Strategic Plan to Prevent and End Homelessness*. Washington, DC: United States Interagency Council on Homelessness. Online at www.usich.gov/opening-doors.

United States Interagency Council on Homelessness. 2018. *Home, Together: The Federal Strategic Plan to Prevent and End Homelessness*. Washington, DC: United States Interagency Council on Homelessness. Online at www.usich.gov/home-together.

United States President's Commission. 2011. *Serve, Support, Simplify: Report of the President's Commission on Care of America's Wounded Heroes*. Memphis, TN: Books LLC.

Urban Indian Health Commission. 2007. *Invisible Tribes: Urban Indians and Their Health in a Changing World*. Seattle, WA: Urban Indian Health Commission.

US Census Bureau. 2012. *The American Indian and Alaska Native Population: 2010*. Washington, DC: Economics and Statistics Administration, US Department of Commerce.

US Commission on Civil Rights. 2004. *Broken Promises: Evaluating the Native American Health Care System*. Washington, DC: US Commission on Civil Rights.

US Department of Health and Human Services. 2000. *Healthy People 2010: Understanding and Improving Health*. Washington, DC: Government Printing Office.

US Department of Housing and Urban Development. 2017. *The 2017 Annual Homeless Assessment (AHAH) Report to Congress*. Washington, DC: US Department of Housing and Urban Development. Online at www.hudexchange.info/.

US Government Accountability Office. 2005. *Indian Health Service: Health Care Services are Not Always Available to Native Americans*. Report to the Committee on Indian Affairs, US Senate. Washington, DC: US General Accountability Office.

"VA History in Brief." n.d. Washington, DC: US Department of Veterans Affairs. Online at www.va.gov/.

"VA Services for Military Sexual Trauma: Help, Hope, Healing." n.d. Washington, DC: US Department of Veterans Affairs. Online at www.mentalhealth.va.gov/.

"VA Utilization Profile: FY 2016." 2017. Washington, DC: US Department of Veterans Affairs. Online at www.va.gov/vetdata/.

Vandenberg, Patricia, Linda R. Bergofsky, and James F. Burris. 2010. "The VA's System of Care and the Veterans under Care." *Journal of American Society on Aging*, 34, no. 2 (Summer): 13–19.

"Veteran Population Projections 2017–2037." n.d. Washinton, DC: US Department of Veterans Affairs. www.va.gov/vetdata/.

"Veterans Access, Choice, and Accountability Act of 2014." n.d. Washington, DC: US Department of Veterans Affairs. Online at www.va.gov/.

Veterans Benefits Administration. 2018. *Denied Posttraumatic Stress Disorder Claims Related to Military Sexual Trauma*. Washington, DC: Office of Inspector General, Department of Veterans Affairs. Report # 17-05248-241.

"Veterans Health Benefits." n.d. Washington, DC: US Department of Veterans Affairs. Online at www.va.gov/.

"Veterans Medical Benefits Package." n.d. Military.com. Online at www.military.com/.

"Veterans Population Projections: FY 2000 to FY 2036." 2010. Washington, DC: National Center for Veterans Analysis and Statistics, Washington, DC: US Department of Veterans Affairs. Online at www.va.gov/vetdata/.

"VHA Program Offices." n.d. Washington, DC: US Department of Veterans Affairs. Online at www.va.gov/health/orgs.asp.

"Visualizing Health Policy: The Washington Post/Kaiser Family Foundation Survey of Iraq and Afghanistan Active Duty Soldiers and Veterans." 2014. Kaiser Family Foundation. Online at www.kff.org/.

Warne, Donald. 2007. "Policy Challenges in American Indian/Alaska Native Health Professions Education." *Journal of Interprofessional Care*, 21, Supplement 2 (October 7): 11–19.

Warne, Donald. 2009. "The State of Indigenous America Series." *Wicazo Sa Review*, 24, no. 1 (Spring): 7–23.

Warne, Donald and Linda B. Frizzell. 2014. "American Indian Health Policy: Historical Trends and Contemporary Issues." *American Journal of Public Health*, 104, no. 53 (Supplement): 5263–5267.

Washington, Donna L. 2004. "Challenges to Studying and Delivering Care to Special Populations—The Example of Women Veterans." Guest Editorial. *Journal of Rehabilitation Research and Development*, 41, no 2: vii–ix.

Waxman, Jay M. 2018. "The VA Mission Act of 2018 and Potential Opportunities for Providers." Foley & Lardner LLP. Online at www.healthcarelawtoday.com/.

Wax-Thibodeaux, Emily. 2018. "When VA Needed Landscaping and Snow Removal, One Employee Hired Her Own Brother for $1 Million." *Stars and Stripes*. Online at www.stripes.com/.

Welty, T.K. 1991. "Health Implications of Obesity in American Indians and Alaska Natives." *American Journal of Clinical Nutrition*, 53, no. 6 Supplement (June): 1616–1620.

"What Is Affordable Care Act?" n.d. Washington, DC: US Department of Veterans Affairs. Online at www.va.gov/health/aca/.

White, L. 2017. "5 Common Problems Facing Military Veterans." *Newswire*. Online at https://newswire.net/.

"Who Do Americans Blame for the VA Scandal?" 2014. *CBS News*. Online at www.cbsnews.com/.

Wilensky, Gail R. 2016. "The VA Continues to Struggle—Especially in Terms of Improved Access." Milbank Memorial Fund. Online at www.milbank.org/.

Woellert, Lorraine, Eliana Johnson, and Connor O'Brien. 2018. "Trumps VA Pick Blindsides Staff, Deepens Agency Disarray." *Politico*. Online at www.politico.com/.

Yen, Hope and Zeke Miller. 2018. "Trump Outs Shulkin from Veterans Affairs, Taps His Doctor." Yahoo. Online at www.yahoo.com/.

Young, T. Kue. 1997. "Recent Health Trends in America Indian Population." *Population Research and Policy Review*, 16, nos. 1–2 (April): 147–167.

Zoroya, Gregg. 2012. "Army Suicide Rate in July Hits Highest One-Month Tally." *USA Today*, August 16. Online at http://usatoday30.usatoday.com/.

Section III
PROBLEMS OF THE HEALTHCARE SYSTEM

7

FALLING THROUGH THE SAFETY NET

The Disadvantaged

By 1970, healthcare policy in the United States had reached its maturity. Medicare and Medicaid were passed in 1965; private insurance covered most of working America. But healthcare costs grew dramatically beginning in the mid-1960s, and portions of the population were left out of the system. Two of the major problems of the healthcare system are cost increases and access. We consider the problem of cost increases in the next chapter. This chapter focuses on the problem of access and the disadvantaged.

We concentrate on issues of access to the healthcare system, the problem of the uninsured and the underinsured, low-income groups, minorities (including immigrants), and women. To some extent, these problems overlap. While a good portion of the uninsured are low-income people, some are not. While minorities in general have lower incomes than whites, not all the problems of minorities and healthcare result from lower incomes. Rural areas have access problems with healthcare in the same way that inner cities do: lack of providers. We spell out these interrelationships as we go along.

Perhaps the underlying issue in looking at the disadvantaged and healthcare is equality and equity. We begin this chapter by considering this issue.

EQUALITY AND EQUITY

Equality means that we should treat people who are in the same situation the same way or treat people who are in different situations differently. That is, we should not discriminate against someone on account of race, religion, age, sex, ethnic group, and so forth. One reality of the healthcare system, to be discussed later in the chapter, is that there is discrimination based on income or at least based on health insurance. Those with private insurance plans, especially very generous ones, tend to get better service than those on public plans (such as Medicaid); those without health insurance tend to get the worst care (Berk and Schur 1998). Some have argued that the United States has a two-tiered healthcare system, one for most of us and another for the poor. In Krause's words,

> we have, combining the doctors and the office and hospital settings, a two-class medical care system. On the one hand, few practitioners and a few public settings for the poor in either the ghetto or rural areas; on the other hand, many practitioners and voluntary nonprofit hospitals for the middle class and the upper class in the suburbs.
>
> (Krause 1977, 146)

This leads us to the notion of equity, an extension of the concept of equality. Equity is related to another concept, social justice. Both ideas suggest that, given that some are disadvantaged in the healthcare system, an extra effort should be made to help overcome those disadvantages. This is, in a sense, the idea behind Medicaid (and to a lesser extent, Medicare). Medicaid recipients pay a minimal amount in co-payments, if anything, for their healthcare. To compensate, their healthcare is subsidized by the larger community (taxpayers) and to some extent by providers and their patients, in the sense that Medicaid reimbursements are lower than for privately insured patients and Medicare beneficiaries, and costs are shifted to privately insured patients. Education programs such as Head Start, where more resources are devoted to children from impoverished backgrounds, are another example of equity-based programs.

A number of philosophical concepts support extending access to healthcare services to those who do not have it. Daniels, Light, and Caplan (1996) argue that the appropriate philosophical ground is *fairness*. To the authors, fairness is related to social justice and equal opportunity, or what they call fair equal opportunity. This concept—not especially well defined, in our opinion—sees healthcare as instrumental in that it allows people to function normally. The lack of healthcare services, according to their reasoning, shortens people's lives or makes it more difficult for them to function normally and therefore to live on a level playing field with other people. They write:

> A commitment to fair equality of opportunity thus recognizes that we should not allow people's prospects in life to be governed by correctable, morally arbitrary, or irrelevant differences between them, including those that result from disease and disability ... By designing a health care system that keeps *all* people as close as possible to normal functioning, given reasonable resource constraints, we can in one important way fulfill our moral and legal obligations to protect equality of opportunity.
>
> (Daniels, Light, and Caplan 1996, 22)

Notice at the end of the quote the reference to resource constraints. Their view of fairness is balanced by a concern for liberty, social productivity, and efficiency (Daniels, Light, and Caplan 1996).

The bulk of their book develops ten benchmarks of fairness to evaluate healthcare policy and then applies those benchmarks to the system as it existed at the time, the Clinton plan in 1993 and 1994, and managed care. Their benchmarks include universal access, equitable financing, value for money, public accountability, comparability, and degree of consumer choice. Their evaluation of the 1993–1994 proposals gives the highest marks to the single-payer plan, lower marks to the Clinton proposal, and lowest marks to a market-oriented plan. Daniels et al. also conclude that the trend toward managed care and system integration would move the United States further away from fairness than any of the proposals considered in the 1993–1994 period.

Baird (1998) uses the concept of justice, in this case gender justice, to evaluate the US healthcare system. Baird summarizes the gender justice framework as follows:

> The framework of gender justice includes the principles of self-determination, which is composed of the criteria of self-development, recognition, and democratic freedom; equality of gendered consequences; and diversity.
>
> (Baird 1998, 114)

Self-development refers to a policy's ability to help people develop their capabilities. Recognition is accepting women's needs and experiences as legitimate, and respecting women. Democratic freedom refers to participating in or determining actions that affect one's life. Equality of gendered consequences asks whether public policies, even those that are seemingly neutral, promote equality. Diversity recognizes differences between men and women, but also differences among women (i.e., minority versus white).

Others argue for the concept of a *right to healthcare*. Cust (1997) contends that there is a moral right to healthcare, what he calls a just minimum. He writes that the moral right to healthcare is based on the fact that it can mean the difference between living and dying, and that it also affects a person's quality of life. The notion of rights, he continues, asserts an obligation to fulfill those rights. However, Cust, like Daniels, Light, and Caplan (1996), notes that because of resource constraints and the ever-increasing demand for healthcare, the right is not unlimited. Thus, he balances the moral right to healthcare with the notion of a just minimum.

One aspect of this underlying issue is whether healthcare is a right, in the same way that there is a right to education (a state mandate). In most industrialized countries, healthcare is indeed considered a right. The United States is the only Western industrialized country without a national healthcare system (see Graig 1999; Reid 2009; White 1995) and, as we shall see, one of the problems to be discussed is the large number of people without health insurance.

Watson (1994) argues that, at least for minorities, civil rights issues are at the base of healthcare inequities. He points to significant noneconomic barriers that lead to less access to healthcare and thus poorer healthcare and healthcare outcomes for minorities. Thus, he advocates new civil rights legislation that would forbid discriminatory practices, including unintentional ones, "if they are not necessary to the provision of health care and if their goals cannot be substantially accomplished through less discriminatory alternatives" (Watson 1994, 132).

A human rights approach to healthcare, with similarities to the ideas discussed above, also provides justification for expanding access to health insurance and healthcare services. Chapman (1994) defines human rights as those rights people inherently have because they are human. Human rights exist within the context of a community (see the discussion of community below) and are given high, though not absolute, priority. Chapman writes that these rights are "regarded as essential to the adequate functioning of the human being within the context of community, and (society) accepts responsibility for its promotion and protection" (Chapman 1994, 5).

Thus, there is the obligation on the part of society to fulfill those rights, though again there are limits to how much those rights, like some of the others we have discussed, are fulfilled. Like Daniels, Light, and Caplan (1996), Chapman holds that healthcare as a human right would be limited to those services that would allow a person to function in society and to achieve his or her potential. Chapman goes further when she states:

> The litmus test in this model of human rights is the extent to which the rights of the most vulnerable and disadvantaged individuals and groups are assured by these arrangements. A human rights standard assumes a special obligation or bias in favor of the needs and rights of the poor, the disadvantaged, the powerless, and those at the periphery of society.
>
> (Chapman 1994, 7)

Aday (1993) argues that we should not base our healthcare system on a right to healthcare, which is within the individualistic, liberal tradition of American politics (see Chapter 1). Instead, we should employ the notion of the common good, that it is in the best interest of the community, of society, not just the individual, that all its members have access to healthcare. Kari, Boyte, and Jennings (1994) argue that healthcare should be seen as a civic question, where all participate in policy deliberations and emphasis should be placed on preventing disease and promoting health.

Stone (1993) contends that in recent years, and for good financial reasons, the private insurance market has moved away from notions of community embodied in the civics and communitarian approach of Kari, Boyte, and Jennings (1994). Insurance was originally intended as a means to spread the risk of individual misfortune among the larger community. Private insurers have increasingly sought to fragment the market, however, searching for those who are good health risks and placing more of the burden of financing care on those who are poor risks. This undermines the idea of community. The Affordable Care Act (ACA) attempts to restore community by forbidding insurance companies from refusing to cover people because of preexisting health conditions and reducing differences in the cost of insurance among age groups.

The debates over national health insurance, Medicare, Medicaid, and healthcare reform are, in a sense, marked by notions of community. Do we help those who are vulnerable or disadvantaged, or is everyone on his or her own? The implications of the two choices are not trivial.

Jecker (1993), likewise, suggests that the link between employment and health insurance itself creates injustices, an argument that Enthoven (2003) makes in a different context. Jecker argues that there is discrimination in the distribution of jobs, focusing on gender-based discrimination, and that this creates discrepancies in the availability of health insurance. As one example, consider that women are less likely to be employed in jobs that offer health insurance than men.

Thus, access to healthcare raises important ethical issues. What we must do now is document that the problems indeed do exist.

IMPORTANT CONSIDERATIONS

Before we do that, there are several other factors to consider. One is that having access to healthcare, including insurance coverage, is important, but not the only factor that affects the health of the individual and the community. The United Health Foundation (2017) employs a model of the factors that impact health outcomes, similar to the discussion below: behaviors, community and environment, policy, and clinical care.

One such factor is *public health*. Public health focuses on the health of the larger community, whether it is a municipality, such as the lead in water problem in Flint, Michigan, or the larger nation (such as the flu epidemic in 2017 or the obesity epidemic or the opioid epidemic or the health effects of tobacco), or the global community (such as the AIDS or Zika epidemics). Its focus is on prevention and understanding of disease/sickness patterns and the cause(s) of those patterns. Public health is also concerned about assessing and mitigating problems, such as the possibility of biological attack by terrorists (see Institute of Medicine 2008; Patel and Rushefsky 2005; Schneider 2000). In the aftermath of the September 11, 2001 attacks by Al Qaeda on the United States, public health, at least for a while, gained some prominence.

Public health has had dramatic achievements that have led to increases in human longevity. These include sanitation services, the development of vaccines, clean drinking water, development of antibiotics, safe automobiles, and so forth. There is a massive public health infrastructure (Patel and Rushefsky 2005), particularly at the local level (county health departments), up to federal agencies such as the Centers for Disease Control and Prevention (CDC). But much of the work and achievements of public health are overlooked and funding for public health by all sectors is dwarfed by funding for medically related services. Medical care is estimated to prevent between 10 and 50 percent of premature deaths (Woolf and Aron 2013). Public health is responsible for some portion of the remainder, though estimates vary widely.

A second consideration is *personal responsibility*. The basic idea here is the health of a person is at least partly a result of decisions that the person makes. This would include, for example, taking appropriate medications and following a doctor's recommendations. There are also lifestyle factors that affect a person's health. These include smoking, diet, drinking, use of drugs, extent of exercise, and so forth (see, for example, Li et al. 2018). The ability to follow directions, such as taking medications, may be a function of the cost of the medication. Similarly, eating a healthy diet is affected by advertising and the availability of healthy alternatives. Nevertheless, Li et al. (2018) find that not smoking, a heathy diet, moderate amounts of exercise, and a low body mass index (BMI) leads to fewer premature deaths and greater life expectancy.

Social Determinants of Health

The third factor that affects the health of the population apart from the medical care system is what has been called the *social determinants of health*, and its related aspect, the importance of geography. The impact of social determinants is captured very nicely in a 2013 book by Bradley and Taylor (2013), *The American Health Care Paradox*. They point out that the United States spends more on healthcare than any other country (see chapters 2 and 8), but, based on numerous studies, does not get as good results as other Westernized industrial countries. Bradley and Taylor (2013) report on studies from the Institute of Medicine and on papers going back as far as the 1960s that point to this paradox of high spending but few improvements. Studies from the Commonwealth Fund find that in terms of quality of care, which includes access, the United States rank pretty low (see, for example, Schneider et al. 2017).

The argument behind a social determinants perspective is that there are factors beyond the control of an individual that will affect that person's health in the present and in the future. For example, children who suffer from child abuse or other adverse events (*adverse childhood events* or ACE) often have effects that show up in poor quality of health in later life (see Flaherty et al. 2006; Wegman and Stetler 2009).

Table 7.1 lists the variety of social determinants that might affect the quality of one's health. Income is one of the major determinants. Combining it with education and occupation allows us to talk about socioeconomic differences. In the case of income, those at higher income levels experience better health than those at lower incomes. Interestingly, Woolf and Braveman (2011) note that the relationship holds beyond the obvious rich and poor. Those at middle-class levels have better health than those at lower-income levels, but worse than those at higher levels. Woolf and Braveman (2011) point to research suggesting that lower income is related to higher

Table 7.1

Social Determinants of Health

- Availability of resources to meet daily needs (e.g., safe housing and local food markets)
- Access to educational, economic, and job opportunities
- Access to healthcare services
- Quality of education and job training
- Availability of community-based resources in support of community living and opportunities for recreational and leisure-time activities
- Transportation options
- Public safety
- Social support
- Social norms and attitudes (e.g., discrimination, racism, and distrust of government)
- Exposure to crime, violence, and social disorder (e.g., presence of trash and lack of cooperation in a community)
- Socioeconomic conditions (e.g., concentrated poverty and the stressful conditions that accompany it)
- Residential segregation
- Language/literacy
- Access to mass media and emerging technologies (e.g., cell phones, the Internet, and social media)
- Culture

Source: US Department of Health and Human Services (2012).

premature death rates. Similar results are found when considering education. Those with lower levels of education have higher premature death rates than those at higher levels of education.

Woolf and Braveman (2011) also look at community effects on health. The quality of food available in low-income communities makes it difficult to lead a healthy lifestyle. Low-income neighborhoods tend to have more environmental problems, such as exposure to lead and other toxic substances, than more affluent communities (see, for example, Zubrzycki 2012). Living in poor neighborhoods, which have multiple chronic problems (high unemployment, poverty, and crime, for example), creates stresses on residents, especially children (Woolf and Braveman 2011). Woolf and Braveman (2011) strongly argue that improving the health of people and communities requires focusing on the social determinants. Healthcare reform such as the ACA by itself will not work. Budget cuts to programs that focus on determinants would likely make matters worse. And it is unlikely that the healthcare system can, should, or will on its own address the social determinants of patients. A 2018 survey of physicians by Leavett Partners found that while a majority of physicians had some concern about social determinants issues, such as housing or transportation, they also felt that it was not their responsibility to do anything about it. Other resources would have to be used (Castelucci 2018).

Heiman and Artiga (2015) and Artiga and Hinton (2018) provide an estimate of how much various factors affect the possibility of premature death based on a 2007 study. In order of most to least important: individual behavior accounts for 40 percent, genetics 30 percent, social determinants 20 percent, and healthcare 10 percent of premature death.

Geography is Destiny

Where an individual chooses to live can have a profound effect on their short- and long-term health.
(Institute of Medicine 2008)

While many of the determinants and disparities mentioned above (see Table 7.1) and in other places (see, for example, Artiga and Hinton 2018; Patel and Rushefsky 2008) are intertwined, the issue of geography or place deserves a separate consideration. And in that spirit, we take a bit of exception to the quote that opened up this section. While many people choose to live in a particular place, many others do not. Children are a good example of this. But people who lack the resources to move also make up a certain percentage of the population. To that we can add people who cannot move to certain places because of discrimination or lack of income. America remains very much a segregated community. One way of looking at this is the idea that "a ZIP code is at least as important as race, age and genetics in determining a person's health" (Walker 2011). A study conducted by the Johns Hopkins Bloomberg School of Public Health found that whites who lived in racially integrated neighborhoods had pretty much the same health outcomes as blacks in those neighborhoods. A study by the US Department of Housing and Urban Development found that when women moved from high-poverty to low-poverty neighborhoods with the help of federal housing vouchers, the levels of obesity fell (Walker 2011).

One way of looking at the importance of place is regions of the country. Some regions, especially in the South and in the Appalachian area, have higher rates of premature death than, say, the Upper Midwest (see, for example, Halverson and Bischak 2008).

Rural areas, in particular, tend to suffer from lack of appropriate healthcare facilities. Part of this is due to the small populations in rural areas. While primary care seems to be adequate, more specialized care and hospitals require larger populations to work with. Transportation is often a barrier to obtaining care. Rural residents are thus less likely to use the healthcare system and less likely to obtain use of preventive services than people in more populous areas. Rural residents also tend to be poorer and older than urban residents (Patel and Rushefsky 2008; Agency for Healthcare Research and Quality 2011). Using 2010 data, Probst et al. (2011) found that rural blacks and whites had higher rates of mortality than did their urban counterparts. While education and income were higher in urban than in rural areas, accounting for some of the disparities, access to health insurance was also greater in urban than in rural areas.

Some statistics will help make the point (data from National Rural Health Association 2012). Rural areas have almost one-quarter of the country's population—about 62 million people. But only 10 percent of all physicians are located in rural areas, and the number of specialists per 100,000 population in rural areas is less than one-third that in urban areas. Average per-capita income levels in rural areas are about three-quarters of what they are in urban areas. The poverty rate in rural areas is 14 percent, compared to the 11 percent in urban areas. Sixty-four percent of rural residents are covered by private insurance, compared to 69 percent in urban areas. Medicare spending per capita in rural areas is 85 percent of the national average, compared to 106 percent in urban areas. Finally, only 45 percent of the rural poor are covered by Medicaid, compared to almost 50 percent in urban areas.

As an illustration of the problems rural communities face, rural hospitals have been closing down. Such hospitals not only provide for the healthcare needs of the community, but also provide jobs. When such hospitals close down, those communities are hurt (Weber and Miller 2017). Many rural hospitals are in the southeast portion of the United States. These are states that for the most part have not expanded Medicaid and have the highest rates of uninsured population. Their populations have high levels of chronic health problems, such as obesity, diabetes, and hypertension (Weber and Miller 2017).

An example of the problems rural communities face when a hospital closes down comes from the authors' home state of Missouri ("Missouri Hospital's Sudden Closure Problematic for Expectant Mothers" 2018). A hospital, Twin Rivers Regional Medical Center, closed in July 2018. It was located in the southeast part of the state in one of the state's poorest counties. A hospital in a neighboring county, also impoverished, is having trouble staying open. The nearest hospital that residents can go to for childbirth delivery is an hour away and many of the residents do not have cars (the transportation issue).

The problems were also demonstrated in a *PBS News Hour* story in 2016 that took place in Grundy, Virginia, population 958. Located in the Appalachian Mountains near Kentucky, it is one of the poorer towns and counties (Buchanan County) in the country. The *News Hour* segment, which aired in November 2016, focused on a charitable clinic, Remote Area Medical, that comes to Grundy once a year to provide free medical care to the population. The clinic is set up in the town's middle school. People come from miles around to this town, which was once a coal town. Dental and medical services are provided and for many residents that is the only formal medical care they may receive until the next year (*PBS News Hour* 2016; see also Khazan 2015). The problems of lower-class, white, rural residents became a focus of the 2016 presidential elections, particularly the Trump campaign, and of a number of books, such as *White Trash* (Isenberg 2016), *Hillbilly Elegy* (Vance 2016), and *White Rage* (Anderson 2017).

The problems of rural hospitals are many. One is the population size of the surrounding communities. Another is that many of the hospitals are outdated. A third is financial issues. Such hospitals often have to treat patients in emergency rooms and bills for services are not paid. The federal government has cut back on payments to hospitals, including for bad debt (Weber and Miller 2017). The result is that getting to a hospital means a longer trip to a more urban hospital. Recall from the Preface the story of the birth of Rushefsky's second child. Had there not been a rural hospital in Rocky Mount, VA, the child may well have been born on the side of the road to Roanoke.

Residents of urban inner-city areas, where the makeup is mostly ethnic minorities, also face health access and outcome problems (Patel and Rushefsky 2008; Smedley et al. 2008). These problems include lack of insurance, lack of a regular provider, and exposure to environmental insults. Smedley et al. (2008) point, as an example, to the neighborhood of South Camden, New Jersey, a largely minority neighborhood, which has a disproportionate number of facilities that pollute, as well as abandoned waste sites. The prevalence of providers within urban areas depends on the type of community. Higher-income neighborhoods have a higher ratio of physicians to population than lower-income neighborhoods do. Hospitals in inner-city areas tend to have more financial problems than those in more affluent areas. Even within urban areas, there are often transportation issues (Patel and Rushefsky 2008).

Addressing Social Determinants

The problem of social determinants helps explain much of the disparities in health and care for portions of the US population. How we address this problem may have more impact on the health of these groups than just increasing access and health insurance coverage (which we discuss below). Bradley and Taylor (2013) point out that while the US spends a great deal on healthcare relative to other Westernized industrial countries (see Chapter 8), it spends near the bottom on social services that would address the social determinants that address these problems. Hacker (2002) argues that social welfare benefits in the US approach other countries' levels if we count what the private sector does. His data, however, focus on health insurance and pension benefits, not encompassing the kinds of social services that Bradley and Taylor (2013) mention. Bradley and Taylor's focus is on three large factors: housing, employment, and education. Our focus, as mentioned above, is somewhat broader, encompassing income, geography, and racial/ethnic/gender factors.

Bradley and Taylor (2013) see the need for more, and better, programs in the social services area, using Sweden as a model. They do note that there are some cultural differences between the two countries that prevent the US from undertaking the scope of actions found in other countries. Without going into detail on this element, one important aspect of cultural differences is the role of individualism in a society. The US is much more individualistic than other Westernized, industrial countries and likely to see lifestyle factors, such as smoking and using seatbelts, as more decisions of individuals than affected by larger cultural factors (such as advertising).

One set of institutions that can meld the health and social determinants elements, mentioned by Bradley and Taylor (2013), are community health centers. Such centers can link patients/people with other services, such as mental health services.

Related to community health centers are *community health workers.* The Community Health Workers section of the American Public Health Association defines a community health worker as follows:

> A community health worker is a frontline public health worker who is a trusted member of and/or has an unusually close understanding of the community served. This trusting relationship enables the worker to serve as a liaison/link/intermediary between health/social services and the community to facilitate access to services and improve the quality and cultural competence of service delivery.
>
> A community health worker also builds individual and community capacity by increasing health knowledge and self-sufficiency through a range of activities such as outreach, community education, informal counseling, social support and advocacy.
>
> (Community Health Workers n.d.)

Community health workers can help people apply for health benefits, such as Medicaid. They can perform health screenings on people, make sure they get and take needed medications, and also help people get other services, such as nutrition and transportation services (Crum 2018).

Artiga and Hinton (2018) and Heiman and Artiga (2015) discuss different ways that the social determinants can be addressed. Heiman and Artiga (2015) mention Health in All Policies. Health in All Policies would bring in health considerations to decisions involving education, transportation, food, and economic development. Artiga and Hinton (2018) note that under Medicaid Section 1115 waivers, states link the healthcare system with some of these other factors. Medicaid has been prompting some providers to look at housing issues. Medicaid could also be used to support employment. The federal government has begun requiring Medicaid managed-care organizations to look at the social determinants of their clients, through screenings and then referrals to appropriate agencies.

The Affordable Care Act requires non-profit hospitals to engage in periodic community needs assessments. Some providers have begun screening their patients for the various social determinant factors.

THE UNINSURED AND UNDERINSURED

Most people in the United States with health insurance, a majority of the population, have it through their jobs. In 2016, the uninsured rate, or the percentage of the population without health insurance, stood at 8.8 percent (Barnett and Berchick 2017; US Census Bureau 2017). In 2008, the uninsured rate was about 15 percent. About 58 percent of those with insurance were covered by their employer, compared to 64.1 percent of people with employer-based insurance in 1999 and 59.7 percent in 2007, the year the Great Recession began. Part of the decline in employer-based insurance was due to the recession, but the numbers show a continued decline in such coverage, especially among smaller businesses. A little over 16 percent of the population purchased their health insurance directly from insurers (the individual market). Just over 36 percent of the population were on either Medicare or Medicaid, or both—as we saw in Chapters 4 and 5 (Barnett and Berchick 2017; US Census Bureau 2017) (see Table 7.2). The decline in the uninsured rate is partially due to the recovery from the recession, which ended in 2009. But much of the decline is due to the Affordable Care Act.

Table 7.2 also presents data about the number and percentage of uninsured persons. Note that the percentage of persons without insurance increased from 1999 to 2003. For 2010, the number of uninsured persons was almost 50 million. These numbers give an incomplete picture of the uninsured problem. The data are, in a sense, a snapshot, a picture of those without insurance. A number of people experience spells of uninsurance during the year. According to the Centers for Disease Control and Prevention, about 59 million people lacked health insurance for some part of the year (Fox 2010). More recent figures are not available, though given the impact of the Affordable Care Act, that number in 2017 was lower than in 2010.

Table 7.2

Sources of Health Insurance Coverage, 1999–2016

	Percent of Population Insured by All Sources	Percent of Population Insured by Employer	Percent of Population Insured by Public Insurance	Percent of Population with Nongroup Insurance	Percent of Population without Insurance	Number of People Uninsured (in Millions)
2016	91.2	55.7	37.3	16.2	8.8	28.1
2015	90.9	56.7	37.1	16.3	9.1	28.9
2014	89.6	56.4	36.5	14.6	10.4	32.9
2013	86.7	56.7	34.6	11.4	13.3	41.8
2012	84.6	54.9	32.6	9.8	15.4	47.9
2011	84.3	55.1	32.2	10.0	15.7	48.6
2010	83.7	55.3	31.0	9.8	16.3	49.9
2009	83.9	56.1	30.6	9.6	16.1	48.9
2008	85.1	58.9	29.1	9.5	14.9	44.8
2007	85.3	59.8	27.8	9.5	14.7	44.1
2006	84.8	60.3	27.1	9.8	15.2	45.2
2005	85.4	60.7	27.3	9.9	14.6	43.0
2004	85.7	61.1	27.3	10.0	14.3	41.8
2003	85.4	61.5	26.4	10.0	14.8	41.9
2002	86.1	62.8	25.5	10.2	13.9	39.8
2001	86.5	63.8	24.9	10.1	13.5	38
2000	86.9	65.1	24.4	10.2	13.1	36.6
1999	86.4	64.1	24.2	10.6	13.6	37.7

Note: public insurance includes Medicare, Medicaid, military and military family, and veterans
Some people have coverage under more than one type of insurance (i.e., Medicare and Medicaid, Medicare plus retiree insurance)
Source: US Census Bureau, "Health Insurance Historical Tables–HIB Series." 2017. Online at census.gov.

One of the unique features of the US healthcare system is the prevalence of employer-sponsored insurance (ESI), though some countries, such as Germany, also have a strong ESI presence (Reid 2009). Indeed, the development of private health insurance in the 1930s and its tie to employment, which became much stronger during World War II, set the US on a course that has largely continued (Starr 1982).

While employers remain the single-largest source of health insurance (US Census Bureau 2017), Table 7.2 shows a precipitous decline in such coverage. The question is why this has occurred. This is an important question, given two facts. One is that much health insurance coverage, as noted earlier, is linked to jobs. This is the uniqueness of healthcare in the United States, a combination of public and private coverage, what Hacker (2002) calls the "divided welfare state." Second, such coverage decreased in the 1990s, even as job expansion was impressive. As noted above, job growth in the 2000s has been slower, with slow recoveries from the two recessions (2001–2002, 2007–2009). Coverage has continued to decline (Foutz et al. 2017). An important related factor is the cost of healthcare and its reflection in the cost of health insurance. Employers try to shift more costs to employees or not cover employees at all (see Hacker 2006). The individual market is so expensive that many either cannot afford it or are discouraged from getting it.

The answer also lies partly in the restructuring of the American economy. Insurance coverage is linked to size and type of firm (Claxton et al. 2017; Employee Benefits Research Institute 2016). The largest firms, those with 100 or more employees, are much more likely to offer health insurance to their employees than smaller firms are. During the period from 1999 to 2017, an average of nearly 97 percent of larger firms offered the health insurance benefit in good times and bad (authors' calculation from Claxton et al. 2017). About 50 percent of the small firms, those with 3–49 workers, offered health insurance to their employees. Most of the decline in employer-sponsored insurance came from the smallest companies (Claxton et al. 2017). The major reasons that smaller firms are less likely to cover their employees are the cost of the coverage and the greater inability of such firms to absorb these costs (Employee Benefits Research Institute 2016). Another reason for the erosion in employer-based health insurance has to do with the sectors of the economy that are growing and shrinking. Manufacturing firms and unionized firms (with much overlapping) are more likely to offer health insurance (and other benefits) than service-based or agricultural firms (Holahan and Ghosh 2004; Mishel 2012). For example, 96 percent of unionized firms offer health insurance to their employees compared to 61 percent of non-union firms (Claxton et al. 2004). The service sector has experienced considerable growth, while the manufacturing sector and unionization have shrunk. In the 2006–2016 period, work in the manufacturing sector declined by 1.8 million jobs, a decline of nearly 13 percent. By contrast, the retail service sector saw an increase of over 467,000 workers, over the same period of time—an increase of about 3 percent (authors' calculations from Bureau of Labor Statistics, n.d.).

Consider the following numbers. In 1970, some 20.7 million workers were in the manufacturing sector. In 2010, the number had shrunk to 14.1 million; by 2016, that number was down to 12.3 million workers. By contrast, 20.4 million workers were in the service sector in 1970; in 2010 that number had jumped to almost 76 million; by 2016 there were 125 million workers in the service sector. Another way of looking at this is to compare the relative shares of manufacturing and service workers. In 1970, the share of workers in manufacturing was 26.4 percent; in 2010, that share had declined to 10.1 percent; by 2016, it was down to 9.5 percent. The share of workers in the service sector in 1970 was 25.9 percent, a little less than the manufacturing share. But by 2010, the service-sector share of jobs had increased to 54.6 percent (calculated from US Census Bureau 2012; Bureau of Labor Statistics, n.d.). Thus, if there is less likelihood that the service sector will offer health insurance than the manufacturing sector will, it is understandable why fewer workers have health insurance.

Walmart, the largest employer in the United States, is a good example of these tendencies and problems (as are Target and Home Depot) (Scheiber and Corkery 2017). Walmart's website (www.corporate.walmart.com/our-story/working-at-walmart) lists the benefits it offers both part-time and full-time workers. Walmart offers a pretty standard health insurance policy, including company contributions to health savings accounts. This includes healthcare insurance for its employees and their dependents (domestic partners). Depending on who one asks, the health insurance offered can be cheap but with high deductibles. Further, Walmart ended coverage for some part-time workers (Tabuchi 2014). Walmart has been buying up online retailers and employees of those companies have found that their cost-sharing has increased significantly (Scheiber and Corkery 2017).

A related problem concerns retirees, especially younger retirees, those between 55 and 65. In 2017, 66 percent of large firms offered health insurance to early retirees, down from 80 percent in 2005 (Claxton et al. 2017). Larger firms (and unionized firms) are more likely to offer health insurance to their retired workers than are smaller and non-unionized firms.

As we have seen, the uninsured rate has gone down dramatically (though, as we note below, it has crept up). The decline is due partially to the recovery from the Great Recession and more strongly from the Affordable Care Act. With the Affordable Care Act, the mechanisms for increased coverage have been the insurance exchanges and Medicaid expansion (see Chapters 3 and 4). Medicaid expansion has had the larger impact—17 million new enrollees through the middle of 2017, with more than 10 million enrollees in the exchanges ("Key Facts about the Uninsured Population" 2017). The numbers would have been larger, especially for Medicaid, if more states had expanded Medicaid and implementation of the exchanges had been smoother (see Chapters 3 and 4).

While the decline in the uninsured rate has been dramatic (see Table 7.2), there is still a sizable portion of the population (over 28 million people in 2017) that does not have health insurance (Foutz et al. 2017; "Key Facts about the Uninsured Population" 2017). The first question we should ask is why these people do not have health insurance. Collins et al. (2016) offers six reasons. First, many of the uninsured were not citizens. This was especially true of the Latino population. Illegal or undocumented persons are not eligible for coverage under the ACA (see the discussion below). A second reason is that some states have not expanded Medicaid as called for under the Affordable Care Act. As of April 2018, 18 states had not expanded their Medicaid programs ("Status of State Medicaid Expansion Decisions" 2018)—states controlled by Republicans, who as we saw in Chapters 3 and 4 have opposed the ACA since its inception in 2010.

A third reason for being uninsured, according to Collins et al. (2016), is that the groups most likely to be uninsured are the least aware about the exchanges or marketplaces. That lack of awareness means that people in these groups do not know that the exchanges are available and that there are subsidies to help them with the costs. Fourth, there is concern among the uninsured about whether they are eligible and whether they can afford the plans. Some had incomes that made them ineligible for either Medicaid or the exchange subsidies, but this was a relatively small portion of the population. The fifth reason is that many of the uninsured who visited the exchanges (on computers) had difficulty in comparing plans. A related point, the sixth reason, is that those who visited the exchanges but did not enroll in a plan did not have any kind of personal assistance or help. Some states, such as the authors' home state of Missouri, refused to pay for navigators to help people find appropriate plans. The federal government during the Trump administration also cut back on paying navigators or offering other help (Soffen 2017) (see Chapter 3).

Another reason people may be uninsured is that they lose their job. A law passed in 1986, the Consolidated Omnibus Budget Reconciliation Act (COBRA), allows workers who lose their jobs to maintain their health insurance for up to 18 months after their job ended (Kreidler, n.d.). While this does help some workers and their families, the insurance is expensive. Under COBRA, the displaced worker pays both the employee's and the employer's share of the costs, including any increases that might occur over the 18-month period. The costs are substantial. In 2017, an employer-covered family health insurance plan cost, on average, $18,764 of which the employee contributed $5,714 (Claxton et al. 2017). The worker with family coverage who lost his or her job would be paying $18,764, more than three times what he or she previously paid, but without the job to pay for it.

The second question that needs to be asked is what the profile is of those uninsured. One such characteristic is that much of the uninsured group is low-income; about 49 percent of the uninsured have incomes lower than 200 percent of the federal poverty (Foutz et al. 2017). Second, many of the uninsured live in households where at least one person is employed; 75 percent of such households have at least one full-time worker and another 11 percent have a part-time worker; 15 percent of the uninsured live in households with no workers (Foutz et al. 2017). One implication of this is that linking employment (or job training, etc.) to Medicaid eligibility as some states have done and the Trump administration has encouraged (see Chapters 3 and 4) will have a minimal effect. Not all employers, as we have seen, offer insurance, and for many workers, the cost of insurance was prohibitive ("Key Facts About the Uninsured Population" 2017).

A third important characteristic of the uninsured is the racial/ethnic breakdown. The largest single block of uninsured people is whites (44 percent). Blacks comprise 15 percent of the uninsured, Hispanics 33 percent, and Asian or Native Hawaiian/Pacific Islander about 5 percent. Having said this, Whites have a lower insurance rate (8 percent) than Hispanics (17 percent) or Blacks (12 percent). (Artiga et al. 2016; Foutz et al. 2017). To quote Foutz et al. (2017, 9): "Differences in coverage by race/ethnicity likely reflect a combination of factors, including language and immigration barriers, income and work status, and state of residence."

Adults are more likely than children to be uninsured. Immigration is also an issue here (we discuss immigration in more detail below). Immigrants, whether legal or undocumented, have a much higher uninsured rate (27 percent) than citizens (about 9 percent) (Foutz et al. 2017).

Above we discussed the importance of geography, where a person lives. Uninsured rates are higher in the South than elsewhere. The states with the highest uninsured rates in 2017 were Texas, Oklahoma, Georgia, Florida, and Mississippi (Quinn 2017). Given the large population in Texas and Florida, those two states have the largest population of uninsured people. The states with the lowest uninsured rates were Massachusetts, Vermont, Hawaii, and Minnesota (Quinn 2017).

Finally, most of the uninsured are adults. Medicaid and the Children's Health Insurance Program (CHIP) provide more coverage for children than adults ("Key Facts about the Uninsured Population" 2017). We should also point out in our discussion of the uninsured that when we refer to adults we are referring to those adults under the age of 65. Most seniors (65 and older) are covered by Medicare, effectively a form of national health insurance for this group (see Chapter 5).

One last aspect remains. The section heading refers to the uninsured and the underinsured. The *underinsured* are those who have health insurance but whose insurance is inadequate for their present or future needs. A commonly used measure of underinsurance is when family healthcare costs exceed 10 percent of family income; for low-income families, the underinsurance threshold is 5 percent (Collins et al. 2014). This refers especially to those who may have illnesses such as AIDS or multiple sclerosis, chronic diseases that are potentially expensive to cover. Adding in the underinsured to the uninsured, one estimate is that as many as 81 million people are at some financial risk (Schoen et al. 2011). Underinsurance rates were highest among the disabled covered by Medicare and those who bought insurance on the individual market (Collins et al. 2014). The association health insurance plans that the Trump administration is pushing may add to the ranks of the underinsured (see Chapter 3).

A major cause of underinsurance is the presence of high deductibles, what the holder has to pay before the insurance company will pay. Employers are increasingly offering high-deductible policies to their employees

(Claxton et al. 2017). Such policies are cheaper for employers and, at least at first, cheaper for employees. Think of car insurance. The higher the deductible, the lower the premiums. The same is pretty much true with health insurance, including those plans purchased on the ACA exchanges. Claxton et al. (2017) present data showing the change in types of plans offered: in 1988, 73 percent of employer health insurance plans were conventional, indemnity insurance. The rest were some variant of managed-care plans, such as health maintenance organizations or preferred-provider plans. By 2006, only 3 percent of plans were conventional, 80 percent were managed-care, and high-deductible plans made their appearance at 4 percent. By 2017, about 1 percent of plans were conventional, 62 percent were managed-care, and 28 percent were high-deductible. The people most likely to be underinsured were those whose income was low and/or with serious medical problems (Collins et al. 2014).

Two other points about underinsurance need to be made. First are what have come to be called *skinny plans*. Such plans, increasingly emphasized in the wake of attempts to repeal the Affordable Care Act (see Chapters 3 and 11), are characterized by low premiums and minimal benefits. For example, such plans can deny applicants for pre-existing conditions and coverage might not include prescription drugs or maternity care (Hansard 2018). Those likely to choose such plans are younger, healthy people. Such plans are attractive to people who do not need those benefits and would like a cheaper plan. But the coverage is limited. Think again of auto insurance. A skinny auto insurance plan might cover liability (costs associated with those hurt in an accident) but not collision (costs associated with repairing one's car).

The second point is one that is likely not mentioned enough. In Chapter 5, we noted that a substantial sector of the Medicare population had fairly low incomes. If we compared the cost of premiums and deductibles to income, we would find that many Medicare recipients are underinsured. Cubanski et al. (2018) found that Medicare households spent an average of 14 percent of their income on healthcare, and about 33 percent spent more than 20 percent of their income on healthcare. While there are supplements available to Medicare recipients, such as medigap policies, those too are expensive.

CONSEQUENCES OF UNINSURANCE AND UNDERINSURANCE

There is a simple and easy, though not pleasant, answer to the question of what the consequences are of inadequate or no insurance. That answer is that such people are at higher risk of disease and death and are less likely to receive the services that they need when they need them than are those who have insurance. Such people are also subject to financial stress. This section documents that claim.

One clearly important consequence is the linkage between health insurance coverage and mortality. In 2002, the Institute of Medicine (IOM) estimated that nearly 18,000 people died in 2000 because of lack of health insurance coverage, what is called excess deaths (Committee on the Consequences of Uninsurance 2002; Dorn 2008). Updating the IOM study, Dorn (2008) estimated the number of excess deaths between 2000 and 2006 at between 137,000 and 165,000 (the different numbers reflect somewhat different methodologies).

The uninsured are far less likely than the insured to have a regular physician (Committee on the Consequences of Uninsurance 2002; Foutz et al. 2017). Forty-nine percent of those without insurance did not have a primary-care physician, compared to 12 percent for those on Medicaid and with private insurance (Foutz et al. 2017). Those with chronic health conditions who are uninsured are also less likely than those with health insurance to get the care they need, including the preventive care that would keep the chronic condition from worsening (Hoffman and Schwartz 2008; "Key Facts about the Uninsured" 2017). In general, the uninsured are less likely to get preventive care than the insured (Foutz et al. 2017).

Foutz et al (2017, 11) note that even when the uninsured are hospitalized, they get fewer services than those with insurance:

> Because uninsured patients are less likely than those with insurance to receive necessary follow-up screenings, they have an increased risk of being diagnosed at later stages of diseases, including cancer, and have higher mortality rates than those with insurance. In addition, when uninsured people are hospitalized, they receive fewer diagnostic and therapeutic services and also have higher mortality rates than those with insurance.

One interesting question focuses on the use of hospital emergency departments (EDs) by the uninsured. There are political aspects to the question, because if the uninsured are crowding emergency departments, care becomes extremely costly. Based on our reading of the literature, we conclude the following. The uninsured are much more likely to make use of emergency departments for care than the insured. According to a study by the Center for Healthcare Research and Transformation (cited by Greene 2011), about 10 percent of the uninsured (Michigan data) use EDs for primary care compared to only 3 percent of the insured. Further, the uninsured are much more likely to utilize walk-in urgent-care centers than the insured. But some have argued that it is insured patients, whether privately insured or on Medicaid, who really crowd the EDs and that blaming the uninsured is a myth. Data from the National Center for Health Statistics seem to support this finding (Garcia, Bernstein, and Bush 2010; LaCalle and Rabin 2010). Both statements appear to be correct.

The seemingly contradictory findings are easily reconcilable. The key is that the uninsured are a small portion, about 17 percent, of the population. While the uninsured are more likely to use EDs than the insured, the insured population is more than five times as large. We would expect that most of the people using ED services would be insured. Further, there is a convenience factor involved. While waiting times may be long for those going to EDs with non-life-threatening issues, it is still easier to see a doctor there than to see a family's regular family physician. Consider a family with a young child who develops an ear infection late Friday night. The parents are more likely to take the child to the ED on Saturday than to wait until Monday to call the child's pediatrician and hope to get in that day.

One result of delaying needed physician visits is that Medicaid patients and those without insurance are more likely than those with private insurance to be hospitalized for conditions that could have been avoided or treated outside hospitals (Foutz et al. 2017). Uninsured hospital patients are more likely to enter hospitals sicker and to have shorter stays and fewer procedures performed on them than privately insured patients. They also have a higher death rate than insured patients (Committee on the Consequences of Uninsurance 2002; Foutz et al. 2017).

Perhaps the most important impact is on children. Children whose families lack health insurance are less likely to see a physician than children in families with insurance and are less likely to get the same quality of care as those who are insured. Typical and treatable maladies of childhood, such as ear and throat infections, may go untreated and worsen (Foutz et al. 2017).

Further, barriers other than lack of insurance may hinder needed physician visits. These include cost-sharing provisions, lack of transportation, and lack of child care (Stoddard, St. Peter, and Newacheck 1994). The General Accounting Office (now the Government Accountability Office) expressed the problem this way:

> But having health insurance is no guarantee that children will get appropriate, high-quality care. Some children live in families that do not understand the need for preventive care or do not know how to seek high-quality care. Some live in neighborhoods that have few health care providers, where they have to travel further and wait longer for care. Some live in families in which most of the members do not speak English or defer getting care because they have had difficulty getting care previously. Some children have health insurance that does not cover some of the services they need the most—such as dental care or physical therapy for the developmentally disabled ... Such barriers can reduce the likelihood that even insured children will get the care they need.
>
> (General Accounting Office 1997)

Lack of insurance may affect the most helpless of people, newborn babies. Uninsured women are less likely to receive prenatal care than are privately insured women and more likely to have underweight children and premature births (Families USA 2010). Private health insurance coverage for pregnant women is spotty. Prior to the Affordable Care Act, insurers could refuse to cover pregnant women, treating pregnancy as a preexisting condition, or could charge higher premiums for pregnant women.

There are public programs to cover pregnancy, especially for low-income women. Federal law requires states under Medicaid to cover pregnant women with incomes under 133 percent of the federal poverty line. There is also an option to cover women with incomes under 185 percent of that indicator. As a result, Medicaid pays for about 50 percent of all births in the United States. New Mexico has the highest rate, covering 72 percent of all pregnancies, and New Hampshire has the lowest rate, covering just 27 percent ("Births Financed by Medicaid" 2017; Kodjak 2017).

Legislation in 2009 and 2010 extended insurance coverage for pregnant women. In 2009, the Children's Health Insurance Program (CHIP) was reauthorized, allowing states to cover pregnant women over the age of 18. The law provides for three options. The newest option is called the Pregnant Woman State Plan Amendments. It provides prenatal care and up to 60 days of care after delivery. Fifteen states make use of the Unborn Child State Plan Amendment, which originated with an administrative decision in 2002 by the Department of Health and

Human Services to define a child from the point of conception and therefore as eligible for benefits under the CHIP program. This program covers only the child and not the mother for non-pregnancy- related health problems. The third option is the Section 1115 waiver, also a result of administrative action, in this case in 2000. Eighteen states had taken part in this program as of 2014. States can design their own benefit programs, which could match those in the Pregnant Woman State Plan Amendments (March of Dimes 2014).

The Affordable Care Act provided new benefits for pregnant women, though some did not start until 2014. One example is that coverage of pregnancy will be part of the package of essential benefits for state health exchanges, something that is not in the skinny plans. Further, insurers will not be able to charge higher premiums to pregnant women nor be able to refuse them coverage. The ACA also provided for a new program of home visitations for pregnant women by nurse practitioners and others (Andrews 2010).

The presence of health insurance also has an impact on the diagnosis of breast cancer. Women who have no health insurance or are covered by Medicaid are more likely to have breast cancer diagnosed later in the progression of the disease and are more likely to die as a result than women with breast cancer who have private health insurance (Committee on Health Insurance Status and Its Consequences 2009).

Those without health insurance also perceive themselves as less healthy than those with insurance. Death rates may be higher for those who lack health insurance than for those with it. This may be caused by both lack of access to medical care and lower quality of care when it is received (Committee on the Consequences of Uninsurance 2002).

Further, the lack of health insurance coverage results in low-income families having to make difficult choices in how to allocate their budgets. The competing demands of housing, food, clothing, and so forth lead lower-income families to forgo purchasing health insurance (Long 2003). Healthcare is expensive, but lack of healthcare coverage can be brutal on families.

Ironically, those without insurance are often charged more for healthcare services than those with coverage. This especially happens compared to employer-sponsored insurance, because employers can negotiate with providers for lower prices (discounts). The uninsured do not have that kind of leverage. The uninsured are often asked to pay prior to receiving services or make arrangements to pay (say, via credit cards) ("The Uninsured: A Primer" 2011; "Key Facts about the Uninsured" 2017). The combination of delaying treatment and lack of insurance coverage often results in the incursion of large amounts of debt and bankruptcy (see Seifert and Rukavina 2006; "Key Facts about the Uninsured" 2017).

Uninsurance and underinsurance have impacts beyond those of the individual. In 1986, Congress passed the Emergency Medical Treatment and Active Labor Act (EMTALA). The legislation was passed, at least partially, in response to instances of what were known as "dumping," whereby hospitals would either refuse to treat uninsured patients or transfer them to other hospitals. Under the EMTALA, hospitals receiving federal funds (through programs such as Medicare and Medicaid) are required to screen and treat anyone showing up at an emergency room with threatening healthcare conditions. Hospitals are required to, at a minimum, stabilize the patient before releasing him or her (Furrow 1995; Rosenbaum 2013). The legislation has sometimes been used to show that people can get care even if uninsured. For example, President Bush in July 2007 said: "The immediate goal is to make sure there are more people on private insurance plans. I mean, people have access to health care in America. After all, you just go to an emergency room" (quoted in Froomkin 2007).

The law has been somewhat limited. Its penalties are fairly light. And in 2003, the Bush administration issued regulations loosening the requirements and downsizing enforcement ("Emergency Medical Treatment and Active Labor Act" n.d.; Rosenbaum et al. 2012). Rosenbaum et al. (2012) document several instances of violations of the EMTALA and suggest that a better system of reporting and monitoring is necessary.

Because uninsured people are more likely to use expensive emergency rooms than a regular physician, the cost of that care is shifted to others. Indeed, hospitals in particular engage in considerable cost-shifting, given service to the uninsured and the low reimbursement rates for Medicaid patients. Those with private insurance are charged more (and pay higher premiums) because of such cost-shifting. Because of the Medicare hospital Prospective Payment System (PPS), discussed in Chapter 5, shifting costs to Medicare patients is virtually impossible. Given this cost-shifting, portions of the community pay for uninsured care, but not on an explicit basis. One way of dealing with this cost issue is the *Disproportionate Share Hospital* (DSH) program. The program, created first in Medicaid in 1981 and then in Medicare in 1985, provides extra funds to hospitals that have a high proportion (a disproportionate share) of Medicaid and uninsured patients. The minimum proportion of such patients is 15 percent (LaCouture 2014). While there are suggestions that the formula used does not target well the appropriate population (LaCouture 2014), DSH payments have proven to be important to hospitals. The ACA called for the reduction of DSH payments, because of Medicaid expansion and the exchanges; however, the cuts were delayed by Congress at least until 2020 (Catron 2018; Sollenberger 2018).

Another aspect of the uninsurance problem is the consequences for communities where a significant percentage of the population lack health insurance. Such communities face what are called "negative spillover effects" (Gresenz and Escarce 2011). Gresenz and Escarce (2011) note that people who were insured, but lived in communities with high uninsured rates, had difficulty accessing the system and lower satisfaction with access to care. This appeared to be the case even among seniors who had Medicare.

INSURANCE AND THE IDEA OF COMMUNITY

This brings us back to the issue of equity. Many health insurance provisions are put in place regardless of income. Consider a company that offers a health insurance plan covering dependents. The premiums are $650 a month for family coverage, and there are cost-sharing provisions. All employees are offered the same plan. The general manager of the company makes $215,000 a year (before taxes) and the janitor makes $20,000 (before taxes). Both have to pay the $650 monthly premium. The premium is less than 1 percent of the general manager's income but is about 3.3 percent of the janitor's income (though the GM may have a more a more generous policy and, in some cases, not have to pay premiums). Now extend this example to those who try to buy health insurance as individuals rather than as part of a group. Typically, premiums for individual policies are not as high as family group policies but are also not as generous. Further, in the case of individual plans, the holder pays all the cost of the premiums, whereas in group (employer-based) plans, the employer will pay some of the premium costs. Cost-sharing provisions (deductibles, co-payments) tend to be larger for individual policies (Kaiser Family Foundation 2004a; Pollack and Kronebusch 2004). The result is that, from 2004 to 2007, about 73 percent of those shopping on the individual health insurance market either could not afford the plan or were turned down because of a preexisting condition (Doty et al. 2007).

There is another way in which ethical issues play a role in the uninsurance and underinsurance problem. This is the problem of changes in insurance company policies. To simplify, health insurance policies can take two forms. On the one hand is *community rating*, by which everybody in the insurance pool pays the same premiums (though there may be differences based on age and other such factors, a practice known as risk adjustment). That way, the risk of using the insurance (needing healthcare) is spread over a larger population. Larger firms are more likely than smaller firms to have a community rating plan. Because the pool of employees is large, there is a large group of workers over which to spread the risk. Smaller firms, with fewer workers, have a smaller group over which to spread the risk. Insurance companies could handle the problem by treating all those they insure as the community, so it would not matter whether the firm was large or small, or the policy was for an individual or a group. Note that pooling risk for individual policies by definition cannot be done.

Prior to 2014, there was an increasing tendency for insurance companies to write policies based on *experience rating*, under which the premiums are adjusted based on the likely risk of needing healthcare. A person with a chronic heart problem, for example, is more likely to need healthcare than one in good health with no chronic problems. Automobile insurance is written on this basis. Premiums are higher for those in the highest-risk groups, which includes those who have been in accidents and those in groups most likely to have accidents. For example, young single males have the highest auto insurance premiums of any group. Someone who was at high risk of needing substantial medical care might be denied coverage, or coverage might be canceled when needed, with the argument being that some preexisting condition was not indicated in the application form, a policy known as rescission.

Such a practice makes sense from the standpoint of the insurance company, as well as policyholders in low-risk groups. Those more likely to need the service should pay more. Having community rating in auto insurance would mean higher rates for those in the low-risk groups and lower rates for those in the high-risk groups, pretty much what we see with the Affordable Care Act (see Chapter 3). Further, such practices were an inherent part of health insurance policies. While the purpose of health insurance companies is to pay for healthcare for their subscribers, the more a company paid out, the smaller its profits were. This issue is known as the *Medical Loss Ratio* or MLR. The higher the ratio, the more an insurance company paid out to subscribers. The lower the ratio, the more of subscriber premiums the company retained. The lower the ratio, the higher the value of the stock of an insurance company. These kinds of motivations put companies in the paradoxical position of having an incentive not to provide services.

There is another insurance practice, very much related to experience rating, that leads to some people being uninsured and others being underinsured. This is the practice of insurance underwriting. Underwriting occurs when an insurance company refuses to insure workers in an entire firm (a practice known as "redlining"), or individuals with preexisting conditions. Examples of redlined firms included "those characterized by an older work force (over age fifty-five) or high employee turnover, those engaged in seasonal work or exposed to hazardous working conditions, those lacking an employer-employee relationship, and those 'known to present frequent claims submissions'" (Zellers, McLaughlin, and Frick 1992, 174–175). Those with preexisting conditions, such as cancer, diabetes, or AIDS, and those with conditions that are likely to result in costly claims in the future may be denied insurance either permanently or during a specified time. In addition, limits may be placed on payments to such individuals. An alternative practice is to raise all the premiums for the groups significantly, sometimes to prohibitive levels. It is not just insurance companies that engage in this practice. Employers that self-insure, and thus do not come under state regulation as do insurance companies, can also deny claims. Another thing companies can do is simply fire workers with high healthcare costs. This apparently happened with workers with disabilities as firms sought to limit their healthcare costs (see Pereira 2003).

Another problem with insurance policies prior to implementation of the Affordable Care Act were policies that had yearly or lifetime limits on payments. Such a policy might have, for instance, a million-dollar lifetime limit. While $1 million is a lot of money to most of us, it is not all that difficult to exceed when a person has an expensive chronic condition or expensive treatment. For example, a premature baby may spend several months in a neonatal intensive-care unit. The cost for that could easily exceed the million-dollar level.

The Affordable Care Act addressed all four of these issues. First, it limited experience rating to four factors ("Health Insurance Reforms: Rate Restrictions" 2012): Whether the policy is for an individual or a family, the geographic area (some places, such as New York and California, have higher medical costs than other places), age (the ACA limited companies to charging up to three times as much for an older person as for a younger one), and whether the subscriber smokes.

Second, the ACA addressed the MLR issue. It requires that insurance companies spend at least 80 percent of their premiums on their subscribers for "health care claims and quality improvement" ("Explaining Health Care Reform: Medical Loss Ratio" 2012). For plans with a large group of subscribers, generally larger firms, the minimum percentage is 85 percent ("Explaining Health Care Reform: Medical Loss Ratio" 2012).

Third, the ACA eliminates pre-existing conditions limitations on obtaining health insurance. Companies cannot refuse to cover someone with a preexisting condition, nor can they charge more because of that condition, with the exception of the four conditions mentioned above (Giled and Jackson 2017).

Finally, there is the issue of annual and lifetime limits. Under the Affordable Care Act, both limits are eliminated, with a few exceptions ("Lifetime and Annual Limits" n.d.).

Stone brings the debate of community versus experience rating out into the open, looking at its philosophical underpinnings:

> Actuarial fairness—each person paying for his own risk—is more than an idea about distributive justice. It is a method of organizing mutual aid by fragmenting communities into ever-smaller, more homogeneous groups and a method that leads ultimately to the destruction of mutual aid. This fragmentation must be accomplished by fostering in people a sense of their differences, rather than their commonalities, and their responsibility for themselves only, rather than their interdependence. Moreover, insurance necessarily operates on the logic of actuarial fairness when it, in turn, is organized as a competitive market.
>
> (Stone 1993, 290)

Such a view was incorporated in President George W. Bush's "ownership society" perspective. Each person would buy his or her own health insurance using money put away in tax-deferred health savings accounts (Vieth 2004).

The important idea here is that the insurance practice of experience rating breaks down the idea of community. The community argument would support, at a minimum, insurance reform and, at a maximum, national health insurance. In-between policies might include tax subsidies and employer mandates.

A CLOSER LOOK: THE POOR, MINORITIES, AND WOMEN

Your healthcare depends on who you are. Race and ethnicity continue to influence a patient's chance of receiving many specific healthcare procedures and treatments. A thorough review of health quality data shows that racial and ethnic minorities continue to receive lower-quality care than whites. These differences persist even when insurance status and socioeconomic factors like education and income are taken into account.

(Robert Wood Johnson Foundation 2014, 1)

In this section, we consider the healthcare problems of the disadvantaged, focusing on the poor, minorities, women, and immigrants. To some extent, the material in this section overlaps with that in the previous section on the uninsured and the underinsured. But as we have noted, a sizable portion of the uninsured are not poor and do work. There are thus other problems that need to be addressed.

Pollack and Kronebusch identify four factors or dimensions that make some groups likely to be uninsured (or underinsured) and therefore suffer the consequences that we have discussed above. These factors are: "needs that hinder access to insurance, general economic disadvantage, discrimination, and impaired and proxy decisionmaking" (2004, 206).

Minorities and Low-Income Groups

In general, minorities and low-income groups do not have the same access to healthcare, or do not compare in health statistics on the same level as those who are white and/or wealthier. This is not a new phenomenon, as Byrd and Clayton (2003) make clear in their historical discussion of disparities in healthcare. In drawing this portrait of low-income and minority groups, we should point out that this is a statistical portrait. It applies in general to the groups discussed.

In looking at the health status of minority and low-income groups, we should note several important features. First, minority groups tend to have lower educational achievement, higher unemployment rates, higher crime rates, lower incomes and therefore higher poverty rates, higher proportions of female-headed families, and higher proportions of out-of-wedlock births. All of this seems to be correlated with health status. One of the confusing aspects of these data is that they are very much related to income and education (Beckles and Truman 2011). That is, many of these characteristics may be a result of poverty (socioeconomic class) rather than ethnicity (race) (Committee on the Consequences of Uninsurance 2002; Patel and Rushefsky 2008).

One issue related to low-income groups suggests that their poorer health status is largely attributable to "risky" behaviors that they engage in, such as smoking, drinking, being overweight, and not exercising. In a sense, this is an argument that can be labeled "blaming the victim" (Ryan 1971; see also the discussion in Levy and Meltzer 2004). That is, this hypothesis suggests that higher mortality rates are due to actions taken (or not taken) by each person. A study reported in the June 3, 1998 issue of the *Journal of the American Medical Association* found that even considering such behaviors, low-income groups had higher mortality rates than higher-income groups. Changing the behaviors would certainly help some, but mortality differences would remain (Lantz, House, and Chen 1998).

African-Americans

McBride argues that healthcare policy toward African-Americans went through three stages. The first stage was engagement (mid-1960s to late 1970s), when healthcare services and financing for the black community were increased, and discrimination was lessened. The second phase, submersion, from the late 1970s to the mid-1980s, saw a cutback in social programs. For example, as a result of the 1981 Omnibus Budget and Reconciliation Act, the working poor were taken off AFDC and Medicaid rolls. The third phase, crisis recognition, began in the mid-1980s. This is a recognition that there is a problem, particularly in the large urban cities. But McBride (1993) points out that this last phase has not yet resulted in changed policies. Thus, the healthcare problems of minorities and low-income groups remained. Indeed, a study of Chicago, Houston, and Los Angeles noted "the progressive deterioration in the delivery of healthcare to the poor and the indigent since the beginnings of the 1980s" (Ginzberg 1994).

There is a fourth, newer stage: those who benefited from provisions of the Affordable Care Act. As we have seen and discussed in Chapter 3, extension of health insurance coverage was largely through Medicaid and, to a lesser extent, through the exchanges or marketplaces. The greatest gains were for people of color—blacks, Hispanics, and Asians. The uninsured rate for Hispanics saw the greatest decline, by 35 percent, from 26 to 17 percent. For African-Americans, the decline was over 29 percent, from 17 to 12 percent. For Asians, the decline was over 46 percent, from 15 to 8 percent. For the white population, the decline was about 33 percent, from 12 to 8 percent. In terms of sheer numbers, the largest uninsured population decline was among whites, because they represent a larger proportion of the population (authors' calculations from Artiga, Foutz, and Damico 2018).

Blacks who remain uninsured tend to live in states that did not expand Medicaid. Therefore, they are more likely to be in the coverage gap than whites (Artiga, Foutz, and Damico 2018). Uninsured Asians and Hispanics face a different problem: lack of citizenship. Forty-four percent of Asians and 50 percent of Hispanics are not citizens (Artiga, Foutz, and Damico 2018).

African-Americans, like many ethnic and racial minorities, remain more likely to be uninsured than the white population. We should thus expect the consequences of uninsurance to be higher among minorities than among the white population (Agency for Healthcare Research and Quality 2010).

The death rate for African-Americans declined by 25 percent from 1999 to 2015. The decline was particularly apparent for the three major causes of death: heart disease, cancer, and strokes. Having said that, death rates for African-Americans continue to be higher than for whites. African-Americans have higher rates of high blood pressure, diabetes, and stroke (Centers for Disease Control and Prevention 2017). Looking at social determinants and personal behaviors, the Centers for Disease Control and Prevention (2017) finds that African-Americans have higher rates of unemployment, lower income, are less likely to own a home, have higher rates of smoking, greater lack of exercise, and higher obesity rates compared to whites. African-Americans report higher levels of fair or poor health (20.5 percent) than whites (15.7 percent) ("State Health Facts" n.d.). The life expectancy at birth of blacks is lower than for whites, with black males having the lowest, at 71.8 years. The comparable figure for black females is 78.1 years. For whites, the respective figures are 73.1 percent (males) and 81.1 percent (for females) (National Center for Health Statistics 2017).

African-American women tend to have less access to prenatal care and to give birth at earlier ages (Grant 2016). African-Americans have higher premature or preterm birth rates (13.4 percent) than whites (8.9 percent). African-Americans have higher rates of low-weight babies and infant mortality (13.3 percent of all births; 11.3 per 1,000 live births, respectively) than whites (6.9 percent of all births; 5.1 deaths per 1,000 live births, respectively) ("State Health Facts" n.d.; see also National Center for Health Statistics 2015, 2017). African-Americans are less likely than whites to have employer-sponsored insurance (48 versus 58 percent) ("State Health Facts" n.d.).

Issues surrounding pregnancy also show problems in the black community. Maternal deaths of black women are up to four times higher than for white women. Many of these deaths are preventable. Black women suffer higher levels of health complications than white women. The quality of care for black pregnant women is lower than for white women ("Black Women's Maternal Health" 2018). Black women have less access to high-quality birth control than white women and thus have a higher rate of unintended pregnancies than white women ("Black Women's Maternal Health" 2018; Grant 2016). Black women also have a higher rate of cesarean births than white women (Grant 2016; National Center for Health Statistics 2015). In general, black women come to pregnancy less healthy than white women and have higher levels of diabetes, hypertension, heart disease, and obesity (Grant 2016). Grant (2016) points to the impact of racism and discrimination on childbirth:

> Perhaps most distressing, racial and socio-economic factors also have a disproportionate effect on the quality of care mothers receive during childbirth. A report titled "Discrimination and Racial Disparities in Health" from the Harvard School of Public Health found that bias, prejudice and stereotyping by health care providers contribute to delivering lower-quality care—affecting how mothers are treated during childbirth and the outcomes. "Assumptions are made about you when you walk through the door, based on how you walk, how you dress, whether you sound educated or not," says Chanel Porchia-Albert, founder and executive director of the Brooklyn-based Ancient Song Doula Services. "That affects the level of support you get."

As noted, overall, African-Americans have worse health status than most other ethnic/racial groups (Artiga et al. 2016b). African-Americans tend to have higher rates of chronic conditions or disability than other ethnic groups (Centers for Disease Control and Prevention 2017). Blacks have high rates of obesity, as well as high rates of heart disease, cancer, and diabetes (Centers for Disease Control and Prevention 2017; Noonan, Velesco-Mondragon, and Wagner 2016).

Much the same can be said for African-American children. African-American children are more likely (by 43 percent) to be obese. Obesity is linked to other diseases, such as "coronary heart disease, high-blood pressure, stroke, Type 2 diabetes and cancer" (Schumaker 2017). African-American children also have higher rates of asthma (by 63 percent) than white children (Schumaker 2017).

Another public health problem of African-Americans, though it may not be typically viewed as a health problem, is homicide. Homicide death rates of African-American males are three times higher than for other ethnic/racial groups. African-American females also have a higher homicide rate than females in other ethnic/racial groups (Noonan, Velesco-Mondragon, and Wagner 2016). Noonan et al. (2016, 9) describe the importance of the violence disparity:

> Homicide is the absolute measurement of violence, revealing the unquestionable ethnic disparity. However, violence affects African Americans in many other ways. In 2013, higher rates of aggravated assault, child maltreatment, and fights among high school students were reported. In 2011, African American women reported higher rates of experiencing rape and physical violence by an intimate partner.

The role of firearms and gun control is about as politically contentious an issue as can be found. The pro-gun lobbies are immensely powerful and have been able to suppress much discussion about this public health issue (see Klein 2012; Murphy 2012). Absent any discussion or action, guns and violence will continue to be a plague, especially in the African-American community (Levine et al. 2012).

AIDS is another health problem that affects ethnicity differently. While a majority of AIDS victims are whites, the relative proportion of AIDS victims is disproportionately much higher among African-Americans and Latinos. For Whites, the AIDS rate is 3 per 100,000. For blacks, the rate is 31 per 100,000. The death rate from AIDS was eight times higher for blacks than for whites (Artiga et al. 2016b). Blacks account for a disproportionate share of HIV/AIDS cases, though in recent years, the death rate from AIDS has declined for all groups, though more whites have AIDS than blacks (Agency for Healthcare Quality and Research 2011). Blacks account for almost 43 percent of those living with HIV. Having said that, the death rate from AIDS is higher for blacks than for whites, especially for black women ("The HIV/AIDS Epidemic in the U.S." 2018).

African-American women are especially hard-hit by the epidemic (see Auerbach 2004; Clemetson 2004; Fears 2005). Indeed, a study released in 2012 suggests that the HIV/AIDS rate among African-American women is about five times higher than the CDC had estimated ("HIV Among Black Women 5 Times Higher than Previously Thought" 2012). In 2016, black women made up 60 percent of new cases, whereas white women made up 19 percent of new cases ("The HIV/AIDS Epidemic in the United States" 2018).

The Centers for Disease Control and Prevention (2011) suggests four reasons why HIV infections are so much higher among African-Americans than other racial or ethnic groups; each of them presents challenges for reducing incidence and consequences. One set of reasons, almost tautological, is that there is a high prevalence of the disease in the African-American community and so sex among African-American partners creates high risks of contracting HIV. A second reason is socioeconomic: high incidence of poverty, lack of access to healthcare, poor housing, and lack of prevention information. The third reason is lack of awareness of one's HIV status. The CDC estimates that 20 percent of those infected with HIV in the United States (and not just in the black community) do not know that they are carrying the infection. This creates a greater possibility of transmitting the virus as well as later diagnosis and thus poorer outcomes. The fourth reason is stigma. HIV is often associated with homosexuality, so that finding out or admitting that one has HIV implies that one is a homosexual. There is, also, fear that someone with HIV or AIDS will be discriminated against.

Quality of care for African-Americans is lower than for whites. Blacks are less likely than whites to receive screenings for possible health threats such as colorectal cancer. As a result, when blacks are diagnosed with that cancer, the disease is more likely to be at an advanced stage than is the case for whites. Whites with diabetes are more likely to receive various services for that chronic disease than blacks. As a result, blacks are much more likely than any other group to be admitted to a hospital with complications related to diabetes (Agency for Healthcare Research and Quality 2010). The pattern is quite clear: African-Americans receive fewer services for various diseases and suffer higher rates of adverse effects from them than whites. It is no wonder that 13 percent of African-Americans report they are not in good health (Russell 2010).

Pearl (2015) provides several examples of poorer quality of health for African-Americans as compared to whites. White women have higher rates of screenings for breast cancer than African-American women. African-American women are more likely to have more radical surgery for breast cancer than white women. African-Americans are more likely to be hospitalized for diabetes than whites. This is likely due to the poorer access to healthcare for African-Americans. Blacks are less likely to be screened for high cholesterol than whites and thus more likely to have heart attacks.

Schumaker (2017) points to the report by the Agency for Healthcare Research and Quality (2016b) that documents the lower level of quality for blacks (and Latinos). The title of Schumaker's (2017) article sums up a critical point of this and other sections in this chapter: "The Quality of Care You Receive Likely Depends on Your Color."

Latinos

There is much variation within the Latino population, coming from Puerto Rico, Mexico, Cuba, and Central America, and so their health issues vary somewhat. Hispanics make up almost 17 percent of the population and are the largest minority group. By 2035, Latinos will likely comprise 25 percent of the population (Centers for Disease Control and Prevention 2015). About 34 percent of Latinos are foreign-born (authors' calculations from Flores 2017); we will discuss immigrants and healthcare below.

Hispanics saw the largest percentage decline (11 percent) of uninsurance of any ethnic/racial group thanks to the Affordable Care Act. Having said that, one-third of the remaining uninsured are Hispanic (2017 data) ("Key Facts about the Uninsured Population" 2017). In 2016, the uninsured rate for Latinos was 29 percent (Collins et al. 2016).

A major access problem for Latinos is language. Those who speak only Spanish have a more difficult time getting needed care (Centers for Disease Control and Prevention 2015; Patel and Rushefsky 2008; Russell 2010). Overall, 69 percent of Hispanics are proficient in English. Of those born in the United States, that percentage rises to almost 90 percent. For those Hispanics not born in the US, only about 35 percent were fluent in English (Flores 2017). As is typical of immigrant groups, English proficiency has risen among American-born Hispanics. People with limited English proficiency (LEP) are more likely than those who are proficient to live in poverty and also have lower educational levels. Forty-nine percent of those with LEP are uninsured compared to 18 percent of those who are proficient. Similarly, people with LEP are less likely than people with English proficiency to have employer-based or private insurance and more likely to be on Medicaid or another public insurance program. People with limited English proficiency have less access to care and less access to preventive services and are more likely to be dissatisfied with the care they receive. LEP patients are more likely to have an adverse outcome (such as contracting an infection while in a hospital) than English speakers, are more likely to have longer hospital stays and delays in procedures, and are more likely to be readmitted to hospitals (Joint Commission 2013). And as with many of the factors we are discussing in this chapter, there is a cumulative effect of having many different barriers to care. These barriers or factors include "race/ethnicity, citizenship status, low education, and poverty" ("Overview of Health Coverage for Individuals with Limited English Proficiency" 2012). The LEP population experiences many of these problems.

As part of its attempt to increase insurance coverage and access to care, the Affordable Care Act addresses the language issues. Section 1557 requires entities receiving Medicare and Medicaid funding, such as hospitals, doctors, exchanges, community health centers, etc., to provide what the section calls "meaningful access" to persons with limited English proficiency. This means that translators need to be available when an LEP person sees a provider and that important documents are available in the patient's language. In addition to Section 1557, assuring access for LEP patients is required under several other sections of the ACA: Section 1331 requires that communications between provider and patient be in "plain language" that is easily understandable, especially for LEP patients. Section 1001 requires insurers to use language that is "culturally and linguistically appropriate." Title VI of the Civil Rights Act of 1964 forbids discrimination based on national origin. A 2000 Executive Order (#13,166) by President Clinton requires federal agencies to look at their policies and provide meaningful access to LEP persons ("A Quick Primer on Affordable Care Act Language Service Requirements" n.d.).

One of the interesting findings in the disparities literature is what is known as the Hispanic paradox. Latinos have a longer life span and lower infant mortality rate than any other group, including whites (Patel and Rushefsky 2008; Russell 2010). The death rate among Hispanics is 20-percent lower than for whites (Centers for Disease Control and Prevention 2015). Hispanic death rates from disease is similar to that of whites, with the exception of diabetes and liver disease (Centers for Disease Control and Prevention 2015). Health status is lower and risks are greater for Hispanics who were born outside of the US compared to those who were born in the US (Centers for Disease Control and Prevention 2015). In 2014, half of the Hispanic population were noncitizens (Artiga et al. 2016b). No accepted explanation has been offered for this paradox, though a small number of possible explanations have been given. It may be that Latino migrants who come to the United States are healthier than those of other groups. Another possibility, which has been called the "salmon-bias," suggests that Latinos who are terminally ill return to their home country. A third possibility is that the available data are inadequate (Patel and Rushefsky 2008).

In 2010, 61 percent of births to Latinas were covered by Medicaid (Curtin et al. 2013). Latinas are less likely to receive early prenatal care than almost any other ethnic or racial group (Mead et al. 2008). This is particularly evident among younger Latinas, what Torres (2016) calls teenagers and emerging adults, because their pregnancy rate is the highest of all ethnic/racial groups. Further, Torres (2016) notes that health risks for the baby are greater when the mother is younger than for adult pregnant women. Why do disadvantaged women not get full prenatal care? One reason is financial barriers. Minority and low-income women are less likely than the general population to have health insurance (Agency for Health Care Research and Quality 2010; Garner et al. 1996; Mead et al. 2008). Another barrier for Latinas, especially young Latinas, is a lack of trust in the healthcare system (Torres 2016). Even if financial barriers did not exist, there are not enough doctors willing to work in low-income areas or with high-risk mothers (Thomas 2014). The federal government uses two designations to delineate this problem: health professional shortage areas (HPSA) and medically underserved areas/populations (MUA/P) ("HPSA and MUA/P" n.d.). There is some tendency in these medically underserved areas for nurse practitioners to be primary-care providers.

American Indians/Alaska Natives

American Indians and Alaska Natives (AIs/ANs) have some of the worst health indicators of any of the racial/ethnic groups we are considering (Artiga et al. 2016b; Burhansstipanov and Krebs 2016). Twenty-one percent do not have health insurance (Artiga et al. 2016b). Compared to whites, AIs/ANs have a 37-percent-higher rate of depression, a 900-percent-higher rate of tuberculosis, and a 350-percent-higher rate of liver disease. They are more likely than whites to die from AIDS, kidney disease, and diabetes (Families USA 2018). The infant mortality rate for American Indians/Alaska Natives is 60-percent higher than for whites (Weinstein et al. 2017). This population also has a high percentage of smokers (Burhansstipanov and Krebs 2016; Mead et al. 2008). AIs/ANs are also less likely than whites to be physically active (Burhansstipanov and Krebs 2016).

Where homicide is a major health issue within the African-American community, suicide is a very serious problem within the American Indian and Alaska Native communities (Leavitt et al. 2018). According to Russell (2010, 5), suicide "is the second leading cause of death for those age 10 to 34 years" (see also Agency for Healthcare Research and Quality 2010; Leavitt et al. 2018). As a related point, mental health problems, including the use of drugs, are also higher for this group than for any other group.

Breast cancer incidence and mortality rates are lower for AIs/ANs than for any other group except Asian/Pacific Islanders (Mead et al. 2008). Fifty-three percent of American Indians and Alaskan Natives report their health condition as fair or poor compared to 42 percent among whites (Mead et al. 2008).

The Agency for Healthcare Quality and Research (2016b) issues a periodic report on disparities among different ethnic racial groups. Among other things, the report looked at changes in core measures of quality of care from 2013–2015. For American Indians/Alaska Natives, 12 of the core measures showed improvement, 50 saw no change, and 31 got worse.

Women

> Research has shown that many diseases and conditions, including heart disease, smoking, and lung cancer, affect women and men very differently. There are also several diseases, such as breast cancer and osteoporosis, that primarily affect women, and another range of conditions, including pregnancy, menopause, and certain reproductive-related cancers, that only affect women. Sex-based differences have been identified on several levels, including treatment efficacy, medication side effects, prevention strategies, and disease etiology.
> (Kaiser Family Foundation 2004b)

> The issues of women's health cannot be understood only in biological terms, as simply the ills of the female of the species. Women and men are different, but we are also similar—and we both are divided by the social relations of class and race/ethnicity. To begin to understand how our social constitution affects our health, we must ask, repeatedly, what is different and what is similar across the social divides of gender, color, and class. We cannot assume that biology alone will provide the answers we need; instead, we must reframe the issues in the context of the social shaping of our human lives—as both biological creatures and historical actors. Otherwise, we will continue to mistake—as many before us have done—what is for what must be, and leave unchallenged the social forces that continue to create vast inequalities in health.
> (Krieger and Fee 1996, 27)

To a degree, women's health issues overlap those of minorities (race/ethnicity) and low-income groups (class). To the extent that women's income is low, especially in families headed by women, all the health problems associated with low income show up here. For example, issues surrounding prenatal care, while obviously a concern for women, are generally associated with low income. If programs aimed at low-income people are cut, as was done in the early 1980s and in the 2000s, then women will be affected.

On the other hand, there are certain issues that are unique to women, though of concern to men as well:

> Women have unique reproductive health care needs, have higher rates of chronic illnesses, and are greater users of the health care system. In addition, women take the lead on securing health care for their families and have lower incomes than men, both of which affect and shape their access to the health system.
>
> (James et al. 2009)

In some ways, there have been impressive improvements in health issues related to women; 59 percent of both women and men were covered by employer-sponsored insurance in 2016. Of those, 35 percent had insurance from their own job and another 25 percent were covered as a dependent. Nine percent of women are covered by insurance on the individual market, 17 percent by Medicaid, and 11 percent were uninsured in 2016 (the numbers are for women aged 19–64) ("State Health Facts" 2016; "Women's Health Insurance Coverage" 2017). The uninsured percentage for women (2016 data) was lower than for men (13 percent) ("State Health Facts" 2016). The heavy reliance on women as a dependent for health insurance creates a risk for women in the event that the spouse loses a job or dies or there is a divorce ("Women's Health Insurance Coverage" 2017). Single women are more likely to be uninsured than women in two-parent families ("Women's Health Insurance Coverage" 2017).

Belluz (2016) argues that there has been a decline in women's health in four areas, and that there are no good explanations for why that is the case. The first area is obesity. A larger percentage of women (40 percent) than men (35 percent) are obese. At greater levels of obesity, women's rate was twice as high as men.

A second factor that Belluz (2016) points to are death rates. The death rate for middle-aged white women has been increasing, while the death rate for similarly aged white men has been decreasing. Further, women are dying at higher rates than in other Westernized industrial countries (Aron et al. 2015).

A third factor is the increasing rate of suicide among women, moving closer to the suicide rate for men.

The final factor discussed by Belluz (2016) is the rise of maternal mortality rates, which we will consider below.

Belluz (2016) does point to advances in women's health. The teen pregnancy rate has declined. The abortion rate has declined, and the use of contraceptives has increased (see discussion below). Cancer rates for breast and cervical cancers have declined due to increases in screenings (preventive care).

Minority women are more likely to be uninsured than white women (Ranji and Salganicoff 2011; "Spotlight on Women of Color" n.d.). Baird (1998) notes that married men have higher rates of employer-provided insurance than married women do. She also notes, as mentioned above, that divorce has a devastating effect on private health insurance for unemployed women. Women's employment careers tend to be intermittent (women may take time off for childbearing, or they may make job changes because their husbands move), and women are more often in lower-paying jobs that are less likely to offer health insurance. Medicaid coverage is sporadic. Fewer than half of those eligible are covered, and doctors do not have to accept Medicaid patients. Further, because women, on the average, live longer than men, issues of long-term care and chronic illnesses are critical ("Role of Medicaid and Medicare in Women's Health" n.d.; Salganicoff et al. 2002). Racial and ethnic minority women and low-income women (there is considerable overlap here) are more likely to experience chronic health conditions than are white women (Ranji and Salganicoff 2011). Medicaid is especially important for women. A majority of people covered by Medicaid and/or Medicare are women. Those on Medicaid tend to be poorer and sicker than women covered by private insurance. Medicaid is a major source of coverage for family planning and birth, as well as long-term care (along with Medicare). Women on Medicare are more likely than men to be widowed, have lower incomes, and more chronic conditions ("Role of Medicaid and Medicare in Women's Health" n.d.).

The above paragraph probably understates the problem. First, the percentage of workers covered by employer-based health insurance has declined. Further, there is a growing trend toward using part-time or temporary workers, also unlikely to have health insurance benefits. The result is that about 25 percent of women had no health insurance for all or part of the year prior to the implementation of the ACA (Ranji and Salganicoff 2011).

The lack of insurance affects access to the healthcare system; 24 percent of women have delayed getting care because of the costs, with higher percentages for those without insurance or with incomes below the federal poverty line. Even women on Medicaid found cost barriers sufficient to delay seeking care. Other barriers women face to obtaining care include lack of transportation or lack of childcare or inability to take time off from work (Ranji and Salganicoff 2011).

Women, like others facing barriers to obtaining healthcare, make trade-offs. In 2004, 8 percent of women said that they cut back on other basic needs because of the costs of healthcare. By 2008, that number had doubled (Ranji and Salganicoff 2011).

Women of whatever race or ethnic group face unique problems related to their role in the family. They are often the primary caregiver for their children. If a child becomes sick, they may have to take off from work because of lack of childcare. Women are less likely than men to work in jobs that provide paid sick leave. Women also tend to be the primary caregiver for family members who are chronically ill or disabled (Ranji and Salganicoff 2011).

The basic federal legislation covering these issues is the Family and Medical Leave Act (FMLA), passed in 1993, the first year of the Clinton administration. It is also the last time that the federal government addressed this issue. The FMLA requires employers to give their employees 12 weeks of unpaid leave because of a family illness or the birth of a child and provides that the employee will have her job when the time period is up. The first thing to note about the legislation is that the leave is unpaid. Therefore, there is a sacrifice the employee makes if she takes leave. Second, the legislation applies to larger companies (50 or more employees). Given this, the FMLA covers about 60 percent of the workforce ("Paid Family Leave and Sick Days in the U.S." 2017).

The Obama administration pushed for paid family leave. In 2015, a presidential memorandum required federal agencies to offer up to six weeks (240 hours) of paid leave for childbirth or adoption (Obama 2015; "Paid Family Leave and Sick Days in the U.S." 2017). An executive order by President Obama in 2015 required federal contractors to provide up to seven days of paid leave to their employees (White House 2015). The Trump administration has expressed interest in the issue. During the 2016 campaign, candidate Donald Trump called for six weeks of paid maternity leave to be paid for with unemployment benefits if the employer does not offer such leave. The administration's 2018 and 2019 budgets called for a similar program. No proposals, however, were offered (Vasel 2018).

There is a federalism aspect to this issue. "California, New Jersey, New York, Rhode Island, and Washington—as well as the District of Columbia (D.C.) have enacted laws offering paid family leave" ("Paid Family Leave and Sick Days in the U.S." 2017, p. 2). The states administer the leave through their disability programs funded by payroll taxes ("Paid Family Leave and Sick Days in the U.S." 2017). Twenty-one states require businesses to have maternity leave policies, though these are not paid policies (Handrick 2017). Additionally, the Pregnancy Discrimination Act, passed in 1978, forbids discrimination based on pregnancy. For example, if a business provides for sick leave, then it must also do so for pregnancy. If a business allows some workers to work from home, then it must do the same for pregnant women (Handrick 2017).

Having said that, the evidence is that becoming pregnant hurts women's future careers. A study by *The New York Times* (Kitroeff and Silver-Greenberg 2018) found considerable discrimination against women who become pregnant. Kitroeff and Silver-Greenberg (2018) describe the situation women face:

> Many of the country's largest and most prestigious companies still systematically sideline pregnant women. They pass them over for promotions and raises. They fire them when they complain.
>
> In physically demanding jobs—where an increasing number of women unload ships, patrol streets and hoist boxes—the discrimination can be blatant. Pregnant women risk losing their jobs when they ask to carry water bottles or take rest breaks.
>
> In corporate office towers, the discrimination tends to be subtler. Pregnant women and mothers are often perceived as less committed, steered away from prestigious assignments, excluded from client meetings and slighted at bonus season.

The *New York Times* study found that having a child results in lower wages, while becoming a father results in higher wages for men. Complaints of employment discrimination based on pregnancy to the Equal Employment Opportunity Commission have increased over the last several decades. While a portion of women voluntarily pull back from their work commitments after pregnancy, those who wish to continue in their career face discrimination. This discrimination occurs in both the public and private sectors (Kitroeff and Silver-Greenberg 2018).

A 2015 report by the US Department of Labor (2015) examined the costs of not having a paid leave program. One set of costs focuses on workers. Women without paid leave programs are less likely than women with paid leave programs to have jobs after childbirth. Or to put it another way, paid leave programs increase women's labor force participation. Such women have less income over a lifetime and are more likely to go on public assistance than women with paid leave programs. Such women are also more likely to experience stress and other health issues.

A second cost is to families. Children born into families without paid leave programs are more likely to have poorer outcomes than other children, including lower birth rates and higher rates of prematurity. For children with special healthcare needs, having paid leave provides better emotional health for children and parents, better physical health for children, and less financial stress for parents. Fathers are less likely to take leave or cut short leave if it is unpaid. Such leave also provides support for caring for elderly relatives.

A third cost is to the country as a whole. The report argues that if there were paid leave programs, labor participation would be higher among women. The report estimates that the higher labor force participation could add as much as $500 billion annually to our gross domestic product.

The bottom line is that this is a patchwork of policies, which largely affect women, for some businesses and in some states. Even the paid leave, especially maternity leave policies, creates financial hardship for women because the paid leave is lower than their salary.

The Battle over Birth Control

Reproductive issues, such as abortion and family planning, are much older than the current debates over abortion acknowledge. From ancient civilizations through the twentieth century, ways were sought and used to control reproduction (Knowles 2012). We can see the volatility, intensity, and controversy surrounding healthcare in the passage of the Affordable Care Act as well as the elections of 2012. The issues of abortion and reproductive rights touch upon the values of order, including the protection of traditional social values, and liberty, including the right of privacy. In this section, we examine issues related to contraception. While the issue of contraception overlaps the issue of abortion, we discuss abortion as well as assisted reproductive technology in Chapter 9.

Advances in the biological sciences produced new means of birth control, such as pills originally developed in the 1950s. A major court case, *Griswold v. Connecticut* (1965), addressed the question of whether the state, in this case Connecticut, could forbid the sale of birth control pills to married couples. The US Supreme Court ruled that the state could not and, in the process, developed the doctrine of a "right to privacy." The next year, the Court ruled that bans on sales of oral contraceptives to unmarried people were also unconstitutional.

Contraception evokes religious values. Catholic Church doctrine holds that any artificial contraceptive, such as the pill, violates the principles of the Church. There are two caveats to this. One is that the practice and beliefs of many American Catholics concerning birth control violate Catholic doctrine (see, for example, Lipka 2013; for a discussion of the Catholic doctrine against birth control, see "Birth Control" n.d.). Second, Pope Francis has said that the use of condoms is acceptable to avoid pregnancy for a woman infected with the Zika virus. This raised much speculation that the Church was making some changes to its doctrine. It is clear, however, that that is not the case ("What Did Pope Francis Actually Say about Contraception?" 2016).

Because there are so many denominations of Protestantism, there is no overall hierarchical organization for Protestants (the hierarchy does exist within some Protestant denominations). There is, thus, no one stance on birth control. Evangelical Protestants have, relatively recently (see Burton 2017) taken a stance opposed to much contraception and have moved closer to the Catholic position. Much of the change may be attributable to opposition to some of the social changes such as the so-called sexual revolution and the *Roe v. Wade* (1973) case, which effectively legalized abortion (Burton 2017).

The Jewish view on birth control, like the Protestant view, varies. Orthodox Jews tend to oppose the use of contraceptives. At the other end, Reform Jews are more supportive. The Islamic view of birth control, as with Christianity and Judaism, varies. But there are some interesting nuances in the Islamic perspective, which can also be found in other religions. Ajani (2013, 121) writes:

> First and foremost, the primary aim of birth control is to bring about wanted births. Many people hold a wrong view of birth control. What comes to their mind anytime they hear or come across birth control is that it refers to an attempt not to give birth to children or that pregnancy should be aborted. This is not correct. Birth control is an attempt to plan for wanted or expected births to make adequate preparation for the incoming child. This preparation includes what the mother will need, how to take care of the pregnancy to ensure its gradual and progressive development.

> How to ensure that the pregnancy will not result into premature birth. To prepare for the safe delivery of the baby, its clothing and feeding, how the baby will be nursed and the likes. It is part of the preparation to make plan for the educational carriers of the child so that at every stage of the child's development, the child will not lack anything. It is this planning that Islam refers to as birth control or family planning.
>
> When a family has made this kind of plan for a child, it is not enough. The family should equally plan for the good health of the mother, i.e., giving the mother some space intervals between one birth and another.
>
> Another reason for birth control in Islam is to guide against unwanted births. Some families do get into unwanted births which they did not adequately prepare for. This at times they say is as a result of mistake or carelessness on their part or on the part of their wives. When they find themselves in this situation, it affects everything they do and may alter their other plans completely. It may sometimes lead to losing golden opportunities which they may not have the opportunity of gaining again.

This quote captures much of the rationale for the use and availability of birth control. The purpose is to allow the family and especially the mother to plan for childbirths. Related to that, contraception avoids unplanned pregnancies, a point to which we return below. A second is to protect the life of the mother. A third is to protect the life of the child (i.e., avoiding prematurity). A fourth purpose, though not explicit in the above quote, is to give women the ability to control their own bodies. In the title of a book published by the Boston Women's Health Book Collective, we are talking about *Our Bodies, Our Selves* (Boston Women's Health Book Collective and Norsigian 2011).

In general, public opinion is supportive of the use and availability of birth control. A Gallup Poll (Newport 2012) finds that a huge majority, including 90 percent of Catholics, find birth control morally acceptable. This is not an issue that divides Republicans and Democrats. There are some, especially among Catholics, who object to some kinds of contraceptives, because they believe the procedure is the equivalent of abortion (i.e., takes place after conception). There seems to be pretty widespread acceptance of the use of birth control.

The issue of reproduction became part of the controversy over the Affordable Care Act. Now the question was whether the insurance plans issued under the state exchanges were required to cover contraception pills, devices, etc. The Obama administration issued a rule that required the coverage of reproductive technologies as part of the "essential benefits" that all plans should cover (see Chapter 3). And that prompted the larger question of whether to cover birth control in insurance policies at all, as well as the defunding of Planned Parenthood. Again, the pro-life forces squared against the pro-choice forces. In this case, the pro-life forces added the religious argument that requiring institutions that objected to birth control to fund it violated religious freedom. The administration's compromise was to permit companies to refuse to pay for birth control coverage, but to allow insurance plans to offer it. This did not satisfy the pro-life groups (Aizenman 2012). While a bill to this effect submitted to Congress failed, a number of states, including the authors' home state of Missouri, have passed such religious exemption bills.

The opposing sides broke down along party and ideological lines, with the Democratic Party in 2012 declaring that the Republicans had declared a "war on women" (see, for example, People for the American Way 2012). Efforts by the Republicans included the defunding of Planned Parenthood, which does provide abortion services but spends most of its funding on providing healthcare, including breast cancer screenings, to low-income women.

The contraceptive coverage mandate, like other parts of the Affordable Care Act (Chapter 3), was challenged in court. In *Burell v. Hobby Lobby* (2014), the US Supreme Court ruled by a 5–4 vote that certain types of corporations, privately held corporations, that had religious objections to providing contraceptives to their employees were exempted from the mandate. The Court majority used the Religious Freedom Restoration Act of 1993 as the basis for its decision (Liptak 2014). Hobby Lobby argued that it objected to some kinds of contraception, such as the "intrauterine device and so-called morning-after pills" (Liptak 2014). The assertion, which is controversial, is that these devices effectively cause abortions. Hobby Lobby said it did not object to other forms of contraception. The minority argued, first, that contraceptive coverage was vital to a woman's health (more about this below) and second, that some corporations might object to any contraceptive coverage. The minority also saw the decision as much more sweeping than the Court majority. Justice Ruth Bader Ginsberg argued that the decision could be applied to all corporations and that the religious freedom argument could be used to refuse to cover things like vaccines or following the minimum wage. Justice Alito, who wrote the majority opinion, argued that he did not foresee a flux of such kinds of cases. He wrote, in the majority opinion, that government had an interest in seeing that women had access to contraceptives. He also noted that there were alternatives: government could pay for the contraceptives, or insurance companies could be required to pay for them, rather than the companies they insured (Liptak 2014).

In attempts to repeal (and replace) the Affordable Care Act (Chapter 3), Republicans looked at the essential benefits portion and focused particularly on contraceptives (Kliff 2017). One of the proposals from 2017, the American Health Care Act, would let states decide whether to require coverage of maternity care in health insurance plans. Giving birth is expensive. In 2017, a normal (i.e., vaginal birth) averaged $28,000 and a cesarian-section birth averaged $50,000. Private insurers paid a little bit more than $18,000, on average, for a normal birth and nearly $28,000 for a cesarian birth (Rovner 2017). Prior to the passage of the Affordable Care Act only about 12 percent of private insurers covered childbirth, and when they did, riders costing as much as $1,000 a month were added to the policy (Kliff 2017; Rovner 2017).

Why would Republicans, who often argue that they are pro-life, want to eliminate the maternity benefit? One reason is that Republicans uniformly oppose the Affordable Care Act. They are trying to dismantle it—if not altogether, then piece by piece (Rovner 2017; Chapter 3). A second reason is that the mandate places restrictions on individuals, who purchase insurance plans, employers who have to provide the benefit, and health insurance companies that offer them. Third, requiring the maternity coverage mandate means that subscribers will pay more for their plans in higher premiums even if they do not use it. The benefit is bundled in with the other essential benefits. The argument is similar to one made about cable and satellite TV. They offer a large variety of channels, most of which we would never watch. Some systems and other enterprises, such as Sling and Facebook, are offering packages that can be tailored to the viewer's interests or let the viewer pick. Of course, the less-popular channels would likely disappear. And the cost to the consumer would go down. In the case of maternity care, cutting back on coverage would be very costly for families both in premiums for the coverage, if they could obtain it, and the actual cost of the pregnancy/delivery. For women with no contraceptive coverage, the expense of prescription contraceptives ranges comprise a substantial portion of out-of-pocket expenses (estimates from Sobel, Salganicoff, and Rosenzweig 2017). After the implementation of the ACA, the percentage of women who had out-of-pocket expenses for oral contraceptives dropped from 20.9 percent in 2012 to 3.6 percent in 2014. This saved women now covered by the ACA about $1.4 billion a year (Sobel, Salganicoff, and Rosenzweig 2017).

Reproductive issues are more than about freedom of choice or moral or religious stances. They are also about economics. The ability to control how many and when to have children has an impact on a woman's ability to help her family economically. A study by Frost and Lindberg (2012; see also Marcotte 2012) for the Guttmacher Institute makes this point very strongly. The study of over 2000 women who used family planning clinics that were funded by tax dollars found many reasons why women used birth control. We quote the summary of the study's results:

> A majority of respondents reported that birth control use had allowed them to take better care of themselves or their families (63 percent), support themselves financially (56 percent), complete their education (51 percent), or keep or get a job (50 percent). Young women, unmarried women, and those without children reported more reasons for using contraception than others. Not being able to afford a baby, not being ready for children, feeling that having a baby would interrupt their goals, and wanting to maintain control in their lives were the most commonly reported very important reasons for using birth control.
>
> (Frost and Lindberg 2012, 2)

A University of Michigan study supports this result; a sizable percentage of the decreased income disparity between men and women is due to access to birth control (Lowder 2012).

Another element that must be considered is the linkage between availability of contraceptives and abortion. A 2012 study of women in St. Louis and Kansas City, Missouri, found that the availability of contraception at no cost to women led to a decrease in unintended pregnancies and abortions (Peipert et al. 2012). A sizable portion of pregnancies were unintended (about 45 percent in 2011) and the abortion rate (number of abortions per 1,000 women) declined dramatically, from 29.3 to 14.6 ("Induced Abortions in the United States" n.d; "U.S. Unintended Pregnancy Rate" 2016).

Having said that, there are disparities in the rate of unintended pregnancies ("U.S. Unintended Pregnancy Rate" 2016). Women with income below poverty levels (measured by the Federal Poverty Level or FPL) and at near-poverty levels (between 100 percent and 199 percent of the FPL) have much higher unintended pregnancy rates than women with incomes greater than 200 percent of the FPL. Black and Hispanic women tend to have higher unintended pregnancy rates than white women.

Further, having contraception covered by insurance enables women to use the more expensive, but more effective, birth control technologies (Andrews 2012). The federal nature of the issue comes in also, because 29 states, as of 2018, require health insurance policies to cover contraception. Six of the state mandates, prior to the enactment of the Affordable Care Act, were signed by Republican governors, including 2012 Republican presidential nominee Mitt Romney in Massachusetts (Geiger and Levey 2012). Further, much of the public supports the Obama rule, including many Catholics (Sobel, Salganicoff, and Rosenzweig 2017).

The linkage between abortions and contraception are clearest in events surrounding Planned Parenthood. Planned Parenthood was founded in 1916 as a clinic to provide information and services about birth control. Established in Brooklyn, New York, it was the first clinic of its kind in the country (Alter 2016). The founder of Planned Parenthood, Margaret Sanger, helped fund research to develop a birth control pill, which first became available in 1960. Planned Parenthood supported the legalization of abortions and began providing abortions after the *Roe. v. Wade* case (Alter 2016).

Pro-life groups' first successful effort to defund Planned Parenthood came in Texas. The Texas Womens Health Program, set up by the state in 2011, forbids funding for any organization that provides abortions. In Texas a failed sting operation, which suggested, falsely, that Planned Parenthood sold fetuses (see "The Planned Parenthood Witch Hunt" 2016), led to cutbacks in funding for the organization. From our perspective, an important impact of the closing of Planned Parenthood offices was the increase in unplanned births, especially among low-income women (Paquette 2016). Other states also cut funding for the organization.

We close this section with a brief examination of Trump administration policies regarding the availability of publicly funded birth control. We should note that this issue is very much tied to views on abortion (i.e., pro-life). We have already discussed the cuts in Title X. But the administration, largely through administrative/regulatory action, is moving toward sex education that is focused on abstinence-only approaches and funding family planning grants that emphasize "'natural family planning' and abstinence" (Alonso-Zaldivar and Crary 2018).

A 2016 survey by the Urban Institute (Johnston and Schartzer 2018) found that "31.6 percent of women of reproductive age, or about 18.6 million women, say they've ever used a safety net family planning clinic." This was especially true of low-income women (the point of having a safety net in the first place). Very importantly, these safety net clinics provided primary healthcare services beyond reproduction needs, including for sexually transmitted diseases. For some women, such clinics were a major source of healthcare. The rule proposed by the Trump administration in 2018 would make it more difficult for women to access such clinics.

Maternal Mortality

Related to issues of the availability of contraceptives is maternal mortality. We noted earlier that African-American women had higher maternal mortality rates than white women. But the problem encompasses all races and ethnic groups. Historically, childbirth has been one of the most important causes of women's death. Maternal deaths have declined significantly. In 1900, the maternal death rate per 100,000 live births was approximately 825. By 2000, the rate was 15 per 100,000 live births (Helmuth 2013). The reasons for the dramatic decrease were better professionals, better care (including better nutrition), the development of antibiotics, and better understanding of pregnancy and childbirth (Helmuth 2013). The development of birth control technology, such as the pill, meant that women could limit the number of children they had and plan for pregnancy. This, too, had a dramatic effect on the declining rate of maternal mortality.

In 2016 and 2017, however, stories appeared stating that the US had a high maternal mortality rate (MMR), especially compared to other Westernized, industrial countries. For example, ProPublica and NPR (Martin et al. 2017) published a series of articles on maternal mortality, called "Lost Mothers." Martin et al. (2017) point out that between 700 and 900 women in 2016 died because of complications related to pregnancy and childbirth. They researched 120 of these women and found them to be a diverse collection of people on many factors, including race/ethnicity, age, geography, and so forth. The ages of the women ranged from 16 to 43.

A study by MacDorman et al. (2016) estimated that the maternal mortality rate doubled between 2000 and 2014. A problem with their very thorough survey was the lack of good, consistent data. To quote the authors (MacDorman et al. 2016, 1): "the United States has not published an official maternal mortality rate since 2007." The problem lies with states that had not produced information on a consistent basis.

Not all thought that the alarm raised about maternal mortality was completely justified. Loftis (2017a, 2017b) makes three important points. The first is that it is difficult to make comparisons between nations, because nations define maternal mortality differently. Second, statistics on maternal mortality across countries are not very good (Loftis 2017a). As noted by MacDorman et al. (2016), even US statistics could be stronger.

Loftis does not deny that the maternal mortality rate has increased in recent years. But she argues, and here is her third point, that a major reason for the increase in the MMR is that there are more high-risk births because the age of expectant mothers has increased. For example, there was a 23-percent increase in the number of women over 35 with their first births from 2000 to 2014 (see also Caplan-Bricker 2017). The older the mother, the greater the risk to her health.

Heuser and Karkowsky (2017) offer another reason for the increasing MMR: poverty and access. The two work together—poverty means having less access to vital prenatal care. Sifferlin (2016) argues that the uptick might be due to poor record keeping, as Loftis points out, higher rates of obesity during pregnancy, poor or inconsistent access to services, the racial disparities that we have already mentioned, a rise in cesarean births, and women having children later in life.

Another reason for the increase and concern about maternal mortality is that there is a shortage of professionals, such as OB/GYN doctors and nurse midwives, especially in rural areas. About half of counties in the US do not have an OB/GYN and more than half do not have a nurse practitioner (Ollove 2016; see also Andrews 2016). There are ways to address this issue. One is to provide more financial incentives to doctors to enter this field. A related concern is that OB/GYNs have some of the highest malpractice insurance rates in the country. A second policy would be to loosen or remove regulations requiring that nurse practitioners work under the direct supervision of physicians (Ollove 2016).

As with many issues, state and local governments have taken the lead in trying to reduce the maternal mortality rate (Martin and Fields 2018). Thirty-nine states now have maternal mortality review committees to examine maternal deaths and research the causes. Such committees, similar to child fatality review teams that exist in all 50 states, have the responsibility to ensure that all such fatalities are identified and then to investigate causes. Emphasis is also put on examining disparities in maternal mortality rates among racial/ethnic groups. Publicity, such as the ProPublica/NPR stories and the work of a multi-source national project funded by the pharmaceutical company Merck and led by the Centers for Disease Control and Prevention, AMCHP, and the CDC Foundation, provided the momentum for more states to set up the committees (Martin and Fields 2018). Martin and Fields (2018) note that having the committee is not a panacea for solving the problem; there are limitations. These include lack of funding and personnel, limited powers to gather more thorough information, and requirements that the individual deaths not be identified.

Aron et al. (2015) sum up the factors that produce disadvantages for women's health:

> The causes and consequences of the US health disadvantage, especially among women, are much more complex and serious than this analysis suggests. We should not be prepared to write-off any generation as lost. In order to tackle the underlying causes of rising mortality among women of reproductive age, the nation needs to take a much broader perspective on health and survival, one that encompasses the social determinants of health of *all* women because women's health and survival have profound implications for the health and wellbeing of children, families, and entire communities.
>
> Men and women have different experiences in the labor market, different responsibilities for caring for children and aging parents, and different economic realities. Improving the conditions of life that shape the health of women and their families and social networks and that are contributing to the "epidemic of pain" is critical. Many systemic and environmental factors are likely at work behind these mortality trends, including unstable and low-paying jobs, a fraying social safety net, and other stressors. When life conditions undermine health or one's ability to make healthy choices, we all suffer.

The Affordable Care Act has had important impacts on protecting women's health (Sun 2018). First, the percentage of uninsured women has declined significantly, from 18 percent of women to 12 percent, a decline of 33 percent (Ranji, Rosenzweig, and Salganicoff 2018). The ACA required coverage of maternity benefits and contraception (though modified by the *Hobby Lobby* case discussed above).

Having said this, two points need to be made. First, women still face many of the barriers of access and cost discussed earlier in this chapter. Second, the ACA, as discussed in Chapter 3, remains under political attack and its long-term political viability remains a question.

The Special Case of Dental Care

Most discussions of healthcare needs focus on the traditional idea of health and medicine but ignore dental care issues. Paradise (2012, 1) notes that cavities remain "the most common chronic disease among children 6–18." Further, this disease is completely preventable. The impact of chronic dental problems in children and adults goes beyond just cavities. Dental issues are linked with diseases such as sinus infection, heart and lung disease, and diabetes. Dental disease can lead to poor school performance, developmental issues among children, and poor speech (Paradise 2012). Oral diseases can lead to poor work performance and chronic pain (Licata and Paradise 2012). McGinn-Shapiro (2008) points to other needs that oral diseases would affect: employability, poor dental habits in children if there are dental problems with adults, worsening diseases (such as stroke, diabetes, and heart diseases), problems in pregnancy (such as low-weight births), oral cancer, preventing HIV from transforming to AIDS, and dealing with adults with special needs. In 2000, the US Department of Health and Human Services (2000) issued a report by the Surgeon General focusing, for the first time, on dental health issues. The report noted that oral health was something that could be achieved, but for too many it was not. The report especially looked at vulnerable populations, such as members of minority groups, the elderly, and children. In the words of the report (US Department of Health and Human Services 2000, 2): "Oral diseases are progressive and cumulative, and become more complex over time."

Access to good dental care for those at the lower end of the socioeconomic scale may be even less than for regular medical care. Interestingly, because of changes to programs such as Medicaid and the Children's Health Insurance Program, low-income children may have better dental coverage than higher-income children. However, as Paradise (2012) points out, insurance coverage and access are not the same things. Medicaid covers dental needs for children but not for adults.

There are disparities in access to dental care based on income, race, and ethnicity. For example, 42 percent of those with income under the federal poverty line had untreated cavities compared to 12 percent of those with incomes greater than 400 percent of the federal poverty line. Hispanic adults were the least likely to have seen a dentist in 2010 (Licata and Paradise 2012).

There are also disparities in dental healthcare related to geography. Rural areas, in particular, tend to have a shortage of dentists. People living in residential facilities or nursing homes also lack dental care (Hinton and Paradise 2016). Further, there is a national shortage of dentists and especially the more specialized ones, such as pediatric dentists (Paradise 2012). Hinton and Paradise (2016) note that about 15 percent of the population (about 49 million people) live in areas where there is a shortage of dental providers. Dentists are also in a much different situation than medical professionals. Dentistry is an essential benefit for children required of the exchanges by the Affordable Care Act. Dentists do not have to accept Medicaid patients, and some dentists do not accept any insurance (Hinton and Paradise 2016). According to Hinton and Paradise (2016, 5): "The reasons dentists generally cite for not participating in Medicaid are low reimbursement rates, administrative burden, and high no-show rates among Medicaid patients." Thus, while covered, for children, at least, access may be limited.

There are policies that address some of the issues discussed above. One such policy would increase reimbursement for dentists who treat Medicaid patients. Another policy would allow the equivalent of physicians' assistants (dental assistants) to provide some treatment. A third possibility is to increase access to community health centers, which do provide dental services (Hinton and Paradise 2016; "Children and Oral Health" 2012).

IMMIGRANTS AND HEALTHCARE

In 2017, over 44 million immigrants were living in the United States, accounting for 13.7 percent of the total population ("Snapshot of U.S. Immigration 2017" 2017). Immigrants are defined as foreign-born individuals living in the United States, including naturalized citizens, lawfully present noncitizens, and undocumented immigrants. Of the 44.1 million immigrants, 20 million (6.2 percent of the US population) were naturalized citizens, while another 13.1 million (4 percent of the US population) were lawfully present noncitizens and 11.1 million were undocumented immigrants (3.4 percent of the US population) ("Snapshot of U.S. Immigration 2017" 2017). Lawfully present noncitizens are those who have been granted permission to remain in the United States because they are permanent residents (have a green card) or have work authorization, refugee status, or political asylum. Undocumented immigrants are those who entered the United States without permission or who initially entered with permission but subsequently lost their lawful status (e.g., foreign students who entered the United States on student visa and stayed past their student visa expiration date) ("Immigration Reform and Access to Health Coverage" 2013).

In 2015, over half of immigrants in the United States were from the Western Hemisphere—Canada, Mexico, Central and South America, and the Caribbean. Over 2 percent were born in Asia or the Pacific Islands, and the remaining quarter were of European, African, and Middle Eastern descent ("Snapshot of U.S. Immigration 2017" 2017). In contrast to immigrants from Europe, Canada, and Australia, who not only have higher educational attainment but also are culturally more similar to citizens of the United States, Hispanics generally enjoy a lower socioeconomic status and have lower levels of employment due to their young age, language difficulty, and lower levels of education. They are also more likely to be employed in sectors such as agriculture, construction, and industries that employ contract and seasonal workers, and thus increase their chances of job loss ("How Does Health Coverage and Access to Care for Immigrants Vary by Length of Time in the U.S?" 2009).

Many of the immigrants live in mixed immigrant-status families that include two or three of the categories of immigrants discussed in the previous paragraph. For example, in 2010, there were over 4 million US-born children whose parents were undocumented ("Immigration Reform and Access to Health Coverage" 2013). Thus, immigrants as a group constitute a very complex mix of individuals who vary by country of origin, number of years they have stayed in the United States, ethnicity/race, socioeconomic and health status, as well as acculturation and assimilation ("How Does Health Coverage and Access to Care for Immigrants Vary by Length of Time in the U.S.?" 2009).

A majority of immigrants who are naturalized citizens of the United States receive their healthcare the same way native citizens do—through their employer or through other private coverage. Those who are low-income and meet eligibility criteria can receive healthcare through safety net programs such as Medicaid or the Children's Health Insurance Program (CHIP).

In general, immigrants are more likely to be uninsured than US-born citizens, and they face increased barriers to accessing needed healthcare. Even immigrants who have lived in the United States for a longer period of time are significantly less likely to be insured than recent immigrants (Artiga and Damico 2016). Given the fact that immigrants have a greater problem accessing care and obtain less physician care, they are more likely to utilize emergency care in hospitals, which is much more expensive. Noncitizen immigrants are more likely than US natives to have a healthcare visit classified as uncompensated care (Stimpson, Wilson, and Su 2013). The higher uninsured rate among immigrants is due to their limited access to private coverage because they work in low-wage jobs and firms that often do not offer health coverage ("How Does Health Coverage and Access to Care for Immigrants Vary by Length of Time in the U.S.?" 2009).

Lawful Noncitizen Immigrants and Healthcare

Lawfully present noncitizen immigrants can obtain health insurance coverage in the United States either through their employer or through private insurance. However, when it comes to public health programs, they are subject to Medicaid and CHIP eligibility restrictions. The Personal Responsibility and Work Opportunity Reconciliation Act (PRWORA) of 1996 decoupled social welfare benefits from health insurance safety-net programs such as Medicaid. The law placed complex restrictions on social welfare and health insurance benefits for legal immigrants who are not citizens, implementing a five-year waiting period before they can access many social safety-net programs such as Medicaid and the CHIP (Scotch and Loganathan 2011).

Under the Children's Health Insurance Program Reauthorization Act (CHIPRA) of 2009, state governments were given the option to eliminate this five-year waiting period for lawfully residing noncitizens who are pregnant women, or children. Since 2002, states have also had the option to use federal CHIP funds to cover prenatal care for pregnant women regardless of their immigration status ("Immigrants' Health Coverage and Health Reform: Key Questions and Answers" 2009). As of 2017, 30 states had elected the CHIPRA option for lawfully present immigrant children (Center for Children and Families 2017). As of 2018, 25 states had adopted the option of covering lawfully residing immigrant pregnant women ("Medicaid/CHIP Coverage of Lawfully-Residing Immigrant Children and Pregnant Women" 2018).

Under the Affordable Care Act, lawfully present noncitizen immigrants will continue to face the five-year waiting period for Medicaid. They will, however, be able to purchase health insurance coverage in the healthcare exchanges and receive tax credits without a waiting period, which could significantly help to expand their coverage and access to healthcare ("Key Facts on Health Coverage for Low-Income Immigrants Today and Under the Affordable Care Act" 2013).

One can see some of the politics involved with immigration and healthcare reform in an incident that occurred in September of 2009. President Obama addressed a televised joint session of Congress urging Congress to pass what would become the Affordable Care Act. During his speech, the President said that illegal immigrants would not be eligible for coverage. At that point, Joe Wilson (R-SC) yelled out "You lie!" to the President. All eyes, Republican and Democratic, turned in his direction. Wilson called the White House and apologized to the President. Wilson was later rebuked by the House (Nasaw 2009).

Two years later, it appeared that illegal immigrants might indeed be covered, though not necessarily through the ACA. The US Department of Health and Human Services (HHS) made a major grant ($28.8 million) to a number of community health centers. A portion of that money, $8.5 million, was aimed specifically at "migrant and seasonal farm workers" (Sink 2011). Wilson maintained that he was right all along because there were undoubtedly undocumented immigrants in this category. HHS maintained that there was nothing new in this policy and that community health centers are concerned only about the health of people who come to them for care. Further, subsidies to purchase plans on the ACA exchanges remain unavailable to undocumented immigrants. Wilson, however, continued to maintain that available healthcare helped this group of people (Sink 2011).

Under the immigration reform proposals presented by both President Obama and a bipartisan group of eight senators, individuals who are granted provisional lawful status will not be eligible for federal public assistance benefits, including health coverage. This is similar to when in June 2012 the Obama administration announced a new program referred to as Deferred Action for Childhood Arrivals (DACA), under which certain undocumented youths would be given temporary permission to stay in the United States. However, in August 2012, the Department of Health and Human Services (DHHS) announced policy that would exclude these youths from the health coverage options that are available to other lawfully present immigrants ("Immigration Reform and Access to Health Coverage" 2013). It remains to be seen if Congress will pass a comprehensive immigration reform bill, and, even if it does, what provisions would be included in the final legislation. Immigration has become one of the most controversial public policy issues during the Trump administration. The administration would like to end illegal immigration and severely curtail lawful immigration.

Undocumented Immigrants and Healthcare

An estimated 11.1 million immigrants living in the United States are undocumented ("Unauthorized Immigrants" 2013; Yee, Davis, and Patel 2017). The Federation for American Immigration Reform (FAIR) estimates that, in 2017, there were 12.5 million undocumented immigrants (Raley 2017). Regardless of the number, illegal immigrants represent a major challenge to the US healthcare system. They are ineligible for most of the federal social and health benefits programs, yet they cost the US healthcare system in numerous ways.

Under federal law, undocumented immigrants are prohibited from enrolling in Medicaid and the CHIP. However, Medicaid payment for emergency services may be made on behalf of undocumented immigrants who would otherwise qualify for Medicaid. Since 2002, state governments also have had the option to use federal CHIP funds to cover prenatal care for pregnant women regardless of their immigration status ("Immigrants' Health Coverage and Health Reform: Key Questions and Answers" 2009). As of January 2018, 17 states and the District of Columbia had elected this option ("Medical Assistance Programs for Immigrants in Various States" 2018; see also "Key Facts on Health Coverage for Low-Income Immigrants Today and Under the Affordable Care Act" 2013). Under the ACA, undocumented immigrants will continue to remain ineligible for Medicaid and will be prohibited from purchasing health insurance coverage through state exchanges and to receive tax credits ("Immigration Reform and Access to Health Coverage: Key Issues to Consider" 2013).

According to the Pew Hispanic Center, most undocumented immigrants in the United States are employed in the agriculture sector (17 percent), followed by construction (13 percent), leisure/hospitality (7 percent), and manufacturing (6 percent) (Passel and Cohn 2017). Most undocumented immigrants, given their immigration status and employment concentration in certain sectors of the economy, earn close to minimum wage and fall below the federal poverty line. However, given their status as undocumented immigrants they are ineligible for Medicaid and the CHIP ("Medicaid/CHIP Coverage of Lawfully-Residing Immigrant Children and Pregnant Women" 2018).

In 1986, Congress barred undocumented immigrants from the federal health benefits generally available to the poor with one major exception—emergencies (Zarembo and Gorman 2008). The Emergency Medical Treatment and Active Labor Act of 1986 guarantees emergency medical treatment to anyone, regardless of their legal status or ability to pay. In return, hospitals receive federal reimbursement for care provided to undocumented immigrants in emergency rooms. Since undocumented immigrants are otherwise ineligible for federal health benefits and are more likely to be uninsured, chronic care for undocumented immigrants often turns into emergency room visits for dialysis or diuretics. Such treatments in hospital emergency rooms are much more expensive compared to outpatient clinics. Acute-care services of emergency rooms are among the most expensive way to pay for healthcare services (Garg 2010). In addition, the federal definition of what constitutes an emergency as well as when an emergency starts and ends is open to interpretation, leaving in place an ambiguous federal policy (Zarembo and Gorman 2008). The result is an irrational public policy that, on the one hand, prohibits federal health benefits such as Medicaid and the CHIP to undocumented immigrants, but, on the other hand, pays for more expensive emergency room services to the same undocumented immigrants. Dialysis offers a striking example. US taxpayers covered the entire cost of dialysis treatment (about 2000 times over a 17-year period) for Marguerita Toribio, an undocumented immigrant from Mexico, including a kidney transplant in 1993. In California alone, undocumented immigrants account for about 1350 of the 61,000 people on dialysis, costing the taxpayer $51 million in 2007 (Zarembo and Gorman 2008).

Health services and other benefits available to illegal immigrants can vary from state to state. Local government and local public hospitals are often responsible for implementing the provision of health services to the medically indigent and uninsured. Many public and private hospitals bear the burden of substantial costs in providing undocumented immigrants care that is often uncompensated (Scotch and Loganathan 2011). State and local governments are generally the ones that bear the cost of undocumented immigrants. During the recession of 2007–2009, many states and local governments facing state budget deficits cut back on health services provided to the uninsured and the indigent, and undocumented immigrants often constitute a sizable portion of such populations (Wood 2009).

Communities with large numbers of undocumented immigrants face considerable financial strain in trying to meet the healthcare needs of the undocumented immigrants. For example, California, which has the nation's largest population of undocumented immigrants, spent an estimated $1.2 billion in 2011 through Medicaid to care for 822,500 undocumented immigrants. The New Jersey Hospital Association in 2010 estimated that it cost between $600 million and $650 million annually to treat 550,000 undocumented immigrants. Texas, in 2010, provided $96 million in benefits to undocumented immigrants (Sherman and Plushnick-Masti 2012). Presented with a high financial burden, public hospitals are often faced with the option of closing down clinics and services. For example, in 2010, two large public hospitals—Grady Hospital in Atlanta, Georgia and Jackson Memorial Hospital in Miami, Florida—closed the doors of their outpatient dialysis clinics to nonpaying patients, most of whom were undocumented immigrants, due to inability to cover the costs. Ironically, many of these same patients now access dialysis in the emergency room of the same hospitals, even though it is a more expensive way to treat the same patients, because hospitals get federal dollars for care provided in the emergency room (Garg 2010).

Conover (2018) estimates that the US spends, despite the restrictions mentioned above, about $18.5 billion a year on healthcare for undocumented immigrants. Medicaid, as mentioned above, will pay for emergency services on a limited basis. States can use their share of Medicaid money (state-only) to pay for healthcare for this group. As of 2018, four states (California, New York, Massachusetts, and Illinois) and the District of Columbia had such programs (Conover 2018).

Another way of providing funding for unauthorized immigrants is through the Disproportionate Share Hospitals Program (DSH; see Chapters 4 and 5). DSH payments go to hospitals that have a high percentage of Medicaid and uninsured patients. Because undocumented immigrants do not have health insurance, DSH payments include treating them at hospitals. Conover (2018) also points out that federally qualified community health centers treat patients who present themselves regardless of their status.

Some of Conover's (2018) estimates, which he admits to being classic "back-of-the-envelope" calculations, could be challenged. For example, he suggests that some portion of the tax exemption for employer-provided health insurance is attributable to undocumented immigrants, but their coverage is less than for legal immigrants and citizens. And while $18.5 billion is a lot of money, it represents about one-half of 1 percent of total healthcare spending in 2017 (calculated from Conover 2018 and "New Government Data" 2017). Further, as we discuss in Chapter 8, some of the spending on healthcare is invisible. For example, the tax deduction for employer-sponsored insurance is not covered in national healthcare expenditures (on the use of tax expenditures, see Mettler 2011); therefore, the percentage spent on healthcare for undocumented immigrants, by this reasoning, is lower than the one-half of 1 percent.

The often confusing, contradictory, and ambiguous federal healthcare policy toward immigrants in general and undocumented immigrants in particular reflects the ambivalent attitudes Americans have about immigration. The plight of undocumented immigrants elicits strong feelings on both sides of the debate. On the one side are those who strictly take an anti-immigration policy position and oppose undocumented immigrants' being able to access publicly financed social welfare and healthcare programs. Those who favor providing access to health services for undocumented immigrants justify their position from a social justice and human rights perspective, that every human being is entitled to basic rights, and that social justice demands that everyone has access to healthcare. This argument has generally failed to win over many converts (Okolec 2009).

Another perspective that advocates providing undocumented immigrants access to healthcare take is a public health approach. Here, advocates argue for changing the perspective or frame on healthcare from an individual level to a community level by appealing to the larger community to take preventive action to avoid disease. This view helps move health from a personal, individual arena to the arena of healthcare as a social good. The reason for this is that Americans are often described as compassionate people when thinking about community as a whole. Framing healthcare as a public—that is, common or social—good rather than an individual good also acknowledges the role of public health in monitoring community health, preventing illness, and living up to one of its ethical principles, which is to advocate for the empowerment of the disenfranchised community members and ensure that resources and conditions necessary for health are accessible to everyone (Okolec 2009). Whether such a perspective takes hold in the long run in the United States remains to be seen. What is clear in the short term is that the current confusing, ambiguous, and irrational healthcare policy with respect to undocumented immigrants is likely to continue. Progress in this area, if any, is likely to come in small, incremental steps.

One can see how these ideas play out in the events that occurred in the Spring of 2018. Donald Trump campaigned for the presidency partly on the promise to reduce immigration to the United States and to build a wall along the border with Mexico (which, he promised, would be funded by Mexico). By executive order, President Trump sought to limit immigration from specified Muslim-majority countries. Though the bans were overturned by federal courts, the US Supreme Court upheld the travel ban in June 2018 (the ban included North Korea) (Liptak and Shear 2018).

The administration then moved to a "zero-tolerance" policy dealing with migrants crossing the US-Mexican border. As part of the implementation of this policy, children were separated from their parents and kept in various places, such as an abandoned Wal-Mart. From the standpoint of this chapter, with its focus on the disadvantaged and healthcare, keeping children away from their parents can cause both physical and psychological harm (Sanchez 2018). "Based on past research ... children who are forcibly taken from their parents have demonstrated links to asthma, obesity and cancer, in addition to tendencies toward substance abuse, developmental delays and mental health issues" (Sanchez 2018).

The policy or practice, which is part of the larger policy issue surrounding immigration, produced considerable opposition in both parties (Collinson and Fox 2018), including former first ladies and, in a subtle statement, First Lady Melania Trump (Ebbs 2018). Interestingly, public opinion opposed forced separation, except among Republicans, particularly Trump's base within the Republican Party (Blake 2018). The President and his supporters argue that the separation policy is intended to discourage immigration. In May 2018, President Trump signed an executive order ending the family separation policy. Two problems remain. One is reuniting families. The other is whether there will be any lasting health effects in the children who were separated.

CONCLUSION: THE PROBLEMS OF THE DISADVANTAGED REMAIN

In this chapter we have considered one of the major problems of the US healthcare system: access. The uniquely American mix of public and private insurance programs, a post-World War II development, covers about 90 percent of the population but leaves over 20 million people without any insurance at all. Especially in the case of private insurance, it also leaves a portion of the population underinsured and vulnerable to catastrophic medical expenses.

One reason why the issue of access and the safety net has been so difficult is that perceptions about the problem differ. White Americans are less likely than African-Americans or Latinos to think there are disparities in coverage, quality, and access. The lack of awareness of disparities exists even within the minority communities (Benz et al. 2011; Lillie-Blanton et al. 2000). The importance of this is that differential perceptions on lack of access make it difficult to deal with a problem and get it on the policy agenda.

Incremental reforms, the kind that generally characterize public policy in the United States, have begun to address some of these problems. The CHIP program focuses on children. The Health Insurance Portability and Accountability Act addresses the "job lock" issue.

The passage of the ACA resulted in an increase in insurance coverage. But hostility to the Act on the part of Republicans meant that the potential of the ACA in covering the population was diminished. As we saw in Chapter 3, the repeal of the tax penalty for not being insured in December 2017 and actions taken by the Trump administration have decreased the potency of the legislation. Not all states expanded Medicaid and the administration has carved out ways to allow people to avoid being covered under the ACA.

Even if the ACA meets its objectives, the problems of the disadvantaged would remain. Having insurance coverage is important. We know from a considerable body of evidence that those without health insurance have more health problems and receive less and poorer-quality service than those with health insurance. But if the providers are not in the geographical area, such as inner cities or rural areas, having insurance by itself is insufficient.

We also know that poverty, ethnicity, and gender play important and intermixing roles in health outcomes. We know that blacks and Latinos on average have poorer health outcomes than whites. We know that minority women and their babies have poorer health outcomes, more troubling pregnancies, low birth weights, and so forth. Additionally, one concern about the ACA, if it meets its access goals, is whether there would be a sufficient increase in the number of providers to meet the anticipated increased demand for services. Even with the comprehensive reform promised by the new legislation, it is likely that the problems of the disadvantaged will remain.

An important consideration in the debate about expanding coverage is what the costs would be. The United States has been and is facing considerable health cost pressures, a topic we address next.

STUDY QUESTIONS

1. The policy process begins with the problem-identification stage. This means getting the political system to recognize that a problem exists. This stage, perhaps the most important in the policy process, is very contentious. There are disagreements over whether a problem that should be addressed by the political system exists, and, if so, what the nature of the problem is. This chapter focuses on the disadvantaged, people and families who lack health insurance. There are estimates that 20 million or more people in the United States lack health insurance. Do you think this is a problem that should be addressed by the political system? Why? Republicans and Democrats disagree on both points (whether it is a problem and the nature of the problem). What are their positions? Why do they take those positions?
2. There are an estimated 10–12 million undocumented immigrants in the United States. While the president and Congress have considered immigration reform legislation, the fact remains that these immigrants do not have health insurance or a regular source of healthcare. When they do need healthcare, they go to hospital emergency departments, though they cannot pay. Hospitals shift some of those costs to insured payers. The Affordable Care Act does not cover the undocumented. Given the impact that they have, should undocumented immigrants be covered? Why or why not?
3. Having a federal system means that some states have a higher percentage of uninsured people than other states do. States with high percentages of uninsured people also tend to be the least generous in their safety net policies. Do you think a more national system would be an appropriate response to this? Or should it be left to the states to decide how much to cover the uninsured?
4. As we note in the chapter, not all disparities are income-based. Some are geographically based. People in inner cities and rural areas have less access to healthcare providers than do those in suburban areas and more affluent parts of cities. Why do you think this is the case? What policies, if any, have been adopted to address these disparities? What additional policies, if any, do you think should be adopted?
5. A major goal of the Affordable Care Act is to cover more of the uninsured. What are the mechanisms for doing so? How well do you think the ACA is working in this respect? To what extent are perspectives on this question influenced by ideology?

REFERENCES

Aday, Lu Ann. 1993. "Equity, Accessibility, and Ethical Issues: Is the U.S. Health Care Reform Debate Asking the Right Questions?" *American Behavioral Scientist*, 36, no. 6 (July/August): 724–740.
Agency for Health Care Research and Quality. 2010. *National Healthcare Disparities Report*. Washington, DC: US Department of Health and Human Services.
Agency for Health Care Research and Quality. 2016a. *National Healthcare Quality and Disparities Report*. Washington, DC: US Department of Health and Human Services.
Agency for Health Care Research and Quality. 2016b. *Chartbook on Health Care for Blacks: National Healthcare Quality and Disparities Report*. Washington, DC: US Department of Health and Human Services.
Aizenman, N.C. 2012. "New Front in Birth Control Rule Battle: The Courts." *The Washington Post*, March 7.
Ajani, Salako Taofiki. 2013. "Islamic Perspectives on Birth Control." *American International Journal of Contemporary Research*, 3, no. 1 (January): 117–127.
Alonso-Zaldivar, Ricardo and David Crary. 2018 "Trump Remaking Federal Policy on Women's Reproductive Health." Associated Press, May 30.
Alter, Charlotte. 2016. "How Planned Parenthood Changed Everything." *Time*, October 14. Online at www.time.com.
"America's Shocking Maternal Deaths." 2016. *The New York Times*, September 3.
Anderson, Carol. 2017. *White Rage: The Unspoken Truth of Our Racial Divide*. New York: Bloomsbury USA.
Andrews, Becca. 2016. "The Biggest Threat to Women's Health that No One Talks About." *Mother Jones*, August 16.
Andrews, Michelle. 2010. "Pregnant Women and New Mothers Will Get Benefits, Services under Health Care Law." *Kaiser Health News*, June 8.
Andrews, Michelle. 2012. "Insurance Coverage Might Steer Women to Costlier—But More Effective—Birth Control." *Kaiser Health News*, February 20.

Aron, Laudn et al. 2015. "To Understand Climbing Death Rates among Whites, Look to Women of Childbearing Age." *Health Affairs*, November 10. Online at www.healthaffairs.org.

Artiga, Samanatha, Julia Foutz, and Anthony Damico 2018. *Health Coverage by Race and Ethnicity: Changes under the ACA*. Menlo Park, CA: Kaiser Family Foundation.

Artiga, Samantha et al. 2016. *Health Coverage by Race and Ethnicity: Examining Changes under the ACA and Remaining Uninsured*. Menlo Park, CA: Kaiser Family Foundation.

Artiga, Samantha et al. 2016b. *Key Facts on Health and Health Care by Race and Ethnicity: A Chartbook*. Menlo Park, CA: Kaiser Family Foundation.

Artiga, Samantha and Anthony Damico 2016. *Nearly 20 Million Children Live in Immigrant Families that Could Be Affected by Evolving Immigration Policies*. Menlo Park, CA: Kaiser Family Foundation.

Artiga, Samantha and Elizabeth Hinton 2018. *Beyond Health Care: The Role of Social Determinants in Promoting Health and Health Equity*. San Francisco, CA: Kaiser Family Foundation.

Auerbach, Judith. 2004. "The Overlooked Victims of AIDS." *Kaiser Health News*, August 6.

Baird, Karen L. 1998. *Gender Justice and the Health Care System*. New York: Garland Publishing.

Barnett, Jessica C. and Edward R. Berchick. 2017. *Health Insurance Coverage in the United States: 2016*. Washington, DC: US Census Bureau, US Department of Commerce.

Beckles, Gloria and Benedict I. Truman 2011. "Education and Income—United States, 2005 and 2009." *Morbidity and Mortality Weekly Report, Special Supplement*, 60 (January 14): 13–17.

Belluz, Julia. 2016. "Women's Health in the U.S. Is Declining in 4 Key Ways, and Researchers Can't Explain Why." *Vox*, June 6.

Benz, Jennifer et al. 2011. "Awareness of Racial and Ethnic Health Disparities Has Improved Only Modestly over a Decade." *Health Affairs*, 30, no. 10 (October): 1860–1867.

Berk, Marc L. and Claudia L. Schur 1998. "Access to Care: How Much Difference Does Medicaid Make?" *Health Affairs*, 17, no. 3 (May/June): 169–180.

"Birth Control." n.d. *Catholic Answers*. Online at www.catholic.com/tract/birth-control.

"Births Financed by Medicaid." 2017. Menlo Park, CA: Kaiser Family Foundation.

"Black Women's Maternal Health: A Multifaceted Approach to Addressing Persistent and Dire Health Disparities." 2018. Washington, DC: National Partnership for Women and Families.

Blake, Aaron. 2018. "The GOP Backs Trump on Separating Families at the Border—Which Is All He Cares About." *The Washington Post*, June 18.

Boston Women's Health Book Collective and Judy Norsigian. 2011. *Our Bodies, Ourselves*. New York: Touchstone.

Bradley, Elizabeth H. and Lauren A. Taylor 2013. *The American Health Care Paradox: Why Spending More Is Getting Us Less*. New York: Public Affairs.

Bureau of Labor Statistics. n.d. *Employment by Major Industry Sector*. Washington, DC: US Department of Labor, US Bureau of Labor Statistics. Online at www.bls.gov.

Burhansstipanov, Linda and Linda A. Krebs 2016. *Health Disparities among American Indians and Alaska Natives: Enormous Hurdles and Opportunities*. Bethesda, MD: National Institute on Minority Health and Health Disparities, National Institutes of Health.

Burton, Tara Isabella. 2017. "How Birth Control Became Part of the Evangelical Agenda." *Vox*, October 7.

Byrd, W. Michael and Linda A. Clayton 2003. "Racial and Ethnic Disparities in Healthcare: A Background and History." In *Unequal Treatment*, eds Brian D. Smedley, Adrienne Y. Stith, and Alan R. Nelson, 455–527. Washington, DC: National Academies Press.

Caplan-Bricker, Nora. 2017. "For the First Time Ever, Thirty-Something Women are Having More Babies than Their Twenty-Something Counterparts." *Time*, May 17.

Catron, David. 2018. "Hospitals Get Reprieve from Obama Pay Cuts." *The American Spectator*, February 7. Online at www.spectator.org.

Center for Children and Families. 2017. *The Children's Health Insurance Program*. Washington, DC: Georgetown University Health Policy Institute.

Centers for Disease Control and Prevention. 2011. *HIV Among African Americans*. Washington, DC: US Department of Health and Human Services.

Centers for Disease Control and Prevention. 2015. *Vital Signs: Hispanic Health*. Washington, DC: US Department of Health and Human Services.

Centers for Disease Control and Prevention. 2017. *Vital Signs: African American Health*. Washington, DC: US Department of Health and Human Services.

Chapman, Audry R. 1994. "Introduction." In *Health Care Reform: A Human Rights Approach*, ed. Audrey R. Chapman, 1–32. Washington, DC: Georgetown University Press.

"Children and Oral Health: Assessing Needs, Coverage, and Access." 2012. Menlo Park, CA: Kaiser Family Foundation.

Chakraborty, Ranjani. 2018. "How More Midwives May Mean Healthier Mothers." ProPublica, May 29.

Claxton, Gary, Isadora Gil, Ben Finder, and Erin Holve. 2004. *Employer Health Benefits 2004 Annual Survey*. Menlo Park, CA: Henry J. Kaiser Family Foundation and Chicago, IL: Health Research and Educational Trust.

Claxton, Gary et al. 2017. *Employer Health Benefits 2017 Annual Survey*. Menlo Park, CA: Henry J. Kaiser Family Foundation, and Chicago, IL: Health Research and Educational Trust.

Clemetson, Lynette. 2004. "Links between Prison and AIDS Affecting Blacks Inside and Out." *The New York Times*, August 6.

Collins, Sara et al. 2014. *The Problems of Underinsurance and How Rising Deductibles Will Make It Worse*. New York: The Commonwealth Fund.

Collins, Sara et al. 2016. *Who are the Remaining Uninsured and Why Haven't They Signed up for Coverage?* New York: The Commonwealth Fund.

Collinson, Stephen and Lauren Fox. 2018. "Outrage Grows as Families are Separated. Will Trump Change His Policy?" CNN, June 18.
Committee on Health Insurance Status and Its Consequences. 2009. *America's Uninsured Crisis: Consequences for Health and Health Care*. Washington, DC: National Academy Press.
"Community Health Workers." n.d. Washington, DC: American Public Health Association. Online at www.apha.org.
Conover, Chris. 2018. "How American Citizens Finance $18.5 Billion in Health Care for Unauthorized Immigrants." *Forbes*, February 26.
Crum, Brooke. 2018. "Grant to Help Jordan Valley Serve Thousands in Springfield." *Springfield News-Leader*, May 7.
Cubanski, Juliette et al. 2018. *The Financial Burden of Health Care Spending: Larger for Medicare Households than for Non-Medicare Households*. Menlo Park, CA: Kaiser Family Foundation.
Curtin, Sally C. et al. 2013. "Source of Payment for the Delivery: Births in a 33-State and District of Columbia Reporting Area, 2010." *National Vital Statistics Reports*, 62, no. 5 (December 19).
Cust, Kenneth F.T. 1997. *A Just Minimum of Health Care*. New York: University Press of America.
Daniels, Norman, Donald W. Light, and Ronald L. Caplan. 1996. *Benchmarks of Fairness for Health Care Reform*. New York: Oxford University Press.
Dorn, Stan. 2008. *Uninsured and Dying because of It: Updating the Institute of Medicine Analysis on the Impact of Uninsurance on Mortality*. Washington, DC: Urban Institute.
Doty, Michelle et al. 2007. *Failure to Protect: Why the Individual Insurance Market Is Not a Viable Option for Most U.S. Families*. Washington, DC: Commonwealth Fund.
Ebbs, Stephanie. 2018. "All Five First Ladies Speak Against Family-Separation Immigration Policy." ABC News, June 18.
"Emergency Medical Treatment and Active Labor Act (EMTALA)" n.d. Ascension Health. Online at www.ascensionhealth.org/index.php?option=com_content&view=article&id=146&Itemid=172.
Employee Benefits Research Institute. 2016. "Fewer Smaller Employers Offering Health Coverage; Large Employers Hold Steady." *EBRI Notes*, 37, no. 8 (July).
Enthoven, Alain C. 2003. "Employment-Based Insurance Is Failing: Now What?" *Health Affairs* (May 23): W3-237–W3-249.
"Explaining Health Care Reform: Medical Loss Ratio." 2012. Menlo Park, CA: Kaiser Family Foundation.
Families USA. 2010. *Covering Pregnant Women: CHIPRA Offers New Option*. Washington, DC: Families USA.
Families USA. 2018. "American Indian and Alaskan Native Health Inequities Compared to Non-Hispanic Whites." Washington, DC: Families USA.
Fears, Darryl. 2005. "U.S. HIV Cases Soar Among Black Women." *The Washington Post*, February 7.
Flaherty, E.G. et al. 2006. "Effect of Early Childhood Adversity on Child Health." *Archives of Pediatric and Adolescent Medicine*, 160, no. 12 (December): 1232–1238.
Flores, Antonio. 2017. *Facts on U.S. Latinos, 2015*. Washington, DC: Pew Research Center. Online at www.pewhispanic.org.
Foutz, Julia et al. 2017. *The Uninsured: A Primer*. Menlo Park, CA: Kaiser Family Foundation.
Fox, Maggie. 2010. "Nearly 59 Million Lack Health Insurance: CDC." Reuters, November 10.
Froomkin, Dan. 2007. "Mock the Press." *The Washington Post*, July 11.
Frost, Jennifer and Laura Duberstein Lindberg. 2012. "Reasons for Using Contraception: Perspectives of U.S. Women Seeking Care at Specialized Family Planning Clinics." *Contraception*, 87, no. 4 (September 27): 1–8.
Furrow, Barry R. 1995. "An Overview and Analysis of the Impact of the Emergency Medical Treatment and Active Labor Act." *Journal of Legal Medicine*, 16, (September): 357–352.
"Gaping, Painful Holes Remain in U.S. Health Care despite Coverage Gains." 2016. *PBS News Hour*, November 4. Online at www.youtube.com/watch?v=LzPCEgc7s_s&feature=youtu.be.
Garcia, Tamyra, Amy B. Bernstein, and Mary Ann Bush 2010. *Emergency Department Visitors and Visits: Who Used the Emergency Room in 2007?* Hyattsville, MD: US Department of Health and Human Services, National Center for Health Statistics.
Garg, Megha. 2010. "It Pays to Provide Health Care: A Case for Including Undocumented Immigrants." *Kennedy School Review*, 10, 25–28.
Garner, M.O., S.P. Cliver, S.F. McNeal, and R.L. Goldenberg 1996. "Ethnicity and Sources of Prenatal Care; Findings from a National Survey." *Birth*, 23, no. 2: 84–87.
Geiger, Kim and Noam N. Levey. 2012. "Before Birth-Control Fight, Republicans Backed Mandates." *Los Angeles Times*, February 15.
General Accounting Office. 1997. *Health Insurance: Coverage Leads to Increased Health Care Access for Children*. Washington, DC: General Accounting Office.
Giled, Sherry and Adlan Jackson 2017. *Access to Coverage and Care for People with Preexisting Conditions: How Has It Changed under the ACA?* Washington, DC: Commonwealth Fund.
Ginzberg, Eli. 1994. "Improving Health Care for the Poor." *Journal of the American Medical Association*, 271, no. 6 (February): 464–465.
Graig, Laurene A. 1999. *Health of Nations: An International Perspective on U.S. Health Care Reform*. Washington, DC: CQ Press.
Grant, Rebecca. 2016. "Pregnant Women's Medical Care Too Often Affected by Race." Newsweek, July 3.
Greene, Jay. 2011. "Report: Uninsured Patients 3 Times More Likely to Use Emergency Departments, are Sicker." *Crain's Detroit Business*, June 19.
Gresenz, Carole Roan and Jose J. Escarce 2011. "Spillover Effects of Community Uninsurance on Working- Age Adults and Seniors." *Medical Care*, 49, no. 9 (September): e14–e21.
Hacker, Jacob S. 2002. *The Divided Welfare State: The Battle over Public and Private Social Benefits in the United States*. New York: Cambridge University Press.

Hacker, Jacob S. 2006. *The Great Risk Shift*. New York: Oxford University Press.
Halverson, Joel A. and Greg Bischak 2008. *Underlying Socioeconomic Factors Influencing Health Disparities in the Appalachian Region*. Washington, DC: Appalachian Regional Commission.
Handrick, Laura. 2017. *Small Business Maternity Leave Policy & Laws—With Examples*. New York: FitSmall Business, November 20. Online at www.fitsmallbusiness.com.
Hansard, Sara. 2018. "Would 'Skinny' Health Plans End up Raising Premiums for Some?" *Bloomberg BNA*, February 23. Online at www.bna.com.
"Health Insurance Market Reforms: Rate Restrictions." 2012. Menlo Park, CA: Kaiser Family Foundation.
Heiman, Henry J. and Samantha Artiga. 2015. "Beyond Health Care: The Role of Social Determinants in Promoting Health and Health Equity." Menlo Park, CA: Kaiser Commission on Medicaid and the Uninsured.
Helmuth, Jane. 2013. "The Disturbing, Shameful History of Childbirth Deaths." *Slate*, September 10.
Heuser, Cara and Chavi Eve Karkowsky. 2017. "Why Is U.S. Maternal Mortality So High?" *Slate*, May 23.
Hinton, Elizabeth and Julia Paradise 2016. *Access to Dental Care in Medicaid: Spotlight on Nonelderly Adults*. Menlo Park, CA: Kaiser Family Foundation.
"HIV among Black Women 5 Times Higher than Previously Thought." 2012. *Huffington Post*, March 10.
"The HIV/AIDS Epidemic in the United States: The Basics." 2018. Menlo Park, CA: Kaiser Family Foundation.
Hoffman, Catherine and Karyn Schwartz 2008. "Eroding Access among Nonelderly U.S. Adults with Chronic Conditions: Ten Years of Change." *Health Affairs*, 27, no. 5 (July 22): W340–W348.
Holahan, John and Arunabh Ghosh. 2004. *The Economic Downturn and Changes in Health Insurance Coverage, 2000–2003*. Washington, DC: Kaiser Commission on Medicaid and the Uninsured.
"How Does Health Coverage and Access to Care for Immigrants Vary by Length of Time in the U.S?" 2009. Washington, DC: Kaiser Commission on Medicaid and the Uninsured.
"HPSA and MUA/P." n.d. St. Paul, MN: Minnesota Department of Health.
"Immigrants' Health Coverage and Health Reform: Key Questions and Answers." 2009. Menlo Park, CA: Kaiser Family Foundation.
"Immigrants' Health Coverage and Health Reform: Key Questions and Answers." 2013. Menlo Park, CA: Kaiser Family Foundation.
"Immigration Reform and Access to Health Coverage: Key Issues to Consider." 2013. Washington, DC: Kaiser Commission on Medicaid and the Uninsured. Henry J. Kaiser Family Foundation.
"Induced Abortion in the United States." n.d. New York: Guttmacher Institute.
Institute of Medicine. 2008. *Challenges and Successes in Reducing Health Disparities: Workshop Summary*. Washington, DC: National Academy Press.
"Insurance Coverage of Contraceptives." 2018. New York: Guttmacher Institute.
Isenberg, Nancy. 2016. *White Trash: The 400-Year Untold History of Class in American*. New York: Viking.
James, Cara V. et al. 2009. *Putting Women's Health Care Disparities on the Map: Examining Racial and Ethnic Disparities at the State Level*. Menlo Park, CA: Kaiser Family Foundation.
Jecker, Nancy S. 1993. "Can an Employer-Based Health Insurance System Be Just?" *Journal of Health Care Politics, Policy and Law*, 18, no. 3 (Fall): 657–673.
Johnston, Emily M. and Adele Schartzer. 2018. *Changes to Title X Funding Could Affect Access to Health Care for Millions of Women*. Washington, DC: Urban Institute.
Joint Commission. 2013. "Overcoming the Challenges of Providing Care to LEP Patients." Washington, DC: The Joint Commission. Online at www.joincommission.org.
Kaiser Family Foundation. 2004a. *Update on Individual Health Insurance*. Menlo Park, CA: Kaiser Family Foundation.
Kaiser Family Foundation. 2004b. *Health Care and the 2004 Elections: Women's Health Policy*. Menlo Park, CA: Kaiser Family Foundation.
Kari, Nancy, Harry C. Boyte, and Bruce Jennings. 1994. "Health as a Civic Question." Prepared for the American Civic Forum Madison, WI. Online at www.cpn.org/topics/health/healthquestion.html.
"Key Facts about the Uninsured Population." 2017. Menlo Park, CA: Kaiser Family Foundation.
"Key Facts on Health Coverage for Low-Income Immigrants Today and under the Affordable Care Act." 2013. Washington, DC: Kaiser Commission on the Uninsured.
Khazan, Olga. 2015. "The Sickest Town in America." *The Atlantic*, January 22. Online at www.theatlantic.com.
Kliff, Sarah. 2017. "Rolling Back the Birth Control Mandate Is Part of a Much Larger GOP Strategy." *Vox*, May 31.
Kitroeff, Natalie and Jessica Silver-Greenberg. 2018. "Pregnancy Discrimination Is Rampant inside America's Biggest Companies." *The New York Times*, June 15.
Klein, Joel. 2012. "How the Gun Won." *Time*, August 4, 26–32.
Knowles, Jon. 2012. *A History of Birth Control Methods*. New York: Planned Parenthood Federation of America.
Kodjak, Allison. 2017. "From Birth to Death, Medicaid Affects the Lives of Millions." *NPR*, June 27. Online at npr.org.
Krause, Elliott A. 1977. *Power and Illness: The Political Sociology of Health and Medical Care*. New York: Elsevier.
Kreidler, Mike. n.d. *Your Rights under the U.S. COBRA Law*. Olympia, WA: Office of the Insurance Commissioner.
Krieger, Nancy and Elizabeth Fee 1996. "Man-Made Medicine and Women's Health." In *Man-Made Medicine*, ed. Kary L. Moss, 17–35. Durham, NC: Duke University Press.
LaCalle, Eduardo and Elaine Rabin 2010. "Frequent Uses of Emergency Departments: The Myths, the Data, and the Policy Implications." *Annals of Emergency Medicine*, 56, no. 1 (July): 42–48.
LaCouture, Brittany. 2014. *Primer: The Disproportionate Share (DSH) Program*. Washington, DC: American Action Forum.

Lantz, Paul M., J.S. House, and J. Chen 1998. "Socioeconomic Factors, Health Behaviors, and Mortality." *Journal of the American Medical Association*, 279, no. 21 (June): 1703–1708.

Leavitt, Rachel A. et al. 2018. "Suicides among American Indian/Alaskan Natives—Violent Death Reporting System, 18 States, 2003-2014." *Morbidity and Mortality Weekly Reports*, 67, no. 8 (March 2): 237–242.

Levine, Robert S. et al. 2012. "Firearms, Youth Homicide, and Public Health." *Journal of Health Care for the Poor and Underserved*, 23, no. 1 (February): 7–19.

Levy, Helen and David Meltzer 2004. "What Do We Really Know About Whether Health Insurance Affects Health?" In *Health Policy and the Uninsured*, ed. Catherine G. McLaughlin, 179–204. Washington, DC: Urban Institute Press.

Li, Yanping et al. 2018. "Impact of Healthy Lifestyle Factors on Life Expectancies in the US Population." *Circulation*, April 30.

Licata, Rachel and Julia Paradise 2012. *Oral Health and Low-Income Nonelderly Adults: A Review of Coverage and Access*. Menlo Park, CA: Kaiser Commission on Medicaid and the Uninsured.

"Lifetime and Annual Limits." n.d. Washington, DC: US Department of Health and Human Services. Online at www.hhs.gov.

Lillie-Blanton, Marsha et al. 2000. "Race, Ethnicity, and the Health Care System: Public Perceptions and Experiences." *Medicare Care Research and Review*, 57, Suppl 1: 218–235.

Lipka, Michael. 2013. *Majority of U.S. Catholics' Opinions Run Counter to Church on Contraception, Homosexuality*. Washington, DC: Pew Research Center..

Liptak, Adam. 2014. "Supreme Court Rejects Contraceptives Mandate for Some Corporations." *The New York Times*, June 30.

Liptak, Adam and Michael D. Shear. 2018. "Trump's Travel Ban Is Upheld by Supreme Court." *The New York Times*, June 26.

Loftis, Leslie. 2017a. "No, America Doesn't Have the Highest Maternal Mortality Rate in the Developed World." *The Federalist*, July 11. Online at www.thefederalist.com.

Loftis, Leslie. 2017b. "U.S. Maternal Mortality Is Rising, but Not for the Reason the Left Claims." *The Federalist*, July 13. Online at www.thefederalist.com.

Long, Sharon K. 2003. "Hardship among the Uninsured: Choosing among Food, Housing and Health Insurance." *New Federalism*, Series B, no. B-54. Washington, DC: Urban Institute.

Lowder, J. Bryan. 2012. "Study Finds that Access to Birth Control Increases Women's Wages, but Do Conservative Women Care?" *Salon*, March 29. Online at www.salon.com.

MacDorman, Marian F. et al. 2016. "Recent Increases in the U.S. Mortality Rate." *Journal of Obstetrics and Gynecology*, 128, no. 3 (September): 447–455.

March of Dimes. 2014. *CHIP Coverage for Pregnant Women*. Washington, DC: March of Dimes.

Marcotte, Amanda. 2012. "Contraception Is an Economic Issue." *USA Today*, September 28.

Martin, Nina et al. 2017. "The Last Person You'd Expect To Die in Childbirth." ProPublica, May 12. Online at ProPublica.org.

Martin, Nina and Robin Fields. 2018. "Here's One Issue Blue and Red States Agree On: Preventing Deaths of Expecting and New Mothers." ProPublica, March 26.

McBride, David. 1993. "Black America: From Community Health Care to Crisis Medicine." *Journal of Health Politics, Policy and Law*, 18, no. 2 (Summer): 319–337.

McGinn, Shapiro. 2008. "Medicaid Coverage of Adult Dental Services." *State Health Policy Monitor*. Washington, DC: National Academy of State Health Policy.

Mead, Holly et al. 2008. *Racial and Ethnic Disparities in U.S. Health Care: A Chartbook*. Washington, DC: Commonwealth Fund.

"Medicaid/CHIP Coverage of Lawfully-Residing Immigrant Children and Pregnant Women" 2018. Menlo Park, CA: Kaiser Family Foundation.

"Medical Assistance Programs for Immigrants in Various States." 2018. Cambridge, MA: National Immigration Law Center, Harvard University.

Mettler, Suzanne. 2011. *The Submerged States: How Invisible Government Policies Undermine American Democracy*. Chicago, IL: University of Chicago Press.

Mishel, Lawrence. 2012. "Unions, Inequality, and Faltering Middle Class Wages." Issue Brief #342. Washington, DC: Economic Policy Institute.

"Missouri Hospital's Sudden Closure Problematic for Expectant Mothers." 2018. *Springfield Neww-Leader*, May 28.

Murphy, Jarrett. 2012. "Fear: The NRA's Real Firepower." *The Nation*, 295, no. 11 (September 10): 11–15.

Nasaw, Daniel. 2009. "House Chastises South Carolina Representative Who Called Obama a Liar." *Guardian*, September 15.

National Center for Health Statistics. 2015. "Health, United States, 2016." Hyattsville, MD: Centers for Disease Control and Prevention, US Department of Health and Human Services.

National Center for Health Statistics. 2017. "Health, United States, 2016." Hyattsville, MD: Centers for Disease Control and Prevention, US Department of Health and Human Services.

National Rural Health Association. 2012. *What's Different About Rural Health Care?* Washington, DC: National Rural Health Association.

"New Government Data Result in a Downward Revision to Recent Health Care Spending Estimates." 2017. Washington, DC: Center for Sustainable Health Care Spending, Altarum Institute.

Newport, Frank. 2012. *Americans, Including Catholics, Say Birth Control Is Morally OK*. Washington, DC: Gallup.

Noonan, Allan S., Hector Eduardo Velesco-Mondragon, and Fernando A. Wagner. 2016. "Improving the Health of African Americans in the USA: An Overdue Opportunity for Social Justice." *Public Health Review*, 37, no. 12 (December): 1–20.

Obama, Barack. 2015. *Presidential Memorandum: Modernizing Federal Leave Policies for Childbirth, Adoption, and Foster Care to Recruit and Retain Talent and Improve Productivity*. Washington, DC: The White House. Online at www.obamawhitehouse.archives.gov.

Okolec, Jeanne E. 2009. "Health Care for the Undocumented: Looking for a Rationale." *Journal of Poverty*, 13, no. 3: 254–265.
Ollove, Michael. 2016. "A Shortage in the Nation's Maternal Health Care." Washington, DC: Pew Charitable Trusts. Online at www.pewtrusts.org.
"Overview of Health Coverage for Individuals with Limited English Proficiency." 2012. Menlo Park, CA: Kaiser Family Foundation.
"Paid Family Leave and Sick Days in the U.S.: Findings from the 2017 Kaiser/HRET Employer Health Benefits Survey." 2017. Menlo Park, CA: Kaiser Family Foundation.
Paquette, Danielle. 2016. "After Planned Parenthood Closures, Poor Women Started Having More Babies." *The Washington Post*, February 5.
Paradise, Julia. 2012. *Children and Oral Health: Assessing Needs, Coverage, and Access*. Menlo Park, CA: Kaiser Commission on Medicaid and the Uninsured.
Passel, Jeffrey S. and D'Vera Cohn. 2017. *Size of U.S. Unauthorized Workforce Stable after the Great Recession*. Menlo Park, CA: Kaiser Family Foundation.
Patel, Kant and Mark E. Rushefsky. 2005. *The Politics of Public Health in the United States*. Armonk, NY: M.E. Sharpe.
Patel, Kant and Mark E. Rushefsky. 2008. *Health Care in America: Separate and Unequal*. Armonk, NY: M.E. Sharpe.
Pearl, Robert. 2015. "Why Health Care Is Different if You're Black, Latino, or Poor." *Forbes*, March 5.
Peipert, Jeffrey F. et al. 2012. "Preventing Unintended Pregnancies by Providing No-Cost Contraception." *Obstetrics and Gynecology*, 120, no. 6 (December): 1291–1297.
People for the American Way. 2012. *How the War on Women Became Mainstream: Turning Back the Clock in Tea Party America*. Washington, DC: People for the American Way.
Pereira, Joseph. 2003. "To Save on Health-Care Costs, Firms Fire Disabled Workers." *The Wall Street Journal*, July 14.
"The Planned Parenthood Witch Hunt." 2016. *The Washington Post*, February 20.
Pollack, Harold and Karl Kronebusch 2004. "Health Insurance and Vulnerable Populations." In *Health Policy and the Uninsured*, ed. Catherine G. McLaughlin, 205–255. Washington, DC: Urban Institute Press.
Probst, Janice et al. 2011. "Higher Risk of Death in Rural Blacks and Whites than Urbanities Is Related to Lower Incomes, Education and Health Coverage." *Health Affairs*, 30, no. 10 (October): 1872–1879.
"Publicly Funded Family Planning Services in the United States." 2016. New York: Guttmacher Institute.
"A Quick Primer on Affordable Care Act Language Service Requirements." n.d. Medford, MA: Language Scientific, Inc. Online at www.languagescientific.com.
Quinn, Mattie. 2017. "States with the Highest and Lowest Uninsured Rates." *Governing*, September 13. Online at governing.com.
Raley, Spencer. 2017. *How Many Illegal Aliens are in the United States*. Washington, DC: Federation for American Immigration Reform.
Ranji, Usha, Caroline Rosenzweig, and Alina Salganicoff. 2018. *Women's Coverage, Access and Affordability: Key Findings from the 2017 Kaiser Women's Health Survey*. Menlo Park, CA: Kaiser Family Foundation.
Ranji, Usha and Alina Salganicoff. 2011. *Women's Health Care Chartbook*. Menlo Park, CA: Kaiser Family Foundation.
Reid, T.R. 2009. *The Healing of America: A Global Quest for Better, Cheaper and Fairer Health*. Farmington Hills, MI: Gale Group.
Robert Wood Johnson Foundation. 2014. *Reducing Disparities in the Quality of Care for Racial and Ethnic Minorities Improves Care*. Princeton, NJ: Robert Wood Johnson Foundation.
"The Role of Medicaid and Medicare in Women's Health." n.d. Menlo Park, CA: Kaiser Family Foundation.
Rosenbaum, Sara et al. 2012. "Case Studies at Denver Health: 'Patient Dumping' in the Emergency Department despite EMTALA, the Law that Banned It." *Health Affairs*, 31, no. 8 (August): 1749–1756.
Rosenbaum, Sara. 2013. "The Enduring Role of the Emergency Medical Treatment and Active Labor Act." *Health Affairs*, 32, no. 12 (December): 2075–2081.
Russell, Lesley. 2010. *Fact Sheet: Health Disparities by Race and Ethnicity*. Washington, DC: Center for American Progress.
Ryan, William F. 1971. *Blaming the Victim*. New York: Pantheon Books.
Salganicoff, Alina et al. 2002. "Women's Health in the United States: Health Coverage and Access to Care." Menlo Park, CA: Kaiser Family Foundation.
Sanchez, Luis. 2018. "Doctors Group Warns of Health Risks for Migrant Children Separated from Parents." *The Hill*, June 16.
Scheiber, Noam and Michael Corkery. 2017. "As Walmart Buys Online Retailers, Their Health Benefits Suffer." *The New York Times*, November 27.
Schneider, Eric C. et al. 2017. *Mirror, Mirror 2017: International Comparison Reflects Flaws and Opportunities for Better U.S. Health Care*. Washington, DC: Commonwealth Fund.
Schneider, Mary-Jane. 2000. *An Introduction to Public Health*. Gaithersburg, MD: Aspen Publishing.
Schoen, Cathy et al. 2011. "Affordable Care Act Reforms Could Reduce the Number of Underinsured U.S. Adults by 70 Percent." *Health Affairs*, 30, no. 9 (September): 1762–1771.
Schumaker, Eric. 2017. "The Quality of Health Care You Receive Likely Depends on Your Skin Color." *Huffington Post*, December 6.
Scotch, Richard K. and Sai Loganathan 2011. "Local Government's Role in Health Care for Undocumented Immigrants: Three Counties in North Texas." *Journal of Public Management & Social Policy*, 17, no. 2 (Fall): 11–24.
Seifert, Robert W. and Mark Rukavina 2006. "Bankruptcy Is the Tip of a Medical-Debt Iceberg." *Health Affairs*, 25 (February 28): W89–W92.
Sherman, Christopher and Ramit Plushnick-Masti. 2012. "Fewer Health Care Options for Illegal Immigrants." *Associated Press*, December 14.

Sifferlin, Alexandra. 2016. "Why U.S. Women Still Die During Childbirth." *Slate*, September 27.

Sink, Justin. 2011. "Wilson: 'You Lie' Has Been Vindicated." *The Hill*, August 17.

Smedley, Brian D. et al. 2008. *Unequal Health Outcomes in the United States: Racial and Ethnic Disparities in Health Care Treatment and Access, the Role of Social and Environmental Determinants of Health, and the Responsibility of the State.* New York: Opportunity Agenda.

"Snapshot of U.S. Immigration 2017." Denver, CO: National Conference of State Legislatures.

Sobel, Laura, Alina Salganicoff, and Caroline Rosenzweig. 2017. *The Future of Contraceptive Coverage.* Menlo Park, CA: Kaiser Family Foundation.

Soffen, Kim. 2017. "These are the Steps the Trump Administration Is Taking to Undermine the ACA." *The Washington Post*, October 2017.

Sollenberger, Donna. 2018. "Delay DSH Cuts and Find a Sustainable Fix for Uncompensated Care." *The Hill*, January 12. Online at thehill.com.

"Spotlight on Women of Color." n.d. Washington, DC: Institute for Women's Policy Research. Online at www.statusofwomen.org.

Starr, Paul. 1982. *The Social Transformation of American Medicine.* New York: Basic Books.

"State Health Facts." 2016. Menlo Park, NJ: Kaiser Family Foundation. Online at www.kff.org.

"Status of State Medicaid Expansion Decisions." 2018. Menlo Park, NJ: Kaiser Family Foundation. Online at www.kff.org/health-reform/slide/current-status-of-the-medicaid-expansion-decision/.

Stimpson, Jim P., Fernando A. Wilson, and Dejun Su. 2013. "Unauthorized Immigrants Spend Less than Other Immigrants and US Natives on Health Care." *Health Affairs*, 32, no. 7 (July): 1313–1318.

Stoddard, Jeffrey J., Robert F. St. Peter, and Paul W. Newacheck 1994. "Health Insurance Status and Ambulatory Care for Children." *New England Journal of Medicine*, 330, no. 20 (May 19): 1421–1425.

Stone, Deborah A. 1993. "The Struggle for the Soul of Health Insurance." *Journal of Health Politics, Policy and Law*, 18, no. 2 (Summer): 287–317.

Sun, Adriana Belmonte. 2018. "Obamacare Was Revolution for Women's Health. The Progress Is Now in Danger." *Yahoo Finance*, December 30. Online at www.yahoo.com\finance.

Tabuchi, Hiroko. 2014. "Walmart to End Health Coverage for 30,000 Part-Time Workers." *The New York Times*, October 7.

Thomas, Lillian. 2014. "Hospitals, Doctors Out of Poor City Neighborhoods to More Affluent Areas." *Milwaukee Journal Sentinel*, June 14.

Torres, Rosamar. 2016. "Access Barriers to Prenatal Care in Emerging Adult Latinas." *Hispanic Health Care International*, 14, no. 1 (March): 10–16.

US Census Bureau. 2017. *Historical Health Insurance Tables.* Washington, DC: US Department of Commerce.

US Department of Health and Human Services. 2000. *Oral Health in America: A Report of the Surgeon General.* Rockville, MD: US Department of Health and Human Services, National Institute of Dental and Craniofacial Research, and National Institutes of Health.

US Department of Health and Human Services. 2012. "Social Determinants of Health." *Healthy People 2020.* Washington, DC: US Department of Health and Human Services.

US Department of Labor. 2015. "The Cost of Doing Nothing: The Price We All Pay without Paid Leave Policies to Support America's 21st Century Working Families." Washington, DC: US Department of Labor.

"U.S. Unintended Pregnancy Rate Falls to 30-Year Low." 2016. New York: Guttmacher Institute.

"Unauthorized Immigrants: How Pew Research Center Counts Them and What We Know about Them." 2013. Washington, DC: Pew Research Center.

"The Uninsured: A Primer." 2011. Menlo Park, CA: Kaiser Family Foundation.

United Health Foundation. 2017. *America's Health Rankings: A Call to Action for Individuals and Their Communities.* Minnetonka, MN: United Healthcare Foundation.

Vance, J.D. 2016. *Hillbilly Elegy: A Memoir of Family and Culture in Crisis.* New York: Harper.

Vasel, Kathryn. 2018. "Calls for Paid Family Leave are Getting Louder." February 13. Online at www.money.cnn.com.

Vieth, Warren. 2004. "Bush Makes His Pitch for 'Ownership Society'." *Los Angeles Times*, September 5.

Walker, Andrea K. 2011. "Where You Live Can Help Determine Your Health, Studies Say." *Baltimore Sun*, November 18.

Watson, Sidney Dean. 1994. "Minority Access and Health Reform: A Civil Right to Health Care." *Journal of Law, Medicine and Ethics*, 22, no. 2 (Summer): 127–137.

Weber, Lauren and Andy Miller. 2017. "A Hospital Crisis Is Killing Rural Communities. This State Is Ground Zero." *Huffington Post*, September 27.

Wegman, Holly and Cinnamon Stetler. 2009. "A Meta-Analytic Review of the Effects of Childhood Abuse on Medical Outcomes in Adulthood." *Psychosomatic Medicine*, 71, no. 8 (October): 805–812.

Weinstein, James N. et al., eds. 2017. *Communities in Action: Pathways to Health Equity.* Washington, DC: National Academies Press.

"What Did Pope Francis Actually Say about Contraception?" 2016. *Catholic News Agency.*

White House. 2015. *Fact Sheet: Helping Middle-Class Families Get Ahead by Expanding Paid Sick Leave.* Washington, DC: White House.

White, Joseph. 1995. *Competing Solutions: American Health Care Proposals and International Experience.* Washington, DC: Brookings Institution.

"Women's Health Insurance Coverage." 2017. Menlo Park, CA: Kaiser Family Foundation.

Wood, Daniel B. 2009. "In Hard Times, Illegal Immigrants Lose Healthcare." *Christian Science Monitor*, March 24.

Woolf, Steve H. and Laudan Aron, eds. 2013. *U.S. Health in International Perspective: Shorter Lives, Poorer Health.* Washington, DC: National Academy Press.

Woolf, Steven H. and Paula Braveman 2011. "Where Health Disparities Begin: The Role of Social and Economic Determinants—And Why Current Policies May Make Matters Worse." *Health Affairs*, 30, no. 10 (October): 1852–1859.

Yee, Vivian, Kenan Davis, and Jugal K. Patel. 2017. "Here's the Reality about Illegal Immigrants in the United States." *The New York Times*, March 6.

Zarembo, Alan and Anna Gorman. 2008. "Dialysis Dilemma: Who Gets Free Care?" *Los Angeles Times*, October 29.

Zellers, Wendy K., Catherine G. McLaughlin, and Kevin D. Frick 1992. "Small-Business Health Insurance: Only Healthy Need Apply." *Health Affairs*, 11, no. 1 (Spring): 174–175.

Zubrzycki, Jaclyn. 2012. "Detroit Studies Illuminate Problem of Lead Exposure." *Education Week*, 32, no. 4 (September 26): 6.

8

THE PROBLEM OF RISING HEALTHCARE COSTS AND SPENDING

The 1960s saw a dramatic expansion in social programs. Civil rights, women's rights, educational opportunities, and improved housing and healthcare for citizens were the battle cries of a social revolution as the federal government attempted to enlarge individual opportunities. In the health field, providing access to decent healthcare became the primary goal of the federal government. The role of the government—that is, the public sector—in healthcare expanded considerably as it created public health insurance programs as a social safety net to provide coverage to those who, for one reason or another, lacked health insurance in the private sector.

In 1965, the federal government established Medicare and Medicaid to provide increased access to healthcare for the elderly and the poor. These programs were very successful in increasing healthcare access for large numbers of people (Davis and Schoen 1978). The creation and implementation of such programs was made possible by a healthy economy, a Democratic president (Lyndon Johnson) dedicated to social issues, and large Democratic majorities in the House and the Senate. Additionally, the Comprehensive Health Planning Act and Public Health Services Amendments of 1966 (PL 89–749) established the goal of providing the highest level of healthcare attainable to every person. Between 1985 and 1990, via congressional mandates, health coverage was expanded significantly in the Medicaid program, especially for women and children. Following the failure of healthcare reform during the Clinton administration in 1993–1994, Congress passed several incremental reforms to further increase access to healthcare. The Health Insurance Portability and Accountability Act (HIPAA) placed some limits on insurance companies' authority to deny coverage or to impose preexisting-condition exclusions and guaranteed portability of insurance coverage. In 1997, Congress created the State Children's Health Insurance Program (SCHIP), now called the Children's Health Insurance Program (CHIP), to extend health insurance coverage to uninsured children. The Medicare Modernization Act (MMA), created in 2003 and implemented in 2006, added prescription drug benefits for Medicare recipients. In 2010, Congress passed, and President Obama signed into law, the Affordable Care Act (ACA).

With the establishment of public health insurance programs, total national healthcare expenditures increased dramatically beginning in the 1960s and have become a major area of concern for policymakers. In this chapter we examine the problem of healthcare costs, factors that have contributed to their escalation, and attempts to restrain costs.

RISING HEALTHCARE COSTS/EXPENDITURES

Healthcare expenditures in the United States have been rising faster than the general growth rate of the economy (see Tables 8.1 and 8.2). Table 8.1 provides data on national healthcare expenditures from 1960 to 2016.

Several observations about healthcare expenditures can be made from the data in Table 8.1. National healthcare expenditures have increased dramatically, from $27.3 billion in 1960 to $3.3 trillion in 2016.

The significant increase in national healthcare expenditures from $41.9 billion in 1965 to $133.5 billion in 1975 can be explained by the establishment of Medicare and Medicaid in 1965, which provided health insurance coverage to millions of elderly and poor people. By 1970 Medicare and Medicaid accounted for 17.4 percent of the total national healthcare expenditures. By 1975, they accounted for 22.4 percent of national healthcare expenditures. By 2016, Medicare and Medicaid accounted for 37 percent of national healthcare expenditures. In fact, Medicare expenditures as a percent of national healthcare costs nearly doubled from 10.3 percent in 1970 to 20.1 percent in 2016. Similarly, Medicaid expenditures as a percent of the national total more than doubled from 7.1 percent in 1970 to 16.9 percent in 2016.

Compared to private insurance, both Medicare and Medicaid have a higher percentage of expenditures dedicated to chronic health conditions. Medicaid also has a higher percentage than private insurance in spending for dedicated health services related to pregnancy and birth (Conway et al. 2011). This is not surprising, considering

Table 8.1

Selected National Healthcare Expenditures by Sources of Funds and Types of Services, 1960–2016 (in $ billions)

	1960	1965	1970	1975	1980	1985	1990	1995	2000	2005	2010	2016
Total National Health Expenditures (NHE)	27.4	41.9	74.9	133.6	255.8	444.6	724.3	1,027.5	1,377.2	2,029.1	2,598.8	3,337.2
Sources of Funds												
Out-of-pocket	13.1	18.3	25.0	37	58.4	96.0	138.7	146.4	201.8	263.4	299.7	352.5
% of total NHE	47.7	43.5	33.4	28	22.8	21.6	19.1%	14.2%	14.7%	13%	11.5%	10.6%
Medicare	0	0	7.7	16.3	37.4	71.8	110.2	184.4	224.3	338.8	519.8	672.1
% of total NHE	0	0	10.3	12.2	14.6	16.2	15.2%	17.9%	16.3%	16.7%	20.0%	20.1%
Medicaid (Title XIX)	0	0	5,289.7	1,345.6	26,032.5	40,937.4	73,660.8	1,44,862.2	2,00,482.8	3,09,538.5	397.2	565.5
% of total NHE	0	0	7.1	10.1	10.2	9.2	10.2%	14.1%	14.6%	15.3%	15.3%	16.9%
CHIP (Title XIX ad Title XXI)	0	0	0	0	0	0	0	0	3.0	7.6	5.9	3.9
% of total NHE									0.2%	0.4%	0.2%	0.1%
Veterans Health Administration	0.9	1.3	1.8	3.7	6.5	10	12.1	16.4	19.5	28.8	45.7	65.2
% of total NHE	3.28	3.10	2.40	2.77	2.54	2.14	1.67%	1.60%	1.42%	1.42%	1.76%	1.95%
Indian Health Service	0.060	0.071	0.120	0.283	0.637	0.872	1.2	2.0	2.4	3.1	4.4	4.1
% of total NHE	0.22	0.17	0.16	0.21	0.25	0.20	0.17%	0.19%	0.17%	0.15%	0.17%	0.12%
Types of Services												
Hospital	8.9	13.5	27.2	51.2	100.5	164.6	250	339.3	415.5	609.4	822.3	1,082.5
% of total NHE	32.8	32.3	36.3	38.4	39.3	37.0	34.6%	33.0%	30.2%	30.0%	31.6%	32.4%
Physician and clinical	5.6	8.6	14.3	25.3	47.7	91	158.9	222.3	290.9	416.9	512.6	664.9
% of total NHE	20.6	20.5	19.1	18.9	18.7	20.4	21.9%	21.6%	21.1%	20.5%	19.7%	19.9%
Prescription drug	3	4	6	8	12	21.8	40.3	59.8	120.9	204.8	253.1	328.6

% of total NHE	9.8	8.9	7.3	6.0	4.7	4.9	5.6%	5.8%	8.8%	10.1%	9.7%	9.8%
Nursing care facilities and CCRC	0.8	1.4	4.0	8.0	15.3	26.3	44.9	64.5	85.1	112.5	143.1	162.7
% of total NHE	3.0	3.4	5.4	6.0	6.0	5.9	6.2%	6.3%	6.2%	5.5%	5.5%	4.9%
Dental services	1.9	2.8	5	8	13.4	21.8	31.7	44.8	62.3	87.0	105.9	124.4
% of total NHE	7.3	6.7	6.3	0	5.2	4.9	4.4%	4.4%	4.5%	4.3%	4.1%	3.7%
Home healthcare	0.6	0.9	0.2	0.6	2.4	5.7	12.6	32.4	32.5	48.7	71.6	92.4
% of total NHE	0.2	0.2	0.3	0.5	0.9	1.3	1.7%	3.1%	2.4%	2.4%	2.8%	2.8%

CCRC = Continuing-care retirement facilities
Sources: National Center for Health Statistics, Centers for Medicare & Medicaid Services. 2016. Baltimore, MD. Online at cms.gov; Office of Management and Budget (2018).

that most of the expansion of the Medicaid program over the years has been designed to provide coverage to poor women who are pregnant or have children.

Both Medicare and Medicaid expenditures are likely to continue to rise for a number of reasons. Medicaid's increase will be the result of its extended eligibility, under the Affordable Care Act (ACA), for health insurance coverage by as many as an additional 15 million individuals (see Chapters 3 and 4). The ultimate number may depend on how many states opt out of Medicaid expansion under the ACA (currently 17 states have opted out) and the future of the Affordable Care Act (see Chapters 3 and 4). However, compared to Medicare, Medicaid has more expenditure restrictions because of very low reimbursement payments to providers, as well as paying for fewer services (Moon 2005). Compared to private insurance, Medicare was more successful in holding the line on growth in healthcare costs during the 1980s and 1990s (Moon 2005). But Medicare expenditures are likely to continue to rise for three reasons. First, since Medicare recipients are elderly and/or disabled, they suffer not only from more health problems but also more serious ones. Many recipients have multiple chronic conditions requiring continual medical care. Second, the number of people eligible for Medicare is expected to increase significantly as more individuals from the Baby Boomer generation reach retirement age over the next decade. Third, because of better medical care, people are also living longer. It is estimated that healthcare for the elderly alone could consume 10 percent of the nation's gross domestic product (GDP) by 2020.

The public sector's role in providing health coverage to individuals has expanded considerably since the 1960s. In 1970, public-sector health programs constituted about 19.7 percent of the national health expenditures. In 2016, public-sector health programs—Medicare, Medicaid, the Children's Health Insurance Program, the veterans' health program, and the health program for American Indians/Alaska Natives (AIs/ANs)—accounted for about 39.12 percent of the national healthcare expenditures, with Medicare and Medicaid responsible for 37 percent.

This actually understates the federal role in healthcare. The federal government uses the tax system to subsidize the purchase of healthcare. For example, employer contributions to health insurance premiums for their employees are considered a tax deduction, dating back to World War II (Starr 2013). Employee contributions to health insurance premiums may also be deducted. Under the Affordable Care Act, subsidies for people to purchase insurance plans on state and federal exchanges (see Chapter 3) are another example. Health savings accounts, where people deposit money to help pay for medical expenses, are a fourth example. In 2015, these tax expenditures totaled nearly $250 billion (Tax Policy Center n.d.; see also Joint Committee on Taxation 2018). Unlike public programs such as Medicare and Medicaid, tax expenditures (of all kinds, not just healthcare-related) are difficult for the public to see; using Suzanne Mettler's (2011) language, they are part of the "submerged state."

Table 8.2 provides annual data about the sources of funds and expenditures by types of services from 2007 to 2016. It provides some insight about recent trends in healthcare expenditures. Out-of-pocket expenditures as a percentage of total national health expenditures have dropped every year down to 10.6 percent in 2016. To understand how low this number has become, in 1960, out-of-pocket expenses were 47.7 percent of total national health expenditures (see Table 8.1). This vast decrease indicates the importance of public programs as well as private insurance. Tables 8.1 and 8.2 show the growing importance of Medicare and Medicaid. Expenditures for the CHIP, veterans, and American Indians/Alaska Natives continue to be a very small percentage of national health expenditures.

Expenditures by Type of Health Service

Table 8.1 also provides data on healthcare expenditures by type of service. Again, several observations are warranted. Slightly over half of the total national healthcare expenditures in 1960 occurred in two service areas—hospital and physician/clinical services. Together these services accounted for the majority of healthcare spending—53.4 percent, with 32.8 percent for hospital services and 20.6 percent for physician/clinical services. The overall expenditure patterns for these two services have pretty much remained the same over the years. Hospital services have consistently remained the top expenditure category, followed by physician/clinical services. Their relative percentages have fluctuated a little over the years, and the growth in these two areas has slowed slightly from the high of the 1980s, but their rates of increase have generally outstripped the rate of inflation (Siegel, Mead, and Burke 2008). Expenditures for inpatient hospital services have increased despite the increase in outpatient care. Medicare paid about 28 percent of the cost of hospital inpatient services; Medicaid paid 17.5 percent of hospital services; and private insurance paid 39.4 percent of such services (authors' calculations from National Center for

Table 8.2

Selected National Healthcare Expenditures by Sources of Funds and Types of Services, 2007–2016 (in $ billions)

	2007	2008	2009	2010	2011	2012	2013	2014	2015	2016
Total National Health Expenditures (NHE)	2,295.3	2,399.1	2,496.4	2,598.8	2,689.3	2,797.3	2,879.0	3,026.2	3,200.8	3,337.2
Sources of Funds										
Out-of-pocket	290.0	295.2	293.7	299.7	310.0	318.3	325.2	330.1	339.3	352.5
% of total NHE	12.6	12.3	11.8	11.5	11.5	11.4	11.3%	10.9%	10.6%	10.6%
Medicare	432.8	467.0	498.9	519.8	544.7	569.6	590.2	618.9	648.8	672.1
% of total NHE	18.9	19.5	20.0	20.0	20.3	20.4	20.5%	20.5%	20.3%	20.1%
Medicaid (Title XIX)	325.7	344.2	37.4	397.2	406.7	422.7	445.4	496.7	544.1	565.5
% of total NHE	14.2	14.3	1.5	15.3	15.1	15.1	15.5%	16.4%	17.0%	16.9%
CHIP (Title XIX ad Title XXI)	6.0	6.9	7.6	7.9	8.6	9.1	9.5	9.3	9.2	14.3
% of total NHE	0.26	0.29	0.30	0.30	0.32	0.33	0.33%	0.31%	0.29%	0.43%
Veterans Health Administration	32.3	37.0	41.9	45.7	50.1	50.6	52.5	56.2	61.9	65.2
% of total NHE	1.41	1.54	1.68	1.76	1.86	1.81	1.82%	1.86%	1.93%	1.95%
Indian Health Service	3.3	3.3	3.6	4.4	4.2	4.5	4.3	4.5	4.6	4.1
% of total NHE	0.14	0.14	0.14	0.17	0.16	0.16	0.15%	0.15%	0.14%	0.12%
Types of Services										
Hospital	691.9	725.6	779.6	822.3	851.9	902.5	937.6	978.1	1,033.4	1,082.5
% of total NHE	30.1	30.2	31.2	31.6	31.7	32.3	32.6%	32.3%	32.3%	32.4%
Physician and clinical	457.5	481.9	497.7	512.6	535.9	557.1	569.6	596.7	631.0	664.9
% of total NHE	19.9	20.1	19.9	19.7	19.9	19.9	19.8%	19.7%	19.7%	19.9%
Prescription drug	235.7	241.5	252.7	253.1	258.8	259.2	265.2	298.0	324.5	328.6
% of total NHE	10.3	10.1	10.1	9.7	9.6	9.3	9.2%	9.8%	10.1%	9.8%
Nursing care facilities and CCRC	124.9	130.5	135.2	140.5	145.4	147.4	149.0	152.4	158.1	162.7
% of total NHE	5.4	5.4	5.4	5.4	5.4	5.3	5.2%	5.0%	4.9%	4.9%
Dental services	97.7	102.7	103.1	105.9	108.0	109.7	111.1	113.8	118.9	124.4
% of total NHE	4.3	4.3	4.1	4.1	4.0	3.9	3.9%	3.8%	3.7%	3.7%
Home healthcare	57.5	62.3	67.7	71.6	74.6	78.1	80.5	84.0	88.8	92.4
% of total NHE	2.5	2.6	2.7	2.8	2.8	2.8	2.8%	2.8%	2.8%	2.8%

CCRC = Continuing-care retirement facilities

Sources: National Center for Health Statistics, Centers for Medicare & Medicaid Services. 2016. Baltimore, MD. Online at cms.gov. Office of Management and Budget (2018).

Health Statistics 2016). The higher expenditures for physician services are generally attributed to greater administrative costs (see, for example, Frakt 2018), higher physician income, more facilities/amenities, and low-capacity utilization of physicians and equipment for specialized diagnostic and therapeutic procedures (Fuchs 1986). Ironically, the Association of American Medical Colleges (AAMC) has been predicting a shortage of physicians over the upcoming decades due to demographic changes, leading to a dramatic increase in demand for and reduction in physician supply through retirement. The AAMC has called for a 30-percent increase in US medical school enrollment, an expansion of graduate medical education (GME) positions to accommodate increased enrollment, and more federal funding for GME (Latham 2005). However, the real problem is the geographic maldistribution of physicians in the country. In fact, the increased supply of physicians may exacerbate the problem because research shows that physician supply follows an "inverse care law," that is, supply of physicians being lowest in highest-need areas, because most newly trained physicians end up practicing in areas that already have the most physicians (Latham 2005). Also, a higher supply of physicians could also lead to increased spending on healthcare. While it is true that regions with proportionately more general practitioners seem to enjoy lower healthcare costs, it does not necessarily follow that a bigger physician supply will reduce healthcare costs further or even slow the rate of growth. The reason is that primary care could be provided more economically by foreign medical school graduates, nurses, physician assistants, and other allied health professionals (Latham 2005).

Expenditures for prescription drugs have been the third-largest category of national healthcares expenditure over the years. The percent of national healthcare expenditures on prescription drugs has varied from a low of 4.7 percent in 1980 to a high of 10 percent in 2010. Since 1990, expenditures on prescription drugs have increased by over 700 percent (see Table 8.1) and likely will continue to grow due to the aging of the population. The fastest increase in healthcare expenditures in 2006 was an 8.5-percent increase in prescription drug expenditures, because of the addition of the new Medicare Part D benefits, which added prescription drug coverage to 25 million Medicare beneficiaries (Siegel, Mead, and Burke 2008) (see Chapter 5).

In 2016, spending on hospital and physician/clinical services and prescription drugs accounted for 62.2 percent of overall national healthcare expenditures. Another 11.4 percent of spending was for nursing home, dental, and home healthcare services. The remainder consisted of administrative costs, durable and nondurable medical products and devices, public health services, research, and other professional services.

Table 8.2 provides data about the sources of funds and expenditures by types of services from 2007 to 2016. During this time period, expenditures for hospital services, physicians/clinical services, and prescription drugs as a percent of total national health expenditures has remained relative stable at around 30, 20, and 10 percent respectively. Between 2007 and 2016, expenditures for nursing and continuing-care facilities and dental services slightly decreased as a percentage of total national health expenditures, while expenditures for home healthcare have increased slightly as a percent of total national health expenditures. This is not too surprising given the emphasis on a policy of deinstitutionalization with respect to long-term care.

Growth in Public-Sector Expenditures and Decline in Out-of-Pocket Expenditures

Expansion of third-party payers as a result of an increase in government and other private health insurance programs has resulted in a dramatic reduction in out-of-pocket payments by consumers. In 1960, prior to the introduction of Medicare and Medicaid, 47.7 percent of all personal healthcare spending was paid out-of-pocket by the patient. In 2016, that percentage had dropped to only 10.6 percent (see Tables 8.1 and 8.2). The introduction of Medicare and Medicaid in 1965, combined with expansion of private health insurance coverage, led to a dramatic decline, relatively, in out-of-pocket expenditures by the patient as a percentage of total national healthcare expenditures (Baicker and Goldman 2011). In terms of actual dollars, there was a significant increase. From 2000 to 2016, out-of-pocket healthcare expenditures increased by nearly 75 percent (authors' calculations from Table 8.1).

Healthcare Expenditures and GDP

Tables 8.3 and 8.4 provide additional data on the growth of national health expenditures, per-capita expenditures, US population, GDP, and national health expenditures as a percentage of GDP. Table 8.3 provides data for five-year intervals from 1960 to 2016, while Table 8.4 provides annual figures from 2001 to 2016.

Total national healthcare expenditures have increased steadily over the last 50 years in the United States. The rate of growth in national healthcare expenditures has been much higher than the growth in GDP over the same time period, and it has been dramatically higher than growth in the US population. Between 1960 and 2016,

Table 8.3

National Healthcare Expenditures and the Economy, 1960–2016

	1960	1965	1970	1975	1980	1985	1990	1995	2000	2005	2016
National healthcare expenditures in $ billions	27	42	75	134	256	445	724	1,027	1,377	2,029	3,337
% change from previous year listed		55.6	78.6	78.7%	91.0%	73.8%	62.7%	41.9%	34.1%	47.3%	64.5%
National healthcare expenditures per capita	$146	$210	$356	$607	$1,110	$1,840	$2,843	$3,825	$4,855	$6,854	$10,348
% change from previous year listed		43.8	69.5	70.5%	82.9%	65.8%	54.5%	34.5%	26.9%	41.2%	51.0%
US population (in millions)	187	200	210	219	230	241	253	266	282	295	324
% change from previous year listed		7.0	5.0	4.3%	5.0%	4.8%	5.0%	5.1%	6.0%	4.6%	9.8%
GDP in $ billions	543	744	1,076	1,698	2,863	4,347	5,980	7,664	10,285	13,094	18,624
% change from previous year listed		37.0	44.6	57.8%	68.6%	51.8%	37.6%	28.2%	34.2%	27.3%	42.2%
National healthcare expenditures as % share of GDP	5.0	5.6	7.0	7.9%	8.9%	10.2%	12.1%	13.4%	13.4%	15.5%	17.9%
Consumer Price Index	29.6	31.5	38.8	53.8	82.4	107.7	130.7	152.4	172.2	195.3	240.0
% change from previous year listed		6.4	23.2	38.7%	53.2%	30.7%	21.4%	16.6%	13.0%	13.4%	22.9%

Sources: worldometers.info/world-population/us-population\ World Bank ND GDP United States data.worldbank.org Federal Reserve Bank of Minneapolis, Consumer Price index, 1913-base year is changed 1982-1984=100 minneapolisfed.org

growth in the US population ranged from a high of 9.8 percent to a low of 4.5. Similarly, GDP growth has ranged from a high of 68.9 percent to a low of 27.3 percent during the five-year intervals. During the same time frame, the growth in national healthcare expenditures has ranged from a high of 91 percent to a low of 34.1 percent. It should be noted from Table 8.3 (and Table 8.4) that during virtually the entire time period, growth in healthcare expenditures exceeded growth in the economy (GDP). Per-capita expenditures on healthcare increased from $146 in 1960 to $10,348 in 2016.

In 1960, national healthcare expenditures accounted for 5 percent of the GDP, but by 2016 it had increased to 17.9 percent. The United States spends more money on healthcare overall and per capita than any other country in the world. Similarly, no other country even comes close to the United States in spending 17.9 percent of its GDP on healthcare. Yet, many of these countries rank higher on several indicators of health status and/or outcomes than does the United States (see below).

The calculation of healthcare expenditures is a function of prices multiplied by the quantity or volume of consumption of healthcare services. Rising growth in healthcare expenditures relative to GDP can be explained by two factors. Either prices are rising faster in the healthcare sector than in any other sector of the economy, and/or the volume of healthcare produced (quantity/volume of consumption) is rising more rapidly than output in other sectors of the economy (McGuire and Serra 2005). In the United States, both of these factors—higher prices and increased consumption—have contributed to increased healthcare expenditures.

As the data in Table 8.4 show, there is some good news with respect to rising healthcare expenditures. They have been growing at a slower rate since 2001, from 9.6 percent in 2001 to a low of 2.9 percent in 2013 (Hartman et al 2018). These drops in annual growth rate of national healthcare expenditures and per-capita expenditures coincide with a drop in the GDP growth rate. The national healthcare expenditure growth rate exceeded the inflation rate for most of these years. The growth rate started to increase in 2014, likely because of the implementation of the Affordable Care Act. One of the aims of the ACA was to increase insurance coverage of the population. If more people have insurance, more people will seek care, and more money will be spent. Table 8.4 shows similar trends with national healthcare expenditures per capita.

However, it is important to keep in mind that lower increases in spending on healthcare in recent years (short-term trends) cannot say anything about long-term trends. Often economic downturn and recession tends to depress health spending for several years. Thus, it is reasonable to assume that the recession of 2007–2009 contributed to the recent decline in healthcare spending growth rates (Kamal and Sawyer 2018).

Another way of looking at healthcare expenditures is to consider projections. Cuckler et al. (2018) present projections for 2017–2026. The reasonable assumption of the projections is that current law and policy will stay in place. Given that, they project (and we should compare these numbers to 2016 figures presented in Table 8.4) that total national healthcare expenditures in 2026 will be $5.7 trillion dollars and the per-capita amount will be $16,167.60. National healthcare expenditures as a percentage of gross domestic product will be 19.7 percent. This certainly suggests that something should be done about continued increases in healthcare spending.

Concentration of Expenditures

When discussing national healthcare expenditures, it is important to note that they are concentrated heavily among certain segments of the population. Looking at 2014 data, 1 percent of the US population accounted for 22.5 percent of healthcare spending; the top 5 percent accounted for just over 50 percent of healthcare spending. The bottom 50 percent accounted for only 2.8 percent of total healthcare spending (Mitchell 2014; Cohen 2016). This holds true for overall spending as well as spending in the Medicaid and Medicare programs. In the case of Medicare, 10 percent of beneficiaries account for 42 percent of Medicare spending (2015 data) (Cubanski et al 2015). Looking at 2009 data, 5 percent of Medicaid recipients account for 42 percent of Medicaid spending ("Medicaid, a Primer" 2013).

Having said this, and the phenomenon is well-documented, a few things should be kept in mind. First, there is some turnover or churning in the top 5 percent (Johnson et al. 2018). In 2015, only 39 percent of those who were in the top 5 five percent were in the top 5 percent the previous year. About 15 percent of those new to the top 5 percent had very little if any healthcare expenditures in the previous year. For example, somebody in good health might need an emergency appendectomy. That might cost around $20,000 and put that person in the top 5 percent. The next year that person would likely not be in the top 5 percent, or what *The Atlantic* magazine refers to as "Platinum Patients" (McGill 2017). Second, Miller (2017–2018; see also Cohen 2016) makes the case that the concentration of healthcare spending has decreased over the years. Much of this is due to the increased use of pharmaceuticals to treat medical conditions. A related point is that a sizable portion of the low spenders are

Table 8.4

National Healthcare Expenditures, 2001–2016 (in $ billions)

	2001	2002	2003	2004	2005	2006	2007	2008	2009	2010	2011	2012	2013	2014	2015	2016
National healthcare expenditures (in $ billions)	1,486.2	1,628.6	1,767.6	1,895.7	2,023.7	2,156.2	2,295.3	$2,399.1	$2,495.4	$2,598.8	$2,689.3	$2,797.3	$2,879.0	$3,026.2	$3,200.8	$3,337.2
% change from previous year		9.6	8.5	7.2	6.8%	6.5%	6.5%	4.5%	4.0%	4.1%	3.5%	4.0%	2.9%	5.1%	5.8%	4.3%
National healthcare expenditures per capita	$5,218	$5,666	$6,096	$6,479	$6,854	$7,232	$7,627	$7,897	$8,143	$8,412	$8,644	$8,924	$9,121	$9,515	$9,994	$10,348
% change from previous year		8.6	7.6	6.3	5.8%	5.5%	5.5%	3.5%	3.1%	3.3%	2.8%	3.2%	2.2%	4.3%	5.0%	3.5%
Gross domestic product (in $ billions)	10,621.8	10,977.5	11,510.7	12,274.9	13,093.7	13,855.9	14,477.6	14,718.6	14,418.7	14,964.4	15,517.9	16,155.3	16,691.5	$17,427.6	$18,120.7	$18,624.5
% change from previous year		3.3	4.9	6.6	6.7	5.8	4.5	1.7	-2.0	3.8	3.7	4.1	3.3	4.4	4.0	2.8
National health expenditures as % share of GDP	14.0	14.8	15.4	15.4	15.5%	15.6%	15.9%	16.3%	17.3%	17.4%	17.3%	17.3%	17.2%	17.4%	17.7%	17.9%
Inflation rate (change in CPI, %)	2.8	1.6	2.3	2.7	3.4%	3.2%	2.9%	3.8%	-0.4%	1.6%	3.2%	2.1%	1.5%	1.6%	0.1%	1.3%

Federal Reserve Bank of Minneapolis, Consumer Price index, 1913-base year is changed 1982-1984=100 minneapolisfed.org
Sources: National Center for Health Statistics, Centers for Medicare & Medicaid Services. Baltimore, MD 2016. Online at cms.gov.

people who are uninsured. Only 2.1 percent of those in the top 5 percent, or Platinum Patients, are uninsured (McGill 2017). Those who are uninsured tend to make less use of the healthcare system because of the cost factor.

One aspect of the concentration of healthcare expenditures is age. Those 65 and older (using 2014 data) comprised 15.1 percent of the population but accounted for 33.6 percent of healthcare expenditures (Mitchell 2014). McGill (2017) notes that 42.3 percent of platinum patients are over 65 years of age. Children (ages 0–17) comprised 23.2 percent of the population and accounted for only 10.6 percent of healthcare expenditures (Mitchell 2014). Declining health after the age of 65 results in significant increases in the use of prescription drugs, hospital admissions, repair and replacement of body parts, and rehabilitative and physical therapy ("Technology and Longer Lives Leading to Higher Health Bills" 1998). In addition, costs at the end of life disproportionately contribute to healthcare expenditures in the United States (Greer and Danis 2011). Two factors—an aging population and healthcare technology—are likely to continue to drive healthcare expenditures higher (McGuire and Serra 2005). As the elderly develop more health problems, their use of healthcare services increases. The elderly's higher use of services is also related not just to the number of treatments but also to the type and complexity of healthcare services, that is, intense use of new medical technologies that drive healthcare costs upward (Moon 2005).

Similar to the concentration of health expenditures among the population, there is a concentration of health expenditures among medical conditions. Looking at 2012 data, the costliest medical conditions were heart disease, trauma-related disorders, cancer, mental disorders, and COPD/asthma (Cohen 2014). Spending on these five conditions totaled $276 billion, nearly 10 percent of total spending (authors' calculations from Cohen 2014 and Table 8.2). A large proportion of the Platinum Patients, 63.2 percent, have one or more chronic conditions of the type mentioned above (McGill 2017).

The top ten causes of death in the United States accounted for 75 percent of the nearly 2.5 million deaths in 2010. In 2007, overall costs of the ten leading causes of death were over $1.1 trillion ("$1.1 Trillion: What the Top 10 Leading Causes of Death Cost the U.S. Economy" 2012). In order of importance, the top ten causes of death were cardiovascular disease, cancer, chronic lung disease, stroke, accidental death, Alzheimer's disease, diabetes mellitus, renal disease, flu and pneumonia, and suicide ("$1.1 Trillion: What the Top 10 Leading Causes of Death Cost the U.S. Economy" 2012).

While data about the cost of the 2010 leading causes of death have not been updated by the Centers for Disease Control and Prevention at present, *24/7 Wall St* reviewed the leading causes of death to determine how much each of them cost the US economy. It is important to note that the figures provided are for costs to the US economy and not necessarily just health-related costs. Thus, these figures also include indirect costs associated with diseases, such as lost wages, productivity, and the like. The breakdown is as follows: heart disease—$190 billion; cancer—$227 billion; chronic lung disease—$65 billion; stroke—$34 billion; accidental death—$308 billion; Alzheimer's—$70 billion; diabetes mellitus—$112 billion; renal disease—$61 billion; pneumonia and flu—$40 billion; and suicide—$36 billion. The total cost to the US economy in 2010 was estimated to be slightly over $1 trillion dollars ("$1.1 Trillion: What the Top 10 Leading Causes of Death Cost the U.S. Economy" 2012).

Chronic Health Conditions

A study by the Rand Corporation (Buttorff, Ruder, and Bauman 2017) found that 60 percent of the population had at least one chronic health condition and 42 percent had more than one chronic health condition. Not surprisingly, older generations are more likely to have multiple chronic health conditions than younger generations: 81 percent of older adults (65+) versus 18 percent of persons age 18–44. A majority of people with multiple chronic conditions are women and a higher percentage of whites have multiple chronic conditions than other racial/ethnic groups. The most common chronic conditions were hypertension (high blood pressure) and high cholesterol, followed by mood disorders and diabetes (Buttorff, Ruder, and Bauman 2017). One estimate suggests that chronic conditions are responsible for the overwhelming majority of healthcare spending—about 84 percent overall and 99 percent of Medicare spending (Ginsburg 2012).

Having a chronic health condition and, especially, having multiple chronic health conditions means greater use of healthcare services and, thus, higher levels of healthcare expenditures. The more chronic conditions a person has, the more likely that person is to visit the emergency department, have a hospital stay, take more prescription medications, and visit the doctor. The 40 percent of the population (2014 data) with no chronic conditions accounts for 10 percent of healthcare spending. The 12 percent with five or more chronic conditions accounts for 41 percent of healthcare spending (Buttorff, Ruder, and Bauman 2017).

Buttorff, Ruder, and Bauman (2017, 1) sum up the implications of the prevalence of chronic conditions:

chronic disease is a burden not only for these patients but also for the health care system overall. Those with multiple chronic conditions have poorer health, use more health services, and spend more on health care—trends that have been stable since 2008.

In the previous chapter, we devoted a section to health problems in rural America. It should not be surprising, therefore, to observe that rural residents suffer from chronic conditions at a higher rate than those in metropolitan areas ("Chronic Conditions in Rural America" n.d.). Rural residents have higher rates of the most common chronic conditions and are more likely to have multiple chronic conditions than those in metropolitan areas. The reasons for the discrepancies, some of which are discussed in Chapter 7, include an older population, greater prevalence of behaviors that lead to chronic conditions (such as smoking, obesity, and lack of exercise), greater exposure to occupation hazards in occupations such as mining and farming, lack of access to healthcare services, and lower screening rates for chronic diseases ("Chronic Conditions in Rural America" n.d.).

Two health issues related to chronic health conditions deserve further discussion. One is the opioid epidemic, which we discuss in detail in Chapter 10. Opioids are part of a class of drugs that derive from opium poppy. Other derivatives in the class include morphine, heroin, codeine, OxyContin, and fentanyl. Opioids are prescribed for people suffering from chronic (and/or severe) pain. Such products can become addictive and give the patient a high that becomes irresistible (National Institute of Drug Abuse 2018).

Opioids in the form of morphine as a pain reliever were used in the Civil War. The marketing of opioids as a pain reliever began in the mid-1990s. Opioids such as fentanyl and OxyContin were pushed by pharmacy companies and overprescribed by doctors. As a result, addictions increased, as did overdosing. Nearly 67 percent of drug overdoses in 2016 were from opioids ("Opioid Fast Facts" 2019). Lopez (2017b) spells out the implications of the overdose deaths:

> That's a higher death toll than *guns, car crashes, and HIV/AIDS ever killed in one year in the US*, and a higher death toll than all US military casualties *in the Vietnam and Iraq wars combined.*
> And the opioid epidemic was *a key contributor* to American life expectancy dropping for two years in a row in 2015 and 2016—the first time there's been a two-year drop in US life expectancy *since the early 1960s.*

While there is much that can be said about the opioid epidemic, our concern here is the costs of the epidemic. While there have been a number of estimates as to the costs of the opioid epidemic (Council of Economic Advisers 2017; Lopez 2017a), a recent estimate by the Council of Economic Advisers (CEA) (2017) suggests the costs, and this refers to costs to the economy as whole, exceed $500 billion a year. The CEA estimates include non-health costs as well as health costs. These include loss of productivity, decline in labor force participation, criminal activity (to pay for the prescriptions and for those who move from prescription opioids to heroin), and mental health issues (Lopez 2017b).

The second health issue related to chronic conditions is obesity. Close to 40 percent of adults are obese and 7.7 percent of adults were severely obese according to 2015–2016 data, significantly higher than in the 2007–2008 period (Blumenthal and Seervai 2018). Blumenthal and Seervai (2018) argue that the obesity epidemic is more serious than the opioid epidemic, though the nature of the two epidemics means more publicity for the latter than for the former.

Obesity is linked to other diseases such as cancer, hypertension, stroke, diabetes, and heart attacks. Obesity is one of the major causes of preventable deaths. Obesity costs the healthcare system nearly $150 billion and also leads to lost productivity (Blumenthal and Seervai 2018). Obesity and overweight also plague children (nearly 33 percent of children). "The rates are even higher among ethnic minorities, rural populations, and those with low income or education" (Hammond 2012). Hammond (2012) notes that obesity may be responsible for over one-fifth of healthcare spending and especially affects Medicare and Medicaid.

In the United States, the traditional method of reporting healthcare costs is reporting costs by healthcare setting or by healthcare payer. Another way to examine healthcare costs is to categorize national medical expenditures into patient-centered care categories such as chronic conditions, acute illness, trauma/poisoning, and the like. A study that analyzed data from the 2007 Medical Expenditure Panel Survey (MEPS) collected by the Agency for Healthcare Research and Quality (AHRQ) and categorized into patient-centered categories of care concluded that nearly half of expenditures were for chronic conditions and another 25 percent were for acute-care categories (Conway et al. 2011).

Healthcare Expenditures in the United States Compared to Other Countries

How do healthcare expenditures in the United States compare with other industrialized countries? The United States spends more money on healthcare than any other member country in the Organisation for Economic Cooperation and Development (OECD) (Congressional Research Service 2007). Papanicolas et al. (2018; see also Kamal and Cox 2018; Squires and Anderson 2015) compared national health spending in the United States to healthcare spending in ten other industrialized countries. Looking at 2016 data, the US had the highest percentage of healthcare spending (17.8 percent) of GDP than any of the other countries. Switzerland was the next highest at 12.4 percent of GDP followed by Sweden (11.9 percent), Germany (11.3 percent), and France (11 percent).

Looking at public spending as a percentage of GDP, the US ranked seventh (at 8.3 percent), behind Sweden, the Netherlands, Denmark, Germany, France, and Japan (Papanicolas et al. 2018). It should be noted that the figures do not include the tax expenditures we discussed above. That would raise the US public spending percentage, though would not put the US in first place. Average spending per capita in the US in 2016 was $9,403, more than 38 percent higher than the second-ranked country, Sweden (authors' calculations from Papanicolas et al. 2018). Looking at 2013 data, the US spent 250 percent more per capita on healthcare than the average of 13 OECD countries (Squires and Anderson 2015).

Three things stand out with respect to healthcare costs when we compare the United States with other OECD countries. First, most OECD countries use a common fee schedule under which hospitals, doctors, and health services are paid similar rates for most of the patients they see. In the United States, how much a healthcare service is paid depends on the kind of insurance a patient carries and where the service is delivered (both geographically and by provider). Second, payment rates in OECD countries are continuously monitored and more flexible. It is easier to lower payment rates if prices are rising too fast. In the United States payment rates are less flexible. Third, in the United States there are fewer methods for lowering rising costs in the private sector than in the OECD countries (Kane 2012). The United States also uses more of the newest medical technologies and performs several invasive surgeries more frequently than in other OECD countries (Congressional Research Service 2007; Kumai and Cox n.d.). For example, the US has, relatively speaking, more MRIs (magnetic resonance imaging machines) and makes, again, relatively speaking, more use of them than most other OECD countries (Kamal and Cox 2018).

Despite the United States spending so much more money on healthcare, some have argued that the health status of Americans trails that of other industrialized countries. Among the most highly industrialized countries, the United States ranks 11th overall out of 11 countries (Schneider et al. 2017), and bottom on the important indicators of low birth rate and neonatal and infant mortality (Squires and Anderson 2015; Papanicolas et al. 2018). The US healthcare system has higher rates of medical errors than other industrialized countries (Sawyer and Gonzales 2017). A survey of adults with recent healthcare problems in six countries found that "The United States often stands out with high medical errors and inefficient care and has the worst performance for access/cost barriers and financial burdens" (Schoen et al. 2005).

It should be noted that not all see the types of studies mentioned in the above as completely accurate. For example, Scandlen (2018) argues that the Commonwealth Fund, in its series of comparative quality reports, tends to "cherry pick" their questions. Coletta (2018) notes that wait times for things like knee replacement surgeries tend to be higher in Canada than in the US.

WHO IS AFFECTED BY HIGH AND INCREASING HEALTHCARE COSTS?

Having looked at the data on healthcare spending, our next question is who that spending affects. The simple answer is everyone. In this section we look closely at different sectors that are affected.

Households

The first group affect by healthcare costs and expenditures are individuals and families—in other words, households. Households are affected in a variety of ways. First, taxes pay for public programs such as Medicare, Medicaid, the Veterans Health Administration, and the Children's Health Insurance Program (CHIP).

Second, households have out-of-pocket costs for healthcare; these include premiums for health insurance plans, deductibles (how much has to paid for a service before the health insurance plan kicks in), co-payments (an amount paid by the patient in addition to the deductible), and coinsurance (a percentage of the remaining bill after the deductible). While out-of-pocket costs have decreased as a percent of total national healthcare expenditures, down to 10.6 percent in 2016, those costs are still substantial, totaling $352.5 billion in 2016 (Table 8.1; see also Hartman et al. 2018).

But healthcare costs do not affect households evenly. Looking at 2012 data, 26.8 percent of households were unable to pay their medical bills, 21.4 percent were paying their bills over time, and 16.5 percent had problems paying their bills in the previous year (Cohen and Kirzinger 2014). Those with lower incomes suffered more financial burdens than those with higher incomes. The same is true for households with children: 36 percent of households with children experienced financial burdens from healthcare costs compared to 25.2 percent of households with two or more adults but no children. Households where some or all members did not have insurance experienced financial burdens from healthcare costs (Cohen and Kirzinger 2014). For people with medical bill problems, the difficulty was likely to be with the cost-sharing, even for those with insurance. In a fair number of cases, the provider was not in the insurer's network and so insurance would cover only some or none of the costs (Hamel et al. 2016). An adverse event, such as a hospital stay, or the use of an ambulance, can cost in the tens of thousands of dollars (if not more)—beyond what most people can pay (Dobkin et al. 2017). A recent story published by *Kaiser Health News* illustrates this problem. In the story's first case (Bebinger 2018), Kristina Cunningham suffered a stroke while attending a wedding in Wichita, Kansas. Because of continuing issues related to the stroke, the decision was made to airlift her to Massachusetts General Hospital in Boston, near her home. The bill for the flight came to over $474,000, a small portion of which was paid for by her insurance plan.

A related point is that increases in cost-sharing have exceeded increases in wages (Claxton et al. 2018). We can see this in the case of the elderly. Inflation has been fairly low in recent years and, as a result, cost-of-living increases in Social Security payments to beneficiaries have been low. In some years, there have been no increases. But the premiums for Medicare Part B have continued to increase. So, even if Social Security benefits remained the same, beneficiaries would have less income because of the premium increases (which come out of Social Security benefits).

The same thing is true for workers. In a study of workers in large companies (Claxton et al. 2018), deductibles accounted for 51.7 percent of cost-sharing in 2016 (up from 28.8 percent in 2006), co-payments accounted for 17.4 percent (42.9 percent in 2006), and coinsurance accounted for 30.9 percent in 2016 (28.4 percent in 2006). Much of this change is due to moves by employers to high-deductible plans.

The annual cost of employer-sponsored insurance per capita for a family plan increased by almost 55 percent from 2007 to 2017. Employers' costs during this same time period increased by 48 percent. The employees' cost increased by 74 percent from 2007 to 2017 (authors' calculations from Claxton et al. 2017). Employees were clearly picking up more of their insurance costs.

Another way of looking at the impact of healthcare spending on household finances is to think about wage growth in the United States. Adjusting for inflation, wages have seen little growth (DeSilver 2014). In current dollars, wages increased from $2.50 an hour in 1969 to $20.67 in 2014. That is an increase of over 700 percent. But adjusting for inflation, the increase is a bit over 7 percent (authors' calculations from DeSilver 2014). The cost of health insurance has an impact on wages. DeSilver (2014), using data from the Bureau of Labor Statistics, found that wages and salaries increased by 37 percent from 2001 to 2014, but health benefits costs increased over the same period by close to 60 percent (not accounting for inflation). American households saw their financial situation falling behind the cost of living and healthcare was one of the reasons for that (DeSilver 2014).

The high cost of medical care has many impacts on American individuals and households. One, discussed in Chapter 7, is that people will postpone getting needed care or medications because of the cost. A related impact is medical debt and medical bankruptcy.

For those who have had a costly medical procedure, the costs can create great pressure on family finances. And Americans are not necessarily prepared for such expenditures. Gabler (2016) cites a study by the Federal Reserve Board about consumer finances:

> But the answer to one question was astonishing. The Fed asked respondents how they would pay for a $400 emergency. The answer: *47 percent* of respondents said that either they would cover the expense by borrowing or selling something, or they would not be able to come up with the $400 at all. *Four hundred dollars!* Who knew?

If a family has difficulty meeting a $400 emergency expense, say for an auto repair, then meeting the costs of medical care would present many more problems. In some cases, the medical expenses are extraordinary. Someone with multiple sclerosis might have pharmaceutical expenses that exceed $10,000 a month. A child in a neonatal intensive-care unit for an extended period of time might see a bill close to $1 million. Insurance, with Medicare or some other form, will cover some, but not all, of these expenses. One not-often-discussed impact of a serious medical event, what Dobkin et al. (2018) call an adverse shock, is not just the expense of the event or shock but the decline in the economic status of the patient and family. Earnings decline, income declines, and access to credit declines. The financial burden of medical care is considerable.

Having insurance certainly helps. But insurance does not cover everything. As we noted above, deductibles can easily reach $1,000. Recall the discussion above about the ability of middle-class families to have money for emergencies. The $1,000 deductible is difficult to meet for many of those families. Other policies, including those on the ACA exchanges, have deductibles higher than $1,000. For a family, the deductible might be $2,300 (Olen 2017). As employers move more to high-deductible plans (Claxton et al. 2017), workers and their families will see much higher deductibles. Insurance plans may also limit the providers a subscriber can see (in-network providers) and pay less for out-of-network providers (Olen 2017). Olen (2017) also points out that expenses associated with a medical event include things like transportation and childcare costs, none of which are covered by insurance plans.

Pollitz et al. (2014) found that 32 percent of non-elderly adults had one or more problems paying medical bills. Some were unable to pay at all; others had worked out arrangements to pay bills off over time. Of those (2012 data), 30 percent were uninsured, so it made sense that they would have trouble with their medical bills. But 54 percent had employer-sponsored insurance. Other were on Medicare or Medicaid. Again, people had problems with various kinds of cost-sharing, such as deductibles and co-payments. Pollitz et al. (2014) observed that even families with incomes greater than 400 percent of the federal poverty level found that their liquid assets were less than their medical bills (see also Rae, Claxton, and Levitt 2017). Pollitz et al. (2014) note the complexities of cost-sharing. For example, a health problem that extended past a calendar year meant that the deductible for the same health problem had to be met twice. Plans may have a separate deductible for each person. For those with chronic ailments, the cost-sharing multiplies over a period of years. As mentioned above, Pollitz et al. (2014) point out the higher cost-sharing that occurs with out-of-plan use, sometimes double the in-network cost-sharing.

To add to all this, there is also a problem with what Pollitz et al. (2014) call "inadvertent out-of-plan care." In this case, care may be given to a patient by a physician who is not in the plan and was not chosen by the patient. This might happen when someone goes in for surgery and the anesthesiologist, who the patient might not even have met, is not part of the plan. Or the patient may be sent to recuperate in a part of the hospital that runs independently of the hospital and is not part of the plan (Pollitz et al. 2014).

A related aspect of medical debt is medical bankruptcy. Bankruptcies increased in the 2000s as a result of the housing crisis, the Great Recession (2007–2009), and the slow recovery from the recession. Some portion of those bankruptcies were due to extremely high medical costs. The percentage of bankruptcies due to medical costs is in some dispute. At the high end was a prominent study that appeared in 2009 in *The Journal of the American Medical Association*. The authors estimated that 62.1 percent of bankruptcies in 2007 (the first year of the Great Recession) were due to medical debts (Himmelstein et al. 2009). One reason importance has been attached to this study is that one of the co-authors was Elizabeth Warren, at the time a law professor at Harvard and later a very strong consumer advocate and US senator from Massachusetts, and contender for the 2020 Democratic presidential nominee.

While medical debt may contribute to bankruptcy, there is controversy over how large that contribution is. Dobkin et al. (2018) point out, first, that about 20 percent of the population have medical debt, but only about 1 percent file for bankruptcy because of that debt. Second, the researchers looked at people who were admitted to a hospital (often the cause of medical debt) and find that while bankruptcies increased among those people, only about 4 percent filed for bankruptcy. Dobkin et al. (2018) acknowledge that they did not look at people who did not have hospitalizations but still had high medical costs. And they also noted, as mentioned above, other impacts of adverse health events, such as loss of income.

One can see how people faced with high healthcare costs dealt with it in two ways. One is *medical tourism*. Medical tourism occurs when someone decides to go to another country for medical treatment. While this is not a widespread phenomenon, it does exist. There is a medical tourism association. There are a number of countries where people in the US go for medical care. These include Costa Rica, Colombia, Mexico, Malaysia, and Thailand, among others ("Save Thousands as a Medical Tourist in These Five Countries" 2016). In 2016, a coronary bypass surgery would cost $88,000 in the United States, but only $31,500 in Costa Rica ("Save Thousands as a Medical Tourist in These Five Countries" 2016). Of course, this is not for everyone and certainly not for every, even most, conditions. Care must be taken to ensure that the medical procedures are of high quality. The ability to come up with the funds for this, often not covered by insurance, would preclude medical tourism as an option.

The second example of people looking for ways to pay for or reduce the cost of medical care is through *crowdsourcing*. While crowdsourcing can be used by healthcare professionals to diagnose conditions, here we consider just the cost issue. In this case, crowdsourcing is going on websites such as Facebook and asking people to contribute money to help pay for treatment of a medical condition. The use of crowdsourcing in this way has been increasing (Belmonte 2018).

The bottom line remains that those experiencing adverse health events, as small as an ambulance ride, find themselves with medical debt.

Businesses

The business sector is also affected by healthcare expenditures. It should be noted, first, that not all businesses offer a health benefit to their employees. The larger the company, the more likely it is to offer a health benefit. Ninety-six percent of large companies, with 100 or more employees, offered the health benefit in 2017. Ninety percent of mid-size companies, with 50–99 workers, offered the benefit in 2017. For the smallest companies, 3–49 workers, only 50 percent offered the benefit (Claxton et al. 2017).

Second, the number of companies offering a health benefit has been decreasing. In 1999, 66 percent of all companies offered a health benefit. By 2017, that was down to 53 percent, a decrease of about 25 percent (Claxton et al. 2017). While there have been some ups and downs in the proportion of companies offering a health benefit—for example, the percentage increased for a while after the recovery from the Great Recession—the trend is clear. Fewer businesses, especially those in the two smaller categories, were offering a health benefit.

Despite the decline in the number of companies offering a health benefit, employer-sponsored insurance (ESI) remains the single-largest source of health insurance for Americans. In 2016, over 178 million people, or 55.7 percent of the population, were covered by ESI (Bureau of the Census 2017). If we looked at just those under 65 years of age, the proportion of those with ESI is nearly 66 percent (authors' calculations from the US Bureau of the Census 2017).

Data on national health expenditures (National Center for Health Statistics 2018) show the importance of employer-sponsored insurance. In 2000, businesses spent $334.9 billion on healthcare for their employees, 24.5 percent of total national health expenditures. In 2016, businesses spent $664.6 billion on healthcare, 19.9 percent of total national health expenditures. As we shall see below, the percentage of government spending on healthcare grew while the percentage of business spending declined (the same is true for household spending). Still, $664.6 billion is a lot of money. Employer costs for employee insurance were 7.5 percent of total employee compensation (US Bureau of Labor Statistics 2018).

It can been argued that the costs of providing healthcare for employees puts businesses in an unfavorable competitive position compared to businesses in other countries that have national health insurance systems, such as Japan. It is not clear that this is actually the case (Johnson 2012). In any event, there have been policy proposals from all ends of the ideological spectrum to do away with employer-sponsored insurance. We will take this issue up in Chapter 11.

Government

A third group strongly affected by healthcare costs is government, at all levels. We begin by looking at some aspects of the federal budget. We have already seen that the two giant healthcare programs, Medicare and Medicaid, account for a substantial portion of total national healthcare expenditures, about 37 percent (see Table 8.1 and Chapters 4 and 5). Those two programs also account for a large percentage of federal spending. In 2010 spending on Medicare and Medicaid comprised 20.8 percent of total federal spending; by 2016, that percentage had increased to 24.8 percent (Office of Management and Budget 2018). It should also be pointed out that both programs have permanent appropriations. That is, spending on Medicare and Medicaid do not have to go through the regular appropriations process as do almost all other federal programs, such as defense spending. Spending on these two programs is mandatory: it depends on the rules of the program, the number of recipients, prices, and their use. Only by changing one of the four factors mentioned in the previous sentence can spending be controlled.

The continued increase in spending for these two programs puts pressure on the rest of the budget and has led some to call for significant changes to ease the pressure. Ezrati (2018), for example, points that out entitlement programs (which include Medicare and Medicaid plus Social Security and payments for the Affordable Care Act, among other programs) take up as much as 70 percent of the federal budget, with the likelihood that they will consume ever-larger portions of the budget. Paul Ryan (R-WI), the Speaker of the US House of Representatives, said that Republicans would look to cut entitlements to reduce federal spending and the federal deficit (Stein 2017). Of course, Democrats point out that the very large tax cut that was passed in December 2017 cut federal revenues and exacerbated the federal deficit (see, for example, Zelizer 2017).

All of this understates the federal role in financing healthcare in the United States. Two studies take a deeper look at the federal contribution to spending on healthcare. The first study (James and Hughes 2015) includes a whole range of programs (see Table 8.5). According to James and Hughes (2015), by 2013 the public sector accounted for over 50 percent of total healthcare spending. Using their figures, Table 8.5 shows that in 2013, federal spending accounted for almost 56 percent of total healthcare spending.

A similar result was found by Himmelstein and Woolhandler (2016). Using similar items as James and Hughes (2015), they found that for 2013, public spending accounted for 64.3 percent of total national health expenditures; in 2015, that percentage had increased to 65 percent. Under current law, Himmelstein and Woolhandler (2016) predict that public spending will account for 67.1 percent of total national healthcare spending by 2024. Himmelstein and Woolhandler (2016) also look at US spending compared to other Westernized, industrialized countries. They find, as we discussed above, that the US spends more than any other country. Somewhat surprising is that US tax-supported spending on a per-capita basis was also much higher than the other nine countries in their study. The US spends more than twice as much as the OECD average (excluding the US) on tax-supported spending. The other countries all have some type of national healthcare system; the US does not. Perhaps, it might be surmised, that is why the US spends so much, and so much more than other countries.

As we have discussed in previous chapters, states play a substantial role in healthcare. Healthcare spending and budgeting issues are no different. In fiscal year 2016, looking at all state funds, Medicaid, which is run by the states (see Chapter 4), comprised 28.7 percent of total state budgets (which include federal and local government funding, plus dedicated taxes), the largest single item. If we looked at only the part of Medicaid funded solely by states, Medicaid comprised 15.9 percent of state budgets (Medicaid and CHIP Access Commission n.d.). In terms of total spending, the federal government pays for the bulk of Medicaid spending, especially for the expansion portion of Medicaid. In 2016, Medicaid expenditures were $565.5 billion. The federal share was 63 percent and the state and local share was 37 percent (see Table 4.3). The ACA Medicaid expansion did not necessarily directly lead to more spending by states because, at least in the first few years, the federal government paid for 100 percent of the costs of the expansion (Somers and Gruber 2017). States may have seen increased spending for two other reasons. First, in

Table 8.5

Federal Spending on Healthcare (in $ billions)

Medicare	585.70
Medicaid	449.40
Medicaid Expansion	47
CHIP	13.50
Veterans Health Administration	56
TRICARE	39
Federal Employees Health Benefits Program	32.40
Indian Health Service	3.70
Federal Refugee Health Promotion Program	0.05
Prisons (includes state and federal)	8.30
Substance Abuse and Mental Health Services Administration	3.30
Tax exemptions for purchase of employer-sponsored insurance	250
Affordable Care Act exchange subsidies	17
Public health, research, and infrastructure	101
Total federal spending	1606.35
Total health expenditures (2013)	2879
Federal spending as percent of total health expenditures	55.8

Source: National Center for Health Statistics (2018).

what is known as the "woodwork effect," people who were already eligible for Medicaid but had not applied decided to apply. This would be true in both states that expanded Medicaid and those that did not. The other reason for increased spending on Medicaid is increases in prices for medical services (Sommers and Gruber 2017).

AMERICANS' VIEWS ABOUT HEALTHCARE COSTS/EXPENDITURES

As we have just seen, the United States spends more money on healthcare (total amount, per capita, and share of the GDP) than any other country in the world. It is clear from surveys that the public's primary concern about healthcare is the cost of that care. In a February 2018 poll (Kirzinger, Wu, and Brodie 2018b), participants were asked what they wanted candidates in the 2018 elections to talk about. The largest single item by far was healthcare costs. Twenty-two percent of registered voters in the survey picked costs. No other topic exceeded 9 percent.

A 2018 study by the Pew Research Center (Milanez and Strauss 2018) found that while Americans differed on the value of various medical treatments, costs were a significant issue. Eighty-three percent of respondents agreed that "Cost of treatments makes quality care unaffordable" (Milanez and Strauss 2018).

Kirzinger et al. (2017) found that costs were on Americans' minds. Sixty-seven percent felt that lowering costs should be the top priority of candidates, including lowering the cost of medications. There was a bit of a partisan divide: Democrats were more likely than Republicans to worry about the cost issues.

A poll by the Commonwealth Fund (Collins et al. 2018) reinforces the research on the public's concern about healthcare costs. The survey found that the percentage of people who were confident "they could afford their healthcare" had declined by about 8 percent over the 2015–2018 period. Interestingly, this was during implementation of the Affordable Care Act. Having a good insurance plan appears to positively affect confidence. Those who bought insurance on the individual market were less confident than those who had employer-sponsored insurance. Again, a sizable portion of the population (around 50 percent) did not have sufficient funds to pay for emergency bills (Collins et al. 2018). "Women, people of color, people who are uninsured, those covered by Medicaid or Medicare, and those with incomes under 250 percent of poverty were among the most likely to say they couldn't pay the bill" (Collins et al. 2018).

As we have seen in this chapter and in the previous chapter, healthcare costs can negatively impact a person's or family's financial situation, especially if someone in the family has a chronic illness. Having cancer is especially costly. Treatment can easily exceed $150,000 and will, as mentioned previously, likely result in loss of income (Moore 2018). The cost-sharing that accompanies health insurance policies, including those on the ACA exchanges, represents a hurdle for many. And costs can lead to people not seeking treatment or not taking needed medications (see above and Chapter 7).

FACTORS RESPONSIBLE FOR RISING HEALTHCARE COSTS/EXPENDITURES

> Exactly why Americans spend so much on health care is not well understood. Some unknown proportion of higher U.S. spending supports economic rents—payments larger than necessary to keep health care resources in their current use. Some goes for superior quality. Some goes for low- or no-benefit services. Some results from inefficient production methods, including wasteful spending. Administrative complexity has been much studied, but how much administrative spending is wasteful and how much it may contribute to the growth of overall health care spending remain controversial.
>
> (Aaron and Ginsburg 2009, 6)

There are many causes for increases in healthcare costs. To some, the increases are the result of higher public expectations about the healthcare system, advances in healthcare technology and their success, and the prevailing sentiment that healthcare is a right (McGregor 1981). Others see healthcare cost increases in the fee-for-service reimbursement system, a medical arms race among hospitals, insurance companies, and third-party payers, and the purchasers of healthcare, such as the federal government and industries, who for a long time ignored the cost problem (Latham 1983). Others argue that virtually all the medical-care price inflation can be accounted for by general inflation, the labor intensity of health industries, the behavior of wage rates during inflation, and the pattern of labor-productivity changes (Virts and Wilson 1984). Still others attribute rising healthcare costs to: an aging population; unhealthy behavior and lifestyle choices such as tobacco consumption, a sedentary lifestyle, and being overweight, leading to diseases that are preventable; the costs of caring for the uninsured; and the practice of defensive medicine (Siegel, Mead, and Burke 2008).

The problem of rising healthcare costs is not a new one. The Committee on the Costs of Medical Care (CCMC) was formed in the late 1920s because of the high cost of hospital care at a time when health insurance had not yet come into existence (Ross 2002; Starr 1982). If there is any agreement among policymakers, healthcare practitioners, researchers, and healthcare consumers and purchasers, it is that healthcare costs too much. There also appears to be a growing consensus that at least some portion of healthcare spending does not produce much value in terms of patient quality of life. Healthcare costs continue to rise despite numerous efforts made by both the public and private sectors to contain them. Over the years, healthcare costs have risen at a much higher rate than the general rate of inflation and rate of growth in GDP. The key question is why spending on healthcare is consistently rising more rapidly than spending on other goods and services. What factors are most responsible for the problem of rising healthcare costs?

As mentioned above and as can been seen in the quote that opened this section, several explanations have been offered. Given the highly interactive nature of factors that contribute to healthcare cost increases, sometimes it may not be possible to isolate each factor and calculate the precise contribution of each. However, there does appear to be a consensus among many healthcare experts and economists that one of the most important factors responsible for driving healthcare costs upward is the rapid development and spread of medical technology (Goyen and Debatin 2009; Hobson 2009; "How Changes in Medical Technology Affect Health Care Costs" 2007; Kumar 2011; Moon 2005; Siegel, Mead, and Burke 2008; Valletta 2008).

The Role and Growth of Medical Technology

In this section we discuss the role of technology in the US healthcare system, focusing on the cost of medical technology and its relation to overall healthcare costs. Medical technology is defined as the procedures, equipment, and processes by which medical care is delivered. Thus, it can include new medical/surgical procedures such as angioplasty and joint replacements; drugs such as biologic agents; and medical devices such as CT scanners and implantable defibrillators ("How Changes in Medical Technology Affect Health Care Costs" 2007).

Americans in general adore technology—iPods, iPads, Kindles, TiVos, Xboxes, smartphones, and so on. Thus, it is not surprising that Americans' infatuation with technology extends to the healthcare system (Hobson 2009). Medicine in the twenty-first century has become increasingly dependent on technology (Kumar 2011). Today the scope of medical intervention includes kidney dialysis, organ transplantation, laser surgery, arthroscopic surgical techniques, computerized tomography scanners, nuclear magnetic resonators, and much more.

Surgical techniques have undergone dramatic changes in the past 40 to 50 years. Organ transplants have become increasingly common, especially with respect to the heart, liver, and kidney. Replacement of human body parts with artificial parts has become a reality. Today it is possible to replace a human arm or hand with a realistic artificial arm or hand that can perform almost the same functions. Soon it may be possible to replace eyes, ears, bones, and other vital organs.

The new digital age is transforming American medicine as well as the practice of medicine. Telemedicine is acting as a bridge between doctors and hospitals, making geographic distances irrelevant (Belluck 2012). Medicine and its practice are being redefined with apps and smartphones and tablets (Hafner 2012; Richtel 2012). The digital age is making e-health opportunities available to seniors to live well (Brody 2012).

New miracle drugs are being marketed each year. Progress in genetic science has created the potential to customize pharmacotherapy; for example, genetic tests could be routinely given to patients and a drug therapy tailored to a patient's drug-response profile. Pharmacogenetics will raise a host of legal, ethical, and policy challenges for major actors in the healthcare system (Patel and Rushefsky 2002; Robertson et al. 2002).

Three emerging technologies—personalized medicine, regenerative medicine, and remote patient monitoring—will significantly alter the role of hospitals in the healthcare delivery system (Goldsmith 2004).

In addition, the practice of online medicine, because of advances in communications and information technologies, will also change medical practice (Miller and Derse 2002). Computerized physician-order entry systems (physicians can prescribe medications by computer) will have the potential to reduce medical errors in hospitals (Doolan and Bates 2002).

Lewis Thomas (1975) provides another useful way of classifying technology in medicine. "Nontechnology" is offered to patients with diseases that are not well understood. It mainly involves reassuring patients and providing nursing and hospital care but offers little hope for recovery. Nontechnology is applied in cases such as incurable cancer, multiple sclerosis, and stroke. The second level of technology is called "halfway technology." This represents the kinds of things that must be done after the fact, as efforts to compensate for the incapacitating effects of certain diseases whose course one is unable to do very much about. It is a technology designed to make up for disease or to postpone death.

(Thomas 1975, 37)

Examples include organ transplants and the use of artificial organs. Halfway technology for chronic kidney failure means dialysis or kidney transplant. For heart disease, halfway technology can mean open heart surgery, a pacemaker, a transplant, or an artificial heart. Such halfway technologies are generally very expensive (Morris 1984). The final level of technology, "high technology," is exemplified by immunization, antibiotics for bacterial infections, and prevention of nutritional disorders. High technology "comes as a result of genuine understanding of disease mechanisms, and when it becomes available it is relatively inexpensive to deliver" (Thomas 1975, 40).

Skinner (2013, 69) distinguishes between technologies "according to their health benefit per dollar of spending." The first category is low-cost, high-benefit technologies including aspirin for heart attack patients and antibiotics for people with bacterial infections. The second category "includes procedures where benefits are substantial for some patients but not all" (Skinner 2013, 69). An example of this category of technology is angioplasty. Skinner (2013) argues that it is often given to patients who do not need it. The third category, treatments of lowest value, "includes treatments whose benefits are small or supported by little scientific evidence" (Skinner 2013, 69). This category includes some surgeries for people with back pain. Skinner (2013) argues that there are alternative treatments that are equally as good or better and less costly. Skinner (2013, 69) states that

it's not just "technology" that is driving our rising health-care costs; it's the type of technology that is developed, adopted, and then diffused through hospitals and doctor's offices.

What accounts for the growth of medical technology in general and halfway (lower-benefit) technologies in particular? Many factors have influenced the dramatic growth in medical technologies in the United States. They include increased public- and private-sector funding for biomedical research, an increase in medical specialties, the third-party insurance payment system, competition among hospitals to attract the best physicians by stocking hospitals with the best technology, physicians' overuse of medical technology, lack of technology assessment and regulation, a culture that values technology, consumer awareness of and demand for new technologies, and the commercial/economic interests of the biotechnology industry (Bozic, Pierce, and Herndon 2004; Davidson 2010; Ernst & Young 2012; Goyen and Debatin 2009; Hobson 2009; "How Changes in Medical Technology Affect Health Care Costs" 2007; Pauly and Burns 2008; Schur and Berk 2008). All parties in healthcare—hospitals, clinics, physicians, consumers, insurers/payers, and manufacturers of medical devices—have a stake in the development and diffusion of medical technology.

The rapid proliferation of healthcare technologies has raised concerns in many quarters about their cost and the strain they put on the nation's resources. It also raises issues about the cost-effectiveness of such technologies.

Medical Technology and Costs/Expenditures

CBO [the Congressional Budget Office] defines technological advances as changes in clinical practice that enhance the ability of providers to diagnose, treat, or prevent health problems. Technological advances take many forms. Examples include new drugs, devices, or services, as well as new clinical applications of existing technologies (providing a particular service to a broader set of patients, for example). Other technological changes are newly developed techniques or additions to knowledge.

(Skinner 2008, 12)

A great deal of modern technology—medical equipment, medical techniques, and pharmaceuticals—is very expensive. More important, the overuse of such technologies and continuous use of some technologies that have shown to be not very effective has helped drive healthcare costs upward (McClellan 1996; Nitzkin 1996). One of the most significant advances in medical technology, and one of the costliest, is the spread and increased use of such diagnostic tools as magnetic resonance imaging (MRI), computed tomography (CT), and positron emission tomography (PET) scans. Since such new diagnostic therapies are simpler and safer than exploratory surgery, they are used at a much higher rate, adding to healthcare costs. MRI, CT, and PET scan equipment costs as much as $3 million. The cost of scans using imaging equipment varies depending on where the equipment is. A hospital-based MRI could cost as much as $4,000, while one in a free-standing clinic might be a tenth of that cost (Taylor 2018). All of this depends on location and what kind of scan one is receiving. A scan in an emergency would likely be much more expensive. A 2012 story by *Consumer Reports* ("That CT Scan Costs How Much?" 2012) mentioned a woman who was charged over $9,000 for a CT scan at an emergency room. Depending on the person, insurance will cover some of those costs.

The United States has a lot of imaging devices and makes much use of them. One way to get a picture of this is to compare the US with other OECD countries. Here we will use MRIs as our example, using 2015 data. The average OECD country has 22 MRIs per million population. The United States has 39 per million population, more than 50-percent higher than the OECD rates. Only Japan, at 52 MRIs per million population, has a higher rate. In terms of usage, the OECD rate is 83 MRIs performed per 1,000 population. In the US, the usage rate is 118 per 1,000 population. Only Germany, at 131 per 1,000 population, has more (Kamal and Cox 2018).

The use of imaging technologies has increased over the years. To take just one example, in 1980, about 3 million CT scans were performed in the United States. By 2011, that number had risen to 85 million (Boodman 2016). For MRIs, the rate of use (number performed) in 1997 was 40 per 1,000 Americans. By 2015, that number had increased to 120.7 per 1,000 Americans (Kincaid 2018). From the very beginning, critics of CT scans had voiced concern that this technology was proliferating more rapidly than it should (Fineberg 1977). MRI equipment has proved to be so popular that today it is available not only in hospitals and doctors' offices but also in roadside facilities and shopping centers. In 2017, there were over 36 million MRIs performed in the United States, half in hospitals and half outside of hospitals (authors' calculations from Organization for Economic Cooperation and Development 2017).

There are two aspects of imaging devices that need to be mentioned. First, and this will be the focus of a section below, an MRI in the United States is much more expensive than elsewhere. Second, technology can lead to overuse of that technology. This is an argument made by Silver and Hyman (2018) and Welch, Schwartz, and Woloshin (2011). Overuse is costly and can be dangerous as some technologies, such as CT scans, emit fairly high doses of radiation. The field of neonatology is another example of how technology has allowed us to save lives at increased cost. Due to numerous medical breakthroughs—incubators, intravenous feeding, advances in cesarean sections, controls for infection—that were made during the 1950s and 1960s, doctors have succeeded in saving the lives of babies with increasingly lower birth weights. However, the cost has been very high. Looking at mid-2000s data, each day a baby stays in a neonatal intensive-care unit (NICU) cost over $3,500; extended stays, say over two or three months, could cost $1 million (Muraskas and Parsi 2008). Looking at 2009 data, a healthy baby will spend two days in the hospital, while a premature baby will spend, on average, 15 days in the hospital. For businesses, the cost of caring for a low-weight, premature baby (including the first year of care) amounts to $12 billion of spending over the cost of a full-term baby (March of Dimes 2014). Of course, insurance pays for most of these costs. And we would be remiss in not saying that there is much good that comes from the use of emerging healthcare technologies. The concern is overuse.

Skinner (2013) points out that unlike many other sectors of the economy, technological advances in healthcare are not cost-saving. Think of what personal computers were like and cost in the 1980s when they first became a consumer item. The capabilities were limited, and the costs were high. Now come back to the 2010s: computers are much more capable and the prices in current dollars, let alone in inflation-adjusted dollars, are lower than 30 years ago. This is known as Moore's Law, where the cost of computing declines every year. But in healthcare, costs (spending) increase each year (Regalado 2013). Regalado (2013) writes that the United States needs a Moore's Law for healthcare.

Sorenson, Drummond, and Khan's (2013) careful review of the literature on technology and costs suggests some caution in examining how much technology impacts healthcare spending. They point to the limits in the data available, the difficulties in measurement, and the lack of complete understanding of the relationship between technologies and increasing costs. Figuring the impact of technologies also depends on the type of technology and whether, as Skinner (2013) also points out, the technology is low-tech (simpler) or high-tech (more complex). Sorenson, Drummond, and Khan (2013, 226–227) write:

> Whether a particular technology increases or decreases costs depends on whether a given technology: substitutes for an existing service; expands the number of treatable conditions, in that it allows providers to treat conditions they previously could not treat or could not treat effectively or aggressively; intensifies level of use of the technology for the same condition; impacts the delivery of care (e.g., improves the capacity of the system to treat more patients); broadens the definition of diseases; and extends life, for which each patient bears (or induces) additional years of health care consumption.

Given the caution of the previous paragraph, the authors do not provide an estimate of the impact of technology on healthcare. Their answer is that it depends. Colin (2008) is similarly cautious about making such estimates and, like Sorenson, Drummond, and Kahn (2013), notes the complexities of the effort. Others have been more willing to make estimates. According to Henry Aaron, medical technologies account for most of the rise in healthcare spending in the United States (Aaron 1991). He argues that developments in medical technology affect outlays in two ways: new technology adds new treatments, and because of its less intrusive nature, many more patients benefit from it, resulting in increased use and costs (Aaron 1991). Cutler and McClellan (2001) have argued that medical technology affects the healthcare system in different ways. Some new technologies often substitute for older ones in therapy of established patients, which is called the treatment substitution effect. Such new technologies often bring health improvements and are valued highly, leading to more people being treated for diseases. This is called the treatment expansion effect. A study that examined the relationship between the supply of new technologies, healthcare utilization, and spending for diagnostic imaging and cardiac, cancer, and newborn care technologies concluded that more availability of medical technology is associated with higher use and more spending (Baker et al. 2003). Of course, it can also be argued that new medical technologies also lead to over-diagnosis and over-treatment that drive up healthcare costs (Brownlee 2007; Welch, Schwartz, and Woloshin 2011; Silver and Hyman 2018).

The hospital is the major center of high-tech medicine, and hospital care constitutes the single-largest component of our healthcare spending, about 32.4 percent in 2016 (see Table 8.2). The most important factor stimulating hospital cost increases is the rapid adoption of new medical technology. Competition among hospitals combined with a third-party reimbursement system provides incentives for rapid installment of new technologies in hospitals. Since hospitals do not compete for patients on the basis of price, they try to gain market advantage by offering the most up-to-date services, and the cost of these technologies is passed on to the third-party payers—insurance companies.

Efforts at healthcare cost-containment produce a conflict with the nation's commitment to medical innovation, which receives widespread support from both elites and the general public (Goyen and Debatin 2009; Hobson 2009; "How Changes in Medical Technology Affect Health Care Costs" 2007; Rettig 1994; Schur and Berk 2008). Furthermore, attempts to control costs associated with medical technology immediately produce a confrontation between two powerful interests in the healthcare system: insurance companies and manufacturers of medical devices. The manufacturers argue that they are unfairly singled out and that many new inventions provide less costly alternatives for diagnosis and treatment. They argue that any technology that allows us to produce existing goods or services at a lower cost while maintaining or increasing quality is to be welcomed. Nevertheless, rapid cost escalation related to wasteful technologies deserves scrutiny.

Insurance companies generally try to limit coverage to care that is "reasonably necessary" or "medically necessary." These terms are generally interpreted broadly to cover any nonexperimental technology accepted by the medical community that is not considered unsafe or ineffective. Furthermore, courts have often expanded the scope of insurance coverage by relying on the notion that all ambiguities should be interpreted against the insurer and in favor of the beneficiary. Courts have often forced insurance companies to cover technologies and treatments still considered to be in an experimental stage.

Of course, not all technology is completely good or bad. On the positive side, technology can play a significant role in supporting the provision of adequate care in the areas of prevention and rehabilitation. Mobile healthcare units can help overcome the challenge of geographic maldistribution by helping to extend service areas and making medical service distribution more equitable (Jaros and Boonzaier 1993). On the negative side, technology can be unsafe, ineffective, and inefficient.

Most healthcare economists and other healthcare experts do seem to agree that medical technology is the most significant factor driving up annual healthcare cost in the United States (Aaron 1991; Baker et al. 2003; Baker 2008; Cutler and McClellan 2001; Fuchs 1986; Gelijns and Rosenberg 1994; Goyen and Debatin 2009; Hobson 2009; "How Changes in Medical Technology Affect Health Care Costs" 2007; Newhouse 1992; Schwartz 1987; Weisbrod 1991). There also appears to be a general consensus among health policy experts that new medical technology has been the largest contributor to the rapid increase in healthcare costs since the 1960s (Valletta 2008).

Some have argued that new medical technology may account for about one-half or more of real long-term growth in healthcare spending ("How Changes in Medical Technology Affect Health Care Costs" 2007). Lubitz (2005) has argued that as a percentage of GDP, health spending rose from 5.7 percent in 1965 to 14.9 percent in 2002, with medical technological changes accounting for at least half of the growth. Smith et al. (2009) estimated that medical technology explains 27–48 percent of health spending growth since the 1960s.

Others have argued that spending on new health technology—machines/devices, drugs, procedures—makes up as much as two-thirds of the more-than-6-percent annual increases in healthcare costs (Hobson 2009). A study by the Advanced Medical Technology Association placed medical technology's share of national health expenditures for 2010 at 6 percent (McCarthy 2012).

However, just because technological change may contribute to growth in healthcare spending, it does not follow that all such changes are bad, because they can bring benefits in addition to costs (Skinner 2013). Thus, the real question is this: are the benefits derived from new technological innovations worth the costs? Do the benefits outweigh the costs? If so, technological change is good, despite the fact that it brings increased costs. Similarly, if the costs outweigh the few marginal benefits produced by a new technology, one can argue that the cost is not worthwhile. Cutler and McClellan (2001) analyzed technological change in five medical conditions—heart attacks, low-birth-weight infants, depression, cataracts, and breast cancer. They concluded that in four of the five conditions examined—heart attacks, low-birth-weight infants, depression, and cataracts—the estimated benefits of technological change were far greater than the costs. In the fifth condition, breast cancer, costs and benefits were about equal in magnitude. Thus, they concluded that medical spending as a whole is worth the increased cost of care.

The introduction of new diagnostic or treatment therapy can increase costs considerably but result in improved health. In other words, some technologies are both high-cost and high-benefit. Some technologies may decrease costs by allowing care to be given in a lower-cost setting, replacing expensive procedures, keeping people healthier, reducing hospital stay and recovery time, and returning people to work sooner. Such technologies may be both low-cost and high-benefit. In contrast, some technologies may be very costly but produce only marginal benefits. It is these technologies—the high-cost and low-benefit technologies—that raise serious concerns among critics of the US healthcare system. Some technologies are unsafe, while others are ineffective. Some technologies are medically effective but are not cost-effective. Technologies that are unsafe, ineffective, or not cost-effective are called "wasteful technologies" (Kalb 1990).

Furthermore, the diffusion of these technologies has outpaced our ability to evaluate their value and their cost-effectiveness. Despite regulatory and competitive strategies to control the diffusion of technology, excessive supply and overuse exists.

Medical Errors and Costs

There are two themes to this section. The first is "First do not harm," popularly but incorrectly attributable to the Hippocratic Oath. The second comes from a 1709 essay by Alexander Pope: "To err is human." As a side note, the rest of the line reads "to forgive, Divine."

The first theme suggests that healthcare providers, when treating their patients, should at a minimum not cause any harm. One should not come back from a visit to a provider worse than when one goes in. The second suggests that mistakes of various kinds are part of human nature. The two together imply that healthcare providers should make efforts and create systems to cause as little harm as possible. According to the Institute of Medicine's (2000) report *To Err Is Human,* as many as 98,000 people die in hospitals each year as a result of medical errors that could have been prevented. In addition, thousands more are injured because of mistakes made in doctors' offices, nursing homes, and outpatient clinics in a complex system of care that is designed for efficiency and not necessarily patient safety (Lieberman 2004). The Institute of Medicine (IOM) defines medical error as the failure to complete a planned action as intended or the use of a wrong plan to achieve a given goal. According to the IOM report (Institute of Medicine 2000), medical errors typically include such mistakes as wrong or delayed diagnosis, an adverse drug event (prescribing the wrong drug, inaccurate dosage, etc.), improper transfusion, surgical injuries (including wrong site surgery), restraint-related injuries or deaths, falls, burns, and mistaken medical identities. Medical errors are generally divided into three categories—preventable and negligent, preventable but not negligent, and other adverse events.

More recent analysis suggests that adverse events happen in one-third of hospital admissions and thus adverse events may be ten times greater than previously measured (Classen et al. 2011). Another analysis suggests that medical interventions that harm or injure patients separate from the underlying medical condition may cause as many as 187,000 deaths in hospitals each year and 6.1 million injuries (Goodman, Villarreal, and Jones 2011). An example of this is hospital-acquired infections, such as MRSA (methicillin-resistant Staphylococcus aureus).

The Heartland Health Research Institute, located in Clive, Iowa, published a series of reports about medical errors, what the institute calls preventable adverse events or PAEs, in seven Midwest states: Illinois, Iowa,

Minnesota, Missouri, Nebraska, South Dakota, and Wisconsin (Lind 2016). The report points out, as others have, that PAEs are the third-leading cause of death in the United States (see also Shanfelt, Sinsky, and Swensen 2017). The statistics on PAEs are not nearly as strong as we would like. Part of the reason is that some states collect data on adverse events and others do not. Death certificates do not list errors as a cause of death, which means that the Centers for Disease Control and Prevention have limited data. And, as Lind (2016) points out, there is the problem that errors occur on an incident basis and thus, unlike, say, an epidemic, there is little publicity. The Heartland Health Research Institute as a result entitled its report "Silently Harmed."

Lind (2016) provides some estimates as to the percentage of patients experiencing adverse events. Using 2012 data, the range is from 19 percent to 33 percent. Using these estimates produces another estimate as to how many people were harmed in 2012: 6.6 million to 11.5 million. The next question addressed by Lind (and others) is how many people die because of PAEs. Again, the estimates are on the soft side. Lind (2016) cites the 1999 Institute of Medicine study that estimated that 98,000 people die a year from PAEs. Lind (2016) cites a second study, which suggests that as many as 440,000 die annually because of PAEs. A third cited study focused on Medicare. That study, from the US Department of Health and Human Services, found that about 14 percent of hospitalized Medicare patients suffer an adverse event, and that, as a result, 180,000 beneficiary deaths annually are at least partially attributable to PAEs. Lind (2016) writes that if the Department's estimate is current, then the number for the nation as a whole is much higher than usually estimated.

Lind (2016, 10) then presents a list of the most common adverse events that occur. We quote this to present a feel for the kinds of assumptions that are used in these estimates:

> Using 2012 U.S. hospital admissions of 34.8 million, we applied the BMJ high-income country adverse event rate of 14.2 per 100 admissions for U.S. hospitals. We further assumed similar break-out percentages for each of the seven common adverse events as reported for all high-income countries shown below:
> 1. Adverse Drug Events—34.5%^p2. Venous Thromboembolisms—23.2%^p3. Decubitus Ulcers—17.3%^p4. Catheter-Related UTI—8.3%^p5. Falls in the Hospital—7.7%^p6. Nosocomial Pneumonia—6.0%^p7. Catheter-Related Bloodstream Infection—3.0%.

Lind (2016) then provides an estimate of total deaths related to PAEs in 2012: 4.9 million events.

Lind (2016) moves on to consider the costs of preventable injuries and deaths. He first lists the types of costs (social and economic) that can occur: "loss of life or functionality, lost wages, lost or reduced worker productivity, impact on family and dependents, malpractice lawsuits, inefficient and wasteful care as a result of poor facility operations, etc." (Lind 2016, 12).He cites an estimate of the social costs of PAEs: $348 billion to $938 billion in 2012. These numbers, if accurate, are about 16–42 percent of total healthcare spending. One of the major costs is in repeated visits to providers; an example of this is hospital readmissions.

We have looked at the Heartland Health Research Institute report in some detail for two reasons. First, it shows that available data are not as strong as we would like. The numbers cited by Lind (2016) are about as good can be found. Second, even if the data are soft, the report indicates there are a fair number of adverse events that occur and that they are costly to individuals, families, the workplace, payers, and society as a whole. There have been several attempts to measure the cost of medical errors. Aside from the cost in human life, the Institute of Medicine's (2000) report placed the cost of preventable medical errors between $17 billion and $29 billion per year in hospitals nationwide. A more recent analysis placed the total direct cost of measurable medical errors in the United States at $17.1 billion in 2008. This figure amounts to only about 0.72 percent of the total $2.4 trillion spent on healthcare in 2008 (Van Den Bos et al. 2011). Thus, the cost of medical errors as a percentage of total national spending on healthcare is rather minor. Of course, when medical error causes the death of a patient, the cost of human life is not easy to measure, since it raises the question of how much a human life is worth. According to Goodman, Villarreal, and Jones (2011), a patient's risk of dying in a US hospital from an adverse medical event is 1 in 200.

Regardless of the wide variance in cost measurement of medical errors, it is clear that the problem has received considerable attention, including several books, such as *Catastrophic Care* (Goldhill 2013); *Epidemic of Medical Errors and Hospital-Acquired Infections* (Charney 2012); *Medical Errors and Patient Safety: Strategies to Reduce and Disclose Medical Errors and Improve Patient Safety* (Kalra 2011); *Medical Errors and Medical Narcissism* (Banja 2005); *Internal Bleeding: The Truth Behind America's Terrifying Epidemic of Medical Mistakes* (Wachter and Shojania 2004); *Wall of Silence: The Untold Story of the Medical Mistakes That Kill and Injure Millions of Americans* (Gibson and Singh 2003); *Medical Error: What Do We Know? What Do We Do?* (Rosenthal and Sutcliffe 2002); and *Anatomy of Medical Errors: The Patient in Room 2* (Crisp 2017).

However, meaningful reforms designed to reduce medical errors are often difficult to achieve because of politics ("Politics Keeps Real Remedies Off Radar" 2004). If medical errors are as widespread as many of the recent reports and publications suggest, compensating patients who have suffered as a result of medical errors is important, whether it is done through the current tort litigation system or some other mechanism (Sage 2004).

Medical Malpractice Liability and Costs

Medical malpractice can be defined in a broad sense as "any unjustified act or failure to act on the part of a doctor or other healthcare professional that results in harm to the patient" (Stauch 1996, 247). Within the legal framework of medical injury, negligence is conduct that fails to achieve accepted standards of professional healthcare, and malpractice is negligent conduct that does harm to a patient. Under the current tort system, negligence is treated as a civil wrong (tort), not a crime or breach of contract (Mullis 1995). In order for a patient (plaintiff) to win a malpractice case in a court, it must be reasonably demonstrated that (1) the healthcare provider deviated from generally accepted medical practice, and (2) the medical injury/harm caused to the patient was the result of the healthcare provider's action or failure to act. It must be shown that the patient's injury resulted from negligence and not from other causes such as the normal risk of medical treatment or the patient's prior health condition (Eastburn 1999; Farber and White 1991; Fielding 1995).

The defenders of the present fault-based system argue that the system promotes values of fairness and acts as a deterrent, because the prospect of being sued and having to pay for losses deters physicians from providing substandard care (Weiler et al. 1993). Critics argue that the current fault-based tort system leaves too many victims of medical malpractice uncompensated or undercompensated (Sugarman 1985) and it fails to act as a deterrent because very few victims of medical injury actually file lawsuits, and of those who do, only about half have any chance of success. Also, very few cases actually go to trial because many cases are dropped by plaintiffs, dismissed by judges, or settled out of court (Golann 2011; Pickert 2009). Critics of the current system also argue that part of the problem is that lawyers often file frivolous lawsuits—that is, malpractice cases that have no merit—because when they win a case, they generally receive 30 percent of the jury award as contingency fees. Thus, lawyers have an incentive for filing lawsuits.

The current tort system is criticized for contributing to rising healthcare costs. Critics point to the high costs of medical malpractice insurance premiums, the current tort system, and the practice of defensive medicine (Brennan and Howard 2004; Howard 2002, 2003) as major factors that contribute to rising healthcare costs. However, it is not easy to estimate the costs of the medical liability system. This is demonstrated by the fact that the US Chamber of Commerce claims that meaningful medical malpractice reform can save from $120 billion to $500 billion over a decade ("Medical Liability Reform Must Have Teeth to Be Effective" 2009). This is a rather large range of estimates, amounting to savings of anywhere from about $12 billion per year to $50 billion a year, but a rather small percent of total national healthcare spending of $2.6 trillion in 2010.

There is also some question as to whether malpractice insurance and defensive medicine are major healthcare cost drivers. First, we should note that malpractice claims have decreased over the years. In 2003, there were about 19,000 paid claims. By 2015, there were about 12,000 (Belk 2018b). In inflation-adjusted dollars, there has been a significant decline in the total amount paid from malpractice claims, from about $5.5 million in 2003 to about $3.4 million in 2015 (Belk 2018b).

A related point is that, for the most part, malpractice premiums are much lower than commonly thought. For many specialties, the premiums are under $10,000 a year. For certain specialties, such as obstetricians/gynecologists, the premiums are in the $30,000 range (Belk 2018a).

The Practice of Defensive Medicine and Costs

Physicians often argue that the fear of medical malpractice suits forces them to practice defensive medicine, which in turn drives up the cost of healthcare (Seabury and Jena 2016; Thomas, Ziller, and Thayer 2012). Thus, they often argue for tort reform (Carrier et al. 2010). Practitioners of defensive medicine are physicians who, in order to protect themselves from potential malpractice lawsuits, overtreat a patient. They often over-prescribe diagnostic and treatment procedures as a defense against possible malpractice lawsuits. The most commonly used definition of defensive medicine was proposed by the now-defunct Office of Technology Assessment (1994, p. 36). It defined defensive medicine as occurring when "doctors order tests, procedures, or visits, or avoid certain high-risk patients or procedures, primarily (but not solely) because of concern about malpractice liability."

Surveys of healthcare professionals do lend some credence to the argument that fear of medical liability lawsuits leads to the practice of defensive medicine, impairs the doctor-patient relationship, and lowers job satisfaction among doctors. In a nationwide Harris Interactive survey of 300 practicing physicians, 100 hospital administrators, and 100 nurses, health professionals said that fear of malpractice leads to defensive medicine and lack of openness in discussing medical errors, and has had a negative impact on their practice. A majority of physicians (94 percent), hospital administrators (84 percent), and nurses (66 percent) believed that unnecessary or excessive care is provided to patients because of fear of malpractice lawsuits. The survey also found that 43 percent of doctors in active practice had considered leaving medicine because of the malpractice liability system. Fifty-nine percent of doctors indicated that liability concerns were a significant factor in discouraging medical professionals from openly discussing and thinking about ways to reduce medical errors and in discouraging hospitals from sharing the results of inquiring into patient injury cases ("Doctors and Other Health Professionals Report" 2003).

A study based on a sample of 824 physician specialists most affected by the malpractice insurance crisis in Pennsylvania concluded that it has led to a decrease in specialist physicians' satisfaction with their own medical practice in ways that may affect quality of care (Mello et al. 2004). In a more recent national survey of US physicians, a majority believed that unnecessary procedures and testing can result from fear of malpractice issues (Bishop, Federman, and Keyhani 2010). Another survey reported an increase in the number of physicians practicing defensive medicine; 92.5 percent of surgeons indicated that they had ordered imaging tests to protect themselves from lawsuits, and they attributed 34 percent of overall healthcare costs to defensive medicine (Hettrich et al. 2010). According to a survey of 3344 practicing members of the American Association of Neurological Surgeons, 72 percent ordered additional imaging tests, 67 percent ordered laboratory tests, and 66 percent referred patients to consultants. Sixty-four percent of respondents considered malpractice premiums a major or extreme burden, and 45 percent stated that the fear of malpractice led them to eliminate high-risk procedures from their practice (Nahed et al. 2012). Finally, in an informal survey on the *Urology Times* website, 93 percent of respondents said they believe urologists practice defensive medicine (Nash 2012).

The estimates of how much the practice of defensive medicine adds to the overall cost of healthcare and the rise in healthcare spending vary considerably because of the difficulty of precise measurement. Some estimates include the cost of the medical malpractice system and the cost of defensive medicine in their calculations, while some have tried to calculate the cost separately.

Some of the critics of defensive medicine have claimed its cost to be in excess of $100 billion (Howard 2003). However, others have questioned that figure (Hyman and Silver 2004). Harvard researchers estimated that the nation's medical liability system accounted for $55.6 billion or 2.4 percent of the total healthcare spending in 2008, with almost $45.6 billion of that figure being spent on the practice of defensive medicine (Robeznicks 2010). Others have concluded that defensive medicine costs account for 5–9 percent of the total healthcare costs (Dove et al. 2010), while others have placed the number in the range of only 1–2 percent (Hermer and Brody 2010).

A recent study (Frakes and Gruber 2018; see also Sanger-Katz 2018) looked at a limited group of patients to estimate the cost of defensive medicine. The group were military families who obtained care from military facilities. The importance of this is that there can be no malpractice suits against military doctors on the part of active military, though a family that receives care on a base can sue. Frakes and Gruber (2018) looked at what happened to the members when a base closes and the military member or member's family receives care in a civilian hospital where lawsuits are certainly a possibility. Their answer is that those seeking care in civilian hospital were given more tests and healthcare spending increased. Frakes and Gruber (2018) found that the increase amounted to 5 percent of healthcare spending. While there are limitations to the study (for example, outpatient services were not looked at), this does suggest that while defensive medicine does occur and does result in increased spending, the increase is fairly small.

A 2014 study (Rothenberg et al. 2014) had a similar result. The researchers looked at three hospitals. Physicians at those hospitals were asked to rate whether services they had ordered were defensive (that is, to avoid a lawsuit). Based on the results, the researchers estimated that completely defensive medicine added just a bit less than 3 percent to the cost of care. Thomas, Ziller, and Thayer (2012) find that both the cost of malpractice premiums and the cost of defensive medicine are fairly small.

It is pretty clear from the above discussion that results of studies seeking to quantify the cost of defensive medicine vary considerably and no definitive answer exists about its cost.

Would Tort Reforms Help Reduce Healthcare Spending?

The criticisms of the current tort system have generated a great deal of debate about the reform of the current system and/or alternatives in order to reduce healthcare costs. Such reforms include placing a cap on noneconomic damages; rapidly compensating victims for medical injury with fair compensation without the need to prove negligence; offsetting payments received by the plaintiff from collateral sources; shortening the statute of limitations; limiting attorney contingency fees; using expert panels or special courts; using alternate dispute resolution methods; establishing medical practice guidelines; and moving to enterprise liability or a no-fault-based system (Greene 1996; McMillen 1996; Sage 2003; Struve 2004; Thorpe 2004).

Would tort reform lead to a reduction in healthcare spending? Proponents argue that it would. This argument is based on the notion that the threat of lawsuits has made medical care costlier (Sloan and Shadle 2009).

However, a great deal of the literature suggests that the impact of savings on overall healthcare cost/spending from tort reform may be overstated (Thomas, Ziller, and Thayer 2012). The Congressional Budget Office in 2008 indicated that it had not found sufficient evidence to conclude that practicing defensive medicine has a significant effect on spending (Pickert 2009). A panel on discussion of tort reform at the Georgetown University School of Law in 2009 concluded that a change in the current tort system is likely to have very little impact on the overall cost of healthcare because medical malpractice, including defensive medicine, adds at most very few percentage points in spending, and medical torts do not make a significant contribution to the annual rate of increase in healthcare costs (McCarthy 2009). According to one of the panelists, David Hyman, there is a mismatch between what we actually know about medical malpractice and the political and public perceptions about it. He further stated that the claim that vast sums are to be saved by enacting tort reform is not borne out (McCarthy 2009). Finally, as Amitabh Chandra of Harvard's Kennedy School of Government, one of the participants in a study that highlighted the $55-billion cost impact of medical malpractice liability on the US healthcare system, stated, the amount of defensive medicine is not trivial, but it is also unlikely to be a source of significant savings (Fox 2010).

Costs of Waste, Fraud, and Abuse in the US Healthcare System

Another explanation proffered for the high costs and spending on healthcare in the United States is that there is a considerable amount of waste in the system and eliminating waste can help reduce healthcare spending. Waste is often defined as healthcare spending that can be eliminated without reducing the quality of care (Kelley 2009). Waste in the healthcare system can result from overtreatment, failure to coordinate care, failure to execute care processes, administrative complexity/inefficiency, pricing failure, and fraud and abuse (Berwick and Hackbarth 2012). Others have categorized waste into administrative, operational, and clinical waste (Bentley et al. 2008).

In addition, misuse, overuse, and underuse of medical services can directly or indirectly add to healthcare costs. Misuse refers to the inappropriate use of services, while overuse refers to providing services that, while appropriate, may not provide much value for a specific patient. Underuse of services can result when a failure to diagnose an illness early and provide preventive and maintenance services can lead to a medical condition becoming more severe/complex, resulting in higher spending to treat the condition. Fraud and abuse are situations in which reimbursement claims are made by providers to third-party payers for services that are not provided and include providers receiving kickbacks, patients seeking treatments that are potentially harmful to them, and physicians prescribing services that are known to be unnecessary (Kelley 2009).

This issue of waste, fraud, and abuse is a major contributor to high healthcare costs and spending in the United States. Table 8.6 presents an estimate of the costs of the various types of waste, etc. Using 2009 data, an Institute of Medicine report (Smith et al. 2013; see also Kelley 2009) estimates that the total cost of waste, etc., is about $750 billion. If we divide the $750 billion from Table 8.6 by total healthcare expenditures of $2.496 trillion dollars for 2009 (see Table 8.2), we find that waste, etc., accounts for about 30 percent of total healthcare expenditures. If we could eliminate all waste and fraud and abuse, an unlikely occurrence, US healthcare expenditures would be closer to that of other advanced, industrialized countries. A more recent study by the Robert Wood Johnson Foundation (2012) placed the range of total waste in the US healthcare system between $558 billion and $1.263 trillion annually. If we were to take the average of the low and high amounts of the total waste estimate in both studies, waste in the US healthcare system contributes to about one-third of the total spending on healthcare.

Perhaps the best discussion of the waste, fraud, and abuse in the American healthcare is Silver and Hyman's 2018 book, *Overcharged: Why Americans Pay Too Much for Health Care*. Their basic argument is that the incentives that exist within the US healthcare system allow for such activity to occur. They attribute the incentives to the presence of insurance and what they call "political control" over much of healthcare. Whether one agrees with their reasoning, their discussion of waste and fraud creates a nasty picture of the American healthcare system. We should also add that much of what they discuss is providers taking advantage of payment systems, sometimes in some venal ways.

Similarly, Rosenthal (2017) explores how healthcare became a big business and how the market is dysfunctional, a point strongly made by Silver and Hyman (2018). Rosenthal, the editor-in-chief of *Kaiser Health News*, presents ten maxims of how the market does not work well. These include the lack of a fixed price for a medical procedure and the lack of standardized billing.

Federal regulators have aggressively prosecuted healthcare fraud since the early 1990s (Kesselheim and Studdert 2008). Patterns of fraud and abuse are strongly connected to the fee-for-service nature of most third-party payment programs. Under such a system, healthcare providers are compensated for each service or product they supply. This gives fiscal incentives to providers to bill for as much as possible. Examples of fraud and abuse that have resulted from such a system include a physician billing Medicaid for services that actually were sexual liaisons, another doctor billing for abortion services on a woman who was not pregnant, and a doctor who charged the program $3,000 for an office visit while he was on an African safari (Jesilow, Geis, and Harris 1995). Silver and Hyman (2018) tell the story of a doctor administering medication. In this case, the dose given to the doctor was to be used on one patient and there was leftover medication. For four patients, four vials of the medication should have been used. In this case, the doctor used one vial for four patients but billed as if he had used four. The rewards to the doctor for doing so were fairly large.

In the public sector, both Medicare and Medicaid are highly susceptible to waste, fraud, and abuse since they are governed by a very complex and interlocking array of state, federal, civil, criminal, and administrative antifraud laws, administered by multiple investigative and enforcement agencies (Hyman 2001; Olson 2010). Medicare providers are reimbursed per unit of service provided, and because the "medical necessity" concept triggers Medicare coverage, providers have an incentive to not only increase service volume but also to increase service intensity. Since Medicare payment is proportional to the complexity of the service, providers also have an incentive to give more complex and thus more remunerative services (Rai 2001; see also Rosenthal 2017). According to Etzioni (2012), bilking Medicare is much easier and the risk of getting caught and punished is much smaller than selling controlled substances. Some of this might change under the Affordable Care Act, as the Centers for Medicare and Medicaid Services are implementing a bundle payment system, where there is a single reimbursement for patient treatment across all providers. The incentive to overtreat and thus receive high reimbursements lessens.

In 1997, Medicare alone lost $20 billion to waste, fraud, and abuse, translating to a loss of 11 cents of every dollar spent on Medicare (Cruise 2002). By 2017, that number had risen to $60 billion. Audits of the Medicare program have estimated that improper payment rates amount to 7–14 percent of total Medicare fee-for-service payments (Hyman 2001). One estimate is that fraud equals about 10 percent of Medicare and Medicaid spending, about $98 billion. That same estimate suggests that fraud in the overall healthcare system could amount to as much as $270 billion ("The $272 Billion Swindle" 2014).

The federal government's war on healthcare fraud began in 1993 when then attorney general Janet Reno made pursuing healthcare-fraud perpetrators a top priority through aggressive use of the False Claims Act. The law made filing whistleblower suits much easier (Cruise 2002). In 1995, the Clinton administration launched a new initiative called Operation Restore Trust (Cruise 2002; Hyman 2001). The antifraud efforts were enhanced by the

Table 8.6

Estimates of the Cost of Waste, Fraud, and Abuse in Healthcare in the United States, 2009

Unnecessary services	$210 billion
Inefficiently delivered services	$130 billion
Excess administrative costs	$190 billion
Prices that are too high	$105 billion
Missed prevention opportunities	$55 billion
Fraud	$75 billion
Total	$765 billion

Source: Smith et al. (2013).

Health Insurance Portability and Accountability Act (HIPAA) of 1996, which created a national Health Care Fraud and Abuse Control Program and provided dedicated funding to pursue healthcare fraud.

Three specific fraud control provisions added were anti-kickback, self-referrals, and civil false claims. The anti-kickback provision criminalizes the solicitation or receipt of remuneration in connection with items or services for which payment could be made under Medicare or Medicaid. Self-referral provisions prohibit physicians from referring Medicare and Medicaid patients to ancillary providers in which they or their families hold financial interests and also prohibit service providers from billing for services performed as a result of such referrals. The civil false claims provision creates a cause of action against individuals or entities who knowingly present a false claim to the government (Rabecs 2006; Hyman 2001).

Under the Health Care Fraud and Abuse Control program, the federal government won or negotiated $605 million in judgments and settlements in 2004 related to Medicare and Medicaid (Rabecs 2006). Funds recovered through healthcare fraud enforcement are distributed to the Medicare Trust Fund, to other federal agencies that investigate and prosecute healthcare fraud, as well as to private parties who initiate suits on the government's behalf under the False Claims Act. However, patients who may have been harmed by such conduct do not receive any benefits (Krause 2006). While $605 million is a lot of money, it is very small compared to the total amount of fraud and abuse.

Despite some success, many obstacles hinder the successful investigation, prosecution, and sanctioning of healthcare providers who engage in fraudulent activities. One of the major obstacles is the hidden nature of the offenses. The old practice of insurance payers mailing to patients copies of bills that healthcare providers submit to third-party payers has been largely abandoned. Thus, the patients rarely know what healthcare providers submit for healthcare services for reimbursement. Second, when medical procedures are carried out on a patient while he/she is unconscious or heavily medicated, the patient is not in a position to determine whether services were actually performed. Third, few patients examine the bills, let alone understand them. Fourth, it is often difficult, even when a fraud is discovered, to obtain the cooperation of prosecutors, given their heavy caseload. Finally, the very nature of medicine effectively limits the possibility of catching a criminally errant practitioner because it is left up to each individual physician to diagnose illness and prescribe remedies, making it difficult to question a physician's diagnosis or treatment decisions (Jesilow et al. 1995). Despite the best efforts, healthcare fraud has continued to grow. As healthcare expenditures have risen over time, so has the amount of fraud and abuse (Iglehart 2010).

Lifestyle Choices and Costs/Expenditures

In Chapter 7, we briefly mentioned personal lifestyle as a factor in the health of individuals. Some observers attribute skyrocketing employee healthcare costs to poor health caused by unhealthy lifestyle choices and argue that almost 87.5 percent of healthcare claims are due to an individual's lifestyle, and thus, these costs are potentially preventable ("Primary Reason Why Health Care Costs Continue to Rise" 2012). By developing healthy habits, Americans can avoid largely preventable diseases such as diabetes, high blood pressure, and heart disease, and billions of dollars can be saved (Mendoza 2009).

According to this view, unhealthy lifestyle choices and behavior by Americans contribute to overall healthcare spending as well as increases in healthcare spending. The argument here is that while some illnesses are unavoidable, other illnesses are caused by unhealthy choices and behaviors and can be prevented by following a healthy lifestyle. Thus, illnesses/diseases caused by unhealthy choices and lifestyle unnecessarily add to spending on health. Circulatory diseases, diabetes, and certain cancers are linked to unhealthy eating, obesity, smoking, drinking, physical inactivity, and psychological stress. For example, the epidemic of obesity, mentioned earlier in this chapter, particularly among young people, is related to diabetes and circulatory diseases. Similarly, the consequences of tobacco smoking include chronic obstructive pulmonary disease; coronary, cerebral, and peripheral pulmonary disease; and a variety of cancers. Lack of physical activity/exercise is related to obesity, risk of coronary heart disease, risk of stroke, and hypertension (Phillip 2002).

Diseases of the heart, cancer, and diabetes are three of the leading causes of death in the United States. Obesity is closely related to diabetes. Obesity levels in the United States have increased significantly over many years and represent a substantial health burden. Obesity leads to 36 percent more total healthcare consumption and 77 percent more pharmaceutical consumption. It is estimated that 9.1 percent of total US medical expenditures are due to obesity and/or being overweight (Comanor, Freech, and Miller 2006). Obesity is also associated with a 36-percent increase in inpatient and outpatient spending and a 7.7-percent increase in medication (Sturm 2002). It is estimated that the increased prevalence of obesity was responsible for almost $40 billion of increased medical spending through 2006, including $7 billion in Medicare prescription drug costs (Kelley 2009). In 2008, obesity costs an estimated $147 billion in healthcare spending (Belluz 2014). The good news is that after the number of obese children more than tripled since the 1980s, the epidemic of obesity among children may have begun to decline. Childhood obesity rates have been dropping in several US cities (Harmon 2012). Also, according to data from the Centers for Disease Control and Prevention, the number of low-income preschoolers who qualify as obese or extremely obese has dropped over the last decade (Pittman 2012).

The impact of cigarette smoking on morbidity and mortality is well established. The socioeconomic status or material position, and lifestyle choices such as cigarette smoking, have an independent influence on health in the United States. Smoking inflicts greater harm among disadvantaged groups (Pampel and Rogers 2004). According to one analysis, smoking costs the country $150 billion each year in health costs and lost productivity (Kelley 2009). The good news here is that US smoking rates are lower than those found in most other countries (Comanor, Freech, and Miller 2006).

Overall, while the United States is the wealthiest nation in the world, it is not the healthiest. Although Americans' life expectancy and health have improved, those gains have lagged behind those of other high-income countries (Institute of Medicine 2013). According to the study, the reasons why Americans are unhealthy compared to other affluent countries include a large number of uninsured people, unhealthy behavior and lifestyle choices, a higher level of poverty, and a built-in physical environment that discourages physical activity.

Both the public and private sector can help reduce their healthcare spending by addressing problems related to unhealthy lifestyle choices of their employees by offering more health and wellness promotion programs (Heinen and Darling 2009). However, it is important to keep in mind that because of the complex pattern of interaction between lifestyle choices, environment, and genetics, it is difficult to separate out the individual contribution of each of these factors to some of the leading causes of morbidity and mortality in the United States. Thus, health and wellness promotion programs may help but not completely solve these problems.

Administration

Table 8.6 lists excessive administrative costs as an important component of waste, fraud and abuse, amounting to $190 billion in 2009. Consider how healthcare has changed over the last 70 years. Let us say that in 1955, a patient needed to see a doctor for some malady. The doctor might have made a home visit, though by the 1950s that had become rarer (see Starr 1982). More likely the patient went to her doctor's office. In many cases, the only person working in that office was the doctor himself (almost all doctors were male at that time). There was no secretary, administrative assistant, nurse, or appointments person. There was no dedicated person who processed insurance claims.

How times have changed. Now a doctor is likely to work in a clinic owned by a hospital. There are nurses and nurse practitioners. There are scheduling clerks and processing clerks. The non-medical doctor staff likely outnumbers the medical staff. Processing claims is more difficult, because there are so many different payers. Patients are on Medicare or Medicaid or have a private insurance policy. Each of these payers has different forms and different levels of reimbursement.

The result is that administrative costs in the United States are higher than in other industrialized countries (Frakt 2018). One estimate suggests that administrative costs are about 17 percent of total healthcare expenditures (Frakt 2018). If that were indeed the case, then, again looking at Table 8.2, administrative costs in 2012 amounted to an estimated $474 billion. If we use the 17-percent number, then administrative costs in 2016 amounted to $567 billion.

One of the controversial questions underlying administrative costs is the comparison between Medicare and private insurance. Archer (2011) argues that Medicare is much more efficient than private insurance. Archer cites estimates suggesting that administrative costs for Medicare were "about 2 percent of operating expenditures." For private insurance, Archer (2011) cites an estimate of "17 percent of revenue." Archer (2011) points out that studies funded by the insurance industry do not include marketing costs, nor the profits the insurance companies make on their plans. She also notes that Medicare spending increases more slowly than insurance premiums.

Roy (2011) argues that Medicare does not have an advantage in administrative costs over the private sector. He notes that other agencies help administer program. The Internal Revenue Service collects Medicare taxes and the Social Security Administration collects premium payments. The Department of Health and Human Services also helps with marketing, fraud detection, and so forth. Finally, Roy (2011) notes that Medicare has an advantage over the private sector because it is so much larger, what economists call economies of scale. Finally, Roy

(2011) states that the appropriate way to measure administrative costs is per beneficiary. Using this measure, Roy (2011) cites a study using 2005 numbers and finds that Medicare administrative costs per beneficiary are actually higher by about 12 percent (authors' calculations from Roy 2011).

The debate over administrative costs is important because advocates of a single-payer system, such as Bernie Sanders' Medicare for All plan, argue that there would be considerable savings from such a plan over the current system (see Chapter 11).

The Overpriced American Healthcare System

> Virtually all healthcare expenditures, including hospital stays, drugs, devices, physician and nurse salaries, and insurance administration, cost more in the United States than in other countries.
>
> (Bauchner and Fontanarosa 2018)

Critics of the American healthcare system have often argued that one of the reasons for the rising spending on healthcare is that it is overpriced, charging too much for health services compared to what other countries charge for similar services. Not only do we spend more on healthcare, our healthcare system also costs more and charges more for services than any other country. Spending in almost every area of healthcare is higher in the United States than any other countries. In recent years, many studies have documented these trends.

Evidence suggests that both higher prices and the provision of more services are important factors, but higher prices have greater influence on higher healthcare spending in the United States (Lind 2012). In fact, it is argued that the central problem with healthcare in the United States is not that it spends too much in general or spends too much on the elderly in particular but that it spends far more than other industrialized countries for similar services and results. The most important cause of America's healthcare inflation is the overcharging of non-elderly Americans by physicians, hospitals, and drug companies (Lind 2012).

A 2003 article in the health policy journal *Health Affairs* (Anderson et al. 2003) argues that the major reason why the US spends so much more on healthcare than other countries is that the prices are higher in the United States. The title of the article states it plainly: "It's the Prices, Stupid." This is a play on the 1992 presidential campaign of Bill Clinton. The Clinton campaigned decided that the most important issue that year was the state of the economy, which was then in a slow recovery from a recession. The campaign's motto became "It's the Economy, Stupid!"

Data suggest that price is, indeed, a major cost driver in the US. Here are some examples of prices of medical procedures in 2014 (Kamal and Cox 2018). An angioplasty cost over $78,000 in the US compared to about $34,000 in Switzerland. A cesarean-section birth costs, on average, over $16,000 in the US compared to just under $10,000 in Switzerland. An average MRI costs $1,119 in the US compared to $788 in Great Britain. The average price for an appendectomy in the US was nearly $16,000 compared to just over $8,000 in Great Britain. The average knee replacement surgery costs over $28,000 in the US compared to just over $20,000 in Great Britain. The average hip replacement surgery costs just over $29,000 in the US compared to over $19,000 in Australia. Looking at 2008 data, spending per capita on physician services was five times higher in the United States than the average of other industrialized countries (Ginsburg 2012). Medical tourism, discussed above, shows even wider spreads between the United States and other countries (Silver and Hyman 2018). A kidney transplant in the Philippines is one-sixth the cost of a transplant in the US. A hysterectomy in Thailand is one-eighth the cost in the United States. Silver and Hyman (2018) further note that the quality of care and expertise of providers is about as good as can be found in the US. We will consider the importance of medication costs below.

The Health Care Cost Institute (Frost, Hargraves, and Rodriguez 2018) issues an annual report that focuses on the largest portion of the insured population, those with employer-sponsored insurance (ESI), with policies offered by four major insurance companies (Aetna, Humana, Kaiser, and UnitedHealthcare). The report notes that spending is a function of utilization of services and prices. In the 2012–2016 period, total spending among this group increased by 15 percent. Utilization of services during this period was pretty much flat. Therefore, the bulk of the spending increases were due to price increases, especially for prescription drugs and inpatient services (Frost, Hargraves, and Rodriguez 2018).

A 2011 study (Roehrig and Rousseau 2011) came to a similar conclusion. In their study of a number of disease conditions, the authors found the growth in cost per case was the major factor in increased spending.

US primary-care physicians receive higher fees than their counterparts in other countries (Papanicolas, Woskie, and Jha 2018; Reid 2009) due to a shortage of primary-care physicians in the United States (see also Baker 2017; Silver and Hyman 2018). For example, public and private payers paid much higher fees to US primary-care physicians for office visits—27 percent more by public and 70 percent more by private payers. US primary physicians also earned a higher average income—$186,582—than their counterparts (Laugesen and Glied 2011). Similarly, the average US physician specialist earns 78 percent above the average in other countries (Cutler and Ly 2011). US orthopedic physicians earn a much higher income than their counterparts in other countries (Laugesen and Glied 2011). For example, the average income (adjusted for differences in cost of living) for orthopedic physicians in the United States is around $442,450 compared to $324,138 in Great Britain, $208,634 in Canada, $202,771 in Germany, $187,609 in Australia, and $154,380 in France (Squires 2012). According to a report by the International Federation of Health Plans (2011), physicians' fees per routine office visit in the United States (in US dollars) are $162 on average compared to $64 in Switzerland, $45 in Chile, $40 in Germany, $30 in Canada, and $23 in France. Similar differences are found in physicians' fees for a variety of medical procedures. For example, physicians' fees for a normal delivery in the United States are around $7,222 compared to $1,639 in Australia, $1,048 in Chile, $460 in Canada, $449 in France, $340 in Spain, and $226 in Germany. For more highly specialized medical services, the differences are even more striking. Physicians' fees for hip replacement in the United States are about $5,379 compared to $2,513 in Australia, $2,500 in Chile, $1,123 in Spain, $1,011 in France, $872 in Canada, and $644 in Germany. Similarly, Papanicolas, Woskie, and Jha (2018) find that providers (family physicians, specialists, and nurses) make considerably more than their counterparts in other countries.

The United States also has higher overall hospital spending because of higher health services cost; that is, they charge more for services. According to the Organization for Economic Cooperation and Development (OECD), the United States spends 60 percent more on hospitalization than other comparable countries (Lind 2012). The average price for hospital services (both medical and surgical) in the United States is about 85 percent higher than the average in other OECD countries. For example, a hospital stay in the United States costs over $18,000 on average, compared to the OECD average of $6,200 (Kane 2012). In 2009, hospital spending per discharge, adjusted for differences in cost of living, was $18,142 in the United States compared to $13,483 in Canada, $11,112 in Denmark, $8,350 in Australia, $5,204 in France, and $5,072 in Germany (Squires 2012). Average cost per hospital stay in the United States is about $15,734, compared to $5,004 in Germany, $3,396 in France, and $2,479 in Australia (International Federation of Health Plans 2011).

Hospital costs are also much higher in the United States for a variety of scanning and imaging services. The average cost of an MRI scan in the United States is about $1,080 in the United States compared to $903 in Switzerland, $599 in Germany, $478 in Chile, $281 in France, and $245 in Spain (International Federation of Health Plans 2011).

Not only are hospital costs higher in the United States compared to other countries, the cost for the same medical procedures also varies widely within the United States. For example, according to Medicare hospital data released by the Centers for Medicare and Medicaid Services, average inpatient charges for services that hospitals provide in connection with a joint replacement range from a low of $5,300 at a hospital in Ada, Oklahoma, to a high of $223,000 at a hospital in Monterey Park, California. Hospital charges for similar services vary significantly within the same geographic area. For example, Bayfront Medical Center in downtown St. Petersburg, Florida, charges $75,739 for a hip replacement, but a patient can pay 30 percent of that amount at St. Anthony's Hospital less than two miles away (Stein 2013). Similarly, Beth Israel Medical Center in New York charges $51,580 to treat a blood clot in a lung, while just down the street, New York University Hospital Center charges $29,869 for the same treatment (Cass and Neergaard 2013).

Finally, prescription drug prices are much higher in the United States compared to most other countries. We address this below.

The above discussion clearly documents much higher physicians' fees and income, hospital prices, and prescription drug prices in the United States compared to many other countries. These are major factors accounting for the higher level of healthcare spending in the United States. However, as we mentioned above, another factor could be that the United States provides more healthcare services—diagnostic services and medical procedures—and has more medical technology compared to other countries. How does the United States compare with other countries with respect to these factors?

The results here are mixed. While it is true that, overall, the United States does provide more health services than many other countries, it is not true with respect to all healthcare services. For example, in the United States hip and knee replacements are performed almost entirely for the elderly. The United States performs 184 such operations per 100,000 residents compared to 296 in Germany, 287 in Switzerland, 236 in Denmark, 232 in Norway, 224 in France, and 214 in Sweden. On the other hand, the United States leads the world in advanced diagnostic tests—91.2 per 1,000 compared to 55.2 in France and 43 in Canada (Lind 2012; Kamal and Cox 2018).

The United States' health system also does less than other countries in certain other areas—practicing physicians (2.4 per 1,000 in the United States compared to the OECD average of 3.1); hospital beds (3.1 per 1,000 population compared to the OECD average of 4.9); average length of hospital stay (4.9 days in the United States compared to the OECD average of 7.1 days); and doctor consultations (3.9 per capita in the United States compared to the OECD average of 6.4 per capita) (Kane 2012).

In other areas, the United States does more than OECD countries. The US health system has more MRI units and CT scanners (31.6 and 40.7 per 1 million population respectively) compared to the OECD average of 12.5 MRI units and 22.6 CT scanners per 1 million population. The United States also performs more MRI exams (97.7 per 1,000 population) and CT exams (265 per 1,000 population) compared to the OECD average of 46.3 MRI exams and 123.8 CT exams per 1,000 population. Also, the US health system performs 254.4 tonsillectomies, 79 coronary bypasses, and 32.9 caesarean sections per 100,000 population, compared to the OECD average of 130.1 tonsillectomies, 47.3 coronary bypasses, and 26.1 caesarean sections per 100,000 population (Kane 2012; Kamal and Cox 2018).

Apart from the fact of higher prices, there are two other concerns that consumers have. One is the cost-sharing, being able to pay the deductibles and co-payments or coinsurance. There have been complaints about cost-sharing associated with the ACA exchanges.

The related issue is surprise medical bills. Many of us belong to plans that have networks of providers. A person may belong to a plan that has a hospital system as part of its networks, but not necessarily all of the physicians who work in the hospital. Two examples follow. First, someone undergoing surgery may find that one of the attending physicians, say a radiologist or anesthesiologist, may not actually be part of the patient's network. In that case, the out-of-network provider will charge the patient the full amount (no plan discount) and the plan may not cover it.

A second example is balanced billing, especially associated with emergency departments. Emergency departments are often not be part of a hospital system; instead, hospitals contract out the services. In that case, the emergency room company charges the patient the full price and the plan may not pay it, or may pay it at a low reimbursement level. The patient is then faced with sizable surprise bills. In neither case is the patient in a position to question whether a provider is in his or her plan. Emergency department doctors are paid at higher rates than other specialties. If the doctor is out-of-network, as is often the case, the payment is about 240 percent higher than if the doctor were in-network (Cooper, Morton, and Shekita 2018).

It is clear that the public does not like surprise medical bills. An August 2018 survey by the Kaiser Family Foundation (Kirzinger et al. 2018a; see also Altman 2018b) found that, not surprisingly, healthcare costs are an important concern. Of the various types of health cost issues, surprise or unexpected bills topped the list. Sixty-seven percent of those sampled were concerned or somewhat concerned about unexpected medical bills. Second on the list, at 53 percent, was concern about deductibles.

About 20 states have laws that at least partially address the surprise bills (which occur in other parts of the emergency department as well) (Lucia, Hoadley, and Williams 2017). Lucia, Hoadley, and Williams (2017) point out that as plans increasingly rely on narrow networks, and as those networks shrink, balance billing will become more of an issue.

Prescription Drugs and Costs/Expenditures

When Medicare was enacted in 1965, the program did not cover outpatient prescription medications. The development of pharmaceuticals since then has been astonishing. In 2003, as we saw in Chapter 5, after several attempts, Congress passed the Medicare Modernization Act, recognizing the growing importance of pharmaceuticals. Use of pharmaceuticals increased and so did prices. In 1965, the United States spent about $4 billion on pharmaceuticals, 8.9 percent of total national healthcare expenditures (see Table 8.1). By 2016, the US spent $328.6 billion on pharmaceuticals, nearly 10 percent of total national healthcare expenditures. Drug prices also accounted for 19 percent of employer health insurance benefits (Altman 2015). Altman (2015) makes the important point that the discussion of prices and expenditures for drugs understates the problem:

> Even that 19% figure is understated. It includes prescriptions that patients fill at pharmacies but not many of the expensive drugs administered in physicians' offices or hospitals. In Medicare, for example, retail prescription drugs represent 13% of overall spending while drugs administered mainly by physicians add an additional 6%.

We look first at US pharmaceutical prices compared to other nations. Based upon the discussion above, it should come as no surprise that the price of pharmaceuticals in the US is dramatically higher than in other countries (Kamal and Cox 2018; International Federation of Health Plans 2016). Here are some examples.

Humira, which is used for arthritis and skin conditions, costs nearly $2,700 in the United States. In Switzerland, the cost $822. Harvoni, used for hepatitis C, costs $43,114 in the US—$10,000 more than in the United Kingdom. The cancer drug Avastin costs $3,930 in the US and $470 in the United Kingdom. Xarelto, used to treat blood clots, costs $292 in the US, and $126 in the UK. Per-capita retail drug spending in the United States in 2014 was $1,112. The average of seven other industrialized countries was $591 per capita. Canada was second on the list, at $772 (authors' calculation from Olson and Sheiner 2017).

Comparative pricing is one element. Another is the increase in prices within the United States. Consider EpiPen. It is the brand name for the drug epinephrine. EpiPen is given via injection to reverse allergic reactions. In 2007, Mylan Pharmaceutical acquired the delivery system from Merck KGaA, which owned the company that developed it, Dey LP. The cost to make the drug and delivery system is about $1, and each unit was sold for $57 in 2007 (Willingham 2016). By 2017, the price for the drug and the delivery system had soared to $600 (Silver and Hyman 2018). Turing Pharmaceutical sold Daraprim, used to treat people with AIDS. The price increased from $13.50 to $750 a pill (Silver and Hyman 2018). Ambien, a sleep aid, increased by 843 percent in 2018 (Rockoff 2018).

If the question becomes why pharmaceutical companies can raise prices like this, the answer is because they can (Silver and Hyman 2018; Willingham 2016). What is interesting about these and other medications is that many of them no longer have patent protection.

Silver and Hyman (2018, 31) quote from a Senate report that sets forth one method for a drug company to increase prices this way.

1. Identify a "sole-source" drug—a drug that has only one manufacturer.
2. Verify that the drug is the "gold standard" for treating an illness. This ensures that doctors will keep prescribing it if the price rises.
3. Determine that the market for the drug is small. Competitors are unlikely to enter small markets even if the prices are high. Plus, small patient populations lack political power and can't protect themselves from price gouging.
4. Acquire the rights to produce the drug and close the distribution network. This prevents patients from acquiring the medicine other than via approved outlets. It also makes it hard for potential competitors to acquire the samples they need in order to gain US Food and Drug Administration (FDA) approval for generic equivalents, in the event the market is large enough to justify entry.
5. Maximize profits by raising prices, and keep prices high as long as possible. When challenged, deflect criticism by emphasizing the value the drug has for patients and cite the high cost of research and development (R&D).

Other strategies include paying off generic manufacturers to keep them out of the market, making minor changes to a pharmaceutical to keep it in patent protection, and so forth (Silver and Hyman 2018).

One reason, as the quote above suggests, for high prices is that often the pharmaceutical is produced and distributed by one company, a monopoly. An easy way to think of why monopolies lead to higher prices is to consider the price of food at concession stands in sports stadiums or in movie theaters. Customers are not allowed to bring in their own food and drinks and thus have to purchase from a concession stand. The candy bar or hot dog purchased there is much more expensive than outside the stadium or theater.

Another way of thinking about the high prices of pharmaceuticals in the United States is the economic concept of *rent-seeking*. In this case, producers seek to squeeze excess profits from their products (see Frank and Zeckhauser 2018; Hacker and Pierson 2016; and Silver and Hyman 2018).

The cost of prescription medications may depend on where a patient lives, even for generic drugs (Thomas 2018a). For example, a drug to treat diabetes varies from $11.16 in Columbus, OH to $66.23 in New York City. The cost-of-living difference between Columbus and New York explains a portion, but not all of the difference.

A sizable portion of Americans regularly take prescription medications and many also take non-prescription medications. The percentages vary depending on the year and the study. According to a comprehensive report on the nation's health issued by the federal government in December 2004, more than 44 percent of Americans take at least one prescription drug, while 16.5 percent take at least three (Pear 2004; Schmid 2004). A 2013 study by the Mayo Clinic found that about 70 percent of the population were regularly taking at least one prescription medication, nearly 50 percent were taking two prescription medications, and about 20 percent were taking at least five prescription medications. The most common medications were for chronic conditions such as heart disease and diabetes, antidepressants, and opioids for pain ("Study Shows 70 Percent of Americans" 2013).

A 2017 survey by *Consumer Reports* found that over half of those surveyed took at least one prescription medication and on average took four (Carr 2017). The report also points out the massive increase in prescription drug use. In 1997, over 2.4 billion prescriptions were filled. Twenty years later, 2017, that number had increased to 4.5 billion filled prescriptions. The increase in the number, 85 percent, dwarfs the increase in the population over the same time, 21 percent (Carr 2017).

One reason for the increase is direct-to-consumer advertising on the part of pharmaceutical companies. In 2016, more than 770,000 ads for prescription medications were on television, about a 65-percent increase from 2012 (Kaufman 2017). This does not count ads for prescription medications in print media. Advertisements work—or the companies paying for them would not continue to do so. The ads are most likely to be seen in television drama series and on news programs. The diseases the ads have targeted in recent years have been the more serious types, such as cancer, heart disease, and diabetes. The target groups tend to be the elderly population, the demographic group most likely to watch television (Kaufman 2017).

Prescription drug overdoses are now the number-one cause of accidental deaths in the United States, surpassing deaths from car crashes and accounting for more than 20,000 deaths per year (Gupta 2012). Since 1990, deaths from unintentional drug overdoses in the United States have increased by over 500 percent. Most of this increase is attributed to prescription pain killers, which now kill more people than heroin and cocaine combined (Meisel and Perrone 2012).

Increased prescription drug consumption in the United States automatically increases spending on prescription drugs. Table 8.7 presents data on national prescription drug expenditures by sources of funds from 1970 to 2016 at ten-year intervals. As the data show, national expenditures for prescription drugs have increased from $5.5 billion in 1970 to $328.6 billion in 2016. The five-year expenditure growth rate for prescription drugs reached a high of a 235-percent increase in the 1980s. As Table 8.7 shows, the growth rate of expenditures for retail prescription drugs has decreased, which is also true of overall healthcare expenditures. The data also show that the growth rate in consumers' out-of-pocket share of prescription drug expenditures declined during this period as the health insurance market started growing considerably in the 1960s, and prescription drug coverage was added as a benefit in private as well as government health insurance programs over the years.

Table 8.8 provides data on prescription drug expenditures from 2000 to 2016. Several trends are discernible. First, the growth rate in prescription drug expenditures declined during this period, from 14.9 percent in 2000 to 1.3 percent in 2016. Third, the overall growth rate for prescription drug expenditures has declined for out-of-pocket expenses as well as for private and public health insurance expenses. Finally, prescription drug expenditures have increased two to three times more than the annual inflation rate.

Rapidly rising prescription drug costs, growing concern about the affordability of needed drugs due to high prices, and high profits earned by drug manufacturers have helped to elevate this issue onto the national policy agenda. Although prescription drug spending is a relatively small proportion of total national healthcare spending, nearly 10 percent in 2016, it is one of the fastest-growing components (see Table 8.1).

The Medicare and Medicaid programs were created in 1965. Medicare did not provide prescription drug coverage for the first 40 years of its existence, except for drugs administered in hospitals and other institutional settings and selected drugs administered in doctors' offices (largely for cancer therapy). In contrast, prescription drugs have been a very important and widely used benefit in the Medicaid program from the beginning of its creation. Prescription drugs play an important role in the treatment of chronic health conditions suffered by Medicaid patients. The data in Tables 8.7 and 8.8 reflect each program's share of prescription drug expenditures.

The Medicare Prescription Drug Improvement and Modernization Act of 2003 created a voluntary outpatient prescription drug benefit known as Medicare Part D (see Chapter 5). The program took effect in 2006. As Table 8.8 shows, Medicare's prescription drug expenditures grew over 900 percent between 2005 and 2006 and began to level off beginning in 2009 to single-digit percentage increases. It should also be noted that this 900-percent increase between 2005 and 2006 paralleled an almost 48-percent decline in Medicaid's expenditures for prescription drugs because Medicaid enrollees over the age of 65 (dual eligible) started receiving prescription drug coverage through Medicare Part D. In 2017, Medicare provided drug benefits to 42 million beneficiaries, costing the federal government $92 billion for an average of just under $2,200 per individual enrolled in the program. The cost is expected to grow as per-capita healthcare costs continue to outpace GDP growth and as the Baby Boomer generation reaches retirement age and more individuals are enrolled in the program. The program accounts for 15.5 percent of Medicare spending ("The Medicare Part D Prescription Drug Benefit" 2017). Thus, Part D has

Table 8.7

National Retail Prescription Drug Expenditures by Sources of Funds, 1965–2016 (in $ billions)

	1970	1980	1990	2000	2005	2010	2016
Total national health expenditures	74.9	255.8	724.3	1,377.2	2,029.1	2,598.8	3,337.2
% increase from previous year listed		241.5	183.2	90.1	47.3	28.1	28.4%
Total prescription drug expenditures	5.5	12.0	40.3	121.0	205.2	253.1	328.6
% increase from previous year listed		118.2	235.8	200.2	69.6	23.3	29.8%
Out-of-pocket expenditures	4.5	8.6	22.9	33.6	51.3	45.2	45.0
% increase from previous year listed		91.1	166.3	46.7	52.7	-11.9	-0.4%
Health insurance	0.9	3.2	16.2	85.1	150.0	204.5	281.7
% increase from previous year listed		255.6	406.3	425.3	76.3	36.3	37.8%
Private health insurance	0.5	1.8	10.9	61.1	102.1	116.1	142.6
% increase from previous year listed		260.0	505.6	460.6	67.1	13.7	22.8%
Medicare	0	0	0.2	2.1	3.9	58.9	95.4
% increase from previous year listed				190.0	180.0	5500.0	3650.0%
Medicaid	0.4	1.4	5.1	19.8	36.5	20.4	33.4
% increase from previous year listed		250.0	264.3	288.2	84.3	-44.1	63.7%
CHIP and VHA	0	0	0.1	2.1	7.4	9.1	10.2
% increase from previous year listed				2000.0	252.4	23.0	12.1%

Source: National Center for Health Statistics (2018).

significantly increased government spending on healthcare. In the long run, it is hoped that Medicare Part D will control spending by allowing private insurance plans to compete with the traditional Medicare program for enrollees by negotiating with drug manufacturers for lower prices, covering treatments valued by Medicare recipients, and empowering consumers to select the most economical plan that best fits their healthcare needs by giving them a large menu of plans to choose from. However, critics are pessimistic about cost controls because they argue that under the plan, the government is not allowed to negotiate drug prices with manufacturers as the Veterans Health Administration does and that the program is too large and generous.

Prescription drug spending in Medicaid was strongly affected by the passage of the Medicare Modernization Act of 2003. When the Act was fully implemented in 2006 spending by Medicaid on prescription medications plummeted (see Table 8.8). But, as with almost everything associated with healthcare, expenditures started growing in 2007. By 2017, Medicaid spending on prescription medications had increased by almost 75 percent over the 2006 figure (calculated from Table 8.8). The increases in spending are due to increased claims and the very high costs of name-brand medications compared to generics, while over 81 percent of drug claims in Medicare were for generic medications (Park 2015).

The biggest factor in slowing the drug spending growth rate has been the increased use of generic drugs in the United States since many of the most prescribed name-brand drugs lost their patent protections starting in mid-2000s. The cost of generic prescription drugs averages about one-fourth that of an equivalent name-brand drug. As of 2016, about 89 percent of prescriptions were filled by generic drugs, compared to about 63 percent in 2006 ("Proportion of Branded versus Generic Prescriptions" n.d.). Thus, aggressive generic substitutions helped bring down increases in total drug expenditures (Hoadley 2012). According to an analysis by the generic drug industry, the use of generic drugs saved the US healthcare system $253 billion in 2006 and $1.67 trillion from 2007 to 2016. In 2016 generics saved the Medicare program an estimated $77 billion (Association for Accessible Medicines 2017).

The slower rate of growth in prescription spending is likely to continue in the short run because many popular prescribed name-brand drugs have already lost or will lose patent protection over the next few years, making generic equivalents available in the market. For five of the top ten drugs—Lipitor, Nexium, Abilify, Seroquel, and Crestor—generics were already available in 2010. Of the other five drugs, Actos, Singulair, and Plavix lost their patent in 2012, making generics available as substitutes (Hoadley 2012). The use of generic drugs in prevention of chronic diseases has been found to be far more cost-effective than previously thought. Increased access to essential generic medication can be an effective tool in controlling prescription drug costs (Shrank et al. 2011). However, this masks the real problem of the rising costs of complex specialty medicines that treat cancer and other diseases. In the long run, prescription drug prices are going to rise again (Thomas 2013).

In recent years, private third-party insurers have also attempted to control rising drug expenditures by steering patients toward preferred drugs on the insurer's list of approved medications, imposing higher copayments for a branded drug in the same therapeutic class, implementing differential co-payments among the various branded drugs within a given therapeutic class under "three tier" formularies, and providing a more attractive co-payment structure to encourage mail order dispensing for certain drugs (Berndt 2002).

However, there is no reason to believe that the slower rate of growth in prescription expenditures will continue. Federal actuaries project the growth rate to accelerate modestly over the next decade and again exceed overall healthcare spending growth due to higher use resulting from expansion of prescription drug coverage (Keehan et al. 2012).

What Accounts for Increased Costs and Expenditures on Prescription Drugs?

According to the Kaiser Family Foundation (2004), three factors have contributed to the increased spending for prescription drugs. One is increased use. The second is the proliferation of different kinds of drugs, with newer and higher-priced drugs replacing older ones. The third factor is the almost-25-percent increases in manufacturers' prices for existing drugs—what we described above as rent-seeking (Silver and Hyman 2018). Others have pointed to an aging population, growth in obesity rates in the country, and an increase in real income as additional contributors to increased spending on drugs during the 1990s. For example, Vandegrift and Datta (2006) have argued that about 8 percent of the increase in spending on prescription drugs during 1990–1998 can be explained by the increase in obesity, as obesity is associated with high-risk factors for cardiovascular disease such as hypertension, elevated cholesterol, and type-2 diabetes as well as an increased risk of cancer, stroke, osteoarthritis, and other diseases. Rising real income accounted for another 55 percent of the increase in prescription drug expenditures. They have also argued that the higher percentage of the population over 65 and new drugs exert an influence on increases in per-capita prescription drug expenditures.

Price increases and the large profits of the pharmaceutical industry have contributed to increased expenditures on prescription drugs. Price variation is also a problem. For generic drugs, the price of the medication can depend upon the residence of the consumer (Thomas 2018a). In some cities, such as New York, drug prices are pretty high, as are most things in the city. But drug prices in Cleveland are higher than in Columbus, Ohio, two cities that are fairly close to each other. Here are two examples (Thomas 2018a). Tamiflu is a medication used for the flu. The highest cost of the five cities in the study cited by Thomas (2018a) was $201.61 in San Francisco; the lowest was $155.46 in New York. For the muscle relaxant Baclofen, New York had the highest price, $301.46, and Columbus had the lowest at $124.53.

One can see drug price increases in New Jersey, where a number of pharmaceutical companies are located (Banco 2018). At the high end, the drug Zetia, a cholesterol-lowering medication, increased by almost 21 percent from 2016 to 2018. The price of Celgene, used to treat certain cancers, increased by almost 20 percent during this same time period, from $16,168 for 28 pills to $19,370 for 28 pills.

A way of looking at price increases of branded drugs is to consider the Medicare Part D program (discussed in Chapter 5). The minority staff (Democratic) of the US Senate Homeland Security & Governmental Affairs Committee (2018) issued a report looking at prices for 20 of the most common prescriptions that Medicare subscribers used. One point the report makes is that the price increases dwarfed overall prices increases during the 2012–2017 period of the study. For example, in the 2013–2014 period, average prices of the 20 brand-name drugs increased 15.1 percent, while inflation increased by only 1.6 percent. A second point is that the average increases

Table 8.8

National Retail Prescription Drug Expenditures by Sources of Funds, 2000–2016 (in $ billions)

	2000	2001	2002	2003	2004	2005	2006	2007	2008	2009	2010	2011	2012	2013	2014	2015	2016
Total national health expenditures	1,369.1	1,486.2	1,628.6	1,767.6	1,895.7	2,023.7	2,156.2	2,295.3	2,399.1	2,495.4	2,598.8	2,689.3	2,797.3	2,879.0	3,026.2	3,200.8	3,337.2
% increase from previous year listed		8.6	9.6	8.5	7.2	6.8	6.5	6.5	4.5%	4.0%	4.1%	3.5%	4.0%	2.9%	5.1%	5.8%	4.3%
Total prescription drug	121.0	139.0	157.9	176.7	192.8	205.2	224.1	235.7	241.5	252.7	253.1	258.8	259.2	265.2	298.0	324.5	328.6
expenditures % increase from previous year listed		14.9	13.6	11.9	9.1	6.4	9.2	5.2	2.5%	4.6%	0.2%	2.3%	0.2%	2.3%	12.4%	8.9%	1.3%
Out-of-pocket expenditures	33.6	36.4	40.6	45.5	48.1	51.3	51.2	52.2	49.6	49.1	45.2	45.2	45.1	43.5	44.8	45.5	45.0
% increase from previous year listed		8.3	12.1	11.5	5.7	6.7	-0.2	2.0	-5.0%	-1.0%	-7.9%	0.0%	-0.2%	-3.5%	3.0%	1.6%	-1.1%
Health insurance	85.1	99.9	114.0	127.6	141.0	150.0	168.9	179.8	188.3	200.2	204.5	210.7	211.6	219.3	251.2	277.1	281.7
% increase from previous year listed		17.4	14.1	11.9	10.5	6.4	12.6	6.5	4.7%	6.3%	2.1%	3.0%	0.4%	3.6%	14.5%	10.3%	1.7%
Private health insurance	61.1	71.2	79.8	87.0	95.1	102.1	102.0	106.9	109.7	116.2	116.1	117.0	112.9	113.6	128.1	141.5	142.6
% increase from previous year listed		16.5	12.1	9.0	9.3	7.4	-0.1	4.8	2.6%	5.9%	-0.1%	0.8%	-3.5%	0.6%	12.8%	10.5%	0.8%
Medicare	2.1	2.4	2.5	2.5	3.4	3.9	39.6	46.0	50.6	54.5	58.9	63.3	67.6	74.1	84.9	92.8	95.4
% increase from previous year listed		14.3	4.2	0.0	36.0	14.7	915.4	16.2	10.0%	7.7%	8.1%	7.5%	6.8%	9.6%	14.6%	9.3%	2.8%
Medicaid	19.8	23.4	27.5	32.2	35.8	36.5	19.1	18.3	19.2	20.3	20.4	21.0	21.6	22.4	28.0	31.7	33.4
% increase from previous year listed		18.2	17.5	17.1	11.2	2.0	-47.7	-4.2	4.9%	5.7%	0.5%	2.9%	2.9%	3.7%	25.0%	13.2%	5.4%
Overall annual inflation rate*	3.40%	2.80	1.60	2.30	2.70	3.40	3.20	2.90	3.8	-0.40%	1.60%	3.20%	2.10%	1.50%	1.60%	0.10%	1.30%

*Consumer Price Index-U

Sources: National Center for Health Statistics (2018); Federal Reserve Bank of Minneapolis (2018).

for these medications has decreased, from the high of the 2013–2014 to 7.6 percent in the 2016–2017 period. Even then prescription medication prices increased by more than three times that of inflation.

A third point is that there is variation in price increases. Again, for the 20 most prescribed brand-name medications for people in Medicare D, the highest increase from 2012 to 2017 was nitrostat, used to relieve chest pain, whose price increased by 477 percent. In second place was lantus solostar, used to treat people with diabetes, whose price increased by 146 percent over the 2012–2017 time period. The smallest increase was for Zostavax, used for preventing shingles in older adults, whose price increased by 31 percent (US Senate Homeland Security & Governmental Affairs Committee 2018). Finally, it should be noted that the title of the report, "Manufactured Crisis," suggests who the committee's minority staff think is responsible for the dramatic increases.

Critics have argued that the drug industry makes too high a profit at the expense of patients. The global market in pharmaceuticals was $1.1 trillion. The US pharmaceutical market is the world's largest market and was estimated to be at $446 billion in 2016 (The Statistical Portal 2018). US companies have about 45 percent of the world market. The six largest US companies ranked by revenue—Pfizer, Merck, Johnson and Johnson, Amgen, Gilead, and AbbVie—had a combined revenue of $200.9 billion in 2017 (authors' calculations from Ellis 2018). The pharmaceutical industry's profits skyrocketed in the 1980s and 1990s. Drug manufacturers have high profit margins, almost 28 percent, compared to the healthcare industry as a whole at 15.4 percent (Kliff 2015). Operating profit margins for drug manufacturers are considerably higher than in other major American industries. Looking at 2016 data, Amgen, at the top end, has an operating profit margin of almost 43 percent. Merck, at the low end, has an operating profit margin of 15.1 percent. By comparison, Walt Disney has an operating profit margin of over 25 percent and Ford Motor Company has an operating margin of just under 3 percent ("Why Drugs Cost So Much" 2017).

Another reason for the increased use of and spending on prescription drugs is aggressive advertising and marketing by the pharmaceutical industry. For every dollar spent on basic research, $19 is spent by the drug companies for self-promotion and marketing (Eichler 2012). In 1985 the FDA lifted its moratorium on direct-to-consumer (DTC) advertising but emphasized that DTC advertising must include a detailed "brief summary" of risks and other information, while the broadcast advertisements are required to have a much shorter "major statement" of risks. In 1997, the FDA issued final guidance on DTC advertising: that in addition to being nondeceptive, prescription drug advertising must present fair and balanced information about effectiveness as well as risks, and include a "major" statement conveying the most important risk information and all relevant information about the product's indications and limitations for use in consumer-friendly language.

In the wake of the FDA's 1997 guidelines, DTC advertising accelerated from $1.3 billion in 1998 to $2.7 billion in 2001 (Calfee 2002). By 2005, spending on DTC advertising had reached $4.2 billion and made up about 40 percent of total promotional spending by the pharmaceutical industry (Donohue 2006). In 2006, spending on drug advertising reached $4.8 billion (Appleby 2008). By 2016, that number reached $6.4 billion ("Why Drugs Cost So Much" 2017).

Additionally, pharmaceutical companies (and medical device companies) rely heavily on direct marketing to doctors, who are, after all, the companies' real consumers because they recommend the medications to their patients. In 2016, pharmaceutical companies spent $24 billion on such activities, dwarfing the amount spent on direct-to-consumer advertising.

The advertising efforts by pharmaceutical companies are effective, if for no other reason than if they were not than the companies would cease to spend that much money on them. A 2016 study by ProPublica (Ornstein, Tigas, and Grochowski 2016) found that the more doctors took from a drug company, the more likely the doctor was to prescribe that company's drugs. The authors make clear that they are not attributing causation, but the correlation or association is strong. Another study (DeJong et al. 2016) found that even a single meal was enough to convince a physician to use an expensive name-brand drug (see also Groningen 2017). A third study (Larkin et al. 2017; see also Groningen 2017) found that when hospitals, in this case academic medical centers, limited such gifts and visits to doctors on the part of pharmaceutical company representatives, there was a tendency for doctors to prescribe much-less-expensive generic drugs than name-brand drugs.

Research on the pharmaceutical industry's advertising expenditures also shows that DTC advertising is highly concentrated on a small subset of new drugs. Furthermore, the decision to advertise a specific product to the public is not based on the superior safety or efficacy of a drug but rather more on the basis of likely returns on investment (Lexchin and Mintzes 2002). Other studies of drug advertising have shown that very few advertisers presented any quantitative data to support claims of benefits—87 percent described the benefits of medication with vague, qualitative terms and only 13 percent used data. Thus, patients have no way to judge a medication's effectiveness for themselves (Lexchin and Mintzes 2002). The rise of drug marketing throughout the pharmaceutical industry has been blamed on the integration of pharmaceutical firms' marketing efforts with their formerly semiautonomous research and development divisions, starting in the 1990s (Applbaum 2009).

Jerry Avron, a Harvard Medical School researcher and clinician and chief of the division of pharmacoepidemiology and pharmacoeconomics at Brigham and Women's Hospital in Boston, argues that millions of dollars a year are wasted on prescription drugs that are excessively priced, poorly prescribed, or improperly taken (Avron 2004). According to John Abramson (2004), a former family practitioner who teaches at Harvard Medical School, Americans are overmedicated and overmedicalized as a result of the commercialization of healthcare. Jerome Kassirer (2005), a former editor-in-chief of the *New England Journal of Medicine,* has argued that the US healthcare system has been turned into a commercial enterprise because of the drug industry's huge expenditures for courting doctors to use their products and for recruiting physicians to tout their drugs. Marcia Angell (2004), another former editor-in-chief of the *New England Journal of Medicine,* has argued that prescription drugs are very expensive because the pharmaceutical industry is fraught with corruption. She contends that a huge portion of the revenue generated by big drug companies goes not into research and development (R&D) but into aggressive marketing campaigns to sell their products, while most of the actual R&D work is done by universities funded by the government. Drug companies offer high-priced junkets to doctors as educational opportunities, but in reality, they are nothing more than bribes to get doctors to prescribe their drugs (Angell 2004).

A number of critics have questioned the honesty and integrity of the pharmaceutical industry (Goozner 2004; Greider 2003; Harris 2004a, 2004b; Harris and Berenson 2005; Kitsis 2009; Maier 1997). Even when drug companies are found guilty of criminal conduct and fines are levied against them, their profits far outweigh the penalties (Evans 2010; Lipton and Sack 2013).

Another major factor cited for increased spending on drugs is the growth of health insurance and prescription drug coverage (Silver and Hyman 2018). An unprecedented spread of insurance coverage for outpatient drugs occurred in the 1990s. Danzon and Pauly (2002) placed the direct effect of the growth in insurance coverage somewhere around one-fourth to one-half of total drug spending during the 1990s. The significant expansion of the Medicaid program under the Affordable Care Act also contributes to higher prescription drug expenditures.

Patent protection and the lack of market competition in the pharmaceutical industry is also responsible for increased spending on prescription medications (Silver and Hyman 2018). The patent system enables protection from price competition. The Food and Drug Administration, a federal agency, is responsible for approving all drugs to make sure they are safe and effective before they are allowed to be sold in the marketplace. After successful clinical trials are completed, the drug company typically files an application for patent certification and exclusivity. The US Patent and Trademark Office grants a patent, which typically expires 20 years from the date of the filing. "Exclusivity" means the FDA grants an exclusive marketing right to a drug company upon FDA approval of the drug, and it can run concurrently or not with a patent ("Development and Approval Process: Drugs." n.d.). Thus, a drug company essentially gets a monopoly on marketing and selling that drug in the marketplace until its patent runs out, at which point other drug manufacturers can enter the market by offering the generic equivalent of that drug. The pharmaceutical industry justifies the patent/exclusivity system on the grounds that they take high investment risks in research and development to discover new drugs.

A further factor attributed to increased spending on drugs is public opinion. Polls suggest that DTC advertising by drug manufacturers works. In a nationwide survey conducted in 2008 by *USA Today*/the Kaiser Family Foundation and the Harvard School of Public Health (2008), one third of respondents stated that prescription drug ads prompted them to ask their doctor about the advertised medicine, and 82 percent of those who asked said their physicians recommended a prescription; 44 percent of this segment said their physician gave them a prescription for the drug they asked about, while slightly more than half said their doctor prescribed a different drug. According to the survey, the percentage of people getting a drug after asking about an ad is on the increase.

The public is unhappy about the high prices of prescription medications. A 2015 survey (DiJulio, Firth, and Brodie 2015) found that large majorities of the public thought that the prices of prescription medications were too high and that profits of drug companies were also too high. About a quarter of those sampled had trouble paying for prescription medications, with higher percentages among those at the low end of the income strata and those who were in poorer health (DiJulio, Firth, and Brodie 2015).

The high price of drugs in the United States is also blamed on the lack of regulation of the pharmaceutical industry in the United States compared to European countries. The reason Americans pay more than their counterparts in Europe for the same prescription drugs is that in the United States, the government does not regulate prescription drug prices and profits made by pharmaceutical companies. As we have discussed previously, the

Centers for Medicare and Medicaid Services (CMS) is prohibited by law from negotiating drug prices with drug companies for their patients. Only the Department of Defense and the Veterans Health Administration negotiate drug prices with drug companies. Thus, veterans pay much less for the same prescription drugs than do other Americans, including Medicare and Medicaid beneficiaries.

In contrast, European governments not only regulate drug pricing, they also regulate and control drug manufacturers' profits, using a variety of tactics including reference pricing, negative lists, price freezes, price cuts, regulation of profits, general practitioner budgets, pharmaceutical expenditure ceilings, and promotion of generic drugs (Jonsson 2001; Nuijten et al. 2001). Also, all Western European countries have some form of universal health insurance system. As a result, about 75 percent of pharmaceutical expenditures are publicly reimbursed. This gives the governments of these countries an opportunity to impose a wide range of pricing policies on drug companies (Ess, Schneeweiss, and Szucs 2003). None of these strategies are used in the United States, where instead the efforts to control rising prescription drug spending are focused more on consumers via tools such as patient co-payments and cost-sharing, medical practice guidelines, and formularies.

A final consideration is the structure of healthcare system as it pertains to prescription medication. The overall US healthcare system is highly fragmented with different payers (government and private), different organization of providers (some in independent practices and many within hospital systems), and so forth. In the case of pharmaceuticals, there are as many five participants in getting the medication to the patient (note that this discussion is about outpatient care). The five participants are the drug manufacturer, the wholesaler, the pharmacy, pharmacy benefit management (PBMs) companies, and the health plan or plan sponsor. There are all kinds of fees and administrative costs and rebates associated with this structure (PhRMA n.d.).

COST DRIVERS

To sum up what has been discussed so far, we consider what factors explain higher prices and spending on healthcare in the United States compared to other countries. There are at least ten possible explanations for this. First, in the United States health services are overpriced and patients are charged more for similar services than in other countries. Second, other countries have a system for rationing care. For example, in countries such as Great Britain, Australia, and New Zealand, the government can decide not to pay for certain services (Lind 2012). Third, the United States has been slow to embrace the advantages of information and communication technology in improving administration of its systems and cutting down waste (Freudenheim 2012). In the United States, about $900 per person per year goes toward administrative costs, compared to $300 per person per year in France (Kane 2012). Fourth, many OECD countries use strong regulations to set/control prices that hospitals can charge for different services. This is not the case in the United States.

Fifth, in America's private health sector, medical providers are allowed to charge different prices for the same goods or services to different customers or insurers in order to maintain predetermined incomes or sales revenues. Such a privilege is not enjoyed by physicians, hospitals, and drug companies in other countries (Lind 2012). Sixth, since most OECD countries have some form of universal health coverage, the government is able to negotiate drug prices. In the United States only the VHA and Defense Department do so. In fact, the Centers for Medicare and Medicaid Services are prohibited by congressional legislation from negotiating drug prices for Medicare and Medicaid patients. Seventh, the market for many medical goods and services in the United States is inherently monopolistic or oligopolistic (for example, the drug industry) and thus market competition often does not work to reduce costs except in a few areas (Lind 2012).

Eighth, there is a fundamental lack of price transparency in the US healthcare system that often acts as an impediment to understanding price and cost differences (Laugesen and Glied 2011; Brill 2015; Makary 2012; Silver and Hyman 2018). Ninth, in several OECD countries, medical professions and health policymakers have developed "clinical guidelines" to promote more rational use of MRI and CT exams. In the United States, medical procedures and the use of expensive diagnostic tests are all largely based on individual physicians' opinions/judgments about desirable procedures and tests. Physicians in the United States are more likely to order more procedures and diagnostic tests to avoid blame and to protect themselves against potential medical malpractice lawsuits. Tenth, since in the United States physicians are paid for the services and procedures they provide regardless of medical necessity or medical outcome, it creates an incentive to provide more services and surgical procedures.

In summary, the old saying that you get what you pay for does not necessarily apply to the US health system (McLaughlin 2011). As we have stated before, the United States spends more money on healthcare (total and per capita), performs more diagnostic tests and medical procedures, and charges more for health services than any other country in the world, yet it does not rank very high on several indicators of healthcare access, health status, and health outcomes.

HEALTHCARE COST-CONTAINMENT: BENDING THE COST CURVE

The cost of healthcare and its continued growth underlie much of the other problems of the healthcare system. Increasing the percentage of the population with insurance, one part of the access issue discussed in Chapter 7, is relatively easy. But all efforts to expand access, whether to insurance or to providers in underserved areas, is costly. If more people have access to the system, more people will use the system, and expenditures will rise.

The cost issues affect individuals and families, providers, insurers, employers, and governments at all levels. Healthcare, especially Medicaid, costs the states as least as much as education, one of the core functions of state governments. Medicare's trust fund, which affects some but not all parts of Medicare, is projected to run out by 2026 (Goldstein 2018). Entitlements, such as Medicare, Medicaid, and Social Security, are a significant portion of the federal budget. Reducing the federal budget deficits from the expenditure or spending side means addressing healthcare costs. The healthcare sector takes up more and more of our country's economy, as measured by gross domestic product (GDP). Clearly there is a problem—really a set of problems—that needs to be addressed.

One way of understanding what many think should be done is to consider the phrase that is the subtitle of this section, "bending the cost curve," a metaphor that lends itself to graphs and pictures (Safire 2009). An illustration of bending the curve can be seen in Figure 8.1. As the figure shows, we are talking about reducing increases in spending, not reducing spending, which is a much more difficult proposition. One could ask the question of whose cost curve should be bent (Elmendorf 2009): overall health expenditures, government health expenditures, insurance premiums, etc. A related point is that a certain proportion of cost-containment is really cost-shifting, moving costs from government or the private sector to consumers/beneficiaries. The question in that case becomes whether costs are really contained.

THEORETICAL FRAMEWORK: GOVERNMENT REGULATION AND MARKET COMPETITION

The debate over how to contain rising healthcare costs centers on two broad approaches or strategies, one that we see again in discussions of healthcare reform in Chapter 11. One strategy relies on government regulation, while the other relies on increasing competition in the healthcare market (see, for example, Enthoven and Singer 1997; Etheredge 1997; Evans 1997; Goldhill 2013; Goodman 2012; Moran 1997; Rice 1997; Silver and Hyman 2018; Zatkin 1997). The federal government has tried both regulatory and competitive strategies to contain health costs. Similarly, state governments and the private sector have undertaken many initiatives in an attempt to contain rising healthcare costs.

The Regulatory Strategy

One of the most important assumptions of the regulatory strategy is that the healthcare market suffers from too many shortcomings, that it does not follow the model of perfect competition. The seminal work in this field is an article published by economist Kenneth Arrow (1963; see also Relman 2005; Stone 2005, 2012). For a retrospective discussion of Arrow's article, see "Special Issue" 2001). Government regulation, it could be argued, can therefore help improve the performance of the market. Thus, one motivation for economic regulation of the system is the premise that the system suffers from serious market failures, including information disparities, or asymmetries, between providers and consumers of health services and an insurance system (third-party financing) that masks the costs of health services (Arrow 1963). This situation in turn produces excessive expenditures, inefficiency, and maldistribution of labor power and resources. A related market failure is that the healthcare system has a severe equity problem in differential access to services and financing (see Morone and Jacobs 2005 and Chapter 7). Thus, the government must play a role, under this assumption, in providing greater access to the healthcare market for those who cannot afford it (McClure 1981).

The second assumption of the regulatory strategy is that the healthcare market is different from other economic markets (Relman 2005). In healthcare, physicians control both supply and demand because the physician is both the patient's consultant on what services are needed and the provider of these services. Physicians are not trained to think in terms of aggregate costs. Physicians influence not only cost decisions regarding individual patients but also the growth and expansion of healthcare institutions, thus affecting hospital costs. In addition, the third-party-payment system, based on private health insurance and government payment, tends to remove the patient from the effects of healthcare costs, a perspective that colors some of the policy proposals of the twenty-first century (Silver and Hyman 2018; see Chapter 11).

Another important potential difference between medical care and other goods and services is the absence of consumer information about appropriate price and quality levels (Arrow 1963; Pauly 1978), an issue we labeled transparency. The role of information in facilitating choices about healthcare goods and services is crucial (Varner and Christy 1986). Some have argued that the medical market is on the verge of remedying the information deficit and that the determination of whether medical care is different from other goods and services is ultimately a political question (Pauly 1978). It might be argued that with the advent of the Internet, more medical information is available to consumers through websites such as WebMD.

The third assumption of the regulatory strategy is that public regulation promotes important values of political accountability, public access to information, and public participation (Weiner 1982). The regulatory process is characterized by a high degree of formal due process. The requirements of public notices, public meetings, adversary procedures, formal recordkeeping, and limits on appeals help inform consumers by providing access to information and extending to them an opportunity to participate in the policymaking process (Eisner, Worsham, and Ringquest 2006).

Thus, government regulation of the healthcare system is justified on many grounds: As a way of improving the workings of the healthcare market, increasing equity, and promoting crucial public values with the hope that it will help contain healthcare costs. Some advocates of a regulatory strategy argue that a pure market in healthcare is unattainable and thus regulation is the second-best choice (Altman and Weiner 1978). Others argue for a more tightly regulated healthcare system as the best policy (Vladeck 1981, 1984).

Critics of the regulatory strategy charge that examples of past regulatory failures suggest that government regulation does not work (see, for example, Breyer 1979). These critics argue that too many fundamental structural and incentive problems are stacked against good regulatory performance (McClure 1981) and that comprehensive regulation will raise, not lower, the true cost of medical care (Davidson 2010; Goodman 1980, 2012), thus contributing to healthcare cost inflation (Durenberger 1982). Regulation, it is asserted, is not cost-effective; it produces inefficiency and prevents technological innovations. Regulation often produces a cartel-like situation resulting in a monopoly on prices because regulatory agencies become captured by the regulated industry (Noll 1975). Wolf (1979) has argued that government programs, including regulation, are also subject to failures, analogous to market failures. To the critics of a regulatory strategy the answer is a competitive market strategy. Competition and market reform are the buzzwords for many health policymakers and healthcare providers (see, for example, Antos, Pauly, and Wilensky 2012; Cannon and Tanner 2005; Herzlinger 1997; Silver and Hyman 2018).

The Market Strategy

Those who support a market/competitive strategy argue that all three assumptions that underlie the regulatory strategy can be addressed.

The market strategy begins with a consideration of some classic works in economics. The "bible" of capitalist economics is Adam Smith's *The Wealth of Nations*, published in 1776. Smith argued that unfettered, competitive

Figure 8.1 **Bending the Cost Curve**

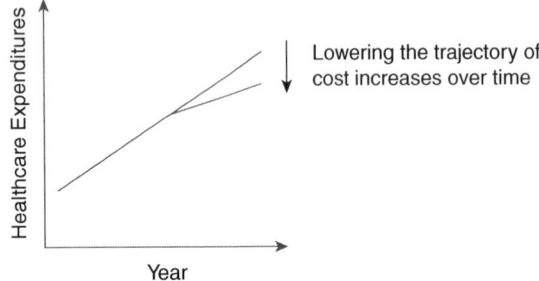

markets, free from government or monopoly interference, would produce the greatest benefits for humankind. Such markets were the most efficient, producing precisely the amounts of a good or service that producers want to sell and that consumers want to buy through the price mechanism. Anything that impeded the price mechanism would lower efficiency.

Smith's work formed the basis for classical (and neoclassical) economics and remains an important part of American ideology. The American bias has always been toward free markets and away from government control, though, as we saw above, in healthcare (as in other areas) the viability of free, competitive markets is questionable.

Frederich Hayek (1944), writing near the end of World War II, warned the country of moving toward more government control. Most influential was Milton Friedman's (1962) *Capitalism and Freedom*. Friedman argued that economic freedom supported political freedom. He discussed a number of policy issues showing how free markets would work better than government intervention or control.

The fundamental premise of the economic critique of the healthcare system is that the incentive structure of healthcare moves the system toward inefficiencies. It does this in several ways. Consider the traditional fee-for-service, third-party payment system.

There are four parts to the transaction: the patient with health insurance seeks a service; the patient sees a doctor, who provides that service; the doctor's charges depend on the amount of services provided; the more services, the higher the charge (that is why it is called fee-for-service). The doctor knows that the patient is covered by health insurance provided by the employer through an insurance company. The patient pays the bill and then files a claim with the insurance company for reimbursement. In some instances (but rarer than it used to be), the health insurance policy is so generous that the patient does not have to pay anything. In other cases, the doctor's office files the claim and bills the patient for the balance after the claim is paid. Depending on the policy, the patient may have met the deductible (the amount the patient has to pay before the insurance pays) for the year and may have limited co-payments (the percentage of the remaining part of the bill, after the deductible, that the patient pays). The insurance company processes the claim and either pays the provider or reimburses the patient. The employer may pay the premiums on the employee's health insurance and may also (if the policy is especially generous) pay premiums for dependents. If not, then the employee pays the dependents' premiums, but at a group rate.

Who is concerned about the cost of care and the quality and efficiency of care (whether a particular test or treatment is really necessary) under such a system? If the doctor and the patient both know that third-party insurance will cover the cost, they have little concern. As long as the premiums cover the reimbursements (plus a profit), the insurer does not care. As long as premium costs are reasonable, and the federal government allows a business tax deduction for premiums (an incentive to cover or continue coverage), the employer does not care. The same situation is true for hospital care.

Under this kind of situation, the cost and the price of service are irrelevant. Economists argue that in the absence of paying the true cost of care, consumers will demand more healthcare than they really need, a problem labeled *moral hazard* (Davidson 2010; Goodman 2012; Pauly 1978).

Healthcare suffers from another problem that impedes the operation of free, competitive markets: *imperfect information*. Providers have considerable information and expertise (though not complete information) and are in a power position compared to other actors, especially consumers/patients. Thus, additional treatments, so the critique goes, are not the result of consumer demand for them but of provider requests. In that sense, healthcare is provider driven rather than consumer driven. Furthermore, consumers do not shop around comparing service and price at critical times (e.g., during a heart attack). Imperfect information, power asymmetries, and lack of a clear price mechanism work together to create market failures in healthcare. The classic discussion of these asymmetries in healthcare, as we have seen, was by the Nobel Prize-winning economist Kenneth Arrow (1963). The question is how to solve these problems.

Not everyone agrees that Arrow's analysis still holds. Roy (2012) argues that Arrow's discussion of the healthcare system's problems is not unique to healthcare. Arrow mentioned five problems or distortions in that system: unpredictability, barriers to entry, importance of trust, asymmetrical information, and idiosyncrasies of payment (patients do not see the full costs of services provided) (Roy 2012). Roy (2012) states that each of these distortions is antiquated and, again, not unique to healthcare. Insurance, warranties, and other mechanisms have been created to deal with the problem of unpredictability in various markets (consumer electronics, homeowners' insurance, etc.). There are also barriers to entry in other fields, such as law and airlines. Other industries or transactions involve trust. When we eat a food product, we trust that it is safe and that it contains the ingredients listed on the label. Auto mechanics know more about cars than most of us do, especially as cars have become more electronically sophisticated. Finally, Roy (2012) notes that the Internet has websites that provide information about medical conditions.

Roy (2012) then looks at liberals' argument that shopping for healthcare is different from shopping for other items. For example, someone suffering a heart attack is not going to shop around for the best cardiologist; he or she will want and need rapid treatment. But Roy points out that much healthcare is not needed on this immediate basis. Those needing knee replacement surgery or routine examinations and care can shop around. Thus, Roy's suggestion is a hybrid system, similar to what others have advocated (see, for example, Silver and Hyman 2018):

> So, it seems to me, those who strongly believe in the shopping argument for socialized medicine should adopt a hybrid approach. Let's have a free market for the 70-plus percent of healthcare where market forces can most directly apply, and let's have universal catastrophic insurance for those situations where market forces work less well.
>
> This way, we might get the best of both worlds: an efficient, affordable, high-quality market for chronic and routine healthcare, and a universal system for those who get hit by a bus, or have a stroke, or get cancer. Such a system would leave no one behind. But it would also allow our health-care system to benefit, as much as possible, from the forces of choice, competition, and innovation.
>
> (Roy 2012)

Goodman (2012) likewise provides an economic critique of the healthcare system. He argues that the reason the system is more complex than other markets is that it is "institutionalized, bureaucratized, and extensively regulated" (2012, 1). A major problem for Goodman is that insurance covers so much of the costs that patients/consumers do not realize or experience the true expense of their healthcare. Indeed, Goodman (2012) makes the important point that the purpose of insurance, whether public or private, is to reduce the burden of costs on consumers. Further, he points to the transparency issue: that it is difficult to find out what something actually costs (on the problem of transparency in healthcare, see Makary 2012).

On one side of the exchange, Goodman (2012) notes that providers are paid based on various reimbursement schedules, which are different depending on the payer: Medicare, Medicaid, various health insurance plans, and so forth. Therefore, markets cannot work as they are supposed to, and the economic incentives are all wrong. Consumers would use the healthcare system more than necessary because costs to them were low; in some cases, there were none at all. Providers make more money by doing more for their patients, knowing that someone else would be footing much of the bill.

Perverse incentives are the focus of Stephen Davidson's 2010 book, *Still Broken*. The incentives facing all elements of the healthcare system—providers, payers, consumers, employers—all move toward creating conditions that allow high healthcare costs, and thus higher healthcare spending, and access problems (individuals and families increasingly unable to afford healthcare coverage and services). What follow from this economic critique are market reforms. The purpose of the reforms is to change the incentives that face all those involved in receiving, delivering, and paying for healthcare services.

In summary, advocates of the competitive strategy argue that improving structural mechanisms and changing incentives through introduction of competition in the healthcare market will result in better economic performance and reduced healthcare costs. Critics of the competitive strategy are skeptical of the results of market competition. To some, the prospects of a competitive strategy are promising but uncertain technically and politically (McClure 1983). Others argue that markets in healthcare are usually pseudo-markets dominated by one side of the transaction (Evans 1983), and that the supporters of competition may be grossly overemphasizing the beneficial results (Ginzberg 1982). It would take more than the stimulus from increased consumer cost-sharing or reduced tax subsidies to produce competitive behavior on the part of healthcare providers (Gabel and Monheit 1983).

In the pages that follow, we examine and evaluate various attempts to control healthcare costs and spending employing different combinations of the regulatory and competitive strategies by the federal government, state governments, and the private sector. We follow that up with looking at cost-containment efforts in the twenty-first century. While the strategies discussed below focus on bending the cost curve, all these strategies also affect access to healthcare and the quality of care (Ginzberg 1977). Some of the plans mentioned are very comprehensive and will be further discussed in Chapter 11, which focuses on overall healthcare system reform.

PAST EFFORTS AT CONTROLLING HEALTHCARE COSTS

Healthcare Planning and Cost-Containment

During the late 1960s and early 1970s, the federal government responded to the concerns of rising healthcare costs by adopting various regulatory mechanisms. Health planning emerged as one of the leading methods for controlling healthcare costs. While the federal government had always engaged in some planning, not until the late 1960s and early 1970s did healthcare planning become a dominant theme. Planning relies on a regulatory strategy and uses centralized decision-making to guide the allocation of resources and ensure access to services.

The rationale for healthcare planning is based on the argument of excess capacity in the healthcare system in general, and in the hospital industry in particular, as a significant contributor to rising healthcare costs. The argument was that there were too many hospitals, beds, and medical equipment, which not only created unnecessary expansion and duplication of expensive resources but also led to overutilization of medical facilities (Goodman 1980). Supply creates its own demand, following Roemer's (1961) argument that hospital beds tend to be filled (for a dissenting opinion on the validity of what is called Roemer's law, see Scandlen 2011). This excess capacity, expansion, and duplication were encouraged by factors such as the third-party payment system, the inability of the market to induce inefficient hospitals to reduce the number of beds or go out of business altogether, and competition among hospitals for prestige and physicians (Havighurst 1973).

Healthcare planning took the form, for the most part, of *certificate-of-need* (CON) legislation. It began at the state level and was adopted by the federal government with the Section 1122 program in 1972 and by the National Health Planning and Resource Development Act of 1974. The 1974 Act required all states to adopted CON legislation and to set up a planning process beginning at the local level, with agencies known as health systems agencies, or HSAs.

CON laws required hospitals to document community need to obtain approval for major capital expenditures for expansion of physical plants, equipment, and services. The primary purpose of these laws was to prevent unnecessary investment in facilities and services. The laws were also designed to prevent the entry of new providers in the healthcare market unless a clear need was demonstrated.

For a variety of reasons, the program had limit impact on healthcare spending, including lack of public support and capture of the health systems agencies by providers. The 1974 legislation was dismantled by the Reagan administration. As of 2018, 35 states had such programs (Cauchi and Noble 2018).

Professional Standards Review

One of the factors often cited as responsible for rising healthcare costs is overutilization of healthcare resources. The rise in healthcare costs since the enactment of Medicare and Medicaid programs in the mid-1960s created concern in Congress about the cost and quality of these programs, concerns that are still present more than 50 years after those two programs were created. The Social Security Amendments of 1972 established the Professional Standards Review Organization (PSRO) program. The PSRO was designed as a peer-review mechanism to promote effective yet efficient and economical delivery of healthcare services for government-financed programs such as Medicare and Medicaid. Under the law, more than 200 local PSROs were created and staffed by local physicians to review and monitor care provided to Medicare and Medicaid patients by hospitals, extended-care facilities, and skilled nursing homes. The PSROs were responsible for determining whether the care provided was medically necessary, of professional quality, and delivered in an appropriate healthcare facility. They also had the authority to deny approval of payment for services to physicians who provide care to Medicaid and Medicare patients. Two of the stated goals of the program were to eliminate unnecessary medical treatment and unnecessary institutionalization. Thus, the PSRO program was created as a regulatory mechanism for reducing the cost of federal healthcare programs.

As with the certificate-of-need program, the PSROs program had little impact on healthcare costs. The programs were controlled by local physicians and self-policing rarely works (Rosenberg 1984). Again, as with the CON program, the Reagan administration opposed the PSRO program. In 1982 it was transformed into the Peer Review Program and then eventually became Quality Improvement Organizations (QIO) in 2002. As the name suggests, the focus was no longer on cost-containment but on quality issues (Centers for Medicare and Medicaid Services 2006).

Price Regulation

The most interventionist of cost-containment strategies is price regulation. Here a government agency reviews prices and particular requests for increases, or sets them. Price regulation can include setting hospital rates, reviewing requests for increases in premiums on the part of health insurance companies, or, in some cases, setting levels that are charged by different providers. There has been experience with this at both the state and federal level.

At the state level, an example of price regulation is approvals required by states for health insurance companies' premium increases. Indeed, states have exercised considerable regulatory authority over health insurance companies beyond prices, such as quality and access. Price regulation encompasses some of the things we discussed in Chapter 7 on access. States might require community rating, where premiums may not be charged according to health status (Fish-Parcham 2006; Kofman and Pollitz 2006).

As we discussed in Chapters 1 and 3, states have an important role in many policy areas. Emanuel et al. (2016, 2) lay out all the different ways that states can affect healthcare, especially costs:

> States also have considerable authority over the regulation of health insurance and the provision of health care within their borders. States control their own insurance markets: They run their Medicaid and CHIP programs and state employee plans, and certain states run the exchanges for individual health insurance. States also control the rate review process, scope-of-practice regulations, physician licensing, antitrust laws, and provider and insurer regulations. Lastly, states and governors have considerable convening power to bring together diverse stakeholders, making reform efforts more politically feasible.

Under the Affordable Care Act (Chapter 3), insurance companies have to submit their requests for rate increases to the federal government. The legislation requires a certain percentage of premiums gathered to be spent on healthcare (the medical loss ratio) and prohibits higher premiums for people with preexisting conditions. States also have the authority to approve insurance premium requests, though this varies from state to state. In recent years, as health insurance companies had to deal with uncertain exchanges, whether federal or state (see Chapter 3), insurance premium requests have been in the double-digit range. For example, in 2018, New Jersey, based on a law passed in May 2018, approved insurance premium rate increases of 5.8 percent. Without the new law, health insurance companies might have requested a nearly-13-percent increase. In 2017, insurers raised premiums by 20 percent. New Jersey also created a reinsurance program that provides extra funds for insurance companies facing particularly high costs (Stainton 2018). Other states were faced with much larger premium requests. Stainton (2018) points to New York (about a 24-percent increase) and Maryland (about a 30-percent increase).

Another element that states could regulate is hospital charges. Seven states enacted such programs, though only one remains, in West Virginia. Atkinson's (2009) review found that when states regulated hospital rates, costs went up less than the national average. Such hospital rate regulation is politically difficult to maintain. And mandates to increase access tend to drive up costs. New (2005) found that the more mandates states imposed on health insurers, the higher the premiums.

States have also attempted to restrain costs through provider reimbursements in Medicaid. Under Medicaid, as we discussed in Chapter 4, states set the levels of reimbursements for physicians, hospitals, nursing homes, and so forth. This kind of control on provider reimbursements does have its tradeoffs. Physicians are not required to take Medicaid patients, so may choose not to serve such patients or may limit the percentage of their practice dedicated to Medicaid patients. It can also cause financial distress to hospitals that find that the cost of treating patients is considerably higher than the reimbursements.

The federal government briefly engaged in price regulation. In 1971, in response to what was considered high inflation, the Nixon administration imposed a wage-and-price control program. For that period of time, costs, though not necessarily spending, slowed down. The difference is that in response to the controls, providers, especially physicians, began to unbundle their services. Rather than charge for treating the patient during a visit, the health services delivered were broken down into its components—a blood test, an injection, etc., with each service billed separately. Thus, the more services delivered, the more income, even if prices and costs remained the same.

In 1974, the price control program was eliminated, with the healthcare industry promising to keep costs down. That did not happen, and the Carter administration proposed legislation in 1977 and 1979 that focused on hospital costs, the single-largest component of healthcare spending. The industry then proposed a "voluntary effort" as a substitute for government controls. When the Carter administration was unable to get such legislation passed, the voluntary effort, not surprisingly, had no volunteers and costs continued to rise (Altman and Levitt 2003; Davis and Stremikis 2009).

Davis and Stremikis (2009, 2) argue that had measures proposed by presidents Nixon, Carter, and Clinton been effective (the key problem in their analysis), we would be spending much less on healthcare than we do today:

> Each set out regulatory restraints on the growth in provider payment or insurance premiums, or both. All had significant mechanisms to control costs, including changing provider payment, increasing competition in the insurance market, and controlling the growth in private insurance premiums.

Assuming the programs would have worked, if the Nixon proposals had been adopted and there had been a 1.5-percent annual decrease in the rate of healthcare spending (for example, if spending increases in a given year were equal to 5 percent of GDP, under this scenario spending increases as a share of GDP would have been 3.5 percent), we would have spent 10.7 percent of our GDP on healthcare in 2010 instead of the 17.7 percent it turned out to be. If we started with the Carter proposal, then healthcare spending as a share of GDP in 2010 would have been an estimated 11.5 percent; if we had adopted the Clinton Health Security proposal, it would have been 14.2 percent (Davis and Stremikis 2009). Of course, that is assuming effectiveness of the proposals.

The Special Case of Maryland

We mentioned above that Maryland was the only state that regulated healthcare prices. In 2011, Maryland began an all-rate-payer model for hospital payments based on a program begun in 1971. It set up the Hospital System Cost Review Commission to set hospital rates for the states. In 1977, Maryland negotiated an agreement to bring in Medicare and Medicaid. The legislature and the Commission saw hospitals as public utilities, though with some modifications, with the idea that private markets would not engage in cost-containment. Further reforms occurred in 1993 and 2014 (Cohen n.d.; Anderson, Chaulk, and Fowler 1993; Sabatini et al. 2017; Huelskoetter 2018). Interestingly, and vital for its success, the Maryland Hospital Association (MHA) supported the program at its onset and continues to support it (Cohen n.d.). The 2014 agreement with the Centers for Medicare and Medicaid Services (CMS) allows the cost commission to set global budgets for hospitals. Hospitals, therefore, know in advance what their budget for the year will be and will have to live with it. How well has the Maryland program worked?

According to Cohen (n.d.), the successes have been impressive. Before the program began, hospital costs in Maryland were considerably higher than the national average. In 2005, the costs were more than 5 percent below the national average. From 1975 to 2005, hospital costs per admission were the lowest in the country. Huelskoetter (2018, 6) writes:

> According to the state Health Services Cost Review Commission (HSCRC), by the end of 2016, the new model had already generated $586 million in Medicare savings from reduced hospital spending growth, significantly exceeding the 2018 target of $330 million. On a per-capita basis, Maryland's all-payer annual hospital spending growth has been held to an average of 1.53 percent, beating the 3.58 percent target rate.

Other studies cited by Huelskoetter (2018) confirm the savings. Further, the quality of care for hospital patients has not been adversely affected, nor has there been any cost-shifting (Huelskoetter 2018; see also Sabatini et al. 2017).

Because they are the largest portion of healthcare expenditures, the focus of Maryland and some other states (Huelskoetter 2018), has been on hospitals. While there has been some discussion, the all-payer model has not been used for physician payments. Some states, such as Massachusetts, Oregon, and Arkansas, are looking at alternative models to restrain healthcare costs and the impact of those costs on state budgets.

Controlling Drug Prices

As discussed above, prescription drug prices are an important factor in growing healthcare expenditures and there is concern about continuing and very high prices. If we look at other Westernized, industrial countries, we see that their prescription medication prices, even for the same drugs used in the US, are much lower than in the US. The major reason for this that there is price regulation in those countries. In the United States, the Department of Defense and the Veterans Health Administration are allowed to negotiate with pharmaceutical companies. Medicare is explicitly forbidden from such negotiation, nor does Medicaid engage in it (Sarnak et al. 2017).

In the case of Medicare, there is some negotiation (Roy 2018), but it is with the Part D insurers and pharmaceutical companies (Congressional Budget Office 2014). The Congressional Budget Office (CBO) (2014) points out that competition among Part D insurers has an impact on drug prices. Where there are more competitors, there is some restraint in pricing. The result of the negotiations is that spending on Medicare Part D has come in below projections, though there are additional reasons why that happened. The other reasons include expiration of patents on name-brand drugs and the slowing down of new name-brand drugs. A third reason for spending below CBO projections was that enrollment in Part D was less than anticipated (Congressional Budget Office 2018).

Having said that, there is negotiation on drug prices in the private sector. Pharmacy benefit managers (PBM) can negotiate prices. Insurance companies generally do accept the prices. Where they can save money is in the formularies that insurers use. Formularies are a list of medications that the company will cover. Regulations are in place so that there is some choice of drugs and that every condition with a Food and Drug Administration (FDA)-accepted medication will have some drug on the list.

Pricing in this area, as in the larger healthcare system, tends to be opaque and confusing. Consider the following: patients with insurance often have co-payments, amounts they have to pay for the medication. But there are cases in which the co-payment is greater than the total cost of the payment. The patient/consumer would be better off buying the drug entirely out of pocket. The difference, known as a clawback, is kept by either the insurance company or the PBM or both. In many cases, pharmacists are not allowed to tell the buyer that she would save money by not using the insurance (Van Nuys et al. 2018).

What are possible policies that might limit drug prices? One is to let Medicare and Medicaid negotiate drug prices with the companies. Another is to allow imports of medications from other countries, which have lower prices. This is similar to the medical tourism discussed above. As might be expected, pharmaceutical companies oppose both policies because they would hurt their revenue stream (i.e., profits).

Another policy possibility is to focus on the patent issues. As Silver and Hyman (2018), among others, point out, patent protection effectively gives a drug company a monopoly on the newly developed, approved drug. Generic drugs, as we have seen, are considerably cheaper. Pharmaceutical companies argue that their pharmaceutical development costs are quite high, $500 million or more per drug, and the revenue from the price helps fund their continued research efforts. The companies also point out that other countries pay so much less for the drugs that prices in the US must be kept high to compensate.

A third possible policy, which applies to the larger healthcare system as well, is to increase price transparency. AARP ("Why Drug Prices Are So High" 2017) argues that it is difficult for consumers to understand the basis for drug costs, particularly the research and development costs. Perhaps the high costs are justified, but it is not clear that is the case.

A fourth possible policy is drug comparison ("Why Drug Prices Are So High" 2017). Is the new, more expensive drug better than an older drug? Is the new drug really different from a previous drug? Perhaps the new drug just adds some ingredient that seems to make it better (Silver and Hyman 2018). Such a proposal suggests the use of cost-effective analysis, where different alternatives are evaluated on the basis of cost and how well they work.

A fifth policy, a difficult one, is value-based pricing ("Why Are Drug Prices So High?" 2017). In this case, drugs that are proven to be more effective, that is, have more value, will be priced higher than drugs that are less effective, that is, have little value. Such decisions would be made by the payer, such as an insurance company. Other countries have used value-based pricing (Docteur and Lopert 2017) with some positive (i.e., cost-saving) results. An example of such a policy in the United States occurred in 2012 (Docteur and Lopert 2017). The Memorial Sloan Kettering Cancer Center decided not to use the cancer drug Zaltrap because its price was very high and there was no evidence that it was better than a drug the Center was already using. Interestingly, the manufacturer dramatically lowered the price of the drug, which raised its cost-effectiveness ratio.

Pharmaceutical Costs and the Trump Administration

The Trump administration, facing calls for addressing the issue of high drug prices, has moved, if slowly, toward some policy changes. One thing that has been done is that President Trump has called out some companies for their high prices, an example of "public shaming" (Mukherjee 2018). In the summer of 2018, the President called out two pharmaceutical companies, Novartis and Pfizer, for their price increases. As a result, both companies announced they would (temporarily) freeze prices (Thomas 2018b). In January 2019, pharmaceutical companies announced that they were raising prices on their products for the new year (Hopkins 2019).

Mukherjee (2018) drew three lessons that he said illustrated "the convoluted nature of American health policy." First, "Drug prices are arbitrary, companies hold the power." Second, and this is the case for many prices in the American healthcare system (Brill 2015), "List prices aren't the same as what patients pay." Think of a person considering the purchase of a new car. When going to a showroom, the prospective buying looks at the sticker price of the vehicle, what is called the manufacturer's suggested retail price or MSRP. What the buyer actually pays is most likely some amount less than that. The MSRP becomes a starting bargaining price. It is worth quoting Mukherjee (2018) at some length on this point:

> Following the setting of a list price, drug companies engage in a complicated dance with pharmacy benefits managers (PBMs) and insurance companies. These overwhelmingly opaque negotiations are what eventually determine what a patient pays for his or her medicine at the point of sale. And, often times, as recent reporting has shown, the various middlemen up and down the pharmaceutical supply chain pocket the rebates they negotiate with drug makers without necessarily passing the savings onto consumers.
>
> This is part of the reason pharma companies set high list prices in the first place—they know that they'll have to engage in a war of attrition with PBMs and insurers to get their products covered at all in the first place. But Americans who are uninsured may easily be left out to dry and face the full brunt of a list price.

Mukherjee's third point is that pharmaceutical companies are making less profit on their efforts. Rates of return on research and development costs were 3.2 percent in 2017. In 2009, they were 10.1 percent. Much of this has to do with, as mentioned previously, the expiration of important brand-name products. The incentive, Mukherjee (2018) continues, is to raise prices to make up for lost revenue. Because price regulation is lax or nonexistent, prices have gone up.

The Trump administration issued a proposal, a blueprint, to address the question of high and increasing drug costs (Department of Health and Human Services 2018). One part of the proposal is to limit the increases in medication prices administered in physician offices paid for Medicare Part B to overall inflation, as measured by the consumer price index (CPI). If that could be done, a considerable amount of money would be saved both for Medicare and patients. A second proposal is to move some medications from Medicare Part B coverage to Medicare Part D coverage. It should be pointed out here that under Medicare Part D, there is no limit on out-of-pocket spending. Another possibility is limited costly medications from Medicare Part D formularies (Department of Health and Human Services 2018; Roy 2018).

The blueprint makes other suggestions. These include requiring PBMs to give rebates to consumers, rather than retain them. Another proposal is to require direct-to-consumer television drug ads to include prices of the drugs. Other suggestions include allowing Medicare to bulk-purchase high-priced medications and to push for more biosimilars, essentially "genetic biotechnology drugs" (Department of Health and Human Services 2018; Roy 2018).

The blueprint is a series of proposals that need to be adopted by Congress or administratively. How likely are they work? Some have argued that the biggest element missing from the proposal is to allow Medicare to negotiate with manufacturers. Despite Roy's (2018) reassurance, the negotiations that do go on within Part D, but not Part B, are limited. Trump pledged during the 2016 campaign to allow Medicare to negotiate with the pharmaceutical companies (Perrone and Colvin 2018). Whether because of the administration's friendliness to industry of all kinds, or opposition from the industry lobbying group, the Pharmaceutical Research and Manufacturing Association (PhRMA), this was not included. Perhaps the most important part of the administration plans is to eliminate the kickbacks or rebates to PBMs (Goldman and Jena 2018).

HEALTH MAINTENANCE ORGANIZATIONS, HEALTHCARE RATIONING, MANAGED CARE, AND COST-CONTAINMENT

Health Maintenance Organizations

The CON, HSA, and PSRO programs are examples of behavioral regulations. These programs were designed to scrutinize decisions about utilization, expansion, and acquisition of healthcare resources by providers. They were based on the assumption that changing behavior and cutting waste could contain healthcare costs (Brown 1986). They were not very successful. There was more success with the Medicare prospective payment system. The Maryland rate regulation system also seems to have successfully restrained cost increases in that state. But overall healthcare costs and spending continued to increase.

During the early 1970s, the federal government also tried a competitive market strategy to contain healthcare costs through prepaid group plans (PGPs), commonly known as *health maintenance organizations* (HMOs). The concept of PGPs was not new. Such plans had existed in the healthcare system without any federal assistance since the 1920s. During the early 1970s, the number of HMOs grew as a result of favorable market conditions and rhetorical support provided by the Nixon administration.

Dr. Paul M. Ellwood Jr., a key health adviser to President Richard Nixon, is credited with bringing the competitive market strategy in the form of HMOs to the attention of national health policymakers (Falkson 1980). In 1970 the Nixon administration asked Congress to create a new HMO option for Medicare recipients. In 1971 the administration began to use discretionary funds to plan the development of about 100 HMOs around the country and asked Congress to create a special HMO development plan. The Department of Health, Education, and Welfare (now the Department of Health and Human Services) argued that there could be as many as 1700 HMOs within a few years, with perhaps as many as 40 million people enrolled (US Department of Health, Education, and Welfare 1971). After long debate, Congress passed the Health Maintenance Organization Act of 1973 (PL 93–222).

The federal government assumed the role of venture capitalist (Iglehart 1980). It encouraged the development of HMOs in an attempt to induce competition in the healthcare market with the hope of containing health costs. This market strategy was designed to eliminate, or at least reduce, centralized healthcare bureaucracy and replace it with decentralized market building. This was to be accomplished through the use of federal funds to support efforts in developing new healthcare organizations and alternative means of healthcare delivery. It promised pluralism, choice, efficiency, and reorganization through competition, markets, and incentives (Ellwood 1971; Havighurst 1970). The expectation was that HMOs would contain costs by (1) creating incentives for channeling health service utilization from costly inpatient settings (hospitals, skilled nursing homes, etc.) to less-costly outpatient settings (visits to doctors' offices), (2) promoting competition with traditional healthcare delivery systems, and (3) exercising market power by obtaining preferential prices from various healthcare providers (Falkson 1980–1981).

An HMO is a prepaid medical practice delivering a comprehensive set of healthcare services to enrollees for a fixed fee (capitation) paid in advance. The Health Maintenance Organization Act of 1973 provided for an expenditure of $375 million over five years. Most of these funds were used to encourage development of HMOs by providing start-up costs. The law offered federally qualified HMOs three basic benefits: (1) money for development of HMOs; (2) overriding of certain restrictive state laws; and (3) a mandate to employers, covered by the Fair Labor Standards Act of 1938, that employ 25 or more employees to offer HMO coverage as an alternative to whatever other health plans they provide. This was designed to provide healthcare consumers with at least a dual choice in health plans. In return, to qualify for federal funds, HMOs were to deliver a comprehensive package of benefits to a broadly representative population on an equitable basis with consumer participation. This was to be done at the same price as, or at a lower price than, traditional forms of health insurance (Rosoff 1975).

The original legislation was burdensome and limited the development of HMOs. Amendments in the late 1970s removed some of the burdens and deregulated much of this sector. In 1981, the federal government stopped providing grants, dropping its venture capital role. Since then, the federal government has focused its attention on the promotion of competition in general, incentives designed to increase private-sector involvement in HMO development, and risk contracts to HMOs that agree to enroll Medicare beneficiaries (Medicare Advantage plans). The health maintenance strategy morphed or transformed into the managed-care strategy (see below).

Healthcare Rationing

One way of addressing rising healthcare costs is rationing. The major concept behind rationing is that there are limits to what we can expect and afford in the way of healthcare. It is based on the notion that healthcare costs are rising disproportionately compared to the small or marginal gains in overall national health. Therefore, we must establish priorities in health services and become more rational in our healthcare spending.

Advocates of this school of thought argue that healthcare costs are out of control and that regulatory controls on spending or competitive approaches based on economic incentives are doomed to fail. Regulatory approaches are, it is asserted, based on the faulty assumption that medical care produces health, and more care produces more health. The only realistic solution, therefore, is the rationing of healthcare resources. If the United States is serious about containing healthcare costs, society will have to forgo some medical benefits, and patients should not expect to receive all the care they want regardless of the costs (Aaron and Schwartz 1984, 1990). Proponents argue that healthcare rationing already exists in the actions of insurance companies, legislatures, hospitals, physicians, and individual premium payers, and we need to get on with the public business of determining how healthcare rationing should be carried out ethically (Menzel 1990). Observers call the existing de facto rationing "silent rationing," "under-the-table rationing," "rationing by finance," or "rationing by wallet" (Mechanic 1997).

Hoffman (2013) examines rationing in the United States and notes that the term is rarely used, and when it is, it is in a pejorative sense. The disputes over so-called "death panels" and comparative effectiveness analysis in the debate over the Affordable Care Act underscore Hoffman's observation. But she also notes that in the United States there is no right to healthcare, and healthcare is rationed on the basis of price. The US has done this kind of rationing since 1930.

All countries engage in some form of rationing (Patel and Rushefsky 2002). In the United States, the major example of rationing is in organ transplantation. There are many more people who need new lungs, kidneys, hearts, and so forth than there are available organs. Both state and federal laws govern the process of deciding who will receive the organs (see President's Council on Bioethics 2003). These include the Uniform Anatomical Gift Act of 1968 and the Organ Transplantation Act of 1984.

As Porter (2012) points out, rationing is inevitable because of limited resources (such as the number of providers). In the United States, we tend to ration depending on financial capability: "You get care if you have the money to pay for it; if not, you probably won't" (Porter 2012). Porter notes that various healthcare proposals from different sides of the political spectrum include, implicitly, some type of rationing. Paul Ryan (R-WI), then chair of the House Budget Committee and the Republican vice-presidential candidate in 2012, offered a plan that would limit spending on Medicare but would give seniors money to purchase their own health insurance plans.

The Affordable Care Act, Porter (2012) notes (see also Nix 2012), also contains provisions that are effectively a form of rationing:

> by levying a tax on "Cadillac" insurance plans, and in turn pushing employers to seek cheaper options and lower costs. It creates an advisory board to cut costs from Medicare if spending rises above a set rate. And it finances an institute to evaluate which therapies are most clinically effective. Careful to avoid political blowback, the president's plan forbids Medicare to base its reimbursement decisions on the institute's findings.

Managed Competition

Some proposals to address the cost problems, such as rationing, focus on the demand for healthcare services. Others focus on the supply of such services. The first attempt at a supply-side, market-reform solution came in the 1960s and 1970s. This was the health maintenance strategy discussed above. The strategy, the brainchild of Dr. Paul Ellwood, was an elegant concept (Bauman 1976; Falkson 1980). Based on already existing prepaid group plans (PGPs), the idea was to limit the money available to providers through a capitation system. The health maintenance organization enrolls subscribers, who pay a monthly premium. The premiums constitute the total budget for the HMO. Providing more services does not produce more revenues. As a result, the incentive was not to overtreat, as market reformers argue is done in the fee-for-service system, but to treat only as necessary. The HMO became the prototype of a *managed-care organization* (in 1990s language), one that would review services and try to eliminate unnecessary care (see below).

There was a further hope behind the HMO strategy: HMOs would create competitive pressures on the fee-for-service system so that all providers and insurers would begin to look at costs. As HMOs penetrated a market, competitive pressures would increase. This idea was embodied in the 1973 Health Maintenance Organization Act to promote, with federal assistance, the development of HMOs. Into the 1980s, at least, the competitive impact of the strategy was questionable.

The second stage came in the late 1970s and early 1980s. Alain Enthoven (1978a, 1978b, 1980) took the competitive strategy a step further by suggesting a complete reorganization of the healthcare system, in essence national health insurance. Originally writing in the 1970s in the *New England Journal of Medicine* (and other journals) and then in his book *Health Plan*, Enthoven wanted to eliminate the employment-based health insurance. Enthoven's plan, originally called the Consumer-Choice Health Plan or CCHP, was a form of a voucher or premium support plan (Rushefsky 1981). Providers and insurers would organize into competitive healthcare plans. Each plan would then determine what its premiums would be. The federal government would estimate the average cost of care in various geographical areas and pay a percentage of that average cost through tax credits or 100 percent of the average cost for the poor via vouchers. CCHP featured an open-enrollment period, community rating (see Chapter 7), and a limit on out-of-pocket costs. Consumers would then choose among the competing plans, which could include a traditional fee-for-service plan, an HMO, a plan with a very high deductible, and so forth. Each plan would charge a different premium, but the federal government would pay the same amount regardless of the plan chosen. Thus, consumers would face the decision of what plan to choose depending on the financial consequences for them. The newly regained place of price signals plus open enrollments would create the competition among the plans and (it was hoped) restrain costs. Healthcare would be consumer-driven rather than cost-driven.

A less ambitious version of the CCHP built on the employment-based insurance system already in place. For those with work-based insurance, the employer would pay the same premium for each employee regardless of which plan was chosen. Employees would have a choice of plans, with similar features, as mentioned above. For the poor or those without employment-based insurance, vouchers from the federal government could be used.

Two developments among public employers provided some experience with choosing among competitive plans. The Federal Employees Health Benefits Program (FEHBP) allows federal employees to choose among competing plans, while the federal government provides level premium contributions. A similar program established in California, the California Public Employees' Retirement System (CalPERS), enrolls nearly 1 million public employees at all levels of government. CalPERS is a purchasing cooperative that negotiates with a number of different plans, such as HMOs, preferred-provider organizations (PPOs), and traditional fee-for-service plans.

The most recent development is the creation of healthcare markets. The 2003 Medicare Modernization Act (see Chapter 5) created the Part D prescription drug benefit. Medicare recipients would choose from among a number of plans and could, during enrollment periods, choose the plan that best met the beneficiary's needs in terms of availability of needed medications and prices. Presumably, lower-price plans will lead other plans to lower their prices. A second development, again in Medicare, is medigap policies. These are policies through which beneficiaries chose plans in a similar manner as the Part D plans, hopefully with a similar impact. The third development began in Massachusetts, with the passage of a health reform act in 2006. It created health insurance connectors or exchanges where people could purchase a plan, with subsidies for those who are eligible ("Massachusetts Health Care Reform: Six Years Later" 2012). As we saw in Chapter 3, the Massachusetts plan became the model for the Affordable Care Act with its federal and state exchanges.

Managed Care

> By managed care, we mean forms of coverage that integrate financing and delivery, as well as the organizations that provide this coverage—health maintenance organizations (HMOs), preferred-provider organizations (PPOs), and point-of-service (POS) plans.
>
> (Gold and Hurley 1997, 29)

> The bottom line is that the American public doesn't want to give too much power to *any bureaucrats*. It doesn't matter whether they work for the federal government or for the insurance industry.
>
> (Schneider 1998, 1714)

Definitions

One important and confusing aspect of policy debates and experiences with managed care is definitional. In this section, we offer some definitions.

We define *managed care* broadly as any health insurance plan that seeks to restrain the use of healthcare services. Such restraint can be as simple as requiring preauthorization for a nonemergency hospital stay (Weinder and de Lissovoy 1993; for a discussion of the symbolic significance of definitions, particularly in regard to managed care, see Hacker and Marmor 1999). Plans can also encompass more organized forms of provider delivery.

The classic type of managed-care organization is the *health maintenance organization* (HMO), which we discussed above. An HMO is an organization whose providers, generally primary-care physicians, are prepaid through monthly subscriber premiums (known as *capitation*) to deliver a comprehensive set of services. The HMO assumes the financial risk of providing those services. The original label for such an organization was *prepaid group plan* (PGP). PGPs were developed to provide healthcare services to employees in areas where medical services were thin. Kaiser-Permanente is typical of such plans.

HMOs come in various forms. A *staff-model HMO* is one in which the physicians are on a salary and members obtain services primarily from the HMO. In a *group-model HMO*, a multispecialty group of doctors works primarily for the HMO's members. There are hybrid versions of these HMOs.

Another type of managed-care organization, the most common, is the *preferred-provider organization* (PPO). Here the employer or insurer contracts with physicians for discount rates on services. Consumers can use providers outside the PPO but must pay higher co-payments.

The Development of Managed Care

The push in the 1980s and 1990s came from the private sector, particularly large employers. The impetus was partly the drastically increasing cost of health insurance and partly the decreases in corporate profits and a weak economy (Bodenheimer and Sullivan 1998; Leyerle 1994). For example, the cost of employee healthcare for General Motors in the mid-1980s was twice the cost of steel, a problem that remains for the giant corporation, 30 years later.

Buchanan (1998) has outlined five cost-containment techniques that are commonly identified with the concept of managed care. One technique is payment limits. An example of such a technique is the use of DRGs by the federal government to reimburse hospitals for Medicare patient fees. A second technique is a requirement of pre-authorization for medical services, such as surgeries. A third technique is the use of primary-care physicians as "gatekeepers" to control access to specialists. A fourth technique is "de-skilling" (i.e., using less-trained providers to provide certain services). A fifth technique is to provide financial incentives to physicians to limit utilization of care. Another technique used by MCOs is provider networks. In this case, the insurer (MCO) includes some but not all of the providers in a network. If a subscriber uses an out-of-network provider, the MCO will cover less of the costs of the service and, in some cases, none of the costs. Managed care is a fancy name for rationing.

The first significant move by a large employer into managed care came in 1988, when Allied-Signal canceled its healthcare plans and transferred its employees into Cigna's HMO (Bodenheimer and Sullivan 1998; see also Anders 1996). Other large companies soon followed. The trend toward managed care can be easily shown. In 1988, 73 percent of workers who had employer-based health insurance were enrolled in conventional fee-for-service plans. Sixteen percent were enrolled in health maintenance organizations, and another 11 percent in preferred-provider organizations. By 2017, less than 1 percent of covered workers were in conventional plans, while about 72 percent of covered workers were in some form of managed-care plan (Claxton et al. 2017).

The public plans, Medicare and Medicaid, as discussed in Chapter 4, have also seen growth in enrollment in managed-care organizations. In the case of Medicare, recipients can choose whether to enroll in private plans through the Medicare Advantage (Part C) program. As we saw in Chapter 5, by 2017 about one-third of Medicare recipients were enrolled in Medicare Advantage plans. Much of the increase in enrollment began in 2005 (Gold et al. 2013).

Medicaid recipients often do not have the luxury of choosing whether to enroll in a managed-care plan. Thus, such enrollment is higher for Medicaid than for Medicare. In 2016, 81 percent of Medicaid recipients were so enrolled ("Medicaid Managed Care Enrollment and Program Characteristics 2016" 2018; see Chapter 4).

One of the important changes in managed care is the rise of preferred-provider organizations (PPOs). Part of this change was due to a backlash on the part of consumers and doctors against more stringent, controlling managed plans. PPOs differ from traditional health insurance plans in two ways. In PPOs, the insurer takes an active role in negotiating payment rates or selecting providers, and the providers are on notice to comply with aggressive utilization review procedures.

Has the use of managed care helped to contain healthcare costs? The success of such a strategy depends on the creation of healthcare delivery systems that are more efficient than the traditional system, and that are able to compete on price, benefits, access, style of medical care, and the existence of sufficient numbers of such systems throughout the country (Moran 1997).

Pinkovskiy (2013) finds that there was, indeed, a positive impact of the managed care revolution. That is, healthcare cost increases decreased in the 1993–2001 period. When the backlash came, led by physicians and consumer groups, healthcare costs rose. The backlash was due to the restrictions that MCOs placed on physicians, such as requiring pre-authorization by the MCO before a treatment was allowed, or restrictions on the allowable number of treatments for a given condition. Health maintenance organizations, the most common type of MCO at the time, took a beating for their cost-control measures. Anders (1996), among others, took HMOs to task for refusing to cover services because it saved the HMO money, even if it adversely affected the health of subscribers. The 1997 movie *As Good as It Gets* contains a scene where a mom, trying to keep medical care for son, curses out an HMO, with the doctor she is talking to pretty much in agreement. As Lesser, Ginsburg, and Devers (2003) point out, in the period of the late 1990s and early 2000s, a number of states passed what were called patient bill-of-rights laws that limited the ability of MCOs to engage in the strict cost control. MCOs backed off and preferred-provider organizations, a less-strict MCO model, became more prevalent. While the federal government did not pass a patient bill-of-rights law, the Affordable Care Act incorporated many of the ideas of such laws (Chapter 3). Pinkovskiy (2013) finds that the easing of the managed-care revolution led to higher spending on healthcare, what he estimates as about a 2-percent higher portion of GDP.

Both Medicare and Medicaid have, as we have seen, turned to increasingly to managed care for their recipients. The data on savings are mixed.

It is clear that managed care, if strictly implemented, can save money. The pain or perceived pain caused by the restrictions (rationing), however, make the stricter policy more politically difficult.

WELLNESS PROGRAMS

Another set of initiatives consists of employee wellness programs. Larger employers are increasingly promoting programs designed to encourage healthier lifestyles and behavior. By 2015, about 70 percent of employers offered such a program (Valet 2015). Many employers offer risk assessment screenings (Claxton et al. 2017). The emphasis is on preventive care to reduce the need for healthcare services. The assumption here is that prevention will lead to healthier workers and therefore reduced healthcare costs. The focus is on such lifestyle issues as smoking and obesity, as well as disease management related to chronic diseases (see Fleming 2005). Wellness programs can include financial incentives to join a fitness club and encouraging employees to provide biometrics testing (for example, of cholesterol and blood-sugar levels). The Affordable Care Act contains incentives for employers to offer such programs. By 2014, 16 states had adopted wellness programs for their employees and another 16 had adopted laws that regulated such programs in the private sector (Pomeranz et al. 2016). Medicare Advantage plans will pay for their subscribers to join fitness centers (the Silver Sneakers program).

As with many programs, there are variations in the details. One plan might penalize someone for not participating, while another might reward such a participant (Mitts 2012). But the big question for this chapter is: do such programs save on healthcare costs? In one sense it is difficult to tell because the results of preventive activities are often not apparent for decades (smoking cessation programs are a good example). Given that it is much rarer that an employee will stay with the same company for all of her worklife, employers may not actually experience any benefits. The evidence overall is unclear, though the impact on the larger healthcare system could be dramatic (Appleby 2012; Draper, Tynan, and Christianson 2012; Mattke et al. 2013).

COST-SHARING

A major strategy for reducing employer healthcare costs, in both the public and private sectors, is cost-sharing or cost-shifting. The patient shares in the direct cost of healthcare services for his or her own coverage, or that of dependents. Cost-sharing includes deductibles, coinsurance, or co-payments, as well as increased premiums. A deductible is the fixed amount that must be paid by the patient before the insurance benefits begin. Coinsurance is the percentage contribution that patients pay once the deductible is exceeded. Co-payments are a fixed contribution, rather than a percentage contribution, toward each unit of service. This strategy helps reduce the cost to the employers by shifting part of the cost to the patient. It is based on the belief that when patients are made to share a higher cost for treatment (negative incentive), they will reduce health service utilization. Some studies have demonstrated that cost-sharing in the form of deductibles or coinsurance reduces the use of healthcare services (Lee and Tollen 2002; Newhouse et al. 1981; Robinson 2002). Others have argued that increased cost-shifting is not in the best interest of the workers, that some of the cost savings are illusory, and that such savings are likely to be one-time savings (Davis et al. 1990). Whatever the case, more and more employers are seeking to reduce costs through cost-sharing.

When a deductible is charged, the average amount for family coverage (2017 data) was $4,527. Preferred-provider organizations tend to require their subscribers to have a deductible; the average amount was $2,503. For those enrolled in high-deductible health plans (HDHP), all members pay a deductible; the average deductible amount for those in a small firm was $6,633; for a large firm, the average deductible was $3,898 (Claxton et al. 2017). In the 2006–2012 period, HMOs experienced the largest annual average increase in deductibles, 12.8 percent, and high-deductible health plans saw the smallest average increase in deductibles, 2 percent (calculated from Claxton et al. 2012). Premiums are also lower for HDHP plans than for the other types (Claxton et al. 2012).

That is the tradeoff the high-deductible health plans make—lower premiums but higher deductibles. It is the same trade-off with the ACA exchanges: the lower premium-cost plans (bronze plans) have higher cost-sharing, the higher-cost plans (such as the platinum plans) have lower cost-sharing. Of course, with the ACA exchanges, there are subsidies for subscribers depending on income (Chapter 3).

Public employers are also increasingly engaging in cost-sharing/shifting. This is partly because of fiscal issues facing governments and because Republican governors have been increasingly successful in cutting back on benefits to state employees (Cauchon 2012).

COST-CONTAINMENT IN THE TWENTY-FIRST CENTURY

The cost of healthcare in the United States is certainly of pressing concern. Some of the policies enacted in the twentieth century had an impact but, for various reasons, were not sustainable. The large federal deficits are driven, in part, by the huge Medicare and Medicaid programs. Employers are looking for ways to decrease the cost of health benefits for their employees. Medicaid takes a big bite out of state budgets. Healthcare costs are a significant portion of family budgets.

A study by the Urban Institute (Holahan et al. 2011) examined different strategies for cost-containment and estimated their impact. One strategy that they examined was to cap the tax exclusion for health insurance premiums paid by employers. The argument here is that insurance protects consumers from the cost of their care, which is, of course, the point of insurance. By lowering the cost at the point of service, the argument goes, consumers will utilize more healthcare than if they had to pay the full cost, or more of the cost. This is the moral hazard argument. Holahan et al. (2011) estimate that reducing the tax exclusion would lower national health expenditures in the 2014–2023 period by about 1.5 percent. This would also have an impact on federal deficits, as it would lower a tax expenditure (income excused from taxation), resulting in increased revenue.

Several of the strategies focus on patient care. These include disease prevention, coordination of care, and end-of-life care. Disease-prevention strategies include raising taxes on cigarettes as a means of reducing consumption, a set of strategies to reduce the onset of asthma attacks at home (such as reducing the amount of dust in homes, plus education), and taxing sweetened beverages (again to reduce consumption and the obesity that may result at least partially from such consumption). Holahan et al. (2011) estimate that such actions could save more than $224 billion over the ten-year period, about 0.6 percent of national health expenditures.

The second patient care strategy is better coordination of care. This is especially important for those with chronic conditions, such as asthma, diabetes, disabilities, and so on. Patients may have multiple chronic conditions. Medicaid and Medicare fund many patients with these conditions and the costs are high. Holahan et al. (2011) estimate that people in these categories account for about 30 percent of healthcare spending. Another estimate is that 84 percent of the population have at least one chronic disease (Ginsburg 2012).

Goetzel et al. (2012) found that there is a significant relationship between health risks and healthcare spending. The ten health risks are depression, high blood glucose levels, high blood pressure, high body weight, tobacco use, physical inactivity, stress, high cholesterol levels, poor nutrition and eating habits, and high alcohol consumption. They argue that workplace programs to reduce the risks from these factors could reduce healthcare spending.

The US healthcare system is fragmented. Patients with multiple chronic conditions will see different providers for each of their chronic conditions. No single provider or provider organization may be in charge or responsible for patient care. Medicare and Medicaid share patients (dual eligibles) but pay for different aspects of healthcare (Medicare focuses more on short-term care and Medicaid more on long-term care). While the cost savings from care coordination are uncertain, Holahan et al. (2011, 16) note that the more successful programs have the following characteristics:

> Targeting interventions to those most likely to benefit, in-person contact, access to timely information on hospital admissions and emergency room visits, close interaction between care coordinators and primary care physicians, and emphasis on teaching self-management skills.

Savings from care coordination would come from reductions in spending on long-term care and from less use of hospitals and pharmaceuticals (Holahan et al. 2011). Holahan et al. (2011) estimate that coordination based on these principles and better coordination between the two giant public insurance programs would save an estimated 0.9 percent on national health expenditures over a ten-year period. It is important to note the uncertainty in this estimate. The estimate of savings could be as much as $331.1 billion over this period, but the low estimate of savings is close to zero.

An important strategy for cost-containment focuses on end-of-life care. As we discussed above, one of the cost issues is the concentration of expenditures (Berk and Monheit 2001). A small proportion of the population accounts for a very large percentage of national healthcare expenditures. This is as true within Medicare as well as the overall healthcare system. Holahan et al. (2011) observe that as much as 30 percent of Medicare spending went for those in the last year of their life, about 5 percent of the Medicare population. Further, much of the healthcare given to those near the end of their life is unwanted by patients and family and often reduces the quality of the patient's life (see Chapter 9). One solution is not to engage in undesired or undesirable heroic but futile treatment.

The alternative is to provide palliative care, care that eases the discomfort of the dying patient, either at home or in a hospice setting. Here is where end-of-life counseling would come in. Holahan et al. (2011) estimate modest savings from focusing on end-of-life care, about 0.3 percent of healthcare spending.

Of course, there are ethical issues related to these kinds of considerations. Physicians have an inbred desire to do all they can to help their patients. We certainly should not allow people to die just to save money. And end-of-life counseling became part of the debate over the Affordable Care Act as critics asserted, falsely, that the proposed legislation required so-called "death panels" for Medicare patients (Starr 2013).

Fraud, Waste, and Cost Control

One of the interesting targets for controlling costs is fraud and waste in healthcare spending. Shortly after the demise of the Clinton plan in 1994, the authors conducted a survey of health policy experts about the problems of the healthcare system and appropriate remedies (Patel and Rushefsky 1998). The policy experts saw problems such as the fee-for-service payment system and overall fragmentation of the healthcare system. We then compared our findings with public opinion polls and found disagreement between the experts and the general public. For the public, the major problem was fraud and waste in the healthcare system. As a side note, we should point out that the public's view of the problems of the healthcare system required virtually no changes on their part, unlike those of the experts.

To a certain extent, the public's view on waste and abuse was fairly accurate. Recent studies, as we saw above, attribute much of US spending to waste and abuse of the system (Goldman 2012; Lallemand 2012b; Silver and Hyman 2018). One estimate is that waste, separate from fraud and abuse, can cost as much as $650 billion a year, much higher than the savings estimated by Holahan et al. (2011) for all their strategies. The Institute of Medicine (Smith et al. 2012) estimates that waste in the American healthcare system is about $765 billion a year.

Waste can be defined as:

> spending on services that lack evidence of producing better health outcomes compared to less-expensive alternatives; inefficiencies in the provision of healthcare goods and services; and costs incurred while treating avoidable medical injuries, such as preventable infections and hospitals.
>
> (Lallemand 2012b, 1)

Fraud and abuse may be defined as below.

> "Fraud" refers to illegal activities in which someone gets something of value without having to pay for it or earn it, such as kickbacks or billing for services that were not provided. "Abuse" occurs when a provider or supplier bends rules or doesn't follow good medical practices, resulting in unnecessary costs or improper payments. Examples include the overuse of services or providing unnecessary tests.
>
> (Goldman 2012, 1)

In addressing the waste, fraud, and abuse issues, and indeed constraining costs in general, it is highly useful to remember that every dollar spent on healthcare is a dollar of revenue for someone. Reducing payments to providers, as has been done in Medicare and Medicaid, means less revenue for those providers. Cutting back on waste or profits means less revenue for someone.

Let us address the waste issue first. Earlier we mentioned the malpractice issue and tort reform. The study by Holahan et al. (2011) and others (Kelly and Fabius 2010; Van Den Bos et al. 2011) suggests more can be saved by reducing medical error than by tort reform. For example, hospital-acquired infections cost over $4 billion a year (Van Den Bos et al. 2011; "Medical Errors Cost Health Care System Billions" 2011; Wachter and Shojania 2004). Van Den Bos et al. (2011) found that most of the medical errors, including hospital-based infections, could be accounted for by ten types, suggesting that preventive efforts should be focused on those.

One way to reduce the number of medical errors (and increase the quality of care) is to develop systems and processes that focus on areas where medical errors are likely to occur. Atul Gawande (2007) offers a series of checklists that limit, if not eliminate, medical errors (see also Pearl 2017). Gawande (2007) points out that there is resistance to such checklists based on medical culture. Pearl (2017) adds to that idea the insights of cognitive psychology about the continued resistance to such changes (obviously not on the part of all providers).

Goodman, Villarreal, and Jones (2011) offer an intriguing, market-based idea. They write that patients should be offered voluntary no-fault insurance against the possibility of an error. By doing so, patients would give up their rights to sue. Patients could also enhance the insurance policy by making additional payments. The premiums would be paid by physicians and hospitals and be experienced-rated. That is, providers with a record of medical errors would pay higher premiums. Providers would naturally wish to avoid the higher premiums and thus put the appropriate systems into place. These include "electronic health records, error-reducing software, and other safety innovations" (Goodman, Villarreal, and Jones 2011, 594). Goodman, Villarreal, and Jones (2011) state that quality would be overseen by insurance companies and that the higher premiums paid would lead consumers to search for alternative providers; here is the use of prices and markets to achieve a goal.

Another set of policies in this area focuses on overuse or overdiagnosis (Brawley and Goldberg 2011; Brownlee 2007; Rosenthal 2017; Silver and Hyman 2018; Welch, Schwartz, and Woloshin 2011). Lallemand (2012a) estimates that overdiagnosis or overtreatment costs as much as $226 billion in unnecessary spending. She defines overtreatment as "care that is rooted in outmoded habits, that is driven by providers' preferences rather than those of informed patients, that ignores scientific findings, or that is motivated by something other than provision of optimal care for a patient." One example Lallemand (2012a, 2) provides is defensive medicine, based on the medical error/malpractice problem. Providers may do additional testing of patients to ensure that all that could possibly be done has been done and to avoid a lawsuit.

Welch, Schwartz, and Woloshin (2011) attribute much of the problem of overtreatment/overdiagnosis to a paradigm of early prevention and diagnostic screening. They argue that by doing early screenings, using advances in technology, more people are categorized as having a condition or potential condition that requires some kind of treatment (on this point, see the discussion of numbers in Stone 2012). Two of their examples are screenings for prostate and breast cancer. Their recommendation is a paradigm shift away from early screening.

While the idea behind these concepts is fairly straightforward and should be noncontroversial, in fact it is not (Patashnik, Gerber, and Dowling 2017). Practitioners see themselves as already utilizing evidence-based medicine based on experiences with their patients, as well as keeping up with the scientific literature. Timble et al. (2012) suggest five sets of reasons why the results of such research may not be adopted or might be delayed in clinical practice. The first is financial incentives that discourage such adoption. As one example, insurance coverage of various treatments may vary. More traditional treatments may be covered, while alternatives or even counseling about alternatives may not be. The following quote will give a taste of the problems that comparative effective and evidence-based medicine face:

> Under fee-for-service payment systems, however, invasive treatments ... are generously reimbursed, while counseling patients about treatment options goes most unreimbursed. Meanwhile, most payers impose few coverage or payment obstacles for many invasive procedures, either because their appropriateness cannot be monitored or because payers are likely to face organized challenges from pharmaceutical or device manufacturers, professional societies, or patient advocates when they attempt to use comparative effectiveness evidence to modify coverage policies.
>
> (Timble et al. 2012, 2169)

Even something like the interpretation of evidence from scientific trials is subject to economic incentives. Pharmaceutical companies will take measures to control the message or frame the meaning of the results of scientific studies, including television advertising, educating practitioners, and so forth (Timble et al. 2012; on framing and interpretation, see Stone 2012). George Lakoff (2008; see also Bai 2005) has written about the importance of framing in politics. Pharmaceutical companies have a financial stake in promoting the efficacy of their products over alternatives (see Abramson 2004).

A second problem is the ambiguity of evidence (Timble et al. 2012). Because scientific evidence is frequently nonconclusive or problematic, it lends itself to interpretation and criticism. Much of this takes the form of a methodological critique, focusing on the methods used in a particular study. This is often the case in scientific disputes, say, over global warming (for a discussion of this, see Patel and Rushefsky 2005).

The third barrier is cognitive biases (Pearl 2017). Timble et al. (2012) point to several such biases. One is confirmation bias: favoring evidence that confirms what someone believes and then rejecting alternative studies. A second bias is to prefer doing something, even if the effectiveness of that something is limited, to doing nothing. A third is a bias in favor of newer over older technology.

The fourth barrier is the failure to think about how and when practitioners need and want the information and for what purpose. The final barrier is limited use of tools, particularly information technologies, to support the use of evidence-based medicine and comparative effective research.

Such research faces other barriers. Comparative effectiveness research has been linked to rationing. For example, Nix (2012) argues that comparative effectiveness research can be used by government bureaucrats to affect decisions made by practitioners and their patients. Nix states, for example, that in an effort to control the costs of Medicare, rationing is occurring through "so-called improvements in value and efficiency" (2012, 5). Indeed, Nix takes exception to the whole idea of quality measures. For one thing, she notes that providers cannot by themselves improve patient outcomes. At least some of the outcome is based on patient behavior (a lesson that those who would put all the responsibility for student achievement on teachers might wish to pay attention to).

On the other hand, Volsky (2009) argues that comparative effectiveness research will not lead to rationing. Rather, the government will provide information and, recognizing the ambiguity of such research, not impose guidelines on doctors. He also notes that the Affordable Care Act prohibits the government agency that examines comparative effectiveness research, the Center for Health Outcomes, from mandating changes in practice or coverage.

Another possible place for savings, at least in theory, is in administrative costs, discussed above. A much higher percentage of healthcare spending is accounted for by administrative costs in the United States than in countries with national healthcare systems. Woolhandler, Campbell, and Himmelstein (2003) found that administrative costs in the United States were about three times as much as in Canada (see also Bartlett 2012). Papanicolas et al. (2018) point to administrative costs as an important driver of high healthcare costs. The United States had the highest administrative costs of eight Westernized, industrial countries (Papanicolas et al. 2018). Himmelstein et al. (2014) found that just over 25 percent of hospital expenditures in the US were attributable to administrative costs. They attribute the high costs to the complexity and fragmentation of payment systems and to difficulties in raising capital.

A related point is whether Medicare's administrative costs are lower than those of private insurance companies. This turns out to be very much an ideological debate. Tyson (2012), for example, makes the argument that they are. She points out, additionally, that Medicare can negotiate for prices better than private insurance because of the size of the program and the number of enrollees. Private insurance also garners profits, which Medicare obviously does not. This is one of the arguments behind Senator Bernie Sanders' (I-VT) Medicare for All plan (see Chapter 11). Not having a large number of payers should save money.

Pearson (2018; see also Frakt 2018) reviewed the literature on administrative costs, focusing on three elements: "billing and insurance-related (BIR) costs, hospital administration, and physician practice administration." Her review produced estimates of BIR costs as high as 25 percent of healthcare expenditures. Administrative costs for the other two elements provided estimated revenue for hospitals of over 12 percent and 10 percent for physicians. Pearson (2018) cites the figure from Himmelstein et al. (2014) that administrative costs might be as high as 25 percent of total healthcare expenditures. Pearson (2018) also notes that the administrative costs are increasing.

Part of the debate is how one measures administrative costs. Liberals such as Krugman (2009) and Hacker (2009) point to the lower overhead cost of Medicare and use as their measure of administrative costs the ratio of such costs to overall expenditures. In that case, Medicare wins: 3 percent compared to as much as 40 percent in the individual insurance market.

Conservatives take great exception to this. As mentioned above, Roy (2011) argues that Medicare is assisted by other agencies, such as the Internal Revenue Service, the Social Security Administration, and the Department of Health and Human Services. Roy also points out that private insurers pay state taxes on the premiums collected, which Medicare does not (see also Silver and Hyman 2018). He also notes the importance of the size of Medicare with its economies of scale that give it an advantage (a point also made by Klein 2009). Roy (2011) asserts that the appropriate measure for comparing administrative costs is cost per patient. In that case, Medicare's administrative costs are higher than private insurance.

Klein (2009) argues that there are difficulties in measuring administrative costs. In any event, he thinks that any savings from reducing administrative costs would be fairly small and not touch upon the real drivers of overall healthcare costs.

Pearson (2018), while supportive of a single-payer plan, is dubious as to its political viability. Instead, she offers two solutions. The first is "standardization and simplification." Using the same form for all payers would help and streamlining certain activities ("credentialing, quality measure, or benefit eligibility") would help. The second suggestion is to automate more; using computer technology such as health information technology (HIT) and electronic health records (EHR). Pearl (2017) strongly advocates the use of technology, not only for records but for doctor/patient interactions.

The Affordable Care Act and Cost Control

As we saw in Chapter 3, the full name of the ACA is the Patient Protection and Affordable Care Act. Affordable, from the standpoint of the legislation, can mean different things. One part is making healthcare and, particularly, health insurance more affordable for patients. For those on the exchanges (whether federal- or state-run), there is a sliding scale of subsidies for insurance premiums (up to 400 percent of the federal poverty line) and subsidies for cost-sharing. The ACA also has provisions for subsidies to insurance companies to offer cheaper policies. The ACA also reduced the cost-sharing in Part D of Medicare by shrinking the "doughnut hole."

In addition, the ACA contained some policies to reduce overall healthcare costs. Some of this involved reduction of payments to providers. For example, the payments to Medicare Advantage plans were supposed to be reduced.

In this section, we will briefly consider policies affecting payments to providers. One is accountable care organizations; the other is bundled payments. *Accountable care organizations* or ACOs can be defined as "a network of doctors and hospitals that shares financial and medical responsibility for providing coordinated care to patients in hopes of limiting unnecessary spending. At the heart of each patient's care is a primary care physician" (Gold 2015). Most the ACOs are aimed at Medicare beneficiaries. The most predominant ACO model is the Medicare Shared Savings Program or MSSP. Under this model, there are incentives for ACOs to save money and then the savings can be shared between the model and Medicare ("Medicare Delivery System Reform: The Evidence Link" n.d.). ACOs can be found in Medicaid programs as well as with private insurers. As of 2018, there are an estimate 32 million people enrolled in an ACO (Dartmouth Institute for Health Policy & Clinical Practice 2018).

The main question, from the standpoint of this chapter, is whether ACOs generated savings, and if so, how much. Here we discuss the Medicare program (Blesser et al. 2018a, 2018b; "Medicare Delivery System Reform: The Evidence Link" n.d.). The evidence is mixed. In 2016, Medicare spent $47 million more because of ACOs ("Medicare Delivery System Reform: The Evidence Link" n.d.). The first year in which Medicare ACOs produced savings was 2017, when the savings amounted to more than $313 million. Blesser et al. (2018a) point out that ACOs tend to produce savings the longer they have been around, suggesting learning is taking place. In any event, the impact of ACOs has been modest.

The second program to achieve savings, also in Medicare, is *bundled payments*. Bundled payments and ACOs share a basic idea: moving away from the fee-for-service model of provider payment to more value-based payments with a set budget. In the case of bundled payment, a total budget is set for a particular medical episode. If the costs come in at less than the set budget, Medicare and providers share in the savings. If the costs exceed the budget, the providers generally take the loss ("Medicare Delivery System Reform: The Evidence Link" n.d.). Bundled payments are similar in some sense to ACOs, except that ACOs are responsible for the total care of the patient and bundled payments are episodic. Bundled payments are also similar to earlier Medicare reforms, such as diagnostic-related groups (DRGs) (see Chapter 5), except that DRGs focus on hospitals and there are other pre-payment systems for physicians. Again, our question is whether bundled payments produce savings. And, as with ACOs, there have been savings, but the savings are small ("Medicare Delivery System Reform: The Evidence Link" n.d.). These two changes plus other reforms in the ACA have a limited impact on cost control (Weiner, Marks, and Pauly 2017).

The Federal Budget and Healthcare Costs

Medicare and Medicaid are two of the largest federal programs (along with Social Security and defense spending). The two public health programs, if their costs are not constrained, will continue to put pressure on federal spending and make deficit reduction more difficult. We address some of these issues in Chapters 4 and 5. Here we look at two related proposals that likely would reduce spending increases, in this case by cost-shifting. Both proposals can be seen in a plan (Ryan 2016) proposed by Speaker of the House Paul Ryan (R-WI). Both of these proposals are based on traditional Republican ideas.

The first, discussed in Chapter 5, focuses on Medicare. This would transform Medicare into a premium support program. In such a program, recipients would be given funds, usually a refundable tax credit, to purchase plans on the market. The tax credit would cover much, though not all, the cost of the plan. The recipient would pay the differences. Those with low incomes would be given subsidies. This transforms Medicare into a budgetable item. The federal government knows how many Medicare recipients there are and there would be a set amount spent for each recipient. The amount of the tax refund could be raised or lowered as needed. There is no question that if the point is to control Medicare spending, premium support would do it.

The Medicaid proposal is a block grant (Ryan 2016). As we saw in Chapter 4, a block grant can either be a set amount of dollars given to each state for its Medicaid program (obviously higher or lower depending on the state) or the block grant could be a per-capita amount. As with the Medicare premium support proposal, a block grant would limit federal (and state) funding to the size of the grant. Again, if the point is to control Medicaid spending, block grants would do it.

A STRATEGY FOR CONTROLLING COSTS

Controlling healthcare costs is never going to be easy, nor, like the "Global War on Terror," is there an end in sight. But there are some promising strategies. One such strategy has been offered by Davis (2005), president of the Commonwealth Fund. She suggests ten steps that concentrate on the supply side of health, which, she argues, have been successfully implemented in other countries.

The first step is better management of people with chronic conditions. One of several examples she provides is that better management of people with diabetes could reduce hospitalizations. The second step is to note that there is strong regional variation in how medical conditions are treated. Reducing the variations could save considerable funds. It would require better record keeping and sharing of data about such things as provider charges and patient outcomes.

Third, Davis suggests that there is overuse of medical procedures. More education for both providers and patients would help. The fourth step is very intriguing: Davis recommends that insurers and public programs stop reimbursing providers for medical errors, what she calls "comorbidity adjustments." This could save billions of dollars and also signal the need to providers to be more careful.

The fifth step is a simple one, which we have briefly mentioned in this chapter and in Chapter 4: negotiate prices for pharmaceuticals. Davis recommends allowing Medicare to negotiate prices. Sixth is to reduce administrative costs by standardizing insurance procedures. She writes:

> Private insurance companies have "overhead" of about 12 to 15 percent of revenues. Simplifying and standardizing private insurance could reduce administrative expenses. Hospitals, physicians, and other healthcare providers incur major administrative expenses as a result of variations across insurers and public programs in terms of benefits covered, payment regulations, conditions of provider participation, and coverage policies. Standardizing products and promoting common practices across all private and public insurers could save hospital and physician administrative costs.
>
> (Davis 2005)

The seventh recommendation, which follows from some of the earlier ones, is to make use of evidence-based medicine in making medical decisions. The eighth step is to make sure that every person has a regular provider who will be responsible for the care of the patient. This is known as primary-care management, and Davis cites studies indicating savings from such programs.

The ninth step, again related to some of the earlier recommendations, is to reduce duplication of tests and paperwork. And the last recommendation is to implement information technology that would help avoid duplication and errors and assist in continuity of care.

Davis notes that the changes would save money while at the same time reducing provider income and possibly reducing jobs. This statement suggests, again, one of the major problems of reform in the healthcare field: every dollar spent on healthcare is a dollar of revenue or income for someone. Nevertheless, Davis suggests that the savings from these changes could be used to improve the system: cover the uninsured, pay for new information technology, expand screening programs, and so forth. Perhaps some combination of demand and supply controls might be the way to go.

CONCLUSION

The United States spends a lot of money on healthcare. It spends more than any other nation, either in total figures or per capita. We know that the public (Kirzinger et al. 2018a) is concerned about costs, as are those in the private and public sectors. We know that healthcare spending as a portion of the economy, measured by gross domestic product, has been increasing, even if at a slower rate recently. We are concerned about waste and whether we are getting value for all the money we are spending. The answers are not clear.

Aaron and Ginsburg (2009) identify a number of factors that lead to ever-increasing healthcare expenditures, many of which we have discussed in this chapter. They identify 14 such factors in four categories: demand, supply, institutional, and research. All these have potential remedies. If we were to pick a couple of factors or drivers, we would pick prices, waste, and incentives. Prices are higher than in other countries, there is much waste and inefficiency/ineffectiveness, and the incentives are in the wrong places.

But addressing these issues is difficult. The United States lacks a strong enough mechanism to make the changes necessary. It also lacks the will and the culture (see Chapter 1 and Pearl 2017) to make the changes some think are necessary. Cutting services (i.e., rationing) leads to an outcry. Cutting prices, whether on pharmaceuticals or hospitals or doctors, leads to an outcry by providers. Pearl (2017) points to the four sets of legacy actors that move to protect themselves: insurers, hospitals (and hospital systems), physician specialty societies, and drug and device companies. These four sets of actors are, understandably, concerned about maintaining their status and incomes. And when their future is threatened in some way, they act to protect, generally speaking focusing on the political system. Change is difficult, as we have seen and will address again in Chapter 11.

Another aspect of the cost problem is that we really do not know how much we should spend to achieve the best healthcare results (Aaron and Ginsburg 2009; Savedoff 2007). If we do not know how much to spend, it is difficult to defend any position, whether to cut, maintain the current level, or increase spending.

We do know that while costs continue to increase, the increases have slowed. Altman (2018b) presents the data. In the 1970s, healthcare spending grew 2.8 percent faster than GDP. In the 1980s, that percentage was 3.3 percent. In the 1990s, healthcare spending was 1 percent higher than GDP growth. In the 2000s, the percentage increase was 2.8 percent. From 2010 to 2016, the percentage increase was 0.5 percent. The projection for the 2016–2016 period is a 1-percent increase (for similar numbers, see Cuckler et al. 2018). Cuckler et al. (2018) point to what they call the fundamentals of healthcare spending increases: prices, an aging population, and the growth of the economy.

Ryu et al. (2013) suggest that health reform may have had an impact, as changes in payment and organization may also have been a factor. It leads them to be cautiously optimistic.

What if cautiously optimistic turns out to be correct? The implications could be profound. Cutler and Sahni (2013) estimate that if the slowdown continues, we would spend about $770 billion less on healthcare in the 2013–2022 period than is being projected. That would mean less pressure on federal and state budgets and businesses and that households would have more money to spend on other things, or to save, which would also positively affect the overall economy.

If this is correct, then we should not worry about healthcare costs (Baumol 2012). If healthcare spending per capita and overall continues to increase at a slower rate, then we have less to be concerned about. In the words of that famous philosopher, Alfred E. Neuman, "What, me, worry?"

STUDY QUESTIONS

1. Discuss the problem of rising healthcare costs and expenditures in the United States. How have sources of healthcare expenditures changed over the years? In what specific areas do we find a high concentration of healthcare expenditures?
2. Discuss the concentration of healthcare expenditures by population characteristics, medical conditions, chronic health conditions, and major causes of deaths in the United States.
3. How do US national healthcare expenditures compare to expenditures in other countries, especially member countries of the Organisation for Economic Cooperation and Development (OECD)?
4. What do public opinion polls show about Americans' views and attitudes about healthcare expenditures and costs in the United States?
5. Discuss the major factors that have contributed to high and rising healthcare expenditures and costs in the United States.

6. What role has medical technology played in rising healthcare expenditures in the United States? Explain different types of medical technologies, and which of these have contributed to rising costs and expenditures.
7. What factors have contributed to growth of medical technologies in the United States?
8. Discuss the history and current state of medical technology assessment in the United States. What are some of the problems with medical technology assessment in the United States?
9. What factors explain the (a) increased use of prescription drugs and (b) increased spending on prescription drugs in the United States?
10. How does the regulation of the pharmaceutical industry in the European countries differ from that in the United States?
11. How do medical errors, the practice of defensive medicine, and medical liability insurance contribute to rising healthcare costs?
12. Compare and contrast costs of healthcare services in the United States and OECD countries.
13. Discuss how waste, fraud, and abuse contribute to excessive healthcare expenditures and costs in the United States.
14. Discuss the role of lifestyle choices in contributing to healthcare expenditures and costs.

REFERENCES

"$1.1 Trillion: What the Top 10 Leading Causes of Death Cost the U. S. Economy." 2012. New York: 24/7 Wall St. Online at http://247wallst.com/2012/01/18/1-1-trillion-what-the-10-leading-causes-of-death-cost-the-u-s-economy.
"The $272 Billion Swindle." 2014. *The Economist*, May 31. Online at economist.com.
Aaron, Henry J. 1991. *Serious and Unstable Condition: Financing America's Health Care*. Washington, DC: Brookings Institution.
Aaron, Henry J. and Paul B. Ginsburg. 2009. "Is Health Care Spending Excessive? If So, What Can We Do about It?" *Health Affairs*, 28, no. 5 (September/October): 1260–1275.
Aaron, Henry J. and William B. Schwartz. 1984. *The Painful Prescription: Rationing Hospital Care*. Washington, DC: Brookings Institution.
Aaron, Henry J. and William B. Schwartz. 1990. "Rationing Health Care: The Choice Before Us." *Science*, 247, no. 4941 (January 26): 418–422.
Abramson, John. 2004. *Overdosed America: The Broken Promise of American Medicine*. New York: HarperCollins.
Altman, Drew E. 2015. "Prescription Drugs' Sizable Share of Health Spending." *Wall Street Journal*, December 13.
Altman, Drew E. 2018a. "The Shrinking Health Spending Gap." *Axios*, May 11. Online at www.axios.com.
Altman, Drew E. 2018b. "Surprise Medical Bills Could Be a Powerful Campaign Issue." *Axios*, September 24. Online at www.axios.com.
Altman, Drew E. and Larry Levitt. 2003. "The Sad History of Health Care Cost Containment as Told in One Chart." *Health Affairs* (October 25): W83–W84.
Altman, Stuart H. and Sanford L. Weiner. 1978. "Regulation as a Second Best Choice." In *Competition in the Health Care Sector: Past, Present, and Future, Bureau of Economics*, ed. Warren Greenberg, 421–427. Washington, DC: US Federal Trade Commission.
Anders, George. 1996. *Health against Wealth: HMOs and the Breakdown of Medical Trust*. Boston: Houghton Mifflin.
Anderson, Gerald, Patrick Chaulk, and Elizabeth Fowler. 1993. "State Model: Maryland." *Health Affairs*, 12, no. 2 (Summer): 40–47.
Anderson, Gerard R. et al. 2003. "It's the Prices, Stupid: Why the United States Is So Different from Other Countries." *Health Affairs*, 22, no. 3 (May/June): 89–105.
Angell, Marcia. 2004. *The Truth about the Drug Companies: How They Deceive Us and What to Do about It*. New York: Random House.
Antos, Joseph R., Mark V. Pauly, and Gail R. Wilensky. 2012. "Bending the Cost Curve Through Market-Based Incentives." *New England Journal of Medicine*, 367, no. 10 (September 6): 954–958.
Applbaum, Kalman. 2009. "Is Marketing the Enemy of Pharmaceutical Innovation?" *Hastings Center Report*, 39, no. 4 (August): 13–17.
Appleby, Julie. 2008. "As Drug Ads Surge, More Get Rx's Filled." *USA Today*, March 4. Online at http://usatoday30.usatoday.com/news/health/2008-02-29-drugs-main_N.htm.
Appleby, Julie. 2012. "Employers Tie Financial Rewards, Penalties to Health Tests, Lifestyle Choices." *Kaiser Health News*, April 2.
Archer, Diane. 2011. "Medicare Is More Efficient than Private Insurance." *Health Affairs*, September 20.
Arrow, Kenneth J. 1963. "Uncertainty and the Welfare Economics of Medical Care." *American Economic Review*, 53, no. 5 (December): 851–883.
Association for Accessible Medicines. 2017. *Generic Drug Access and Savings in the U.S.* Washington, DC: The Association for Accessible Medicines.

Atkinson, Graham. 2009. *State Hospital Rate-Setting Revisited*. New York: Commonwealth Fund.
Avron, Jerry. 2004. *Powerful Medicine: The Benefits, Risks, and Costs of Prescription Drugs*. New York: Alfred A. Knopf.
Bai, Matt. 2005. "The Framing Wars." *The New York Times*, July 17.
Baicker, Katherine and Dana Goldman. 2011. "Patient Cost-Sharing and Healthcare Spending Growth." *Journal of Economic Perspectives*, 25, no. 2 (Spring): 47–68.
Baker, Colin. 2008. *Technological Change and the Growth of Health Care Spending*. Washington, DC: Congressional Budget Office.
Baker, Dean. 2017. "The Problem of Doctors' Salaries." *Politico*, November 7.
Baker, Laurence, Howard Birnbaum, Jeffrey Geppert, David Mishol, and Erick Moyneur. 2003. "The Relationship between Technology Availability and Health Care Spending." *Health Affairs, Web Exclusive* (November 5): W3-537–W3-551.
Banco, Erin. 2018. *Some N.J. Drug Prices Are Skyrocketing. Here's How Much More You're Paying*. NJ Advanced Media for NJ.com, July 29. Online at nj.com.
Banja, John D. 2005. *Medical Errors and Medical Narcissism*. Sudbury, MA: Jones and Bartlett.
Bartlett, Bruce. 2012. "A Conservative Case for the Welfare State." *The New York Times*, December 25.
Bauchner, Howard and Phil B. Fontanarosa. 2018. "Health Care Spending in the United States Compared with 10 Other High-Income Countries What Uwe Reinhardt Might Have Said." *Journal of the American Medical Association*, 319, no. 10 (March 13): 990–992.
Bauman, Patricia. 1976. "The Formulation and Evolution of the Health Maintenance Organization Policy, 1970-1973." *Social Science and Medicine*, 10, nos. 3–4 (March–April): 129–142.
Baumol, William J. 2012. *The Cost Disease: Why Computers Get Cheaper and Health Care Doesn't*. New Haven, CT: Yale University Press.
Bebinger, Martha. 2018. "Massachusetts Stroke Patient Receives 'Outragous' $474,725 Medical Flight Bill." *Kaiser Health News*, December 21.
Belk, David. 2018a. "Medical Malpractice: Myths and Realities." The True Cost of Health Care. Online at truecostofhealthcare.org.
Belk, David. 2018b, "Malpractice Statistics." The True Cost of Health Care. Online at truecostofhealthcare.org.
Belluck, Pam. 2012. "With Telemedicine as Bridge, No Hospital Is an Island." *The New York Times*, October 8. Online at www.nytimes.com/2012/10/09/health/nantucket-hospital-uses-telemedicine-as-bridge-to-mainland.html?
Belluz, Julia. 2014. "21 Maps and Charts that Explain the Obesity Epidemic." *Vox*, November 17.
Belmonte, Adriana. 2018. "'Troubling and Shocking': Americans are Increasingly Crowdfunding Medical Bills." Yahoo! Finance. Online at finance.yahoo.com, August 18.
Bentley, Tanya G.K., Rachel M. Effros, Kartika Palar, and Emmett B. Keeler. 2008. "Waste in the U.S. Health Care System: A Conceptual Framework." *Milbank Quarterly*, 86, no. 4 (December): 629–659.
Berk, Marc L. and Alan C. Monheit. 2001. "The Concentration of Health Care Expenditures, Revisited." *Health Affairs*, 20, no. 2 (March/April): 9–18.
Berndt, Ernst R. 2002. "Pharmaceuticals in U.S. Health Care: Determinants of Quality and Price." *Journal of Economic Perspectives*, 16, no. 4 (Autumn): 45–66.
Berwick, Donald M. and Andrew D. Hackbarth. 2012. "Eliminating Waste in U.S. Health Care." *Journal of the American Medical Association*, 307, no. 14 (April): 1513–1516.
Bishop, Tara F., Alex D. Federman, and Salomeh Keyhani. 2010. "Physicians' Views on Defensive Medicine: A National Survey." *Archives of Internal Medicine*, 170, no. 12 (June): 1081–1083.
Blendon, Robert J., Mollyann Brodie, John M. Benson, Drew E. Altman, and Tami Buhr. 2006. "Americans' View of Health Care Costs, Access, and Quality." *Milbank Quarterly*, 84, no. 4: 623–657.
Blesser, William et al. 2018a. "Half a Decade In, Medicare Accountable Care Organizations are Generating Net Savings, Part 1." *Health Affairs*, September 20.
Blesser, William, et al. 2018b. "Half a Decade In, Medicare Accountable Care Organizations are Generating Net Savings, Part 2." *Health Affairs*, September 21.
Blumenthal, David and Shanoor Seervai. 2018. *Rising Obesity in the United States Is a Public Health Crisis*. New York: The Commonwealth Fund.
Bodenheimer, Thomas. 2003. "The Not-So Sad History of Medicare Cost Containment as Told in One Chart." *Health Affairs* (October 25): W88–W90.
Bodenheimer, Thomas and Kip Sullivan. 1998, "How Large Employers are Shaping the Health Care Marketplace." *New England Journal of Medicine*, 338, no. 14 (April 12): 1003–1007.
Boodman, Sandra G. 2016. "Should You Worry about Radiation from CT Scans?" *The Washington Post*, January 4.
Bozic, Kevin J., Read G. Pierce, and James H. Herndon. 2004. "Health Care Technology Assessment." *Journal of Bone and Joint Surgery*, 86, no. 6 (June): 1305–1314.
Brawley, Otis Webb, and Paul Goldberg. 2011. *How We Do Harm: A Doctor Breaks Ranks about Being Sick in America*. New York: St. Martin's Press.
Brennan, Troyen A. and Philip K. Howard. 2004. "Heal the Law, Then Health Care." *The Washington Post*, January 25.
Breyer, S. 1979. "Analyzing Regulatory Failures: Mismatches, Less Restrictive Alternatives and Reform." *Harvard Law Review* 92, no. 1: 549–609.
Brill, Steven. 2015. *America's Bitter Pill: Money, Politics, Backroom Deals, and the Fight to Fix Our Broken Healthcare System*. New York: Random House.
Brody, Jane E. 2011. "Tackling Care as Chronic Ailments Pile Up." *The New York Times*, February 21. Online at www.nytimes.com/2011/02/22/health/22brody.html?_r=0.

Brody, Jane E. 2012. "E-Health Opportunities for Seniors." *The New York Times*, October 8. Online at http://well.blogs.nytimes.com/2012/10/08/e-health-opportunities-for-seniors/.

Brown, Lawrence D. 1986. "Introduction to a Decade of Transition." *Journal of Health Politics, Policy and Law*, 11, no. 4 (Winter): 569–583.

Brownlee, Shannon. 2007. *Overtreated: Why Too Much Medicine Is Making Us Sicker and Poorer*. New York: Bloomsbury.

Buchanan, Allen. 1998. "Managed Care: Rationing without Justice, but Not Unjustly." *Journal of Health Politics, Policy and Law*, 23, no. 4 (Winter): 617–634.

Bureau of Labor Statistics. 2018. *Employer Costs for Employee Compensation—March 2018*. Washington, DC: US Department of Labor.

Bureau of the Census. 2017. *Health Insurance Historical Tables*. Washington, DC: Department of Commerce.

Buttorff, Christine, Teague Ruder, and Melissa Bauman. 2017. *Multiple Chronic Conditions in the United States*. Santa Monica, CA: RAND Corporation.

Caitlin, Aaron C. and Cathy A. Cowan. 2015. *History of Health Spending in the United States, 1960–2013*. Washington, DC: Centers for Medicare and Medicaid Services.

Calfee, John E. 2002. "Public Policy Issues in Direct-to-Consumer Advertising of Prescription Drugs." *Journal of Public Policy & Marketing*, 21, no. 2 (Fall): 174–193.

Cannon, Michael F. and Michael D. Tanner. 2005. *Healthy Competition: What's Holding Back Health Care and How to Free It*. Washington, DC: Cato Institute.

Carr, Teresa. 2017. "Too Many Meds? America's Love Affair with Prescription Medication." *Consumer Reports*, August 3. Online at consumerreports.org.

Carrier, Emily R., James D. Reschovsky, Michelle M. Mello, Ralph C. Mayrell, and David Katz. 2010. "Physicians' Fear of Malpractice Lawsuits are Not Assuaged by Tort Reform." *Health Affairs*, 29, no. 9: 1585–1592.

Cass, Connie and Lauran Neergaard. 2013. *High Hospital Bills Go Public, but Will It Help?* Associated Press, May 8. Online at http://news.yahoo.com/high-hospital-bills-public-help-211625086.html.

Cauchi, Richard and Ashley Noble. 2018. *CON-Certificate of Need State Laws*. Denver, CO: National Conference of State Legislatures. Online at www.ncsl.org.

Cauchon, Dennis. 2012. "States Rein in Health Insurance Expenses." *USA Today*, October 24.

Centers for Medicare and Medicaid Services. 2006. *Report to Congress: Improving the Medicare Quality Improvement Organization Program—Response to the Institute of Medicine Study*. Woodlawn, MD: US Department of Health and Human Services.

Charney, William. 2012. *Epidemic of Medical Errors and Hospital-Acquired Infections: System and Social Causes*. Boca Raton, FL: Taylor & Francis.

Chronic Disease in Rural America. n.d. Grand Forks, ND: Rural Health Information Hub. Online at ruralhealthinfo.org.

Classen, David C., Roger Resar, Frances Griffin, Frank Federico, Terri Frankel, Nancy Kimmel, John C. Whittington, Allan Frankel, Andrew Seger, and Brent C. James. 2011. "'Global Trigger Tool' Shows that Adverse Events in Hospitals May Be Ten Times Greater than Previously Measured." *Health Affairs*, 30, no. 4: 581–589.

Claxton, Gary et al. 2017. *Employer Health Benefits: Annual Survey 2017*. Chicago: Health Research and Educational Trust. Menlo Park, CA: Kaiser Family Foundation.

Claxton, Gary et al. 2018. *Increase in Cost-Sharing Payments Continue to Outpace Wage Growth*. Peterson-Kaiser Health System Tracker. Menlo Park, CA: Kaiser Family Foundation.

Cohen, A. Harold. n.d. "Maryland's All-Payor Hospital Payment System." The Maryland Health Services Cost Review Comission. Online at www.hscrc.state.md.us.

Cohen, Robin A. and Whitney K. Kirzinger. 2014. "Financial Burden of Medical Care: A Family Perspective." NCHS Data Brief # 142 (January).

Cohen, Steven B. 2014. *The Concentration of Health Care Spending and Related Expenses for Costly Medical Conditions, 2012*. Statistical Brief # 455 (October). Rockville, MD: Agency for Healthcare Research and Quality.

Cohen, Steven B. 2016. "The Concentration of Health Care Spending and Predictions of Future Spending." *Journal of Economic and Social Measurement*, 41, no. 2: 167–180.

Coletta, Amanda. 2018. "Canada's Health-Care System Is a Point of National Pride. But a Study Shows It's at Risk of Becoming Outdated." *The Washington Post*, February 23.

Collins, Sara et al. 2018. *Americans' Confidence in Their Ability to Pay for Health Care Is Falling*. New York: Commonwealth Fund.

Comanor, William S., H.E. Freech, III, and Richard D. Miller. 2006. "Is the United States an Outlier in Healthcare and Health Outcomes? A Preliminary Analysis." *International Journal of Health Care Finance and Economics*, 6, no. 1 (March): 3–23.

Congressional Budget Office 2014. *Competition and the Cost of Medicare's Prescription Drug Program*. Washington, DC: Congressional Budget Office.

Congressional Budget Office. 2018. *The Budget and Economic Outlooks: 2019–2029*. Washington, DC: Congressional Budget Office.

Congressional Research Service. 2007. *U.S. Health Care Spending: Comparison with Other OECD Countries*. CRS Report for Congress. Washington, DC: Congressional Research Service.

Conway, Patrick, Kate Goodrich, Steven Machlin, Benjamin Sasse, and Joel Cohen. 2011. "Patient-Centered Care OuCategorization of U.S. Health Care Expenditures." *Health Research Services*, 46, no. 2 (April): 479–490.

Cooper, Zack, Fiona Scott Morton, and Nathan Shekita. 2018. *Surprise! Out-of-Network Billing for Emergency in the United States*. Cambridge, MA: National Bureau of Economic Research.

"The Cost of Generic and Name-Brand Drugs." 2016. *Harvard Men's Health Watch*, August. Online at www.health.harvard.edu/drugs-and-medications/the-cost-of-generic-and-name-brand-drugs.

Coukell, Allan. 2017. "Other Countries Control Drug Prices. The U.S Could, Too." *The Hill*, December 7.

Council of Economic Advisers. 2017. *The Underestimated Cost of the Opioid Epidemic*. Washington, DC: Executive Office of the White House.

Crisp, Donna Helen. 2017. *Anatomy of Medical Errors: The Patient in Room 2*. Indianapolis, IN: Sigma Theta Tau International.

Cruise, Peter L. 2002. "Are There Virtues in Whistleblowing? Perspectives from Health Care Organizations." *Public Administration Quarterly*, 25, no. 4 (Winter): 413–435.

Cubanski, Julie et al. 2015. *A Primer on Medicare*. Menlo Park, CA: Kaiser Family Foundation.

Cuckler, Gigi et al. 2018. "National Health Expenditure Projections: 2017–2026: Despite Uncertainty, Fundamentals Primarily Drive Spending Growth." *Health Affairs*, 37, no. 3 (March): 482–492.

Cutler, David M. and Dan P. Ly. 2011. "The (Paper) Work of Medicine: Understanding International Medical Costs." *Journal of Economic Perspectives*, 25, no. 2 (Spring): 3–25.

Cutler, David M. and Mark McClellan. 2001. "Is Technological Change in Medicine Worth It?" *Health Affairs*, 20, no. 5 (September-October): 11–29.

Cutler, David M. and Nikhil R. Sahni. 2013. "If Slow Rate of Health Care Spending Growth Persists, Projections May Be off by $770 Billion." *Health Affairs*, 32, no. 5 (May): 841–850.

Danzon, Patricia M. and Mark V. Pauly. 2002. "Health Insurance and the Growth in Pharmaceutical Expenditures." *Journal of Law and Economics*, 45, no. 52 (October): 587–613.

Dartmouth Institute for Health Policy & Clinical Practice. 2018. *National Survey of Accountable Care Organizations*. New Haven, CT: Dartmouth Institute for Health Policy & Clinical Practice.

Davidson, Stephen M. 2010. *Still Broken: Understanding the U.S. Health Care System*. Stanford, CA: Stanford Business Books.

Davis, Karen. 2005. *Taking a Walk on the Supply Side: 10 Steps to Control Health Care Costs*. New York: Commonwealth Fund.

Davis, Karen and Cathy Schoen. 1978. *Health and the War on Poverty: A Ten-Year Proposal*. Washington, DC: Brookings Institution.

Davis, Karen, et al. 1990. *Health Care Cost Containment*. Baltimore, MD: Johns Hopkins University Press.

Davis, Karen and Kristof Stremikis. 2009. *The Costs of Failure: Economic Consequences of Failure to Enact Nixon, Carter, and Clinton Health Reforms*. New York: Commonwealth Fund.

DeJong, Collette et al. 2016. "Pharmaceutical Industry-Sponsored Meals and Physician Prescribing Patterns for Medicare Beneficiaries." *Journal of the American Medical Association Internal Medicine*, 176, no. 8 (August): 1114–1122.

Department of Health and Human Services. 2018. *American Patients First: The Trump Administration Blueprint to Lower Drug Prices and Reduce Out-of-Pocket Costs*. Rockville, MD: US Department of Health and Human Services.

DeSilver, Drew. 2014. *For Most Workers, Real Wages Have Barely Budged for Decades*. Washington, DC: Pew Research Center.

Development and Approval Process: Drugs. n.d. Washington, DC: Food and Drug Administration. Online at www.fda.gov/Drugs/DevelopmentApprovalProcess/default.htm.

DiJulio, Bianca, James Firth, and Mollyann Brodie. 2015. *Kaiser Health Tracking Poll: August 2015*. Menlo Park, CA: Kaiser Family Foundation.

Dobkin, Carlos et al. 2017. *The Economic Consequences of Hospital Admissions*. Cambridge, MA: National Bureau of Economic Research.

Dobkin, Carlos et al. 2018. "Myth and Measurement—The Case of Medical Bankruptcies." *New England Journal of Medicine*, 378, #12 (March 22): 1076–1078.

Docteur, Elizabeth and Ruth Lopert. 2017. *Payment Policies to Manage Pharmaceutical Costs: Insights from Other Countries*. Philadelphia, PA: Pew Charitable Trusts.

"Doctors and Other Health Professionals Report that Fear of Malpractice Has a Big, and Mostly Negative, Impact on Medical Practice, Unnecessary Defensive Medicine, and Openness in Discussing Medical Errors." 2003. *Health Care News*, 3, no. 2 (February 7): 1–5.

Donohue, Julie. 2006. "A History of Drug Advertising: The Evolving Roles of Consumers and Consumer Protection." *Milbank Quarterly*, 84, no. 4: 659–699.

Doolan, David F. and David W. Bates. 2002. "Computerized Physician Order Entry System in Hospitals. Mandates and Incentives." *Health Affairs*, 21, no. 4 (July–August): 180–188.

Dove, James T., John E. Brush, Richard A. Chazal, and William J. Oetgen. 2010. "Medical Professional Liability and Health Care System Reform." *Journal of the American College of Cardiology*, 55, no. 25 (June): 2801–2803.

Draper, Debra A., Ann Tynan, and Jon B. Christianson. 2012. "Health and Wellness: The Shift from Managing Illness to Promoting Health." Brief no. 121, June. Washington, DC: Center for Health System Change.

Duggan, Mark, Patrick Healy, and Fiona S. Morton. 2008. "Providing Prescription Drug Coverage to the Elderly: America's Experiment with Medicare Part D." *Journal of Economic Perspectives*, 22, no. 4 (Fall): 69–92.

Durenberger, David F. 1982. "The Politics of Health." In *Competition in the Marketplace: Health Care in the 1980s*, eds. James R. Gay and Barbara J. Sax Jacobs, 4. New York: Spectrum Publications.

Eastburn, Larry. 1999. "Medical Malpractice Update." *Modern Medicine*, 67, no. 7 (July): 58–62.

Eichler, Alexander. 2012. "Pharmaceutical Companies Spent 19 Times More on Self-Promotion than Basic Research: Report." *Huffington Post*, August 8. Online at www.huffingtonpost.com/2012/08/09/pharma-ceutical-companies-marketing_n_1760380.html.

Eisner, Marc Allen, Jeff Worsham, and Evan J. Ringquest. 2006. *Contemporary Regulatory Policy*, 2nd edn. Boulder, CO: Lynne Rienner.

Ellis, Monique. 2018. *What are the Top Ten Pharmaceutical Companies in the World? (2018)*. New York: ProClinical. Online at proclinical.com.
Ellwood, Paul M., Jr. 1971. "Health Maintenance Strategy." *Medical Care*, 9 (May/June): 291–298.
Elmendorf, Douglas W. 2009. *Letter to Honorable Max Baucas, Chairman, Committee on Finance, United States Senate*. Washington, DC: Congressional Budget Office.
Emanuel, Zeke et al. 2016. *State Options to Control Health Care Costs and Improve Quality*. Washington, DC: Center for American Progress.
Enthoven, Alain C. 1978a. "Consumer Choice Health Plans (First of Two Parts)." *New England Journal of Medicine*, 298 (March 23): 650–658.
Enthoven, Alain C. 1978b. "Consumer Choice Health Plans (Second of Two Parts)." *New England Journal of Medicine*, 298 (March 30): 709–720.
Enthoven, Alain C. 1980. *Health Plan: The Only Practical Solution to the Soaring Cost of Medicare Care*. Reading, MA: Addison-Wesley.
Enthoven, Alain C. and Sara J. Singer. 1997. "Markets and Collective Action in Regulating Managed Care." *Health Affairs*, 16, no. 6 (November/December): 26–32.
Ernst & Young. 2012. *Beyond Borders: Global Biotechnology Report 2011*. Washington, DC: Ernst & Young.
Ess, Silvia M., Sebastian Schneeweiss, and Thomas D. Szucs. 2003. "European Healthcare Policies for Controlling Drug Expenditures." *Pharmacoeconomics*, 21, no. 2: 89–103.
Etheredge, Lynn. 1997. "Promarket Regulation: An SEC-FASB Model." *Health Affairs*, 16, no. 6 (November/December): 22–25.
Etzioni, Amitai. 2012. "Cut Medicare? Cut Fraud." *Huffington Post*, December 12.
Evans, David. 2010. "When Drug Makers' Profits Outweigh Penalties." *Washington Post*, March 21. Online at www.washingtonpost.com/wp-dyn/content/article/2010/03/19/AR2010031905578.html.
Evans, Robert G. 1983. "Incomplete Vertical Integration in the Health Care Industry: Pseudomarkets and Pseudopolicies." *Annals of the American Academy of Political and Social Science*, 468 (July): 60–87.
Evans, Robert G. 1997. "Going for the Gold: The Redistributive Agenda behind Market-Based Health Care Reform." *Journal of Health Politics, Policy and Law*, 22, no. 2 (Summer): 427–466.
Ezrati, Milton. 2018. "Entitlements Threaten the Entire Federal Budget)." *Forbes*, February 9.
Falkson, Joseph L. 1980. *HMOs and the Politics of Health Service Reform*. Chicago: American Hospital Association and Robert J. Brady.
Falkson, Joseph L. 1980–1981. "Market Reform, Health Systems, and HMOs." *Policy Studies Journal*, 9, no. 2: 213–220.
Farber, Henry S. and Michelle J. White. 1991. "Medical Malpractice: An Empirical Examination of the Litigation Process." *RAND Journal of Economics*, 22, no. 2 (Summer): 199–217.
Federal Reserve Bank of Minneapolis. 2018. *Consumer Price Index, 1913–*. Minneapolis, MN: Federal Reserve Bank of Minneapolis.
Fielding, Stephen L. 1995. "Changing Medical Practice and Medical Malpractice Claims." *Social Problems*, 42, no. 1 (February 1): 38–55.
Fineberg, H.V. 1977. "Computerized Tomography: Dilemma of Health Care Technology." *Pediatrics*, 59, no. 2 (February): 147–149.
Fish-Parcham, Cheryl. 2006. *Understanding How Health Insurance Premiums Are Regulated*. Washington, DC: Families USA.
Fleming, Sibley. 2005. "Wellness Programs Lighten Health Costs." *American City & County*, 120, no. 3 (March): 8–10.
Fox, Maggie. 2010. "Malpractice Liability Costs U.S. $55.6 Billion: Study." *Romanian Journal of Medical Practice*, 5, no. 3: 191.
Frakes, Michael D. and Jonathan Gruber. 2018. *Defensive Medicine: Evidence from Military Immunity*. Cambridge, MA: National Bureau of Economic Research.
Frakt, Austin. 2018. "Hidden from View: The Astonishing High Administrative Costs of U.S. Health Care." *The New York Times*, July 16.
Frank, Richard G. and Richard J. Zeckhauser. 2018. *High-Priced Drugs in Medicare Part D: Diagnosis and Prescription*. Washington, DC: Hutchins Center on Fiscal and Monetary Policy, Brookings Institution.
Freudenheim, Milt. 2012. "The Ups and Downs of Electronic Medical Records." *The New York Times*, October 8.
Friedan, Joyce. (2018). "States Seek to Refine 'All-Payer Hospital Payments System.'" *MedPage Today*, March 13.
Friedman, Milton (with the assistance of Rose D. Friedman). 1962. *Capitalism and Freedom*. Chicago, IL: University of Chicago Press.
Friedman, Milton. 1993. *The Future of Health Care Policy*. Cambridge, MA: Harvard University Press.
Friedman, Milton. 2005. "Health Care Expenditures Reexamined." *Annals of Internal Medicine*, 143, no. 4 (July): 76–78.
Frost, Amanda, John Hargraves, and Sally Rodriguez. 2018. *2016 Health Care Cost and Utilization Report*. Washington, DC: Health Care Cost Institute.
Fuchs, Victor R. 1986. *The Health Economy*. Cambridge, MA: Harvard University Press.
Gabel, Jon R. and Alan C. Monheit. 1983. "Will Competition Plans Change Insurer-Provider Relationships?" *Milbank Memorial Fund Quarterly/Health and Society*, 61, no. 4 (Fall): 614–640.
Gabler, Neal. 2016. "The Secret Shame of Middle-Class Americans." *The Atlantic*, May. Online at theatlantic.com.
Gawande, Atul. 2007. "The Checklist." *The New Yorker*, December. Online at www.newyorker.com/magazine/2007/12/10/the-checklist.
Gelijns, Annetine C, Lawrence D. Brown, Corey Magnell, Elettra Ronchi, and Alan J. Moskowitz. 2005. "Evidence, Politics, and Technological Change." *Health Affairs*, 24, no. 1 (January–February): 29–40.
Gelijns, Annetine C. and Nathan Rosenberg. 1994. "The Dynamics of Technological Change in Medicine." *Health Affairs*, 13, no. 3 (Summer): 28–46.

Generic Pharmaceutical Association. 2012. *Savings $1 Trillion over 10 Years: Generic Drug Savings in the U.S.* Washington, DC: Generic Pharmaceutical Association. Online at www.fdalawyersblog.com/GPhA%202012%20Generic%20Drug%20Savings%20Study.pdf.

Gibson, Rosemary and Janardan Prasad Singh. 2003. *Wall of Silence: The Untold Story of the Medical Mistakes that Kill and Injure Millions of Americans.* Washington, DC: LifeLine Press.

Ginsburg, Paul. 2012. *What Is Driving U.S. Health Care Spending?* Washington, DC: Bipartisan Policy Center.

Ginzberg, Eli. 1977. *The Limits of Health Reform: The Search for Realism.* New York: Basic Books.

Ginzberg, Eli. 1982. "Procompetition in Health Care: Policy or Fantasy?" *Milbank Memorial Fund Quarterly/Health and Society*, 60, no. 3 (Summer): 386–398.

Goetzel, Roy Z. et al. 2012. "Ten Modifiable Health Risk Factors are Linked to More than One-Fifth of Employer-Employee Health Care Spending." *Health Affairs*, 31, no. 11 (November): 2474–2484.

Golann, Dwight. 2011. "Dropped Medical Malpractice Claims: Their Surprising Frequency, Apparent Causes, and Potential Remedies." *Health Affairs*, 30, no. 7: 1343–1350.

Gold, Jenny. 2015. "Accountable Care Organizations, Explained." *Kaiser Health News*, September 14.

Gold, Marsha and Robert Hurley. 1997. "The Role of Managed Care 'Products' in Managed Care Plans." *Inquiry*, 34, no. 1 (Spring): 29–37.

Gold, Marsha et al. 2013. *Medicare Advantage 2013 Spotlight: Enrollment Market Update.* Menlo Park, CA: Kaiser Family Foundation.

Goldhill, David. 2013. *Catastrophic Care: How American Health Killed My Father—And How to Fix It.* New York: Alfred A. Knopf.

Goldman, Dana and Anupam Jena. 2018. "Surprise! Trump Might Actually Lower Drug Prices." *The Washington Post*, August 28.

Goldman, T.R. 2012. "Health Policy Brief: Eliminating Fraud and Abuse." *Health Affairs*, July 31.

Goldsmith, Jeff. 2004. "Technology and the Boundaries of the Hospital: Three Emerging Technologies." *Health Affairs*, 23, no. 6: 149–156.

Goldstein, Amy. 2018. "A Crucial Medicare Trust Fund Will Run Out Three Years Earlier than Predicted, New Report Says." *The Washington Post*, June 5.

Goodman, John C. 1980. *The Regulation of Medical Care: Is the Price Too High?* San Francisco: Cato Institute.

Goodman, John C. 2012. *Priceless: Curing the Healthcare Crisis.* Oakland, CA: Independent Institute.

Goodman, John S., Pamela Villarreal, and Biff Jones. 2011. "The Social Cost of Adverse Medical Events, and What We Can Do about It?" *Health Affairs*, 30, no. 4: 590–595.

Goozner, Merrill. 2004. *The $800 Million Pill: The Truth behind the Cost of New Drugs.* Berkeley, CA: University of California Press.

Goyen, Mathias and Jorg F. Debatin. 2009. "Healthcare Costs for New Technologies." *European Journal of Nuclear Medicine & Molecular Imaging*, 36, Supplement no. 1 (March): 139–143.

Greene, Risa B. 1996. "Federal Legislative Proposals for Medical Malpractice Reform: Treating the Symptom or Effecting a Cure?" *Cornell Journal of Law and Public Policy*, 4, no. 2: 563–607.

Greer, Donley and Marion Danis. 2011. "Making the Case for Talking to Patients about the Costs of End- Of-Life Care." *Journal of Law, Medicine, and Ethics*, 39, no. 2 (Summer): 183–193.

Greider, Katharine. 2003. *The Big Fix: How the Pharmaceutical Industry Rips off American Consumers.* New York: Public Affairs.

Groningen, Nicole Van. 2017. "Big Pharma Gives Your Doctor Gifts. Then Your Doctor Gives You Big Pharma's Drugs." *The Washington Post*, June 13.

Gupta, Sanjay. 2012. "Let's End the Prescription Drug Death Epidemic." CNN, November 15. Online at www.cnn.com/2012/11/14/health/gupta-accidental-overdose/index.html.

Hacker, Jacob S. 2009. *The Case for Public Plan Choice in National Health Reform: Key to Cost Control and Quality Coverage.* Berkeley, CA: Institute for America's Future, Center on Health Economic & Family Security, University of California, Berkeley School of Law.

Hacker, Jacob S. and Theodore R. Marmor. 1999. "The Misleading Language of Managed Care." *Journal of Health Politics, Policy, and Law*, 24, no. 5 (October): 1033–1043.

Hacker, Jacob S. and Paul Pierson. 2016. *American Amnesia: How the War on Government Led Us to Forget What Made America Prosper.* New York: Simon & Schuster.

Hafner, Katie. 2012. "Redefining Medicine with Apps and iPads." *The New York Times*, October 8. Online at www.nytimes.com/2012/10/09/science/redefining-medicine-with-apps-and-ipads-the-digital-doctor.html?

Hamel, Liz et al. 2016. *The Burden of Medical Debt: Results from the Kaiser Family Foundation/New York Times Medical Bills Survey.* Menlo Park, CA: Kaiser Family Foundation.

Hammond, Ross A. 2012. *Obesity, Prevention, and Health Care Costs.* Washington, DC: The Brookings Institution.

Harmon, Katherine. 2012. "Early Childhood Obesity Rates Might Be Slowing Nation-Wide." *Scientific American*, December 25. Online at http://blogs.scientificamerican.com/observations/2012/12/25/early-childhood-obesity-rates-might-be-slowing-nation-wide/.

Harris, Gardiner. 2004a. "F.D.A. Failing in Drug Safety, Official Asserts." *The New York Times*, November 19.

Harris, Gardiner. 2004b. "At F.D.A., Strong Drug Ties and Less Monitoring." *The New York Times*, December 6.

Harris, Gardiner. 2005. "F.D.A. To Create Advisory Board on Drug Safety." *The New York Times*, February 16.

Harris, Gardiner and Alex Berenson. 2005. "10 Voters on Panel Backing Pain Pills Had Industry Ties." *The New York Times*, February 25.

Hartman, Micah et al. 2018. "National Health Care Spending in 2016: Spending and Enrollment Growth Slow after Initial Coverage Expansion." *Health Affairs*, 37, no. 1 (January): 150–160.

Havighurst, Clark C. 1970. "Health Maintenance Organizations and the Market for Health Services." *Law and Contemporary Problems*, 35, no. 1 (Autumn): 716–795.

Havighurst, Clark C. 1973. "Regulation of Health Facilities and Services by 'Certificate of Need'." *Virginia Law Review*, 59, no. 7 (October): 1143–1233.

Hayek, Friedrich A. 1944. *The Road to Serfdom*. Chicago, IL: University of Chicago Press.

Heinen, Luann and Helen Darling. 2009. "Addressing Obesity in the Workplace: The Role of Employers." *Milbank Quarterly*, 87, no. 1 (March): 101–122.

Hermer, Laura D. and Howard Brody. 2010. "Defensive Medicine, Cost Containment, and Reform." *Journal of General Internal Medicine*, 25, no. 5 (May): 470–473.

Herzlinger, Regina. 1997. *Market Drive Health Care: Who Wins, Who Loses in the Transformation of America's Largest Service Industry*. Cambridge, MA: Perseus Books.

Hettrich, Carolyn M., Richard C. Mather, III, Manish K. Sethi, Ryan M. Nunley, and Amir A. Jahangir. 2010. "The Cost of Defensive Medicine." *American Academy of Orthopedic Surgeons Now*, 4, no. 12 (December): 29.

Himmelstein, David U. et al. 2009. "Medical Bankruptcy in the United State, 2007: Results of a National Study." *Journal of the American Medical Association*, 122, no. 8 (August 19): 741–746.

Himmelstein, David U. et al. 2014. "A Comparison of Hospital Administrative Costs in Eight Nations: US Costs Exceed All Others by Far." *Health Affairs*, 33, no. 9 (September): 1586–1594.

Himmelstein, David U. and Steffie Woolhandler. 2016. "The Current and Projected Taxpayer Shares of US Health Costs." *American Journal of Public Health*, 106, no. 3 (March): 449–452.

Hoadley, Jack. 2012. *Adapting Tools from Other Nations to Slow U.S. Prescription Drug Spending*. Washington, DC: Center for Studying Health System Change, National Institute for Health Care Reform. Online at www.nihcr.org/Drug_Spending.

Hobson, Katherine. 2009. "Critics Take Aim at High-Tech Care." *U.S. News & World Report*, 146, no. 7 (August): 76–78.

Hoffman, Beatrix. 2013. *Health Care for Some: Rights and Rationing in the United States since 1930*. Chicago, IL: University of Chicago Press.

Holahan, John et al. 2011. *Containing the Growth of Spending in the U.S. Health System*. Washington, DC: Urban Institute.

Hopkins, Jared S. 2019. "Drugmakers Raise Prices on Hundreds of Medicines." *Wall Street Journal*, January 1.

How Changes in Medical Technology Affect Health Care Costs. 2007. Washington, DC: Kaiser Family Foundation. Online at www.kff.org/insurance/snapshot/chcm030807oth.cfm.

Howard, Philip K. 2002. *The Collapse of the Common Good: How America's Lawsuit Culture Undermines Our Freedom*. New York: Ballantine Books.

Howard, Philip K. 2003. "Legal Malpractice." *Wall Street Journal*, January 27.

Huelskoetter, Thomas. 2018. *Evaluating State Innovations to Reduce Health Care Costs*. Washington, DC: Center for American Progress.

Hyman, David A. 2001. "Health Care Fraud and Abuse: Market Change, Social Norms, and the 'Trust Reposed in the Workmen'." *Journal of Legal Studies*, 30, no. S2 (June): 531–567.

Hyman, David A. and Charles Silver. 2004. "Believing Six Impossible Things: Medical Malpractice and Legal Fear." *Harvard Journal of Law and Public Policy*, 28, no. 1 (Fall): 107–118.

Iglehart, John K. 1980. "The Federal Government as Venture Capitalist: How Does It Fare?" *Milbank Memorial Fund Quarterly/Health and Society*, 59, no. 4 (Fall): 656–666.

Iglehart, John K. 2009. "Finding Money for Health Care Reform—Rooting Out Waste, Fraud, and Abuse." *New England Journal of Medicine*, 363, no. 3 (July): 229–231.

Iglehart, John K. 2010. "The Supercharged Federal Effort to Crack down on Fraud and Abuse." *Health Affairs*, 29, no. 6: 1093–1095.

IMS Institute for Healthcare Informatics. 2013. *Declining Medicine Use and Costs: For Better or Worse?* Parsippany, NJ: IMS Institute for Healthcare Informatics. Online at www.imshealth.com/deployedfiles/ims/Global/Content/Insights/IMS%20Institute%20for%20Healthcare%20Informatics/2012%20U.S.%20Medicines%20Report/2012_U.S.Medicines_Report.pdf.

Institute of Medicine. 2000. *To Err Is Human: Building a Safer Health System*. Washington, DC: National Academy Press.

Institute of Medicine. 2013. *U.S. Health in International Perspective: Shorter Lives, Poorer Health*. Washington, DC: National Academies Press.

International Federation of Health Plans. 2011. *Comparative Price Report: Medical and Hospital Fees by Country*. London: International Federation of Health Plans.

International Federation of Health Plans. 2016. *2015 Comparative Price Report: Variations in Medical and Hospital Prices by Country*. London: International Federation of Health Plans.

Jacobson, Gretchen et al. 2017. *Medicare Advantage 2017 Spotlight: Enrollment Market Update*. Menlo Park, CA: Henry J. Kaiser Family Foundation.

James, Everette and Meredith Hughes. 2015. "Government-Sponsored Programs Make up 52% of What We Spend on Healthcare." *Forbes*, July 29.

Jaros, G.G. and D.A. Boonzaier. 1993. "Cost Escalation in Health-Care Technology—Possible Solutions." *South African Medical Journal*, 83, no. 6 (June 1): 420–422.

Jesilow, Paul, Gilbert Geis, and John C. Harris. 1995. "Doomed to Repeat Our Errors: Fraud in Emerging Health-Care System." *Social Justice*, 22, no. 2 (Summer): 1995: 125–138.

Johnson, Toni. 2012. *Healthcare Costs and U.S. Competitiveness*. New York: Council on Foreign Relations.

Johnson, William C. 2018. "Consistently High Turnover in the Group of Top Health Care Spenders." *NEJM Catalyst*, February 1.
Joint Committee on Taxation. 2018. *Estimates of Federal Tax Expenditures for Fiscal Years 2017–2021*. Washington, DC: Joint Committee on Taxation.
Jonsson, B. 2001. "Flat or Monotonic Pricing of Pharmaceuticals: Practice and Consequences." *European Journal of Health Economics*, 2, no. 3: 104–112.
Kaiser Family Foundation. 2004. *Prescription Drug Trends*. Fact sheet #3057-03. Washington, DC: Henry J. Kaiser Family Foundation. Online at www.kff.org/rxdrugs/upload/Prescription-Drug-Trends-October-2004-UPDATE.pdf.
Kalb, Paul E. 1990. "Controlling Health Care Costs by Controlling Technology: A Private Contractual Approach." *Yale Law Journal*, 99, no. 4 (March): 1109–1126.
Kalra, Jay. 2011. *Medical Errors and Patient Safety: Strategies to Reduce and Disclose Medical Errors and Improve Patient Safety*. Berlin: De Gruyter.
Kamal, Rabah and Cynthia Cox. 2018 *How Do Healthcare Prices and Use in the U.S. Compare to Other Countries?* Peterson-Kaiser Health System Tracker. Menlo Park, CA: Kaiser Family Foundation.
Kamal, Rabah and Bradley Sawyer. 2018. *How Much Is Health Care Spending Expected to Grow?* Peterson-Kaiser Health System Tracker. Menlo Park, CA: Kaiser Family Foundation.
Kane, Jason. 2012. *Health Costs: How the U.S. Compares with Other Countries*. Arlington, VA: Public Broadcasting Corporation. Online at www.pbs.org/newshour/rundown/2012/10/health-costs-how-the-us-compares-with-other-countries.html.
Kassirer, Jerome P. 2005. *On the Take: How America's Complicity with Big Business Can Endanger Your Health*. New York: Oxford University Press.
Kaufman, Joanne. 2017. "Think You are Seeing More Drug Ads on TV? You Are, and Here's Why." *The New York Times*, December 24.
Keehan, Sean P., Gigi A. Cuckler, Andrea M. Sisko, Andrew M. Madison, Sheila D. Smith, Joseph M. Lizonitz, John A. Poisal, and Christian J. Wolfe. 2012. "National Health Expenditure Projections: Modest Annual Growth until Coverage Expands and Economic Growth Accelerates." *Health Affairs*, 31, no. 7 (July): 1600–1612.
Kelley, Robert. 2009. *Where Can $700 Billion in Waste Be Cut Annually from the U.S. Healthcare System?* New York: Thomson Reuters.
Kelly, Robert and Raymond Fabius. 2010. *A Path to Eliminating $3.6 Trillion in Wasteful Healthcare Spending*. Ann Arbor, MI: Thomson Reuters.
Kesselheim, Aaron S. and David M. Studdert. 2008. "Whistleblower-Initiated Enforcement Actions." *Annals of Internal Medicine*, 149, no. 5 (September): 342–350.
Kincaid, Ellie. 2018. "Want Fries with That? A Brief History of Medical MRIs, Starting with A McDonald's." *Forbes*, April 16. Online at forbes.com.
Kirzinger, Ashley et al. 2017. "U.S. Public Opinion on Health Care Reform, 2017." *Journal of the American Medical Association*, 317, no. 15 (April 18): 1516.
Kirzinger, Ashley et al. 2018a. *Kaiser Health Tracking Poll – Late Summer 2018: The Election, Pre-Existing Conditions, and Surprises on Medical Bills*. Menlo Park, CA: Kaiser Family Foundation.
Kirzinger, Ashley, Bryan Wu, and Mollyann Brodie. 2018b. *Kaiser Health Tracking Poll – February 2018: Health Care and the 2018 Midterms, Attitudes toward Proposed Changes to Medicaid*. (May) Menlo Park, CA: Kaiser Family Foundation.
Kitsis, Elizabeth A. 2009. "Rx for the Pharmaceutical Industry: Call Your Doctors." *Hastings Center Report*, 39, no. 4 (August): 18–21.
Klein, Ezra. 2009. "Administrative Costs in Health Care: A Primer." *The Washington Post*, July 7.
Kliff, Sarah. 2015. "8 Facts that Explain What's Wrong with American Health Care." *Vox*, January 20.
Kliff, Sarah and Oh, Soo 2018. "America's Health Care Prices are Out of Control. These 11 Charts Prove It." *Vox*, May 10.
Kofman, Mila and Karen Pollitz. 2006. *Health Insurance Regulation by States and the Federal Government: A Review of Current Approaches and Proposals for Change*. Washington, DC: Health Policy Institute, Georgetown University.
Krause, John H. 2006. "A Patient-Centered Approach to Health Care Fraud Recovery." *Journal of Criminal Law and Criminology*, 96, no. 2 (Winter): 579–619.
Krugman, Paul. 2009. "Administrative Costs." *The New York Times*, July 6.
Kumar, Krishna R. 2011. "Technology and Healthcare Costs." *Annals of Pediatric Cardiology*, 4, no. 1 (January–June): 84–86.
Lakoff, George. 2008. *The Political Mind: Why You Can't Understand 21st-Century American Politics with an 18th-Century Brain*. New York: Viking.
Lallemand, Nicole C. 2012a. *Reducing Waste in Health Care*. Health Policy Brief, Washington, DC: Robert Wood Johnson Foundation.
Lallemand, Nicole C. 2012b. "Health Policy Brief: Reducing Waste in Health Care." *Health Affairs*, December 13.
Larkin, Ian, et al. 2017. "Association between Academic Medical Center Pharmaceutical Detail Policies and Physician Prescribing." *Journal of the American Medical Association*, 317, no. 17 (May 2): 1785–1795.
Latham, Bryan W. 1983. *Health Care Costs: There Are Solutions*. New York: American Management Association.
Latham, Stephen R. 2005. "Two Few Physicians, or Too Many?" *Hastings Center Report*, 40, no. 1 (January/February): 11–12.
Laugesen, Miriam J. and Sherry A. Glied. 2011. "Higher Fees Paid to U.S. Physicians Drive Higher Spending for Physician Services Compared to Other Countries." *Health Affairs*, 30, no. 9 (September): 1647–1656.
Lee, Jason S. and Laura Tollen. 2002. "How Low Can You Go? the Impact of Reduced Benefits and Increased Cost-Sharing." *Health Affairs* (June 19): W229–W241.
Lesser, Cara S., Paul B. Ginsburg, and Kelly J. Devers. 2003. "The End of an Era: What Became of the 'Managed Care Revolution' in 2001?" *Health Services Research*, 38, no. 1, Part II (February): 337—355.

Lexchin, Joel and Barbara Mintzes. 2002. "Direct-to-Consumer Advertising of Prescription Drugs: The Evidence Says No." *Journal of Public Policy and Marketing*, 21, no. 2 (Fall): 194–201.
Leyerle, Betty. 1994. *The Private Regulation of American Health Care*. Armonk, NY: M.E. Sharpe.
Lieberman, Trudy. 2004. "Your Health: Fatal Mistakes." AARP Bulletin Online. Online at www.aarp.org/bulletin/yourhealth/Articles/a2004-10-27-fatal_mistakes.html.
Lind, David P. 2016. *Silently Harmed: Hospital Medical Errors in the Heartland*. Clive, IA: Heartland Health Research Institute.
Lind, Michael. 2012. *America Doesn't Need Health Care Rationing*. Salon.com, October 2. Online at www.salon.com/2012/10/02/america_doesnt_need_health_care_rationing.
Lipton, Eric and Kevin Sack. 2013. "Fiscal Footnote: Big Senate Gift to Drug Maker." *The New York Times*, January 19. Online at www.nytimes.com/2013/01/20/us/medicare-pricing-delay-is-political-win-for-amgen-drug-maker.html?
Lopez, German, 2017a. "White House: One Year of the Opioid Epidemic Cost the U.S. Economy More than $500 Billion." *Vox*, November 20.
Lopez, German. 2017b. "The Opioid Epidemic Explained." *Vox*, December 21.
Lubitz, James. 2005. "Health, Technology, and Medical Care Spending." *Health Affairs*, Web Exclusive 24, no. 2 (Supplement): R81–R85.
Lucia, Kevin, Jack Hoadley, and Ashley Williams. 2017. *Balance Billing by Health Care Providers: Assessing Consumer Protections across States*. New York: The Commonwealth Fund.
Maier, Timothy W. 1997. "Pharmaceuticals: What Do They Buy?" *Insight on the News*, 13, no. 25 (July 7): 14–15.
Makary, Marty. 2012. *Unaccountable: What Hospitals Won't Tell You and How Transparency Can Revolutionize Health Care*. London: Bloombury Press.
March of Dimes. 2014. "Premature Babies Cost Employers $12.7 Billion Annually." March of Dimes. Online at www.marchofdimes.org/news/premature-babies-cost-employers-127-billion-annually.aspx.
Massachusetts Health Care Reform: Six Years Later. 2012. Menlo Park, CA: Kaiser Family Foundation.
Mattke, Soeren et al. 2013. *Workplace Wellness Programs Study: Final Report*. Santa Monica, CA: RAND Corporations.
McCarthy, Mark. 2009. "Panel: Tort Reform Is Likely to Have Very Little Effect on Cost." *Medical Device Daily*, 13, no. 193 (October): 1, 7.
McCarthy, Mark. 2012. "Study Says Med Tech Inflation at 1% Share of NHE Still 6%." *Medical Device Daily*, 16, no. 207 (October): 1–8.
McClellan, Mark. 1996. "Are the Returns to Technological Change in Health Care Declining?" *Proceedings of the National Academy of Sciences of the United States*, 93, no. 23 (November 12): 12701–12709.
McClure, Walter. 1981. "Structural and Incentive Problems in Economic Regulation of Medical Care." *Milbank Memorial Quarterly/Health and Society*, 59, no. 2 (Spring): 107–144.
McClure, Walter. 1983. "The Competitive Strategy for Medical Care." *Annals of the American Academy of Political and Social Science*, 469 (July): 30–47.
McGill, Andrew. 2017. "The Platinum Patients." *The Atlantic*. Online at www.theatlantic.com.
McGregor, Maurice. 1981. "Hospital Costs: Can They Be Cut?" *Milbank Memorial Fund Quarterly/Health and Society*, 59, no. 1 (Winter): 89–98.
McGuire, Alistair and Victoria Serra. 2005. "The Cost of Care: Is There an Optimal Level of Expenditure?" *Harvard International Review*, 27, no. 1 (Spring): 70–73.
McLaughlin, Neil. 2011. "Pricey Healthcare: Studies Show U.S. Costs are Higher, Benefits Lower—With Blame for All." *Modern Healthcare*, 41, no. 39 (September): 17.
McMillen, Scott R. 1996. "The Medical Malpractice Statute of Limitations: Some Answers and Some Questions." *Trial Lawyers Forum*, 70, no. 2: 44–47.
Mechanic, David. 1997. "Muddling through Elegantly: Finding the Proper Balance in Rationing." *Health Affairs*, 16, no. 5 (September/October): 83–92.
Medicaid and CHIP Access Commission. n.d. *Medicaid's Share of State Budgets*. Washington, DC: Medicaid and CHIP Access Commission.
Medicaid Managed Care Enrollment and Program Characteristics 2016. 2018. Online at www.medicaid.gov/.
Medicaid, A Primer: 2013. 2013. Washington, DC: Kaiser Commission on Medicaid and the Uninsured.
"Medical Errors Cost Health Care System Billions." 2011. *National Journal*, April 7.
Medical Liability Reform Must Have Teeth to Be Effective. 2009. Press release, September 17. Washington, DC: US Chamber of Commerce.
Medicare Delivery System Reform: The Evidence Link. n.d. Menlo Park, CA: Kaiser Family Foundation.
The Medicare Part D Prescription Drug Benefit. 2017. Menlo Park, CA: Kaiser Family Foundation, October 2.
Meisel, Zachary F. and Jeanmarie Perrone. 2012. "The Pain Game: Are Doctors to Blame for Prescription- Drug Abuse?" *Time*, 180, no. 24 (December 10). Online at http://ideas.time.com/2012/11/26/viewpoint-prescription-drug-abuse-is-fueled-by-doctors/.
Mello, Michelle M., David M. Studdert, Catherine M. DesRoches, Jordan Peugh, Kinga Zapert, Troyen A. Brennan, and M. Sage William. 2004. "Caring for Patients in a Malpractice Crisis: Physician Satisfaction and Quality of Care." *Health Affairs*, 23, no. 4 (July–August): 42–53.
Mendoza, Allie. 2009. "Staggering Health Care Costs Due to Unhealthy Lifestyle Pose a Major Threat to U.S. Economy." Examiner.com, July 2. Online at www.examiner.com/article/staggering-health-care-costs-due-to-unhealthy-lifestyle-pose-major-threat-to-u-s-economy.
Menzel, Paul T. 1990. *Strong Medicine: The Ethical Rationing of Health Care*. New York: Oxford University Press.
Mettler, Suzanne. 2011. *The Submerged States: How Invisible Government Policies Undermine American Democracy*. Chicago, IL: University of Chicago Press.

Milanez, Isadora and Mark Strauss. 2018. *Americans are Closely Divided over Value of Medical Treatments, but Most Agree Costs are a Big Problem.* Washington, DC: Pew Research Center, July 9.

Miller, Tom. 2017–2018. "The Concentration and Persistence of Health Care Spending." *Regulation*, 40, no. 4 (Winter): 28–34.

Miller, Tracy E. and Arthur R. Derse. 2002. "Between Strangers: The Practice of Medicine Online." *Health Affairs*, 21, no. 4 (July–August): 168–179.

Mitchell, Emily M. 2014. *Concentration of Health Expenditures in the U.S. Civilian Noninstitutionalized Population, 2014.* Rockville, MD: Agency for Healthcare Research and Quality, US Department of Health and Human Services.

Mitts, Lydia. 2012. *Wellness Programs: Evaluating the Promises and the Pitfalls.* Washington, DC: Families USA.

Moon, Marilyn. 2005. "Confronting the Rising Costs of Healthcare in Medicare and Medicaid." *Generations*, 29, no. 1 (Spring): 59–64.

Moore, Peter. 2018. "Broke from Cancer." *AARP The Magazine*, 61, #4C (June/July): 50–53.

Moran, Donald W. 1981. "HMOs, Competition, and the Politics of Minimum Benefits." *Milbank Memorial Fund Quarterly/Health and Society*, 59, no. 2 (Spring): 190–208.

Moran, Donald W. 1997. "Federal Regulation of Managed Care: An Impulse in Search of a Theory?" *Health Affairs*, 16, no. 6 (November/December): 7–21.

Morone, James A. and Lawrence R. Jacobs, eds. 2005. *Healthy, Wealthy, & Fair: Health Care and the Good Society.* New York: Oxford University Press.

Morris, Jonas. 1984. *Searching for a Cure: National Health Policy Considered.* New York: Pica Press.

Mukherjee, Sy. 2018. "3 Key Lessons from Trump's Price Feud with Pfizer." *Fortune*, July 11.

Mullis, Jeffrey. 1995. "Medical Malpractice, Social Structure, and Social Control." *Sociological Forum*, 10, no. 4 (March 1): 135–163.

Muraskas, Jonathan and Kayhan Parsi. 2008. "The Cost of Saving the Tiniest Lives: NICUs versus Prevention." *American Medical Association Journal of Ethics*, 10, no. 10 (October): 655–658.

Nahed, Brian V., Maya A. Babu, Timothy R. Smith, and Robert F. Heary. 2012. "Malpractice Liability and Defensive Medicine: A National Survey of Neurosurgeons." *Public Library of Science One*, 7, no. 6 (June): 1–7.

Nash, Karen. 2012. "Urologists Often on the 'Defensive' When Ordering Tests." *Urology Times*, June 12: 59–60.

National Center for Health Statistics. 2016. *National Health Expenditures Data.* Baltimore, MD: Centers for Medicare & Medicaid Services.

National Center for Health Statistics. 2018. *National Health Expenditures Data.* Baltimore, MD: Centers for Medicare & Medicaid Services, 2012. Online at www.cms.gov/Research-Statistics-Data-and-Systems/Statistics-Trends-and-Reports.

National Institute of Drug Abuse. 2018. *Prescription Opioids.* Rockville, MD: US Department of Health and Human Services.

New, Michael J. 2005. *The Effect of State Regulations on Health Insurance Premiums: A Preliminary Analysis.* Washington, DC: Center for Data Analysis, Heritage Foundation.

Newhouse, Joseph P. et al. 1981. "Some Interim Results, Form a Controlled Trial of Cost-Sharing in Health Insurance." *New England Journal of Medicine*, 305, no. 5 (December): 1501–1507.

Newhouse, Joseph P. 1992. "Medical Care Costs: How Much Welfare Loss?" *Journal of Economic Perspectives*, 6, no. 3: 3–21.

Nitzkin, Joel L. 1996. "Technology and Health Care—Driving Costs Up, Not Down." *IEEE Technology and Society Magazine*, 15, no. 3 (Fall): 40–46.

Nix, Kathryn. 2012. *Comparative Effectiveness Research under Obamacare: A Slippery Slope to Health Care Rationing.* Backgrounder no. 2679. April 12. Washington, DC: Heritage Foundation.

Noll, Roger G. 1975. "The Consequences of Public Utility Regulation of Hospitals." In *Controls on Health Care*, ed. Institute of Medicine, 32–48. Washington, DC: National Academy of Sciences.

Nuijten, M.J.C., P. Berto, G. Berdeaux, J. Hutton, F.U. Fricke, and F.A. Villar. 2001. "Trends in DecisionMaking Process for Pharmaceuticals in Western European Countries: A Focus on Emerging Hurdles for Obtaining Reimbursement and A Price." *European Journal of Health Economics*, 2, no. 4: 162–169.

Office of Management and Budget. 2018. *Historical Budget Statistics FY2019.* Washington, DC: Office of Management and Budget.

Office of Technology Assessment. 1994. *Defensive Medicine and Medical Malpractice.* Washington, DC: US Office of Technology Assessment.

Olen, Helaine. 2017. "Even the Insured Often Can't Afford Their Medical Bills." *The Atlantic*, June 18. Online at theatlantic.com.

Olson, Laura Katz. 2010. *The Politics of Medicaid.* New York: Columbia University Press.

Olson, Peter and Louise Sheiner. 2017. *The Hutchins Center Explains: Prescription Drug Spending.* Washington, DC: Brookings Institution.

"Opioid Fast Facts." 2019. CNN, April 11. Online at cnn.com.

Organization for Economic Cooperation and Development. 2017. *Magnetic Resonance Imaging (MRI) Exams.* Online at https://data.oecd.org/healthcare/magnetic-resonance-imaging-mri-exams.htm.

Ornstein, Charles, Mike Tigas, and Ryann Grochowski. 2016. *Now There's Proof: Docs Who Get Company Cash Tend to Prescribe More Brand-Name Meds.* New York: ProPublica. Online at propublica.org.

Pampel, Fred C. and Richard G. Rogers. 2004. "Socioeconomic Status, Smoking, and Health: A Test of Competing Theories of Cumulative Advantage." *Journal of Health and Social Behavior*, 45, no. 3 (September): 306–321.

Papanicolas, Irene et al. 2018. "Health Care Spending in the United States and Other High-Income Countries." *Journal of the American Medical Association*, 319, no. 10 (March 13): 1024–1039.

Park, Chris. 2015. *Trends in Medicaid Spending for Prescription Drugs.* Washington, DC: Medicaid and CHIP Payment and Access Commission.

Patashnik, Eric M., Alan S. Gerber, and Conor M. Dowling. 2017. *Unhealthy Politics: The Battle over Evidence-Based Medicine*. Princeton, NJ: Princeton University Press.

Patel, Kant and Mark Rushefsky. 2002. *Health Care Policy in an Age of New Technologies*. New York: M.E. Sharpe.

Patel, Kant and Mark Rushefsky. 2005. *The Politics of Public Health in the United States*. Armonk, NY: M.E. Sharpe.

Patel, Kant and Mark E. Rushefsky. 1998. "The Health Policy Community and Health Care Reform in the United States." *Health: an Interdisciplinary Journal for the Social Study of Health, Illness and Medicine*, 2, no. 4 (October): 459–484.

Pauly, Mark V. 1978. "Is Medical Care Different?" In *Competition in the Health Care Sector: Past, Present and Future*, ed. Bureau of Economics, US Federal Trade Commission, 19–48. Washington, DC: Government Printing Office.

Pauly, Mark V. and Lawton R. Burns. 2008. "Price Transparency for Medical Devices." *Health Affairs*, 27, no. 6: 1544–1553.

Pear, Robert. 2004. "Americans Relying More on Prescription Drugs, Report Says." *The New York Times*, December 3.

Pearl, Robert. 2017. *Mistreated: Why We Think We're Getting Good Health Care – And Why We're Usually Wrong*. New York: Public Affairs.

Pearson, Elsa. 2018. "How Much Is Too Much. What Does the US Actually Spend on Health Care Administration?" *The Incidental Economist*, April 4. Online at https://theincidentaleconomist.com.

Perrone, Mathew and Jill Colvin. 2018. "Trump's Plan to Reduce Drug Prices Doesn't Include Campaign Pledge to Allow Medicare to Negotiate Prices." *Chicago Tribune*, May 11.

Phillip, Peter. 2002. "The Rising Cost of Health Care: Can Demand Be Reduced through More Effective Health Promotion?" *Journal of Evaluation in Clinical Practice*, 8, no. 4: 415–419.

PhRMA. n.d. *Follow the Dollar: Flow of Payment for $3,000 HIV Medicine*. Washington, DC: Pharmaceutical Manufacturers of America.

Pickert, Kate. 2009. "Malpractice Reform." *Time*, 174, no. 12 (September 28): 16.

Pinkovskiy, Maxim. 2013. *The Impact of the Managed Care Backlash on Health Care Costs: Evidence from State Regulation of Managed Care Cost Containment Practices*. New York: Federal Reserve Bank of New York.

Pittman, Genevra. 2012. "Obesity Declining in Young, Poorer Kids: Study." *Huffington Post*, December 26. Online at www.huffingtonpost.com/2012/12/26/childhood-obesity-rate_n_2365422.html.

"Politics Keeps Real Remedies Off Radar." 2004. *USA Today*, September 14.

Pollitz, Karen et al. 2014. *Medical Debt among People with Medical Insurance*. Menlo Park, CA: Kaiser Family Foundation.

Pomeranz, Jennifer L. et al. 2016. "Variability and Limits of US State Laws Regulating Workplace Wellness Programs." *American Journal of Public Health*, 106, no. 6 (June): 1028–1031.

Porter, Eduardo. 2012. "Rationing Health Care More Fairly." *The New York Times*, August 21.

Prescription Drug Trends. 2010. Washington, DC: Kaiser Family Foundation, May. Online at www.kff.org/rxdrugs/upload/3057-08.pdf.

President's Council on Bioethics. 2003. *Organ Transplantation: Ethical Dilemmas and Policy Choices*. Staff background paper. Washington, DC: Executive Office of the President.

Primary Reason Why Health Care Costs Continue to Rise. 2012. Gaithersburg, MD: Potomac Companies, May 2. Online at www.potomacco.com/general/wellness-general/primary-reason-why-health-care-costs-continue-to-rise-employee-lifestyle-choices/.

"Proportion of Branded Versus Generic Drug Prescriptions Dispensed in the United States from 2005 to 2016." n.d. Statista. Online at statista.com.

Rabecs, Robert N. 2006. "Health Care Fraud under the New Medicare Part D Prescription Drug Program." *Journal of Criminal Law and Criminology*, 96, no. 2 (Winter): 727–756.

Rae, Matthew, Gary Claxton, and Larry Levitt. 2017. *Do Health Plan Enrollees Have Enough Money to Pay Cost Sharing?* Menlo Park, CA: Kaiser Family Foundation.

Rai, Arti K. 2001. "Health Care Fraud and Abuse: A Tale of Behavior Induced by Payment Structure." *Journal of Legal Studies*, 30, S2 (June): 579–587.

Regalado, Antonio. 2013. "We Need a Moore's Law for Medicine." *MIT Technology Review*, 116, no. 6 (October 3): 67–69.

Reid, T.R. 2009. *The Healing of America: A Global Quest for Better, Cheaper, and Fairer Health Care*. New York: Penguin Press.

Relman, Arnold S. 2005. "The Health of Nations." *New Republic*, 232, no. 4703 (March 7): 23–30

Rettig, Richard A. 1994. "Medical Innovation Duels Cost Containment." *Health Affairs*, 13, no. 3 (Summer): 7–27.

Rice, Thomas. 1997. "Can Markets Give Us the Health System We Want?" *Journal of Health Politics, Policy and Law*, 22, no. 2 (1997): 383–426.

Richtel, Matt. 2012. "Apps Alert the Doctor When Trouble Looms." *The New York Times*, October 8. Online at http://well.blogs.nytimes.com/2012/10/08/apps-alert-the-doctor-when-trouble-looms.

Robert Wood Johnson Foundation. 2012. *Health Policy Brief: Reducing Waste in Health Care*. Princeton, NJ: Robert Wood Johnson Foundation. Online at www.rwjf.org/content/dam/farm/reports/issue_briefs/2012/rwjf403314.

Robertson, John A., Baruch Brody, Allen Buchanan, Jeffrey Kahn, and Elizabeth McPherson. 2002. "Phar- Macogenetic Challenges for the Health Care System." *Health Affairs*, 21, no. 4 (July–August): 155–167.

Robeznicks, Andis. 2010. "The Fear Factor." *Modern Healthcare*, 40, no. 37 (September): 6–7.

Robinson, James. 2002. "Renewed Emphasis on Consumer Cost Sharing in Health Insurance Benefit Design." *Health Affairs* (March 20): W139–W154.

Rockoff, Jonathan D. 2018. "This Form of Ambien Now Costs over 800% More." *Wall Street Journal*, July 14.

Roehrig, Charles S. and Donald M. Rousseau. 2011. "The Growth in Cost per Case Explains Far More of US Health Spending Increases than Rising Disease Prevalence." *Health Affairs*, 30, no. 9 (September): 1657–1663.

Roemer, Milton I. 1961. "Hospital Utilization and the Supply of Physicians." *Journal of the American Medical Association*, 178, no. 1 (December): 933–989.

Rosenberg, Charlotte L. 1984. "Why Doctor-Policing Laws Don't Work." *Medical Economics*, 61 (March 5): 84–96.
Rosenthal, Elisabeth. 2017. *An American Sickness: How Healthcare Became a Big Business and How You Can Take It Back*. New York: Penguin Press.
Rosenthal, Marilyn M. and Kathleen M. Sutcliffe, eds. 2002. *Medical Error: What Do We Know? What Do We Do?* San Francisco, CA: Jossey-Bass.
Rosoff, Arnold J. 1975. "Phase Two of the Federal HMO Development Program: New Directions after a Shaky Start." *American Journal of Law and Medicine*, 1, no. 2 (Fall): 209–243.
Ross, James S. 2002. "The Committee on the Costs of Medical Care and the History of Health Insurance in the United States." *Einstein Quarterly Journal of Biological Medicine*, 19: 129–134.
Rothenberg, Michael B. et al. 2014. "The Cost of Defensive Medicine on 3 Hospital Medical Services." *Journal of the American Medical Association Internal Medicine*, 174, no. 11 (November): 1867–1868.
Roy, Avik. 2011. "The Myth of Medicare's 'Low Administrative Costs'." *Forbes*, June 30.
Roy, Avik. 2012. "Liberals Are Wrong: Free Market Health Care Is Possible." *The Atlantic*, May 18. Online at www.theatlantic.com.
Roy, Avik. 2018. "The Trump Plan to Reduce Prescription Drug Prices Will Have a Major Impact." *Forbes*, May 14.
Rushefsky, Mark E. 1981. "A Critique of Market Reform in Health Care: The Consumer-Choice Health Plan," *Journal of Health Politics, Policy and Law*, 5 (August): 720–741.
Ryan, Paul. 2016. "A Better Way: Our Vision for A Confident America." Better Off Now. Online at www.better.gop, June 22.
Ryu, Alexander et al. 2013. "The Slowdown in Health Care Spending in 2009–2011 Reflected Factors Other than the Weak Economy and Thus May Persist." *Health Affairs*, 32, no. 5 (May): 835–840.
Sabatini, Nelson et al. 2017. "Maryland's All-Payer Model—Achievements, Challenges, and Next Steps." *Health Affairs Blog*, January 31.
Safire, William. 2009. "Bending the Curve." *The New York Times*, September 11.
Sage, William M. 2003. "Medical Liability and Patient Safety." *Health Affairs*, 22, no. 4 (July–August): 26–36.
Sage, William M. 2004. "The Forgotten Third: Liability Insurance and the Medical Malpractice Crisis." *Health Affairs*, 23, no. 4 (July–August): 10–21.
Sanger-Katz, Margot. 2018. "A Fear of Lawsuits Really Does Seem to Result in Extra Medical Tests." *The New York Times*, July 23.
Sarnak, Dana O., David Squires, and Shawn Bishop. 2017. *Paying for Prescription Drugs around the World: Why Is the U.S. An Outlier?* New York: The Commonwealth Fund.
"Save Thousands as a Medical Tourist in These Five Countries." 2016. *Huffington Post*, August 26.
Savedoff, William D. 2007. "What Should a Country Spend on Health Care?" *Health Affairs*, 26, no. 4 (July/August): 962–970.
Sawyer, Bradley and Selena Gonzales. 2017. *How Does the Quality of the U.S. Healthcare System Compare to Other Countries?* New York: Peterson Center on Health Care; Menlo Park, CA: Kaiser Family Foundation.
Scandlen, Greg. 2011. "Myth Busters #1: Roemer's Law." Health Policy Blog. Online at http://healthblog.ncpa.org/myth-busters-1-roemer%E2%80%99s-law/.
Scandlen, Gregg. 2018. *Health Care in America: The Commonwealth Fund's Deceptive Research*. Washington, DC: The Federalist Society.
Schmid, Randolph E. 2004. "40 Percent in U.S. Use Prescription Drugs." *The Washington Post*, December 2.
Schneider, Eric C. et al. 2017. *Mirror, Mirror: International Comparison Reflect Flaws and Opportunities for Better U.S. Health Care*. New York: Commonwealth Fund.
Schneider, William. 1998. "Fear of Bureaucrats Strikes Again." *National Journal* 30, no. 29 (July 18): 1714.
Schoen, Cathy et al. 2005. "Taking the Pulse of Health Care Systems: Experiences of Patients with Health Problems in Six Countries." *Health Affairs* (November 3): W5-509–W5-525. Online at healthaffairs.org.
Schur, Claudia L. and Marc L. Berk. 2008. "Views on Health Care Technology: Americans Consider the Risks and Sources of Information." *Health Affairs*, 27, no. 6 (November/December): 1654–1664.
Schwartz, William B. 1987. "The Inevitable Failure of Current Cost-Containment Strategies: Why They Can Provide Only Temporary Relief." *Journal of the American Medical Association*, 257, no. 2 (January 9): 220–224.
Seabury, Seth and Anupam B. Jena. 2016. "Why Do so Many Doctors Practice Defensive Medicine? Maybe because It Works." The Evidence Base. Online at evidencebase.usc.edu.
Shanfelt, Tait, Christine A. Sinsky, and Stephen Swensen. 2017. "Preventable Deaths in American Hospitals." *NEJM Catalyst*, January 23. Online at catalyst.nejm.org.
Shrank, William H., Niteesh K. Choudhry, Joshua N. Liberman, and Troyen A. Brennan. 2011. "The Use of Generic Drugs in Prevention of Chronic Disease Is Far More Cost-Effective than Thought, and May Save Money." *Health Affairs*, 30, no. 7 (July): 1351–1357.
Siegel, Bruce, Holly Mead, and Robert Burke. 2008. "Private Gain and Public Pain: Financing American Health Care." *Journal of Law, Medicine, and Ethics*, 36, no. 4 (Winter): 644–651.
Silver, Charles and David A. Hyman. 2018. *Overcharged: Why Americans Pay Too Much for Health Care*. Washington, DC: Cato Institute.
Skinner, Jonathan. 2013. "The Costly Paradox of Health-Care Technology." *Technology Review*, 116, no. 6 (October 7): 69–70.
Sloan, Frank A. and John H. Shadle. 2009. "Is There Empirical Evidence for "Defensive Medicine"? A Reassessment." *Journal of Health Economics*, 28, no. 2 (March): 481–491.
Smith, Mark et al., eds. 2013. *Best Care at Lower Cost: The Path to Continuously Learning Health Care in America*. Washington, DC: National Academy Press.

Smith, Sheila, Joseph P. Newhouse, and Mark S. Freeland. 2009. "Income, Insurance, Ad Technology: Why Does Health Spending Outpace Economic Growth?" *Health Affairs*, 28, no. 5 (September/October): 1276–1284.

Smith-Bindman, Rebecca, Diana L. Miglioretti, Eric Johnson, Choonsik Lee, Heather S. Feigelson, Michael Flynn, Robert T. Greenlee, Rendell L. Kruger, Mark C. Hornbrook, Douglas Roblin, Leif I. Solberg, Nicholas Vanneman, Sheila Weinmann, and Andrew E. William. 2012. "Use of Diagnostic Imaging Studies and Associated Radiation Exposure for Patients Enrolled in Large Integrated Health Care Systems." *Journal of American Medical Association*, 307, 22 (June 13): 2400–2409.

Sommers, Benjamin D. and Jonathan Gruber. 2017. "Federal Funding Insulated State Budgets from Increased Spending Related to Medicaid Expansion." *Health Affairs*, 36, no. 5 (May): 938–944.

Sorenson, Corinna, Michael Drummond, and Beena Bhiyan Khan. 2013. "Medical Technology as a Key Driver of Rising Health Expenditure: Disentangling the Relationship." *ClinicoEconomics and Outcomes Research*, 5 (May 29): 223–234.

"Special Issue: Kenneth Arrow and the Changing Economics of Health Care." 2001. *Journal of Health Politics, Policy, and Law*, 26, no. 5 (October): 823–1204.

Squires, David and Chloe Anderson. 2015. *U.S. Health Care from a Global Perspective: Spending, Use of Services, Prices, and Health in 13 Countries*. New York: Commonwealth Fund.

Squires, David A. 2012. *Explaining High Health Care Spending in the United States: An International Comparison of Supply, Utilization, Prices, and Quality*. Washington, DC: Commonwealth Fund.

Stainton, Lilo H. 2018. "State Actions Help Keep Lid on Health Insurance Rate Hikes in NJ." *NJSpotlight*, August 13.

Starr, Paul. 1982. *The Social Transformation of American Medicine*. New York: Basic Books.

Starr, Paul. 2013. *Remedy and Reaction: The Peculiar American Struggle over Health Care Reform*. New Haven, CT: Yale University Press.

The Statistical Portal. 2018. "U.S. Pharmaceutical Industry – Statistics and Facts." Statista. Online at statista.com.

Stauch, Marc S. 1996. "Causation Issues in Medical Malpractice: A United Kingdom Perspective." *Annals of Health Law*, 5: 247–258.

Stein, Jeff. 2017. "Ryan Says Republicans to Target Welfare, Medicare, Medicaid Spending in 2018." *The Washington Post*, December 6.

Stein, Letitia. 2013. "Tampa Bay Hospital Charges Vary Widely, Medicare Data Shows." *Tampa Bay Times*, May 8. Online at www.tampabay.com/news/health/tampa-bay-hospital-charges-vary-widely-medicare-data-show/2119958.

Steinberg, Earl P. and Bryan R. Luce. 2005. "Evidence Based? Caveat Emptor!" *Health Affairs*, 24, no. 1 (January–February): 80–92.

Stone, Deborah. 2005. "How Market Ideology Guarantees Racial Inequality." In *Wealthy, Healthy, & Fair*, ed. James A. Morone and Lawrence R. Jacobs, 65–89. New York: Oxford University Press.

Stone, Deborah. 2012. *Policy Paradox: The Art of Political Decision Making*, 3rd edn. New York: W.W. Norton.

Struve, Catherine T. 2004. "Improving the Medical Malpractice Litigation Process." *Health Affairs*, 23, no. 4 (July–August): 33–41.

"Study Shows 70 Percent of Americans Take Prescription Drugs." 2013. *CBS News*, June 20. Online at cbsnews.com.

Sturm, Roland. 2002. "The Effects of Obesity, Smoking, and Drinking on Medical Problems and Costs." *Health Affairs*, 21, no. 2: 245–253.

Sugarman, Stephen D. 1985. "Doing Away with Tort Law." *California Law Review*, 73: 555–664.

Tax Policy Center. n.d. *Briefing Book: A Citizen's Guide to the Fascinating (Though Often Complex) Elements of the Federal Tax System*. Washington, DC: Urban Institute and Brookings Institution.

Taylor, Mikil. 2018. "How Much Does an MRI Cost." *Healthcare Bluebook*, March 13. Online at healthcarebluebook.com.

"That CT Scan Costs How Much?" 2012. *Consumer Reports*, July. Online at consumerreports.org.

Thomas, Katie. 2013. "U.S. Drug Costs Dropped in 2012, but Rises Loom." *The New York Times*, March 18. Online at www.nytimes.com/2013/03/19/business/use-of-generics-produces-an-unusual-drop-in-drug-spending.html?pagewanted=all&_r=0.

Thomas, Katie. 2018a. "What Does a Drug Cost? It Depends on Where You Live." *The New York Times*, July 6.

Thomas, Katie. 2018b. "Bowing to Trump, Novartis Joins Trump in Freezing Drug Prices." *The New York Times*, July 18.

Thomas, Lewis. 1975. *The Lives of a Cell*. New York: Bantam Books.

Thomas, J. William, Erika C. Ziller, and Deborah A. Thayer. 2012. "Low Costs of Defensive Medicine, Small Savings from Tort Reform." *Health Affairs*, 29, no. 9: 1578–1584.

Thorpe, Kenneth E. 2004. "The Medical Malpractice 'Crisis': Recent Trends and the Impact of State Tort Reforms." *Health Affairs*, Web Exclusive W-4 (January–June): 20–30.

Timble, Justin W. et al. 2012. "Five Reasons that Many Comparative Effectiveness Studies Fail to Change Patient Care and Clinical Practice." *Health Affairs*, 31, no. 10 (October): 2168–2175.

Tyson, Laura D'Andrea. 2012. "Evidence Vs. Ideology in the Medicare Debate." *The New York Times*, August 24.

US Department of Health, Education, and Welfare. 1971. *Toward a Comprehensive Health Policy for the 1970s: A White Paper*. Washington, DC: US Government Printing Office.

US Senate Homeland Security & Governmental Affairs Committee, Minority Office. 2018. *Manufactured Crisis: How Devastating Drug Price Increases Are Harming America's Seniors*. Washington, DC: US Congress.

USA Today/Kaiser Family Foundation/Harvard School of Public Health. 2008. *The Public on Prescription Drugs and Pharmaceutical Companies*. Menlo Park, CA: Kaiser Family Foundation.

Vale, Luke. 2010. "Health Technology Assessment and Economic Evaluation: Arguments for a National Approach." *Value in Health*, 13, no. 6 (September/October): 859–861.

Valet, Vicky. 2015. "More than Two-Thirds of U.S. Employers Offer Currently Offer Wellness Programs, Study Sats." *Forbes*, July 8.

Valletta, Robert G. 2008. "The Cost and Value of New Medical Technologies: Symposium Summary." *Federal Reserve Bank of San Francisco Economic Letter*, 2007, no. 18 (July): 1–3.

Van Den Bos, Jill, Karan Rustagi, Travis Gray, Michael Halford, Eva Ziemkiewicz, and Jonathan Shreve. 2011. "The $17.1 Billion Problem: The Annual Cost of Measurable Medical Errors." *Health Affairs*, 30, no. 4: 596–603.

Van Nuys, Karen et al. 2018. *Overpaying for Prescription Drugs: The Copay Clawback Phenomenon*. Los Angeles, CA: Leonard Schaeffer for Health Policy & Economics, University of Southern California.

Vandegrift, Donald and Anusua Datta. 2006. "Prescription Drug Expenditures in the United States: The Effects of Obesity, Demographics, and New Pharmaceutical Products." *Southern Economic Journal*, 73, no. 2 (October): 515–529.

Varner, Theresa and Jack Christy. 1986. "Consumer Information Needs in a Competitive Health Care Environment." *Health Care Financing Review* (Annual Supplement): 99–104.

Virts, John R. and George W. Wilson. 1984. "Inflation and Health Care Prices." *Health Affairs*, 3, no. 1 (Spring): 88–100.

Vladeck, Bruce C. 1981. "The Market Vs. Regulation: The Case for Regulation." *Milbank Memorial Fund Quarterly/Health and Society*, 59, no. 2 (Spring): 209–223.

Vladeck, Bruce C. 1984. "Variation Data and the Regulatory Rationale." *Health Affairs*, 3, no. 2 (Summer): 102–119.

Volsky, Igor. 2009. "Why Comparative Effectiveness Research Will Not Ration Care." *ThinkProgress*, June 19. Online at https://tfhinkprogress.org/why-comparative-effectiveness-research-will-not-ration-care-66dc80b98dfd/.

Wachter, Robert M. and Kaveh G. Shojania. 2004. *Internal Bleeding: The Truth behind America's Terrifying Epidemic of Medical Mistakes*. New York: RuggedLand.

Weiler, Paul C., Howard H. Hiatt, Joseph P. Newhouse, William G. Johnson, Troyen A. Brennan, and Lucian I. Leape. 1993. *A Measure of Malpractice: Medical Injury, Malpractice Litigation and Patient Compensation*. Cambridge, MA: Harvard University Press.

Weinder, Jonathan P., and Gregory de Lissovoy. 1993. "Razing A Tower of Babel: A Taxonomy for Managed Care and Health Insurance Plans." *Journal of Health Politics, Policy and Law*, 18, no. 1 (Spring): 75–103.

Weiner, Janet, Clifford Marks, and Mark Pauly. 2017. *Effects of the ACA on Health Care Cost Containment*. Philadelphia, PA: Leonard Davis Institute of Health Economics, University of Pennsylvania.

Weiner, Stephen M. 1982. "On Public Values and Private Regulation: Some Reflections on Cost Containment Strategies." *Milbank Memorial Fund Quarterly/Health and Society*, 59, no. 2 (Spring): 269–296.

Weisbrod, Burton A. 1991. "The Health Care Quadrilemma: An Essay on Technological Change, Insurance, Quality of Care, and Cost Containment." *Journal of Economic Literature*, 29 (June): 523–555.

Weisbrod, Burton A. and C.L. LaMay. 1999. "Mixed Signals: Public Policy and the Future of Health Care R&D." *Health Affairs*, 18, no. 2 (March–April): 112–125.

Welch, Gilbert H., Lisa M. Schwartz, and Steven Woloshin. 2011. *Overdiagnosed: Making People Sick in the Pursuit of Health*. Boston: Beacon Press.

Wolf, Charles, Jr. 1979. "A Theory of Non-Market Failures." *Public Interest*, 55 (Spring): 114–123.

"Why Drugs Cost So Much." 2017. Washington, DC: AARP. Online at aarp.org.

Willingham, Emily. 2016. "Why Did Mylan Hike EpiPen Prices 400%? because They Could." *Forbes*, August 21.

Woolhandler, Steffie, Terry Campbell, and David U. Himmelstein. 2003. "Costs of Health Care Administration in the United States and Canada." *New England Journal of Medicine*, 349, no. 8 (August 21): 768–775.

Zatkin, Steve. 1997. "A Health Plan's View of Government Regulation." *Health Affairs*, 16, no. 6 (November/December): 33–35.

Zelizer, Julian. 2017. "Blowing up the Deficit Is Part of the Plan." *The Atlantic*, December 19.

Section IV
CONTEMPORARY CHALLENGES IN AMERICAN HEALTHCARE

9

THE ROLE OF BIOMEDICAL TECHNOLOGY

The Beginning and the End of Life

MEDICAL TECHNOLOGIES: LAW, POLITICS, RELIGION, AND ETHICS

Technology assessment has been highly fragmented and sporadic in the United States. American society has failed to make systematic decisions about research and development of medical technologies such as: who should determine whether a particular technology should be developed and funded? On what basis should individuals be provided access once a technology is available in the marketplace? What level of technological intervention is appropriate for a specific medical problem? What is the total impact of the rapid spread of high-cost medical technologies on society in general and on the US healthcare system in particular (Blank 1989)?

New medical discoveries and advances in medical technologies are happening often at a much faster pace than society's ability to understand the implications of such developments and to formulate public policies designed to address complex legal, ethical, and political questions raised by them. Consider the following developments in the field of biomedical technologies in recent years.

- Scientists are closer to growing human organs in animals and the National Institute of Health (NIH) is considering lifting a moratorium that blocked funding for experiments involving human stem cells and animal embryos. This can open up federal research funds for chimera (organisms composed of cells or genes obtained from two or more different species) research and could help create organs like kidneys for transplants (Imam 2016).
- Scientists have developed a new approach to keep donated organs "alive" for a longer time period by keeping the donated organs in a device that maintains their temperature rather than being packed in ice. This could help increase the supply of donated organs (Bernstein 2016).
- Scientists at the University of Bristol were able to produce large quantities of artificial blood in the lab. This could revolutionize the blood transfusion process and can help address the shortage of donated blood in the future (Gregoire 2017).
- Australian scientists have discovered a key to stopping incurable child brain cancer with a malaria drug (Hansen 2017).
- Advances in 3D printing technology have paved the way for pharmaceutical companies to print prescription drugs that can tailor the form of medication to the specific needs of patients. For the first time ever, the FDA recently approved a 3D printed drug—prescription pill Spritam levetiracetam—used to treat certain types of seizures in epilepsy patients (Baker 2015; King 2015).
- In 2015, Nicklaus Children's Hospital in Miami got a 3D printer that makes exact replicas of organs that doctors can use to plan surgery and do practice operations (Storrs 2015).
- Scientists in the United States have developed a new drug capsule that stays in the patient's stomach for up to two weeks after being swallowed and gradually releases its payload (Kelland 2016).
- At London's Royal Free Hospitals scientists are growing noses, ears, and blood vessels in the laboratory in an attempt to make body parts using stem cells, in the hope that they will be able to transplant more types of body parts into patients (Zolfagharifard 2014).
- Scientists have created the first monkey clones in the laboratory in China in the hope of using them for research into human diseases such as cancers and metabolic and immune disorders. Critics say the work raises ethical concerns about bringing the world closer to human cloning (Briggs 2018).
- An international team of researchers announced the creation of a part-human and part-pig embryo, raising the possibility of interspecies organ transplants (Kaplan 2017).
- An artificial womb successfully grew baby sheep. The artificial womb could eventually help premature human babies to term outside of the uterus, eliminating the health risks of pregnancy (Becker 2017).

- Scientists in Japan recently announced that they had made progress in creating the precursor to a human egg cell in a dish from nothing but a woman's blood cell. The reproductive cell they created is not a mature egg and cannot be fertilized to create an embryo, but this puts them a step closer to one day creating a human baby "in vitro gametogenesis," i.e., a method of creating eggs and sperm in a dish in a laboratory. This could become a game-changing technology that could transform reproductive technology (Johnson 2018).
- Great Britain became the first country to allow a "three-parent" IVF technique. The first three-parent baby was born in 2016 to a couple in New York after they underwent a new IVF procedure at a clinic in Mexico (Kolata 2016). A second three-parent baby was born to an infertile couple using a slightly different three-parent procedure called pronuclear IVF (Roberts 2017). Critics see this as a step toward creating designer babies (Kelland and MacLellan 2015).

The above list is just a sampling of some of the rapid developments taking place in the field of biomedical research and technology. The rapid proliferation of medical technologies and spiraling healthcare costs raises many legal, political, and ethical dilemmas that we as a society must confront and address through public policies related to healthcare. The term "dilemma" in the popular sense is understood to mean a difficult choice between two or more alternatives. An ethical dilemma refers to a situation in which all the alternatives are morally problematic, that is, each alternative seems to involve a wrong act or action (Van DeVeer 1987).

Advancements in medical technology and ethical concerns raised by such technologies have given rise to the field of bioethics. "Bioethics is the application of ethical analysis to issues of health care" (Pillar 1992, 419). Debates about ethical issues raised by medical technology start during the developmental stage and continue through the experimental and implementation stages. Arthur Caplan (1989) has argued that society's obligation to provide healthcare exists if four conditions are present. The first is that the person is clearly in need of help. The second condition is that help exists and is available. Third, that the person in need wants help, and our obligation to help is stronger if such help does not harm others. Finally, that there is a reasonable chance of actually providing some help, that is, doing some good.

Any discussion of the ethical uses of medical technology must also take into consideration special concerns about respecting the patient's dignity. Threats to a patient's dignity can arise from a variety of sources, such as substandard conditions of treatment (inadequate space, equipment, etc.), healthcare providers' decisions and behaviors, and the clash of innovative technology with traditional standards (Pillar 1992).

Unfortunately, the use of many new medical technologies raises a complex set of legal, ethical, political, and policy questions that are not easy to resolve. The discussion about medical technology is never purely a matter of science. Political beliefs and ideologies, along with religious values, constantly enter into debates about the use of such technologies.

In this chapter, we focus on two areas of medical technologies and their applications in the field of healthcare—assisted reproductive technologies and the life-sustaining technologies spanning two spectra of human life—the beginning of life and the end of life. Assisted reproductive technologies raise some fundamental questions about who is a parent, what is informed consent, what is contractual surrogacy, and who is legally and financially responsible for a child conceived through assisted reproductive technologies, especially when a child does not have any genetic connection to his/her parents. Similarly, life-sustaining technologies raise questions such as: what is life? What is the quality of life? When does life begin? Does an individual have the right to refuse the use of life-sustaining technologies to prolong his/her life, that is, does an individual have a right to die with dignity? Can religious beliefs and healthcare needs or necessities coexist? The current healthcare market has seen an unprecedented growth in the size and influence of religious health systems, which can affect access to assisted reproductive health services and end-of-life decisions. Religious hospitals are the fastest-growing type of hospital system in the United States. There has also been an expansion of religiously affiliated managed-care plans (Fogel and Rivera 2003). Religiously sponsored managed-care plans often do not provide certain services, such as contraception. Refusal clauses, such as the 1973 Church Amendment, allow healthcare providers to opt out of providing abortion or sterilization services (Fogel and Rivera 2003).

In the following pages, we discuss some of the legal, policy, and ethical dilemmas raised by the application of medical technology. First, we examine the assisted reproductive technologies and women's reproductive health and reproductive rights including abortion. Next, we examine the life-sustaining technologies and the right to die. In both areas, we look at recent developments, court decisions, government regulations, and public opinion.

THE BEGINNING OF LIFE

What are Assisted Reproductive Technologies?

Assisted reproductive technologies (ARTs) are noncoital methods of conception involving manipulation of both eggs and sperm. There is no one commonly accepted definition of ARTs. Instead, various definitions have been used by scholars/researchers and government agencies. "Reproductive technologies include drugs, devices, and medical interventions that control reproduction and/or prevent sexually transmitted infections (STIs), such as contraceptives and products used to enhance fertility, as well as techniques for in vitro and in vivo fertilization" (Woodsong and Severy 2005, 194). In other words, reproductive technologies include those designed to prevent unwanted pregnancies and births as well as those aimed at enabling a couple to conceive and bear children (Beckman and Harvey 2005).

The Centers for Disease Control and Prevention (n.d.) define ARTs to include all fertility treatments in which both eggs and sperm are manipulated. In general, ART procedures involve surgically removing eggs from a woman's ovary, combining them with sperm in the laboratory, and returning them to a woman's body or donating them to another woman. According to the CDC, ARTs do not include treatments in which only sperm are handled or other procedures in which a woman is given medicine to stimulate egg production without the intent of retrieving eggs. However, the National Institutes of Health (NIH) refer to ARTs as any treatment and procedure that aims to achieve pregnancy (National Institutes of Health 2017).

Types of ARTs

ARTs technologies can be grouped in two broad categories. One category of ARTs generally involves two parties. The second category involves a third-party-assisted ART (National Institutes of Health 2017). The first category of ARTs includes techniques such as the following.

Intrauterine Insemination

Intrauterine insemination (IUI) procedure involves the placement of a man's sperm into a woman's uterus using a long, narrow tube like a straw. IUI can be combined with medications that stimulate ovulation to increase the chances of pregnancy. Procedures that involve only the use of fertility drugs or intrauterine insemination (IUI), generally known as artificial insemination (AI), are not considered ARTs since a woman takes medicine to stimulate egg production without the intention of having the eggs retrieved.

In Vitro Fertilization

In this procedure, eggs and sperms from a couple are incubated together in a laboratory to produce an embryo. The embryo is then placed into the woman's uterus, where it may implant and result in a pregnancy. There are four steps involved in the *in vitro* fertilization (IVF) procedure. First, a woman is given medication to stimulate the ovaries to make many mature eggs at one time. The second step involves removing the eggs from the ovaries to fertilize them. In the third step, a man's sperm, if healthy, is centrifuged to concentrate it and reduce its volume and placed in a dish with the egg in an incubator overnight to fertilize the egg. If the sperm fails to fertilize the egg on its own, a single sperm is injected into an egg with a needle to fertilize the egg. In the fourth step, embryos that develop from IVF are inserted into the uterus. Sometimes, the embryos are frozen and thawed at a later date for embryo transfer.

Both IVF and IUI allow a couple to contract with a third-party woman (a surrogate) who carries the child. The child is genetically linked to one or both partners (a couple). The third-party woman relinquishes the child to the couple after the child is born (Beckman and Harvey 2005).

The second category of ARTs involves third-party assistance. When couples fail to achieve pregnancy from infertility treatments or traditional ARTs, couples often opt to use a third-party to assist in achieving pregnancy. Third-party reproduction can take a variety of forms (American Society for Reproductive Medicine 2018).

Sperm Donation

A couple can opt for donated sperm if a man does not produce sperm, produces a low sperm count, or has a genetic defect. Donated sperm can be used with IUI or with IVF to generate a pregnancy.

Egg Donation

When a woman is unable to produce healthy eggs that can be fertilized, egg donation provides another option to an infertile couple. In this procedure, an egg donor undergoes the superovulation and egg retrieval steps of IVF. The donated egg then can be fertilized by sperm from the woman's partner. The resulting embryo then is placed in the woman's uterus, which is receptive for implantation due to hormone treatment.

Embryo Donation

Embryo donation is also often referred to as embryo adoption. Couples who have undergone IVF successfully and have had children often choose to donate their remaining embryos. The donated embryo is transferred to the recipient woman's uterus, allowing her to experience pregnancy and give birth to her adopted child.

Surrogate and Gestational Carriers

When a woman is unable to carry a pregnancy to term, she and her partner can choose to use a surrogate or gestational carrier. In this method, a surrogate is third-party, a woman who is inseminated with sperm from the male partner of a couple. The resulting child will be biologically related to the surrogate and the male partner. Surrogates are also often used when a female partner of a couple is unable to produce healthy eggs that can be fertilized.

A gestational carrier is implanted with an embryo that is not biologically related to her. This is an option when a woman produces healthy eggs but is unable to pregnancy to term. An egg or sperm donation can also be used, if necessary, in such a situation.

The Role of Consent and Contracts in ARTs

It is important to understand the role of consent and contracts in the field of ARTs. The consent forms serve a dual purpose. First, the consent form provides information about the medical risks, benefits, and alternatives. Second, it provides for selection of options regarding the disposition of any excess embryos that may be created. It is this duality and the enforceability of the terms of the consent that have often led to legal disputes between divorcing couples who no longer agree about the disposition of excess embryos remaining after the fertility treatment. In most cases, courts have viewed such consent agreements as contracts between both members of the couple (Elster 2005).

In contractual parenting (surrogacy), the intended parents (couple) contract with a woman to carry a child for them and to relinquish that child after birth. In traditional surrogacy, the surrogate is impregnated with the sperm of the male partner of the intended parents through artificial insemination. This is also called AI surrogacy. In this situation, the impregnated woman is both the genetic and birth mother and the intended father is the genetic father. Gestational surrogacy is the term used when the female partner of the intended parents has viable eggs but is unable to successfully carry a pregnancy to term. Here, the intended mother's eggs are fertilized with her male partner's sperm in a laboratory using IVF, and the embryo is then implanted into the surrogate mother's uterus. In this case, the surrogate has no genetic connection to the child and the intended parents are the genetic parents (Ciccarelli and Ciccarelli 2005).

The use of ARTs produces complicated policy dilemmas that often challenge the social, political, and legal understanding of family, property, and reproductive rights. ARTs have created many challenges to traditional notions of family building and the legal construction of parenthood. Medical technology in this area has advanced much more rapidly than the law's ability to address questions of rights and responsibilities that arise between the parties. It raises questions such as who should control stored embryos when the couple who created them no longer agree on their disposition. Who should be recognized as a child's legal parent or parents when donated gametes or a surrogate are involved in the child's conception? How do we define motherhood when one woman provides an egg to be gestated by another woman once it has been fertilized? Can an intended parent escape liability for child support when a child has been conceived through third-party assisted reproduction if the couple eventually gets a divorce? When a couple has divorced, who has the right to determine if preserved embryos will be used to create a baby after the embryos have been frozen but before they have been implanted (Ciccarelli and Ciccarelli 2005; Elster 2005)?

New Developments in ARTs

Three-Parent IVF

In 2016, after undergoing a fertility procedure at a Mexico clinic, a couple delivered a healthy baby boy in New York. This was the birth of the first three-parent child and thus was viewed as a major new development in the field of assisted reproductive medicine. The method that was used to help the couple is very controversial because it uses genetic material from a donor in addition to that of the couple trying to conceive. The procedure involved removing the DNA from an egg of the mother who had a mutated mitochondrion (which could lead to fatal diseases) and was placed in the egg of a healthy donor after first removing the healthy donor's nuclear DNA from her egg cell. Then the new egg with healthy mitochondria and the mother's DNA was fertilized. In short, the unhealthy DNA from the mother's egg was replaced with healthy DNA from a healthy egg donor to conceive a healthy child. Thus, the child was born with DNA from the couple as well as a third-party egg donor.

In 2017, a baby was born to a previously infertile couple in Ukraine through a slightly different technique than used in Mexico. A team of doctors in Kiev used a method called pronuclear transfer, the first of its kind, in which the team first fertilized the mother's egg with her partner's sperm and then transferred the combined gene into an egg taken from a donor. This child has the genetic identity of the parents, along with a small amount of DNA from the second egg donor.

Mitochondrial replacement therapy (MRT), such as the procedure used in the Mexico clinic, can help women who are at risk of passing on serious genetic disorders called mitochondrial disease to have healthy children. However, this new technique and gene editing to modify an embryo have been very controversial and raise a host of ethical concerns about altering future generations of humans and the potential of state-led eugenics programs, like those of the Nazi movement to create an "Aryan race" by wiping out people with "undesired" traits, or selective breeding to create "perfect" human species or "designer babies" (Achenback 2016; Kolata 2016; Roberts 2017; Stein 2016; Viswanathan 2018).

Great Britain has been at the forefront in MRT. However, it is illegal to perform MRT in the United States. With scientific data backing it up, in 2015 the FDA considered approving MRT in the US. The FDA asked a committee from the National Academy of Sciences to review the procedure and the committee published a report justifying MRT. However, any progress on this front came to a stop when Congress passed the Consolidated Appropriation Act of 2016, which included a rider that prohibited germline modifications. The policy prohibiting germline modification has been reviewed several times but still remains in effect in the United States. The term "germline modification" includes all genetic engineering on eggs, sperm, or early embryos—a modification that could be passed down beyond a single generation. Because of this law, the gene editing technique known as "CRISPR-CAS9" (also called the "cut-and-paste" technique), in which scientists cut out the inherited genes that might cause cancer from the cells and replace them with healthy genes, also remains illegal. While MRT has become popular in the UK, in the US its application remains up in the air despite the fact that most of the original research behind MRT was the result of the work of American scientists and doctors (Viswanathan 2018).

Uterus Transplant

In 2016, the first ever uterus transplant procedure was done as part of a study at Cleveland Clinic. The procedure can help women who have had a hysterectomy, with the resulting scarring, and can give new hope to women who suffer from rare genetic disorders that negatively affect their reproductive system (Mohney 2016). In 2017, the first American baby was born from a transplanted uterus from a living donor. The baby was born to a mother who had been born without a uterus and who had received a uterus transplant at Baylor University Medical Center. The woman suffered from Absolute Uterine Factor Infertility, whereby the uterus is non-functioning or non-existent—a condition from which about 1 in 500 women the US suffer (Hafner 2017; Thorbecke 2017).

Making Babies without Eggs?

In 2016, scientists at the University of Bath in the UK announced that their early experiments suggested that one day it might be possible to make babies without using eggs. They succeeded in creating healthy baby mice by tricking sperm into believing they were fertilizing normal eggs. The scientists started with an unfertilized egg and then used chemicals to trick it into becoming a pseudo-embryo. Next, they injected sperm into mouse pseudo-embryos, resulting in healthy baby mice. Doctors believe that one day it might be possible to achieve a similar result in humans using cells that are not from eggs. If successful in humans, it could mean women can be removed from the baby-making process (Gallagher 2016).

Human Eggs Grown in the Laboratory

In 2018, British scientists announced that they had successfully grown the first human eggs in the laboratory. Women are born with immature eggs in their ovaries that can develop fully only after puberty. Some eggs mature during teenage years, and others develop decades later. Growing human eggs in a laboratory could lead to new ways of preserving the fertility of children undergoing cancer treatment like chemotherapy and radiotherapy, which can lead to sterility. While women can freeze matured eggs or even embryos if they are fertilized with a partner's sperm, children with childhood cancer do not have such options. Being able to make eggs in a laboratory could provide a safer option for such patients (Gallagher 2018).

Perimortem Sperm/Egg Harvesting

The retrieval of sperm from a cadaver is not a new development; the first successful retrieval of sperm from a dead person was reported in the 1970s and the first birth resulting from a postmortem sperm extraction occurred in 1999 when a woman gave birth from sperm extracted 30 hours after her husband died (Morber 2016). In 2010, the first case of harvesting eggs from a comatose woman occurred in 2010. The practice is becoming more common and raises a variety of complex issues. Two examples illustrate the complexities involving such practice.

In 2010, a 36-year-old female patient suffered brain damage after a heart attack. She was on a ventilator and the prognosis was not good. After initially agreeing to scale down her treatment, her husband and his family changed their minds and requested intensified medical treatment to allow for the harvesting of the patient's eggs before she died. The request was ultimately denied because a surrogate would be required to carry the child even though doctors involved in the case agreed that such a procedure was clinically feasible. This case illustrates some of the complex questions, including the fact that there was no advance consent from the patient to do this. Also, the question remains of whether the procedure of harvesting her eggs could have hastened her death (Smajdor 2010). In general, there has been a willingness to allow sperm harvesting from terminally ill, comatose, or deceased patients for the purpose of inseminating a known spouse or partner and women seeking to have children with their now-deceased husband or partner have been able to obtain perimortem sperm harvest. However, what about the situation when the request for perimortem sperm harvesting comes from someone other than the spouse or partner?

Consider the following case study presented by Hanson and Auden (2014), which illustrates this point. A 29-year-old man is hospitalized after cardiac arrest and meets the criteria for classification as brain-dead. The patient's mother claims that her son had said that he wanted to give her grandchildren. Thus, she wants to harvest sperm from her son for future use with an as-yet-to-be determined surrogate mother. The patient has a girlfriend but his mother is his legal healthcare surrogate decision-maker and she does not involve the girlfriend in the decision-making process. The patient's father is never in the hospital and is also not part of the decision-making process. The patient's remark about grandchildren was a vague statement about the future because the patient had not directly discussed sperm harvesting (Hanson and Auden 2014). Should the mother's request be granted?

Globalization of the Fertility Market

Surrogacy has become a global billion-dollar industry (Greenfield 2015). A growing number of infertile heterosexual couples, same-sex couples, and single men and women who desire to have children are traveling abroad to use donor gametes or a surrogate. There has been a dramatic increase in the number of "fertility tourists" from affluent countries crossing national boundaries and traveling to low-income countries for the purpose of achieving conception and childbirth, often referred to as "biocrossing." India has become the surrogacy outsourcing capital of the world in the globalized assisted reproduction industry. However, India is not alone. Clinics in Southern European countries and regions such as Spain and Cyprus offer "IVF holidays" to wealthy Northern Europeans seeking reproductive services. Singapore and Thailand are also popular destinations for such "fertility tourists." A variety of terms are used to describe the phenomena, such as "cross-border reproductive care," "Travel ART/Travel IVF," "reproductive tourism," "fertility tourism," and "procreative tourism" (Gupta 2012).

In 2006, BBC aired a four-part documentary, *A Child Against All Odds*, on television documenting reproductive journeys of several couples crossing national boundaries in their quest to have children. Globalization of reproduction is driven by fast and speedy transportation technologies, making it possible for couples to travel thousands of miles, and communication technologies like the media and the Internet can help disseminate ART information and help bring together couples desiring children and potential surrogates and egg/sperm donors (Gupta 2012).

Infertility and ARTs

Infertility is a significant public health issue in the United States. According to the CDC's National Survey of Family Growth, 1 in 8 couples or 12 percent of married women have trouble getting pregnant or sustaining a pregnancy. During 2006–2010, among all US women ages 15 to 44 (in all marital statuses), 10.9 percent suffered from impaired fecundity according to the Centers for Disease Control and Prevention (CDC). During the same period and in the same age group, 7.4 million women or 11.9 percent received fertility services (Chandra, Copen, and Stephen 2014; "Key Statistics from the National Survey of Family Growth" 2011).

In 2015, there were 499 assisted reproductive technology clinics in the United States. During the same year, 182,111 ART procedures with intent to transfer at least one embryo were performed in 464 fertility clinics that reported the data to CDC. These procedures led to 59,334 live-birth deliveries. Nationwide, the number of ART procedure performed per 1 million women of reproductive age (15–44 years) was 2832 (rough idea of ART utilization rate). ART contributed to 1.7 percent of all infants born in the United States. ART also contributed to 17 percent of all multiple-birth infants, 16.8 percent of all twin infants, and 22.2 percent of all triplets and higher-order infants (Sunderam et al. 2015).

Some studies have suggested that babies born through ARTs might be at higher risk of birth defects and genetic disorders. However, a comparative study of the health of ART babies and naturally conceived babies by a panel of experts from Johns Hopkins University, the American Society for Reproductive Medicine, and the American Academy of Pediatrics found that ART babies do not have a greater risk of birth defects, cancer, or problems with growth or psychological development (Stenson 2005).

In recent years, several newspaper stories have reported some of the problems with fertility clinics and fertility doctors. For example, in 2016 an Indiana fertility doctor was sued for 50 instances of using his own sperm while telling his patients that he was inseminating them with fresh sperm from a medical student or resident (Scutti 2016). In 2018, in Ohio, a storage tank malfunctioned at a fertility center in Cleveland, destroying more than 4000 frozen eggs and embryos (Nestel 2018). Similarly, a couple filed a class-action lawsuit against a fertility clinic after a liquid-nitrogen tank failed and destroyed thousands of frozen eggs and embryos (Brown 2018).

Government Regulation of ARTs and Surrogacy

At present, there is almost no federal regulation of ARTs in the United States. Federal regulatory agencies have also not played any meaningful role in the regulation of reproductive technologies largely because their jurisdictions about what they can do have been limited by Congressional laws. The National Institutes of Health's (NIH) Recombinant DNA Advisory Committee, which has the expertise in this area, is limited in its jurisdiction by the fact that in 1996 Congress passed the Dickey-Wicker Amendment prohibiting the NIH from using federal funds to create human embryos for research or conducting research in which human embryos are destroyed or knowingly subjected to risk, injury, or death. The Food and Drug Administration's (FDA) main focus is on safety regulations, not research. The FDA is responsible for the oversight and regulation of human genetic engineering and regulation of the safety of biologics (gene therapy products or tissue) and medical devices. Thus, technically, regulation of reproductive technologies could fall under its purview, but ARTs are not quite biologics, nor medical devices. Also, the FDA role is to regulate safety and not the moral or legal legitimacy of such technologies. Thus, at the federal level, there is no body or institution that has a clear authority to regulate the development and use of many of the reproductive technologies (Ossareh 2017).

Regulating reproductive technologies could conceivably fall under the state's "police power," which gives states the power to protect the health, safety, and general welfare of its residents. States certainly have, for example, implemented regulations dealing with abortions. However, most state regulation is limited and varies considerably from state to state. Most states have stayed clear of interfering with the practice of reproductive technologies (Ossareh 2017).

The same can be said about the regulation of surrogacy in the United States. Surrogacy has been a growing industry since the 1970s. The practice of surrogacy is largely run by private, for-profit agencies. The biggest change in the practice of surrogacy has been from "traditional surrogacy" to "gestational surrogacy." When legal disputes began to arise in the 1980s with respect to the practice of surrogacy, courts looked to public policy guidelines to resolve such disputes. However, there were no national laws regulating the practice of surrogacy, and such is the case even today (Lollo 2018). During and prior to the 1980s, in most states surrogacy contracts were considered legal but unenforceable.

After the famous Baby M case in 1988 (see next section), states began to adopt more explicit laws dealing with surrogacy. However, state laws vary considerably under a federal system of government in which states enjoy considerable autonomy and freedom. Today, many states have laws that allow surrogacy to take place within their borders. California is the most surrogacy-friendly state. Other states also allow the practice of surrogacy but restrict the practice in some fashion. For example, Florida requires that either the egg or the sperm or both come from intended parents, surrogacy contracting is permitted only if a licensed physician determines that the intended mother cannot carry a baby on her own, and the state has set limits on the amount that can be paid to the birth mother (surrogate) to reasonable expenses. Also, Florida allows only married couples to contract for surrogacy. Utah has similar regulations to those of Florida. In contrast, Delaware and New Hampshire, like California, impose very few restrictions on surrogacy contracts. Some states, such as Washington, New York, and Michigan, prohibit compensated surrogacy and make such practices illegal. Some states treat surrogate contract just like any other commercial contract (Field 2014). Other states have called for more uniformity in surrogacy regulations (Feldman 2018).

In July of 2017, the Uniform Law Commission approved a new version of the Uniform Parentage Act (UPA), which updated the 2002 version of the UPA. It incorporates changes relevant to families formed through assisted reproduction. The UPA acts as model legislation and provides states with the legal framework for establishing parent-child relationships within their own states. The UPA was originally promulgated in 1973 and has been revised several times to accommodate changed circumstances and has helped shape parentage laws in over half of states. The 2017 revised UPA incorporates three major changes designed to address issues raised by families formed through assisted reproduction. First, it seeks to ensure equal treatment of children by permitting and recognizing intended parents without regard to sex, sexual orientation, or marital status. Second, the 2002 UPA surrogacy provisions followed the adoption model requiring pre-pregnancy court validation of agreements. The 2017 UPA revision shifts in favor of gestational surrogacy agreements and streamlining of the process. Third, the 2017 UPA adds a new provision that addresses the right of donor-conceived children through ARTs to access medial and identifying information of a gamete donor. It does not require disclosure of the identity of a gamete donor but requires that the donor is asked whether they would like their identity disclosed. States are encouraged to adopt the UPA model legislation for their individual states (Joslin and Pendersen 2017).

ARTs and reproductive procedures frequently raise complex legal issues and conflicts, and courts are often called upon to resolve such legal disputes. Since it is impossible within this limited space to discuss all state and federal court cases dealing with ARTs, in the next section we highlight some of the major cases and court decisions in the United States.

Courts and the Right to Conceive and Bear Children

Courts have tended to support the premise that intent, as reflected in consent forms or contracts, should define the relationships created through collaborative reproductive arrangements. In the case of *Davis v. Davis* in 1992 in Tennessee, where the issue involved who should have control over stored embryos in the case of a divorcing couple, the court determined that the party seeking to avoid procreation (in this case the husband) should prevail. *Kass v. Kass*, a 1998 New York case, involved a situation in which seven embryos remained frozen when a couple divorced. The wife wanted control over the embryos so she could continue her attempts to have a child, but the husband objected on the ground that he did not want to have a child with his ex-wife. The appellate court enforced a written directive signed by the couple at the time the embryos were created that specified that the embryos should be donated for scientific research. However, in the 2000 case of *A.Z. v. B.Z.* in Massachusetts, the court refused to enforce a prior written disposition agreement, arguing that the consent form did not state that the husband and wife intended it to act as a binding agreement. In a 2001 New Jersey case, *J.B. v. M.B.*, where a husband in a divorce case wanted, over the wife's objection, to exercise control over the stored embryos, the court concluded that the party choosing not to become a biological parent should prevail (Daar 2001; Elster 2005).

In 2016, the Missouri Court of Appeals ruled that a divorced man and woman must mutually consent to use embryos that were frozen and stored while they were married. The court declared that embryos were marital property and not humans with constitutional rights. In this case, the former wife wanted to use the frozen embryos to have more children while the former husband argued that he should not be required to reproduce and he was willing to donate the embryos for research, to another infertile couple, or to have them destroyed (Suhr 2016).

A recent case that received a great deal of media publicity was the case involving Sofia Vergara, star of the TV show *Modern Family*. In 2013, Vergara and her then-fiancé Nick Loeb had created five embryos. The former couple had undergone IVF in California, had signed a California contract, and the planning of their IVF, the granting of the right to parenthood in connection with the IVF, and the surrogacy arrangement had all occurred in California. The remaining frozen embryos were stored at a clinic in California. In addition, the couple had signed a contract stipulating that neither party could use the embryos without the other's consent. Vergara underwent two rounds of IVF but both failed. When they split up in 2014, there were still two frozen embryos left. Loeb sued Vergara in California for custody of the two remaining frozen embryos because he wanted to implant them in a surrogate. Vergara's lawyers had argued that Loeb was using his newfound pro-life stance to gain publicity in his fight for the frozen embryos. In addition, Loeb had impregnated two women who later had had abortions and her lawyer wanted to question both women in court to contradict Loeb's pro-life position. A California judge ruled in favor of Vergara. Loeb appealed the decision but the case was dismissed by an appellate court in California (Crockin 2017; Konstantinides 2016; Smith 2016).

The case took a bizarre turn when Loeb named the two embryos "Emma" and "Isabella" and created a trust for their benefit in the state of Louisiana. Louisiana is the only state that recognizes embryos as "juridical persons," i.e., embryos are juridical people that have a right to sue and be sued and cannot be intentionally destroyed. Loeb filed a lawsuit, *Human Embryo #4B-A v. Vergara*, in Louisiana against Vergara in the name of Emma and Isabella arguing that the embryos needed to be brought to life so they could obtain the trust benefits. In other words, Vergara was being sued by her own embryos. Vergara's lawyers argued that the Louisiana court had no personal jurisdiction over Vergara and had no subject matter jurisdiction over the frozen embryos since they were created and stored in California, and asked that the case be dismissed. A federal district court in Louisiana ultimately dismissed the case, ruling that the court had no personal jurisdiction over Vergara since she had had only a minimum, transient contact with the state of Louisiana while filming a movie (Crockin 2017; Konstantinides 2016; Smith 2016).

In another case, a former couple had undertaken several unsuccessful IVF attempts and had one remaining embryo when they were divorced. The wife wanted to use the embryo as a last chance to have a child and in 2017 a divorce court had awarded her the embryo for that purpose. The couple had signed an agreement with their fertility center in which they had agreed that either spouse could withdraw consent to use their frozen embryo. In 2018, the New York Appellate Court upheld the agreement and reversed the lower-court decision. This decision is consistent with the majority of appellate embryo disposition cases around the country wherein an unequivocal, written agreement among two parties regarding the future disposition of embryos is respected (Crockin 2018).

While the practice of surrogacy has been going on since the 1970s, the legal landscape of surrogacy still remains unsettled. The first formal surrogacy contract was drafted in 1976 and the first successful birth as a result of IVF occurred in 1978. Surrogacy contracts generally clarify the rights and responsibilities of both parties and include a provision that requires the surrogate mother to terminate her parental rights, assuming that the intended parents would take legal custody of the child. Commercial surrogacy also involves payments from intended parents to the surrogate mother that typically focus on living and medical expenses and life insurance coverage. Surrogacy agencies generally charge $30,000 to $40,000 for a child and the surrogate mother generally receives $10,000 to $15,000 plus expenses (Bryant 2015).

With respect to contract and surrogacy, one of the most well-known cases is the 1998 case of Baby M. This case involved a surrogacy arrangement in which the surrogate not only gestated the child but was also the genetic contributor. The surrogate, Mrs. Whitehead, turned over the baby to the intended parents (Mr. and Mrs. Stern). However, the very next day, she changed her mind. Fearing she might commit suicide, the intended parents gave the child back to Mrs. Whitehead. Four months later, the baby was forcibly taken by the police from a home where Mrs. Whitehead was hiding the baby. Mr. Stern filed a complaint seeking possession and custody of the child and enforcement of the terms of the surrogacy contract. The trial court found that the surrogacy contract was valid and granted sole custody to Mr. Stern. The appellate court argued that the surrogacy contract was equal to baby-selling and found the contract to be void and unenforceable. However, the court also concluded that the surrogate was the mother of the child. The court granted custody of the child to Mr. Stern but remanded the case back to the lower court for a determination of the nature and extent of Mrs. Whitehead's visitation rights (Ciccarelli and Ciccarelli 2005; Foote, Reibstein, and Figueroa 1998). The New Jersey Supreme Court ultimately held that the surrogacy contract was in violation of New Jersey's statutes and the surrogacy contract violated New Jersey's prohibition against paying or accepting money in connection with an adoption (Bryant 2015).

In the 1989 case of *In re Marriage of Buzzanca*, a couple—John and LuAnne Buzzanca—had selected an egg donor and a sperm donor and contracted with a gestational surrogate party to carry the resultant embryo. The couple was divorced before the child was born, and the husband argued that he had no child support obligation. The trial court ruled that the child had no legal parents since neither John nor LuAnne had any genetic or biological link to the child nor had they adopted the child. The appellate court, however, reversed the decision on the ground that the child would never have been born without the actions undertaken by the Buzzancas and thus determined that they were the legal parents (Elster 2005).

Five years after the *Baby M* case, the California Supreme Court came to the opposite conclusion in 1993 in *Johnson v. Calvert* to what the New Jersey Supreme Court had ruled in the *Baby M* case. The case involved gestational surrogacy in which a couple, the Calverts, provided the sperm and egg; Johnson had served as the surrogate mother and was paid $10,000. The couple had a falling out. Ms. Johnson threatened that she would not terminate her parental rights unless the Calverts gave her the remaining payment. In the lawsuit both parties sought to declare themselves the legal parents. The court ruled that surrogacy contracts were not contrary to public policy and ruled in favor of the Calverts. The court reasoned that while all three parties were necessary for the child to be born, the Calverts were the primary players in the procreative relationship and it was their intent that brought about the child. The approach the court used in coming to its conclusion is often referred to as the "intent test" for surrogacy contracts, i.e., the "intent" of the parties was the major factor in the court's determination of parentage (Bryant 2015).

Similarly, in 2013 in *Rosecky v. Schissel*, the Wisconsin Supreme Court held that surrogacy contracts were valid and enforceable under Wisconsin Law. The court also stated that such contracts should be considered in determining the custody and placement of a child provided the surrogacy agreement does not conflict with the best interests of the child (Bryant 2015).

In recent years there have also been lawsuits filed against sperm banks involving sperm donation. For example, in 2016, three families filed a lawsuit against the Georgia-based sperm bank Xytex Cryo International claiming that the company had failed to undertake proper vetting of its sperm donors. The controversy involved Sperm Donor 9623, who the company had profiled as handsome and healthy with an IQ of 160 and with multiple degrees in neurosciences. However, after 14 years, when the donor's true identity was revealed it turned out that the donor was a schizophrenic college dropout with a felony conviction. The same year a woman in Florida also filed a lawsuit against the same sperm bank because she thought her child's biological father was a schizophrenic felon, rather than the genius neuroscientist the company had promised. According to the lawsuit filed by the woman, the donor had been hospitalized twice for mental health reasons and was a diagnosed psychotic schizophrenic with narcissistic personality disorder and significant grandiose delusions. Recent research has shown that interactive gene clusters can create between 70 and 80 percent of the risk of developing the disorder. The Florida woman was one of 36 who bore children using the same donor's sperm. A Georgia judge dismissed the case but acknowledged that the law was outdated when it came to reproductive issues. Subsequent appeals were shut down in Georgia after the judge ruled that the case fell under the category of wrongful birth, which is unrecognized in that state (Knothe 2016; Stapleton 2016).

In 2015, the US Supreme Court in the case of *Obergefell v. Hodges* ruled that the fundamental right to marry is guaranteed to same-sex couples by the Due Process Clause and the Equal Protection Clause of the 14th Amendment to the US Constitution. The ruling required all 50 states to recognize the marriage of same-sex couples as having all the rights and responsibilities of marriages of heterosexual couples. As same-sex couples build families through gamete donation, surrogacy, and adoption, states had to confront the matter of issuing a birth certificate listing both spouses as legal parents. Initially, several states refused to issue birth certificates to children born through ARTs or adoption to same-sex couples. Arkansas took the position that while it recognized same-sex marriages, it was constitutionally not required to issue birth certificates listing a non-biological partner in a same-sex couple as the legal parent of the child born to their spouse. In 2015 two married lesbian couples filed a lawsuit against Arkansas for refusing to grant a birth certificate. The state of Arkansas argued that it was using birth certificates simply as a way of recording biological parentage. However, the Supreme Court made note of the fact that a birth certificate is often used for important transactions such a medical decision or school enrollment. In other words, a birth certificate was more than just a tool for recording biological parentage and thus, the US Supreme Court in 2017, in case of *Pavan v. Smith*, ruled that the state of Arkansas had denied the same-sex couples' access to other benefits the state had linked to marriage. Consequent to this decision, most states have come to accept parentage as a constitutional right flowing from the *Obergefell v. Hodges* decision (Crockin 2017).

Judicial resolution of some issues raised by ARTs is incomplete because courts have addressed specific legal issues raised in specific cases. However, not all issues raised by such technologies have been addressed. There exists a wide gap between the incomplete nature of judicial resolutions and the lack of comprehensive public policy in this area at either the national or state levels. For example, the US Supreme Court's due-process jurisdiction has firmly established the right to avoid bearing children via its decisions announcing the right to contraceptive use and right to abortion. However, courts have said little about the right to have children. Often women who have been convicted of a crime and sentenced are required, as a part of probationary conditions, to use specific forms of birth control or to simply avoid procreating, restricting their reproductive rights. In recent years there has been an increased trend toward appellate court acceptance of such probationary conditions by focusing not on the constitutionality of these conditions but rather on their reasonableness in the particular case. This, in turn, has created inconsistencies across courts (Nairn 2010).

Another issue raised is whether children born through ARTs are entitled to information about their biological origins. Child-focused research has begun to address the psychological implications for children conceived through ARTs. The psychological issues related to assisted human reproduction have not been addressed adequately, demonstrating the gap between emerging technologies and law. Some have called for a uniform legal approach that will recognize the right of all children to have access to information about their identity and conception for their psychological well-being (Moyal and Shelley 2010). Even when a donor is known when a child is created using ARTs, legal questions arise such as does the donor have the right to sue for custody or visitation rights? In August 2016, in *Brooke S. B. v. Elizabeth A. C.C.*, New York's highest court overturned the previous precedent and ruled that non-biological and non-adoptive parents had a right to sue for custody and visitation in the state's family court system. However, the court did not specifically address the issue of a known donor's rights to a child he helped bring into the world. This issue came to the court in the case of *Christopher YY v. Jessica ZZ and Nicole ZZ*. Christopher had voluntarily offered his sperm to family friends, Jessica and Nicole, a lesbian couple, as a humanitarian gesture and he expected to be a godparent-type figure. Jessica became pregnant shortly after she and Nicole were married. Christopher was not involved in Jessica's prenatal care, nor did he attend the child's birth. Nor did he pay any child support, though he did give a few clothes. Seven months after the girl's birth, Christopher changed his mind and wanted access to the child. In April 2015, he filed a petition in family court asking the court to order a paternity test. The family court agreed and ordered a paternity test. The couple, Jessica and Nicole, appealed the decision. In 2018, a five-judge panel overturned the 2015 family court's decision on the ground that the paternity test would be against the child's best interests. More importantly, the court asserted that the general legal assumption that a child born to husband and wife is the biological child of both parents also extends to same-sex couples (Zadrozny 2018; "Known Donor Family Law New York—Protecting Lesbian Mothers" 2018).

Another area where laws are needed is embryo donation. When a person or couple uses *in-vitro* fertilization to create embryos, they often end up with more embryos than they need. Most fertility clinics require such people to specify what they want to be done with the remaining embryos. They can elect to destroy them, store them, donate them for research, or donate them to other persons for artificial reproduction. Yet, there are still hundreds of thousands of frozen embryos in fertilization clinics in the United States. Litigation related to embryo donations is limited. As embryo donations increase, the need for legislation that would help predictability for parents and guidance for courts becomes all the more necessary (Miller 2010).

Also, current laws are inadequate to allocate the paternal obligations between two men involved in the artificial insemination process. If a man is financially responsible for a child during his lifetime, that child is generally classified as his heir if he dies intestate. Once an artificially conceived child is allowed to inherit from his/her father, the issue to be resolved becomes: from which father does the child have the legal right to inherit? The child may have the right to inherit from the husband of his/her mother or from the man who donated the sperm that resulted in his/her conception (Lewis 2009). There is also a controversy over whether a child conceived by way of ARTs after the death of one parent is considered a child of that parent for inheritance purposes (Suppon 2010).

Under current laws relating to child support, it is typically presumed that it is in the "child's best interests" to receive financial support from mothers as well as fathers. Thus, those men who never consented to the sexual act that caused the pregnancy are nevertheless liable for the support of the resulting child. These include men who become fathers as a result of statutory rape and also adult males who become fathers as a result of a sexual assault or having their sperm stolen and used by a woman for the purposes of self-insemination.

Consider the following two examples. In the first case, an Alabama man attended a party at the home of a female friend. He arrived at the party intoxicated and shortly thereafter passed out in a bed at the female friend's house. After several months, his female friend boasted to several people that she had engaged in sexual intercourse with this man while he was unconscious and how the evening saved her a trip to the sperm bank. The woman gave birth to a child, and genetic testing confirmed the biological paternity of the man she had intercourse with. Another case involved a Louisiana man who, in 1983, was visiting his sick parents at the hospital. One evening a nurse offered to perform oral sex on him, but only if he wore a condom. At the end of their encounter, the nurse had agreed to dispose of the used condom, but the man never saw her actually do it. Nine months later, the nurse gave birth to a child, and genetic testing revealed a 99.9994-percent probability that the man she had performed oral sex on was the father. In both these cases, courts ordered each man to pay child support for the resulting child. These are examples of men who had been forced into fatherhood and were forced to pay child support despite not having consented to the act that led to insemination. Under the child's-best-interests standard, fathers are strictly liable for any biological child regardless of wrongful conduct by the mother, and courts have been unwilling to allow fathers to even raise lack of consent as a defense against liability (Higdon 2012).

However, this notion of the child's best interests is undermined by laws regulating artificial insemination. In the context of artificial insemination, a man becomes the legal father of an artificially inseminated child only if he affirmatively consents to fatherhood. Few states have comprehensive laws to establish parentage of children born using ARTs, even though thousands of such children are born each year and courts are forced to apply antiquated laws. In 2008, the Uniform Probate Code (UPC) added two sections on complicated parentage and inheritance issues that arise in the field of ARTs. These sections address donation of all reproductive material; apply to all participants in ARTs; and address ARTs, assisted insemination, maternity, and also situations in which the intended parents have divorced or one parent has died before the pre-embryos are implanted. However, it is not clear whether states will enact these new UPC sections because earlier efforts to enact uniform laws (the Uniform Parentage Act) dealing with the parentage of children born through the use of ARTs have met with very little success. Very few states have enacted comparable provisions of the Uniform Parentage Act (Knaplund 2012).

PREVENTING UNINTENDED PREGNANCIES, BIRTHS, AND ABORTIONS

Reproductive technologies are often defined to include those aimed at enabling a couple to conceive and bear children as well as those designed to prevent unwanted pregnancies and births. Reproductive technologies help women control their own bodies and reproductive processes.

Contraceptive Use, Unintended Pregnancies, and Abortions

An unintended pregnancy refers to a pregnancy that is either mistimed or unwanted. Mistimed pregnancy occurs when a woman does not want to become pregnant at the time pregnancy occurs, but does want to become pregnant at some future point in time. Unwanted pregnancy refers to a situation when a woman becomes pregnant without wanting to be pregnant at the time or at any time in the future. Intended pregnancy is pregnancy that is desired at the time it occurs. In 2011, 55 percent of all pregnancies in the United States were intended, 27 percent were mistimed, and 18 percent were unwanted. For a number of social and economic reasons, most individuals or couples want to plan the timing and spacing of their children and to avoid unintended pregnancies ("Unintended Pregnancy in the United States" 2016).

There are 61 million US women of reproductive age, between the ages of 15 and 44, and 43 million of them (70 percent) are at risk of unintended pregnancy because they are sexually active and do not want to become pregnant but could become pregnant if they or their partner fail to use some form of contraceptive method correctly or consistently. About 60 percent of all women of reproductive age use contraceptive methods. Of those who use a contraceptive, the most common method used is the pill (25.3 percent), tubal (female sterilization; 21.8 percent), male condom (14.6 percent), IUD (11.8 percent), and vasectomy (male sterilization; 6.5 percent). The remaining 20 percent consists of other methods of contraception. Couples who do not use any contraceptive method have about an 85-percent chance of experiencing a pregnancy over the course of a year ("Contraceptive Use in the United States" 2018).

A much higher percentage of married women (77 percent) compared to unmarried women (42 percent) use a contraceptive. Ten percent of women at risk of unintended pregnancy do not use any contraceptive method. The proportion of women at risk of unintended pregnancy who do not use any contraceptive method is highest among young women (aged 15–19) ("Contraceptive Use in the United States" 2018).

In 2011, 55 percent of pregnancies in the United States were intended, 27 percent were mistimed, and only 18 percent were unwanted. The unintended pregnancy rate of 45 percent (mistimed and unwanted) is much higher in the US than in most other developed countries. Preventing unintended pregnancies is one of the major goals of public health.

The highest rates of unintended pregnancy tend to be among poor and low-income women aged 18 to 24, and women without a high school degree. Correspondingly, the unintended pregnancy rate among women tends to decrease with higher age and higher income. For example, the unplanned birth rate among poor women is seven times higher than the unplanned birth rate among higher-income women. The percentage of unintended pregnancies increased between 2001 and 2008 slightly from 48 percent to 51 percent. However, by 2011, the unintended pregnancy rate had dropped to 45 percent. In 2011, 42 percent of unintended pregnancies (not including miscarriages) ended in abortion and 58 percent ended in birth, which represented a small increase from 2008, when 40 percent of unintended pregnancies ended in abortion and 60 percent ended in birth ("Unintended Pregnancy in the United States" 2016).

Abortions in the United States

The United States Supreme Court in 1973, in *Roe v. Wade*, legalized abortion. Since then abortion methods have evolved and improved. Today, there are four legal abortion methods—medication, aspiration, dilation and evacuation (D&E), and induction. In 2013, about 68 percent of abortions were performed using the aspiration method. Its use is likely to decline with increased use of the medication method. In 2014, a large majority of abortions were performed in nonhospital settings—59 percent in abortion clinics, 36 percent in clinics offering a variety of medical services including abortion, and about 5 percent in a hospital setting (National Academy of Sciences 2018).

In 2014, there were 272 abortion clinics in the US. Since 2011, their numbers have declined by about 17 percent. The largest proportion of decline has occurred in states that have adopted abortion-specific regulations. Thirty-nine percent of women of reproductive age live in counties that do not have an abortion provider and about 17 percent of women travel more than 50 miles to obtain an abortion (National Academy of Sciences 2018).

Who Has Abortions?

More than 50 percent of abortion patients in 2014 were in their 20s and 12 percent of patients were adolescents. About 46 percent of all abortion patients had never married and were not cohabitating. About 75 percent of all abortion patients were poor or low-income individuals. Of all abortion patients in 2014, 38 percent reported no religious affiliation, 24 percent identified themselves as Catholics, 17 percent Mainline Protestants, 13 percent Evangelical, and another 8 percent reported some other religious affiliation. With respect to race, white patients accounted for 39 percent of all abortion procedures performed in 2014, blacks 24 percent, Hispanics 25 percent, and 9 percent reported other racial/ethnic identities. Thus, in summary, women who get abortions tend to be young, unmarried, and poor or have low-income. Over half of women who have an abortion are racial minorities. Fifty-nine percent of patients had had at least one previous birth while 94 percent were heterosexual. Twenty-eight percent of abortion patients did not have health insurance, and a majority, 53 percent, paid for abortion out of their own pocket ("Induced Abortion in the United States" 2018; Jerman, Jones, and Onda 2016; National Academy of Sciences 2018).

The Decline of Abortions in the US

In 2011, 45 percent of all pregnancies were unintended and about four in ten of these were terminated by abortion. Two-thirds of abortions occur at eight weeks of pregnancy or earlier and 89 percent occur in the first 12 weeks ("Induced Abortion in the United States" 2018; National Academy of Sciences 2018).

About 1.06 million abortions were performed in 2011 and had declined to 926,200 abortions in 2014, a decline of 12 percent. In 2014, around 1.5 percent of women aged 15 to 44 had an abortion. Immediately following the *Roe v. Wade* decision in 1973, legal abortions increased steadily and peaked in 1980. In 1980, there were 29 abortions per 1,000 women aged 15 to 44. Since then, the abortion rate per 1,000 women aged 15 to 44 has declined steadily, from 16.9 in 2011 to 14.6 in 2014 ("Induced Abortion in the United States" 2018). The number and rate of abortion have fallen to their lowest levels in decades ("Abortion Hit New Low in U.S." 2016).

The rate of unintended pregnancy per 1,000 women aged 15 to 44 in the US declined 18 percent between 2008 and 2011, reaching its lowest level in decades. The proportion of unintended pregnancies fell to 45 percent in 2011, down from 51 percent in 2008. Consequently, the rate of abortion and unplanned birth also fell significantly. The unplanned birth rate among women aged 15 to 44 fell from 27 per 1,000 population in 2008 to 22 per 1,000 population in 2011, while the rate of abortion fell from 19 per 1,000 population in 2008 to 17 per 1,000 population in 2001 (Finer and Zolna 2016). In fact, the rates of pregnancy, birth, and abortion among adolescents and young adults have continued to decline and reached a new low in 2013 ("U.S. Rates of Pregnancy, Birth, and Abortion Among Adolescents and Young Adults Continue to Decline" 2017).

What factors account for this decline? Factors such as changes in sexual behavior among women aged 15 to 44, demographic shifts, and a greater desire for pregnancy fail to account for a significant decline in unintended pregnancies and abortion. One factor that may explain this decline is the fact that the use of any contraceptive method increased slightly from 89 percent in 2008 to 90 percent in 2012. More importantly, women's use of more effective contraceptive methods such as IUD and implants have increased dramatically in recent years, increasing from 3.7 percent in 2007 to 11.6 percent in 2012 (Dreweke 2016).

Opponents of abortion argue that contraception reduces neither unintended pregnancies nor abortions. In fact, they argue that contraception may actually increase unintended pregnancies and abortions because it encourages more sexual activity and thus the increased risk of an unintended pregnancy ending in abortion. They have made similar arguments in their push for defunding of Planned Parenthood, a leading provider of contraceptive care. In addition, they attribute the reduction in abortion rates between 2008 and 2011 to more restrictive abortion regulations adopted by states. Many states have indeed adopted more restrictive abortion regulations. However, this argument does not hold any credibility since most of the abortion restrictions adopted by states did not go into effect until 2011 or after. Furthermore, abortion rates declined in 44 states and the District of Columbia, including states such as New York and California, which have very few or any restrictions on abortions. Finally, opponents of abortion also claim that abortions declined between 2008 and 2011 because of growing public sentiment against abortion that prompted younger women to carry an unintended pregnancy to term rather than have an abortion. However, the data contradict this claim because among teenagers aged 15 to 19 the percentage of unintended pregnancies ending in abortion did not decline but rather remained relatively stable between 2008 and 2011—at about 37–38 percent (Dreweke 2016).

Federal and State Regulation of Abortions

Federal Regulations

The *Rose v. Wade* decision by the US Supreme Court in 1973 made abortion legal in the United States. However, merely three years after the decision, the US Congress placed a restriction on women's right to abortion. In 1976, Congress passed the Hyde Amendment prohibiting the use of Medicaid funds for abortion. This put abortion out of reach of many low-income women who cannot afford to pay for an abortion out of their own pocket since in-clinic surgical abortions can cost up to $1,500 in the first trimester and $3,000 in the second trimester. The use of an abortion pill, known as medication abortion, can cost over $900. The Hyde Amendment impacts all federal programs that pay for women's reproductive health services. Thus, it includes federal prisons, ICE detention centers, the Indian Health Service, the Peace Corps, and the military's TRICARE program. In 1990, Congress provided an exception to the prohibition against Medicaid funding of abortion if the woman's life was at risk, or if her pregnancy was the result of a rape or incest. State governments are free to use their own nonfederal Medicaid funds to cover abortion and 17 states have a policy requiring the state to provide abortion coverage under Medicaid ("How Congress has Used the Power of the Purse to Restrict Block Abortion Access" 2017).

Under the Affordable Care Act (ACA), states have the option to restrict abortion coverage in the health insurance marketplaces and for women who receive income-based federal subsidies to buy private health insurance (Donovan 2017).

State Regulations

Many states have adopted laws that limit when and under what circumstances a woman can obtain an abortion. State regulations vary on certain physician and hospital requirements, healthcare providers, time limits and waiting periods, parental involvement, private insurance coverage, and counseling. The following is a brief summary ("An Overview of Abortion Laws" 2018; "Counseling and Waiting Periods for Abortion" 2018).

- Forty-five states allow healthcare providers and 42 states allow institutions to refuse to participate in abortion.
- In 43 states, after a specific time point in pregnancy, abortion can be performed only to protect a woman's life or health.
- A large majority of states (41) require abortion to be performed by a licensed physician. In 19 states, after some specified point in pregnancy, abortion can be performed only in hospitals and/or require the involvement of a second physician.
- Thirty-three states require a woman to receive counseling before an abortion is performed. The nature and type of information provided in the counseling vary by states.
- Thirty-two states and the District of Columbia prohibit the use of public funds for abortion except in cases involving rape, incest, or when a mother's life is in danger. However, 17 states allow the use of public funds for all medically necessary abortions under the Medicaid program.
- Twenty-seven states require a woman seeking an abortion to wait a specified period of time, generally 24 hours, between receiving abortion counseling and the abortion procedure.
- Partial-birth abortion is prohibited by law in 20 states.
- Eleven states restrict coverage of abortions in private insurance plans except in cases where a mother's life might be in danger if the pregnancy is carried to full term.

During the first half of 2018, several states proposed and/or passed laws designed to further restrict access to abortion. However, several of these laws have not yet been implemented because of pending legal challenges in the courts. For example, Iowa passed a new law that bans abortion as early as six weeks of pregnancy based on the detection of a fetal heartbeat while Louisiana and Mississippi have passed laws that ban abortion at 15 weeks after the last menstrual period. A new Kentucky law would ban certain abortion methods such as D&E after 12 weeks of pregnancy. The US Supreme Court has blocked the implementation of restrictions designed to limit access to abortion services in seven states (Nash et al. 2018a).

While many states are adopting more restrictive laws with respect to access to abortion, several states are expanding insurance coverage for contraceptives. In 2018, four states and the District of Columbia (DC) adopted measures related to insurance coverage for contraception. For example, DC and Washington state adopted laws that ensure coverage of all contraceptive methods approved by the Food and Drug Administration (FDA). Washington state's law also ensures coverage of over-the-counter methods. When these new measures take effect, 29 states and DC will guarantee all FDA-approved contraceptive methods (Nash et al. 2018b).

The net effect of abortion restrictions imposed by the states is that in a growing number of states, women face more difficulty in accessing abortion services simply because there are fewer places they can go to obtain an abortion. In many states, more restrictive abortion laws have resulted in the closing of abortion clinics. For example, In Iowa, Louisiana, and Arkansas many abortion clinics have closed in recent years. In Iowa, 11 abortion clinics have closed in the past eight years. The state of Louisiana has only three abortion clinics, while states of West Virginia, Kentucky, Mississippi, North Dakota, South Dakota, Wyoming, and Arkansas have only one abortion clinic (Keneally 2018).

EMERGENCY CONTRACEPTION

Background

In 1999, the FDA approved the emergency contraceptive Plan B as a prescription drug. A citizen petition was filed to sell the drug over the counter without a prescription. The FDA's own advisory panel of experts agreed that such a change made sense to increase access. However, under the George W. Bush administration, FDA officials refused to grant an approval because they feared that if they did, they would be fired (Bazelon 2013). The Bush administration was accused by high-level officials of engaging in ideological meddling for political reasons and ignoring science.

In 2003, an FDA Advisory Panel overwhelmingly voted for the FDA to allow the product to be sold without a prescription (Dooren 2011). That same year, Plan B manufacturer Women's Capital Corporation applied to the FDA to have the status of emergency contraceptive Plan B changed from by-prescription-only to over-the-counter (OTC). In 2004, the FDA overruled the panel recommendation, and Plan B was refused OTC status on the ground of lack of data on the effects that accessible emergency contraceptive would have on the behavior of teenagers; that is, teenagers might engage in riskier sexual behavior if they had easy access to emergency contraception. The ruling had very little to do with the safety and efficacy of the pill itself. The administration was again accused of stonewalling the review process of the emergency contraceptive Plan B for almost two years (2003–2005) to appease the administration's religious base and of ignoring the agency's own procedures and trampling on science (Spencer 2005).

In 2006, the FDA under the Bush administration made a partial concession by allowing the sale of Plan B over the counter to women aged 18 or older while keeping the drug available by prescription only for girls aged 17 and younger (Bazelon 2013). In 2009, the FDA lowered the age at which the pill can be sold without a prescription to 17 (Dooren 2011). This means that a girl under 17 has to go through added steps of getting a prescription from a physician for the emergency contraception and asking the pharmacist for the drug. In addition, some physicians may refuse to write such a prescription or a pharmacist may refuse to dispense emergency contraception on grounds of conscience or ethics. There have been many recorded instances of girls with prescriptions turned away at the pharmacy. Others have also rejected the claim of the right of pharmacists to refuse to dispense an emergency contraceptive for conscience's sake (Card 2011; Kelleher 2010; Lewis and Sullivan 2012).

In 2011, FDA Commissioner Margaret Hamburg was ready to approve a request by the drug's manufacturer, Teva Pharmaceutical Industries, Ltd., to remove the current requirement that girls under the age of 17 need a prescription for the emergency contraceptive drug. She stated that the agency found the drug to be safe and effective in adolescent females. She also stated that younger women could properly use the drug without the intervention of a doctor. However, Health and Human Services Secretary Kathleen Sebelius overrode the decision by the FDA commissioner on the ground that the data submitted by the agency did not prove it was appropriate for girls under the age of 17 to take Plan B without a prescription. President Obama issued a statement supporting Secretary Sebelius's decision (Bazelon 2013).

Sebelius's action met with much negative feedback from the medical and scientific communities as well as supporters of women's rights. Erin Matson, vice president of the National Organization for Women, the largest feminist advocacy group in the United States, criticized the decision and argued that Obama's and Sebelius's statements had no medical evidence to offer against the scientifically based opinion the FDA had about the health effects of Plan B on girls of all ages (Lu 2012). Three scientists writing in the *New England Journal of Medicine* (Bazelon 2013), including the journal's editor, questioned the soundness of Secretary Sebelius's reasoning by pointing out that a 12-year-old girl can buy a lethal dose of acetaminophen (Tylenol) without any prescription and no questions asked. Swallowing a bottle of Tylenol could cause death. The side effects of Plan B, by comparison, are nausea and delayed menstruation. They pointed out that if one were to really apply the reasoning that Secretary Sebelius set, laxatives, cough suppressants, and analgesics would have to be taken off the over-the-counter market (Bazelon 2013).

Left-leaning women's health advocates accused the Obama administration of allowing election-year politics to interfere with a decision the FDA typically makes based on scientific evidence. The FDA's timing was politically bad because it preceded President Obama's reelection, and the administration showed a lack of courage by overruling the FDA's decision. On the other hand, right-leaning organizations praised Secretary Sebelius's decision (Dooren 2011).

In the aftermath of this controversy, several health professional groups publicly took the position that emergency contraceptives should be available over the counter. In November 2012, the nation's largest group of obstetricians and gynecologists stated that birth control pills should be sold over the counter, like condoms. The American College of Obstetricians and Gynecologists declared that birth control pills are safe, women can easily tell if they have risk factors, other over-the-counter drugs are sold despite the fact that they have serious side effects, and there is no need for a pap smear or pelvic exam before using birth control pills (Neergaard 2012). Also, in November 2012, the American Academy of Pediatrics (AAP), after examining the risks and benefits based on available data, called on the nation's pediatricians to counsel all of their adolescent patients about emergency contraception and make advance prescriptions for it available to girls under the age of 17 (American College of Obstetricians and Gynecologists 2012; Begeley 2012).

On April 5, 2013, US District Judge Edward Korman, in his latest ruling in a lawsuit filed back in 2005 by the Center for Reproductive Rights to push for unfettered over-the-counter access to Plan B, ruled that the FDA must remove all age restrictions on the sale of emergency contraception without a doctor's prescription and declared that Plan B would be among the safest drug sold over the counter (Koebler 2013; Neumeister and Neergaard 2013). In a scathing rebuke accusing the Obama administration of letting election-year politics trump science, Judge Korman indicated that it was unclear whether Secretary Sebelius had the power to issue an order overruling FDA decision. He further argued that even if she did have the power, her decision was arbitrary, capricious, and unreasonable. The judge ordered an end to age restriction within 30 days. On April 30, 2013, the FDA announced that it was approving Plan B One-Step—the morning-after pill—to be sold without a prescription to girls 15 and over, in the retail aisle next to other over-the-counter medications. However, girls will have to show an ID to prove their age to purchase Plan B One-Step. The FDA spokesperson insisted that the decision to drop the age to 15 from 17 was made independent of Judge Korman's ruling and was not intended to address the court's ruling.

The Obama Administration initially indicated that it would file an appeal against judge Korman's ruling. However, in June of 2013, the administration abandoned its decision to appeal and agreed to abide by Judge Korman's ruling ("Obama Administration Drops Fight to Keep Age Restrictions on Plan B Sales" 2013).

Types of Emergency Contraception

Emergency contraception, often called the "morning-after pill," is designed to prevent pregnancy after a woman has unprotected sex or if she thinks that the birth control method has failed to work. Some emergency contraceptive pills (ECPs) can work when taken within five days of unprotected sex. ECPs work mainly by preventing or delaying ovulation, i.e., the release of an egg from the ovary. ECPs to a lesser extent may also prevent fertilization of the egg by the sperm if ovulation has already taken place. Some ECPs require a prescription while others do not.

Currently, there are two types of ECPs approved by the FDA available on the market. One is called *Plan B One-Step* (Levonorgestrel [LNG]). There are several generic versions also available. They are available to anyone without a prescription and are recommended to be taken as soon as possible within three days (72 hours) after unprotected sex. There is also a two-dose version available in which one pill is taken as soon as possible within three days and then the second pill is taken 12 hours later. The two-dose versions of ECPs are available to people age 17 and over without a prescription. The second type of emergency contraception pill is called *Ella* (ulipristal acetate), to be taken within five days (120 hours) after unprotected sex. This is available only with a prescription by a doctor, nurse, or family planning clinic. Under the ACA, most insurance plans cover FDA-approved emergency contraception and birth control. Insurance coverage under Medicaid varies from state to state. Those without health insurance coverage may be able to obtain emergency contraception either free or at low cost through local family planning or health clinic like Planned Parenthood ("Emergency Contraception: A Fact Sheet from the Office on Women's Health" 2017).

Use of Emergency Contraception

According to experts, as many as 1.5 million of the over-3 million unintended pregnancies occurring annually in the United States can be prevented by the use of emergency contraception, including as many as 700,000 pregnancies that result in induced abortions ("Emergency Contraceptive Pills" 2004).

In 2000, only 2 percent reported using emergency contraceptives. This number was up to 6 percent in 2003. The increased use of emergency contraception may have accounted for up to 43 percent of the total decline in abortion rates in the United States between 1994 and 2000 ("Emergency Contraceptive Pills" 2004). Ten percent of women between the ages of 15 and 44 reported using emergency contraception at least once between 2006 and 2008 ("Emergency Contraception" 2010). According to the National Center of Health Statistics (NCHS) of the Centers for Disease Control and Prevention, approximately 10 percent of women in the United States have used emergency contraception ("Emergency Contraception State Laws" 2012). According to a report by the NCHS, by 2013, as many as 11 percent of women aged 15 to 44 reported having used emergency contraception at least once. About half of the 11 percent (5.8 million) indicated that they used emergency contraception because they had unprotected sex while the other half used it because they thought their birth control method did not work. The report also showed that the use of emergency contraception was most common among women aged 20 to 24 who were never married, Hispanic or white, and college-educated (Jayson 2013; Tavernise 2013; "National Statistics Reveal that Use of Emergency Contraception is Growing" 2013). According to a new tabulation by the NCHS, between 2011 and 2015, the percentage of women aged 15 to 49 who had ever used emergency contraception after sex had jumped to 20 percent ("Key Statistics from the National Survey of Family Growth" 2017).

The federal Emergency Contraception Education Act of 2010 was designed to fund a national campaign to educate women and healthcare providers and has been credited with increasing awareness of emergency contraception and its use ("Emergency Contraception" 2010).

State Governments and Emergency Contraception

Since 1999 when the FDA approved emergency contraceptive pill Plan B as a prescription drug, states' responses to it have varied. Some states have attempted to expand access to ECPs while others have tried to limit access. Some state governments mandated emergency contraceptive services for women who have been victims of sexual assault. For example, 18 states and DC require hospital emergency rooms to provide emergency contraceptives to women who have been victims of sexual assault. Eight states allow pharmacists to dispense emergency contraceptives without a physician's prescription under certain conditions. Still other states direct pharmacists to fill all valid prescriptions or discourage pharmacists from refusing to fill a prescription on moral or ethical grounds. In contrast, some states have attempted to restrict access to ECPs by excluding emergency contraception coverage from family planning eligibility expansion or contraceptive coverage mandates. Nine states have adopted some restrictions on emergency contraception ("Emergency Contraception: Background" 2018). Some states, like Arizona, Arkansas, Georgia, Mississippi, and South Dakota, have laws that specifically allow pharmacists the right to refuse to fill emergency contraceptive prescriptions. Other states have broader laws that allow healthcare providers to refuse certain types of services but prohibit them from preventing customers from accessing them somewhere else (Weiss 2018).

Emergency Contraception and the Courts

Given the varied regulations and laws adopted by states with respect to access to emergency contraception, it is not too surprising that some of these regulations/laws have been challenged in the courts by either the opponents or the supporters of ECPs.

Oklahoma was one of the nine states that had passed laws restricting women's access to Plan B One-Step or other generic emergency contraceptives. In January 2014, An Oklahoma district court judge permanently struck down this law as unconstitutional. Oklahoma appealed the ruling but in November 2014, the US Supreme Court declined to hear Oklahoma's appeal seeking to reinstate the ban (McDonough 2014). The state of Washington, in contrast to Oklahoma, had passed a law requiring pharmacists to dispense Plan B or other emergency contraceptives. In 2016, the US Supreme Court rejected an appeal from a pharmacy owned by a family from the state of Washington who said they had religious objections to providing the drugs ("Supreme Court Rejects Pharmacists' Religious Rights Appeal" 2016).

Some have argued that in issues involving pharmacists' refusal to dispense emergency contraception too much focus has been placed on health providers' rights and not enough emphasis has been placed on their responsibilities. Some of their obligations and responsibilities are included in laws and others are enshrined in the professional code of ethics that define what it means to be a healthcare professional, which are often supplemented by professional associations' policy statements. The core values that are generally agreed upon across most health professions as well as in the field of bioethics include three important principles. The first is beneficence, which requires the provider to act in the best interest of the patient and her/his welfare including and related to the notion of nonmaleficence, i.e., the obligation to do no harm. The second is the principle of justice, which includes nondiscrimination and the obligation on part of the healthcare provider to promote the public good. Third, the principle of respect for autonomy includes the notions of informed consent, the need for confidentiality, and respect for the decisions of colleagues (Sonfield 2005).

The Politics of Emergency Contraception

As can be seen from the above discussion, the administrations of both George W. Bush and Barack Obama have been accused by critics of playing politics with public policy dealing with emergency contraception and letting political considerations triumph over medical and scientific evidence. The use of and easy access to emergency contraception have been advocated by women's rights groups as well as several groups of health professionals. Morning-after pills are particularly controversial among conservative groups on the ground that emergency contraceptives cause abortion by interfering with the implantation of a fertilized egg that they regard as a person (Tavernise 2013). However, conservative groups have had a harder time making their case since morning-after pills are designed to prevent a pregnancy rather than to abort a pregnancy. Advocates of emergency contraception view the issue as one of empowerment of women and as a sensible public policy to prevent unwanted pregnancies and thus reduce the need for abortion.

RU-486 AND MEDICATION ABORTION

Emergency contraception and morning-after pills should not be confused with the RU-486 medication. Emergency contraception such as Plan B and Ella are designed to prevent a pregnancy, not to terminate a pregnancy.

The FDA approved the use of RU-486 (whose brand name is Mifeprex, while the generic name is mifepristone) for non-surgical abortion in 2000. Sometimes it is referred to as an abortion pill, but this is somewhat misleading since it actually refers to using two different medicines to end a pregnancy. The procedure is also referred to as medical or chemical abortion. The use of this procedure requires three steps. The first step requires a visit to a doctor's office or medical clinic to obtain RU-486. The second step involves taking the RU-486 medication, and after 24–48 hours taking a second medicine called misoprostol under doctor's instructions. The third step involves a follow-up appointment with a doctor after two weeks to make sure that the medication has worked. RU-486 works by blocking the progesterone receptors in a woman's body, i.e., the hormone that causes the uterine lining to build up and prepare for pregnancy (Stacey 2018). RU-486 is considered very effective because, for women who are eight weeks pregnant or less, it works about 98 percent of the time. Between eight and nine weeks of pregnancy, it works about 93 percent of the time, while between nine and ten weeks of pregnancy it works 91 to 93 percent of the time.

A total of 784,507 abortions were reported to the CDC in 2009, of which 16.5 percent were performed by early medical abortion. The use of early medical abortions increased 10 percent from 2008 to 2009 (Pazol et al. 2012). From the time of its introduction in the US market from September 2000 to April 2011, about 1.52 million women have used mifepristone. During the same period, 2207 cases with an adverse event have been reported among patients who took the drug, including 14 deaths ("Mifepristone U.S. Postmarketing Adverse Events Summary Through 04/30/2011" 2011). In 2014, 22.6 percent of all abortions performed were early medical abortions (a nonsurgical abortion at fewer than eight weeks' gestation), while 67.4 percent were surgical abortions. The percentage of reported early medical abortions increased 110 percent from 2005 to 2014 (Jatlaoui et al. 2017).

State Governments and Medication Abortion

Many states have passed laws to limit the use of mifepristone since the FDA's approval. In some states, only licensed physicians can administer the drug, not nurses or physician assistants. Currently, 34 states have such a requirement. Seventeen states require that the clinician providing a medication abortion be physically present during the procedure. This is designed to prohibit the use of telemedicine to prescribe medication for abortion remotely. Three states require that mifepristone be proved in accordance with FDA protocol ("FDA Eases Guidelines for Abortion Pill Use" 2016; "Medication Abortion" 2018). Anti-abortion advocates argue that such precautions are necessary to protect women's health and safety. However, proponents of medication abortion argue that research has demonstrated that medication abortions are safe and attempts to impose and keep such restrictions are disguised attacks on abortion itself (Boonstra 2013).

Medication Abortion and the Courts

In 2011, Oklahoma passed a law that prevented doctors from "off-label" use of the drug mifepristone. Even though the FDA had approved the drug in 2000, the "off-label" use developed later and it allowed less physician oversight when the drug was used. The main purpose behind the banning of the off-label uses of the drug was to prevent medication abortions in the state. In 2012, the Oklahoma Supreme Court declared the state law invalid. The court reasoned that the effect of banning abortion-inducing drugs completely would be to ban all medication abortion in the state. The law was challenged by the Center for Reproductive Rights. The court's decision was appealed in the federal courts. In 2013, in *Cline v. Oklahoma Coalition for Reproductive Justice*, the US Supreme Court, in a one-sentence order, dismissed the case and let the Oklahoma Supreme Court's decision stand, making the decision final (Brandes 2014; Hurley 2013).

The same year, US Supreme Court, in *Humble v. Planned Parenthood Arizona*, also let stand the Ninth US Circuit Court of Appeals' ruling that had prevented the Arizona law from going into effect. Like Oklahoma, the Arizona law had attempted to prohibit "off-label" use of the abortion drug. The state had appealed the state court decision in the federal courts. In Arizona, nearly half of all abortions performed have been without a surgery. In both cases, the US Supreme Court passed up an opportunity to hear the case and issued a ruling about states' authority to strictly limit women's access to medication abortion in favor of letting this issue percolate in state courts before involving itself in the controversy (Denniston 2014; Hurley 2014).

However, in a setback to abortion rights advocates, the US Supreme Court in 2018 declined to hear a case challenging Republican-backed Arkansas law adopted in 2015 that had effectively prohibited medication abortions in the state. The Arkansas law had not been enforced pending its appeal to the US Supreme Court. Planned Parenthood had sued to block the law that set regulation on the use of RU-486 (Wax-Thibodeaux 2018).

The Politics of RU-486

In 2016, the FDA relaxed guidelines for the use of RU-486, allowing women to use the drug further into pregnancy and with fewer visits to the doctor. In supporting the relaxation of guidelines by the FDA, doctors argued that new scientific evidence had demonstrated that lower dosage had fewer side effects and it was safer for women to take the medication over a longer time frame. The American Congress of Obstetricians and Gynecologists issued a statement supporting the FDA's relaxation of guidelines. However, in so doing, the FDA also revived one of the most contentious issues in the abortion debate ("FDA Eases Guidelines for Abortion Pill Use" 2016).

RU-486 has generated a considerable amount of controversy in the United States. On the one side are doctors and patients who see RU-486 as a safe, effective, and private method for terminating a pregnancy and thus consider it to be a major medical breakthrough. RU-486 has been touted as "the gentle abortion" by its supporters (Ebert 2002). On the other side are conservatives who view RU-486 as a "death pill" and an easy way to terminate even more unborn lives. The primary concern of opponents is that easy access to RU-486 discourages self-critical abortion decisions and that abortion will be trivialized by a pill taken at home (Stulac 1991).

Medical abortion has made it more difficult for opponents of abortions to use traditional methods/strategies to protest and to promote their anti-abortion agenda. For example, in the past, the pro-life movement has tended to focus its condemnation on abortion providers—doctors and clinics. In a medical abortion, the perpetrator of abortion is no longer the provider but the pregnant woman herself. The pro-life movement would need to change its legal strategy from trying to criminalize actions of abortion providers to vilifying and criminalizing the actions of the pregnant woman herself. Also, it is difficult to focus demonstrations and picket lines away from abortion clinics since medical abortion can take place within the privacy of a woman's own home (Colb 2013). In summary, access to medical abortion has made it more difficult for pro-life groups to use some of the traditional tools to oppose abortion in the United States. Nevertheless, abortion continues to remain a very controversial issue in the United States.

COURTS AND ABORTION: THE RIGHT TO PREVENT UNWANTED PREGNANCIES AND BIRTHS

In 1943, the US Supreme Court—in the first reproductive rights case, *Skinner v. Oklahoma*, struck down vasectomies as criminal punishment and recognized the right to have offspring as a sensitive and important area of human rights (Northup 2011). However, as we noted earlier, often women who have been convicted of a crime and sentenced are required as a probationary condition to use specific forms of birth control or to simply avoid procreating, restricting their reproductive rights. In individual cases, courts have often declared such probationary conditions/restrictions to be reasonable. Thus, courts have been inconsistent in this area.

In 1965, in *Griswold v. Connecticut*, the US Supreme Court recognized that married couples have a constitutional right to use contraception within a "zone of privacy" that encompasses the marital relationship. The Court's decision focused on the special nature of the marital relationship (Northup 2011). In 1972, in *Eisenstadt v. Baird*, the US Supreme Court extended the right to use contraceptives to unmarried individuals and justified it on the ground that the "right of privacy" includes the right of an individual, married or single, to be free from unwarranted governmental intrusion into matters that fundamentally affect a person such as a decision whether to have a child. Thus, the Supreme Court made a transition from a zone of privacy based on a marital relationship to a zone of privacy protecting all individuals from unwarranted government intrusion into the most private decisions.

The US Supreme Court in 1977, in *Casey v. Population Services International*, relying on the same reasoning, struck down New York State's ban on the sale of contraceptives to minors under 16 years of age. However, the Court did not recognize a right for minors to engage in sexual activity and validated the state's interest in curbing teenage promiscuity. The Court found it unreasonable for the state to prescribe pregnancy (by denying contraceptive) and the birth of an unwanted child as a punishment for fornication (Northup 2011). The Affordable Care Act requires health insurance plans to cover contraceptive services. This has created much controversy and objections by religious organizations that argue that requiring them to provide and/or pay for contraceptive services goes against their religious beliefs and violates their First Amendment right to freedom of religion. The controversy surrounding this issue is discussed more extensively in the chapter on the Affordable Care Act (Chapter 3).

In the 1973 landmark case *Roe v. Wade*, the US Supreme Court made abortion legal for women in the United States. The Court's decision recognized a woman's right to choose an abortion under the constitutional right to privacy (Farmer 2008). The Court stated that not only does the right to privacy include activities related to marriage, family relationships, and childbearing and education, but it is also broad enough to include a woman's decision to terminate a pregnancy (Northup 2011).

Ever since the establishment of abortion rights, the political controversy has continued, as opponents of abortion rights have continuously sought either to get the Supreme Court to overturn the *Roe v. Wade* decision or to at least impose more restrictions on access to abortion (Gerber Fried 2008). While opponents have failed thus far to get the Supreme Court to overturn *Roe v. Wade*, they have succeeded in getting the courts to impose more restrictions on abortion rights. In a major setback to *Roe v. Wade*, the US Supreme Court in 1992, in *Planned Parenthood v. Casey*, adopted an undue burden test under which the plaintiffs have the burden of proof and have to show that they faced a substantial obstacle to getting an abortion in order to win or prevail in their challenge to an abortion restriction (Farmer 2008). In 2003, President George W. Bush signed into law the Partial-Birth Abortion Ban Act. The law was found unconstitutional in the US District Courts for the Northern District of California, the Southern District of New York, and the District of Nebraska. The attorney general of the United States, Alberto Gonzales, appealed the decisions to the US Court of Appeals and ultimately to the US Supreme Court. The Supreme Court in 2007 in *Gonzales v. Carhart* and its companion case, *Gonzales v Planned Parenthood*, overturned the US District Court decisions and upheld the constitutionality of the Partial-Birth Abortion Ban Act of 2003. This was the first time the court had upheld a ban of a specific abortion procedure. Writing for the majority, Justice Kennedy further ruled that the law did not impose an undue burden on the due process right of women to obtain an abortion despite the fact that the law did not provide an exception for when a woman's health was in danger. Justice Kennedy also discussed the potential for women to experience "psychological harm" following an abortion (Farmer 2008).

Encouraged by the ruling in *Gonzales v. Carhart*, several states stepped up efforts to regulate abortion. Ten states enacted laws that require physicians to perform an ultrasound procedure prior to an abortion. Some of these laws have been challenged in the federal courts. A federal court in 2011, in *Texas Medical Providers Performing Abortion Services v. Lackey*, a federal district court ruled that the Texas law requiring abortion providers to perform an ultrasound, describe the ultrasound image, and make the fetal heart sounds audible to the patient was unconstitutional because it violated the First Amendment rights of the physicians and patients by requiring a conversation that neither party may desire. The same year another federal court struck down a similar law passed by North Carolina using the same reasoning.

Nine states passed laws prohibiting abortions at 20 weeks or even earlier. Opponents of abortion in supporting and pushing for such laws argued that a fetus of 20 weeks onward can experience pain from the abortion procedure. The doctors and reproductive rights groups that oppose such law argue that the scientific evidence does not support such "fetal pain" theory since a fetus does not develop neurological structures necessary to experience pain until at least 26 weeks of development. Ultimately, controversies surround ultrasound laws, and fetal pain laws adopted by states to restrict abortions will end up in the US Supreme Court to resolve the constitutionality of such measures ("A History of Key Abortion Rulings of the U.S. Supreme Court" 2013).

In 2012, the US Supreme Court declined to review an Oklahoma Supreme Court decision to block a ballot measure that would have outlawed abortion in the state. The national anti-abortion group was gathering signatures to place an initiative on the ballot that would have amended the definition of "person" in the state constitution to include humans from the moment of conception by granting full constitutional rights and protection to every fertilized egg. The Secretary of State had approved the language of the ballot initiative. The Oklahoma Supreme Court stopped the signature-gathering effort by ruling that the proposed ballot measure was clearly unconstitutional (Malewitz 2012).

In 2016, in *Whole Woman's Health v. Hellerstedt*, the US Supreme Court struck down Texas's requirement that doctors who perform the abortion must have admitting privileges at nearby hospitals and that health/abortion clinics have to meet hospital-like standards for out-patient surgery. The justices rejected Texas's argument that requirements and regulations were necessary to protect women's health. The court ruled argued that Texas's requirements placed a significant obstacle in the path of women seeking an abortion and which constituted an undue burden on women's access to abortion and thus violated the Constitution (DeMillo 2016; "Whole Woman's Health v. Hellerstedt" 2016).

In 2018, in a case called *Jane Doe*, the US Supreme Court dismissed/vacated a lower court's decision that allowed an undocumented immigrant teenager to obtain an abortion. Jane Doe was being held in a government-funded shelter. She was seeking an abortion when she found out after crossing the border that she was pregnant. The Trump administration had refused to facilitate abortion for minors in federal custody. The decision was a victory for the Trump administration. However, by the time of the Supreme Court ruling the issue had become moot because Jane Doe had turned 18, was released to a US sponsor, was no longer in federal custody, and had already obtained an abortion (Barnes and Marimow 2018; Wolf 2018).

Also, in 2018, the Supreme Court in the case of *National Institute of Family and Life Advocacy v. Becerra* ruled in favor of opponents of abortion on free-speech grounds. The case involved a California law that required centers operated by opponents of abortion to provide women with information about the availability of abortion by requiring such centers to post notices that free, low-cost abortions, contraception, and prenatal care are available to low-income women through public programs and to provide a phone number for women to get more information. The centers had argued that the law violated their right to free speech by forcing them to convey messages at odds with their beliefs. The court ruled that the state of California may not require religiously oriented crisis pregnancy centers to provide information about abortion services and the state cannot co-opt licensed facilities to deliver its messages for it (Liptak 2018).

ARTs, Religion, and Politics

Most state laws, in general, consider the husband or male partner, with his consent to insemination, to be the legal father of any child born of the procedure. However, only eight states specifically address the issue of egg donation by women. These statutes recognize the recipient couple as the legal parents of any child born through such an arrangement but do not confer parental rights or obligations upon the donor of the eggs (Elster 2005). Fourteen states have amended their constitutions to prevent gay couples from having the right to marry. However, hundreds of gay couples are finding ways to create families with or without marriage through surrogates. The definition of "parent" varies considerably from state to state ("Definition of 'Parent' and Related Variations in Child Welfare" n.d.). Most state laws also vary with respect to the embryo and gamete disposition ("Embryo and Gamete Disposition Laws" 2007).

In addition to technologies that help overcome infertility problems, a host of technologies make it possible for a woman to prevent unwanted pregnancies and limit unwanted births. These include female hormones delivered via injection or pill, mechanical devices placed in the uterus, and surgical procedures (Beckman and Harvey 2005). These technologies are not high-tech like the ones that help conceive children. Of course, the 1973 *Roe v. Wade* decision established the right to legalized abortion in the United States.

Religious groups have been very active in influencing the public regarding issues such as procreation, infertility treatments, and abortion (Schenker 2005). Birth control technologies such as contraceptives and abortions have been very controversial. Some religious groups view many of these technologies as unacceptable. For example, the Catholic Church characterizes abortion and contraception as immoral (Beckman and Harvey 2005).

Reproductive technologies have received a great deal of public attention and debate because politics and religious belief systems have become intertwined in public policymaking. This is reflected in a very mobilized and well-funded pro-life movement that advocates that legal personhood is conferred at conception (Solinger 1998). Social conservatives have also pushed for more restrictive policies with respect to fertility treatments as well as stem cell research (see Chapter 2).

The fact that these new technologies are often viewed by some as "playing God" brings religious interests to the policy debate (Russo and Denious 2005). Pro-life advocates have lobbied for defunding organizations such as family planning clinics that provide abortions, and pro-life advocates have also pushed for extending the gag rule, which prohibits medical professionals from discussing abortion as an alternative in family planning counseling. Even appointments to scientific advisory panels have become political, and there has been unprecedented interference by politicians, policymakers, and ideological groups with the peer-review process used by government agencies such as the NIH, combined with attempts to distort, misrepresent, and/or suppress scientific findings that run counter to the conservative social agenda (Russo and Denious 2005). The politics of reproductive technologies is characterized by conservative religious groups promoting policies that attempt to limit women's access to these technologies. On the other side of the political spectrum, advocates for women's rights have lobbied for public policies designed to increase access to reproductive technologies (Beckman and Harvey 2005).

In the field of bioethics, a philosophical consensus called the Great Bioethics Compromise was developed in 1970 to keep a close eye on scientific innovations and their social implications, and to apply the brakes now and then through regulations and guidelines (Moreno 2005). The President's Council on Bioethics was founded in November 2001, and as science became politicized, there was a breakdown of this consensus on the council (Moreno 2005). This is reflected in several of the council's reports on cloning, stem cell research, and reproductive technologies, in which it has taken a much more conservative position. The council's report on reproductive technologies recommended that Congress impose unspecified penalties on clinics for not reporting assisted reproduction as required under the federal statute. It urged professional societies to create unspecified enforcement mechanisms to force compliance with ethics and practice guidelines. Furthermore, it recommended that Congress enact eight prohibitions on the practice and research related to assisted reproduction and called for a temporary moratorium on these practices and research but, ironically, proposed no time limit or sunset provisions (President's Council on Bioethics 2004). In effect, the indefinite duration of these prohibitions would make them functionally a permanent ban. However, the council failed to provide any meaningful analysis for its recommendations, and the report failed to address important ethical and policy questions (Wolf 2004). The council's work reflected a shift in balance toward using the law to ban and penalize, and away from a more moderate and rights-oriented approach (Wolf 2004).

The President's Council on Bioethics ceased to exist when, in November 2009, President Barack Obama created a new commission by an executive order, the Presidential Commission for the Study of Bioethical Issues ("History of Bioethics Commissions" n.d.). The commission acts as an advisory panel for the nation's leaders in medicine, science, ethics, religion, law, and engineering. It advises the president on bioethical issues arising from advances in biomedicine and related areas of science and technology ("About the Commission" n.d.). The commission has not issued any new reports or studies on the subject of reproductive health since its creation.

ARTs, Ethics, and Law

Aside from the legal and political issues, ARTs raise a host of ethical issues, reflected in a plethora of literature on this topic (Ansermet 2018; Devine 2004; Feinberg and Feinberg 2010; Gilbert, Tyler, and Zackin 2005; Harwood 2007; Mason and Eckman 2017; Pollard 2009; Ryan 2001; Salzman and Lawler 2012; Shannon 2004; Smith 2015).

The ethical and legal issues are likely to get only more complicated in the future because of several new trends. First, there is a growing movement of surrogate mothers who are choosing to carry children for gay couples over traditional families. Second, many surrogates, whether for heterosexual or gay couples, work as gestational carriers, meaning that they bring children to term but not with their own genetic material (Bellafante 2005). Finally, there is a growing trend of harvesting sperm from cadavers. Ethicists seem to agree that whatever is done should reflect what the dead person would have wanted. When a wife makes the request to extract sperm from the deceased husband because she wants to conceive a child, it raises few questions. But, even in such a case, the issue can get very complex, as demonstrated by an example that arose in Florida. In this case, two weeks after the wedding, the husband was killed in an automobile accident. At the request of the widow and her mother, physicians extracted a sperm sample from the deceased husband. Soon after, the wife met someone new, and she decided not to use her husband's sperm to conceive. However, her mother wanted to carry the child herself, that is, she wanted to give birth to her own grandchild! The sperm bank refused to release the sample (Bauman 1997).

Ethical issues of fertility and reproduction can be examined from two perspectives—that of the infertile individual who wants to have a child and that of the perspective of a community—and these two perspectives do not always coincide. ARTs raise issues not only of autonomy and personal choice but also of malfeasance and justice (Baird 1996). Some of the ethical issues raised by ARTs are the following.

In the United States, the private marketplace plays a major role in this field. One of the important issues is how to control and balance private commercial activity to protect vulnerable consumer interests, since commercial organizations, which are solely interested in making money, have no reason or incentive to balance conflicting interests. What role should government play in protecting consumer interests through regulations and a system of accountability? How should collective resources be allocated in a society? Is there a danger of devaluing human dignity if the process of having children and creating families becomes commercialized? Are ARTs luxury items, or services that should be underwritten by a society? How do we ensure that everyone in society has equal access to ARTs (Baird 1996; Shanner and Nisker 2001)?

Other ethical questions raised by ARTs include: what constitutes informed consent, specifically when it is applied to posthumous assisted reproduction? Is it ethical to retrieve spermatozoa from patients who are in a coma? What is the best way to respect the wishes of the deceased donor and to protect the interests of the unborn child? Could gametes be considered property, and what is the definition of paternity in cases of children born in such circumstances (Bahadur 2004; Benagiano 2003)? Are embryos persons, property, objects, or a unique category (Shanner and Nisker 2001)?

Since, in some ARTs, as many as five adults may play a parenting role (genetic mother and father—ovum and sperm provider; the gestational mother; and the intended social parents) and each is operating in his or her best interest, how do we protect the offspring, who could not consent to an arrangement that may significantly shape their developing identities? In such arrangements, donor anonymity protects the privacy of donors and recipients, but what about the rights of the offspring with regard to having access to their genetic medical history (Shanner and Nisker 2001)?

Finally, one of the most important issues is ensuring equal access to medically necessary and appropriate ARTs and avoiding overuse, both at the micro and macro level. At the macro level, issues of accountability, cost-effectiveness, and justice become important in the distribution of resources. At the micro level, issues of autonomy, personal choice, and responsibility play an important role.

Advocates for ARTs argue that many factors, such as lack of uniform laws governing surrogacy, lack of health insurance coverage for expensive infertility treatment, lack of information about available options, and the like restrict women's access to ARTs. Furthermore, the acceptability of ARTs is influenced by factors such as culture, social class, ethnicity, age, and sexual preference. Some analysts suggest that only a group of well-off white women have access to many of the available options, but not disadvantaged women (Beckman and Harvey 2005). Approximately 12 percent of US women of childbearing age have received assistance for infertility. Since the 1980s, only 15 states have passed laws that require insurers to either cover or offer coverage for infertility diagnosis and treatment ("State Laws Related to Insurance Coverage for Infertility Treatment" 2012).

THE END OF LIFE: THE RIGHT TO DIE AND PHYSICIAN-ASSISTED SUICIDE

The Right-to-Die Movement

The origin of the right-to-die movement in the United States can be traced back to 1975 when Derek Humphry helped his wife, who was dying from cancer, take her own life. In 1980, he founded the Hemlock Society, the first right-to-die organization in the United States. The organization was dedicated to helping terminally ill people die peacefully and it advocated the adoption of laws supporting physician-assisted suicide (PAS). In 1990, a patient suffering from Alzheimer's committed suicide using a suicide machine built by Dr. Jack Kevorkian. Dr. Kevorkian, nicknamed "Dr. Death," acknowledged helping an estimated 130 people to take their lives over the course of eight years. In 1991, a grand jury declined to indict Dr. Timothy Quill, a palliative care physician who had prescribed a lethal dose of barbiturates at the request of a terminally ill patient who was suffering from leukemia and had expressed her wish to die. This case sparked a nationwide debate about the right to die and PAS. In 1993, partly in response to Dr. Kevorkian, Michigan passed a law banning PAS. It also started a movement in some states to pass legislation supporting physician-assisted suicide. In 1994, Oregon became the first state in which voters approved the ballot initiative called Measure 16, which ultimately became the Death with Dignity Act supporting PAS. In 1999, Dr. Kevorkian was convicted of second-degree murder for helping a patient suffering from Lou Gehrig's disease commit suicide by providing him with a controlled substance. He was sentenced to 10–25 years in prison but was released from prison after eight years upon promising not to assist in another suicide. In 2003, the Hemlock Society Changed its name to End-Of-Life Choices and in 2005 it merged with Compassion in Dying, and the new organization became Compassion and Choices. Dr. Kevorkian died of natural causes in 2011 (Childress 2012; Head 2017).

Dr. Jack Kevorkian played a significant but also controversial role in shaping public opinion and public policy on PAS in the 1990s. On the one hand, his many court trials sparked a nationwide public debate about the core issues involving PAS—the role of physicians as well as difficult struggle and hard choices faced by the suffering of persons dying of terminal illness. On the other hand, many question Dr. Kevorkian's motives and argue that he was more interested in drawing attention to himself than patients' rights. His actions had ambiguous effects on the right-to-die movement and generated polarization among the movement's supporters (DeCesare 2015).

The idea of a right to die was born in an environment of informed consent and patients' rights to making autonomous choices. In 1972, three landmark court cases—*Canterbury v. Spence, Cobbs v. Grant*, and *Wilkinson v. Vesey*—recognized informed consent as important and emphasized a patient-oriented standard of disclosure. In the beginning, the right to die was framed as a right to refuse life-prolonging treatments and not as a right to die. This emphasis on the right to refuse life-prolonging treatments led to the passage of laws that permitted the right of the patients to control some features of time and manner of their death through the use of a living will document. The California Natural Death Act of 1976, which allowed patients faced with terminal illness to give an advance directive to their healthcare provider about their medical treatment, led other states to adopt similar laws. The law acknowledged the rights of terminally ill patients to refuse medical treatments and interventions. In 1990, Congress passed the Patient Self-Determination Act, expanding the scope of do-not-resuscitate (DNR) orders (Beauchamp 2006).

Thus, by the early 1990s a social consensus had emerged in the United States centered on how end-of-life decision-making should happen. The consensus was that passive euthanasia, letting a patient die as a result of a patient's or family's valid decision to terminate treatment, was permissible but active euthanasia, active assistance by a physician in hastening a patient's death—perceived as killing—was not permissible even when requested by a patient or the patient's family. However, in the late 1990s, the US Supreme Court ruled that while there is no constitutional right to physician-assisted suicide, each state is free to establish its own policy. This opened the door to active euthanasia by allowing states to permit PAS in their state (Beauchamp 2006). It is also important to note that when it comes to active euthanasia there is a distinction made between one in which a physician himself administers a lethal dose of medication to a patient, and a situation in which a physician simply provides a patient with a prescription for a lethal dose and the patient takes/administer the lethal dose himself or herself. In the first situation, a physician actively participates in hastening a patient's death, while in the second situation a physician's involvement is limited to providing the patient with a means to end his/her own life. In 1994, Oregon became the first state to permit PAS. However, the law did not go into effect until 1997 due to legal challenges.

Life-sustaining technologies and the right-to-die movement raise a number of legal and ethical questions: what constitutes informed consent? Who should live and who should die? Who decides? When is a life worth preserving? Who determines what quality of life is? How does one measure a person's quality of life? Should the courts be involved in making such decisions? Does a patient have a right to demand unending medical treatment in a hopeless case? Does a patient have a right to seek the assistance of a physician to help end his or her own life? Can euthanasia ethically be justified? What should be the ethical role of the physician and other caregivers? Is every life precious no matter how disabled? Do human beings have the right to self-determination and to decide when life has value?

These are the ultimate questions that have been debated throughout the history of Western thought. The answers depend on our understanding of what makes us human beings. Aristotle argued that existence itself is inviolable. Thus, the plea to continue feeding Terri Schiavo against the wishes of her husband or the courts' determination of her expressed inclination is consistent with Aristotle's teaching. On the other side, Rene Descartes, a philosopher of the Enlightenment, defined human life not as biological existence (an inviolable gift of life from God) but as consciousness about which people can make judgments.

Approximately 10,000 patients live in a vegetative state in the United States. The complexities created by life-sustaining technologies have given rise to the "right-to-die" movement across the country. Proponents of the right to die assert that individuals have a right to die with dignity and to determine when to end their lives. They argue that passive, as well as active, euthanasia is justified. They also argue that the right to die, like the right to give informed consent, reflects a triumph of patient autonomy. Opposition to the right-to-die movement has come from many sources, including the right-to-life movement. These opponents argue that suicide is wrong on religious and theological grounds, as well as being harmful to the community and the common good and that it produces harmful consequences for other individuals in society. Others have argued that no human being has a right to decide, for himself/herself or for others, when life is no longer worth living. They posit that there is a danger that such decisions may be based on wrong or ulterior motives. An example would be an agreement to end the life of a patient whose continual stay in the hospital was a financial burden to the family, or of a patient whose family members stood to benefit financially by inheritance. It can be argued that, once a society agrees that at some stage a life is not worth sustaining, society is on a "slippery slope." Once passive euthanasia becomes acceptable, the next step will be active euthanasia, which in turn can easily lead to forced or involuntary euthanasia.

In 2018, the Council on Ethical and Judicial Affairs of the American Medical Association recommended that the AMA maintain its opposition to PAS. Based on this recommendation, at its annual meeting AMA delegates voted to continue to review at regular intervals, but maintain, its long-standing opposition to PAS (Popik 2018).

The Right to Die and Physician-Assisted Suicide in Other Countries

Support for PAS has been slowly growing around the world. The term assisted suicide is also often referred to as assisted dying, death with dignity, and mercy killing. The different terms used often tend to reflect the different assumptions people bring to the debate. As of 2018, PAS was legal in seven countries—Austria, Belgium, Canada, Finland, Germany, Luxembourg, the Netherlands, and Switzerland. However, it is important to note that the specifics of circumstances in which PAS is permitted differ from one country to the next. For example, two countries even recognize a request from minors under strict circumstances, while others do not. Countries such as Switzerland, Germany, Finland, and Austria allow PAS under very specific scenarios, while Belgium, the

Netherlands, and Luxembourg impose fewer restrictions (Bello 2018; "Euthanasia and Physician-Assisted Suicide (PAS) Around the World" 2016). The issue of assisted suicide is a particularly sensitive topic since euthanasia was part of a public policy used by the Nazis to kill more than 200,000 people with physical and mental disabilities. The law passed by Germany in 2015 allows assisted suicide for "altruistic motives" but prohibits such practice in cases where it is conducted on a "business" basis ("Germany Passes Law Allowing Some Types of Assisted Suicide" 2015).

Some countries like Spain, Great Britain, Italy, Hungary, and Norway do not allow PAS but allow only passive euthanasia under strict circumstances such as artificial nutrition or hydration, by allowing patients suffering from the incurable disease to refuse life-prolonging treatments (Bello 2018).

In Canada, suicide had been decriminalized since 1972 but the Criminal Code had retained a provision criminalizing suicide assistance and the Canadian Supreme Court had upheld this provision. In 2014, Quebec Passed a law legalizing euthanasia but not PAS. In 2015 the Canadian Supreme Court struck down a prohibition on assisted suicide and gave the Canadian Parliament a year to pass a law legalizing and regulating PAS. In 2016, Canada passed a law that made assisted suicide legal, effective immediately, and regulating PAS ("Euthanasia and Physician-Assisted Suicide (PAS) Around the World" 2016). The Supreme Court of Canada unanimously found a right to die in the Charter of Rights and Freedom, i.e., under the Canadian Bill of Rights (Kay 2015).

THE RIGHT TO DIE IN THE UNITED STATES

Courts and the Right to Refuse Life-Sustaining Treatments

Today's life-support technologies are capable of keeping patients alive for a long time, even when they have no chance of regaining consciousness. Mechanical ventilators can keep patients breathing, and artificial nutrition and hydration can sustain severely debilitated and dying individuals for many years. This raises the specter of individuals being kept alive in vegetative, helpless states, sustained by a host of tubes and machines (Cantor 1993). The questions of who shall live, who shall die, and who shall decide raise difficult ethical and legal issues (Buckley 1990). Some well-publicized court cases help illustrate the complexities involved in such situations.

The Karen Quinlan Case

One of the early cases to highlight the ethical and legal dilemmas involved a New Jersey woman named Karen Quinlan who, at the age of 21, slipped into a deep coma. She was hooked up to a respirator in a hospital. Her doctor informed her parents that their daughter was never going to come out of her coma because her brain was severely damaged. She might not necessarily die and, kept on a life-support system, might live for many years. Quinlan's parents asked the doctor to turn off the respirator. The doctor refused, and they went to court. The judge in the lower court disagreed with the parents. They then appealed the decision to the New Jersey Supreme Court and, on March 31, 1976, the parents won the right to have the respirator turned off. The state supreme court ruled that Karen had a constitutional right to privacy, which her guardian could assert on her behalf (Peters 1990). Ironically, it turned out that Karen Quinlan was able to breathe on her own. She was moved from a hospital to a nursing home, where she died in June 1985.

The Elizabeth Bouvia Case

A different dilemma was presented in the case of 26-year-old Elizabeth Bouvia, who in September 1983 admitted herself to the psychiatric unit of California's Riverside General Hospital.

She had had a very difficult life and was almost totally paralyzed from cerebral palsy. Once admitted, she asked for assistance in starving herself to death. What was unique about this case is that Ms. Bouvia was not terminally ill but wanted the hospital staff to provide her with pain-killing drugs and hygienic care while she waited to die. The hospital refused. Elizabeth Bouvia went to court and lost; the court ordered that she be force-fed. On April 7, 1984, she left the hospital. The hospital bill for 217 days, excluding physicians' fees, was more than $56,000; it was paid by the hospital and the state of California. After repeated court appeals, the California Court of Appeals found in her favor. The court said that she could refuse life-sustaining medical treatment. The court ruled that the right of a competent adult patient to refuse treatment is a constitutionally guaranteed right. After her victory, Bouvia changed her mind and did not kill herself (Pence 1995; Shreve and Kailes 1990).

The Nancy Cruzan Case

Another case involved 32-year-old Nancy Cruzan of Missouri. She had been in a persistent vegetative state for seven years since a car accident. Her prognosis was hopeless. Her cerebral cortex had atrophied, but she was not dead, and she could have lived in such a vegetative state for many more years. The cost of her medical treatment was about $130,000 a year, paid by the state. In 1987 her parents requested that Nancy's feeding tube be removed so she could die. A lower court granted the request in July 1988, but the state supreme court in November 1988 reversed the decision, agreeing with the state's argument that the state of Missouri had an "unqualified" interest in preserving life. According to the court, the state's interest was not in the "quality" of life—the state's interest was in "life" (Angell 1990).

Nancy's parents appealed the decision to the US Supreme Court. In June 1990, the court, in a 5–4 decision, agreed with the decision of the Missouri Supreme Court. The court found that a competent person has a constitutionally protected right to refuse lifesaving hydration and nutrition. If the person is incompetent, the court ruled, the state is entitled to require rigorous proof that this person, when competent, would have requested removal of a feeding tube in the event of his or her future incompetence. According to the court, the state of Missouri was entitled to require clear and convincing proof that a surrogate decision-maker was choosing what Ms. Cruzan herself, when competent, desired (Meilaender 1990).

It is interesting to note that the court based its ruling not on the ground of a fundamental privacy right, as was the case with Quinlan, but on the ground of a liberty interest. The court argued that the state's interests must be balanced against the interests of the patient (McCormick 1990; Peters 1990). On December 14, 1990, the Circuit Court of Jasper County, Missouri, declared that there was clear and convincing evidence that if Nancy Cruzan were mentally able, she would want to terminate her nutrition and hydration and she would not want to continue her present existence. Her parents were authorized to remove the nutrition and hydration tube. After the removal of the feeding tube, Nancy Cruzan died on December 26, 1990.

On the other side of the ledger was a case in Minnesota in which a public hospital sought permission to remove a respirator from an 87-year-old woman who was in a persistent vegetative state. The hospital argued that continuing treatment was not in the woman's best medical or personal interest; however, the family of the woman opposed the request. The family won, and the woman died a year later (Kamisar 1991).

The Barbara Howe Case

The case of Barbara Howe, who suffered from Lou Gehrig's disease, reflects the complexities involved in such cases. She was admitted to Massachusetts General Hospital in November 1999. She had told her daughter, doctors, and nurses to do whatever was necessary to keep her alive as long as she could appreciate her family. Over the years, Barbara Howe continued to lose control of her body. A ventilator breathed for her and a feeding tube nourished her. She was no longer able to communicate with her caregivers what she wanted. Blue Cross and Blue Shield of Massachusetts had stopped covering her hospital stay in 2003. Howe's longtime doctor and nurses believed that she was in pain and that keeping her alive was tantamount to torture. However, Barbara Howe's oldest daughter, Carol Carvitt, who was her healthcare proxy, disagreed. Barbara Howe had become stuck in a limbo that no one foresaw. Howe's doctors and nurses wanted to withdraw life support, but the probate and family court in February 2005 found that there was no sufficient cause to overturn Carol Carvitt as her mother's healthcare proxy (Kowalczyk 2005a). However, the judge urged Carvitt to think about her mother's best interest. Finally, in March 2005, Carol Carvitt agreed to terminate life support to her mother by June 30, 2005 (Belluck 2005). Barbara Howe passed away on Saturday, June 4, 26 days before a court settlement that would have allowed the hospital to turn off her life support (Kowalczyk 2005b).

One subtle change that has occurred in right-to-die cases is that most of the earlier cases involved a conflict between family members and hospitals in which the families pressed to let their loved ones die, while the hospitals tried to keep the patient alive. However, in the past decade or so, in instances when family members and hospitals have clashed, it is often the family members who want to continue life support and aggressive medical treatment while the doctors believe it is time to stop. This is the case partly because extraordinary medical advances have given hope to families. Patients and families are often skeptical or suspicious of doctors' and hospitals' intentions and believe that a life-support system may be terminated for economic reasons (Belluck 2005). The technology of artificial hydration and nutrition (AHN) that helps prolong life has become common practice. The question has become: who decides when technology actually stops benefiting and becomes harmful to the patient? Drs. Jeffrey Ponsky and Michael Gauderer, who created the current techniques for inserting feeding tubes into patients in

1979, recently stated that the procedure has gone too far because the feeding tubes are often used for patients who do not have any potential for recovery. They never imagined that their procedure would lead to such a massive ethical dilemma. Feeding tubes are used 250,000 times a year and have become a routine part of end-of-life care (Milicia 2005).

The Terri Schiavo Case

No right-to-die case received more national attention and generated more political maneuvering than the tragic case of Terri Schiavo in Florida. On February 25, 1990, she suffered a cardiac arrest, apparently caused by a potassium imbalance. Her heart stopped temporarily, cutting off oxygen to her brain and causing brain damage. In June 1990, a court appointed Terri's husband, Michael Schiavo, as her guardian. Terri's parents, the Schindlers, did not object, because, according to all the reports, Michael and the Schindlers got along splendidly. In November 1992, Michael Schiavo won a malpractice case against one of Terri's doctors for misdiagnosing Terri's medical condition. He was awarded $750,000 for Terri's care and $300,000 for himself.

It is at this point that the relationship between Michael Schiavo and his in-laws, the Schindlers, started to turn sour, and they began to have disagreements over the use of this money and Terri's treatment. In 1993, the Schindlers attempted to remove Michael as Terri's legal guardian, but the state district court refused. On March 1994, a court-appointed guardian said that Michael Schiavo had acted appropriately and attentively toward his wife. In May 1998, Michael Schiavo filed a petition to remove Terri Schiavo's feeding tube. The Schindlers were strongly opposed to the removal. A second court-appointed guardian, in December 1998, reported that Terri Schiavo was in a persistent vegetative state with no chance for improvement. However, he also indicated that Michael Schiavo's decision-making might be influenced by the potential to inherit the remainder of Terri's estate.

The court trial began on January 20, 2000. Terri Schiavo had not left a living will. Her husband Michael testified that in their past conversations, Terri had indicated that she would not want to live her life this way. Based on the testimony of her husband and two other individuals, Judge George Greer ruled on February 11, 2000, that Terri would have chosen to have her feeding tube removed. He ordered the removal of the feeding tube but later stayed his order to give the Schindlers an opportunity to appeal. On January 24, 2001, the Florida Second District Court of Appeals upheld Judge Greer's ruling permitting the removal of Terri's feeding tube. On April 18, 2001, the Florida Supreme Court elected not to review the decision of the second district court of appeals (Cerminara and Goodman 2005; "Indepth: Terri Schiavo, Schiavo Timeline" 2005; "Key Dates in Schiavo Right-to-Die Case" 2005; "Terri Schiavo Timeline" 2005).

For the next several years, the struggle between Michael Schiavo and the Schindlers continued, as appeal after appeal was filed by the two sides. After many appeals, Judge Greer ordered the removal of the feeding tube to take place on October 15, 2003. On October 7, 2003, Florida Governor Jeb Bush filed a brief in federal district court supporting the Schindlers' efforts to stop the removal of the feeding tube. On October 10, 2003, a federal judge ruled that he lacked jurisdiction to hear the case. Terri Schiavo's feeding tube was removed on October 15, 2003 (Cerminara and Goodman 2005).

It was at this point that politics took over. As the Schindlers' legal options dwindled, Catholic, Evangelical, and anti-abortion groups seized on their cause, helping to publicize it and fund it. Starting in 2001, the anti-abortion Life Legal Defense Foundation had paid for the Schindlers' legal costs. All this helped get the attention of politicians eager to show off their pro-life credentials (Campo-Flores 2005).

Within days of the feeding tube removal, the Florida legislature passed a special law, referred to as "Terri's Law," that gave Governor Jeb Bush the power to issue a "one-time stay" in certain cases ("Can States Intervene in Medical Decisions?" 2004). On October 21, 2003, Governor Bush issued an executive order to reinstate the feeding tube. On October 29, 2003, Michael Schiavo, joined by the American Civil Liberties Union, filed a lawsuit in state court arguing that "Terri's Law" was unconstitutional. In September 2004, a unanimous Florida Supreme Court declared "Terri's Law" unconstitutional on the grounds that it violated the principle of separation of powers between the executive, legislative, and judicial branches of government (Hallifax 2004; Sutton 2004). Governor Bush filed a petition seeking US Supreme Court review of the Florida Supreme Court's decision. On January 24, 2005, the US Supreme Court refused to grant such a review (Roig-Franzia 2005).

At this point, conservatives decided to nationalize the issue. Representative Dave Weldon (R-FL) and Senator Mel Martinez (R-FL) pushed for Congress to pass a broadly worded law aimed at due-process law for disabled people like Terri. House Majority Leader Tom DeLay (R-TX) and Senate Majority Leader Bill Frist (R-TN) provided the leadership. The US Senate wanted a narrowly worded bill specifically addressing Terri Schiavo's situation. After compromises, on March 21, 2005, Congress passed a narrowly crafted law that applied only to Terri

Schiavo. The law, called "An Act for the Relief of the Parents of Theresa Marie Schiavo," gave the US District Court for the Middle District of Florida jurisdiction to hear and review the Schiavo case. President Bush signed it into law the same day (Hulse 2005). This set in motion a series of lawsuits filed by the Schindlers in federal district courts and appeals to the US Court of Appeals and the US Supreme Court in an effort to have the feeding tube reinserted in Terri Schiavo. The federal courts consistently rejected the Schindlers' various constitutional claims and refused to reinstate the feeding tube. The US Court of Appeals and the US Supreme Court similarly denied such requests on several appeals (Goodnough 2005a, 2005b; Goodnough and Liptak 2005a, 2005b; Long 2005).

The feeding tube was removed on March 18, 2005. The parents of Terri Schiavo appealed to Governor Bush to intervene further in the case (Lyman 2005). Responding to political pressure from the conservatives, Governor Bush asked the Florida Department of Children and Families (FDCF) to obtain custody of Terri Schiavo in light of allegations of spousal abuse brought against Michael Schiavo. After holding a hearing, Judge Greer, on March 24, 2005, issued a restraining order prohibiting the FDCF from removing Terri Schiavo from the hospice or reinstating the feeding tube. The Schindlers decided to end their federal appeals (Associated Press 2005). Terri Schiavo died on March 31, 2005. President Bush called upon the nation to build a culture of life. The Vatican issued a statement calling Ms. Schiavo's death a violation of the sacred nature of life that shocked the conscience (Goodnough 2005c).

An autopsy of Terri Schiavo backed her husband's contention that she was in a persistent vegetative state. The medical examiner's office stated that Terri Schiavo had suffered massive and irreversible brain damage and was blind. It also found no evidence that she was strangled or otherwise abused as had been alleged by her parents and others ("Schiavo Autopsy Finds No Sign of Trauma" 2005; "Schiavo Autopsy Shows Irreversible Brain Damage" 2005).

While the right of patients to refuse life-sustaining technology is now well established, new and unanticipated events and cases continue to raise a host of legal and ethical issues and demonstrate the limits of laws to deal with any and every conceivable circumstance that arise with respect to life-sustaining technology. The case of a Texas woman, Marlise Munoz, age 33, illustrates the point. She was on life support at John Peter Smith Hospital in Fort Worth, Texas and in November of 2013, she was declared brain-dead following oxygen deprivation related to a possible blood clot in her lungs. However, she was 14 weeks pregnant. Her advance directive, as well as the wishes of her husband and family, called for the removal of life support. But, the Texas law prohibits removing life support from pregnant women. Consequently, the hospital refused to remove her from life support. At $5,000 per day, Munoz's hospital bill would have been $350,000 after 24 weeks of pregnancy, when the baby would have about a 50-percent chance of survival. At 30 weeks of pregnancy, the hospital bill would have been $560,000 and the baby would have had a more-than-92-percent chance of survival. A baby born prematurely could spend anywhere from two to four months in the neonatal intensive-care unit at about $3,500 per day. In sum, even at a conservative estimate, the cost for the baby to be born could have added up to more than $1 million (Baker and Campbell 2014; Merchant 2014; Owens 2014; Wickline 2014; Winter 2014).

Her husband filed a lawsuit in an effort to remove the life support and his lawyer claimed that keeping Munoz on life support violated her Fourteenth Amendment right, which states that a state cannot deprive any person of life, liberty, or property without the due process of the law and a competent person has a constitutionally protected liberty interest in making decisions regarding their own body rooted in common law. In January of 2014, a Texas judge ordered the hospital to declare Marlise Munoz dead and return her body to her family. The hospital complied with the judge's order and brought the case to an end. The 23-week-old fetus Munoz was carrying would not be born. The lawyers for the Munoz family issued a statement describing the fetus as "distinctly abnormal," and indicated that the fetus' lower extremities' were deformed and there were also other abnormalities in the fetus. An attorney who had helped write the law that was used to keep Munoz on life support indicated that lawmakers had never discussed the law being applied to a brain-dead person (Baker and Campbell 2014; Merchant 2014; Owens 2014; Wickline 2014; Winter 2014).

However, the Munoz case was not the only case of its kind. In the 1990s, Medical ethicist Jeffrey Spike was part of a hospital team that had wrestled with a similar case of a brain-dead pregnant woman on life support where the woman was kept alive for 100 days and a healthy baby was eventually delivered by a cesarean section. Dr. Spike called the case among the most difficult of his career. Also, in a survey of international medical literature from 1982 to 2010, German researchers found 19 cases of brain-dead women who were put on life support for the purpose of sustaining a fetus, resulting in 12 viable infants who survived the neonatal period. The researchers acknowledge the ethical and moral conundrum presented by such cases. Some professionals argue that it is ethically unacceptable to maintain the mother's body after brain death to use it as a fetal container or to consider the mother as a cadaveric incubator (Madigan 2014).

Courts and Physician-Assisted Suicide

In the 1981 movie *Whose Life is it Anyway*, actor Richard Dreyfuss portrayed a sculptor's fight to end his own life with the assistance of his doctor after he was paralyzed in a car accident. By early 1990s a consensus had emerged in the United States that passive euthanasia, letting a patient die as a result of a competent patient's or family's valid decision to terminate treatment, was permissible but active euthanasia, assistance by a physician in hastening a patient's death—perceived as killing—was not permissible even when requested by a patient or a patient's family. Reflecting this consensus, several states had laws on their books that explicitly prohibited assisted suicide. The constitutional question raised by such laws was whether a terminally ill patient has a constitutional right to PAS under the US Constitution.

In 1997, the US Supreme Court addressed this question when in two cases it rejected the constitutional challenges to Washington's and New York's state laws prohibiting assisted suicide.

In *Washington v. Glucksberg*, the legal question presented was whether Washington State's law that made promoting a suicide attempt a felony and declared a person guilty of a felony if he knowingly caused or aided another person to attempt suicide violated the Due Process Clause of the Fourteenth Amendment to the US Constitution. The lawsuit challenging the constitutionality of the law was filed by four Washington State physicians and three gravely ill patients who claimed that the state law infringed upon their "liberty" interest protected by the Due Process Clause of the Fourteenth Amendment. The Supreme Court ruled that Washington state's law did not violate the Due Process Clause. The court reasoned that Anglo-American common law for over 700 years had disapproved and punished anyone rendering such assistance and in light of this history, the right to assistance in committing suicide is not a fundamental liberty interest protected by the Due Process Clause (Mariner 1997; "The U.S. Supreme Court's 1997 Decisions on Assisted Suicide" n.d.).

The same year, in *Vacco v. Quill*, Dr. Timothy Quill with some other physicians and three seriously ill patients challenged the constitutionality of New York State's law banning PAS. The law permitted patients to refuse lifesaving treatments on their own but made it a crime for doctors to help patients commit or attempt suicide even if patients were terminally ill or in great pain. The constitutional question raised was whether New York's ban on PAS violated the Fourteenth Amendment's Equal Protection Clause since the law allowed competent terminally ill adults to withdraw their own lifesaving treatment but denied the same right to patients who could not withdraw their own treatment and could only hope that a physician would do so for them. The Supreme Court ruled that New York law did not violate the Equal Protection Clause of the Fourteenth Amendment. The court reasoned that it was both important and logical to make a distinction between withdrawing life-sustaining treatment and assisted suicide because the distinction relates to the legal principle of causation and intent. In the first case, when a patient refuses life-sustaining medical treatment he/she dies from an underlying fatal disease or pathology (death is caused by disease) but if a patient injects a lethal medication prescribed by a doctor he/she is killed by that medication (death is caused intentionally). The court ruled that New York's ban on PAS was rationally related to the state's legitimate interest in protecting medical ethics, preventing euthanasia, and protecting the disabled and terminally ill patients from prejudice that might encourage them to end their own lives, as well as preservation of life (Mariner 1997; "The U.S. Supreme Court's 1997 Decisions on Assisted Suicide" n.d.).

In 1994, Oregon had become the first state to pass the Death with Dignity Act permitting PAS but its implementation was delayed until 1997 due to court challenges. The US Supreme Court's decisions in the above two cases that the US Constitution does not guarantee a right for dying terminally ill patients to seek the assistance of a physician to get lethal medication to end their life came before the Oregon law's provisions went into effect and left states to free to continue to debate about PAS.

On November 8, 1994, Oregon voters approved the Death with Dignity Act by a margin of 52 percent to 48 percent. Known as Ballot Measure 16, the Act allows physicians in the state to write lethal drug prescriptions for terminally ill patients who are expected to die within six months. Opponents of the law took the issue to the federal courts and lost. The Ninth US Circuit Court of Appeals rejected the argument that depressed terminally ill adults would be prevented under the law from making informed decisions. The court stated that the specter of involuntary suicides was merely speculative. The US Supreme Court, in October 1997, refused to hear the challenge and, without comment, issued an order letting the ruling of the Ninth US Circuit Court of Appeals decision stand (Biskupic 1997). On June 9, 1997, the Oregon legislature, declining to either amend or repeal the Act, placed it on the ballot for a second vote. In the November 4, 1997 election, 60 percent of voters voted against the repeal of the law, while 40 percent voted in favor ("Oregon Repeal of 'Death with Dignity,' Measure 51 (1997) n.d.).

In March 2005, the US Supreme Court agreed to hear the George W. Bush administration's challenge to Oregon's law. The Bush administration wanted to revoke the license of doctors who prescribe a lethal prescription on the ground that federal drug laws trump states' rights to regulate medical practice (Eisenberg 2005). However, in a stinging rebuke to the Bush administration, the US Supreme Court in January 2006, in *Gonzales v. Oregon*, by a majority of 6–3, sided with the state of Oregon and upheld the state's Death with Dignity Act and ruled that the federal government did not have the authority to prosecute physicians under the federal drug laws ("Oregon's Right-to-Die Law Upheld by Supreme Court" 2006). The net effect of the ruling was to leave it up to each individual state to deal with the issue of PAS.

In 2009, Montana's highest court in *Baxter v. Montana* legalized the practice of PAS. It ruled that state law prohibiting assisted suicide did not apply to doctors who gave lethal doses of drugs to dying patients. The court reasoned that physicians could not be convicted of violating the homicide statute since physicians could always assert the consent of the patient in question as a defense. Thus, no rule-abiding physician practicing medicine in Montana had any reason to fear prosecution for engaging in PAS. Furthermore, the court pointed to the Montana Rights of the Terminally Ill Act under which a doctor may engage in the death-related action of withdrawing a respirator from a patient dependent on a respirator. The court concluded that since Montana's public policy allows a doctor to withdraw respirator from a respirator-dependent patient that can lead to a patient's death, then it follows that the practice of a doctor engaged in the death-related action of prescribing a lethal dose of medication to be taken by a patient in the hope that it may cause their death cannot be against Montana's public policy (Kardish 2015; Robinson 2010).

In 2014, the case of Brittany Maynard again focused the nation's attention on the issue of PAS. She was a 29-year-old school teacher who was diagnosed with the most lethal form of brain cancer and doctors gave her six months to live. She decided to forgo her aggressive treatment and die with dignity. She announced in a YouTube video that she had decided to utilize Oregon's Death with Dignity Act. The video drew more than 16 million unique visitors. She also became an advocate for death with dignity laws in the last weeks of her life. She and her husband moved from California to Oregon so she could use Oregons' Death with Dignity Act to end her life. In November of 2014, at home with her family and close friends, she ended her life by taking a lethal dose of medication prescribed by a doctor. Today, her case is widely touted by the advocates of PAS. The *New Yorker* called her "the poster child for assisted death" while the *New England Journal of Medicine* called her "the new face of the movement to give dying patients the choice to end their lives humanely." It is important to note that what was unique about Brittany Maynard's case is that she was only 29 years old, compared to the typical 71-year-old who seeks physician-assisted death. Since 1997, when the Oregon law went into effect, among all people who have used the law to end their lives, only seven individuals were under the age of 34 (Kotva 2016; "Brittany Maynard Doesn't Want to Die" 2014; "Death with Dignity Advocate Brittany Maynard Ends Her Life" 2014).

In 2016, New Mexico's Supreme Court ruled that there was no fundamental right to die. In 2017, New York's highest court—the Court of Appeals—in *Myers v. Schneiderman* rejected a challenge by the plaintiff's argument that an individual has a fundamental constitutional right to aid in dying. The plaintiff had challenged the constitutionality of state law that prohibited PAS in the state. The court also rejected the plaintiff's assertion that the state's prohibition against assisted suicide is not rationally related to legitimate state interest. In fact, the court in its decision echoed some of the same reasoning adopted by the US Supreme Court in the *Washington v. Glucksberg* and *Vacco v. Quill* rulings in 1997 (Foster 2017; Niedzwiadek 2017).

In May 2018, California's Fourth District Court of Appeals let stand a lower-court ruling that had overturned California's 2015 End of Life Option Act, which allowed doctors to prescribe lethal drugs for patients with six months or less to live. The court's reasoning was that the California legislature should not have approved the law during the special session because the subject of the law fell outside the grounds for which the special session was called. However, in June of 2018 the same court reinstated the law and ruled that it can stay in effect temporarily until legal challenges by the law's opponents are considered ("An Update on the Status of California's End of Life Option Act" 2018; Denton 2018; Neuman 2018).

States and Physician-Assisted Suicide

A large majority of states do not allow PAS. However, there is a slow movement toward more states approving PAS and several other states are actively considering the issue. Currently, there are seven states and the District of Columbia that allow PAS. They are Oregon, Washington, Montana, Vermont, California, Colorado, Hawaii, and District of Columbia. Table 9.1 provides information about when PAS provisions went into effect and how they came about.

Two primary methods through which states have adopted PAS are citizen-driven ballot initiatives or state legislative action. In three states—Oregon, Washington, and Colorado—PAS laws came about as a result of citizen-initiated ballot initiatives while in two states—Vermont and California—and in the District of Columbia, the initiative came from their respective legislative bodies. Montana is unique in the sense that the state currently does not have a specific law on the book that permits PAS but, as we discussed above, it was the Montana Supreme Court that legalized PAS

Table 9.1

Physician-Assisted Suicide Laws in American States, October 2018

State	Year of Implementation	Name of Law	Method by which Law was Created
Oregon	1997	Death with Dignity Act	Voter-approved ballot initiative
Washington	2009	Death With Dignity Act	Voter-approved ballot initiative
Montana	2009	Court broadened the interpretation of the State's Rights of Terminally Ill Act	State Supreme Court decision
Vermont	2013	Patient Choice and Control at the End of Life Act	State legislature
California	2016	End of Life Action Act	State legislature
Colorado	2017	End of Life Option Act	Voter-approved ballot initiative
District of Columbia	2017	Death with Dignity Act	State legislature
Hawaii	2019	Our Care, Our Choice Act	State legislature

Source: Compiled by the authors from information available at www.deathwithdignity.org/. Death With Dignity National Center, Portland, Oregon.

in Montana. In fact, several attempts to pass legislation supporting PAS have failed in the state legislature. The legislature in California approved PAS in 2015 and the law went into effect in 2016. However, it is being litigated in the court at the present time.

Oregon was the first state to approve PAS in 1994 but its implementation was delayed until 1997 due to legal challenges. Thus, Oregon law has been in effect for over 20 years now. Washington was the second state to approve PAS in 2008 and it went into effect in 2009. Hawaii was the last state to approve PAS in 2018 but the law does not go into effect until 2019.

While specific provisions and procedures outlined in state laws with respect to PAS may vary from state to state, all seven states and DC share certain common requirements with respect to PAS ("Death with Dignity Laws by State" n.d.; "Physician-Assisted Suicide Fast Facts" 2018). They include the following.

- The physician prescribing a lethal dose of medication to a patient to help them end their own life must be a Doctor of Medicine (M.D.) or Doctor of Osteopathy (D.O.).
- The physician must be a willing participant.
- The patient requesting the lethal dose of medication must be at least 18 years of age.
- The patient suffering from terminal illness must be expected to live six months or less.
- The patient must make at least two requests of his/her physician for a lethal dose of prescription two to three weeks apart. One of the requests must be in writing.

In recent years, the right-to-die movement has gained some momentum in the US. In 2018, 23 states were actively considering some form of death-with-dignity proposals, while 20 states were not considering any action with respect to this issue ("Death with Dignity Around the U.S." 2018). However, it is important to note that simply because 23 states are actively considering PAS proposals it does not mean that it would translate into the passage of laws supporting it. For example, in 2017, 27 states debated assisted dying but none approved it. Thus, progress toward laws supporting assisted suicide is likely to continue to be a very slow process ("Assisted-Dying Movement Gathers Momentum in America" 2018; Sandeen 2018).

Physician-Assisted Suicide Statistics

Opposition to PAS has largely come from social conservatives and religious organizations. Some of the opposition is based on religious and moral ground that suicide is immoral. Opponents have also expressed fears that once you go down this path, there will be no stopping. This is the slippery-slope argument. The second fear expressed is that poor, less-educated, and less-well-off individuals may decide to end their life because of financial pressures about the cost of end-of-life care. Third, more minorities are likely to use PAS because of their low socioeconomic status. The data presented in Table 9.2 suggest that such fears have failed to materialize in states that have implemented PAS. Since Oregon and Washington are the two states where PAS has been legal for several years, Table 9.2 presents data regarding PAS for these two states from 2009 to 2016.

One of the first thing that stands out is how similar the data are for both states. Second, while the number of individuals who ended their lives with the physician assistance has increased in both states between 2009 and 2011, the overall number of individuals who have participated in PAS has remained relatively stable. Third, of the total number of patients who requested and received a prescription for a lethal dose to end their lives, about one-third of them did not use/digest the lethal dose. Of this, some may have changed their minds while others may have died due to their underlying illness before they had an opportunity to take the lethal dose. Fourth, for over two-thirds of patients, their underlying illness was some form of malignant neoplasm.

Fifth, in general, male patients used PAS more than female patients. Sixth, over 95 percent of participants in PAS were white. Seventh, with respect to age, in any given year, between 64 and 80 percent of patients were over the age of 65. Finally, on the whole, the largest plurality of patients (often close to 50 percent) who utilized physician assistance in ending their lives had a bachelor's degree or higher compared to less than 10 percent of patients who had less than high school education.

In Oregon's data for 2016, the most frequently mentioned end-of-life concerns by participants in PAS included loss of autonomy (90 percent), being less able to engage in activities that make life enjoyable (90 percent), loss of dignity (65 percent), burden to family, friends, and caregivers (49 percent), losing control of bodily functions (37 percent), and inadequate pain control or concern about it (35 percent). Only 5 percent of participants mentioned financial implications of treatment as their end-of-life concerns ("Oregon Death with Dignity Act: 2016 Data Summary" 2017). The 2016 data for the state of Washington showed a similar pattern. The most frequently mentioned end-of-life concerns included loss of autonomy (87 percent), being less able to engage in activities that make life enjoyable (84 percent), loss of dignity (65 percent), burden on family, friends, and caregivers (51 percent), losing control of bodily functions (43 percent), and inadequate pain control or concern about it (40 percent). Only 8 percent mentioned financial implications of treatment as their end-of-life concerns ("Washington State Death with Dignity Act Report" 2018).

Thus, it is clear from the data that the fear that minorities and the less-educated might feel the pressure to utilize PAS were unfounded. It is not possible to ascertain the economic status of the patients who utilized PAS since neither state collects such data.

No PAS data are available for the state of Montana since it was the state supreme court's decision that legalized PAS in the state. States that have legalized PAS are required to collect and publish data on it on an annual basis. Only limited data are available for Vermont, California, Colorado, and the District of Columbia since their PAS laws have been in effect for only a couple of years, while Hawaii's law only went into effect in 2019. However, the limited amount of data available for 2017 for the states of Colorado, Vermont, and California indicated similar patterns to those demonstrated in Oregon and Washington ("California End of Life Option Act: 2017 Data Report" 2018; "Colorado End-of-Life Options Act, One Year 2017 Data Summary" 2018; "Vermont Report Concerning Patient Choice at the End of Life" 2018).

The End of Life: The Legacy of Terri Schiavo and Brittany Maynard

Two Oscar-winning films released in 2004, *Million Dollar Baby* and *The Sea Inside*, which provided sympathetic views of people seeking to end their own lives, brought the issue of assisted suicide to the center of the national stage. Terri Schiavo's case and her death in 2005 spurred debate in statehouses across the country and prompted many states to examine end-of-life care and decisions surrounding it. All 50 states already have laws that allow people to write advance directives or a living will that specifies their healthcare preferences if they are incapacitated or designates a healthcare proxy to make decisions for them. The new proposed laws are designed to address situations like Terri Schiavo's, in which the incapacitated person has not left a living will or designated a healthcare proxy. Her private ordeal became national news and political battleground for opponents and supporters of the right-to-die movement. In fact, her end-of-life ordeal became a national symbol for how not to die in America. Her case languished inside the courtroom for years. Today, her name has become synonymous with questions about when life ends and who gets to decide it. Perhaps politicians have learned that end-of-life discussions are probably best left to families and not politicians. Terry Schiavo influenced and shaped the right-to-die movement in the United States (Haberman 2014; Sanburn 2015).

Table 9.2

Physician-Assisted Suicide Statistics in Oregon and Washington, 2009–2017

	2009	2010	2011	2012	2013	2014	2015	2016	2017
Oregon									
Number of prescriptions written/dispensed	95	97	114	116	121	155	218	204	NA
Number of patients who ended their lives by taking prescription	59	65	71	85	73	105	135	133	NA
Proportion of patients who ended their lives by taking prescription	62%	67%	62%	73%	60%	68%	62%	65%	NA
Underlying Illness									
Malignant neoplasms	80%	79%	82%	75%	65%	69%	72%	79%	NA
Other	20%	21%	18%	25%	35%	31%	28%	21%	NA
Demographic Characteristics									
Gender									
Male	53%	58%	37%	51%	62%	53%	42%	54%	NA
Female	47%	42%	63%	49%	38%	47%	58%	46%	NA
Race									
White	98%	100%	96%	97%	94%	95%	93%	96%	NA
Non-white	2%	0%	4%	3%	6%	5%	7%	4%	NA
Age									
18–64 years	24%	29%	31%	33%	31%	33%	27%	20%	NA
65–85+ years	76%	71%	69%	67%	69%	67%	73%	80%	NA
Education									
Less than high school	5%	6%	4%	3%	3%	6%	5%	4%	NA
High school graduate	24%	20%	13%	17%	14%	23%	24%	17%	NA
Some college	22%	31%	34%	37%	30%	24%	28%	29%	NA
Baccalaureate or higher	48%	42%	49%	43%	54%	47%	43%	50%	NA
Washington									
Number of prescriptions written/dispensed	63	87	103	121	173	176	213	248	212
Number of patients who ended their lives by taking prescription	36	51	70	83	119	126	166	192	164
Proportion of patients who ended their lives by taking prescription	57%	59%	68%	69%	69%	72%	78%	77%	77%
Underlying Illness									
Malignant neoplasms	79%	78%	78%	73%	77%	76%	72%	77%	72%
Other	21%	22%	22%	27%	23%	24%	28%	23%	28%
Demographic Characteristics									
Gender									
Male	55%	50%	52%	52%	53%	44%	54%	50%	48%
Female	45%	50%	48%	47%	47%	56%	46%	50%	52%
Race									
White (non-Hispanic)	98%	95%	94%	96%	97%	92%	98%	96%	94%
Non-white	2%	5%	6%	4%	3%	7%	2%	4%	6%

(Continued)

Table 9.2 **(Cont.)**

	2009	2010	2011	2012	2013	2014	2015	2016	2017
Age									
18–64 years	26%	29%	36%	33%	26%	29%	27%	30%	26%
65–85+ years	74%	71%	64%	67%	74%	71%	73%	70%	74%
Education									
Less than high school	2%	10%	5%	2%	1%	2%	4%	4%	5%
High school graduate	37%	28%	20%	15%	23%	22%	22%	27%	19%
Some college	22%	18%	28%	27%	26%	24%	26%	35%	22%
Baccalaureate or higher	39%	44%	46%	56%	50%	50%	47%	32%	53%

Note: NA = not available. Percentages may not add to 100 due to rounding.
Sources: Washington State Death with Dignity Act Annual Reports. Washington State Department of Health. www.doh.wa.gov/.
Oregon Death with Dignity Act Annual Reports. Oregon Public Health Division. www.healthoregon.org/dwd.

In 2014, the tragic case of Brittany Maynard again focused the nation's attention on the issue of the right to die and more specifically PAS. Proponents of PAS point to her case for the need to allow PAS. Since the Oregon law went into effect in 1997, only seven individuals under the age of 34 have used Oregon's Death with Dignity Act to end their lives. In addition, 54 percent of those receiving lethal medication fall into the category of widowed, divorced, or never married. In contrast, Brittany Maynard had deep social connections, i.e., loving relationships with her husband, mother, stepfather, and friends (Kotva 2016). Her case reinvigorated the assisted suicide movement and was credited with the passage of California's End of Life Action Act in 2016 (Nirappil 2015) and the introduction of similar legislation in Pennsylvania, Wyoming, and New York (Mathias 2015). The passage of PAS laws in Colorado and the District of Columbia in 2017, and Hawaii in 2018, was also inspired by her case. In addition, the already-strong public support for the right to die grew even stronger following the planned death of Brittany Maynard.

Public Opinion and the Right to Die

A number of polls suggested that Americans had strong feelings about the Terri Schiavo case and that social conservatives had miscalculated public opinion. In a CBS poll of a nationwide random sample of 737 adults (interviewed by telephone between March 21 and 22, 2005), 66 percent said that the feeding tube should not be reinserted into Terri Schiavo. Sixty-one percent said that the case should not be heard by the US Supreme Court. A larger number, 82 percent, indicated that Congress and the president should not be involved in the Schiavo matter. Seventy-two percent said that members of Congress got involved to advance their own political agenda and not because they really cared about Terri Schiavo. Only 34 percent said that they approved of Congress's job performance—the lowest rating Congress had received since December 1997. A strong majority of 75 percent said that the government should stay out of deciding life-support cases ("Poll: Keep Feeding Tube Out" 2005). A poll conducted in 2014 after Brittany Maynard's case found that 74 percent of American adults believe that terminally ill patients who are in great pain should have the right to end their own lives, while only 14 percent were opposed (Thompson 2014).

In a 2004 Gallup poll, 65 percent agreed that a doctor should be allowed to assist a suicide when a person has a disease that cannot be cured and that person is living in pain, while 41 percent opposed physician-assisted suicide on moral or religious grounds. The support for physician-assisted suicide in this 2004 survey actually rose from 52 percent who supported physician-assisted suicide in a 1996 survey (Schwartz 2005). In a survey by *Time* magazine in March 2005, 52 percent of Americans said that they agreed with Oregon's physician-assisted-suicide law, while 41 percent disagreed (Eisenberg 2005). In fact, according to a Harris/BBC World News America poll conducted in August 2010, a majority of Americans, 58 percent, favor physician-assisted suicide for those terminally ill in great pain who want to end their lives ("Large Majorities Support PAS for Terminally Ill Patients in Great Pain" 2011). In fact, after Brittany Maynard's case, support for PAS has increased dramatically. In a 2015 Gallup Poll, 68 percent of respondents stated that doctors should be allowed to assist terminally ill patients in committing suicide. In the same poll, 56 percent of Americans expressed the view that, in general, PAS is morally acceptable (Dugan 2015).

Despite such strong public support for PAS, very few states have actually legalized PAS. Why have many states failed to pass laws legalizing PAS? Drum (2016) provides some possible explanations. One, he argues that assisted suicide has largely been a West Coast movement. Perhaps, outside of the West Coast, this is not a major issue. A second explanation may lie in the demographics. The assisted suicide movement has long been dominated by well-off, educated whites. As Table 9.2 suggests, whites are the ones who have utilized PAS the most in states that allow it. Assisted suicide legislation may be more difficult to pass in more ethnically diverse states. Minority patients have historically been wary of the medical establishment because they have less access to healthcare and they may feel that they will be shortchanged by the same medical establishment by pressing them to forego expensive end-of-life care treatments. Minority groups may feel that they will be disproportionately counseled to opt for PAS. A third reason may be due to moral objections. The fourth factor may have to do with the terminology and the use of the term "suicide." For example, while polls show a majority of Americans support the notion that terminally ill patients should get the help of a physician to hasten the end of their life by painless means, support drops by about ten points when Americans are asked whether doctors should be permitted to assist the patient to commit suicide. Thus, in the debate over PAS, opponents emphasize the word "suicide" with its negative connotation while supporters argue that physician assistance is simply designed to help in the natural process of dying. That is also why states that have legalized assisted suicide use terms such as death with dignity, end-of-life options, patient's choice, and the like.

Living Wills and Durable Power of Attorney

Media publicity surrounding major court cases in the area of the right to die has led to more people contemplating preparing an advance directive to navigate end-of-life care. An advance directive is anything that a person prepares in advance of his/her death. The two main types of advance directives are a living will and a durable power of attorney for healthcare.

A living will must be signed by a competent person in good health and gives permission to his or her doctor to turn off life-support systems in the case of terminal illness or a permanent coma. Thus, the living will gives the person some control over his/her last few days or weeks of life. Because both the National Conference of Commissioners of Uniform State Laws and the American Bar Association have given their stamp of approval to the Uniform Rights of the Terminally Ill Act, the number of persons signing living wills is expected to increase. To prevent abuse, state laws in the area of living wills often stipulate specific conditions that must be met. For example, some states require that at least two physicians certify that the patient's illness is terminal. Some states require that the living will is witnessed by people who are not healthcare providers or beneficiaries of the person's last will.

An alternative to a living will is for an individual to assign a permanent power of attorney for healthcare to another person. In this scheme, another person (for example, a spouse, a family member, or a friend) is designated as a surrogate healthcare decision-maker in case a person is unable or incompetent to make decisions for herself/himself due to serious illness.

The primary difference between a living will and a durable power of attorney for healthcare is that a living will is used to declare a person's desire not to have life-prolonging measures to be taken if there is no hope for recovery such as brain death or terminal illness and it deals only with deathbed concerns. A durable power of attorney for healthcare covers all healthcare decisions made by the designee (healthcare surrogate) and lasts only as long as the individual is incapable of making decisions for himself or herself ("Living Will vs. Durable Healthcare Power of Attorney" n.d.).

Due to publicity surrounding the Terri Schiavo and Brittany Maynard cases, interest in advance directives spiked, with more individuals completing them (Goldbach 2014; Novotney 2010). In 2000, only 47 percent of Americans more than 60 years old had filled out paperwork spelling out their desires regarding their end-of-life care or had designated a person legally empowered to fulfill their wishes. By 2010, 72 percent of that age group had done the paperwork (Maron 2014; "Record Number of Older Adults Completing Living Wills" 2014). However, in 2014, when one considers all Americans, only about 26 percent of Americans had an advance directive like a living will and the number of persons with advance directives for end-of-life care had increased to 37 percent by 2017 (Crist 2017; "Nearly Two-Thirds of Americans Don't Have a Living Will—Do You" 2016). According to another study, many Americans avoid end-of-life care planning (Andrews 2017).

The importance of having a clear living will to avoid unforeseen circumstances is demonstrated in one recent case. An unconscious man with a history of serious health problems and high blood alcohol level was admitted to a Miami, Florida hospital. He had no identification and no family with him. However, on his chest, he had a tattoo, "Do Not Resuscitate." At first, a doctor attending to the man wanted to ignore the tattoo because there was no way to be absolutely certain that the man did not want to be treated with potentially life-saving treatment. Tattoos aren't legally binding and are usually considered too ambiguous to act upon. The hospital sought the counsel of its ethics consultant, who said that the doctor should honor the patient's tattoo because it was reasonable to infer that the tattoo expressed his authentic preference. Supporting the ethical consultant's position was the fact that the hospital's social work department was able to locate a copy of the man's Florida Department of Health "Out-of-Hospital" do-not-resuscitate order, which supported the request on his tattoo. The end result was that a do-not-resuscitate order was issued and the man died (Holt et al. 2017; Willingham 2017).

Physician-Assisted Suicide: Religion, Morality, and Ethics

The debate and arguments for and against PAS center around religious beliefs and questions about morality and ethics. Arguments against PAS include the following.

The opposition to the PAS by the Catholic Church is primarily based on moral grounds. Suicide has always been considered a sin by the Catholic Church and the Vatican reaffirmed this in 1965 when it declared abortion, euthanasia, and other forms of taking life as a poison in human society. In 1980, the Church in its "Declaration on Euthanasia" stated that while the refusal of extraordinary measures when death was imminent was permissible, it opposed any kind of assisted suicide as a violation of the divine law. In 1995, Pope John Paul II condemned the growing acceptance of euthanasia as a personal right. Born-again Christians and evangelicals have opposed abortion and assisted suicide as promoting a culture of death right (Drum 2016). The Catholic Church played a major role in opposing Measure 16 in Oregon, the ballot initiative responsible for the passage of the Death with Dignity Act in 1994 legalizing PAS. The Church solicited donations and urged Catholics to vote against Measure 16. It failed because only 12 percent of Oregon's population is Catholic and the supporters successfully used the Catholic Church's support of an anti-gay measure on the ballot the same election and the anger it generated among voters to argue that this was an attempt by the Church to impose its values on the public. The Catholic Church has opposed similar assisted suicide measures in other states (Hehir 2014; Purvis 2012).

The opposition also comes from within the disability rights community, who often have been apprehensive of the medical establishment and believe that society often holds negative stereotypes about people with disabilities. They fear that if assisted suicide becomes a universal right, the right to die can turn into the duty to die, with minorities, the poor, and disabled individuals pressured by family members, insurance companies, or government to end their lives. Some individuals might view themselves as unproductive and burdensome, and society and the medical profession as a matter of social justice have a duty to safeguard and protect vulnerable members of society such as the disabled, the poor, the elderly, children, minorities, and others. There is certainly a racial/ethnic divide when it comes to views about PAS. In a poll conducted in 2013 by the Pew Research Center, 53 percent of white respondents approved of PAS laws while only 32 percent of Hispanics and 29 percent of blacks approved such laws, reflecting minorities' apprehensions (Kim 2015).

This argument reflects the fear of a slippery slope. The slippery-slope argument is based on the notion that the first step leads to a chain of related steps that can result in a significant and unwanted effect. Thus, some fear that, over time, rules for assisted suicide will become more lenient and relaxed, encouraging more people to end their lives and forgo more expensive end-of-life care. Opponents often point to the Netherlands and Belgium as a classic example of countries that have gone down the slippery slope (Drum 2016; Piana 2015; Sulmasy and Mueller 2017).

The arguments against PAS also come from many in the medical profession itself on grounds of professional ethics. The Hippocratic Oath requires doctors to act in the best interest of the patient and recognize the unique nature of the relationship between a physician and their patient. Physicians have duties to patients based on the ethical principles of beneficence, i.e., acting in the best interest of the patient; nonmaleficence, i.e., avoiding or minimizing harm; and respect for patient autonomy. Physician-assisted suicide requires physicians to breach general duties of beneficence and nonmaleficence and inconsistent with the physician's role as a healer. It is not for a physician to decide the fate of a patient and even if the patient gives his consent to assisted suicide, killing is intrinsically wrong. Proponents of PAS argue that withdrawing treatment on behalf of patients' wishes, such as forgoing a mechanical ventilator, is not any different from prescribing a lethal dose of medicine for a patient to use since both acts lead to the patient's death. However, opponents point out that the two acts are very different because intent and causation are different. Withdrawing life-sustaining technology at the patient's request simply removes an intervention that prevents an underlying illness from running its course. The intent is not to terminate the patient's life. The intent of the patient in refusing life-sustaining technology is freedom from unwanted intervention. However, if a doctor were to withdraw life-sustaining technology without the patient's consent and the patient dies, that act would be considered wrong. In contrast, death by a lethal dose of medication, i.e., PAS, is not a natural death caused by the patient's underlying condition. Rather, the intent of the act is to cause the death of a patient. To deal with the issue of professional ethics, states that have legalized PAS make a distinction between what is legal and what is ethical. States may legalize PAS but it cannot force doctors who oppose the practice on grounds of professional ethics or personal beliefs to participate. Thus, doctors are not required to participate in the practice of PAS, just as they are not required to perform abortions (Jordan 2017; Lagay 2003; Quill and Sussman, n.d.; Sulmasy and Mueller 2017).

The main argument in support of PAS emphasizes the principle of respect for patient autonomy and broad interpretation of the physician's duty to relieve patient's suffering and obligation of non-abandonment. If a patient's pain and suffering cannot be relieved with state-of-the-art palliative care then the physician has an obligation to do everything in their power to relieve that suffering, including hastening death at the patient's request. Since those seeking PAS cite concern about the loss of autonomy and dignity as primary reasons, it follows that physician assistance in assisted suicide is an act of compassion that respects the patient's choice. Others argue that while patient autonomy is important and respected, it must be balanced with other ethical principles such as beneficence and nonmalfience (Quill and Sussman, n.d.; Sulmasy and Mueller 2017).

CONCLUSION

The discussion of reproductive and life-sustaining technologies in this chapter exemplifies the complexities of legal and ethical issues raised by modern medical technology. Ethical objections to artificial insemination are often raised on religious or theological grounds. Objections are also raised on the ground that artificial insemination produces harmful consequences for society when the woman is not married, when the donor is not screened, or when the identity of the donor is concealed. Similar ethical concerns are raised with *in-vitro* fertilization (i.e., test-tube fertilization), surrogate parenthood, embryo transfers, and the use of frozen embryos and sperm banks.

Similarly, end-of-life technologies have produced many legal and ethical concerns as reflected in the right-to-die cases discussed in this chapter. They raised profound questions about what is life, what constitutes quality of life, who should have ultimate control over the end of life choices, and how we balance respect for patients' autonomy versus physicians' professional ethics. The cases of Terri Schiavo and Brittany Maynard and others have highlighted the clash of science, religion, ethics, and politics when it comes to policymaking.

Healthcare technology is developing at a rapid pace, while our capacity and our ability to comprehend and deal with the legal and ethical issues raised by medical technology are lagging behind. Now that we have entered the twenty-first century, policymakers will be increasingly confronted with the challenge of formulating public policies that require an understanding of the legal and ethical implications of rapidly emerging new technologies. Developments in the United States can be best characterized as a patchwork approach to bioethics. Most initiatives have tended to be private rather than government-sponsored. This has the advantage of producing multiple or pluralistic approaches that foster diversity.

Ira H. Carmen (1994) argues that "good" or "ethical" biomedicine cannot be defined in the abstract. According to Carmen, our constitutional and political order requires a delicate weighing and balancing of competing interests by policymakers. The Madisonian model that underlies our political system requires that the people's representatives, not some presidential commission, work through the political branches to formulate national policies. Whether Congress is up to the task remains to be seen.

The same notion is applicable to controversies surrounding issues of emergency contraceptives, RU-486, and healthcare for immigrants, especially for undocumented immigrants. Legal and ethical issues are also present in these issues, though perhaps not as intense as in other reproductive technologies and end-of-life issues. The controversy surrounding emergency contraceptives and RU-486 reflects a clash of moral and religious values in American society, which plays out in the political process along ideological and partisan lines about how such issues are defined and perceived. Low-level ideological and partisan divides sometimes make it possible to arrive at a policy consensus through bargaining and compromises. Under conditions of intense partisan and ideological conflicts, it is much more difficult to achieve policy consensus, resulting in policy paralysis. However, more often than not, policy decisions are based more on partisan and electoral calculations than on science or facts.

STUDY QUESTIONS

1. What is bioethics, and how does it relate to medical technology? Give examples of major developments that have taken place in the field of medical technology.
2. What are different types of assisted reproductive technologies (ARTs)? What kinds of ethical issues do such technologies raise?

3. Discuss some of the major court cases dealing with the right to conceive and bear children, parenthood, and surrogacy.
4. Discuss some of the major court cases dealing with preventing unwanted pregnancy and birth.
5. Discuss major cases dealing with the withdrawal of life-sustaining technologies and the constitutional principles the courts have established.
6. Discuss the evolution of the right-to-die movement in the United States. What do public opinion polls show about Americans' views on this issue?
7. Discuss some of the major court cases and rulings dealing with the issue of assisted suicide.
8. Discuss common elements/provisions in physician-assisted suicide laws adopted by states; what do the statistics for Oregon and Washington demonstrate?
9. What are the major arguments for and against physician-assisted suicide?
10. How did the policy about the use of emergency contraception evolve in the United States? What role did religion, political ideology, and partisanship play in shaping policymaking in this field? Do you agree with the current policy? Why?
11. How does the availability of RU-486 change the debate about abortion?
12. Discuss the intersection of politics, religion, political ideology, and ethics with reproductive technologies and right-to-die issues.

REFERENCES

"Abortion Hit New Low in U.S." 2016. NBC News. Online at www.nbcnews.com/.
"About the Commission." n.d. Presidential Commission for the Study of Bioethical Issues. Online at http://bioethics.gov/.
Achenback, Joel. 2016. "Human Embryo Experiment Shows Progress Toward 'Three-Parent' Babies." *Washington Post*. Online at www.washingtonpost.com/.
"A History of Key Abortion Rulings of the U.S. Supreme Court." 2013. Pew Research Center. Online at www.pewforum.org/.
American College of Obstetricians and Gynecologists. 2012. "Over-the-Counter Access to Oral Contraceptives." *Committee Opinion*, no. 544 (December): 1–5.
American Society for Reproductive Medicine. 2018. *Third Party Reproduction: A Guide for Patients*. Birmingham, AL: American Society for Reproductive Medicine.
Andrews, Michelle. 2017. "Many Avoid End-of-Life Care Planning, Study Finds." NPR. Online at www.npr.org/.
Angell, Marcia. 1990. "Prisoners of Technology: The Case of Nancy Cruzan." *New England Journal of Medicine*, 322, no. 17 (April 26): 1226–1228.
Ansermet, Francois. 2018. *The Art of Making Children: The New World of Assisted Reproductive Technology*. New York: Routledge.
"An Overview of Abortion Laws." 2018. Guttmacher Institute. Online at www.guttmacher.org/.
"An Update on the Status of California's End of Life Option Act." 2018. Death with Dignity. Online at www.deathwithdignity.org/.
"Assisted Reproductive Technology (ART)." n.d. Centers for Disease Control and Prevention. Online at www.cdc.gov/ART/index.htm.
"Assisted-Dying Movement Gathers Momentum in America." 2018. *The Economist*. Online at www.economist.com/.
Associated Press. 2005. "Schiavo's Parents Give Up Their Federal Appeal." *The New York Times*, March 27.
Bahadur, G. 2004. "Ethical Challenges in Reproductive Medicine: Posthumous Reproduction." *International Congress Series*, 1266 (April): 295–302.
Baird, P.A. 1996. "Ethical Issues of Fertility and Reproduction." *Annual Review of Medicine*, 47, no. 1: 107–116.
Baker, Amy. 2015. "3d-Printed Prescription Drugs a Huge Stride Forward for Personalized Medicine." *National Law Review*. Online at www.natlawreview.com/.
Baker, Max B. and Elizabeth Campbell. 2014. "Texas Law Didn't Anticipate Munoz Case, Drafters Say." *Fort Worth Star-Telegram*. Online at www.star-telegram.com/.
Barnes, Robert and Ann E. Marimow. 2018. "Supreme Court Throws Out Lower-Court Decision that Allowed Immigrant Teen to Obtain Abortion." *Washington Post*. Online at www.washingtonpost.com/.
Bauman, Norman. 1997. "Dead Men Conceiving: Trend Raises Ethical, Legal Questions." *Urology Times*, 25, no. 2 (February): 4–5.
Bazelon, Emily. 2013. "The Politics of Prude." *Slate*. Online at www.slate.com/.
Beauchamp, Tom L. 2006. "The Right to Die as the Triumph of Autonomy." *Journal of Medicine and Philosophy*, 31, no. 6 (January): 643–654.
Becker, Rachel. 2017. "An Artificial Womb Successfully Grew Baby Sheep – And Humans Could Be Next." The Verge. Online at www.theverge.com/.
Beckman, Linda J. and S. Marie Harvey. 2005. "Current Reproductive Technologies: Increased Access and Choice?" *Journal of Social Issues*, 61, no. 1 (March): 1–20.
Begeley, Sharon. 2012. "Prescribe Morning-After Pill in Advance, Say, Pediatricians." Reuters News, November 26. Online at www.reuters.com/.

Bellafante, Ginia. 2005. "Surrogate Mothers' New Niche: Bearing Children for Gay Couples." *The New York Times*, May 27.
Bello, Camille. 2018. "Where in Europe in Assisted Dying Legal?" EuroNews. Online at www.euronews.com/
Belluck, Pam. 2005. "Tide Has Turned When Hospitals, Families Clash Over Patient Care." *San Diego Union Tribune*, March 27.
Benagiano, G. 2003. "Public Health and Infertility." *Reproductive Medicine Online*, 7, no. 6 (December): 606–614.
Bernstein, Lenny. 2016. "Donated Organs Kept 'Alive' May Ease the Transplant Shortage." *Washington Post*. Online at www.washingtonpost.com/.
Biskupic, Joan. 1997. "Oregon's Assisted Suicide Law Leaves On." *Washington Post*, October 15: A03.
Blank, Robert H. 1989. "Introduction." In *Biomedical Technology and Public Policy*, ed. Robert H. Blank and Miriam K. Mills, vii–xv. New York: Greenwood Press.
Boonstra, Heather D. 2013. "Medication Abortion Restrictions Burden Women and Providers—And Threaten U.S. Trend toward Very Early Abortion." *Guttmacher Policy Review*, 16, no. 1 (Winter): 18–23.
Brandes, Heide. 2014. "Oklahoma Judge Allows Law on Abortion Pill to Take Effect." Yahoo. Online at www.yahoo.com/.
Briggs, Helen. 2018. "First Monkey Clones Created in Chinese Laboratory." BBC. Online at www.bbc.co.uk/.
"Brittany Maynard Doesn't Want to Die." 2014. CBS News. Online at www.cbsnews.com/.
Brown, Elisha. 2018. "California Fertility Clinic Sued over 'Thousands' of Lost Embryos and Eggs." *The Daily Beast*. Online at www.thedailybeast.com/.
Bryant, J.J. 2015. "A Baby Step: The Status of Surrogacy Law in Wisconsin following Rosecky V. Schissel." *Marquette Law Review*, 98, no. 4 (August): 1729–1758.
Buckley, Jerry. 1990. "How Doctors Decide: Who Shall Live, Who Shall Die." *U.S. News & World Report*, January 11.
"California End of Life Option Act: 2017 Data Report." 2018. California Department of Public Health. Online at www.cdph.ca.gov/.
Campo-Flores, Arian. 2005. "The Legacy of Terri Schiavo." *Newsweek*, April 4.
"Can States Intervene in Medical Decisions?" 2004. *Christian Science Monitor*, August 3.
Cantor, Norman L. 1993. *Advance Directives and the Pursuit of Death with Dignity*. Indianapolis, IN: Indiana University Press.
Caplan, Arthur. 1989. "Hard Data on Efficacy: The Prerequisite to Hard Choices in Health Care." *Mount Sinai Journal of Medicine*, 56, no. 3: 185–190.
Card, Robert F. 2011. "Conscientious Objection, Emergency Contraception, and Public Policy." *Journal of Medicine and Philosophy*, 36, no. 1 (January): 53–68.
Carmen, Ira H. 1994. "Bioethics, Public Policy and Political Science." *Politics and Life Sciences*, 13, no. 1 (February 1): 79–81.
Centers for Disease Control and Prevention. n.d. "What Is Assisted Reproductive Technology?" Centers for Disease Control and Prevention. Online at www.cdc.gov/.
Cerminara, Kathy and Kenneth Goodman. 2005. "Key Events in the Case of Theresa Marie Schiavo." Joint Project of the University of Miami Ethics Programs and the Shepard Broad Law Center at Nova Southeastern University. Online at www.miami.edu/ethics2/schiavo/timeline.htm.
Chandra, Anjani, Casey E. Copen, and Elizabeth H. Stephen. 2014. "Infertility Service Use in the United States: Data from the National Survey of Family Growth, 1982–2010." *National Health Statistics Reports*, no. 73 (January): 1–21.
Childress, Sarah. 2012. "The Evolution of America's Right-to-Die Movement." PBS. Online at www.pbs.org/.
Ciccarelli, John K. and Janice C. Ciccarelli. 2005. "The Legal Aspects of Parental Rights in Assisted Reproductive Technology." *Journal of Social Issues*, 61, no. 1: 127–137.
Colb, Sherry F. 2013. "The U.S. Court of Appeals for the Sixth Circuit Upholds Restrictions on Medical Abortion: Why Should Anyone Care?" *Verdict*, January 9. Online at http://verdict.justia.com/.
"Colorado End-of-Life Options Act: Year One 2017 Data Summary." 2018. Colorado Official State Web Portal. Online at www.colorado.gov/.
"Contraceptive Use in the United States." 2018. Guttmacher Institute. Online at www.guttmacher.org/.
"Counseling and Waiting Periods for Abortion." 2018. Guttmacher Institute. Online at www.guttmacher.org/.
Crist, Carolyn. 2017. "Over One Third of U.S. Adults Have Advanced Medical Directive." Reuters News. Online at www.reuters.com/.
Crockin, Susan. 2017. "Legally Speaking Sept. 2017." American Society for Reproductive Medicine. Online at www.asrm.org/.
Crockin, Susan. 2018. "Embryo Disputes in Both U.S. and Canada." American Society for Reproductive Medicine. Online at www.asrm.org/.
Daar, Judith F. 2001. "Frozen Embryo Disputes Revisited: A Trilogy of Procreation-Avoidance Approaches." *Journal of Law, Medicine and Ethics*, 29, no. 2 (summer): 197–202.
"Death with Dignity Advocate Brittany Maynard Ends Her Life." 2014. CBS News. Online at www.cbsnews.com/.
"Death with Dignity around the U.S." 2018. Death with Dignity. Online at www.deathwithdignity.org/.
"Death with Dignity Data." 2012. Washington State Department of Health. Online at www.doh.wa.gov/.
"Death with Dignity Laws by State." n.d. FindLaw. Online at https://healthcare.findlaw.com/.
DeCesare, Michael. 2015. *Death on Demand: Jack Kevorkian and the Right-to-Die Movement*. Lanham, MD: Rowman & Littlefield.
"Definition of 'Parent' and Related Variations in Child Welfare." n.d. Washington, DC: National Conference of State Legislatures. Online at www.ncsl.org/.
DeMillo, Andrew. 2016. "Analysis: Court Ruling Latest Wrinkle for Anti-Abortion Push." KSL. Online at www.ksl.com/.
Denniston, Lyle. 2014. "Court Passes Up RU-486 Abortion Issue, Again." Supreme Court of the United States Blog. Online at www.scotusblog.com/.
Denton, Joshua. 2018. "Superior Court Judge Overturns California's Physician-Assisted Suicide Law." California Family Council. Online at https://californiafamily.org/.

Devine, Richard J. 2004. *Good Care, Painful Choices: Medical Ethics for Ordinary People.* New York: Paulist Press.

Donovan, Megan K. 2017. "In Real Life: Federal Restrictions on Abortion Coverage and the Women They Impact." *Guttmacher Policy Review*, 20 (January): 1–7.

Dooren, Jennifer C. 2011. "Obama Health Chief Blocks FDA on 'Morning After' Pill." *Wall Street Journal*, December 8. Online at http://online.wsj.com/.

Dreweke, Joerg. 2016. "New Clarity for the U.S. Abortion Debate: A Steep Drop in Unintended Pregnancy Is Driving Recent Abortion Decline." *Guttmacher Policy Review*, 19, 16–22.

Drum, Kevin. 2016. "Assisted Suicide, My Family, and Me." *Mother Jones* (January–February): 27–32.

Dugan, Andrew. 2015. "In U.S., Support up for Doctor-Assisted Suicide." Gallup. Online at https://news.gallup.com/.

Ebert, Martina. 2002. "RU 486 and Abortion Practices in Europe: From Legalization to Access." *Women and Politics*, 24, no. 3: 13–34.

Eisenberg, Daniel. 2005. "Lessons of the Schiavo Battle." *Time*, April 4, 22–30.

Elster, Nanette R. 2005. "Assisted Reproductive Technologies: Contracts, Consents, and Controversies." *American Journal of Family Law*, 18, no. 4 (Winter): 193–199.

"Embryo and Gamete Disposition Laws." 2007. Washington, DC: National Conference of State Legislatures. Online at www.ncsl.org/.

"Emergency Contraception." 2010. Office of Women's Health. Online at www.womenshealth.gov/files/documents/fact-sheet-emergency-contraception.pdf.

"Emergency Contraception: A Fact Sheet from the Office on Women's Health." 2017. Office of Women's Health. Online at www.womenshealth.gov/.

"Emergency Contraception: Background." 2018. Guttmacher Institute. Online at www.guttmacher.org/.

"Emergency Contraceptive Pills." 2004. Washington, DC: Henry J. Kaiser Family Foundation. Online at www.kff.org/womenshealth/.

"Emergency Contraception State Laws." 2012. Washington, DC: National Conference of State Legislatures. Online at www.ncsl.org/.

"Euthanasia and Physician-Assisted Suicide (PAS) around the World." 2016. ProCon.org. Online at https://euthanasia.procon.org/.

Farmer, Ann. 2008. "Roe's Mid-Life Crisis Protecting Reproductive Health Rights." *Perspectives*, 17, no. 2 (Fall): 4–7.

"FDA Eases Guidelines for Abortion Pill Use." 2016. *Tampa Bay Times*. Online at www.tampabay.com/.

Feinberg, John S. and Paul D. Feinberg. 2010. *Ethics for a Brave New World.* Wheaton, IL: Crossway.

Feldman, Eric A. 2018. "Baby M Turns 30: The Law and Policy of Surrogate Motherhood." *American Journal of Law and Medicine*, 44, no. 1 (March): 7–22.

Field, Martha A. 2014. "Compensated Surrogacy." *Washington Law Review*, 89, no. 4 (December): 1155–1184.

Finer, Lawrence B. and Mia R. Zolna. 2016. "Decline in Unintended Pregnancy in the United States, 2008–2011." *New England Journal of Medicine*, 374, no. 9 (March): 843–852.

Fogel, Susan B. and Lourdes A. Rivera. 2003. "Religious Beliefs and Healthcare Necessities." *Human Rights: Journal of the Section of Individual Rights and Responsibilities*, 30, no. 2 (Spring): 8–11.

Foote, Donna, Larry Reibstein, and Ana Figueroa. 1998. "And Baby Makes One." *Newsweek*, 131, no. 5 (February 2): 68–69.

Foster, Catherine G. 2017. "Deciding Death: New York State Is the Latest Train Wreck for Doctor-Aided Death." US News. Online at www.usnews.com/.

Gallagher, James. 2016. "Making Babies without Eggs May Be Possible, Say Scientists." BBC. Online at www.bbc.com/.

Gallagher, James. 2018. "First Human Eggs Grown in Laboratory." BBC. Online at www.bbc.com/.

Gerber Fried, Marlene. 2008. "Thirty-Five Years of Legal Abortion: The U.S. Experience." *IDS Bulletin*, 39, no. 3 (July): 88–94.

"Germany Passes Law Allowing Some Types of Assisted Suicide." 2015. Associated Press. Online at https://apnews.com/.

Gilbert, Scott F., Anna L. Tyler, and Emily J. Zackin. 2005. *Bioethics and the New Embryology: Springboards for Debate.* Sunderland, MA: W.H. Freeman and Sinauer Associates.

Goldbach, Hayley. 2014. "Advance Directives More Popular over Last Decade." Stanford School of Medicine. Online at https://aging.stanford.edu/.

Goodnough, Abby. 2005a. "Appeals Court Refuses to Order Schiavo's Feeding Reinstated." *The New York Times*, March 23.

Goodnough, Abby. 2005b. "Few Options for Schiavo's Parents as U.S. Judge Denies Request." *The New York Times*, March 25.

Goodnough, Abby. 2005c. "Schiavo Dies, Ending Bitter Case Over Feeding Tube." *The New York Times*, April 1.

Goodnough, Abby and Adam Liptak. 2005a. "Schiavo's Parents Appeal to the Supreme Court on Feeding Tube." *The New York Times*, March 24.

Goodnough, Abby and Adam Liptak. 2005b. "Supreme Court Rejects Request to Reinsert Feeding Tube." *The New York Times*, March 24.

Greenfield, Beth. 2015. "Legal Battle Erupts between Surrogate Mom and Gay Dads." Yahoo. Online at www.yahoo.com/news/.

Gregoire, Carolyn. 2017. "In Breakthrough Discovery, Scientists Mass-Produce Artificial Blood." *Huffington Post*. Online at www.huffingtonpost.com/.

Gupta, Jyotsna A. 2012. "Reproductive Biocrossings: Indian Egg Donors and Surrogates in the Globalized Fertility Market." *International Journal of Feminist Approaches to Bioethics*, 5, no. 1 (Spring): 25–51.

Haberman, Clyde. 2014. "From Private Ordeal to National Fight: The Case of Terri Schiavo." *The New York Times*. Online at www.nytimes.com/.

Hafner, Josh. 2017. "Uterus Transplant Results in Successful Birth – The 1st in the US." *USA Today*. Online at www.usatoday.com/.

Hallifax, Jackie. 2004. "Fla. Court Nixes Law Keeping Woman Alive." Associated Press, September 23. Yahoo. Online at story.news.yahoo.com.

Hansen, Jane. 2017. "Scientists Find Key to Stopping 'Incurable' Child Brain Cancer with Malaria Drug but They Need Funding." *Daily Telegraph*. Online at www.dailytelegraph.com.au/.

Hanson, Stephen S. and Annie-Lauri Auden. 2014. "Case Study: Last Chance at Grandchildren: A Request for Perimortem Sperm Harvesting." *Hasting Center Report*, 44, no. 1 (January-February): 13–14.

Harwood, Karey. 2007. *The Infertility Treadmill: Feminist Ethics, Personal Choice, and the Use of Reproductive Technologies*. Chapel Hill, NC: University of North Carolina Press.

Head, Tom. 2017. "The Right to Die Movement: A Timeline History." ThoughtCo. Online at www.thoughtco.com/.

Hehir, Bryan J. 2014. "Physician-Assisted Suicide: Political, Pastoral Challenges Ahead." *Health Progress*, 95, no. 1 (March): 6–10.

Higdon, Michael J. 2012. "Fatherhood by Conscription: Nonconsensual Insemination and the Duty of Child Support." *Georgia Law Review*, 46, no. 2 (Winter): 407–457.

"History of Bioethics Commissions." n.d. The Department of Bioethics. Online at http://bioethics.gov/cms/history.

Holt, Gregory E, Bianca Sarmento, Daniel Kett, and Kenneth W. Goodman. 2017. "An Unconscious Patient with a DNR Tattoo." *New England Journal of Medicine*, 377, no. 22 (November): 2192–2193.

"How Congress Has Used the Power of the Purse to Restrict Block Abortion Access." 2017. Moyers. Online at https://billmoyers.com/.

Hulse, Carl. 2005. "Congress Passes and Bush Signs Legislation on Schiavo Case." *The New York Times*, March 21.

Hurley, Lawrence. 2013. "Supreme Court Lets Stand Ruling Throwing Out 'Abortion Pill' Limits." Yahoo. Online at www.yahoo.com/news/.

Hurley, Lawrence. 2014. "U.S. Top Court Rejects Arizona Appeal over Abortion Drug Law." Reuters News. Online at www.reuters.com/.

Imam, Jareen. 2016. "Feds Open Talks on Growing Human Organs in Animals." CNN. Online at www.cnn.com/.

"Immigrants' Health Coverage and Health Reform: Key Questions and Answers." 2009. Focus on Health Reform. Washington, DC: Henry J. Kaiser Family Foundation. Online at www.kff.org/.

"Indepth: Terri Schiavo, Schiavo Timeline." 2005. *CBC News*, March 31. Online at www.cbc.ca.

"Induced Abortion in the United States." 2018. Guttmacher Institute. Online at www.guttmacher.org/.

Jatlaoui, Tara C, Jill Shah, Michele G. Mandel, Jamie W. Krashin, Danielle B. Suchdev, Denise J. Jamieson, and Karen Pazol. 2017. "Abortion Surveillance—United States, 2014." *Morbidity and Mortality Weekly Report*, 66, no. 24 (November): 1–48.

Jayson, Sharon. 2013. "5.8M Women Have Used 'Morning After' Pill." *USA Today*. Online at www.usatoday.com/.

Jerman, Jenna, Rachel K. Jones, and Tsuyoshi Onda. 2016. *Characteristics of U.S. Abortion Patients in 2014 and Changes since 2008*. New York: Guttmacher Institute.

Johnson, Carolyn Y. 2018. "The 'Game-Changing' Technique to Create Babies from Skill Cells Just Stepped Forward." *Washington Post*. Online at www.washingtonpost.com/.

Jordan, Madeline. 2017. "The Ethical Considerations of Physician-Assisted Suicide." *Dialogue & Nexus*, 4, no. 1 (Fall 2016–Spring 2017): 1–7.

Joslin, Courtney and Jamie Pendersen. 2017. "Updated National Uniform Parentage Act (UPA 2017) Approved." American Society for Reproductive Medicine. Online at www.asrm.org/.

Kamisar, Yale. 1991. "Who Should Live—Or Die? Who Should Decide? An Interview with Professor Kamisar at the University of Michigan Law School." *Trial*, 27, no. 12 (December 1): 20–26.

Kaplan, Sarah. 2017. "Scientists Create a Part-Human, Part-Pig Embryo—Rasing the Possibility of Interspecies Organ Transplants." *The Washington Post*. Online at www.washingtonpost.com/.

Kardish, Chris. 2015. "Courts are Keeping Assisted Suicide Laws Alive." Governing. Online at www.governing.com/.

Kay, Jonathan. 2015. "Will People Go to Canada to Die?" The Daily Beast. Online at www.thedailybeast.com/.

Kelland, Kate. 2016. "New Drug Capsule Delivers Medicine for Weeks after Swallowing." Reuters News. Online at www.reuters.com/.

Kelland, Kate and Kylie MacLellan. 2015. "Britain Votes to Allow World's First 'Three-Parent' IVF Babies." Reuters News. Online at www.reuters.com/.

Kelleher, Paul J. 2010. "Emergency Contraception and Conscientious Objection." *Journal of Applied Philosophy*, 27, no. 3 (August): 290–304.

Keneally, Meghan. 2018. "In Growing Number of States, Women Seeking Abortions Face the Problem of Where to Go." ABC News. Online at https://abcnews.go.com/.

"Key Dates in Schiavo Right-to-Die Case." 2005. Associated Press, May 23. Yahoo. Online at news.yahoo.com.

"Key Statistics from the National Survey of Family Growth." 2011. Centers for Disease Control and Prevention. Online at www.cdc.gov/.

"Key Statistics from the National Survey of Family Growth." 2017. Centers for Disease Control and Prevention. Online at www.cdc.gov/.

Kim, Jennifer. 2015. "Physician Assisted Suicide's Demographic Divide." Brown Political Review. Online at www.brownpoliticalreview.org/.

King, Hope. 2015. "First 3D-Printed Drug Approved by FDA." CNN. Online at https://money.cnn.com/.

Klein, Renate, Janice G. Raymond, and Lynnette Dumble. 2013. *RU 486: Misconception, Myths, and Morals*, 2d edn. North Melbourne, Australia: Spinifex Press.

Knaplund, Kristine S. 2012. "Children of Assisted Reproduction." *University of Michigan Journal of Law Reform*, 45, no. 4 (Summer): 899–935.

Knothe, Alli. 2016. "Tampa Bay Woman Sues after Discovering Sperm Donor Was a Schizophrenic Felon." *Tampa Bay Times*. Online at www.tampabay.com/.

"Known Donor Family Law New York – Protecting Lesbian Mothers." 2018. PFLAG Long Island. Online at www.pflagli.org/.

Koebler, Jason. 2013. "Federal Judge Order FDA to Remove Age Restriction on the over the Counter Morning after Pill." *U.S. News and World Report*, April 15. Online at www.usnews.com/news/articles/2013/04/05/federal-judge-orders-fda-to-remove-age-restriction-on-over-the-counter-morning-after-pill.

Kolata, Gina. 2016. "Birth of a '3-Parent Baby' a Success for Controversial Procedure." *The New York Times*. Online at www.nytimes.com/.

Konstantinides, Anneta. 2016. "Sofia Vergara Sued by Her Own Embryos as Her Ex-Fiancé Continues His Fight for the Fertilized Eggs He Has Already Named Isabella and Emma." *Daily Mail*. Online at www.dailymail.co.uk/.

Kotva, Joseph J., Jr. 2016. "Dying in Oregon: A Critical Look at Death with Dignity." Online at The Christian Century. www.christiancentury.org/.

Kowalczyk, Liz. 2005a. "Hospital, Family Spar over End-of-Life Care." *Boston Globe*, March 11.

Kowalczyk, Liz. 2005b. "Woman Dies at MHG after Battle over Care." *Boston Globe*, June 8.

Lagay, Faith. 2003. "Physician-Assisted Suicide: The Law and Professional Ethics." *Virtual Mentor*, 5, no. 1 (January): 19–21.

"Large Majorities Support Physician Assisted Suicide for Terminally Ill Patients in Great Pain." 2011. Harris/BBC World News America. Online at www.harrisinteractive.com/.

Lewis, Browne. 2009. "Two Fathers, One Dad: Allocating the Paternal Obligations between the Men Involved in the Artificial Insemination Process." *Lewis and Clark Law Review*, 13, no. 4 (Winter): 949–1006.

Lewis, Jeffrey D. and Dennis M. Sullivan. 2012. "Abortifacient Potential of Emergency Contraceptives." *Ethics and Medicine*, 28, no. 3 (Fall): 113–120.

Liptak, Adam. 2018. "Supreme Court Backs Anti-Abortion Pregnancy Centers in Free-Speech Case." *The New York Times*. Online at www.nytimes.com/.

"Living Will Vs. Durable Healthcare Power of Attorney." n.d. Rocket Lawyer. Online at www.rocketlawyer.com/.

Lollo, Samantha. 2018. "Our Baby, Her Choices: The Need for Enforcement of Gestational Surrogate Contracts." *Family Court Review*, 56, no. 1 (January): 180–194.

Long, Mark. 2005. "Federal Judge Nixes Schiavo's Feeding Tube." Associated Press, March 25. Online at news.yahoo.com.

Lu, Kerri. 2012. "Obama Administration Overrules FDA Decision—The Politics of Emergency Contraception." *Yale Journal of Medicine and Law*, May 21. Online at www.yalemedlaw.com/.

Lyman, Rick. 2005. "Governor Is Pressed on Schiavo as Legal Moves Dwindle." *The New York Times*, March 27.

Madigan, Tim. 2014. "Few Precedents Exit in case of Brain-Dead Pregnant Woman." *Fort Worth Star-Telegram*. Online at www.star-telegram.com/.

Malewitz, Jim. 2012. "High Court Declines Oklahoma 'Personhood' Case." The Pew Charitable Trusts. Online at www.pewtrusts.org/.

Mariner, Wendy K. 1997. "Physician Assisted Suicide and the Supreme Court: Putting the Constitutional Claim to Rest." *American Journal of Public Health*, 87, no. 12 (December): 2058–2062.

Maron, Dina F. 2014. "Many More Americans Issue End-of-Life Instructions." *Scientific American*. Online at www.scientificamerican.com/.

Mason, Mary A. and Tom Eckman. 2017. *Babies of Technology: Assisted Reproduction and the Rights of the Child*. New Haven, CT: Yale University Press.

Mathias, Christopher. 2015. "Brittany Maynard's Story Moves New York Lawmakers to Introduce Death with Dignity Bill." *Huffington Post*. Online at www.huffingtonpost.com/.

McCormick, Richard A. 1990. "Clear and Convincing Evidence: The Case of Nancy Cruzan." *Midwest Medical Ethics*, 6, no. 4 (Fall): 10–12.

McDonough, Katie. 2014. "Oklahoma Judge Permanently Striked Down State Resctrictions On Emegency Contraception." Salon. Online at www.salon.com/.

"Medication Abortion." 2018. Guttmacher Institute. Online at www.guttmacher.org/.

Meilaender, Gilbert. 1990. "The Cruzan Decision: 9.5 Theses for Discussion." *Midwest Medical Ethics*, 6, no. 4 (Fall): 3–5.

Merchant, Nomaan. 2014. "Family: Brain-Dead Texas Woman Off Life Support." Yahoo. Online at www.yahoo.com/news/.

"Mifepristone U.S. Postmarketing Adverse Events Summary Through 04/ 30/2011." 2011. Washington, DC: Food and Drug Administration. Online at www.fda.gov/.

Milicia, Joe. 2005. "Doctors: Feeding Tube Goes Beyond Purpose." Associated Press, March 26. Online at news.yahoo.com.

Miller, Molly. 2010. "Embryo Adoption: The Solution to an Ambiguous Intent Standard." *Minnesota Law Review*, 94, no. 3: 869–895.

Mohney, Gillian. 2016. "First Uterus Transplant in US Gives Hope to Women with Rare Condition." ABC News. Online at https://abcnews.go.com/.

Morber, Jenny. 2016. "Inside the Strange World of Harvesting Sperm from Dead Guys." Thrillist. Online at www.thrillist.com/.

Moreno, Jonathan D. 2005. "The End of the Great Bioethics Compromise." *Hastings Center Report*, 35, no. 1 (January–February): 14–15.

Moyal, Dena and Carolyn Shelley. 2010. "Future Child's Rights in New Reproductive Technology: Thinking outside the Tube and Maintaining the Connections." *Family Court Review*, 48, no. 3 (July): 431–446.

Nairn, Joanna. 2010. "Is There a Right to Have Children? Substantive Due Process and Probation Conditions that Restrict Reproductive Rights." *Stanford Journal of Civil Rights and Civil Liberties*, 6, no. 1 (April): 1–39.

Nash, Elizabeth, Rachel B. Gold, Lizamarie Mohammed, Zohra Ansari-Thomas, and Olivia Cappello. 2018a. "Laws Affecting Reproductive Health and Rights: State Policy Trends at Midyear 2018." Guttmacher Institute. Online at www.guttmacher.org/.

Nash, Elizabeth, Lizamarie Mohammed, Zohra Ansari-Thomas, Olivia Cappello, and Rachel B. Gold. 2018b. "Policy Trends in the States: First Quarter 2018." Guttmacher Institute. Online at www.guttmacher.org/.

National Academy of Sciences. 2018. *The Safety and Quality of Abortion Care in the United States.* Washington, DC: The National Academies Press.
National Institutes of Health. 2017. "Assisted Reproductive Technology (ART)." National Institute of Child Health and Human Development. Online at www.nichd.nih.gov/.
"National Statistics Reveal that Use of Emergency Contraception Is Growing." 2013. Relias Media. Online at www.reliasmedia.com/.
"Nearly Two-Thirds of Americans Don't Have Living Wills." 2016. American College of Emergency Physicians. Online at http://newsroom.acep.org/.
Neergaard, Lauran. 2012. "OB/GYN Back Over-the-Counter Birth Control Pills." Associated Press, November 20. Online at http://news.yahoo.com/.
Nestel, M.L. 2018. "More than 4,000 Eggs, Embryos Affected in Storage Tank Failure, Hospital Says." ABC News. Online at https://abcnews.go.com/.
Neuman, Scott. 2018. "Court Upholds Ruling Against California's Assisted Suicide Law." NPR. Online at www.npr.org/.
Neumeister, Larry and Lauran Neergaard. 2013. "Judge Making Morning-After Pill Available to All." *U.S. News and World Report*, April 5. Online at http://health.usnews.com/.
Niedzwiadek, Nick. 2017. "Court of Appeals Rejects Right to 'Aid in Dying'." Politico. Online at www.politico.com/.
Nirappil, Fenit. 2015. "Mother: Aid-in-Dying Bill Carries Brittany Maynard's Legacy." *U.S. News and World Report.* Online at www.usnews.com/.
Northup, Nancy. 2011. "Estranged Bedfellows." *Human Rights*, 38, no. 2 (Spring): 2–22.
Novotney, Amy. 2010. "The Living Will Needs Resuscitation." American Psychological Association. Online at www.apa.org/.
"Obama Administration Drops Fight to Keep Age Restrictions on Plan B Sales." 2013. *Washington Post.* Online at www.washingtonpost.com/.
"Oregon Death with Dignity Act: 2016 Data Summary." 2017. State of Oregon. Online at www.oregon.gov/.
"Oregon Repeal of 'Death with Dignity,' Measure 51 (1997)." n.d. Online at https://ballotpedia.org/Oregon_Repeal_of_%22Death_with_Dignity%22,_Measure_51_(1997).
"Oregon's Right to Die Movement." 1905. Denver, CO: The Hemlock Society, USA. Online at www.compassionandchoices.org/.
"Oregon's Right-to-Die Law Upheld by Supreme Court." 2006. ABC News, January 17. Online at http://abcnews.go.com/.
Ossareh, Tandice. 2017. "Would You like Blue Eyes with That? A Fundamental Rights to Genetic Modification of Embryos." *Columbia Law Review*, 117, no. 3 (April): 729–766.
Owens, Marjorie. 2014. "Husband Sues to Remove Pregnant Wide from Life Support." *USA Today.* Online at www.usatoday.com/.
Pazol, Karen, Andreea A. Creanga, Suzanne B. Zane, Kim D. Burley, and Denise J. Jamieson. 2012. "Abortion Surveillance—United States, 2009." *Morbidity and Mortality Weekly Report*, 61 (November): 1–44.
Pence, Gregory E. 1995. *Classic Cases in Medical Ethics*, 2nd edn. New York: McGraw Hill.
Peters, Philip G., Jr. 1990. "The Constitution and the Right to Die." *Midwest Medical Ethics*, 6, no. 4 (Fall): 13–16.
"Physician-Assisted Suicide Fast Facts." 2018. CNN. Online at www.cnn.com/.
Piana, Ronald. 2015. "Debate over Physician-Assisted Suicide Continues, State by State." *The ASCO Post.* Online at www.ascopost.com/.
Pillar, Barbara. 1992. "Bioethical Issues in the Use of Technology." *Nursing Economics*, 10, no. 6 (November–December): 419–422.
"Poll: Keep Feeding Tube Out." 2005. March 21. CBS News. Online at www.cbsnews.com/.
Pollard, Irina. 2009. *Bioscience Ethics.* New York: Cambridge University Press.
Popik, Jennifer. 2018. "AMA Vote Causes Worry in Fight against Assisted Suicide." National Right to Life. Online at www.nationalrighttolifenews.org/.
President's Council on Bioethics. 2004. *Reproduction and Responsibility: The Regulation of New Biotechnologies. A Report of the President's Council on Bioethics.* Washington, DC: President's Council on Bioethics. Online at www.bioethics.gov.
Purvis, Taylor E. 2012. "Debating Death: Religion, Politics, and the Oregon Death with Dignity Act." *Yale Journal of Biology and Medicine*, 85, no. 2 (June): 271–284.
Quill, Timothy W. and Bernard Sussman. n.d. "Physician Assisted Death." Bioethics Briefings, The Hastings Center. Online at www.thehastingscenter.org/.
Raymond, Janice G, Renate Klein, and Lynette Dumble. 1991. *RU 486: Misconceptions, Myths, and Morals.* Cambridge, MA: Institute on Women and Technology.
"Record Number of Older Adults Completing Living Wills, Trend Had Little Impact on Hospitalization Rates." 2014. University of Michigan. Online at www.uofmhealth.org/.
Roberts, Michelle. 2017. "IVF: First Three-Parent Baby Born to Infertile Couple." BBC. Online at www.bbc.co.uk/.
Robinson, John. 2010. "Baxter and the Return of Physician-Assisted Suicide." *Hastings Center Report*, 40, no. 6 (November–December): 15–17.
Roig-Franzia, Manuel. 2005. "Court Lets Right-to-Die Ruling Stand." *Washington Post*, January 25.
Russo, Nancy F. and Jean E. Denious. 2005. "Controlling Birth: Science, Politics, and Public Policy." *Journal of Social Issues*, 61, no. 1 (March): 181–191.
Ryan, Maura A. 2001. *Ethics and Economics of Assisted Reproduction: The Cost of Longing.* Washington, DC: Georgetown University Press.
Salzman, Todd A. and Michael G. Lawler. 2012. *Sexual Ethics: A Theological Introduction.* Washington, DC: Georgetown University Press.
Sanburn, Josh. 2015. "How Terri Schiavo Shaped the Right-to-Die Movement." *Time.* Online at http://time.com/.

Sandeen, Peg. 2018. "State of the Death with Dignity Movement." Death with Dignity. Online at www.deathwithdignity.org/.
Schenker, Joseph G. 2005. "Assisted Reproductive Practice: Religious Perspectives." *Reproductive BioMedicine Online*, 10, no. 3 (March): 310–319.
"Schiavo Autopsy Finds No Sign of Trauma." 2005. CNN, June 15. Online at www.cnn.com.
"Schiavo Autopsy Shows Irreversible Brain Damage." 2005. Associated Press, June 15. Online at www.msnbc.msn.com.
Schwartz, John. 2005. "New Openness in Deciding When and How to Die." *The New York Times*, March 21.
Scutti, Susan. 2016. "Indiana Fertility Doctor Used His Own Sperm 'Around 50 Times,' Papers Say." CNN. Online at www.cnn.com/.
Shanner, Laura and Jeffrey Nisker. 2001. "Bioethics for Clinicians: 26. Assisted Reproductive Technologies." *Canadian Medical Association Journal*, 164, no. 11 (May 29): 1589–1594.
Shannon, Thomas A., ed. 2004. *Reproductive Technologies: A Reader*. Lanham, MD: Rowan & Littlefield.
Shreve, Maggie and June Isaacson Kailes. 1990. "The Right to Die or the Right to Community Support." *Midwest Medical Ethics*, 6, nos. 2–3 (Spring/Summer) : 11–15.
Smajdor, Anna. 2010. "Should Doctors Harvest Eggs from a Comatose Woman?" BioNews. Online at www.bionews.org.uk/.
Smith, Emily. 2016. "Sofia Vergara Sued by Her Own Embryos." Page Six. Online at https://pagesix.com/.
Smith, Malcolm K. 2015. *Savior Siblings and the Regulation of Assisted Reproductive Technology: Harm, Ethics, and Law*. New York: Routledge.
Solinger, Rickie, ed. 1998. *Abortion Wars: A Half Century of Struggle, 1950–2000*. Berkeley, CA: University of California Press.
Sonfield, Adam. 2005. "Rights Vs. Responsibilities: Professional Standards and Provider Refusals." *Guttmacher Policy Review*, 8, no. 3 (August): 7–9.
Spencer, Naomi. 2005. "Bush Administration Plays to Religious Right in Delaying Contraceptive Approval." World Socialist Web Site. Online at www.wsws.org/.
Stacey, Dawn. 2018. "The Abortion Pill – RU486." Verywell Health. Online at www.verywellhealth.com/.
Stapleton, Anne C. 2016. "Sperm Donor Lied about Criminal and Mental Health History, Lawsuit Alleges." CNN. Online at www.cnn.com/.
"State Laws Related to Insurance Coverage for Infertility Treatment." 2012. Washington, DC: National Conference of State Legislatures. Online at www.ncsl.org/.
Stein, Rob. 2016. "New York Fertility Doctor Says He Created Baby With 3 Genetic Parents." NPR. Online at www.npr.org/.
Stenson, Jacqueline. 2005. "Viva in Vitro." *Health*, 19, no. 2 (March): 77.
Storrs, Carina. 2015. "How a 3-D-Printer Changed a 4-year-old's Hearth and Life." CNN, October 6. Online at www.cnn.com/2015/10/06/health/3d-printed-heart-simulated-organs/index.html.
Stulac, Francine. 1991. "RU 486: The Politics of Choice." *Health Matrix*, 1, no. 1 (Spring): 77–100.
Suhr, Jim. 2016. "Missouri Appeals Court: Frozen Embryos Property, Not People." Springfield News-Leader. Online at www.news-leader.com/.
Sulmasy, Lois S. and Paul S. Mueller. 2017. "Ethics and the Legalization of Physician-Assisted Suicide: An American College of Physicians Position Paper." *Annals of Internal Medicine*, 167, no. 8 (October): 576–587.
Sunderam, Saswati, Dmitry M. Kissin, Sara B. Crawford, Suzanne G. Folger, Sheree L. Boulet, Lee Warner, and Wanda B. Barfield. 2015. "Assisted Reproductive Technology Surveillance – United States, 2015." *Morbidity and Mortality Weekly Report*, 67, no. 3 (February): 1–28.
Suppon, Jenna M. 2010. "Life after Death: The Need to Address the Legal Status of Posthumously Conceived Children." *Family Court Review*, 48, no. 1 (January): 228–245.
"Supreme Court Rejects Pharmacist's Religious Rights Appeal." 2016. WJLA. Online at https://wjla.com/.
Sutton, Jane. 2004. "Florida Court Strikes down Law in Right-to-Die Case." *Reuters News*, September 23. Online at news.yahoo.com.
Tavernise, Sabrina. 2013. "Use of Morning-After Pill Rising, Report Says." *The New York Times*, February 14. Online at www.nytimes.com/.
"Terri Schiavo Timeline." 2005. CBS News, April 1. Online at www.cbs4.com/.
Thompson, Dennis. 2014. "Did Brittany Maynard Change Minds about Right-to-Die Laws?" CBS News. Online at www.cbsnews.com/.
Thorbecke, Catherine. 2017. "Doctors behind 1st US Baby Born a Uterus Transplant Describes the 'Beautiful' Medical Milestone." Yahoo. Online at www.yahoo.com/.
"U.S. Rates of Pregnancy, Birth and Abortion among Adolescents and Young Adults Continue to Decline." 2017. Guttmacher Institute. Online at www.guttmacher.org/.
"U.S. Supreme Court's 1997 Decisions on Assisted Suicide." n.d. United States Conference of Catholic Bishops. Online at www.usccb.org/.
"Unintended Pregnancies in the United States." 2016. Guttmacher Institute. Online at www.guttmacher.org/.
Van DeVeer, Donald. 1987. "Introduction." In *Health Care Ethics: An Introduction*, eds Donald Van DeVeer and Tom Regan, 3–57. Philadelphia, PA: Temple University Press.
"Vermont Report Concerning Patient Choice at the End of Life." 2018. Vermont General Assembly. Online at https://legislature.vermont.gov/.
Viswanathan, Radhika. 2018. "3 Biological Parents, I Child, and an International Controversy." Vox. Online at www.vox.com/.
"Washington State Death with Dignity Act Report." 2018. Washington State Department of Health. Online at www.doh.wa.gov/.
Wax-Thibodeaux, Emily. 2018. "Arkansas Abortion Pill Restriction Seen as Both Protecting Women and a Major Rights Setback." *Washington Post*. Online at www.washingtonpost.com/.
Weiss, Sabrina R. 2018. "Walgreen Pharmacist Denies Women Miscarriage Medication Due to His Beliefs." Yahoo. Online at www.yahoo.com/.

"Whole Woman's Health V. Hellerstedt." 2016. Supreme Court of the United States Blog. Online at www.scotusblog.com/.

Wickline, Sarah. 2014. "A Brain-Dead Mother, A Million-Dollar Baby." MedPage Today. Online at www.medpagetoday.com/.

Willingham, A.J. 2017. "A Man's Tattoo Left Doctors Debating whether to Save His Life." CNN. Online at www.cnn.com/.

Winter, Michael. 2014. "Lawyers: Brain-Dead Woman's Fetus 'Abnormal'." *USA Today*. Online at www.usatoday.com/.

Wolf, Richard. 2018. "Supreme Court Erases Ruling against Government in Illegal Immigrant Teen's Abortion Case as Moot." *USA Today*. Online at www.usatoday.com/.

Wolf, Susan M. 2004. "Law and Bioethics: From Values to Violence." *Journal of Law, Medicine & Ethics*, 32, no. 2 (Summer): 293–306.

Woodsong, Cynthia and Lawrence J. Severy. 2005. "Generation of Knowledge for Reproductive Health Technologies: Constraints on Social and Behavioral Research." *Journal of Social Issues*, 61, no. 1 (March): 193–205.

Zadrozny, Brandy. 2018. "Lesbian Couple's Sperm Donor Sues for Parental Rights." The Daily Beast. Online at www.thedailybeast.com/.

Zolfagharifard, Ellie. 2014. "The Hospital Growing Noses, Tear Ducts, and Blood Vessels: British Scientists Make Custom-Made Body Parts Using Stem Cells." *Daily Mail*. Online at www.dailymail.co.uk/.

10

CHALLENGES FACING THE AMERICAN HEALTHCARE SYSTEM

In this chapter we address some of the challenges facing the American healthcare system. The Affordable Care Act (ACA) increased access to affordable healthcare for millions of Americans and consequently the number of uninsured has declined significantly. However, many challenges remain. We discuss four such challenges. The first is the opioid epidemic and the number of American lives lost annually as a result of an overdose of prescription drugs as well as illegal drugs. The second challenge is the promise and perils of gene therapy. Gene therapy has the potential to unlock the mystery of many diseases and find a cure for them. However, there are also some pitfalls involving high costs and ethical concerns. The third challenge is dealing with new specialty drugs, which promise relief and/or cure for certain diseases, but the cost of such drugs is so high that it raises questions about their affordability and access. Last, we address the problem of shortage of a healthcare workforce as it relates to primary care and certain specialties, lack of ethnic/racial diversity, and whether the current healthcare workforce is prepared to meet the changing healthcare needs of American society.

THE OPIOID CRISIS

The current opioid epidemic in the United States is the latest in a string of such epidemics in US history. During the Civil War, there was a drug crisis when soldiers and others became addicted to morphine, the first of many man-made opioids. Morphine was derived from opium through a chemical process and made battlefield injuries more bearable for Civil War soldiers. During the Civil War, medics also used morphine as a battlefield anesthetic.

Unfortunately, many veterans got hooked on morphine and morphine addiction came to be called "the army's disease" ("Opioid Crisis Fast Facts" 2017; Stobbe 2017). In the 1800s, opium had become an addictive and dangerous drug given to patients for pain who had trouble sleeping. The drug was also used by people to get "high." Ironically, cocaine and heroin were developed in part to help morphine addiction. In the early 1900s cocaine use became epidemic and its recreational use came to be associated with prostitution and violent crimes. In 1914 Congress passed the Harrison Act, which required that cocaine and heroin could be sold only as prescription medicines. The widespread use of cocaine had for the time being been prevented by economics and politics. During the Great Depression, very few individuals had the disposable income to engage in illicit drug habits, and World War II pretty much stopped the supply of drugs from overseas. However, during the 1960s and 1970s, heroin used surged, especially among Vietnam War soldiers who were exposed to it while fighting overseas. President Nixon's "War on Drugs" focused on the "supply" side by attacking the drug problem through beefed-up law enforcement and tougher sentences for users and dealers. By the late 1970s, heroin use faded but cocaine was on its way back in the form of the crack epidemic in the 1980s. The crack epidemic died out in the 1990s ("Opioid Crisis Fast Facts" 2017; Stobbe 2017). During the 1980s, under the Reagan administration, First Lady Nancy Reagan's simplistic "Just Say No" campaign focused on the "demand" side of the drug problem.

The current opioid epidemic started around 1995 with a drug called OxyContin, which, like morphine and heroin, was meant to be a safer, more effective opioid for pain control and management. It was supposed to be effective and safer because the drug was designed to release the medicine slowly over a long period of time and thus was considered effective to use for months to treat chronic pain. However, patients soon became hooked on the drug and wanted more. The abuse of the drug became common when many users discovered that by crushing the tablet and snorting or injecting it, they could deliver the drug to the bloodstream much quicker. The problem was compounded by aggressive marketing and distribution of millions of pills into communities by drug companies. Addicts also turned to cheaper alternatives like heroin and fentanyl, bought illegally, making the situation worse. Fentanyl is an opioid medication that was developed to treat intense end-of-life pain and cancer patients and is 50 to 100 times more powerful than morphine (Stobbe 2017).

According to the Centers for Disease Control and Prevention (CDC), the rise in opioid overdose occurred in three distinct waves. The first wave started with a significant increase in prescriptions written for opioids. This led to an increase, since 1999, in deaths by overdose involving prescription opioids, both natural and semi-synthetic opioids, and methadone. The second wave began in 2010 with the rapid increase in overdose deaths involving heroin. The third wave started in 2013 with a significant increase in overdose deaths involving synthetic opioids, especially illicitly manufactured fentanyl ("Understanding the Epidemic" 2017).

Deaths by drug overdose have been on the rise in the United States. Between 2009 and 2013, a majority of states recorded an increase in deaths by drug overdose, with about 52 percent related to prescription drugs. The CDC have declared prescription drug abuse an epidemic in the United States ("Death from Drug Overdose Rise Across America" 2015). In 2016, the number of overdose deaths involving opioids, including prescription opioids and illegal opioids like heroin and fentanyl, was five times higher than in 1999 ("Understanding the Epidemic" 2017). In 2016, the death of the pop star Prince as a result of an overdose of opioids like fentanyl implicated in his death became a public example of a growing cultural problem. The head of the Drug Enforcement Agency (DEA) stated that synthetic opioids like fentanyl pose an unprecedented threat of overdoes and deaths, especially among youth (Bump 2016; "Synthetic Drugs Pose Alarming US Overdose Risk, DEA Chief Says" 2016). Experts call the current situation the opioid epidemic because more than 2 million Americans have become dependent on or abuse prescription pain pills and street drugs ("Opioid Crisis Fast Facts" 2017).

What Are Opioids?

Opioids, sometimes called opiates, are medicines used to treat acute or chronic (long-term) pain. Some are stronger than others. There are many different types of painkillers, ranging from weak opioids such as codeine and dihydrocodeine, to strong opioids such as methadone, diamorphine, morphine, oxycodone, and fentanyl. Strong opioids differ a lot in their strengths. The weaker opioids are usually taken as tablets while strong opioids can be taken as liquid or syrup, quick-acting tablets or capsules, slow-release tablets and capsules, sachets, tablets held in the mouth, patches for the skin, or injections (Harding 2016).

Opioids are drugs designed to replicate the pain-reducing properties of opium and they include both legal painkillers like morphine, oxycodone or hydrocodone prescribed by doctors for acute or chronic pain, and illegal drugs like heroin or illicitly made fentanyl. Opioids are addictive because they push the buttons of the brain usually triggered by pleasurable activities like eating. However, opioids are more powerful and they prompt the body to release the chemical dopamine, creating a feeling of euphoria or a "high" that encourages more use. Opioids bind the receptors to the brain and spinal cord, disrupting pain signals. Opioids such as morphine and codeine are naturally derived from poppy plants while hydrocodone and oxycodone are semi-synthetic opioids manufactured in labs with both natural and synthetic ingredients. Fentanyl is a totally synthetic opioid. It was originally developed as a powerful anesthetic for surgery and is also often administered to alleviate severe pain associated with a terminal illness such as cancer. Fentanyl is up to 100 times more powerful than morphine (Gander 2017; "Opioid Crisis Fast Facts" 2017). The clinical term used for opioid addiction or abuse is opioid use disorder. Individuals who become dependent on pain pills may switch to heroin because it is less expensive than prescription drugs. The National Institute on Drug Abuse estimates that half of the young people who inject heroin turned to the street drug after abusing prescription painkillers and three in four new heroin users start out using prescription drugs ("Opioid Crisis Fast Facts" 2017).

The most common drugs involved in prescription overdose deaths include methadone, oxycodone such as OxyContin, and hydrocodone such as Vicodin. The risk factors that make individuals vulnerable to prescription opioid abuse and overdose include obtaining overlapping prescriptions from multiple healthcare providers or pharmacies, taking high dosage of prescriptions daily to relieve pain, having a history of mental illness or alcohol and substance abuse, and living in a rural area and having a low income ("Understanding the Epidemic" 2017).

Use of illicit drugs like heroin has increased sharply in the United States among both genders, most age groups, and all income levels. Heroin is a highly addictive opioid drug and people at most risk of addiction are people who are addicted to prescription opioid pain relievers, people addicted to cocaine, marijuana, and alcohol, people living in large metropolitan areas, non-Hispanic whites, the young, and men. Similarly, the rate of overdose death involving synthetic opioids like fentanyl had doubled from 2015 to 2016. Around 19,400 people died from an overdose involving synthetic opioids other than methadone in 2016 ("Understanding the Epidemic" 2017).

The Nature and Scope of the Opioid Epidemic

One of the harsh realities of the opioid crisis in the United States is that majority of overdose deaths are a result of the abuse of prescription medication even though the use of heroin as a cheap substitute for addiction to prescription drugs has also increased significantly. Drug overdose now kills more people in the United States each year than gunshot wounds or car accidents ("Our Drug Overdose Epidemic, and What You Can Do About it" 2015). In 2014, there were about one-and-a-half times more drug overdose deaths in the United States than deaths from motor vehicle crashes. The same year, opioids were involved in 61 percent of all drug overdose deaths (Rudd et al. 2016).

Since 2000, the rate of death from drug overdose increased 137 percent, including a 200-percent increase in the rate of overdose death involving opioid pain relievers and heroin. Drug overdose death increased 6.5 percent, from 13.8 per 100,000 in 2013 to 14.7 per 100,000 persons in 2014. Similarly, the rate of opioid overdose death also increased 14 percent, from 7.9 per 100,000 in 2013 to 9.0 per 10,000 persons in 2014. During the same time frame, the age-adjusted rate of death involving natural and semi-synthetic opioid pain relievers increased 9 percent, death involving heroin increased 26 percent, while overdose death involving synthetic opioids other than methadone, like fentanyl, increased 80 percent. The dramatic increase in overdose death involving synthetic opioids like fentanyl coincided with the increased availability of illicitly manufactured fentanyl, a synthetic opioid. Heroin overdose deaths have more than tripled since 2010 from 1.0 per 100,000 in 2010 to 3.4 per 100,000 in 2014. The increased availability of heroin combined with its relatively low price compared to prescription opioids was the major factor in the upward trend in heroin use and overdose (Rudd et al. 2016).

Sam Quinones (2015), in his book *Dreamland: The True Tale of America's New Opiate Epidemic*, provides an explanation of how during the mid- to late 1990s two developments came together to create the current plague of prescription opioid and black-tar heroin. One development was how the sugar cane farmers on the west coast of Mexico created a unique distribution system that brought black-tar heroin, the cheapest and the most addictive form of opiate, which is two to three times purer that its white-powder cousin, to the United States. It was young men in Mexico, in search of their American Dream of fast and enormous profit and independent of the drug cartels, who brought trafficking of black-tar heroin to America's rural areas. The upsurge in heroin addiction at first did not garner much attention because it happened in what the author describes as "voiceless parts of the country"—Appalachia and rural America, where poverty and despair turned the heartland on to black tar. The second development was that Purdue Pharma in Stamford, Connecticut, cornered the market on pain with its new and expensive miracle drug, OxyContin, an extremely addictive drug in its own right.

OxyContin was approved in December of 1995 by the Food and Drug Administration (FDA) and hit the market in 1996. In its first year, OxyContin accounted for $45 million in sales for Purdue Pharma. By the year 2000, the number had ballooned to $1.1 billion, an increase of over 2000 percent in the span of four years. Ten years later, the profit amounted to $3.1 billion and OxyContin accounted for 30 percent of the painkiller market. The Purdue Pharma's patent for OxyContin did not expire until 2013. Thus, a single, private, family-owned pharmaceutical company controlled nearly a third of the entire US market for painkillers. These two developments fit together as cause and effect. Hooked on expensive OxyContin, American addicts were lured to a much cheaper black-tar heroin (Quinones 2015).

According to the data collected by the CNN from all 50 states, drugs have become the leading cause of accidental death in this country, surpassing shooting deaths and fatal traffic accidents. It took 50 years for the rate of heart disease to double in this country, but when it came to drug deaths, it took a fraction of that time. The rapid growth in the drug epidemic happened out of the national spotlight and media attention, because drug deaths disproportionally hit small towns and rural America largely in the Appalachia and in the Southwest parts of the country and became a dangerous problem for middle-aged white men and women (Christensen and Hernandez 2016).

Heroin-related deaths increased 439 percent from 1999 to 2014, tripling in five years and quintupling in ten years. The CDC noted that data from 2014 reflected two distinct but interrelated trends—a long-term increase in overdose deaths due to prescription opioids and a surge in illicit opioid overdose deaths largely related to heroin (Christensen and Hernandez 2016).

According to the CDC, of 52,404 Americans who died from a drug overdose in 2015, some 80 percent of the drug-related deaths were due to misuse of opioids including not only illicit substances such as heroin and synthetic fentanyl but also legal pain medications such as OxyContin and Vicodin. In fact, the prescription opioids accounted for 17,536 deaths, the largest share of opioid deaths in 2015 ("The Great Opioid Epidemic" 2016).

OxyContin came into the market in 1996. In 2007, the manufacturer Purdue Pharma had pleaded guilty to misleading consumers about the risk of abuse associated with the drug and the company had paid $600 million in fines. OxyContin was prone to abuse because drug users soon discovered that by crushing the pill and chewing, snorting, or injecting, the drug delivered 12 hours of powerful painkiller dosage at once. In response to this concern, Purdue Pharma released a new formulation in 2010 that made it very difficult to crush or dissolve or otherwise abuse the pill. It was hoped that this would help reduce the number of deaths caused by overdose. In fact, it became the first drug to receive an "abuse-deterrent" designation from the FDA. However, according to researchers at the RAND Corporation, and Wharton School, the reformulation of OxyContin in 2010 became the chief driver for the explosion in heroin overdose deaths in subsequent years, as much as 80 percent of the three-fold increase in heroin mortality since 2010. They also found that states with the highest initial rates of OxyContin misuse experienced the largest increase in heroin deaths. In fact, prior to 2010, there was no correlation between OxyContin abuse and heroin mortality. Thus, ironically, while Purdue Pharma was successful at reducing OxyContin abuse, each percentage-point reduction in the rate of OxyContin misuse due to reformulation led to 3.1 more heroin-related deaths per 100,000 persons (Ingraham 2017). This was due to the fact that those addicted to prescription OxyContin switched to a cheaper alternative like heroin. This is an example of how even a well-intended policy may at times produce unintended negative consequences and spillover effects.

In 2017, 72,000 Americans died from drug overdose, an increase of 7 percent from the previous year. According to experts, the primary cause for the continued surge in overdose deaths can be attributed to the presence of the deadly opioid fentanyl in the illicit drug supply market (Vestal 2018).

Finally, Americans are dying earlier and living shorter lives than previous generations and dying earlier compared to their counterparts around the world. According to CDC, the average life expectancy at birth in the US fell by 0.1 a year to 78.6 in 2016, following a similar drop in 2015. This is the first time in 50 years that average life expectancy has fallen for two successive years. The big culprit is the opioid epidemic, which has contributed greatly to an increase in death rates for 15-to-64-year-old Americans. However, drug abuse epidemic overdose deaths have not affected other developed countries as they have the United States. The United States population accounts for only 4 percent of the world's population but it accounts for 27 percent of the world's drug overdose deaths. In 2014, the European Union, with a population of about 507 million, reported 6,800 overdose death compared to 47,055 in the United States, with a population of 317 million (Blumenthal 2018).

From 1999 to 2016, more than 630,000 people died from a drug overdose in the United States. Of the 63,600 drug overdose deaths in the United States in 2016, around 66 percent involved an opioid. On average 115 Americans die every day from an opioid overdose ("Understanding the Epidemic" 2017). The number of people killed by drug overdose tops the death toll of the Vietnam War and both Iraq wars combined (Gander 2017).

A *Washington Post* and Kaiser Family Foundation survey of a random national sample of 809 long-term prescription painkiller users, adults 18 and over and their household members, between October 3 and November 9, 2016 found that one in three (34 percent) of those who had recently used prescription painkillers for at least two months reported that they were addicted or had become dependent on them. A large majority (98 percent) of long-term users reported relieving physical pain as a reason for their use but others reported other reasons as well. Another one-third (34 percent) stated that they had taken painkillers for fun (20 percent) or to get high (14 percent), while one in five (22 percent) said that they took prescription painkillers to deal with day-to-day stress. One in ten (10 percent) said that they took prescription painkillers to relax or relieve tension. Seventy percent of those personally taking prescription painkillers also reported being sick and disabled due to debilitating disability or chronic disease and 57 percent reported taking four or more prescription drugs. Fourteen percent of respondents reported sharing their painkillers with family members or friends. Finally, 97 percent of long-term painkiller users stated that they started taking the painkillers through a prescription from a doctor; however, only 33 percent stated that their doctor discussed with them a plan for getting off the medication (Dijulio, Wu, and Brodie 2016).

The Demographics and Geography of the Opioid Epidemic

The face of the opioid epidemic has changed over the years; black Americans were severely affected by the opioid epidemic of the 1960s and 1970s when heroin addiction ravaged communities and was dominant in urban and large metropolitan areas of the country. Today's opioid epidemic is affecting the white men and women and is to be found largely in rural America.

Drug overdose is driving up the death rates of young, white adults at a rate not seen since the AIDS epidemic. Young white adults, aged 25 to 34, are the first generation since the Vietnam War years of the 1960s to have higher death rates in early adulthood than the generation before. An analysis by *The New York Times* of 60 million death certificates collected by the CDC from 1990 to 2014 found death rates for non-Hispanic whites either rising or flattening for all adults in the under-65 age group, a trend that is also pronounced in women. However, in 2014, the overdose death rates for whites aged 25 to 34 had increased five times the level of 1999, while the rate for 35–44-year-old whites tripled during the same period. The numbers cover both illegal and prescription drugs (Kolata and Cohen 2016). Uneducated, middle-aged whites in rural areas also report the highest levels of stress, worry, and desperation, and—not coincidently—they have experienced the starkest increase in premature mortality due to suicide, and opioid and other drug overdoses (Hoban 2017).

However, it is important to emphasize that people at risk of opioid abuse are not just young people using opioid without a prescription. In 2015, an estimated 2.7 million Americans suffered from opioid dependence or addiction. People aged 45 to 64 accounted for 40 percent of all drug overdose deaths and a majority of these cases involved people who received legitimate prescriptions from their medical providers. According to the CDC, the death rate by opioid overdose including prescription or illegal drugs was greatest among adults aged 55 to 64. In 2015, adults aged 45 to 54 had the highest rate—30 per 100,000 persons (Seegert 2017).

The opioid crisis and its fallout are also very real for the older population in rural areas. Approximately 10 million people aged 65 and over live in rural America. They tend to be older, sicker, have higher rates of poverty, and have less access to healthcare than their urban counterparts. People in their 60s, 70s, and 80s also suffer from chronic pain because of the heavy physical or manual labor they did when younger. For example, those living in the Appalachian Mountains of eastern Kentucky have very high rates of disability and rely on prescription painkillers to deal with chronic physical pain issues. Yet, there are fewer opportunities for non-opiate therapies for pain like physical therapy or acupuncture in rural communities. Thus, to access such facilities would require them to often travel hundreds of miles and many of them do not receive Medicare or Medicaid (Seegert 2017). A study in 2016 found that more than 25 percent of Medicare patients were prescribed opioids upon hospital discharge and the risk of opioid use one year later was four times greater than for those who did not receive an opioid, underscoring the danger of becoming addicted to painkillers (Jena, Goldman, and Karaca-Mandic 2016).

Complicating the issue is the fact that many older Americans are reluctant to seek help out of shame of being an addict at their age, creating what addiction experts call a silent epidemic. The problem is compounded by the fact that drug-related deaths of the elderly are often undercounted because it is assumed on the death certificate that they died of age-related illness and not because of an overdose of painkillers. An analysis by Stanford University found that people covered by Medicare have among the highest and most rapidly growing prevalence of opioid use disorder, with more than 6 out of every 1,000 Medicare patients being diagnosed with an opioid disorder compared to 1 out of every 1,000 patients covered by commercial health insurance plans (Lembke and Chen 2016). Young people may have access to heroin and illicit prescription drugs through their social contacts; many elderly rely on alcohol to deal with physical pain and loneliness and now are increasingly becoming addicted to prescription pain medications such as OxyContin, Vicodin, and Percocet, and sedatives such as Xanax, Valium, and Ativan. In fact, a study by a researcher at Texas State University and the University of Michigan found a significant increase in the abuse of prescription painkillers and sedatives among people aged 65 and over since 2003. Older persons as a group have received a disproportionate share of opioid prescriptions because of age-related pain. In recent years, tighter prescription drug monitoring laws have made it more difficult for seniors to continue taking high doses of opioid medications from their doctors. Many states now require physicians to check patients' prescription drug history to see if they are taking pills prescribed by more than one doctor and if so physicians can limit patient's doses, prescribe fewer pills, or cut them off completely (Vestal 2016).

White men are not the only ones impacted by the opioid epidemic. Death rates have also risen sharply among middle-age white women, especially in rural America. One of the biggest reasons for the dramatic increase in the death rate among middle-aged white women is the combination of prescriptions for opioids and anti-anxiety drugs known as benzodiazepines. Between 1999 and 2014, anti-anxiety drugs contributed to a growing share of 54,000 deaths among middle-aged white women while the number of middle-aged white women dying annually from opiate overdose increased by 400 percent according to an analysis by the *Washington Post* of the data from the CDC. White women are more likely than women of any other race to be prescribed opiates and are more likely to be prescribed both opiates and anti-anxiety drugs. White women who are prescribed opiates are five times more likely than white men to be given the drug combination, putting white women at special risk (Kindy and Keating 2016).

Since middle-age women more likely than men to suffer from a variety of painful conditions such as lupus, migraines, and rheumatoid arthritis, they are more likely to be prescribed opioids and become dependent on them and anti-anxiety drugs. The town of Bakersfield in Kern County, California provides a good example. Accidental overdose among white women has tripled there since 1999 and suicides have doubled. According to the Kern County coroner's records, over a seven-year period, 85 white women between the ages of 35 and 60 killed themselves; about half of them overdosed on prescription drugs. Twenty-one women had some combination of opioids, benzodiazepines, and alcohol in their blood stream. In 2016, the FDA began requiring warning labels on opioids and benzodiazepines with information about the potentially fatal consequences of taking these medications at the same time (Kindy and Keating 2016).

The death rate has risen sharply among white women, spreading an epidemic of self-destruction in small-town and rural America. This is especially the case among those with a high school education or less. They are dying from a rash of pathologies, sicknesses, and addictions that experts have come to call "diseases of despair." Consequently, the suicide rate among middle-aged white women has also risen in parallel with prescriptions for psychiatric drugs for anxiety in combination with painkillers. Nearly one in four white women aged 50 to 64 are being treated with anti-depressants. Binge drinking is also on the rise in this group. Chillicothe, a historic town in Ohio, provides an example. Once it was the first capital of Ohio and a destination on the underground railroad. Today, it has changed dramatically. The theft and violent crime rate has gone up because of the drug problem. The residents of the town blame the drug problem on "the 23 pipeline," a reference to Route 23, the highway that brings drug dealers from Columbus and Detroit to the north. In fact, to the south of Chillicothe, the town of Portsmouth on the Ohio River, once famous for shoe factories, today is better known as the setting of the acclaimed book *Dreamland*, which describes the proliferation of pain clinics also known as pill mills (Achenbach 2016).

Finally, while it is true that the most dramatic increase in opioid-related deaths has occurred for white Americans, the opioid epidemic has also affected communities of color. Opioid deaths, particularly related to heroin overdose, have almost doubled among black Americans since 2000. Also, fentanyl has become a significant contributor to overdose deaths in black communities. However, nationally, the rate of overdose deaths related to synthetic opioids including fentanyl is higher for whites than blacks (James and Jordan 2018).

It should also be clear from the above discussion that the opioid epidemic and drug-related overdose deaths have disproportionately hit small towns and rural America, mainly in Appalachia and in the Southwest. In 2010, West Virginia moved into the top spot on the list of states with the highest number of drug-related deaths. The top ten states for drug overdose deaths per 100,000 people in 2015 were West Virginia, New Hampshire, Kentucky, Pennsylvania, Ohio, New Mexico, Massachusetts, Nevada, Maine, and Utah. This was followed closely by Oklahoma, Missouri, North Carolina, and South Carolina (Christensen and Hernandez 2016). In a recent work by researchers at the Brookings Institute, based on well-being metrics in a Gallup poll and mortality data from the CDC, robust association was found between lack of hope (and high levels of worry) among poor whites and mortality rates both at the individual level as well as metropolitan statistical area (MSA) levels. According to this research, the worst places for poor white worry were Nevada, Utah, Kentucky, West Virginia, Maryland, New Jersey, and Massachusetts. The highest level of pain for poor whites was in Maine, the Appalachian states, Alabama, Arkansas, and Oklahoma. The states with the highest level of desperation were the Dakotas, Wyoming, Montana, Idaho, Wisconsin, Missouri, West Virginia, and Kentucky. It is not a coincidence that states with the highest levels of worry, pain, and desperation also happen to be states with the high levels of opioid-related deaths, suicides, and premature mortality (Graham, Pinto, and Juneau II 2107). Suicide, drug overdoses, and alcohol-related fatalities are often referred to as "death by despair." Suicide rates are the highest they have been in decades in the country, and they are worst in rural America (Maciag 2018).

The idyllic small rural towns of America, romanticized in *The Andy Griffith Show* of the 1960s, are today replaced by the wasteland of despair, hopelessness, and self-destruction brought on by the opioid epidemic.

The Economic and Social Costs of the Opioid Epidemic

The opioid epidemic, aside from the obvious human cost in the number of lost lives, also produces economic and social costs. A study estimated the total US cost of prescription opioid abuse, dependence, and misuse in 2007 to be $55.7 billion. It put the health-related cost attributed to prescription opioid abuse at $25 billion. In addition, the study estimated the workplace cost in the form of lost earnings and employment to be $25.6 billion and $5.1 billion to the criminal justice system (Birnbaum et al. 2011). A hearing before the Joint Economic Committee of Congress put the economic cost of the opioid crisis at $80 billion in 2013 due to increased healthcare costs, higher rates of incarceration, and lost productivity ("Economic Aspects of the Opioid Crisis" 2017).

The President's Council of Economic Advisors, using the "value of a statistical life" (VSL) analytic method, i.e., cost-benefit analysis of regulations and policies including health-related interventions, also estimated the total societal cost of the opioid epidemic to be close to $504 billion in 2015, representing 2.8 percent of the US gross domestic product (GDP) (Council of Economic Advisors 2017). A study by a conservative think tank, the American Enterprise Institute (AEI), estimated the total cost of the opioid epidemic at $504 billion in 2015, which included $72.3 billion in non-fatal cost and $431.7 billion in fatal cost. The study estimated that at the state level, the total cost of the opioid epidemic was highest in the state of West Virginia, at $4793 per resident, and lowest in Nebraska, at $465 per resident (Brill 2018).

There are also indirect costs related to the opioid epidemic, though they are often difficult to quantify, such as the children who become wards of the state after losing one or more parents to an opioid overdose. A recent study by researchers at the University of South Florida concluded that prescription drug abuse is driving more children into Florida's foster care system. The research team found that 2 out of every 1,000 children in Florida were removed from their home due to parental neglect between 2012 and 2015—a 129-percent increase over the three-year period. During the same time frame, the number of opioid prescriptions prescribed by doctors rose 9 percent from 72 prescriptions per every 100 residents in 2012 to 81 prescriptions per every 100 residents in 2012. The authors found that a one-standard-deviation increase in the opioid prescription rate was associated with a 32-percent increase in the removal rate for parental neglect (Quast, Storch, and Yampolskaya 2018). According to the Florida Coalition of Children, which advocates for the state's abused, abandoned, and neglected at-risk children, drug abuse by parent(s) is the number-one reason children enter state care (Griffin 2018).

One silver lining, if it can be called that, is that is the rise in drug-related deaths has coincided with the rise in the number of organ donors who die of drug overdoses. According to Organ Procurement and Transplantation Network data, in 2015 over 848 organ donors died of drug intoxication. In the previous five years, the share of organ donors who died of drug overdose jumped 50 percent. In 2016, one out of every 11 organ donors was a drug-related victim (Izadi 2016).

What is Responsible for the Opioid Epidemic? The Blame Game

The opioid crisis is a uniquely American crisis driven by four factors: a laxed regulatory environment with respect to drugs; physicians' overprescribing of pain medications to their patients; cultural differences related to perceptions about pain; and the influence of drug companies on American healthcare policy and the FDA.

The Different Regulatory Environments of the US and Europe

Facing a backlash in the United States and Canada, drug companies have turned their attention to Asia and Europe for marketing painkillers (Humphreys, Caulkins, and Felbab-Brown 2018). Could the American opioid epidemic go global? In the US, pharmaceutical manufacturers have relied heavily on aggressive marketing of their product. However, marketing of drugs in Western European countries is regulated more strongly and it is generally prohibited to grant, offer, or promise benefits to physicians who prescribe drugs or to the organization that employs the physicians. Such prohibitions include not only monetary benefits but also material benefits such as all-expenses-paid conferences hosted by pharmaceutical companies. In addition, such prohibitions are also rigorously enforced by governments and countries' medical societies and they also implement and enforce such prohibitions against member physicians (Vokinger 2018). In contrast, both the federal and the state governments in the United States have very few, if any, restrictions on marketing and advertising of drugs by manufacturers and on physician behavior.

Cultural Differences and Perceptions about Pain

Why is the United States an outlier when it comes to dependence on powerful and addictive painkillers? Why is it so much easier to get an opioid prescription in the US compared to Europe or Japan? One reason is that in Europe, opioids are generally dispensed by specialists, not primary-care doctors. In contrast, in the United States, primary-care doctors write half of the nationwide prescriptions for opioid pain relievers.

Some observers blame the opioid crisis on a "pill for every ill" American culture. Thus, part of the difference may be cultural. American culture values treating pain at all costs, which, combined with a lax regulatory environment, makes it easier to obtain dangerous and addictive drugs.

In addition, doctors in different cultures view pain differently. The United States and Japan provide a good comparison. The United States ranks number one with respect to the amount of opioid consumed, while Japan does not rank among the top 25 countries (Nilsen 2017).

American and Japanese doctors' perceptions about pain provide a good example. Japan actually has an older population than the United States and still uses fewer opioid than does the United States. However, a survey found that about 50 percent of the 461 Japanese doctors surveyed said they prescribed opioids for patients with acute pain, compared to 97 percent of 198 American doctors who participated in the survey. Similarly, 64 percent of Japanese doctors were willing to prescribe opioids for chronic pain compared to 91 percent of American doctors. Why? The answer is the simple fact that the US and Japan have very different views about treating pain. When *The New York Times* asked why Japanese doctors prescribed so few opioids, the answers ranged from an attitude that pain was something to be endured to concern about the drug' addictive properties. In Japan, opioids are generally used only when patients are in severe pain from a disease like cancer. They are also prescribed largely in a hospital setting and not in community-based clinics (Nilsen 2017).

US Physicians' Overprescribing of Opioids

Some have placed part of the blame for sparking the opioid crisis on physicians for overprescribing highly addictive opioids to treat everyday pain to their patients (Clement and Bernstein 2016). For example, in 2016, Michael Botticelli, the White House Drug Policy Director, placed the blame for the opioid epidemic on both doctors and pharmaceutical companies. He stated that the root cause of the epidemic was the overprescription of pain medications because physicians get little or no training related to addiction in general and opiate prescription in particular (Shedrofsky 2016). The opioid prescriptions dispensed by doctors increased steadily from 112 million prescriptions written in 1992 to a peak of 282 million in 2012. Between 2006 and 2014, the most heavily prescribed opioid was hydrocodone (Vicodin). In 2014, 7.8 billion hydrocodone pills were distributed nationwide. The second-most prescribed opioid was oxycodone (Percocet), with nationwide distribution of about 4.9 billion. In 2015, Americans represented about 99.7 percent of the world's hydrocodone consumption. Since 2012, the number of painkiller prescriptions has declined, falling to 236 million in 2016 ("Opioid Crisis Fast Facts" 2017). This suggests that perhaps healthcare providers have become more cautious in their opioid prescribing practices. Yet, in 2017, there were still almost 58 opioid prescriptions written for every 100 Americans and more than 17 percent of Americans had at least one opioid prescription filled, with an average of 3.4 opioid prescriptions dispensed per patient ("Understanding the Epidemic" 2017). The amount of opioid drugs prescribed annually in the US was enough for every American to be medicated 24/7 for three weeks (McGreal 2017).

According to an analysis by ProPublica, a non-profit organization engaged in investigative journalism in the public interest, in 2012, 269 healthcare providers wrote at least 3000 prescriptions for Schedule 2 drugs. These Schedule 2 drugs include hydromorphone, methadone, oxycodone, fentanyl, and such that have a high potential for abuse and that may lead to severe psychological or physical dependence. They were concentrated in a handful of states. The top eight states were Florida (52 providers), Tennessee (25 providers), North Carolina and Ohio (15 providers each), Georgia (14 providers), Pennsylvania and Alaska (12 providers each), and Kentucky (11 providers). The top three prescribers of Schedule 2 drugs wrote 14,438, 11,493, and 10,705 prescriptions respectively in 2012. One in five doctors who wrote at least 3000 prescriptions for Schedule 2 drugs had faced some kind of sanctions or investigation. Also, in 2012, 12 of the Medicare's top 20 prescribers of drugs such as oxycodone, fentanyl, morphine, and Ritalin faced disciplinary actions by their state medical boards or criminal charges related to their practice. Prescribing a high volume of Schedule 2 drugs can indicate that a doctor is running a pill mill (Ornstein and Jones 2014). It is important to emphasize that such extreme practices are limited to a small percentage of the physician population.

Whether the opioids are overprescribed is difficult to figure out because pain is hard to objectively quantify. Similarly, it is also difficult to quantify the amount of actual pain relief except what the patient says, which could be subjective. The ultimate question is whether reducing access to prescription opioids is the cure for the current opioid crisis. Another question is whether federal and state laws designed to change physicians prescribing practices interfere with physicians' professional autonomy (Cicero 2018; Guevremont, Barnes, and Haupt 2018; Jena, Barnett, and Goldman 2017)

Drug Companies' Influence over American Healthcare Policy

Most observers place a majority of the blame for the opioid crisis in the United States on the pharmaceutical companies and their influence over American healthcare policy. Pushed by the pharmaceutical companies through their aggressive and often deceptive marketing, the idea took hold in America that physical pain can be simply made to disappear by a pill and that there is a right to be pain-free. According to an investigation by the House Energy and Commerce Committee, over the decade, out-of-state drug companies shipped 20.8 million powerful prescription painkillers (hydrocodone and oxycodone) to two pharmacies four blocks apart in the southern West Virginia town of Williamson, with a population of 2,900. Between 2006 and 2016, drug wholesalers shipped 10.2 million hydrocodone and 10.6 oxycodone pills to Tug Valley Pharmacy and Hurley Drug Company, Inc. Pharmacy in Williamson (Eyre 2018).

The FDA also played a role because in 2013, for example, it permitted a powerful opiate, Zohydro, into the market over the near-unanimous objection of its own review committee. It was clear from hearings that doctors understood the danger but the FDA placed commercial considerations first. The opioid epidemic largely is a result of the business model followed in the United States when it comes to opioids (McGreal 2017).

Unfortunately, open and vigorous competition in a free market is not what the prescription drug industry welcomes or wants. The prescription drug market does not operate by the supposed beauty of supply and demand because drug companies game the patent and regulatory system to create monopolies for their products. When a drug company gets a patent approval (generally for 20 years from the patent application date) for their name-brand pharmaceuticals to recoup their research and development costs, it creates exclusivity for those products, which protects them from competition from both generic and other name-brand drugs that treat the same condition. In addition, it also allows the manufacturers to market their drugs for conditions for which they never received regulatory approval. When their patent is about to expire, they often successfully fight off generics, refusing to cooperate with generic companies on safety plans, or they engage in product hopping. Product hopping tactics involve making a small modification to the dosage or formula of a drug as the original patent is about to expire and obtain a brand new patent for their "new and improved" version of the same drug. Finally, an exclusive monopoly also allows pharmaceutical companies to charge whatever they want for their product or engage in indiscrete price hikes to increase their profits. For example, consider the price of Suboxone, a drug for the treatment of addiction. An oral strip costs over $500 for a three-day supply and tablets cost $600 for a 30-day supply (Feldman 2017; Feldman and Frondorf 2017; Parramore 2017).

Martin Shkreli, the infamous former CEO of Turing Pharmaceutical who had bought the rights to a cheap, off-patent lifesaving drug called Daraprim, which treats rare parasitic infection that often strikes babies of HIV/AIDS patients and which had no other generic competitors, hiked the cost of the drug from $13.50 to $750 overnight per pill (a price increase of more than 5,000 percent). He once tweeted that he grieved every time a drug went generic. In August of 2017, he was convicted of three counts of securities fraud related to the two hedge funds he managed and a pharmaceutical company he founded (Feldman 2017). However, the reality is that while the Shkreli conviction helped shed some light on the general problem of high drug prices in the United States, it did not solve the overall problem. If anything, it proved that we as a society and culture are not really interested in fixing the problem of price manipulation and deception by drug companies because other companies have got away with doing similar things. In fact, the tragedy of Daraprim was that a cheaper version of the drug was available overseas and that Congress could have acted to allow importation of off-patent drugs in cases of an extreme price hike, but, it did not (Herper 2018).

Opioids are a potent product from a profit standpoint. Opioids create a vicious cycle for more drug consumption and dependence. For example, many patients who take opioids for pain wind up very sedated, so they are prescribed amphetamines to make them alert, but now they cannot sleep so they get a prescription for Ambien or Lunesta! Thus, many patients end up with three or four prescriptions. The opioid market has expanded to include a growing number of medications aimed at treating side or secondary effects rather than controlling pain and is estimated at nearly $10 billion a year in sales (Cha 2016). For example, studies show that 40 to 90 percent of opioid patients are afflicted by constipation. Drug companies promote opioid-induced constipation (OIC) as a legitimate medical condition that needs more targeted treatment with another pill. Starting in 2010, OIC began appearing in papers in top medical journals and presented at medical conferences. AstraZeneca, the maker of Movantik, that treats opioid-induced constipation, aired a television ad during the Super Bowl 50 in February of 2016, to an audience of more than 100 million people. Each Movantik pill retails for about $10. Since the Super Bowl ad, the prescription for the pill jumped from 6,600 to 8,800 a week. Vermont Governor Peter Shumlin (D) called the ad a shameful attempt to exploit America's addiction crisis to boost corporate profit. The drug industry's answer to the opioid addiction is more pills because more pills and higher sales mean more profit (Cha 2016). Purdue Pharma, the maker of OxyContin and one the largest opioid producers measured by sales, made an estimated $2.4 billion from opioid sales in 2015 alone ("How Big Pharma Lobbyists Make the Opioid Crisis Worse" 2016).

Specialty pharmaceutical companies, to entice investors, often tout "expansion opportunities" that exist in the "opioid use disorder population" and highlight "growth drivers" for the market by noting that millions of additional Americans not yet identified are also likely to become dependent on opioid painkillers. According to analysts each of the submarkets—addiction, overdose, and side effects—is worth at least $1 billion a year in sales. If the addiction epidemic were to be successfully treated and eliminated, it would wipe billions of dollars from the drug companies' bottom lines (Cha 2016).

An investigation by the Center for Public Integrity and the Associated Press found that major drug companies frequently lobbied state legislatures across the country to resist legal restriction on their drugs such as OxyContin, Vicodin, and fentanyl. Between 2006 and 2015, drug companies and their allies spent $800 million nationwide on campaign contributions and their lobbying efforts in state houses. The drug companies and their allies on average employed 1350 lobbyists a year to influence state lawmakers. The opioid lobby has done everything possible to preserve the status quo of aggressive prescribing for painkillers ("How Big Pharma Lobbyists Make the Opioid Crisis Worse" 2016). Companies selling some of the most profitable prescription painkillers also have funneled millions of dollars to advocacy groups that in turn promote opioids' use.

A minority report, *Fueling an Epidemic: Reports One to Three* (2017–2018) chaired by Senator Claire McCaskill (D-MO), revealed that the makers of top five opioid painkillers by worldwide sales in 2015 spent more than $10 billion between 2012 and 2017 to support 14 advocacy groups and affiliated doctors. Fourteen non-profit groups, most representing pain patients and specialists, received near $9 million from drugmakers while doctors associated with those groups received another $1.6 million. According to the report, Purdue Pharma, the maker of OxyContin, contributed $4.7 million while Insys Therapeutics provided more than $3.5 million to interest groups and physicians. In 2012, Insys Therapeutics, which manufactures the fentanyl drug Subsys, largely prescribed to cancer patients, found that insurers reimbursed for Subsys in only about 30 percent of cases. The company set up a special unit to try to get reimbursement numbers up by giving employees significant financial incentives and management pressures including quotas and group and individual bonuses to boost the rate of Subsys reimbursement authorization. The unit, in fact, engaged in shady behavior, including falsifying patients' medical records to help them get prescriptions for Subsys. The company's representatives misled or outright lied about patients' needs and helped pushed the drug for patients who did not need it (*Fueling an Epidemic: Report One to Three* 2017–2018; Lopez 2017).

An investigation by the *Los Angeles Times* found that Purdue Pharmaceutical marketed its OxyContin claiming its supposed ability to provide 12 hours of pain relief. However, before it went on the market in 1996, clinical trials showed that many patients were not getting 12 hours of pain relief and thus it was not any more effective than similar painkillers already on the market. Yet, Purdue stood by its claim for years and told doctors that if patients were not getting 12 hours of pain relief the problem was that the doses were too low. Between 1996 and 2002, Purdue Pharma funded more than 20,000 pain-related educational programs through direct sponsorship or financial grants and launched a multifaceted campaign to encourage long-term use of painkillers. Purdue Pharma and others whisked doctors to stylish retreats to push them to prescribe for uses not approved by US regulators (Parramore 2017). Ultimately, in 2007, the company and several of its chief executives paid more than $600 million in fines (Lopez 2017). In 2018, as a result of several lawsuits, Purdue Pharma said that it will stop marketing opioid drugs to doctors and indicated that the company had eliminated more than half its sales staff and will no longer send sales representatives to doctors' offices to discuss opioid drugs (Jay and Perrone 2018).

In summary, driven by the quest for profit, opioid makers and distributors mislead doctors, insurers, patients, and the general public about their drugs, and through aggressive and often deceptive marketing and lobbying help create and fuel the opioid epidemic in the United States.

Government's Response to the Opioid Crisis

The Federal Response

In response to the opioid epidemic, in March of 2016, the Centers for Disease Control and Prevention (CDC) issued the first national guidelines urging doctors to use more caution and to consider alternatives before prescribing highly addictive narcotic painkillers. The guidelines also urged patients seeking pain treatment to first try non-opioid medications whenever possible. It also suggested that if doctors prescribe opioids, they should be low doses and patients should be provided with less than a week's supply compared to the practice of prescribing for several weeks or a month. Finally, the guidelines encouraged doctors to monitor the effectiveness of the drugs they prescribe. The guidelines are aimed largely at primary-care physicians. However, the guidelines were nonbinding and doctors cannot be punished for failing to comply (Demirjian and Bernstein 2016).

In March of 2017, President Trump signed an executive order establishing the President's Commission on Combating Drug Addiction and Opioid Crisis with a mission to study the scope and effectiveness of the federal response to drug addiction and the opioid crisis and to make recommendations to the president to improve the response. The specific goals included: to identify and describe existing federal funding; to assess the availability and accessibility of drug addiction treatment services; to identify and report best practices for addiction prevention; to evaluate the effectiveness of educational messages for youth and adults; and to make recommendations to improve the federal response ("Combating the Opioid Epidemic" 2018). The Commission was chaired by New Jersey Governor Dough Christie. In August of 2017, the Commission issued a preliminary report urging the president to declare the opioid crisis a national emergency and the use of a public health approach to address the crisis. The Commission called on federal government to do more to combat the opioid crisis, including expanding funding through Medicare and Medicaid to extend treatment options, including medication-assisted treatment such as use of the drugs methadone and buprenorphine to prevent relapses, and for the Secretary of the Department of Health and Human Services (HHS) to negotiate lower prices for drugs like naloxone, which reverses overdoses (Allen 2017).

Initially, President Trump declined to officially declare a state of emergency for the opioid crisis (Wing 2017). However, after two days, he changed his mind and on August 10, 2017, he declared the opioid crisis a national emergency (Vitali and Siemaszko 2017a). Such a declaration would allow the administration to waive some of the federal rules that restrict drug addiction treatment under Medicaid (Vitali and Siemaszko 2017b). However, no concrete plan to deal with the crisis was forthcoming. In October of 2017 he declared that the opioid crisis was a public health emergency and promised to deliver an emergency declaration to combat the crisis. However, there was very little consensus in the administration on how to implement an emergency declaration and administration officials were left to scramble to come up with a plan. No one seemed to be in charge of the emergency declaration effort. The declaration did not include any new funding (Ehley 2017; Ehley and Carlin-Smith 2017; Ehley, Dawsey, and Karlin-Smith 2017).

Part of the problem was that there was a leadership vacuum at top of four key health and law enforcement agencies that would have been responsible for executing any plan. Secretary of the HHS Price had resigned under pressure in September 2017, for spending more than a $1 million in taxpayer money on private and government planes for travel. The acting director of the Drug Enforcement Agency (DEA) had also resigned in September 2017 in protest of President Trump's statements. Trump's nominee to lead the Department of Homeland Security (DHS), critical in stopping the flow of drugs into the United States, had not been confirmed by the Senate. Finally, Trump's nominee to head the Office of National Drug Control Policy, Tom Marino, had to withdraw his nomination amid accusations that he had deep ties to the drug industry and had pushed a bill in Congress making it harder for the DEA to halt drug shipments to different communities. One senior FDA official called the emergency declaration effort a "mess" (Ehley 2017; Ehley, Dawsey, and Karlin-Smith 2017; Shesgreen 2017).

The critics of the administration argued that the president's announcement of the opioid crisis as a public health emergency did very little beyond paying lip service and slapping a label on a crisis. The declaration made it a public health emergency for just 90 days, though this can be renewed. Others argued that Trump's proposed solution to declare a "war on drugs" to solve the opioid crisis made very little sense from a scientific viewpoint. Studies have consistently shown that massive advertising campaigns aimed at children, like Reagan's "Just Say No" campaign, are a waste of time and money because often such campaigns have exactly the opposite impact because of the psychological pull—i.e., when you tell a person that something is forbidden, it makes such a forbidden activity all the more attractive, especially to young people (Basu 2017; Walsh 2017).

On November 1, 2017, the President's Commission Combating Drug Addiction and the Opioid Crisis (2018) issued its final report, which included among many others the following recommendations: the administration and Congress to block grant federal funding for opioid-related activities to states; to fund a private- and public-sector media campaign; to develop model statues, regulations, and policies that enforce informed-consent prior to opioid prescription for chronic pain; to develop a national curriculum and standard of care for opioid prescribers; for federal agencies to collect participation data; to develop model training programs for screening substance use and to identify at-risk patients; and to train pharmacists on best practices to evaluate the legitimacy of opioid prescriptions. It also urged the administration to support the Prescription Drug Monitoring Program (PDMD) Act.

In late March of 2018, President Trump signed a 2018 budget bill that included $3 billion for efforts related to the opioid epidemic. It allocated $500 million in grant funding for research on opioid addiction and the development of opioid alternatives, pain management, and addiction treatment ("The Crisis Continues" 2018). Many health policy experts argued that the amount was not big enough to make a meaningful impact on the opioid epidemic and falls short of what is necessary to combat the crisis. In comparison, the federal budget for HIV care in 2017 was $32 billion (Quinn 2018).

In a rare bipartisan effort, in October 2018, Congress passed, and President Trump signed into law, the Opioid Crisis Response Act of 2018, designed to make it easier for states to expand access to addiction treatment. The bill passed the House by a vote of 393 to 8 and 98 to 1 in the Senate. The law calls for around $8 billion in federal investment over five years. One of the major provisions in the law would allow Medicaid to pay for residential treatment in large facilities. This provision lifts a 53-year-old ban in Medicaid law that prohibits coverage of mental health and addiction treatment services in facilities with more than 16 beds. Fifteen states had already received a federal waiver from this Medicaid rule and others are seeking similar waivers. Another provision would allow Medicare to pay for methadone treatment, one of the three medications considered the gold standard for addiction treatment. Again, critics argue that the law does not go far enough. Several groups, including the Harm Reduction Coalition, recommended $100 billion more in federal spending similar to the Ryan White HIV/AIDS program (Vestal 2018; Zezima and Kim 2018).

In an ironic twist, On November 2, 2018, the FDA approved a powerful new opioid for use in a healthcare setting, rejected criticisms from some of its own advisors, including the head of the FDA advisory committee on painkillers, that the drug would inevitably be diverted to illicit use and cause more overdose deaths. The opioid is five to ten times more potent than the pharmaceutical fentanyl. The manufacturer of the drug, a California company called AcelRx, started marketing the drug in early 2019 under the name Dsuvia at a wholesale price of $50 to $60 per dose. One of the factors that played a major role in the decision was the military's interest in the drug for possible battlefield use. The Pentagon has spent millions of dollars helping to fund AcelRx's research (Bernstein 2018).

State Governments' Response

Many state governments had begun to respond to the opioid epidemic long before the federal government acted. The Medicaid expansion under the Affordable Care Act (ACA) that went into effect in 2014 had already started to shape the states' spending of federal grant money to deal with the opioid epidemic. According to an analysis by the Associated Press, the Medicaid expansion states had a running start on the opioid epidemic since it allowed states to go beyond the basic requirements with the federal grant money. States with Medicaid expansion were able to use the grant money to create new infrastructure to deal with the opioid epidemic. In contrast, states that did not expand Medicaid under the ACA were dealing with populations more likely to be uninsured and more likely to need coverage for drug addiction and without the extra funding available under the Medicaid expansion had to work hard to catch up. Congress in 2016 had approved $1 billion to address opioid addiction under the Twenty-First Century Cures Act and states had begun to spend the money on different services such as treatment, job training, and housing (Johnson and Forster 2018).

State governments were beginning to take action to address the problem of overdose deaths caused by heroin and the illegal use of prescription drugs. For example, by 2014, 17 states and the District of Columbia had passed "Good Samaritan" laws that granted limited immunity to drug users who seek help. The Good Samaritan laws vary slightly from state to state but the basic idea behind them is that anyone who seeks help in the case of an overdose cannot be prosecuted for possession of small amounts of drugs or drug paraphernalia. However, such laws do not grant immunity for other crimes such as drug trafficking. Similarly, 17 states had expanded access to naloxone, known by its brand name Narcan, a medication that quickly reverses the effects of opioid overdose (Ollove 2014). By 2015, 26 states had passed Good Samaritan laws and 34 states had facilitated access to naloxone medication (Chokshi 2015). By 2016, 48 states had authorized some variation of a law that provided access to naloxone medication (Ayers and Jalal 2018).

Also, by 2015, 25 states had passed laws that increased penalties related to the sale and distribution of fentanyl (Bartolone 2018). In addition, other initiatives undertaken by states include initiatives to educate the general public (48 states), prescribers (31 states), patients and families (24 states), and pharmacists (22 states) about the risk of opioids. Twenty-six states have established guidelines for safe opioid prescribing and 14 states have enacted laws to regulate pain clinics (Wickramatilake et al. 2017). In 2016, New York passed a law that limits initial prescription for acute pain to seven days down from 30 days with refills and renewals to be done only after further consultations. The law does make some exception for chronic pain and hospice and palliative care ("New York Sets 7-Day Limit on Initial Opioid Prescriptions" 2016).

Several states have also expanded their Medicaid programs to cover alternative treatments such as acupuncture, massage, yoga, chiropractic manipulation, and various types of physical and behavioral therapies to help manage patients' pain and limit their dependence on opioids. However, some critics have raised concerns about the risk of wasting taxpayer money on an unproven alternative treatment that may not be science-based and taking money away from potentially effective treatments. Acupuncture is at the forefront of this debate because the evidence of its effectiveness remains unclear ("Medicaid's Role in Addressing the Opioid Epidemic" 2018; Ross 2018).

Today, all states except Missouri have passed a law establishing Prescription Drug Monitoring Programs (PDMPs). The objective of these programs is to detect patterns of drug abuse and prevent doctor shopping or prescription duplication by creating and maintaining a database of all prescriptions of controlled substances issued to a patient. Thus, doctors have an opportunity to access past records of patients before prescribing opioids to them. Except for Nebraska, all states with PDMPs require dispensaries to report data on patients (Ayers and Jalal 2018).

The war against opioids has also moved to the courtrooms as more states are filing lawsuits against manufacturers of opioids. Some of the lawsuits are based on the model state governments had followed when they had successfully sued tobacco companies for misleading claims that tobacco products were not addictive. Today, states are making the claim that opioid manufacturers had lied when they claimed that there was less than a 1-percent chance of getting addicted to opioids ("The War on Opioids Moves to the Courtroom" 2018). Some states have filed antitrust lawsuits and others have accused opioid manufacturers of deceptive marketing, and unreasonable drug price hikes. For example, in February of 2018, Alabama filed a lawsuit in federal court against Purdue Pharma, the maker of OxyContin, for fueling the opioid epidemic by deceptively marketing prescription painkillers. The lawsuit claims that marketers persuaded doctors that prescription painkillers were not addictive (Raphelson 2018). Similarly, in May of 2018, six more states—Texas, Florida, Nevada, North Carolina, North Dakota, and Tennessee—also filed a lawsuit against Purdue Pharma on the grounds that the company violated state consumer protection laws by falsely denying or downplaying the risk of addiction while overstating the benefits of opioids (Bellon 2018). The lawsuits show that states are using divergent strategies to sue opioid manufacturers (Fisher 2018; Gluck, Hall, and Curfman 2018; Jackson 2018).

The state of Florida provides an interesting example of a state that where the Republican State Attorney General Pam Bondi is suing opioid makers and distributors of violating the Florida Deceptive and Unfair Trade Practices Act, the Florida RICO Act, and common-law public nuisance while the opioid makers have helped fill the campaign coffers of the same politicians. For example, opioid manufacturers have given more than $1 million to state lawmakers during the opioid crisis. It wasn't until the beginning of 2011 that the Republican legislature decided to fund a prescription drug monitoring program and upon taking office in 2011, the Republican governor Rick Scott wanted to get rid of the prescription drug monitoring program, claiming it was an invasion of privacy. He also eliminated the Office of Drug Control. He also had ties to two of the companies that were sued. The overwhelming majority of opioid companies' campaign contributions have gone to the Republic Party of Florida ($429,550) and the Republican State Leadership Committee ($225,000) ("Opioid Makers Fill State Coffers" 2018).

Early Assessment of Efforts to Address the Opioid Crisis

What impact have the federal and state efforts to address the opioid crisis had thus far? Early indications are positive and suggest limited successes. For example, after years of significant growth, for the first time, the number of opioid prescriptions has declined for several years in the United States, signaling perhaps that doctors who have heard the drumbeat of warnings about the addictive nature of opioids are taking a more cautious approach in prescribing them to their patients. IMS Health, an information firm, found a 12-percent decline in opioid prescriptions nationally since 2012, while another data company, Symphony Health Solutions, reported a drop of 18 percent during the same year. Opioid prescriptions have fallen in almost all states, with Alabama, Oklahoma, and Ohio experiencing some of the biggest declines. The federal government's tightening of prescription rules for painkillers like hydrocodone combined with a second analgesic like acetaminophen has led to a 22 and 16-percent decline, respectively, in dispensed prescriptions for these drugs (Goodenough and Tavernise 2016).

Some of the New England states like Massachusetts, Rhode Island, Vermont, and New Hampshire have experienced a drop in overdose deaths ("States Make Headway on Opioid Abuse" 2017). According to data from the CDC, drug overdose deaths declined in 14 states during the 12-month period ending in July 2017. According to public health experts, this decline is most likely related to a decline in the rate of prescribed opioids and the increased use of the overdose antidote naloxone (Vestal 2018). However, a report issued by the National Safety Council (NSC) also found that while several states had some successes, some states have failed to deal with the opioid crisis and the opioid epidemic remains a costly public health emergency (Cannon 2018).

Despite some early successes, the problem of addiction and overdose is still raging across the United States and it is unclear whether the country has turned a corner on the opioid crisis. While there is some good news with respect to some decline in deaths from overdose, the overall number still remains grim. According to a CDC estimate in September 2017, there were 29,000 synthetic opioid overdose deaths and the use of heroin was also up slightly from the previous year. In summary, it is too early to tell how successful federal and state efforts have been in addressing the opioid crisis (Cunningham 2018).

The Need for Hard Data on thte Opioid Epidemic

How would we know how much progress has been made in addressing the opioid crisis or when the crisis has been resolved? Hard data could help our understanding of the crisis and progress made in addressing it. Relevant data about overdose, addiction, overdose deaths, abuse of legal prescription drugs and illicit drugs, drug arrests, use of naloxone, etc., often come from different sources because they are collected by different agencies, such as the CDC, HHS, public health surveillance, law enforcement agencies, and PDMPs, among others. What are relevant data and what is the quality of the data collected? Also, the much of the data currently available are in data "silos," i.e., data are kept and stored in different repositories that are unable to talk to each other, making it difficult to match and share data and identify trends across different data sources. Furthermore, state regulations regarding health information differ. Some states differ with respect to how data-based programs operate, how long the data can be retained, who is authorized to access them and conditions of access, and how data are shared across states (Martinez 2018).

All states except one, Missouri, have passed legislation establishing prescription drug monitoring program (PDMPs) and in all states, except Nebraska, the PDMPs require dispensers to report data on patients, making it possible to detect a pattern of drug abuse, doctor shopping, and prescription duplication, and to help physicians guide their prescription decisions. However, the problem is that PDMPs are only effective if they obligate doctors to check patient history prior to filling out an opioid prescription, which they are not (Ayers and Jalal 2018). In fact, the use of PDMPs by physicians has been low, because the use of PDMPs is time-intensive and poorly integrated into a physician's daily workflow, i.e., most PDMPs are not embedded within electronic health records. Munch of the routine opioid prescribing that can lead to long-term opioid dependence may not be flagged by a PDMP. Thus, PDMPs may not be a panacea for addressing the opioid crisis (Jena, Barnett, and Goldman 2017).

SPECIALTY DRUGS/PHARMACEUTICALS

A second challenge confronting the American healthcare system is the rapid proliferation and high cost of specialty drugs. Specialty drugs primarily treat complex chronic medical conditions such as cancer, hepatitis C, multiple sclerosis, and a variety of autoimmune conditions such as rheumatoid arthritis, psoriasis, and Crohn's disease. Complex, innovative, and high-priced specialty drugs are entering the US healthcare market at a rapid pace. Specialty drugs offer the most effective and, in some cases, the only treatment for certain illness and medical conditions (Pharmaceutical Care Management Association 2016). In 1990, of all drugs approved by the Food and Drug Administration (FDA), only ten were considered specialty drugs. By 2012, there were almost 300 specialty drugs on the market (National Pharmaceutical Services 2018). The proliferation of specialty drugs had led to increased use and increased spending.

In 2011, spending on specialty drugs accounted for 77.5 billion, 24 percent of all prescription drugs sold in the United States. In 2012, spending on specialty drugs had increased to $87 billion, amounting to 39 percent of all prescription drug spending. By 2015, spending on specialty drugs had reached $150 billion. The spending on specialty drugs is expected to continue to increase and by 2020 reach $402 billion annually, 47 percent of all prescription drug spending (National Pharmaceutical Services 2018). In 2015, only 1 to 2 percent of Americans used specialty drugs but they accounted for around 38 percent of total spending on prescription drugs. The use of specialty drugs increased 6.8 percent in 2015 (Pew Charitable Trusts 2016). In 2015, the top ten specialty therapeutic drug classes were: inflammatory conditions, multiple sclerosis, oncology, hepatitis C, HIV, growth deficiency, cystic fibrosis, pulmonary hypertension, hemophilia, and sleep disorder, with multiple sclerosis, oncology, and inflammatory conditions accounting for 56.3 percent of all spending on specialty drugs (Santye 2016).

The rapid growth of specialty drugs, their increased use, very high costs, and the increase in prices have had implications not only for healthcare spending in general but Medicare spending in particular since the elderly, who are more likely to suffer from chronic medical conditions, rely on specialty drugs to deal with and manage their medical conditions. In addition, the high costs and increased prices raise questions and concerns about the affordability of such drugs and the financial burden they place on payers—patients, employers, government, insurance companies, and ultimately taxpayers.

What are Specialty Drugs?

There is no one commonly agreed definition of specialty drugs. Rather, specialty drugs are often defined by certain unique attributes that set them apart from other drugs. The definition of specialty drugs has continued to evolve to accommodate new complex, innovative drugs, and therapies designed to treat them. According to the Academy of Managed Care Pharmacy (2006), specialty pharmaceuticals/drugs typically are large, unstable, protein-based molecules produced through a biotechnology process. Most common medications are manufactured through synthetic processes or are extracted from biological sources. Specialty pharmaceuticals are drugs and biologics, i.e., medicines derived from living cells cultured in a laboratory, that are complex to manufacture, difficult to administer, may require patient monitoring, and sometimes have FDA-mandated strategies to control and monitor their use ("Specialty Pharmaceuticals" 2013). In addition, most health plans consider high cost a determining factor in identifying specialty drugs. Medicare's definition of specialty drugs is also based on price. Pharmaceuticals costing more than $600 a month are considered specialty drugs (Pew Charitable Trusts 2016).

According to National Pharmaceutical Services (NPS) (2018), general characteristics of specialty drugs include a limited distribution network, close patient monitoring, requirements for special handling, a high cost per unit or treatment course, and use in a unique patient population. Thus, the NPS defines a specialty drug as having at least two or more of the following specific attributes: (1) treats a condition that requires intense patient monitoring; (2) requires special patient training or patient compliance assistance; (3) requires special handling with storage and preparation; (4) requires special administration by a patient or healthcare professional; (5) has a limited distribution network; and (6) has a high total cost.

Similarly, the Pharmaceutical Care Management Association (2016) defines a specialty drug as possessing a number of the following common attributes: (1) prescribed for a patient with a complex or chronic physical, behavioral, or developmental medical condition; (2) treats rare or orphan disease indications; (3) requires additional patient education, adherence, and support beyond dispensing of medication; (4) is an oral, injectable, inhalable, or infusible drug product; (5) has a high monthly cost; (6) has unique storage or shipment requirements such as refrigeration; and (7) is not stocked at a majority of retail pharmacies.

The Management of Specialty Drugs

The unique requirements to handle and manage specialty drugs means that pharmacists need to acquire special expertise. Such expertise is often not available at most community pharmacies or mail-order pharmacies. This has led many healthcare plans and managed-care organizations to develop two approaches to the delivery of specialty pharmaceuticals. One such approach is "insourcing," whereby they hire distinct staff, Pharmacy Benefit Managers (PBMs), to manage high-cost and high-demand areas. The second approach is "outsourcing," in which they contract with licensed pharmacies to develop specialized expertise and services to meet the unique requirements of dispensing and monitoring the use of specialty drugs. Such pharmacies are referred to as "specialty pharmacies" and their numbers have grown with the growth in the number of specialty drugs on the market (Academy of Managed Care Pharmacy 2006).

Healthcare plans and managed-care organization relies on PBMs to manage the use of and payment for specialty drugs. PBMs utilize a variety of strategies to support patients who are prescribed specialty drugs. These strategies include things such as negotiating rebates with drug manufacturers, negotiating discounts from drug stores, offering more affordable pharmacy alternatives, encouraging administration of specialty drugs at the patient's home instead of more expensive sites such as physician offices or outpatient facilities, encouraging patients to use low-cost drug options, reducing waste, and improving compliance with drug prescription regimens (Pharmaceutical Care Management Association 2016).

Specialty pharmacies, in order to offer a full range of clinical and operational services that enhance the safety, quality, and affordability of specialty medications for patients, perform a variety of management functions. They include providing access to specially trained pharmacists, nurses, and clinicians, direct consultation with physicians to deal with concerns about side effects of specialty drugs on patients including adverse reaction and noncompliance, performing disease and drug-specific patient care management services to ensure patient safety, collecting data and tracking outcomes for specific patients, ensuring that patients adhere to drug prescription regimens, ensuring adherence to rigorous storage, shipping, and handling standards for specialty drugs, coordinating patient care with other healthcare providers, navigating on behalf of patients with insurance companies, managing formularies, i.e., continually updating lists of prescription drugs approved for reimbursement by PBMs, utilization management such as prior-authorization and quantity limits, encouraging use of preferred products by patients, and cost management (Academy of Managed Care Pharmacy 2006; National Pharmaceutical Services 2018; Pharmaceutical Care Management Association 2016).

Biopharmaceutical companies find research into specialty drugs attractive from both an innovation as well as a business perspective. The relatively high cost of specialty pharmaceuticals creates a significant economic incentive for companies to research and develop products that help meet serious healthcare needs. Consequently, we can expect continued growth of specialty drugs in the healthcare marketplace.

The Role of the FDA in Specialty Drugs

The Food and Drug Administration (FDA) plays a crucial role in the approval of specialty drugs as well as making sure that those who could benefit from specialty drugs have access to them in a timely fashion. In 1962, amendments to the Federal Food, Drug, and Cosmetic Act gave the FDA authority to require pharmaceutical manufacturers to establish the safety and efficacy of their prescription drugs in clinical trials before marketing the drugs. Given the fact that specialty drugs involve risks, benefits, and complexities, the FDA has come to play an important role in the development and regulation of these drugs. However, once the FDA approves a drug for marketing, it does not regulate the practice of medicine and physicians are generally free to prescribe these drugs as they see fit (Kesselheim et al. 2014). The number of specialty drugs approved by the FDA has continued to grow significantly over the years. In 2013, a majority (19) of all the new drugs (28) approved by the FDA were specialty drugs. In fact, this was the third year in a row that the majority of all new drugs approved by the FDA were specialty drugs (Hogan 2015).

The FDA's drug approval process essentially involves three major components. First is the analysis of the medical condition that is targeted by the proposed new drug and treatment options already available. Second, the assessment of the risks and benefits of the clinical data. Third, establishing strategies for the management of risks involved. This may include FDA-approved drug labels, which clearly describe the drug's benefits and risks, and how the risks can be detected, and requirements for the drug maker to implement risk management and mitigation strategies. It is important to keep in mind that while the FDA uses the best scientific and technological information available in its deliberative process, sometimes risks and benefits may be uncertain and may be difficult to interpret or predict. The FDA and drug makers may reach a different conclusion after analyzing the same data. An approval of a drug for marketing by the FDA means that FDA's Center for Drug Evaluation and Research (CDER) has reviewed the data on the effects of the new drug under consideration for approval, and has determined that the benefits provided by the drug outweigh potential and known risks for the population for which the drug is intended ("Development and Approval Process (Drugs)" 2018).

When a specialty drug shows evidence of potential important benefits in an early clinical trial, the FDA can expedite its availability in two ways—expanded access and accelerated approval. Expanded access allows patients to receive a drug that is undergoing a clinical trial before the formal approval. Under this scenario, an individual patient can receive a drug from a willing physician if the patient cannot enroll in a clinical trial for a valid reason. In 2009, the FDA issued a guideline that expanded access was appropriate only when the disease was serious or life-threatening, no comparable therapy was available, and the potential benefits justified the risk. Some patient advocacy groups have argued that there is a constitutional right to such access. However, the courts have repeatedly rejected such claims (Kesselheim et al. 2014).

Accelerated approval is applied to promising therapies that treat a serious or life-threatening conditions and provide therapeutic benefits over other available therapies. This approach allows for a rapid approval of a drug that demonstrates an effect on a "surrogate endpoint" that is reasonably likely to predict a clinical benefit, i.e., the drug demonstrates potential clinical benefits earlier in the clinical trial that may not be as robust as benefits at the end of the clinical trial ("Development and Approval Process (Drugs)" 2018).

The FDA utilizes three approaches to encourage the development of drugs that represent the first available treatment for an illness, or ones that have significantly more benefits over existing drugs. The FDA uses three designations to a new drug application. A new drug application may receive more than one designation. Each designation is designed to ensure that new therapies for serious medical conditions are made available to patients as soon as the review process concludes that the benefits justify the risk. The three designations are the following ("Development and Approval Process (Drugs)" 2018).

Fast-Track designation puts the approval of a new drug on a fast track based on the promising data based on animal or human clinical trials so the drug gets to the patient earlier than the time it would take to approve a new drug through a regular or normal approval process. The drug company in its application must request the fast-track process.

Breakthrough Therapy designation expedites the development and review of drugs that are intended to treat a serious medical condition and where clinical data indicates that the drug may demonstrate significant improvement over available therapies. A drug with this designation is also available for fast-track designation.

Priority Review designation means that the FDA plans to take action on a drug application within six months compared to ten months under the standard review process.

The FDA expedited review and approval process has been frequently applied to specialty drugs. For example, between 2010 and 2013, 82 new drugs were approved under the fast-track designation and of those 46 (61 percent) were specialty drugs. The FDA also plays a role in limiting the overuse of specialty drugs after it approves them because the high costs of specialty drugs provide incentives for drug companies to promote specialty drugs for off-label uses. However, drug manufacturers have been successful in getting courts to overturn state and federal restrictions on pharmaceutical promotions on the grounds of First Amendment protection of commercial speech (Kesselheim et al. 2014).

The Cost of Specialty Drugs and Price Increases

The United States has entered a new era of specialty drugs and specialty pharmacies. Specialty drugs promise to treat serious medical conditions. Specialty drugs also face the peril of mishandling. The misadministration of such drugs can cause serious adverse effects. Specialty drugs are very costly and their prices have continued to rise often due to lack of competition (Weil 2014).

Specialty drugs have been one of the key factors in driving up healthcare costs. Eleven of the 12 new cancer drugs approved in 2012 were priced above $100,000 annually (Light and Kantarjian 2014). The price of injectable name-brand cancer drugs has risen faster than inflation. According to a study that analyzed the average cost of 24 patented, injectable cancer treatments approved between 1996 and 2012, the average price increase of all drugs was 25 percent over eight years. When the researchers accounted for inflation the average price increase was 18 percent (Gordon et al. 2018).

In 2013, of the 28 drugs approved by the FDA, 19 were specialty drugs. The cost of specialty drugs came into focus when in 2013, Sovaldi, a medication shown to cure about 90 percent of common cases of hepatitis C, highlighted the problem. A 12-week supply of Sovaldi (typical treatment regimen) cost $84,000. About 3.2 million Americans are infected with this condition, which, if left untreated, could lead to liver damage, cirrhosis, liver cancer, and death (Hogan 2015). The retail prices for over 100 widely used specialty prescription drugs surged by nearly 11 percent in 2013, surpassing the median income of an American family. In 2013, the median income of a US household was $52,250, while the average annual cost of a specialty medication used on a chronic basis was over $53,000 ("Report: Rapid Rise in Cost of Specialty Drugs Exceeds Median Family Income" 2015).

The high costs and rising prices of specialty drugs also place a significant financial burden on employers. In 2013, even though only 4 percent of patients take specialty drugs, they represent about 20 percent of total drug costs. At 84 Lumber Co., located in Pennsylvania, spending on specialty drugs went up 94 percent between 2013 and 2014. The annual spending on Sovaldi, which was not approved in 2013, went from zero in 2013 to $178,000 when the drug was approved in 2014. In fact, one employer, the Southeastern Pennsylvania Transportation Authority in Philadelphia, in 2014 filed a lawsuit against Gilead for alleged price gouging. The agency paid more than $2.4 million for Sovaldi prescriptions for its employees that year. Gilead announced a discount of 46 percent on Sovaldi and Harvoni (another drug to treat hepatitis C) for 2015. The primary reason was the introduction of a competing drug—AbbVie's Viekira Pak. This was a game changer because it introduced competition in the market; before this, Sovaldi had faced no competition (Pyrillis 2015).

Most expensive drugs treat rare diseases. Some drugs, while expensive, need to be taken for only a short period of time. For example, some of the specialty drugs that cure hepatitis are taken for a period of 12 weeks. There are other drugs that patients take for life and cost tens of thousands of dollars a month. Some drugs come close to hitting the $1 million mark. For example, the price of the gene therapy drug Luxturna, which can restore sight to children with a rare retinal disease, was set at $850,000. The five most expensive drugs in the United

States are: Actimmune, used to boost the immune system in chronic granulomatous, at about $52,321 for one month; Daraprim, a drug used to treat toxoplasmosis, at about $45,000 for one month; Cinryze, used to prevent attacks in people with a hereditary angioedema, at about $44,140 for one month; Chenodal, a tablet that helps patients with gallstones for whom surgery is risky, at about $42,570 for one month; and finally Myalept, an injectable drug that helps people with leptin deficiency, a rare disorder, at $42,137 per month (Christensen 2018).

Not only do specialty drugs carry high costs, but their prices also have continued to spiral upward. From 2003 to 2014, the proportion of specialty drugs, defined as those reimbursed at a cost of $600 or more for a 30-day fill by third-party payers, has quadrupled in commercial health plans. During this time frame, prescription fills for specialty drugs increased by 198 percent and spending for them increased by 292 percent (Dusetzina 2016). Each year from 2006 to 2013, the average annual increases in the retail prices for name-brand and specialty drug products exceeded the corresponding rate of general inflation. During the same timeframe, price decreases among generic drugs were offset by price increases for name-brand and specialty drugs (AARP Public Policy Institute 2016). In 2015 alone, the retail price for 101 widely used specialty prescription drugs increased by 9.6 percent, compared to general inflation of 0.1 percent—80 times faster. Retail prices increased for 94 of the 101 (93 percent) widely used specialty prescription drug products. In all but 2 of the 22 therapeutic categories of specialty drug products, the average annual retail price increase exceeded the rate of general inflation in 2015 (Schondelmeyer and Purvis 2017).

Medicare and the Cost of Specialty Drugs

Medicare defines specialty drugs as those costing $600 or more a month (Pew Charitable Trusts 2016). Since the elderly are more likely to suffer from chronic health conditions, it stands to reason that Medicare beneficiaries are often prescribed name-brand as well as specialty drugs to deal with their medical conditions. Medicare beneficiaries receive their prescription drug coverage through Part D of the Medicare program and the cost of specialty drugs and their rising prices have a direct impact on the overall cost of the Medicare program. A significant portion of specialty drug users are Medicare beneficiaries and they typically face a co-payment rate of 25 to 33 percent of the price of these drugs (Trish, Joyce, and Goldman 2014).

According to a study by the AARP's Public Policy Institute, retail price increases for specialty prescription drugs widely used by Medicare beneficiaries significantly outstripped price increases for other consumer goods and services between 2005 and 2009. For example, in 2009, the average annual increase in retail prices for 112 name-brand an generic specialty prescription drugs used by Medicare Part D beneficiaries was 8.9 percent while the general inflation rate was 0.3 percent (Schondelmeyer and Purvis 2017). Another study that examined the trends in specialty drug spending among Medicare and Medicare Advantage enrollees using the 2007–2011 pharmacy claim data from a 20-percent sample of Medicare beneficiaries found that annual specialty drug spending per beneficiary who used specialty drugs increased from $2,641 to $8,976 during the study period (Trish, Joyce, and Goldman 2014).

To determine how much a consumer pays for prescription drugs, health insurance plans organized covered drugs by tiers. At the bottom tier 1, a generic drug might require a flat $10 co-payment. But drugs at tier 4 or 5—the specialty tier—might require co-payments for a percentage of the cost, sometimes as much as 33 percent. In Medicare, in 2014, more than 95 percent of all Part D prescription drug plans have at least one drug in the specialty tier up from 50 percent of them in 2006. Unlike Medicaid and Veterans Affairs, Medicare by law is prohibited from using its strength in numbers to negotiate lower prices from drug companies. Consequently, higher specialty drug prices can lead to higher co-payment, i.e., out-of-pocket expenses, for Medicare enrollees even when the drug is covered under the Medicare prescription drug plan. If Medicare enrollees take medication that is excluded from their plan, the out-of-pocket cost can be very high. For example, the out-of-pocket cost fom Enbrel, a rheumatoid arthritis medicine, could reach close to $50,000 a year because it is not covered under the plan (Kodjak 2015).

An analysis of trends in total and out-of-pocket spending among Medicare beneficiaries who take at least one high-cost specialty drug from the top eight specialty drug classes using 2008–2012 pharmacy claim data found that annual total drug spending per specialty drug user studied increased from $18,335 in 2008 to $33,301 in 2012. The proportion of expenditures incurred while in the catastrophic coverage phase (the doughnut hole) increased from 70 to 80 percent (Trish, Xu, and Joyce 2016). Between 2010 and 2015, federal payments for catastrophic coverage more than tripled, growing from $10.8 billion to $32.2 billion. By 2015, high-priced drugs were responsible for almost two-thirds (65 percent) of the total drug spending ($33.4 billion of the $51.4 billion) in catastrophic coverage, i.e., the doughnut hole. During the same period, beneficiaries' out-of-pocket costs for high-priced drugs in catastrophic coverage increased by 47 percent (US Department of Health and Human Services

2017). Even after Medicare Part D enrollees' drug costs have exceeded the catastrophic coverage threshold, they can expect to pay thousands of dollars out-of-pocket for a single specialty drug (Hoadley, Cubanski, and Neuman 2015).

The Affordable Care Act (ACA) had important implications for Medicare beneficiaries' use of specialty drugs and out-of-pocket costs. Beginning in 2011, the ACA enhanced prescription drug coverage for those who were in the coverage gap (the doughnut hole), resulting in 50-percent discounts for name-brand drugs. These discounts will grow over time through 2020, when beneficiaries cost-sharing in the doughnut hole will become subject to a 75-percent discount indefinitely. Thus, this cost-sharing reduction under the ACA should help reduce the out-of-pocket costs for Medicare beneficiaries who take high-cost specialty drugs for the treatment of cancer, rheumatoid arthritis, and other complex and chronic health conditions (Trish, Joyce, and Goldman 2014).

What Accounts for the High Cost of Specialty Drugs?

Drug companies argue that they have no choice but to charge a great deal for specialty drugs in order to recoup their research and development costs. Without it, they cannot innovate and introduce new treatments in the market. In addition, they argue that the average cost of bringing a new specialty drug into the market is estimated to be $2.6 billion per drug. They also point out that they spend about $4 billion a year on programs that provide patients with a significant discount on the price of specialty drugs (Hogan 2015). Another drug industry-sponsored estimate puts the average cost of developing a new drug and getting it approved by the FDA at $1.3 billion, which includes the cost of failures, i.e., research and development costs of drugs that do not make it to the market (Light and Kantarjian 2014). Additionally, it is a mistake to compare the research and development (R&D) cost of marketing a drug to drug companies' profits, given that 90 percent of drugs fail the clinical trial process and thus drug companies that develop a successful drug need to charge a high price to cover the cost of the 90 percent of trials that fail (Goldman, Jena, and Philipson 2015). Thus, the high prices of specialty drugs simply reflect huge research and development costs, including failures.

Some have also argued that there are several myths about specialty drugs that are simply not true. For, example, they argue that it is a myth that growth in specialty drug spending will bankrupt the American healthcare system. They point to the fact that despite the growth in spending for specialty drugs, in 2014, specialty drugs accounted for only 4 percent while cancer drug spending accounted for only 1 percent of the total spending on healthcare in the United States. In addition, they argue that specialty drug prices decline considerably with the introduction of competition from other patented drug or biosimilar drugs after the patents expire (Goldman, Jena, and Philipson 2015).

On the other side of the ledger, opponents of the high cost of specialty drugs argue that there is a total lack of transparency when it comes to the true cost of developing specialty drugs. They argue that the estimated cost of $1.3 billion for developing a new drug and getting it approved is highly misleading because half of it includes not research costs but rather the high figure for-profit companies would have made if they had invested their research in stocks and bonds. While profit forgone may be a common way to estimate whether it is worthwhile to develop a new project, it is not a real cost that should be recouped from customers. In addition, taxpayers already subsidize about half of company research costs through tax credits and deductions that are granted to drug companies. Thus, in reality, no accurate estimate exists because the cost of a new discovery varies considerably and could include anything from an inexpensive lucky break to a costly 30-year research program before a new drug is discovered (Light and Kantarjian 2014).

The reality is that the rise of specialty drugs and their high prices have helped drug companies offset revenues they have lost from the expiration of patents for small-molecule agents like aspirin, beta-blockers, and statins, among others, allowing the entry of generic drugs for many prescriptions. Consequently, the pharmaceutical industry has shifted its focus from blockbuster small molecules to specialty pharmaceuticals (Hirsch, Balu, and Schulman 2014).

Strategies to Reduce the Costs of Specialty Drugs

A study that examined the prevalence of specialty drug coupons offered by manufacturers found that such discount coupons significantly helped reduced patients' out-of-pocket costs. The study found that in 2013 drug coupons accounted for $21.2 million of patients' $35.3 million annual out-of-pocket costs. The proportion of prescriptions for which patients' costs were more than $250 before coupon use was 12 percent, which dropped to only 3 percent after the coupon was applied. In a large majority of cases, coupons reduced patients' out-of-pocket cost-sharing to less than $250, making it less likely that patients would abandon their use of specialty drugs/therapy. Patients with higher out-of-pocket costs are more likely to abandon the use of specialty drugs because they may not be able to afford the cost-sharing burden. For example, the specialty drug abandonment rate among patients was 10 percent when their monthly out-of-pocket costs were less than $500, but the abandonment rate spiked to 52.3 percent for patients whose monthly out-of-pocket expenses were more than $2,000. The discount coupon program for specialty drugs has been a successful strategy to reduce the cost-sharing burden and make them more affordable for patients who need them.

Potential negative side effects of this strategy may be that reducing the cost-sharing burden may undermine PBMs' attempts to keep plan premiums low, tempering moral hazard by discouraging patients from using preferred formulary drugs (Starner et al. 2014). Moral hazard theory posits that the consumption of healthcare services increases since the presence of health insurance shields the patient from the full financial cost of using services. Thus, one way to reduce the impact of moral hazard is to increase cost-sharing of patients. However, the prospect theory stands in sharp contrast to the moral hazard theory. The prospect theory describes the way in which patients weigh the risks and benefits of a decision in the context of gains and losses. According to this theory, a patient making a decision confronted with a loss, i.e., a cancer diagnosis, may, in fact, become risk-seeking in considering treatment options. Emotion can also play a role in a patient's decision-making when facing a loss. Individuals confronted with a life-threatening illness may be willing to bear high out-of-pocket costs for treatment that they feel could save their lives. Thus, specialty pharmaceuticals may be driven not by moral hazard but by more complex decision-making processes that may ignore financial considerations in making treatment choice (Hirsch, Balu, and Schulman 2014).

A second strategy that can help reduce the costs of specialty drugs is for the FDA to play a role in limiting their overuse. Specialty drug manufacturers have successfully fought in courts state and federal restrictions on pharmaceutical companies promoting off-label use of specialty drugs. However, the FDA can limit the overuse of specialty drugs by: (1) further narrowing the scope of FDA-approved indications. Approved indications set the parameters for how insurers will cover a drug in their health plans. Overly broad indications can lead to inappropriate prescribing and payments. (2) Concomitantly approving companion diagnostic tests that can provide information about the patient population more likely to benefit from the drug. (3) Requiring manufacturers to create a risk evaluation and mitigation strategy (REMS) if safety risks are identified at the time the drug is approved (Kesselheim et al. 2014).

A third strategy to control costs of specialty drugs is to increase the use of off-patent agents. Since specialty pharmaceuticals are approved by the FDA under biologics license applications they are not subject to the generic drug provisions under the Drug Price Competition and Patent Term Restoration Act of 1984. Consequently, at present, there is no standard pathway for competitors to enter the market when specialty drugs' patents expire. The Affordable Care Act includes provisions for the approval of biosimilar products with the hope of generating competition in the biologics market to help decrease costs of specialty pharmaceuticals. This is important because between 2013 and 2018 several biologic agents such as Epogen or Procrit, Neulasta, Rituxan, Avastin, and Herceptin will lose their patents. However, the impact of biosimilar drugs in the near future is likely to be limited to generic medications that cost $1 million–$5 million to develop and three to five years for approval. Because of their complexity, biosimilars will cost $100 million–$200 million to develop and eight to ten years to produce. Also, FDA approval will require new clinical data to support the safety of the biosimilars. Since the cost of R&D drives investment and pricing decisions, one potential solution could be to create a new pathway under which drug developers could compete for federal grants to support the cost of developing biosimilars and, in return for this financial support, drug developers would agree to provide concessions on prices (Hirsch, Balu, and Schulman 2014).

Another possible strategy to help reduce the costs of specialty drugs is to reduce the exclusivity time period for their patents. In the United States, biologics approved by the FDA are granted a 12-year period of exclusivity during which time drug developers do not face any competition from biosimilars. This exclusivity period is significantly longer than the five-year exclusivity typically granted to traditional, small-molecule drugs. Many other countries grant a much shorter period of exclusivity than the United States. Also, when all patents and exclusivity period for name brand specialty drugs end, to speed up the entry of biosimilars into the market, the FDA could conceivably create an abbreviated license approval pathway for biosimilars instead of requiring developers of biosimilars to go through the same lengthy approval process as the original specialty drugs ("Policy Proposal: Reducing the Exclusivity Period for Biological Products" 2017).

The Benefits and Effectiveness of Specialty Drugs

Specialty drugs are playing an increasing role in the prescription drug marketplace. Between 1999 and 2012 the FDA approved 279 new molecular entities, of which 154 (55.2 percent) were specialty drugs. Given the growth of specialty drugs, their high costs, rising prices, and the fact that a small number of individuals use these drugs, the questions they raise include what benefits they provide and how effective they are.

A study that examined the literature dealing with published estimates of health gains, costs, and resource use association with 58 specialty drugs and 4 traditional drugs approved by the FDA found that specialty drugs were associated with a greater gain in quality-adjusted life years (QALYs) than traditional drugs. The study found that many specialty and traditional drugs offer relatively modest benefits over preexisting care. However, specialty drugs tended to offer greater health improvements over preexisting conditions than traditional drugs. Specialty drugs were associated with some of the largest health gains since they are often designed to treat diseases such as cancer and multiple sclerosis that have unmet needs. The study concluded that while specialty drugs are often more costly than traditional drugs, they also often confer greater benefits and thus they provide reasonable value for the money (Chambers et al. 2014).

It is generally easier to justify new treatments that produce large improvements in survival or quality of life. Specialty drugs that offer only incremental benefits at a high cost often receive more scrutiny and critiques question their worth. Others argue that in therapeutic areas where the rate of innovation is very high, new therapies that produce only marginal value should not be underestimated because such therapies create "option value" by allowing some patients to live long enough to benefit from future therapies. Such was the case with early HIV treatment. The first drug approved for treating HIV in the early 1990s had only a very modest increase but for some patients, it extended their life long enough to allow them access to "wonder drugs" that emerged in the late 1990s. Additionally, what policymakers value, i.e., costs versus benefits, may be different from what patients' value, i.e., even a modest improvement may be valued highly by patients suffering from chronic and/or life threating diseases (Godman, Jena, and Philipson 2015).

Policy Dilemma: Balancing the Costs and Benefits of Specialty Drugs

The high costs of specialty drugs are placing significant financial burdens on payers, employers, and patients. Payers have often responded by shifting drug costs to patients, making such drugs less affordable to many patients. The question about specialty drugs revolves around their value/benefits relative to their costs. Overall many specialty drugs do offer more value compared to traditional drugs to a small segment of the population that need and use specialty drugs to treat their medical conditions. One can even argue that the development of specialty drugs benefits society as a whole. However, the public policy dilemma that remains unanswered is who should pay, and how much, to receive the benefits of specialty drugs.

The American healthcare system faces the challenge of determining how to pay for effective specialty drugs and determining when benefits are worth the costs and when they are not. As the growth, use, and price of specialty drugs continue to rise, policymakers will be confronted with the dilemma of making sure that the healthcare system and patients are receiving good value relative to their costs, while at the same time ensuring that patients who benefit have access to such drugs at affordable prices.

GENE THERAPY: THE FUTURE OF MEDICINE?

The Evolution of Gene Therapy

The field of gene therapy has evolved from the early 1990s to the present day through many trials and errors, and along the way it has experienced many successes and setbacks. After failing to deliver on early promises of treatment and cure of many diseases during the 1990s, the field of gene therapy has reemerged since the early to mid-2000s with more successes and is beginning to deliver on some of its earlier promises.

The Human Genome Project

By the mid-1980s the scientific community was making important discoveries about the role of genes in diseases and there was excitement about the human genome project. Cancer and heart diseases were increasingly tied to recessive genes or normal genes that went haywire as a result of mutation. Walter Gilbert, American biochemist, physicist, molecular biology pioneer, and Nobel laureate, was an enthusiastic supporter of the human genome project and advocated proceeding with human gene sequencing. In 1986, Charles DeLisi, director of the Office of Health and Environment at the Department of Energy (DOE), advanced a plan for a five-year human genome project that would including physical mapping, development of automated high-speed sequencing techniques, and research into the computer analysis of sequence data. In 1987, the Secretary of the Energy Department ordered the establishment of human genome research centers at three of the department's national laboratories—Los Alamos, Livermore, and Lawrence Berkley. The movement picked up steam as biomedical scientists and representatives of pharmaceutical and biotechnology industries lobbied Congress for support. An added incentive was competition with the US in high technology as other countries in Europe and Japan were moving toward major genome projects of their own.

For the fiscal year 1988, Congress appropriated a significant amount of start-up funds to both the DOE and the National Institutes of Health (NIH). An office for the Human Genome was established within the NIH and Dr. James Watson, the co-discoverer of the structure of DNA, was appointed to head the office. In 1988, Congress awarded the NIH and DOE together $39 million dollars for the genome project for 1989. The same year, the Office of Human Genome Research within the NIH was elevated to the National Center for Human Genome Research. In 1991, the human genome project was inaugurated as a formal federal program and received $135 million; the project moved into high gear (Kevles 1997).

In 1989, in an editorial *The Wall Street Journal* had enthusiastically endorsed the project by arguing that the mapping of the human genome would make possible the techniques of gene identification, separation, and splicing, and would open doors to discovery of basic causes of diseases and cures and precursory treatment that might ward off the onset of illnesses from cancer, to heart disease, to AIDS. In fact, the editorial also warned that the Human Genome Initiative may be attacked by those who are fearful or hostile to the future ("Chromosome Cartography" 1989). Similarly, Dr. James Watson, the most prominent cheerleader for the project, had argued that the project provided an extraordinary potential for human betterment because it would give the scientific community tools to understand human beings on the molecular level. In fact, the Human Genome Project has often been compared to the Manhattan Project and the Apollo Project (Annas 1989).

To be sure, there was opposition to the Human Genome Project from a certain segment of the scientific community. In February 1990, Martin Rechsteiner, a professor in the biochemistry department at the University of Utah, called the Human Genome Project a waste of national resources and sent a letter to colleagues around the US to raise a protest against the project. He further added that ascertaining the sequence of coding regions would not advance biological science. One of the primary reasons for this opposition was the fear that funding of the project would financially squeeze out basic research in biological sciences. The project's technological emphasis created the image of Big Science crowding out small-scale research in the biomedical sciences. Opponents saw favoritism in funding for the Human Genome Project and a threat to smaller-scale experiments. Some questioned the practicality and the reliability of funding a project that may not lead to any plausible conclusions. Still, others worried about potential insurance and employment discrimination based on an individual's genetic makeup and a host of ethical concerns raised by the project. Ultimately, the attacks against the Human Genome Project proved to be largely ineffective and failed to stop it (Hamdoun 2017; Kevles 1997).

The Human Genome Project, funded by the DOE and NIH, became an international research project. The Sanger Institute, the British extension that pioneered pilot sequencing projects, provided integral support to the sequencing efforts. At the same time, Celera Genomics' privately funded gene sequencing efforts, headed by J. Craig Venter, created a healthy competition to finish the project first. In June of 2000, the Human Genome Project announced that it had completed sequencing of a majority of the human genome and in February of 2001 it officially published its results in the February issue of the journal *Nature*. Celera Genomics also published its results the same year. Two years, later, in April 2003, a more accurate version of the human genome was released, with greater precision and more information. Before the launch of the project, estimates concerning the number of genes within the human genome had ranged from 35,000 to 100,000, with protein-based genes numbering up to 40,000. However, the results of the Human Genome Project revealed that protein-coding genes averaged only about 21,000 genes (Hamdoun 2017).

Early Successes and Setbacks: 1990s

Even prior to the successful completion of the Human Genome Project, the early use of gene therapy had met with some initial successes with the treatment of a 4-year-old patient named Ashanti De Silva. She was treated for the fatal inherited disease severe combined immunodeficiency (SCID), caused by mutations in a few different genes. Patients lacking a functional immune system can die from even a mild infection. De Silva's treatment, which had begun in 1990, included isolating her white blood cells and injecting altered T blood cells into her bloodstream, which resulted in an improved immune system (Hamdoun 2017). This was done 11 times over a two-year period, which led to increased white blood cell counts. The skeptics pointed to the fact that the patient had to continue to receive enzyme replacement therapy at a cost of $400,000 per year during the trial and a majority of patients in further safety trials did not exhibit increased enzyme activity (Simon 2002).

By 1999, there were about 40 ongoing clinical human gene therapy trials in the US designed to treat 18 inherited diseases. However, the death of an 18-year old volunteer, Jesse Gelsinger, undergoing gene therapy treatment in a clinical trial in September of 1999 at the University of Pennsylvania Medical Center shocked the scientific community and raised doubts about the promise of gene therapy (Simon 2002). Confidence in the newly emerging field plummeted and new questions arose about the safety and reliability of gene therapy. The situation was made worse because Gelsinger's parents claimed that they were not informed about the serious side effects experienced by previous patients and that three monkeys had died from clotting disorder and liver inflammation—raising the issue of informed consent (Hamdoun 2017). Consequently, the Food and Drug Administration (FDA) faulted the researchers and the university for inadequate oversight and shut down all six clinical trials at the University of Pennsylvania's Institute of Human Gene Therapy (Simon 2002). Soon after the death of Jesse Gelsinger, treatment for another disorder, severe combined immunodeficiency (SCID), triggered five cases of leukemia, including one death, in 20 children. The gene delivery system was identified as a cause for the failure (Lewis 2014).

This put many other clinical trials on hold as the field went through intense scrutiny and peer reviews by outside panels and government agencies. A realistic assessment of the early stage of gene therapy in the 1990s is that despite some of the early advances the promise of gene therapy outweighed its accomplishments (Simon 2002).

The Reemergence of Gene Therapy: 2000–2018

The successful completion of the Human Genome Project in 2003 with the mapping and sequencing of the human genome helped informed analysis and improved our understanding of the relationship between disease-causing agents in humans, ushering in an era of regenerative and personalized medicine and ultimately the reemergence of gene therapy.

Following the death of Jesse Gelsinger in 1999, the field of gene therapy grounded to a halt for almost 15 years. This and other setbacks led scientists to rethink their approaches, prompting them to focus on safer and more efficient means of delivering genes to the target tissue, especially concerning the most common delivery system for gene therapy: engineering a virus to act as a sort of microscopic injection gun (Lewis 2014). The past failures resulting from shortcomings of a variety of vectors led to a search for the optimal gene therapy vector.

The idea took hold that by understating the flow of genetic information within the human biological system any pathology caused by molecular defects can be corrected and normal cell activity at a molecular level can be restored. Gene therapy seeks to treat and often cure the disease by introducing the functional or curative form of the gene into a host to improve the functioning of the existing mutated gene or by replacing it with a healthy gene. Today various approaches are used for the development of gene therapy agents (Zamyatnin 2016).

Gene therapy has finally begun to deliver results on its early promises. For example, experimental procedures for placing healthy genes wherever they are needed in the body has restored sight in dozens of individuals who suffered from a hereditary form of blindness. Similar successes have been recorded in patients with various forms of cancers of the blood—several of whom have remained malignancy free three years after the treatment. Researchers have also had some success in using gene therapy to enable a few men with hemophilia, a bleeding disorder that can be fatal at times, to go long periods of time without incidents, or taking high doses of clotting drugs. In fact, medical researchers are moving beyond treating hereditary diseases to trying to reverse genetic damage that naturally occurs due to the aging process. For example, scientists at the University of Pennsylvania are using gene therapy to treat a common childhood cancer known as acute lymphoblastic leukemia (AAL) (Lewis 2014).

In 2017 the FDA approved three gene therapies to enter the market. One is Luxturna, which is a virus vector-based therapy for the treatment of patients with retinal dystrophy. The other two are CAR T-Cell therapies—Kymriah to treat leukemia and Yescarta to treat lymphoma (Weintraub 2018). This new pioneering cancer drug therapy, called CAR T-Cell, is made by harvesting patients' white blood cells and rewiring them to hone in on tumors. This therapy has produced unprecedented success in patients with rare and deadly cancers (McGinley 2017; Patel 2017). The price tag is $475,000 for a course of treatment (Garde 2017). The cost of first gene therapy for an inherited disorder—a rare condition that causes a progressive form of blindness that usually starts in childhood—is estimated to be around $1 million for each treatment (Stein 2017).

The FDA has also approved several cell and gene therapy products for the treatment of prostate cancer, a cell transplantation procedure for hematopoietic and immunologic reconstitution in patients with disorders affecting the hematopoietic system that are inherited, acquired, or result from myeloablative treatment, and T-cell immunotherapy indicated for the treatment of adult patients with relapsed or refractory large B-cell lymphoma after two or more lines of systemic therapy, and the like ("Approved Cellular and Gene Therapy Products" 2018).

Also, the same year, a team of researchers at Oregon Health and Science University announced the successful elimination of genetic disease from human embryos. Critics argue that this type of genetic manipulation can open the door to other possibilities in human engineering that raise ethical concerns (Garneau 2017).

What are Gene Editing and Gene Therapy?

Gene Editing

Gene editing is a method used by scientists to change the DNA of organisms including plants, animals, and humans. The agricultural industry was the first to start using gene editing in plants to improve crops and develop seedless tomatoes, gluten-free wheat, mushrooms that do not turn brown when older, and host of other modifications to vegetables and fruits. Genetically modified organisms (GMOs) in the field of agriculture have produced some backlash among some segments of the population. Gene editing rewrites the biological code that makes up the instruction manual for living organisms. With gene editing, scientists can disable the defective genes, correct harmful mutations, and change the activity of specific genes. Gene editing can be used to add, remove, or alter the DNA in the genome (Sample 2018). Gene editing is often compared to editing a manuscript in which one corrects a misspelled word, replaces a wrong word with a correct or better word, or rewrites sentences ("Gene Editing" n.d.)

Gene editing in humans is done in the hope of treating or preventing human diseases by rewiring (modifying/repairing or cutting/replacing) the DNA of a defective gene that causes illness. There are many genetic disorders that can be passed on from one generation to the next (inherited diseases), like cystic fibrosis, sickle-cell anemia, and muscular dystrophy. Human gene editing holds the promise of being able to treat such hereditary diseases by rewiring corrupt or defective DNA in a patient's cell. Similarly, gene editing can be used to modify individuals' immune cells to fight cancer or HIV infection. It can also be used to fix defective genes in human embryos to prevent babies from inheriting diseases (Sample 2018).

The first gene editing techniques were developed in the 1990s. There are a number of recognized gene editing methods, and researchers have been experimenting with different methods. A new gene editing tool, called CRISPR/Cas9, has received a great deal of national limelight because it has shown great promise in guiding the targeting mechanism to the desired genetic location to remove the faulty gene and replace it with a normal gene template (cut and paste). The method is faster, cheaper, and more accurate than previous gene editing techniques (Towers 2017; "What are Genome Editing and CRISPR-Cas9?" 2017). In 2017, scientists at Harvard University unveiled a new gene editor that uses the CRIPS/Cas9 technology to target and change a single letter in a string of DNA bases without any cutting. There are billions of letters in the human genome and tens of thousands of diseases can be traced back to tiny mistakes, and converting one letter to another may help find a treatment or cure for thousands of diseases. This new technique is like using a pencil and an eraser (Netburn 2017).

Gene Therapy

Today scientists are developing gene therapies to treat diseases using gene editing techniques. Gene therapy is a technique that uses genes to treat or prevent disease. With rapid advances made in the field of gene therapy, physicians in the future might be able to treat a disorder by inserting a healthy gene into a patient's cells instead of using drugs or surgery. Gene therapy introduces genetic material into human cells to compensate for abnormal genes or to make a beneficial protein ("What is Gene Therapy" 2017). Genes are the functional units of heredity that encode instructions to make proteins that perform most life functions. When genes are mutated the encoded proteins fail to carry out normal life functions resulting in genetic disorder and diseases (Singh et al. 2016).

When a mutated gene causes a necessary protein to become faulty or missing, gene therapy can introduce a normal copy of the gene to restore the function of the protein. Since a gene inserted directly into a cell generally does not function, a carrier called a vector is engineered to deliver the gene. Often certain viruses are used as vector because they can deliver the new gene by infecting the cell. The trick is to genetically modify the virus to carry human DNA and to prevent the virus from causing disease in the patient. The advantage is that a vector can be injected or given intravenously (IV) directly into a specific tissue in the body, and is then taken up by individual cells. Researchers are experimenting with several different approaches to gene therapy such as replacing a mutated gene that causes disease with a healthy one, inactivating or "knocking out" a mutated gene that is functioning improperly, or introducing a new gene into the body to help fight disease. The theory behind gene therapy is to treat a disease through replacement of the abnormal gene with a normal or healthy gene ("Genes and Gene Therapy" 2018; Simon 2002; "What is Gene Therapy" 2017).

There are two basic types of gene therapy. One is somatic gene therapy, where therapeutic genes are transferred into somatic cells of a patient. Here, the modification of the gene and its effects are restricted to the individual patient and will not be inherited by the patient's offspring or later generations. The second type of gene therapy is germline gene therapy, in which germ cells (sperm or eggs) are modified by introducing a functional gene that is integrated into the patent's genome. Under this method, changes made are heritable and would be passed on to later generations (Singh et al. 2016).

One of the challenges in the field of gene therapy is the development of gene transfer tools and today the field has developed a large variety of such tools and has advanced knowledge and understanding of the pathobiology of disease and the application of gene therapy to challenging diseases such as cancer, aging, blindness, and cardiovascular and neurological disorders (Glorioso and Lemoine 2017). Powerful new gene-based therapies are likely to dramatically transform future medical practice, allowing people to live longer and healthier lives. Interventions to replace underdeveloped, faulty, destroyed, or degenerated tissues by actually regenerating tissues is often called regenerative medicine. Regenerative medicine depends on the availability of appropriate cells and cell lines (Trommelmans 2010).

Haseltine (2003) classifies regenerative medicine into four basic types. Type 1 regenerative medicine include recombinant drugs such as human insulin, hormones, and erythro-proteins, a substance that stimulates the formation of red blood cells. Since the body accepts another person's purified substances, protein drugs made from one person's gene can treat anyone. Similarly, some therapeutic proteins can substitute for those that the patients cannot make themselves. For example, recombinant insulin can help compensate for diabetic patients who cannot make insulin themselves, thus allowing them to regain control over blood sugar in their body. In type 2 regenerative medicine, cells are removed from the patient's body, grown in a culture, and then reintroduced into the patient. This is called tissue engineering and can be accomplished by building an organ or tissue outside the body by combining human cells with appropriate material to provide support or growing suitable cells in a lab and then injecting them into a tissue needing repair. For examples, companies now make artificial skin that has helped improve the care of burn victims. Scientists can also grow new blood vessels, cardiac muscles, corneas, and the like. The third type of regenerative medicine is embryonic stem cells, special cells obtained from very-early-stage human embryos. These cells can develop into every major kind of cell in the human body. Embryonic stem cells have been used successfully to treat injury and illnesses in animals. Today, the cloning of several species of animal, like sheep (Dolly), dogs, and monkeys, has been done successfully. However, the use of embryonic stem cells in humans has been a controversial issue in the United States because of fear of creating a potential for human cloning. In the fourth type of regenerative medicine, new materials are engineered to atomic-scale precision to integrate seamlessly with individual patients' own cells without causing rejections. Examples include devices and prosthetics that can fuse with the body.

Stem cell-based gene therapy is a new therapeutic branch of medicine, but is still at the experimental stage at this point in time. Thus far, the FDA has approved very few gene therapies for application. However, stem cell-based gene therapy shows a great deal of promise. Cell-based gene therapies are being studied to treat cartilage repair (Longo et al. 2012), cancer (Kershaw, Westwood, and Darcy 2013), muscular dystrophies (Benedetti, Hoshiya, and Tedesco 2013; Emrani 2017), HIV (Schultz 2018; Zhen and Kitchen 2014), retinal disorder (Garg et al. 2017), spina bifida (Watts 2017), and Parkinson's disease (Loring 2017), among many others.

The Twenty-First Century Cures Act, signed into law in December 2016, is designed to accelerate medical product development and to bring new innovations and advances to patients quickly and efficiently. The law establishes new expedited product development programs for the Regenerative Medicine Advanced Therapy to expedite the process for some biologic products and the Breakthrough Device Program to speed up the review of certain new innovative medical devices ("21st Century Cures Act" 2018). One of the challenges surrounding regenerative medicine, since it depends on the availability of appropriate human cells and cell lines, is the ownership of human material and products derived from it, as well as the rights of cell donors versus the rights of scientists who develop new products from the donated cells (Trommelmans 2010).

The Pros and Cons of Gene Therapy

Despite some of the successes of gene therapy, it has attracted both supporters and critics. Many arguments have been put forward in support and opposition to gene therapy. The supporters of gene therapy point to its many advantages.

The pros and cons of gene therapy are summarized below ("12 Pros and Cons of Gene Therapy"; n.d.; "17 Biggest Pros and Cons of Gene Therapy" 2018; "Playing God? The Pros and Cons of Gene Therapy" 2018; Singh et al. 2016).

The pros are as follows.

- Gene therapy has great untapped potentials and it offers hope to children born with birth defects. One in every 33 babies experiences birth defects of some sort and gene therapy can help correct some of these defects and reduce fatalities.
- Somatic gene therapy could be utilized to not only cure patients that are severely ill but also to prevent the onset of devastating illnesses.
- In contrast to drug therapy that often treats the symptoms of illness, gene therapy can provide a cure for illness.
- Gene therapy has the potential to eliminate and prevent hereditary diseases such as cystic fibrosis, and cure cancer, AIDS, and heart disease.
- While some diseases can be cured by medicine, genetic disorders can be cured only by replacing the defective gene with a healthy one. Rare diseases affect about 10 percent of the general US population and many of them are caused by faulty genetics.
- Gene therapy technology can be applied to plants and animals as well. It can help create healthier food chains and restore the immune systems of plants and animals.
- Gene therapy could help end the stigma of genetic disorders.

The cons are as follows.

- Manipulating the genetic makeup of humans is similar to interfering with nature and amounts to playing God.
- Gene therapy is very costly and raises concerns about affordability and ability to pay, and thus the cost of administering such therapies can make access difficult for low-income individuals.
- Gene therapy can provide false hope.
- It can lead to unethical uses such as gene doping by athletes through the use of performance-enhancing drugs, growth hormones, and blood doping.
- It may not be as effective in the long run and the immune system's negative response to the introduction of a foreign substance into human tissue may make it difficult to repeat gene therapy in patients.
- The best candidates for gene therapy are disorders that arise from a mutation in a single gene. Some of the most commonly occurring disorders such as heart disease, arthritis, high blood pressure, diabetes, and Alzheimer's are caused by the combined effects of variation in several different genes and thus multi-genetic disorders may be difficult to treat with gene therapy.
- Reproductive gene therapy triggers the fear of eugenics and creation of designer babies.

The Cost of Gene Therapy

The European Medicines Agency in 2012 recommended for approval Glybera, a gene therapy used to treat adults with lipoprotein lipase (LEL) deficiency. It is an orphan disease that results in abnormally large particles of fat in the blood and causes inflammation of the pancreas. The therapy consists of LPS, encoded by an adeno-associated virus vector administered through a series of intra-muscular injections. It was the first gene therapy approved in the Western world and went on sale in Germany in 2014 at an initial cost of $1.22 million per treatment ("$1-Million Price Tag Set for Glybera Gene Therapy" 2015).

In the United States, the FDA in 2017 approved a breakthrough therapy for B-cell acute lymphoblastic leukemia. This gene therapy modifies the genetics of a patient's cells so the cells recognize and attack the patient's cancer. The FDA also approved CAR T-Cell therapy marketed as Kymriah by Novartis for treatment of relapsed childhood acute lymphoblastic leukemia for patients 25 years old or younger. Novartis set the price of Kymriah at $475,000 for a single treatment. There are about 3100 patients who suffer from this disease in the US and if every patient were to get this treatment, the total annual cost to patients and insurers in the United States is projected to be $1.5 billion. Furthermore, the therapy can lead to life-threatening side-effects and thus the FDA requires hospitals and physicians to be trained and certified to administer the therapy; they must also inventory the drugs needed to quell severe reactions, adding another $1.5 billion in cost. The introduction of other CAR T-Cell therapies may ultimately lower the cost slightly. For example, Kite Pharma's Yescarta, a CAR T-Cell therapy for adults with certain types of lymphoma, is priced at $375,000. The CAR T-Cell gene therapy in a way represents a double-edged sword—a miraculous treatment mixed with significant clinical risks and costs (Kodish 2017; Webster 2018).

Similarly, an injectable gene therapy treatment for blindness, Luxturna from Spark Therapeutics, will cost about $425,000 per eye or $850,000 for both eyes. The therapy is a one-time treatment and can improve the eyesight of patients with a rare genetic mutation that eventually causes complete blindness by adulthood. It is also the first gene therapy approved by the FDA for an inherited disease. It requires a 45-minute operation in which a tiny needle delivers a replacement gene to the retina, tissue at the back of the eye that converts light into electric signals that produce vision. The cost of the operation itself is about $4,000 to $5,000. Previously, there was no treatment for this condition, which affects a couple of thousand individuals in the United States. Initially, Sparks had suggested that its therapy could be worth more than $1 million but later decided to lower the price after hearing concerns from health insurers about affordability. The company has also offered unconventional payment plans to insurers such as paying for the drug in installments over several years. The company has also suggested offering to refund some of the costs if patients do not experience the expected improvement in their vision (Cortez 2018; Perrone 2018).

Gene therapy, after weathering tragedies and setbacks in the 1990s, has emerged as a beacon of hope for treating and finding cures for many diseases as it has evolved from experimental to applied medicine. However, steep prices for gene therapy treatment have also generated debate and controversy about access and affordability ("Gene Therapy Offer Dramatic Promises but Shocking Costs" 2015). Furthermore, there is a correlation between specific gene therapy and the target patient population, i.e., the fewer the eligible patients, the more expensive the treatment. The smaller the number of individuals afflicted by a disease, the higher the market pricing power of the therapy designed to treat that disease (Mullin 2017). The problem is compounded by the lack of competition in the marketplace for some of the newly approved gene therapies.

If a gene therapy is priced by its value, i.e., value-based drug pricing, the cost of a cure is likely to be very expensive. However, value-based pricing can make the cure unaffordable to patients. Chandra (2017) suggests two possible solutions: the first involves enforcing the same premiums for precision medicine regardless of disease and spreading the risk across more people, i.e., expanding the insurance pool. Second, he proposes government participation in research and development, something akin to NASA for drug development. Under this proposal, a government-funded R&D agency would use private contractors, including universities and current drug companies, to develop and manufacture drugs and run clinical trials. The advantages include the fact that society would owe the patent, not a drug company; an agency can channel R&D into areas of medicine where profits are small but prevalence of disease and suffering are high; and a reduction in R&D cost by learning from failure. However, potential disadvantages include the potential lack of financial discipline by a government R&D agency; the slow pace of R&D; and unwillingness to take "risks" or taking stupid risks at taxpayer expense.

Gene therapy is one of the most significant developments in the history of medicine because of the hope it offers for to those borne with genetic and incurable medical conditions. Gene therapy products that thus far have reached the market are very expensive. Thus, the ultimate question is whether steep and rising prices will prevent patients from accessing new gene therapies (Kent and Spink 2017).

Controversy over Germline Human Gene Editing

One of the most controversial areas of human gene-editing among the world's scientists and governments is what is called germline human gene editing. Germline editing refers to genetic editing on sperm, eggs, or embryo cells. One of the main concerns is that modifications in these cells' genes will alter the DNA not only of that future person but of all of their future descendants. When gene editing is used with adults, genetic changes are not passed down to the next generation. Given the fact that the CRISP-Cas9 technique for gene editing is new, it is also difficult to predict what unforeseen consequences may arise (Almendrala 2018). Yet, at the same time, germline editing has the potential to treat and cure many hereditary diseases.

In 2015, Chinese scientists announced that they had used the CRISP-Cas9 technique on human embryos for the first time. The project was unsuccessful but it caught everyone by surprise and set off a global discussion about the legal and ethical implication of such research (Smaglik 2017). In 2015, at the International Summit on Human Gene Editing held in Washington DC, the world's leading geneticists gave a cautious approval of gene editing of human embryos and called for public discussion by scientists and the general public about what constitutes acceptable use of this technology, following which countries could introduce regulations that outline acceptable and unacceptable use of this technology. For example, germline editing may be acceptable to reduce a person's risk of Alzheimer's, but not acceptable to change a person's skin color (Nowogrodzki and Le Page 2015). After several days of discussion, the members of the organizing committee issued a statement summarizing the conclusions they had reached. One, basic and clinical research is needed and should proceed subject to appropriate legal and ethical rules. Second, many promising applications of gene editing are directed at altering genetic sequence only in a somatic cell, cells whose genomes are not transmitted to the next generation. Third, while each country has the ultimate authority to regulate activities under its jurisdiction, there is a need for an ongoing forum among an international community to discuss norms concerning germline editing. Forth, germline gene editing might be used for introduction of a naturally occurring variant or totally new genetic changes thought to be beneficial but it should avoid enhancement of human capabilities. Challenges facing germline gene editing include the risk of inaccurate editing, difficulty of predicting harmful effects, and obligations to consider implications to both the individual and future generation who would carry the genetic alterations. Once introduced into the human population, genetic alterations are difficult to remove and would not remain in a single community or a nation. There is also the possibility of permanent genetic enhancement to a subset of the population, which could exacerbate social inequality or could be used coercively (Baltimore et al. 2016; Jones 2017).

The same year, a summit held by the US National Academies of Science and Medicine, the Chinese Academy of Sciences, and the United Kingdom's Royal Society issued a statement in which it was argued that human gene-editing research, even on embryos, is needed and should go forward as long as no pregnancy results from such research. However, it was argued that it would be irresponsible to proceed with clinical studies in germline cells that transmit altered DNA to future generations (Saey 2015). In 2017, the National Academies of Science and Medicine changed their earlier position and adopted a new position that altering human embryos, eggs, sperm, or cells that produce eggs and sperm would be permissible, provided it is limited to situations where no other reasonable alternatives are available, editing would prevent serious disease, and edited genes match versions already in the population. In short, altering DNA of germline cells should be permissible to prevent genetic diseases from being passed on to future generations and provided it is done to correct disability or disease and not to enhance individuals' health or abilities (Saey 2017a, 2017b).

In 2016, in the world's first, Chinese scientists injected a human with cells genetically modified to fight cancer. The scientists used the controversial "cut-and-paste" gene editing technique CRISPR-Cas9 in which scientists cut out the inherited genes that might cause cancer from the cells and replace them with healthy genes (Best 2016). In November of 2018, a Chinese researcher, He Jiankui, announced that he had helped make the world's first genetically edited twin baby girls, whose DNA he had altered. He altered the embryos of seven couples during fertility treatment, which thus far has resulted in one pregnancy. He claimed that his goal was not to prevent an inherited disease but rather to resist possible future infection with HIV, the AIDs virus. The gene editing was carried out during IVF via lab-dish fertilization by first washing the sperm to separate it from semen, where HIV can lurk. Then a single sperm was placed into a single egg to create an embryo. When the embryos were three to five days old, 16 of the 22 embryos were edited using the CRISPR-Cas9 editing tool to surgically change one out of 3 billion letters of the embryos' DNA code to build a resistance to HIV infection. Eleven edited embryos were used in six implant attempts, which led to a successful twin pregnancy. Tests suggested that one twin had both copies of the intended altered gene and the other twin had just one gene altered (Marchione 2018; Morgan 2018). However, as of this writing, there was no independent verification of He's claim and the research had not yet been published in any scientific journal where it could be vetted by other experts.

The news set off international controversy over science and ethics. Some condemned the action as premature, unconscionable, and morally or ethically indefensible. Others argued that even if the gene editing worked perfectly, individuals without the normal CCR5 gene face the risk of getting other viruses such as West Nile and dying from flu (Marchione 2018; Morgan 2018). He Jiankui justified his research on the ground that he performed gene editing to protect babies from future infection with the AIDS virus because HIV infection is a big problem in China. He also stated that he had practiced gene editing with mice, monkeys, and human embryos in the lab for several years (Harney and Kelland 2018; Marchione 2018).

He Jiankui, immediately following his announcement, facing a skeptical and incensed audience at the International Summit on Human Gene Editing in November of 2018, offered an apology for the fact that the results were leaked unexpectedly and announced that his study had been submitted to a scientific journal for peer review. He also announced that a potential second gene-edited pregnancy was underway at a very early stage. The summit was organized to try to reach an international consensus on whether, how, and when it might be permissible to create children from genetically modified embryos ("The Latest: Scientist Reports 2nd Gene-Edited Pregnancy" 2018; Stein 2018). Meanwhile, Chinese health officials and medical ethics authorities have started an investigation into the claims. The Southern University of Science and Technology, where He Jiankui is an associate professor, announced that it was unaware of the project, which was a serious violation of academic ethics and standards, and that He Jiankui was on leave without pay (Harney and Kelland 2018). He was ultimately fired by the university in January 2019.

Germline Human Gene Editing and Ethical Concerns

Today there appears to be a consensus among scientists, physicians, legal experts, and ethicists that when it comes to human genome editing, one needs to proceed slowly due to several ethical concerns raised by human germline editing. The need for caution and moving forward very slowly with respect to human germline modification is justified on the following grounds. One, there is a need to consider the interests of future generations, since germline gene modification will be passed on. Second, there is a need to first evaluate the risks and safety concerns involved in germline human gene editing, since any errors, mistakes, and side effects could be passed on to future generations, and they may be irreversible. Third, it could lead to more inequality. Fourth is the importance of the public's trust in science. Fifth, the potential exists for misuse of this technology for human enhancement and eugenics (Mahoney and Siegal 2018).

Mahoney and Siegal (2018) argue that the problem with the "go-very-slow" approach is that fast developments are overtaking such an approach and efforts to constrain the spread of germline human gene editing may not only fail but may drive cutting-edge technology work into the shadows, out of sight of government regulators and scientific organizations. They attempt to debunk all of the arguments in defence of the "go-very-slow" approach. First, they argue that human history demonstrates that humans have always engaged in mate selection with an eye toward the characteristics of their decedents and new gene editing technologies simply help make a better choice of mate by avoiding inherited genetic diseases. Thus, it protects the interests of future generations. The argument that editing human germlines will lead to irreversible consequences is unsatisfactory because current human behavior already has a significant impact on the genotypes of members of the future generations and a go-slow approach ignores the nature of innovation. There is no clear answer to how the current generation should take account of the needs and preferences of future generations. Second, all medical technologies entail some risks and things could always go wrong but equally absurd would be to demand perfect safety since such demand would make any medical progress impossible. Third, the strongest demand for human germline editing will be for modifications that help eliminate heritable diseases. Thus, the argument that germline human gene editing will worsen inequality is not very persuasive. In fact, by eliminating burdensome heritable diseases such as sickle-cell anemia and Huntington's disease, such technology can help create more equality. Fourth, the argument that a lack of a moratorium on germline human gene editing will lead to a loss of public trust in science is speculative. In fact, a 2016 Pew Research Center poll found that a large number of Americans view science and technology as beneficial forces in American society. Finally, the fear that germline human gene editing will lead to human enhancement, i.e., "designer babies," and eugenics, i.e., involuntary sterilization and termination of "unfit" individuals or groups of people, was supported in the past by the belief that alleged collective goods trumped the rights of the individual. The main goal of the heritable genome editing will be to expand the options available to individuals.

Human enhancement could take the form of *pharmacological enhancement*, which includes stimulant drugs that can be used to ward off sleep, to improve concentration, and in blood doping by athletes to increase muscle endurance; *cybernetic enhancement*, which involves the transformation of humans into cyborgs or cybernetic organisms; *genetic enhancement*, which can include sex selection of offspring, the exclusion of offspring with certain genetic diseases by parental screening, selective abortion, *in-vitro* fertilization, or embryo selection; and *nanotechnology enhancement*, which to many holds the greatest promise since the structure of all biological molecules such as proteins, enzymes, and DNA have dimensions on the nanoscale, making it possible to analyze and repair any physical defects in the body. While some forms of enhancement offer many benefits, critics of enhancement put forth the following arguments against human enhancement. First, they argue that new human enhancements are unnatural because they aim to alter human beings in fundamental ways by transforming the structure of the human body or the way it functions, or by transforming the nature of the human mind. Second, new enhancement poses certain definite risks including liver tumors, high blood pressure, and the like, and the risks far outweigh the expected benefits. Third, such enhancements pose risks to the social fabric of society by increasing the divide between the haves and the have-nots, since people of lower socioeconomic status will not have equal access to all these enhancements. Fourth, such enhancements may harm self-esteem and freedom of choice. An industry that is the major funder of enhancement research has a vested interest in making money by promoting the message that no one is ever good enough or happy enough without such enhancements. However, enhancement advocates say that while new enhancements are unconventional there is nothing sacred about our present system of doing things or the current nature of humans. Humans are continually evolving and new enhancements allow society to take full advantage of scientific and technological knowledge to control our own evolution (Kourany 2014).

Rehmann-Sutter (2018) provides counter-arguments to Mahoney and Siegal's (2018) pro-germline human gene editing position. He suggests that the claim that human germline gene editing is in the best interest of the child-to-be who has an interest in being cured is factually incorrect because the embryo, a potential future patient, is brought into existence by the same act that is also the treatment. The act of curing presupposes a person who is ill and will be better off after and an individual who can live well or unwell, which is questionable. The therapeutic assumption behind germline human gene editing is that it aims at producing a future person, not a patient in need and is based on the hope that the treated embryo will, in fact, be born and develop into a healthy child. Without this assumption, it simply becomes an intervention and not a cure. Any deliberate modification into the genome of the germline cannot be evaluated purely on the effect of change itself would have on the subsequent generations. Making germline changes can lead to both potentially beneficial as well as harmful tools at science's disposal. The unchanged parts of the germline DNA, as well as the remaining risks and side effects, would be the result of decisions made by an earlier generation, which could be prone to fallibility. Decisions about the germline human gene editing will in a fundamental way change the structure of the relationship between generations. Germline human gene editing is ethically more complicated than just curing diseases. Thus, the author argues that germline human gene editing could not be justified as a therapeutic imperative or even as a moral obligation.

Some bioethicists and policymakers express fear of genetic enhancement and advocate banning germline human gene editing while others advocate proceeding full-scale because of the prospect of eliminating hereditary disease and the increased level of comfort with the concept of regenerative medicine. A middle or moderate ground is occupied by those who take the position that biomedical enhancement technologies cannot be and should not be banned but instead should be controlled by extending and enlarging mechanisms for regulation of such research, application, and treatment (Mehlman 2009).

The Regulation of Gene Editing and Gene Therapy

The US follows a fairly permissive approach in its regulation of biotechnology as applied to genetically engineered animals and plants. The agriculture industry was quick to jump on gene editing to improve crops. The regulation of genetically modified crops is divided among three federal regulatory agencies—The US Department of Agriculture's Animal and Plant Inspection Service, the US Environmental Protection Service (EPA), and the Food and Drug Administration (FDA) within the Department of Health and Human Services (Alta Charo 2016; "Gene Editing" n.d.).

However, the United States follows a more cautious approach when it comes to biotechnology when applied in the context of human research, clinical trials, and gene therapies. The broader context for ethics involving human subjects was established in 1979 by the National Commission for the Protection of Human Subjects in Biomedical and Behavioral Research in its landmark Belmont Report, which established principles of avoiding harm, accepting the duty of beneficence, and commitment to justice. These principles have come to put emphasis on balancing risks and benefits and respecting individual autonomy (Alta Charo 2016; National Academy of Sciences, Engineering, and Medicine et al. 2017). In general, a great deal of emphasis is placed on self-regulation by the scientific community. Over time, voluntary self-regulatory activities may get incorporated as part of formal government regulation.

In the United States, gene therapy is treated as a biological drug or a device and thus it falls under the purview and regulation of the FDA. The FDA also regulates human genome editing under its existing regulatory framework for biological products. In general, laboratory work and research are subject to local oversight by Institutional Biosafety Committees (IBCs), Institutional Review Boards (IRBs), and the Recombinant DNA Advisory Committee (RAC) established by the National Institutes of Health (NIH) in 1974. The FDA seeks advice and guidance from such advisory bodies to ensure the safety of human subjects and to make sure that human clinical trials are conducted in line with the country's norms and regulations. Clinical genome editing trials cannot commence without permission from the FDA. The FDA performs its oversight function by the monitoring of clinical trials, reviews, and evaluating data related to the safety, effectiveness, and appropriate use of human cells, tissues, and gene-transfer therapies with the help and advice of IBCs, IRBs, and RAC, and other federal advisory committees such as the Cellular, Tissue and Gene Therapies Advisory Committee (National Academy of Sciences, Engineering, and Medicine et al. 2017). Once a drug, device, or biologic is approved by the FDA and is on the market, the regulatory control becomes much weaker. In short, the FDA regulates the products but not the physicians who use the products. Thus, physicians can take a product that was approved for one purpose and use it for a different purpose, dosage, or population (Alta Charo 2016).

Finally, when it comes specifically to the regulation of germline human genome editing, countries utilize many different approaches. Some countries prohibit all germline human genome intervention. Other countries have relied on advisory guidelines. Still, other countries allow limited application of germline human genome editing. The United States follows a complicated regulatory framework under which germline human genome research (editing sperm, eggs, or embryos) is allowed only in the lab. There are strict funding restrictions in place on embryo research and the NIH has restated its ban on gene editing of human embryos (Alta Charo 2016; Marchione 2018; Smaglik 2017).

THE ROLE OF THE HEALTHCARE WORKFORCE

The healthcare workforce consists of people who provide direct patient care and includes staff that support the caregivers and health institutions such as hospitals, clinics, doctors' offices, and nursing homes, and as such the healthcare workforce is the most significant component of a nation's healthcare infrastructure (Salsberg 2014). The healthcare workforce is an important resource to enhance the health of a nation and one of the most important determinants of a nation's health, expenditures, and health outcomes (Constantin 2014). As such it plays a crucial role in the healthcare delivery system. An effective healthcare workforce requires the right mix of essential healthcare providers who have the right skills and training, and are geographically distributed relative to the healthcare needs of the population. The interaction between healthcare providers within multiple care settings requires a team approach to improve healthcare outcomes (Solis 2012).

According to the Bureau of Labor Statistics (BLS), in 2016, 13 of the 30 fastest-growing occupations in the United States are in healthcare, ranging from physician assistants, nurse practitioners, and medical assistants, to home health and personal care aids and genetic Counselors (US Department of Labor 2018). The major factors driving demand for healthcare employment include expansion of healthcare coverage under the ACA, advances in health information technology and medical sciences, changing and increasing healthcare needs due to an aging population, and a push toward improved delivery and quality of care. The American healthcare system is undergoing a major transformation due to new technologies, new competition, new reimbursement methods, demographic trends, and regulatory uncertainties. These changes in turn impact how healthcare is delivered, how healthcare is paid for, and how health systems manage costs and the future of the healthcare workforce (Stevenson 2018). The healthcare workforce is at the center of the American healthcare system's transformation.

The current transformation of the American healthcare system will impact all sectors of healthcare, including how healthcare is delivered and the changing role of the healthcare workforce. It will be important to figure out the changing role of the healthcare workforce in the future as well as how future changes in the healthcare workforce will impact access to care and the quality of care. It will require healthcare providers to understand, anticipate, and prepare for future turnovers and shortages within the healthcare workforce (Stevenson 2018). This will be a crucial factor in the American healthcare system's ability to deliver accessibly and quality care in an increasingly diverse society with complex medical needs. However, accurately predicting or anticipating future changes particularly in healthcare is problematic because of an unpredictable political agenda, unforeseen economic circumstances, and rapidly changing medical technology (Danielson and Wendel 2016).

The Profile of the Healthcare Workforce

The US government's Standard Occupation Classifications list 34 health occupations employing millions of individuals. Some of the largest health occupations are registered nurses, physicians, home health aides, and personal care aides. Recent years have witnessed significant growth in physician assistants and medical assistants ("U.S. Health Workforce Chartbook—In Brief" 2018).

Physicians

Physicians are the most important component of the healthcare workforce. There are 990,688 professional active physicians in the United States. This includes both allopathic (MDs) and osteopathic (DOs) physicians. MDs typically treat disease, while DOs focus on the musculoskeletal system and emphasize preventive medicine and take a more holistic approach to health. Of the total, 518,128 (52 percent) are specialists while 472,560 (48 percent) are primary-care physicians. Of the total primary-care physicians, around 41 percent are concentrated in the field of internal medicine, 29 percent in family or general practice, 18 percent in pediatrics, and 11 percent in obstetrics and gynecology. Primary care is the most fundamental element of the US healthcare system and primary-care physicians act as gatekeepers to specialized care. Primary care is critical in ensuring access to healthcare for all Americans. The top five fields of practice among specialists include psychiatry and emergency medicine (11 percent each), surgery and anesthesiology (10 percent each), and emergency medicine (10 percent). The rest practice in the fields of radiology, cardiology, oncology, endocrinology and others (Kaiser Family Foundation 2018a).

Of the total number of active physicians, 65 percent are male while 35 percent are female (Kaiser Family Foundation 2018a). By race, 67 percent of active physicians are white, 19.7 percent are Asian Native/Hawaiian-Pacific Islander, 6.3 percent are Hispanic, 4.8 percent are black/African-American, 0.1 percent are American Indian/Alaska Native, and 2.1 percent are of multiple races or other races ("U.S. Health Workforce Chartbook Part I: Clinicians" 2018).

Physician Assistants

Physician assistants (PAs), like general internists or doctors, diagnose illnesses, develop and implement treatment plans, provide general guidance to patients, and assist in surgeries. However, by law, they are required to practice under the supervision of a licensed physician or a surgeon. PAs are certified by the National Commission on Certification of Physician Assistants (NCCPA). There are 123,089 certified PAs in the United States and their numbers are growing. Between 2010 and 2017, the PA profession grew 45.8 percent. Of the total number of PAs, 68 percent are females and 38 percent are males. The median age of PAs is around 38. Whites constitute an overwhelming majority (86.9 percent) of PAs, Asians 5.6 percent, blacks/African-Americans 3.7 percent, American Indians/Alaska Natives 0.3 percent, and 3.1 percent make up the other races (National Commission on Certification of Physician Assistants 2017a).

One of the major trends in healthcare is the significant growth in the number of certified PAs driven by changes in technology, the scope of practice and specialization, and its impact on how healthcare is delivered. PAs have also filled the gap created by a shortage of physicians and increased demand for health services created by increased access to healthcare due to the ACA and other reforms. The *U.S. News and World Report* (2018) ranked physician assistants in third place among the 100 best jobs in America. The scope of PAs' practice is expanding as state legislatures look for ways give patients more access to a qualified healthcare provider. Several states already give PAs full authority to prescribe medicine. Some states are considering eliminating the number of PAs that a physician can supervise.

Historically, certified PAs primarily worked in the area of primary care. However, that has changed as more PAs have moved into specialty services prompted by demographic shifts (aging population), increasing demand for more specialty services. Today, more than 70 percent of certified PAs practice in specialty areas outside of primary care. Some of the areas of high growth include surgery, emergency medicine, hospital medicine, and psychiatry. PAs can also earn a Certificate of Added Qualification (CAQ) in seven specialty areas. The prevalence and growth in the number of PAs mean that patients are more likely to encounter a PA for treatment. Some of the top PA practice settings include office-based private practices (40.6 percent), hospitals (40 percent), federal government facilities/hospitals/military facilities (5.6 percent), urgent care settings (3.2 percent), and community health centers (3.1 percent) (National Commission on Certification of Physician Assistants 2017b, 2018).

Nurses

There are 4.2 million professionally active nurses in the United States, of whom 3.1 million (80 percent) are registered nurses (RNs) and 821,298 (20 percent) are licensed practical nurses (LPNs). Of the total, 88 percent are female while 8 percent are male, and 4 percent are unspecified (Kaiser Family Foundation 2018b).

Nurses' role in the United States can be divided into three broad categories: (1) registered nurses (RNs) who provide healthcare in a variety of setting and perform physical exams, health history, health promotion, education, and counseling, and coordinate care with other healthcare professionals. (2) Advance-practice registered nurses (APRNs) hold at least a master's degree and provide primary and preventive care, treat and diagnose illnesses, and manage chronic disease. They also perform a specialist role in areas of mental health, low-risk obstetrical care, prescribe medication, diagnose and treat minor illnesses, and more. (3) Licensed practical nurses (LPNs), also known as licensed vocational nurses (LVNs), work under the supervision of RNs, APRNs, or physicians ("What is Nursing?" n.d.).

Medical Assistants

In 2016, there were 634,400 medical assistants (MAs) in the United States and their numbers are expected to rise 29 percent between 2016 and 2026. They are one of the fastest-growing occupations in the US. MAs generally perform administrative and clinical tasks under the supervision of a physician. They work in primary-care settings, including doctors' offices, hospitals, and a variety of other healthcare facilities. Medical assistants typically have a postsecondary education such as a certificate (Bureau of Labor Statistics 2018). The majority of MA training programs are one year or less in duration. MAs are racially and ethnically diverse—57 percent white, 23 percent Hispanic, 14 percent African-American, and 4 percent Asian.

In the traditional role, MAs escorted patients to an exam room, taking vital signs, and recording patients' description of illness for the physician. However, their role is changing and they are taking on increased duties, responsibilities, and more autonomy, including some new functions that overlap with other occupations such as radiology technician. Medical assistants can be cross-trained in flexible roles (Chapman and Blash 2017).

Community Health Workers

The community health workers include both paid professionals and volunteers. They provide a range of health and social services that include patient education, patient advocacy, community outreach, interpretation services, social support, and connecting patients with resources. Due to the variety of job titles and a large number of unpaid volunteers, estimating the size of the community health workers is problematic. Federal estimates put the number at 115,700 in 2014. The group tends to be more diverse than other groups, with more than 80 percent being women and one-third Hispanic (Whatley et al. 2017).

Community health workers have gained new attention due to their ability to act as a bridge between the community and different healthcare facilities/settings. They have also moved from being employed largely in community-based organizations to being employed by hospitals and health systems (Washkow and Fennell 2017).

Other Healthcare Support Workers

The healthcare support workers include lower-skilled workers such as home health aides, personal care aides, and medical and clinical lab technologists. Largely due to the aging population, the demand for them is expected to grow the most and the fastest through 2025 (Mercer LLC 2018).

The Healthcare Workforce and Challenges Facing the American Healthcare System

Reform to the ACA, combined with other healthcare/insurance and health systems reform, is transforming the American healthcare system in a significant way. The success of the American healthcare system in meeting the future needs of the population will depend on how successfully it meets the challenges it faces.

Healthcare Workforce Shortages

Advances in modern medicine leading to increased life expectancy, overall population growth, increased access to healthcare because of healthcare reforms, and the aging population will increase demand for healthcare workers in years to come.

Being at the heart of the healthcare system, physicians are in high demand. The top ten types of physicians that are in high demand are primary-care/family physicians, internists, pediatricians, psychiatrists, obstetricians and gynecologists, surgeons, anesthesiologists, pathologists, neurologist, and allergists and immunologists ("20 Types of Physicians in High Demand" 2018). Several professional medical organizations have sounded warning alarms about coming future shortages of physicians covering primary care to various subspecialties. However, their projections of shortages tend to vary considerably. Many of the projections cite years 2025 or 2030 as the tipping point when finding a doctor will become very difficult unless something is done to address the future predicted shortages.

The supply of doctors seeing patients full-time is declining as many Baby Boomer-generation physicians are readying for retirement and will be leaving the workforce in the next 10 to 15 years. Some physicians are leaving the profession to pursue other careers. Additionally, young people are becoming less interested in pursuing medical careers with increased opportunities in science, technology, engineering, math, and medicine (STEM) jobs. They also want to live in hip, urban areas, which often is not possible for those coming fresh out of medical school and in need of a residency (Howley 2018; Spector 2018).

The American Academy of Family Physicians (AAFP) projects a shortage of 149,000 physicians by 2020. Twenty-four states have released reports projecting physician shortages and 21 other medical specialties have released reports projecting shortages in their fields (Florence 2018). The Association of American Medical Colleges (AAMC) forecasts that in 15 years, the United States will face a shortage of up to 159,300 physicians. The AAMC also projects that the ACA and increased access to healthcare would increase physician shortage by an additional 31,000. According to the AAMC, by 2030 there would be a shortage of primary-care physicians between 14,800 and 49,300, and a shortfall of between 33,800 and 72,700 non-primary-care physicians, including 20,700 to 30,500 surgical specialists (Association of American Medical Colleges 2018). The general surgeon shortage is expected to become worse since the number of doctors graduating each year is not keeping up with the needs of a growing and aging population. Shortages are also expected in the areas of vascular surgery and neurosurgery (Darves 2017).

One of the most serious problem areas is the shortage of primary-care or general-care physicians. Only one in four medical students select to go into primary care. There are several reasons for this. First, many medical students choose not to go into primary care because of the lower income compared to the income of specialists. Second, there is accelerated demand for more medical care due to increased access and a growing population. Third, few medical schools express interest in community service or primary care in their admission decisions. Fourth, medical school graduates tend to stay and practice in areas where they went to school. Fifth, there is no government oversight over how physicians are sorted into different specialties (Court 2016; DeAngelis 2016).

Some have argued that there is no need to worry about the shortage of physicians, especially primary-care physicians, because of the growing number of PAs and NPs who can fill the gap. However, there are certain limitations to this approach. While around 83 percent of NPs are certified in primary care, only about 24 percent of PAs are in primary care and the rest practice in specialties. Additionally, the PA accreditation process takes a long time—almost three years from the start of the process until initial approval of the class and five years until the first class graduates (Danielson and Wendel 2016).

The problem of the future shortage is not limited to physicians. Nursing is projected to have some of the highest demand over the next 10 to 15 years. While hospitals employ the largest number of nurses, job growth is expected to be fastest for registered nurses in the area of home healthcare, a 61-percent increase by 2024 ("Graphics: The Exploding Health Care Workforce" 2017). Demand is also expected to grow significantly for lower-skilled healthcare workers such as home health aides, nursing assistants, and medical and clinical lab technicians. For example, jobs for home health aides are expected to grow 32 percent by 2025 and experience a shortage of 446,300. Similarly, by 2025, the shortage of nursing assistants is expected to be 95,000 and 58,700 for medical and clinical lab technicians (Mercer LLC 2018).

Geographic Maldistribution

Compounding the problem of the healthcare workforce shortage is the geographic maldistribution of the workforce. There is a long-standing maldistribution of physicians in the United States. This maldistribution is most pronounced between urban and rural areas and inner cities. For example, the Health Services and Resources Administration designates 6200 health professional shortage areas for primary care nationwide and 67 percent of shortage areas are in non-urban areas (Florence 2018). Similarly, it is difficult to attract specialists to rural areas.

Thus, it is important to note that sometimes it is misleading to talk about healthcare workforce shortages as if they are nationwide and spread evenly across all parts of the country. Shortages are dire in some parts (regions or states) of the country while others may have a surplus. For example, the shortage of physicians is most acute in parts of the South since it has many rural areas. It also has many large minority communities. Providing the same amount of medical care to underserved areas would require many more healthcare workers in these areas (Ollove 2016). Similarly, the projection of nurse shortages will be also spread unevenly in the country. In fact, many states are expected to have a surplus of nurses but states such as Texas and Illinois are expected to experience shortages (Mercer LLC 2018). Thus, in the long run, the distribution of the healthcare workforce will be uneven, with large cities and urban areas facing less-severe repercussions in contrast to rural areas (Spanu 2018).

To address the problem of shortages, some states like Georgia and Texas are increasing the number of medical residencies to keep doctors in their states after completion of their residency. Some states are offering grants and stipends to medical students and residents who are willing to do clinical rotations in parts of the state where the need is greatest. Other states have created branches of their medical schools in underserved areas. States like Arkansas, Kansas, and Missouri are enabling medical students to treat patients before completing their residencies. Most states have also embraced telemedicine while others have liberalized state laws to allow NPs and PAs to perform some treatments normally done by physicians (Ollove 2016).

Lack of Racial Diversity

The Institute of Medicine (2008) report *Unequal Treatment: Confronting Racial and Ethnic Disparities in Health Care* not only demonstrated the existence of racial/ethnic disparities in healthcare but also recommended increasing the proportion of underrepresented minority groups in the healthcare workforce and cross-cultural training. Racial and cultural diversity in the healthcare workforce can be an effective tool to help reduce disparities in healthcare. Yet, more than a decade after the report, very little progress has been made in increasing the racial/ethnic diversity in the healthcare workforce. As the US population becomes racially and culturally more diverse, cultural competence of the healthcare providers will become an important factor to better serve patients with diverse racial and cultural backgrounds (Jackson and Gracia 2014).

According to a US Census Bureau projection, by 2050, minority groups will be a numerical majority in the United States. This racial/ethnic demographic transition will have important consequences, including a demand for more minority healthcare workers. According to the American Association of Medical Colleges, blacks, Hispanics, and American Indians/Alaska Natives represented only 12 percent of the physician workforce in 2010 while they accounted for 30 percent of the general population. The same year non-Hispanic whites made up 83 percent of licensed registered nurses, with blacks and Hispanics/Latino people accounting for a combined 9 percent of licensed registered nurses (LaVeist and Pierre 2014).

The primary mission of the Health Resources and Service Administration (HRSA) is to improve health and achieve health equity, and one of the key elements of this mission is to ensure a diverse healthcare workforce to improve healthcare access, quality, outcomes, patient satisfaction, and patient-healthcare provider communication, especially in underserved populations. Diversity in health occupations is measured by the representation of the minority groups in a health occupation relative to their numbers in the general population. The lower representation of minority groups in healthcare occupations relative to their numbers in the general population signifies lack of racial/ethnic diversity in the workforce. The HRSA's 2017 report on the distribution of gender and racial/ethnic distribution among 30 health occupations during the 2011–2015 time period provides some additional insight about healthcare workforce diversity, or the lack thereof. The 30 health occupations are grouped into six major categories: community and social services (e.g., counselors, social workers); life, physical, and social sciences (psychologists); health diagnosing and treating practitioners (physicians, PAs, nurses, therapists, dentists, etc.); health technologists and technicians (emergency medical technicians (EMTs), paramedics, clinical and health information technologists, etc.; healthcare support (MAs, home health aides, dental assistants, etc.); and personal care services (personal care aides) (Health Resources and Services Administration 2017).

According to the report, white workers represent the majority component of all 30 health occupations, representing over 50 percent of almost every occupation, and whites are overrepresented in 23 of the 30 occupations. Whites are heavily concentrated in the life, physical and social sciences, and health diagnosing and treating practitioners' occupations. For example, whites constitute 84 percent of the psychologist workforce, Hispanics 6.3 percent, blacks 4.9 percent, Asians 3.4 percent, and American Indians/Alaska Natives 0.2 percent. Minority groups are also underrepresented in many of the occupations in the health technologies and technicians' category. In contrast, minority groups are well represented in occupations that fall into the category of healthcare support and personal care services. The occupations in which whites are most underrepresented are home health aides and personal care aides. In summary, minority groups are often underrepresented in more high-skill health occupations and overrepresented in lower-skill health occupations.

By 2050, a majority of the population in the United States is expected to be non-white, i.e., racial/ethnic minorities will make up a majority of the population. From 2012 to 2060, the Hispanic population is expected to more than double from 53.3 million (16.6 percent) in 2012 to 128.8 million (33 percent); the African-American population is expected to grow from 41.2 million (13.1 percent) 61.8 million (14.7 percent); the Asian population is expected to double from 15.9 million (5.1 percent) to 34.4 million (8.2 percent); and the size of the American Indian/Alaska Native population is expected to grow from 3.9 million to 6.3 million while Native Hawaiians and other Pacific Islanders are expected to double from a population of 706,000 to 1.4 million. Finally, the number of people who identify themselves as belonging to two or more races is expected to more than triple from 7.5 million to 26.7 million (Phillips and Malone 2014).

Increasing the diversity of the healthcare workforce remains one of the major challenges facing the American healthcare system.

Gender Equity and Discrimination

Although males represent a larger proportion of the US workforce, female workers represent the majority in 25 of the 30 health occupations analyzed by the HRSA. However, women are underrepresented in certain health occupations—Dentists (27.4 percent), chiropractors (28.2 percent), physicians (34.9 percent), and optometrists (40.1 percent). Women are also underrepresented in EMTs, and among paramedics (Health Resources and Services Administration 2017). Similarly, fewer than 6 percent of urologists are women despite the fact that women constitute 30 percent of the patients. The fact that patients often exhibit a preference to receive care from physicians of the same gender, especially in certain subspecialties like urology, tends to contribute to gender disparity (McDevitt and Roberts 2014).

There is a persistent salary gap within the nursing workforce despite the fact that women have predominated the nursing profession. According to a national salary research report, male nurses earn more (average salary of ($79,688) than female nurses ($73,090). The study concluded that gender bias was alive and well in nursing ("Nursing Salary Research Report" 2018). Foreign-born nurses, home aides, and personal care aide workers are also likely to make a lower salary compared to those born in the US (Lowell 2013). Similarly, despite the fact that US healthcare has become more dependent on immigrants, especially women physicians, they are more likely to experience gender as well as race-based discrimination from employers and colleagues (Bhatt 2013).

Gender inequality is more pronounced with respect to women in the top echelon of the executive in the field of healthcare, where they remain underrepresented. Gender difference also exists in the types of leadership roles women obtain as well as salary even when controlling for differences in educational attainment, age, and experience. Ideas and perceptions about leadership are often gender-based. Studies suggest that men and women prefer male leaders even when credentials of male and female candidates are the same. This is often due to stereotypes of female attributes and behavior such as cooperation, modesty, and emotiveness often tending to be viewed as incongruent with strong leadership (Lantz 2008).

More recent data confirm the same findings. Women are underrepresented in leadership positions in the healthcare industry. None of the Fortune 500 healthcare companies had a woman serving as a CEO in 2018 and only 21 percent of companies' board members were women. Furthermore, women who do make it to the executive level are more likely to be in human resources, legal, and marketing functions and less likely to be operations or technology positions. For example, according to the Bureau of Labor statistics, in 2016, 74 percent of human resources managers were women. Among the top 100 hospitals, women make up only about 32 percent of executives and 11 percent of CEOs. The most common hospital executive role for women is chief nursing officer. Despite the fact that the nursing profession is dominated by women, they earn lower salaries than male nurses and they are less likely to end up in management positions. Only about one-third of physicians are women and they make less money than their male counterparts (Joyce 2018; Tecco 2018). To address this problem will require more effective mentoring of women and minorities, attention to leadership succession, and leadership development by healthcare organizations providing better career development opportunities (Lantz 2008; Tecco 2018).

An Aging Population

One of the most significant demographic trends in the United States is the growth of the population aged 65 and older. Planning for and meeting the healthcare needs of the Baby Boomers (those born between 1946 and 1964) will present a unique challenge to the American healthcare system. According to the Population Reference Bureau's 2015 report, "Aging in the United States," the number of Americans 65 and older is projected to more than double from 46 million in 2014 to 98 million by 2060. The proportion of people 65 and older will increase from 15 percent to 24 percent of the total population. The older population is also projected to become racially and ethnically more diverse. About 27 percent of women aged 65 to 74, 41 percent of women aged 75 to 84, and 56 percent of women aged 85 and older lived alone in 2014. The aging of the Baby Boomer generation could fuel a 75-percent increase in the number of people 65 and older requiring nursing home care by 2030. The number of Americans living with Alzheimer's disease could triple by 2050 (Mather, Jacobsen, and Pollard 2015).

This will require retooling the healthcare workforce to meet the healthcare needs of an aging America. The Institute of Medicine (2008), in its report titled *Retooling for an Aging America*, concluded that as the population of seniors grows, they will face a healthcare workforce that will be too small and critically unprepared to meet their healthcare needs. The report called for bold initiatives designed to explore ways to enhance the geriatric competence of the entire healthcare workforce, increase recruitment and retention of geriatric specialists and caregivers, and improve the way healthcare is delivered. Many of the recommendations of the report still remain unfulfilled and eldercare workforce reform has failed to keep pace with eldercare healthcare service demands. The ACA's direct impact on the eldercare workforce has been limited. Grants under the Personal and Home Aides State Training (PHAST) programs have had only a modest impact at the state level (Dawson and Langston 2016).

CONCLUSION

The American healthcare system is undergoing a major transformation as a result of healthcare and insurance reforms, medical and technological advances, market forces, as well as population growth and demographic changes. As a result, American healthcare will face many challenges in the coming decades and how it responds to these challenges will have significant consequences in meeting the future needs of Americans. In this chapter, we have discussed four major challenges facing American healthcare—the opioid crisis, specialty drugs, gene editing and gene therapy, and the healthcare workforce.

Over 100,000 lives are destroyed every year because of prescription and/or illicit drug overdose at a high human and economic cost to the society. While overdose deaths are happening in every age group and every region of the country, they have impacted young and middle-aged whites, both men and women, more than any other age group and have had a disproportionate impact on small-town rural America, more than on urban America. Many factors have contributed to this crisis and it will require a comprehensive strategy to address the problem. Federal funds and state efforts to address the problem have produced some successes but we still have a long way to go in solving the problem.

Specialty drugs have given hope to millions of Americans suffering from debilitating illnesses and the FDA has accelerated its approval process to make these drugs available to the patients as soon as possible. However, the market for such drugs is limited and thus they have high price tags attached to them. The high cost of specialty drugs is driving up overall healthcare costs. Given the high price, they also raise questions about accessibility, affordability, and cost-effectiveness.

Similarly, gene editing has opened up a new field of regenerative medicine and personalized medicine. Gene therapy has the potential to revolutionize the future of medicine and raises the possibility of not only treating but also curing or eliminating certain inheritable diseases entirely. However, like specialty drugs, gene therapy is very expensive and raises questions about who should pay for it. Additionally, gene editing in general and germline human gene editing in particular raises a host of ethical concerns including potential misuse and abuse of such technology.

Finally, population and demographic trends in American society point to a need for a retooling of the American healthcare workforce to meet the healthcare needs of the aging and racially diverse population. The American healthcare system needs to address the problems of healthcare workforce shortages and their geographic maldistribution, lack of racial-ethnic diversity, gender inequity and discrimination, and an aging population.

STUDY QUESTIONS

1. What factors have helped contribute to the problem of the opioid epidemic in American society? Who should bear the responsibility for the problem and why it is not a major problem in other countries?
2. Discuss the nature and scope of the opioid epidemic.
3. Discuss the demographics and geography of the opioid crisis.
4. Why does the pharmaceutical industry have a great deal of influence on American health policy?
5. Discuss the federal and state efforts to address the opioid crisis. How successful are they?
6. What are specialty drugs? What role does the FDA play in their approval?
7. Discuss the cost of specialty drugs; what factors account for their high prices? What are the arguments for and against high prices of specialty drugs?
8. What are some of the strategies to reduce or offset the high price of specialty drugs?
9. Discuss the evolution of gene therapy, including early failures and recent successes.
10. What are the pros and cons of gene therapy?
11. Discuss the controversy surrounding germline human gene editing, including ethical concerns raised by it.
12. Discuss the challenges confronting the American healthcare workforce.

REFERENCES

"$1-Million Price Tag Set for Glybera Gene Therapy." 2015. *Nature*. Online at www.nature.com/articles/nbt0315-217.
"12 Procs and Cons of Gene Therapy." n.d. Vittana Blog. Online at https://vittana.org/.
"17 Biggest Pros and Cons of Gene Therapy." 2018. Brandon Gaille. Online at https://brandongaille.com/.
"20 Types of Physicians in High Demand." St. George's University. Online at www.sgu.edu/.
"21st Century Cures Act." 2018. US Food and Drug Administration. Online at www.fda.gov/.
AARP Public Policy Institute. 2016. "Price Growth for Brand Name and Specialty Drugs More than Offset Substantial Price Decreases for Generic Drugs." AARP Public Policy Institute. Online at www.aarp.org/.
Academy of Managed Care Pharmacy. 2006. "Concept Series Paper on Specialty Pharmaceuticals." Academy of Managed Care Pharmacy. Online at http://amcp.org/.
Achenbach, Joel. 2016. "No Longer 'Mayberry': A Small Ohio City Fights an Epidemic of Self-Destruction." *Washington Post*. Online at www.washingtonpost.com/.
Allen, Greg. 2017. "Should the Opioid Crisis Be Declared a National Emergency?" NPR. Online at www.npr.org/.
Almendrala, Anna. 2018. "The Gene-Editing Babies and CRISPR-Cas9 Controversy, Explained." *Huffington Post*. Online at www.huffingtonpost.com/.
Alta Charo, R. 2016. "The Legal and Regulatory Context for Human Gene Editing." *Issues in Science and Technology*, 32, no. 3 (March): 39–44.
Annas, George J. 1989. "At Law: Who's Afraid of the Human Genome?" *Hastings Center Report*, 19, no. 4 (July–August): 19–21.
"Approved Cellular and Gene Therapy Products." 2018. US Food and Drug Administration. Online at www.fda.gov/.
Association of American Medical Colleges. 2018. *2018 Update: The Complexities of Physician Supply and Demand: Projections from 2016 to 2030*. Final Report. Washington, DC: HIS Markit, Ltd. Online at www.aamc.org/data/workforce.
Ayers, Ian and Amen Jalal. 2018. "The Impact of Prescription Drug Monitoring Programs on U.S. Opioid Prescriptions." *Journal of Law, Medicine & Ethics*, 46, no. 2 (Summer): 387–403.
Baltimore, David et al. 2016. "On Human Gene Editing: International Summit Statement by the Organizing Committee." *Issues in Science and Technology*, 32, no. 3 (March): 55–56.
Bartolone, Pauline. 2018. "Drug Overdose Death Soar Nationally but Plateau in Some States." Governing. Online at www.governing.com/.
Basu, Tanya. 2017. "Trump Foolishly Thinks He Can Solve the Opioid Crisis with Zero Cash and a Dumb Ad Campaign." *The Daily Beast*. Online at www.thedailybeast.com/.
Bellon, Tina. 2018. "U.S. State Lawsuits Against Purdue Pharma Over Opioid Epidemic Mount." Reuters. Online at www.reuters.com/.
Benedetti, Sara, Hidetoshi Hoshiya, and Francesco S. Tedesco. 2013. "Repair or Replace? Exploiting Novel Gene Therapy Strategies for Muscular Dystrophies." *Federation of European Biochemical Society Journal*, 280, no. 17 (February): 4263–4280.
Bernstein, Lenny. 2018. "FDA Approves Powerful Opioid despite Fears of More Overdose Deaths." *Washington Post*. Online at www.washingtonpost.com/.
Best, Shivali. 2016. "China Tests Controversial 'Cut and Paste' Gene-Editing Technique on a Human in World's First." *Daily Mail*. Online at www.dailymail.co.uk/.
Bhatt, Washuda. 2013. "The Little Brown Woman: Gender Discrimination in American Medicine." *Gender & Society*, 27, no. 5 (October): 659–680.
Birnbaum, Howard G., Alan G. White, Matt Schiller, Tracy Waldman, Jody M. Cleveland, and Carl L. Roland. 2011. "Societal Costs of Prescription Opioid Abuse, Dependence, and Misuse in the United States." *Pain Medicine*, 12, no. 4 (March): 657–667.
Blumenthal, David. 2018. "Drop in U.S. Life Expectancy Is an 'Indictment of the American Health Care System'." STAT. Online at www.statnews.com/.
Brill, Alex. 2018. "New State Level Estimates of the Economic Burden of the Opioid Epidemic." American Enterprise Institute. Online at www.aei.org/.
Bump, Philip. 2016. "Prince's Death by Opioid Overdose Is a Very Public Example of a Growing Cultural Problem." *Washington Post*. Online at www.washingtonpost.com/.
Bureau of Labor Statistics. 2018. "Occupational Outlook Handbook: Medical Assistants." US Department of Labor. Online at www.bls.gov/.
Cannon, Lou. 2018. "Some States Progress in Deadly Opioid Crisis." LexisNexis. Online at www.lexisnexis.com/.
Cha, Ariana E. 2016. "The Drug Industry's Answer to Opioid Addiction: More Pills." *Washington Post*. Online at www.washingtonpost.com/.
Chambers, James D., Teja Thorat, Junhee Pyo, Matthew Chenoweth, and Peter J. Neumann. 2014. "Despite High Costs, Specialty Drugs May Offer Value for Money Comparable to that of Traditional Drugs." *Health Affairs*, 33, no. 10 (October): 1751–1759.
Chandra, Amitabh. 2017. "Losing the Genetic Lottery, Bur Winning at a Cure." *NEJM Catalyst*. Online at https://catalyst.nejm.org/.
Chapman, Susan A. and Lisel K. Blash. 2017. "New Role of Medical Assistants in Innovative Primary Care Practices." *Health Service Research*, 52, no. 1 (February): 383–400.
Chokshi, Niraj. 2015. "America's Drug Overdose Problem—And What States Can Do to Fight It—In 4 Charts and Maps." *Washington Post*. Online at www.washingtonpost.com/.
Christensen, Jen. 2018. "The 5 Most Expensive Drugs in the United States." CNN. Online at www.cnn.com/.

Christensen, Jen and Sergio Hernandez. 2016. "This Is America on Drugs: A Visual Guide." CNN. Online at www.cnn.com/.

"Chromosome Cartography." 1989. *Wall Street Journal*, March 16: A16.

Cicero, Theodore J. 2018. "Is Reduction in Access to Prescription Opioids the Cure for the Current Opioid Crisis?" *American Journal of Public Health*, 108, no. 10 (October): 1322–1323.

Clement, Scott and Lenny Bernstein. 2016. "One-Third of Long-Term Users Say They're Hooked on Prescription Opioids." *Washington Post*. Online at www.washingtonpost.com/.

"Combating the Opioid Epidemic." 2018. *Congressional Digest*, 97, no. 2 (February): 22–16.

Constantin, Vlad D. 2014. "The Role of Healthcare Workforce in the Healthcare System." *American Journal of Medical Research*, 1, no. 2 (January): 38–43.

Cortez, Michelle. 2018. "A Breakthrough Blindness Treatment Will Cost $425,000 per Eye, if It Works." Bloomberg. Online at www.bloomberg.com/.

Council of Economic Advisors. 2017. *The Underestimated Cost of Opioid Crisis. The Executive Office of the President*. Washington, DC. Online at www.whitehouse.gov/cea.

Court, Emma. 2016. "America's Is Facing a Shortage of Primary-Care Doctors." MarketWatch. Online at www.marketwatch.com/.

"The Crisis Continues." 2018. American Physical Therapy Association. Online at www.apta.org/.

Cunningham, Paige W. 2018. "The Health 202: Here's How to Tell When the Opioid Crisis Is Starting to Recede." *Washington Post*. Online at www.washingtonpost.com/.

Danielson, Randy D. and O. T. Wendel. 2016. "Who's on First: A Look at Workforce Projections." *Clinician Review*, 26, no. 10 (October): 9–10, 24.

Darves, Bonnie. 2017. "Physician Shortage Spikes in Several Specialties." NEJM Career Center. Online at www.nejmcareercenter.org/.

Dawson, Steven L. and Christopher A. Langston. 2016. "The Eldercare Workforce: Who Cares?" *Generations*, 40, no. 1 (January): 6–9.

DeAngelis, Catherine D. 2016. "Where Have All the Primary Doctors Gone?" *Milbank Quarterly*, 94, no. 2 (June): 246–250.

"Deaths from Drug Overdoses Rise across America." 2015. Yahoo. Online at www.yahoo.com/.

Demirjian, Karoun and Lenny Bernstein. 2016. "CDC Warns Doctors about the Dangers of Prescribing Opioid Painkillers." *Washington Post*. Online at www.washingtonpost.com/.

"Development and Approval Process (Drugs)." 2018. US Food and Drug Administration. Online at www.fda.gov/.

Dijulio, Bianca, Bryan Wu, and Mollyann Brodie. 2016. "The Washington Post/Kaiser Family Foundation Survey of Long-Term Prescription Painkiller Users and Their Household Members." Kaiser Family Foundation. Online at www.kff.org/.

"Drug Overdoes Propel Rise in Mortality Rates of Young Whites." 2016. *The New York Times*. Online at www.nytimes.com/.

Dusetzina, Stacie B. 2016. "Share of Specialty Drugs in Commercial Plans Nearly Quadrupled, 2004–2014." *Health Affairs*, 35, no. 7 (July): 1241–1245.

"Economic Aspects of the Opioid Crisis." 2017. *Hearing Before the Joint Economic Committee, Congress of the United States*, One Hundred Fifteenth Congress, First Session. Washington, DC: US Government Publishing Office.

Ehley, Brianna. 2017. "Marino Out as Trump's Drug Czar Nominee." Politico. Online at www.politico.com/.

Ehley, Brianna and Sarah Carlin-Smith. 2017. "Trump Vows to 'Liberate' Americans from 'Scourge of Drug Addiction'." Politico. Online at www.politico.com/.

Ehley, Brianna, Josh Dawsey, and Sarah Karlin-Smith. 2017. "Blindsided Trump Officials Scrambling to Develop Opioid Plan." Politico. Online at www.politico.com/.

Emrani, Hamidesh. 2017. "Taming an Unruly Immune System: A Risky Stem Cell Transplant that Changed Fate of Some Canadian MS Patients." Knoepfler Lab Stem Cell Blog. Online at https://ipscell.com/.

Eyre, Eric. 2018. "Drug Firms Shipped 20.8 Million Pills to WV Town with 2,900 People." *Charleston Gazette*. Online at www.wvgazettemail.com/.

Feldman, Robin. 2017. "How Big Pharma Is Hindering the Fight against the Opioid Epidemic." PBS. Online at www.pbs.org/.

Feldman, Robin and Evan Frondorf. 2017. *Drug Wars: How Big Pharma Raises Prices and Keeps Generics off the Market*. Cambridge, MA: Cambridge University Press.

Fisher, Daniel. 2018. "Latest Wave of State Opioid Lawsuits Shows Diverging Strategies and Lawyer Pay Scales." *Forbes*. Online at www.forbes.com/.

Florence, Tom. 2018. "Ten Statistics and Trends about Physician Shortage." Merrit Hawkins. Online at www.merritthawkins.com/.

Fueling an Epidemic. Reports One to Three. 2017–2018. Minority Staff Reports. US Senate Homeland Security Government Affairs Committee, Congress of the United States. Online at www.hsgac.senate.gov/.

Gander, Kashmira. 2017. "America's Opioid Crisis: How the Strength of Prescription Drugs Created a Public Health Emergency." *International Business Times*. Online at www.ibtimes.co.uk/.

Garde, Damian. 2017. "Pioneering Cancer Drug, Just Approved, to Cost $475,000 – And Analysts Say It's a Bargain." STAT. Online at www.statnews.com/.

Garg, Aakriti, Jin Yang, Winston Lee, and Stephen H. Tsang. 2017. "Stem Cell Therapies in Retinal Disorders." *Cells*, 6, no. 4 (February): 1–7.

Garneau, Will. 2017. "Groundbreaking Study Demonstrates Promise and Controversy of Gene Editing in Embryos." ABC News. Online at https://abcnews.go.com/.

"Gene Editing." n.d. Purdue University College of Agriculture. Online at https://ag.purdue.edu/.

"Gene Therapy Offer Dramatic Promises but Shocking Costs." 2015. *Washington Post*. Online at www.washingtonpost.com/.

"Genes and Gene Therapy: What are Genes?" 2018. Fighting Blindness. Online at www.fightingblindness.ie/.

Glorioso, J.C. and N. Lemoine. 2017. "Gene Therapy—From Small Beginnings to Here We are Now." *Gene Therapy*, 24, no. 9 (September): 495–496.

Gluck, Abbe R., Ashley Hall, and Gregory Curfman. 2018. "Civil Litigation and the Opioid Epidemic: The Role of Courts in a National Health Crisis." *Journal of Law, Medicine & Ethics*, 46, no. 2 (Summer): 351–366.

Godman, Dana, Anupam Jena, and Tomas Philipson. 2015. "Myths and Facts about Specialty Drugs." *Forbes*. Online at www.forbes.com/.

Goodenough, Abby and Sabrina Tavernise. 2016. "Opioid Prescriptions Drop for the First Time in Two Decades." *The New York Times*. Online at www.nytimes.com/.

Gordon, Noa, Salomon M. Stemmer, Dan Greenberg, and Daniel A. Goldstein. 2018. "Trajectories of Injectable Cancer Drug Costs after Launch in the United States." *Journal of Clinical Oncology*, 36, no. 4 (February): 319–325.

Graham, Carol, Sergio Pinto, and John Juneau, II. 2017. "The Geography of Desperation in America." The Brookings Institution. Online at www.brookings.edu/.

"Graphics: The Exploding Health Care Workforce." 2017. Politico. Online at www.politico.com/.

"The Great Opioid Epidemic." 2016. *Washington Post*. Online at www.washingtonpost.com/.

Griffin, Justine. 2018. "Opioid Crisis Herds Kids to Foster Care." *Tampa Bay Times*. Online at www.pressreader.com/.

Guevremont, Nathan, Mark Barnes, and Claudia E. Haupt. 2018. "Physician Autonomy and the Opioid Crisis." *Journal of Law, Medicine, & Ethics*, 46, no. 2 (June): 203–219.

Hamdoun, Zainab. 2017. "Aftermath of the Human Genome Project: As Era of Struggle and Discovery." *Turkish Journal of Biology*, 41, no. 3 (January): 403–418.

Harding, Mary. 2016. "Strong Painkillers: Opioids." Patient. Online at https://patient.info/.

Harney, Alexandra and Kate Kelland. 2018. "China Orders Investigation After Scientist Claims First Gene-Edited Babies." Reuters. Online at https://in.reuters.com/.

Haseltine, William A. 2003. "Regenerative Medicine: A Future Healing Art." *Brookings Review*, 21, no. 1 (Winter): 38–43.

Health Resources and Services Administration. 2017. *Sex, Race, and Ethnic Diversity of U.S. Health Occupations (2011–2015)*. Washington, DC: US Department of Health and Human Services. Online at https://bhw.hrsa.gov/.

Herper, Matthew. 2018. "You Hate Shkreli. That's Sort of the Problem." *Forbes*. Online at www.forbes.com/.

Hirsch, Bradford, Suresh Balu, and Kevin A. Schulman. 2014. "The Impact of Specialty Pharmaceuticals as Drivers of Health Care Costs." *Health Affairs*, 33, no. 10 (October): 1714–1720.

Hoadley, Jack, Juliette Cubanski, and Tricia Neuman. 2015. "It Pays to Shop: Variation in Out-Of-Pocket Costs for Medicare Part D Enrollers in 2016." Kaiser Family Foundation. Online at www.kff.org/.

Hoban, Brennan. 2017. "The Far-Reaching Effects of the US Opioid Crisis." The Brookings Institution. Online at www.brookings.edu/.

Hogan, Bill. 2015. "Feeling the Pain of Costly Prescription Drugs." AARP. Online at www.aarp.org/.

"How Big Pharma Lobbyists Make the Opioid Crisis Worse." 2016. Yahoo. Online at https://finance.yahoo.com/.

Howley, Elaine K. 2018. "What Can Be Done about the Coming Shortage of Specialist Doctors?" *US News & World Report*. Online at https://health.usnews.com/.

Humphreys, Keith, Jonathan P. Caulkins, and Vanda Felbab-Brown. 2018. "Opioids of the Masses: Stopping an American Epidemic from Going Global." *Foreign Affairs*, 97, no. 3 (May–June): 118–129.

Ingraham, Christopher. 2017. "How an 'Abuse-Deterrent' Drug Created the Heroin Epidemic." *Washington Post*. Online at www.washingtonpost.com/.

Institute of Medicine. 2008. *Retooling for an Aging America: Building the Healthcare Workforce*. Washington, DC: National Academies Press.

Izadi, Elahe. 2016. "So Many People are Dying of Drug Overdose that They're Easing the Donated Organ Shortage." *Washington Post*. Online at www.washingtonpost.com/.

Jackson, Chazeman and J. Nadine Gracia. 2014. "Addressing Health and Health-Care Disparities: The Role of a Diverse Workforce and the Social Determinants of Health." *Public Health Reports*, 128, no. 2 (Supplement) (January–February): 57–61.

Jackson, Liane. 2018. "Opioids, Justice & Mercy: Courts are on the Front Lines of a Lethal Crisis." *ABA Journal*, 104, no. 6 (June): 36–43.

James, Keturah and Ayana Jordan. 2018. "The Opioid Crisis in Black Communities." *Journal of Law, Medicine, & Ethics*, 46, no. 2 (June): 404–421.

Jay, Marley and Matt Perrone. 2018. "Oxycontin Maker Will Stop Promoting Opioids to Doctors." *US News & World Report*. Online at www.usnews.com/.

Jena, Anupam, Michael Barnett, and Dana Goldman. 2017. "How Health Care Providers Can Help and End the Overprescription of Opioids?" Harvard Business Review. Online at https://hbr.org/.

Jena, Anupam, Dana Goldman, and Pinar Karaca-Mandic. 2016. "Hospitals Prescribing Opioids to Medicare Beneficiaries." *Journal of the American Medical Association Internal Medicine*, 176, no. 7 (July): 990–997.

Johnson, Carla K. and Nicky Forster. 2018. "AP Analysis: 'Obamacare' Shapes Opioid Grant Spending." ABC News. Online at https://abcnews.go.com/.

Jones, David A. 2017. "Editing Out the Embryo: The Debate over Genetic Editing in the United Kingdom and the United States." *National Catholic Bioethics Quarterly*, 17, no. 1 (January): 83–105.

Joyce, Trish. 2018. "Does Healthcare Have a Gender Problem?" Health eCareers. Online at www.healthecareers.com/.

Kaiser Family Foundation. 2018a. "Providers and Service Use Indicators: Physicians." Online at www.kff.org/.

Kaiser Family Foundation. 2018b. "Providers and Service Use Indicators: Nurses and Physician Assistants." www.kff.org/.

Kent, A. and J. Spink. 2017. "Will Rising Prices and Budget Constraints Prevent Patients from Accessing Novel Gene Therapy?" *Gene Therapy*, 24, no. 9 (September): 542–543.

Kershaw, Michael H, Jennifer A. Westwood, and Phillip K. Darcy. 2013. "Gene-Engineered T Cells for Cancer Therapy." *Nature Reviews Cancer*, 13, no. 8 (August): 525–541.

Kesselheim, Aaron S., Yongtian T. Tan, Jonathan J. Darrow, and Jerry Avorn. 2014. "Existing FDA Pathways Have Potential to Ensure Early Access to, and Appropriate Use of, Specialty Drugs." *Health Affairs*, 33, no. 10 (October): 1770–1778.

Kevles, Daniel J. 1997. "Big Science and Big Politics in the United States: Reflections on the Death of SSC and the Life of Human Genome Project." *Historical Studies in the Physical and Biological Sciences*, 27, no. 2 (January): 269–297.

Kindy, Kimberly and Dan Keating. 2016. "Opioids and Anti-Anxiety Medications are Killing White American Women." *Washington Post*. Online at www.washingtonpost.com/.

Kodish, Eric. 2017. "What's in a Name? Cart-T Gene Therapy." *Hastings Center Report*, 47, no. 6 (November): inside back cover.

Kodjak, Alison. 2015. "Specialty Drugs Can Prove Expensive Even with Medicare Coverage." NPR. Online at www.npr.org/.

Kolata, Gina and Sarah Cohen. 2016. "Drug Overdoses Propel Rise in Mortality Rates of Young Whites." *The New York Times*. Online at www.nytimes.com/.

Kourany, Jennet A. 2014. "Human Enhancement: Making the Debate More Productive." *Erkenntnis*, 79, no. 5 (special issue) (June): 981–998.

Lantz, Paula. 2008. "Gender and Leadership in Healthcare Administration: 21st Century Progress and Challenges." *Journal of Healthcare Management*, 53, no. 5 (September): 291–301.

LaVeist, Thomas A. and Geraldine Pierre. 2014. "Integrating the 3Ds—Social Determinants, Health Disparities, and Health-Care Workforce Diversity." *Public Health Reports*, 129, no. 2 (Supplement) (January–February): 9–14.

Lembke, Anna and Jonathan H. Chen. 2016. "Use of Opioid Agonist Therapy for Medicare Patients in 2013." *Journal of the American Medical Association Psychiatry*, 73, no. 9 (September): 990–992.

Lewis, Ricki. 2014. "Gene Therapy's Second Act." *Scientific American*, 310, no. 3 (March): 52–57.

Light, Donald W. and Hagop Kantarjian. 2014. "Cancer Drugs' Rising Costs: The 100,000 Myth." AARP. Online at www.aarp.org/.

Longo, Umile G., Stefano Petrillo, Edorado Franceschetti, Alessandra Berton, Nicola Maffulli, and Vincenzo Denaro. 2012. "Stem Cell and Gene Therapy for Cartilage Repair." *Stem Cell International*. NCBI. Online at www.ncbi.nlm.nih.gov/.

Lopez, German. 2017. "Want to Understand How Big Pharma Helped Create the Opioid Epidemic? Read This Report." Vox. Online at www.vox.com/.

Loring, Jeanne. 2017. "On the Threshold of Cell Therapy for Parkinson's Disease." Knoepfler Lab Stem Cell Blog. Online at https://ipscell.com/.

Lowell, Lindsay. 2013. "The Foreign Born in the American Healthcare Workforce: Trends in This Century's First Decade." *Migration Letters*, 10, no. 2 (May): 180–190.

Maciag, Mike. 2018. "Suicide Rate Highest in Decades but Worst in Rural America." Governing. Online at www.governing.com/.

Mahoney, Julia D. and Gil Siegal. 2018. "Beyond Nature? Genomic Modification and the Future of Humanity." *Law and Contemporary Problems*, 81, no 3 (August): 195–214.

Marchione, Marilynn. 2018. "Chinese Researcher Claims First Gene-Edited Babies." Associated Press. Online at www.apnews.com/.

Martinez, Catherine. 2018. "Cracking the Code: Using Data to Combat the Opioid Crisis." *Journal of Law, Medicine & Ethics*, 46, no. 2: 454–471.

Mather, Mark, Linda A. Jacobsen, and Kevin M. Pollard. 2015. "Aging in the United States." *Population Bulletin*, 70, no. 2 (December): 1–18.

McDevitt, Ryan C. and James W. Roberts. 2014. "Market Structure and Gender Disparity in Health Care: Preferences, Competition, and Quality of Care." *RAND Journal of Economics*, 45, no. 1 (Spring): 116–139.

McGinley, Laurie. "Novel Cancer Treatment Wins Endorsement of FDA Advisors." *Washington Post*. Online at www.washingtonpost.com/.

McGreal, Chris. 2017. "Don't Blame Addicts for America's Opioid Crisis. Here are the Real Culprits." *Guardian*. Online at www.theguardian.com/.

"Medicaid's Role in Addressing the Opioid Epidemic." 2018. Kaiser Family Foundation. Online at www.kff.org/.

Mehlman, Maxwell J. 2009. *The Price of Perfection: Individualism and Society in the Era of Biomedical Enhancement*. Baltimore, MD: Johns Hopkins University.

Mercer LLC. 2018. "Demand for Healthcare Workforce Will Outpace Supply by 2025: An Analysis of the US Healthcare Labor Market." Online at https://mercer.healthcare-workforce.us/.

Morgan, David. 2018. "Chinese Researcher Claims to Have Genetically Altered Babies Using CRISPR." CBS News. Online at www.cbsnews.com/.

Mullin, Emily. 2017. "Tracking the Cost of Gene Therapy." *MIT Technology Review*. Online at www.technologyreview.com/.

National Academies of Sciences, Engineering, and Medicine et al. 2017. *Human Genome Editing: Science, Ethics, and Governance*. Washington, DC: National Academies Press.

National Commission on Certification of Physician Assistants. 2017a. "2017 Statistical Profile of Certified Physician Assistants: Annual Report." NCCPA. Online at www.nccpa.net/.

National Commission on Certification of Physician Assistants. 2017b. "2017 Statistical Profile of Certified Physician Assistants by Specialty." NCCPA. Online at www.nccpa.net/.

National Commission on Certification of Physician Assistants. 2018. "PAs in Specialty Practice: An Analysis of Need, Growth and Future." Online at http://prodcmsstoragesa.blob.core.windows.net/.

National Pharmaceutical Services. 2018. "Specialty Medications." CastiaRx. Online at www.pti-nps.com/.

Netburn, Deborah. 2017. "New Gene-Editing Technique May Lead to Treatments of Thousands of Diseases." *Los Angeles Times*. Online at www.latimes.com/.
"New York Sets 7-Day Limit on Initial Opioid Prescription." 2016. Fox News. Online at www.foxnews.com/.
Nilsen, Ella. 2017. "Why It's so Much Easier to Get an Opioid Prescription in the US than in Europe or Japan?" *Vox*. Online at www.vox.com/.
Nowogrodzki, Anna. and Michael Le Page. 2015. "Green Light for Editing Embryos." *New Scientist*, 228, no. 3051 (December): 8–9.
"Nursing Salary Research Report." 2018. Nurse.com. Online at http://mediakit.nurse.com/.
Ollove, Michael. 2014. "States Combat Overdose Deaths." Pew Charitable Trusts. Online at www.pewtrusts.org/.
Ollove, Michael. 2016. "States Attack a Severe Doctor Shortage." Pew Charitable Trusts. Online at www.pewtrusts.org/.
"Opioid Crisis Fast Facts." 2017. CNN. Online at www.cnn.com/.
"Opioid Makers Fill State Coffers." 2018. *Tampa Bay Times*, Saturday, May 19: B1.
Ornstein, Charles, and Ryan G. Jones. 2014. "Doctors Prescribing Most Potent Painkillers Face Scrutiny." *USA Today*. Online at www.usatoday.com/.
"Our Drug Overdose Epidemic, and What You Can Do about It." 2015. *Daily Kos*. Online at www.dailykos.com/.
Parramore, Lynn. 2017. "Worse than Big Tobacco: How Big Pharma Fuels the Opioid Epidemic." Institute for New Economic Thinking. Online at www.ineteconomics.org/.
Patel, V. Neel. 2017. "Car T-Cell Therapy Is Making Untreatable Cancer Treatable." *The Daily Beast*. Online at www.thedailybeast.com/.
Perrone, Matthew. 2018. "Gene Therapy for Rare Form of Blindness Comes with Nearly $1 Million Price Tag." *Time*. Online at http://time.com/.
Pew Charitable Trusts. 2016. "Specialty Drugs and the Health Care Costs." Pew Charitable Trusts . Online at www.pewtrusts.org/.
Pharmaceutical Care Management Association. 2016. "The Management of Specialty Drugs." PCMA. Online at www.spcma.org/.
Phillips, Janice and Beverly Malone. 2014. "Increasing Racial/Ethnic Diversity to Reduce Health Disparities and Achieve Health Equity." *Public Health Reports*, 129, no. 2 (Supplement) (January–February): 45–50.
"Playing God? The Pros and Cons of Gene Therapy." BiologyWise. Online at https://biologywise.com/.
"Policy Proposal: Reducing the Exclusivity Period for Biological Products." 2017. Pew Charitable Trusts. Online at www.pewtrusts.org/.
President's Commission Combating Drug Addiction and the Opioid Crisis. 2018. Washington, DC. WhiteHouse.gov. Online at www.whitehouse.gov/.
Pyrillis, Rita. 2015. "Specialty Drug Costs: Hard Pill to Swallow." Workforce. Online at www.workforce.com/.
Quast, Troy, Eric A. Storch, and Svetlana Yampolskaya. 2018. "Opioid Prescription Rates and Child Removals: Evidence from Florida." *Health Affairs*, 37, no. 1 (January): 134–139.
Quinn, Mattie. 2018. "6 Months since Trump Declared an Opioid Emergency, What's Changed?" Governing. Online at www.governing.com/.
Quinones, Sam. 2015. *Dreamland: The True Tale of America's Opiate Epidemic*. New York: Bloomsbury Press.
Raphelson, Samantha. 2018. "Alabama Targets OxyContin Maker Purdue Pharma in Opioid Suit." NPR. Online at www.npr.org/.
Rehmann-Sutter, Christoph. 2018. "Why Human Germline Editing Is More Problematic than Selecting between Embryos: Ethically Considering Intergenerational Relationship." *New Bioethics*, 24, no. 1 (April): 9–25.
"Report: Rapid Rise in Cost of Specialty Drugs Exceeds Median Family Income." 2015. AARP. Online at https://press.aarp.org/.
Ross, Casey. 2018. "As the Opioid Crisis Grows, States are Opening Medicaid to Alternative Medicine." STAT. Online at www.statnews.com/.
Rudd, Rose A., Puja Seth, Felicita David, and Lawrence Scholl. 2016. "Increases in Drug and Opioid—Involved Orsedose Deaths—United States, 2010–2015." *Morbidity and Mortality Weekly Report*, 65, no. 50–51 (December): 1445–1452.
Saey, Tina H. 2015. "Human Gene Editing Research Gets Green Light." *Science News*, 188, no. 13 (December): 12.
Saey, Tina H. 2017a. "U.S. Panel Backs Human Gene Editing." *Science News*, 191, no. 5 (March): 7.
Saey, Tina H. 2017b. "Gene Editing of Human Embryos Human Embryo Yields Early Results." *Science News*, 191, no. 7 (April): 16–17.
Salsberg, Edward. 2014. "The Health Workforce: A Critical Component of the Health Care Infrastructure." *Health Affairs*, March 24. Online at www.healthaffairs.org/.
Sample, Ian. 2018. "What Is Gene Editing and How Can It Be Used to Rewrite the Code of Life?" *Guardian*. Online at www.theguardian.com/.
Santye, Lauren. 2016. "Top 10 Specialty Drug Therapeutic Classes." *Specialty Pharmacy Times*. Online at www.specialtypharmacytimes.com/.
Schondelmeyer, Stephen W. and Leigh Purvis. 2017. "Trends in Retail Prices of Specialty Prescription Drugs Widely Used by Older Americans, 2006 to 2015." AARP. Online at www.aarp.org/.
Schultz, Kathy J. 2018. "This Doctor's Revolutionary Stem Cell Treatment Could Eradicate HIV." *The Daily Beast*. Online at www.thedailybeast.com/.
Seegert, Liz. 2017. "Opioid Crisis Takes a Toll on Rural Older Adults." nextavenue. Online at www.nextavenue.org/.
Shedrofsky, Karina. 2016. "Drug Czar: Doctors, Drugmakers Share Blame for Opioid Epidemic." *USA Today*. Online at www.usatoday.com/.
Simon, Eric J. 2002. "Human Gene Therapy: Genes Without Frontiers?" *American Biology Teacher*, 64, no. 4 (April): 264–270.

Singh, Shashi P, Awani K. Rai, Pranay Wal, Ankita Wal, Asfa Parveen, and Chitranshu Gupta. 2016. "Gene Therapy: Recent Developments in the Treatment of Various Diseases." *International Journal of Pharmaceutical, Chemical, and Biological Sciences*, 6, no. 2 (April): 205–214.

Smaglik, Paul. 2017. "Regulating the Brave New World of Human Gene Editing." *Discover*, 38, no. 1 (December): 30.

Solis, Amanda R. 2012. "Insights from 'Creating the Healthcare Workforce for the 21st Century' Conference." *Population Health Management*, 15, no. 1 (February): 1–2.

Spanu, Anca. 2018. "Doctor Shortages in the US Is Getting Worse. The American Healthcare System Is at Risk." *Healthcare Weekly*. Online at https://healthcareweekly.com/.

"Specialty Pharmaceuticals." 2013. *Health Affairs Health Policy Briefs* (November). Online at www.healthaffairs.org/.

Spector, Nicole. 2018. "The Doctor Is Out? Why Physicians are Leaving Their Practice to Pursue Other Careers." NBC News. Online at www.nbcnews.com/.

Starner, Catherine I, Caleb Alexander, Kevin Bowen, Yang Qiu, Peter J. Wickersham, and Patrick P. Gleason. 2014. "Specialty Drug Coupons Lower the Out-Of-PocketCosts and may Improve Adherence at the Risk of Increasing Premiums." *Health Affairs*, 33, no. 10 (October): 1761–1769.

"States Make Headway on Opioid Abuse." 2017. *Christian Science Monitor*. Online at www.csmonitor.com/.

Stein, Rob. 2017. "FDA Panel Endorses Gene Therapy for A Form of Childhood Blindness." *NPR*. Online at www.npr.org/.

Stein, Rob. 2018. "Facing Backlash, Chinese Scientist Defends Gene-Editing Research on Babies." *NPR*. Online at www.npr.org/.

Stevenson, Matthew. 2018. "Demand for Healthcare Workers Will Outpace Supply by 2025: An Analysis of the US Healthcare Labor Market." Mercer. Online at www.mercer.us/.

Stobbe, Mike. 2017. "Opioid Epidemic Shares Chilling Similarities with the Past." *Denver Post*. Online at www.denverpost.com/.

"Synthetic Drugs Pose Alarming US Overdose Risk, DEA Chief Says." 2016. Fox News. Online at www.foxnews.com/.

"The Latest: Scientist Reports 2nd Gene-Edited Pregnancy." The Republic. Online at www.therepublic.com/.

Tecco, Halle. 2018. "Women in Healthcare 2017: How Does Our Industry Stack Up?" Rock Health. Online at https://rockhealth.com/.

Towers, Susan L. 2017. "Gene Therapy: What Is It? How Is It Different from CRISPR/Cas9? Why Is CRIPSR//Cas9 Getting So Much Media Hype?" *American Medical Writers Association Journal*, 32, no. 4: 172–175.

Trish, Erin, Geoffrey Joyce, and Dana P. Goldman. 2014. "Specialty Drug Spending Trends among Medicare and Medicare Advantage Enrollees 2007–2011." *Health Affairs*, 33, no. 11 (November): 2018–2024.

Trish, Erin, Jianhui Xu, and Geoffrey Joyce. 2016. "Medicare Beneficiaries Face Growing Out-of-Pocket Burden for Specialty Drugs while in Catastrophic Coverage Phase." *Health Affairs*, 35, no. 9 (September): 1564–1570.

Trommelmans, Leen. 2010. "The Challenge of Regenerative Medicine." *Hastings Center Report*, 40, no. 6 (November–December): 24–26.

US Department of Health and Human Services. 2017. *High-Price Drugs are Increasing Federal Payments for Medicare Part D Catastrophic Coverage*. Office of Inspector General. Online at https://oig.hhs.gov/.

US Department of Labor. 2018. "Fastest Growing Occupations." Bureau of Labor Statistics. Online at www.bls.gov/.

"U.S. Health Workforce Chartbook – In Brief." 2018. Health Resources and Services Administration. Online at https://bhw.hrsa.gov/.

US News & World Report. 2018. "U.S. News Announces the 2018 Best Jobs." *US News & World Report*. Online at www.usnews.com/.

"Understanding the Epidemic." 2017. Centers for Disease Control and Prevention. Online at www.cdc.gov/drugoverdose/epidemic/.

Vestal, Christine. 2016. "Older Addicts Squeezed by Opioid Epidemic." Pew Charitable Trusts. Online at www.pewtrusts.org/.

Vitali, Ali and Corky Siemaszko. 2017a. "Trump Declares Opioid Crisis National Emergency." NBC News. Online at www.nbcnews.com/.

Vitali, Ali and Corky Siemaszko. 2017b. "Trump Calls Opioid Crisis a National Emergency but Still Hasn't Made It Official." NBC News. Online at www.nbcnews.com/.

Vokinger, Kerstin N. 2018. "Opioid Crisis in the US – Lessons from Western Europe." *Journal of Law, Medicine, & Ethics*, 46, no. 1 (Spring): 189–190.

Walsh, Michael. 2017. "Trump Declares 'Public Health Emergency' over Opioid Crisis: We Can Be the Generation that Ends the Epidemic." Yahoo. Online at www.yahoo.com/.

"The War on Opioids Moves to the Courtroom." 2018. CBS News. Online at www.cbsnews.com/.

Washkow, Michelle M. and Mary L. Fennell. 2017. "The Epicenter of Effectiveness and Efficiency: The Evolving U.S. Health Care Workforce." *Health Services Research*, 52, no. S1 (February): 353–359.

Watts, Sarah. 2017. "Spina Bifida Could Vanish with This Experimental Fetal Stem Cell Therapy." *The Daily Beast*. Online at www.thedailybeast.com/.

Webster, Deacon Gregory. 2018. "Financial Toxicity: Treatment Expense and Extraordinary Means." *National Catholic Bioethics Quarterly*, 18, no. 2 (January): 227–236.

Weil, Alan R. 2014. "The Promise of Specialty Pharmaceuticals." *Health Affairs*, 33, no. 10 (October): 1710.

Weintraub, Arlene. 2018. "Rewriting the Faulty Code." *U.S. News and World Report*. September 6. US News & World Report. Online at www.usnews.com/.

"What are Genome Editing and CRISPR-Cas9?" 2017. Genetics Home Reference. Online at https://ghr.nlm.nih.gov/.

"What Is Gene Therapy." 2017. Genetics Home Reference. Online at https://ghr.nlm.nih.gov/.

"What Is Nursing?." n.d. ANA Enterprise. Online at www.nursingworld.org/.

Whatley, Monica, Clese Erickson, Shana Sandberg, and Karen Jones. 2017. "Community Health Workers: An Underused Resource, Rediscovered." *Academic Medicine*, 92, no. 4 (January): 1.

Wickramatilake, Shalini, Julia Zur, Norah Mulvaney-Day, Melinda Campopiano von Klimo, Elizabeth Selmi, and Henrick Hardwood. 2017. "How States are Tackling the Opioid Crisis." *Public Health Reports*, 132, no. 2 (February): 171–179.

Wing, Nick. 2017. "Trump Rebuffs His Opioid Task Force, Declines to Declare State of Emergency." *Huffington Post*. Online at www.huffingtonpost.com/.

Zamyatnin, A.A. 2016. "Special Issue: Genome Editing and Gene Therapy." *Biochemistry* (Moscow), 81, no. 7 (July): 867–869.

Zezima, Katie and Seung M. Kim. 2018. "Trump Signs Sweeping Opioid Bill: Expect to Hear about in on the Campaign Trail." *Washington Post*. Online at www.washingtonpost.com/.

Zhen, Anjie and Scott Kitchen. 2014. "Stem-Cell-Based Gene Therapy for HIV Infection." *Viruses*, 6, no. 1 (January): 1–12.

Section V
THE CONTINUING STRUGGLE FOR HEALTHCARE REFORM IN THE UNITED STATES

11

HEALTHCARE POLITICS AND POLICY IN AMERICA

Moving Toward Reform?

> But there's a reason that, prior to Obama, president after president failed to pass health care reform. To overhaul something as important to people's lives as the health care system, you need the trust of the public; the votes in Congress; and, if you're paying for the plan, a whole lot of money. It's easy to look back on the places Obamacare fell short and imagine how the law could have been more ambitious or more generous, but the compromises written into the Affordable Care Act were written for a reason: The politics of health care reform are hellish, and the modal outcome is failure.
>
> *(Klein 2018)*

The focus of this chapter is reform of the American healthcare system. Reform, generally speaking, means making changes in something that will improve that something. Further, we are considering systemic changes in the healthcare system. Some of the changes/innovations considered in previous chapters meet this definition. Certainly, the Affordable Care Act, whatever its strengths and weaknesses, sought systemic changes, though clearly it left much of the system the way it was. Medicaid and Medicare, while important advances in coverage for specific groups, did not fundamentally change the system. Proposals to increase access and get a handle on costs offer change, but, for the most part, fairly incremental change. So, this is the focus of this final chapter: What kind of policies can we envision that represent improvements in the healthcare system through fundamental changes?

We begin the chapter by examining generic healthcare system goals. Next, we consider values that shape the kind of healthcare system we have and the kind of healthcare system we might like to have.

We follow that up by considering how well the US healthcare system has performed. We do this by examining the value of quality and comparing the US with other Westernized, industrial nations.

We then move on to consider reform proposals. We begin this part by considering what fixes might be made to the Affordable Care Act that get us closer to the kind of healthcare system we would like.

The major part of the chapter considers liberal and conservative health reform proposals. We will point out, among other things, the value differences that underlie these sets of proposals.

We conclude the chapter with some observations about the future of the American healthcare system.

HEALTHCARE SYSTEM GOALS AND VALUES

Goals

The classic formulation of healthcare goals is presented by Ginzberg (1977). Ginzberg discusses four goals, though here we will merge the fourth goal with the first.

The first goal is *access*. As we saw in Chapter 7, access can mean many things. The basic idea of access is the ability of people to obtain the services they need in a timely fashion. We can look at the uninsured rate, the percentage of people who do not have insurance. We can look at differences by demographic group, by income, and by gender in access to services. We can look at differences in access by geography. Healthcare reform should seek to improve access to the healthcare system.

Certainly, the United States has adopted programs to increase access and the capacity of the system. Innovations include the Hill-Burton Act, which provided money to build hospitals, especially in rural areas; funding for medical education to help increase the supply of providers; Medicaid, to provide insurance coverage to people with low incomes; Medicare, to provide insurance coverage for the elderly; the Children's Health Insurance Program (CHIP) to increase coverage for children; the Affordable Care Act, which provided insurance coverage to a larger portion of the population.

All these programs have their problems but did increase access to the healthcare system. But the problem of access remains. There are still millions of people without health insurance. There are still disparities among different groups.

The second goal is *cost*. The ideal is to have a healthcare system that provides access to that system at a reasonable cost. But as we have seen, healthcare costs continue to grow faster than the economy as a whole, faster than inflation, and faster than wages. The US spends far more on healthcare than any other country. One way of looking at this (see Chapter 8) is by comparing health spending as a percentage of gross domestic product (GDP) in the United States with other countries. In 2017, healthcare spending in the US comprised 17.8 percent of GDP. The next-highest was Switzerland at 12.4 percent. Another way of looking at this is to consider healthcare spending per capita. Again, in 2017, the US spent $9403 per capita. The next-highest country was Sweden at $6808 per capita (Papanicolas et al. 2018).

As we have seen earlier in the text, high and increasing cost is a problem for individuals, businesses, and state and federal governments. It underlies many of the problems of the healthcare system.

Ginzberg (1977) points out that there is a trade-off between access and cost. If we decide to cover more people, it is going to cost more. That was certainly the case after Medicaid and Medicare were enacted. By 1970, five years after enactment, healthcare costs in the US began to outstrip costs in other countries.

If we want to control costs, then we either have to limit payments to providers, ask patients/consumers to bear more of the burden of their healthcare, and/or change the incentives in the system. It is these kinds of issues that plague policymakers and differentiate policy proposals.

The third goal is quality, a rather elusive concept. An example of a quality issue are studies that argue that medical errors are a major cause of death in the United States (see, for example, Makary and Daniel (2016). The Institute of Medicine (1999) estimated that between 44,000 and 98,000 people die in hospitals each year because of medical errors. These are all estimates because death certificates do not list errors as a cause of death. Further, there are problems with the estimates (see, for example, Gianoli 2016).

The Commonwealth Fund has produced reports comparing the quality of healthcare in the United States to that of other Westernized, industrial countries. The 2010 report (Davis, Schoen, and Stremikis 2010) evaluated healthcare systems on a number of measures. The quality measures included effective care, safe care, coordinated care, and patient-centered care. The access measures included cost-related access problems and timeliness of care. Other measures included efficiency, equity and long, healthy productive lives. On most measures the US came in last or near-last compared to six other countries. The title of the 2010 study "Mirror, Mirror, On the Wall" concluded, in our words rather than the study's words, that the United States was not the fairest of them all. A more recent study (Schneider et al. 2017) came up with the same conclusion. Their overall ranking placed the US 11th of 11 nations. The measures had changed somewhat since the 2010 report. The US did its best (fifth) on care process measures. Clearly, according to the report, there was much that needed to be done to improve the performance of the American healthcare system. A study by Papanicolas et al. (2018) confirmed much of these findings.

This is not to say that the quality studies are without criticism. First, the US is different from other countries. It is larger (the United States has the third-largest population in the world, behind the People's Republic of China and India) than other nations in the studies, and has a much more diverse population. A second criticism is that the measures used by the Commonwealth Fund are subjectively chosen and perhaps not the best (see, for example, Gur-Arie 2014). A third criticism is that studies such as that from the Commonwealth Fund are based on surveys rather than, according to critics, objective data (Atlas 2011). A final criticism is that for Americans, perhaps more than other industrialized countries, lifestyle is a major factor in healthcare outcomes. The obesity and opioid epidemics (discussed in previous chapters) are indicators of this.

Some have argued that the American healthcare system is quite good. Atlas (2011) takes great exception to studies such as those produced by the Commonwealth Fund and the World Health Organization (WHO). He writes that "the most important role of health care … is the diagnosis and treatment of serious diseases" (xxiii). To take just one example of the kind of argument Atlas makes, infant mortality is one of the measures used to evaluate the performance of a healthcare system. The comparative studies, such as that of Papanicolas et al. (2018), find that the US rate exceeds that of other countries. Atlas argues, however, that the US ranks high, though not the highest, in infant survival rates for those who are premature and severely premature, that is, those infants who require medical attention. Atlas continues by noting that the high infant mortality rate in the US is, to a great extent, a function of the high premature birth rate. Further, Atlas (2011) points out that data systems that various countries employ vary in how they register premature births. Additionally, Atlas notes the great diversity of population in the United States compared to other countries, and that has an impact as well.

To reiterate, the major point that Atlas (2011) makes is that the medical care system in the US is quite good and, when applied, produces generally good outcomes. For Atlas (2011), the Affordable Care Act was the wrong way to go and the real problem of the American healthcare system is costs.

In closing this section, we should note the ideological/value differences between the two perspectives. Both see problems with the US healthcare system, but their understanding of the problems is different and, therefore, so are their proposals for reform. Those who support the idea that the US healthcare system is significantly worse in quality than other countries tend to be liberals; those who argue that those studies are wrong tend to be conservatives. We, therefore, next turn to consider values.

Values

As noted above, differences in values distinguish ideological positions (see Rushefsky 2017 and the citations listed). The value foundation of American political ideological positions rests on three legs.

The first value is *order*. For our purposes, order refers to traditional social mores. Those who oppose abortion and some (if not all) contraceptives cite their moral values, usually based on their religion, and their desire to protect life ("right to life").

The second value is *freedom*. Freedom means the right to be left alone, by both the public and private sectors, without heavy oversight. This value underlies many controversial public policy issues. From the standpoint of abortion and contraceptive technology, those who favor the ready availability of both argue that government should, for the most part, stay out of the picture and let women have the right to choose. Clearly, there is a clash here between the two underlying values.

Freedom as a value also underlies differences in healthcare proposals. Conservatives argue that large government programs, such as the Affordable Care Act, not only misperceive the problems of the system, but also involve considerable government interference with free markets and free-market decisions on the part of patients/consumers and providers. Opposition to the individual mandate was largely, though clearly not entirely, due to what was seen as the heavy hand of government, mandating the purchase of insurance.

The third value is *equality*. This suggests that public policies should work toward reducing inequities in society. This value underlies much social policies, from minimum wage to ACA exchange subsidies to making sure that people with preexisting conditions can get insurance and service. Clearly, there is a clash between the value of freedom and the value of equality. For example, the ACA mandate on preexisting conditions is basically a restriction on health insurance companies' freedom to determine pricing for their insurance policies.

With these value clashes in mind, we turn to healthcare reform proposals.

FIXING THE AFFORDABLE CARE ACT

As we saw in Chapter 3, the Affordable Care Act has survived since its enactment in 2010. This is despite efforts to repeal it by congressional Republicans, and efforts by the Trump administration to undermine it. The most significant change to the law came in December 2017, when Congress added an amendment (a rider) to the tax-cut legislation, to repeal the tax penalty for not having health insurance, the individual mandate. A court case is pending, *Texas v. Azar*, that challenges the constitutionality of the ACA, but unless the courts decide against the ACA, it will remain as a fundamental piece of healthcare legislation (see Chapter 3).

Two other things support the ACA, both discussed in Chapter 3. First, the ACA has gained in public support as it has faced Republican opposition. Second, the Democrats regained control of the US House of Representatives, creating a divided government (see Chapter 1). That division makes it much less likely that the ACA will be legislatively dismantled.

One option for healthcare reform, therefore, is fixing the problems with the ACA. One place to start is with President Barack Obama. In an October 2016 speech, the president defended the legislation that, informally, bears his name (Obamacare) by pointing to the large number of newly insured people and the significant decline in the percentage of uninsured people. He also pointed to consumer protections, the effect of which is much more difficult to quantify than the impact of the law on the uninsured rate (Demko 2016).

Obama then noted some problems with the ACA. The first was that there remained over 20 million Americans without health insurance. The second problem was the affordability of insurance for people who had it (Demko 2016).

The president suggested three reforms. The first is that the remaining states (19 at the time of the speech) expand Medicaid. A second suggestion was to implement within the ACA a public option. The problem Obama was referencing was insurance companies pulling out of the exchanges and the lack of competition as a result. A public option would provide competition to private insurance companies and, hopefully, put pressure on insurance prices. Obama's third option was to expand the tax subsidies for the purchase of insurance on the exchanges and for the cost-sharing that is part of the insurance plans. This would make insurance more affordable (Demko 2016).

The most comprehensive set of ACA fixes were proposed by Jost and Pollack (2015). We will look at their suggestions because they encompass most of the others that have been offered. In this section, we look at some of the proposals.

Their first suggestion is to fix what has become known as the "family glitch" (Jost and Pollack 2015). We quote Jost and Pollack (2015) to describe the problem:

> Under the law, an individual worker and her family are eligible for financial help on the new marketplaces if she lacks access to "affordable" employer-sponsored coverage. Unfortunately, current IRS regulations deem such coverage affordable if the cost of covering only the worker herself is less than 9.5 percent of household income—whatever the cost to that employee of covering the rest of her family. Under this rule, a single mother of three earning $40,000 annually would be excluded from receiving any marketplace assistance as long as her employer offered a policy covering only herself that would cost her less than about $3,800, or 9.5 percent of her income, even though average 2013 private-sector employee contributions for family coverage were about $4,400. The rule would thus leave this worker—by any definition, struggling to get by—ineligible for any financial assistance. Until this glitch is fixed, many low-income workers are effectively denied access to affordable health coverage.

A second idea is to increase tax credits for "moderate-to-middle-income households" (Jost and Pollack 2015). A third, related, suggestion, is to reduce the cost-sharing requirements. Recall in the discussion in Chapter 3 that cost-sharing was a major complaint among those purchasing insurance on the exchanges.

The next two suggestions are intriguing and bring in ideas supported by conservatives. Jost and Pollack (2015) propose making greater use of health savings accounts (HSAs) and health reimbursement accounts (HRAs) as a way to help consumers pay for their insurance. With heath savings accounts, similar in some ways to individual retirement accounts (IRAs), individuals deposit money in the accounts (which are not taxed) and then use that money for paying for healthcare not covered by health insurance policies, such as deductibles and cost-sharing. Jost and Pollack (2015) suggest that small employers be allowed to contribute to the accounts to help pay for the cost of healthcare. A health reimbursement account is similar to HSAs, but, in this case, employers make contributions to the accounts that employees can then use to pay for healthcare.

Another suggest is to simplify the process of determining the tax credit. Jost and Pollack (2015) also propose that the tax credit subsidies be strengthened for middle-income families, many of whom are not eligible for the subsidies because their income exceeds 400 percent of the federal poverty level.

One of the complaints about the ACA is that cost-sharing can be burdensome to families. Jost and Pollack (2015) recommend reducing the cost-sharing provisions and also reducing the total amount of out-of-pocket spending that consumers on the exchange have to pay. They also call for protections against high-balanced billing and surprise medical bills. Jost and Pollack (2015) recommend more support for consumers choosing plans on the exchanges, so that consumers can choose the plans that best meet their needs.

There are many other suggestions that Jost and Pollack (2015) make. Some comments are in order. First, many of their proposals will require that more money be spent. For example, reducing cost-sharing and increasing tax credit subsidies is going to cost more money. Expanding the reach of the ACA (covering more people) will cost more money. Doing so is effectively a societal decision to cover more people and to give them financial protection.

This is related to our second point. The political will needs to be there to do this. While there have been more states willing to expand Medicaid (Chapters 3 and 4), the reality is that the political contours do not favor making improvements to the ACA (nor some of the other reforms discussed below). Jost and Pollack (2015) and others were writing at a time when Republicans, opponents of the ACA, controlled Congress. Following the 2016 elections, Republicans controlled both houses of Congress and the presidency, with a president who was a sworn enemy of the ACA and sought ways to undermine it (Chapter 3). As a result of the 2018 elections, Republicans increased their majority in the Senate and Democrats recaptured the House. Unless things change, this is not a scenario for much change in the ACA except continued administrative actions to weaken the law. Unless there is a significant public demand for improvements, perhaps seen in the 2020 elections, much of this will not be done. But that could be said of other reform proposals.

LIBERAL/DEMOCRATIC REFORM PROPOSALS

Regardless of the political realities mentioned in the previous paragraph, liberal politicians and think tanks have proposed massive health reforms. To simplify, the proposals are based on expansion of Medicaid and Medicare. Depending on how one counts, as of the end of 2018 there were eight or nine proposals (see Kliff and Scott 2018; Neuman, Pollitz, and Tolbert 2018). We will examine a few of the proposals.

Medicaid-Based Plans

We begin with Medicaid, perhaps the least likely source of systemic reform. Medicaid has always been seen as a poor sister to Medicare, though more people are enrolled in Medicaid than in Medicare and Medicaid expenditures are higher than those for Medicare. Medicaid, as we saw in Chapter 4, has been considered more like welfare for poor people than healthcare for deserving people. Some states, such as Kentucky and Arkansas, have instituted work requirements approved by the Trump administration. These are attempts to make Medicaid more like the major cash assistance program Temporary Assistance to Needy Families—a temporary program designed to move people into the work force. Despite efforts to cut the program on the part of the Trump administration, the program remains popular across party lines, though Democrats and independents have more favorable opinions about Medicaid than Republicans. Majorities of both parties oppose a lifetime limit on Medicaid eligibility (Scott 2018a). Still, it seems like an unlikely platform to support health reform.

The basic proposal can be labeled "Medicaid for All" (Sparer 2017). Such a proposal, supported by Senator Brian Schatz (D-HI), would use Medicaid as the foundation for increasing coverage and saving money. One part of the proposal is that states not currently expanding Medicaid via the ACA do so. That would provide coverage to millions of more people. The second feature is to allow people to buy into Medicaid. People would pay premiums for the program.

Sparer (2017) presents some advantages of Medicaid that make it a good platform to expand coverage. Sparer mentions studies that show that people on Medicaid have good access to care, that they are more likely than those without insurance to get screenings that catch diseases at an early stage.

Sparer (2017) also points out that despite the huge costs, largely a function of a large covered population, costs per capita are lower than for either Medicare or those with private insurance. A major reason for this is that Medicaid reimbursement is lower than for the other two sources of health insurance (employers and Medicare). Sparer (2017) also notes that a majority of Medicaid beneficiaries are in managed-care plans, thus run by the private sector (generally insurance companies) rather than a government agency.

A third reason Sparer (2017) gives is that Medicaid is a more generous program than Medicare. Thus the need that most Medicare beneficiaries find to get additional coverage (either through medigap policies or Medicare Advantage policies) would be unnecessary.

A fourth advantage is the federal-state nature of the program. Sparer (2017) writes that there should be some national standards for eligibility (some of which already exist). And a number of states have either begun a Medicaid buy-in program or have considered it.

The fifth advantage is a political one. States are already experimenting with some of the ideas that Sparer (2017) and others have advocated. Much of what needs to be done is already in place and therefore is likely the easiest plan to implement.

The final advantage is that a large segment of the population supports Medicaid for All. A 2018 study found that 48 percent of those surveyed support a single-payer system. But 57 percent supported Medicaid for All (Rainey 2018).

Like any other proposal, there are critics. Pipes (2018) argues that Medicaid provides low-quality care to its recipients and a Medicaid for All would extend that to more affluent populations. Pipes (2018) addresses several of the points made by Sparer (2017).

The first point is that Medicaid is a lower-cost program than private insurance. Pipes does not disagree but does note that one reason providers charge more to their privately insured patients is because Medicaid reimbursement is low, what Pipes calls "underpaid."

Pipes (2018) states that an important problem with Medicaid is that providers (doctors) can refuse to take Medicaid patients, noting that less than 50 percent of doctors will take new patients because of the low reimbursement and also because of administrative requirements. Pipes (2018) notes that only about two-thirds of doctors have Medicaid patients.

Pipes (2018) argues that allowing employees with health insurance to drop their coverage and buy into Medicaid will result in millions moving into a low-quality program and at the same costing more to states and the federal government.

While Sparer (2017) and others have addressed some of the problems that Pipes indicates (see, for example, Krugman 2013), there do remain problems with the program. One is the diversity of Medicaid, which is both a strength and a weakness. It is a strength because it allows states to craft the kind of program they want. It is a weakness because there is significant variation from state to state. Costs are another issue. While Sparer (2017) and Krugman (2013) believe that if Medicaid were more predominant, providers would accept more patients and reimbursements, it is likely that such a program would require higher reimbursements, resulting in fewer savings.

Still, it is an intriguing idea.

Medicare-Based Plans

Another place to look for reform proposals is Medicare. One of the earliest such proposals came in 2007. Jacob Hacker (2007) proposed "Health Care for America" right at the time that considerations of what would eventually become the Affordable Care Act began. The proposal would maintain employer-based insurance and build on Medicare. Hacker writes that the Health Care for America Plan, modeled after Medicare, would be available for those under 65 who did not have insurance. Employers would either provide health insurance for their employees or pay into a fund to help finance the Health Care for America Plan (what is known as play-or-pay). It also contained what is effectively an individual mandate. Hacker's plan called for Medicaid and CHIP (Children's Health Insurance Program) recipients to enroll in Health Care for America. States would no longer have the burden of paying for Medicaid but would have to provide funds for benefits that Medicaid covered but Health Care for America might not. Employers could enroll their workers in Health Care for America. Finally, Hacker argued that Medicare plus Health Care for America could work together and bargain for lower prices while still maintaining high-quality care.

A different Medicare-based policy would allow people aged 55 to 64 to buy in to Medicare, similar to the buy-in to Medicaid discussed above. One version would allow the buy-in to be optional; another version would make people in this age group automatically enrolled (similar to Part A of Medicare; see Chapter 5) and eligible for all the Medicare benefits (Bodenheimer 2017; Glickman 2017). One of the advantages is that it would pull those with higher risk of needing healthcare out of the private markets and into Medicare. It would require some additional taxation, both from the payroll tax and general federal revenue. Such a proposal is a relatively modest one, because it seeks to leave much of the ACA in place and deal with a population with high costs and limited insurance options.

The granddaddy of Medicare reform is Medicare for All. It is closely associated with Senator Bernie Sanders (I-VT), the socialist senator who made a run for the 2016 Democratic presidential nomination. For Sanders, Medicare for All, a single-payer system, is basically a moral issue:

> This is a pivotal moment in American history. Do we, as a nation, join the rest of the industrialized world and guarantee comprehensive health care to every person as a human right? Or do we maintain a system that is enormously expensive, wasteful and bureaucratic, and is designed to maximize profits for big insurance companies, the pharmaceutical industry, Wall Street and medical equipment suppliers?
>
> We remain the only major country on earth that allows chief executives and stockholders in the health care industry to get incredibly rich, while tens of millions of people suffer because they can't get the health care they need. This is not what the United States should be about.
>
> (Sanders 2017)

Sanders (2017) listed the major problems of the American healthcare system: Costs that hinder people from getting care that they need; a complex, fragmented, highly bureaucratized system; healthcare expenditures that dwarf those of other countries; millions of people still uninsured.

To Sanders (2017), the problems were obvious. The system seems designed to create profits for various healthcare industries. There is waste and fraud in the system. The US does not control spiraling pharmaceutical costs.

The solution, for Sanders, is opening up Medicare to everyone. It would be a single-payer system, replacing other payers such as Medicaid and private insurance. It would "expand and overhaul" Medicare (Kurtzleben

2017). It would eliminate cost-sharing and private insurance company participation in Medicare (Parts C and D). It would be phased in over a four-year period, with eligibility to join eventually covering everyone. It would expand the benefits offered to recipients, such as dental and vision coverage. The Veterans Health Administration and the Indian Health Service would remain (Kliff 2017). It would also rely on increased taxes to finance the plan (Kurtzleben 2017). The Sanders plan would be more generous in terms of benefits and cost-sharing than employer-sponsored insurance in the United States or single-payer systems in other countries (Kliff 2017).

As can be imagined, the Sanders plan created a lot of opposition. Clearly insurance companies would be unhappy about effectively losing a major line of business. But there are two other criticisms that can be made of the Sanders plan.

First, Anderson, Liu, and Friedberg (2018), looking at all the Medicare-based proposals, ask "what does Medicare for All" mean. They point out there are a variety of Medicare-based proposals, including a Medicare for All offered by Representative Keith Ellison (D-MN), the Medicare Buy-In Plans, discussed above; and a Medicare-based public option as an addition to the Affordable Care Act (Kaiser Family Foundation 2018). Each proposal is a bit different from the others. And, more importantly for Anderson, Liu, and Friedberg (2018) is that Medicare, as currently formulated, is a complex program, with different parts (A, B, C, and D), with different benefits, financing, and cost-sharing. Additionally, those in traditional Medicare can purchase supplemental insurance (medigap policies). The warning from Anderson, Liu, and Friedberg (2018) is to be clear as to how the proposals are addressing the structure of Medicare as well as its limitations.

Perhaps a more important question is financing. Again, we focus on the Sanders plan, though it is an issue that all reform proposals, including fixing the ACA, face. The cost issue is also one that conservatives raise as a problem with all health reform proposals.

Let us begin by considering how the Medicare for All plan would be financed. The Sanders plan would make use of current federal healthcare spending. This would include the federal portion of Medicaid, the subsidies for the ACA exchanges, the current funding for Medicare, and the amount lost in federal revenue because of tax expenditures for employer-sponsored insurance (Kaiser Family Foundation 2018). The plan also assumes cost savings. Some of that comes because providers would be paid at Medicare reimbursement rates, higher than Medicaid, but lower than employer-sponsored insurance. The rates would be negotiable. The plan also would allow negotiations over drug prices with pharmaceutical companies, which, presumably, would result in savings. It would also establish a global budget for healthcare, unlike the non-budget situation that exists now (Kaiser Family Foundation 2018).

Sanders (n.d.) offers a variety of ways to raise revenue. One addresses employers. Employers would pay a 7.5-percent income-based premium, a payroll tax. Sanders calculates that this would raise $3.9 trillion over a ten-year period. But he points out that businesses would get a net saving. Sanders (n.d.) shows how this would work:

> In 2016, employers paid an average of $12,865 in private health insurance premiums for a worker with a family of four who makes $50,000 a year. Under this option, employers would pay a 7.5 percent payroll tax to help finance Medicare for All—just $3,750—a saving of more than $9,000 a year for that employee.

Sanders' plan would exempt the first $2 million in payroll from the tax, which would protect smaller businesses.

A similar calculation would work for families (Sanders n.d.).

> Last year [2016] the typical working family paid an average of $5,277 in premiums to private health insurance companies. Under this option, a typical family of four earning $50,000, after taking the standard deduction, would pay a 4 percent income-based premium to fund Medicare for All—just $844 a year—saving that family over $4,400 a year. Because of the standard deduction, families of four making less than $29,000 a year would not pay this premium.

The Sanders plan also assumes $4.2 billion per year of savings from the tax expenditure for employer-sponsored insurance.

Another set of revenue options focuses on the federal income tax. Sanders (n.d.) proposes a more progressive income tax system, which means that wealthier people would have their taxes increased. The Sanders proposal estimates $1.8 trillion in extra revenue over a ten-year period. A related proposal would make the estate tax more progressive. Additional taxes would be imposed on corporations. Ellison's Medicare for All makes use of similar revenue proposals.

Blahous (2018) estimates that the cost of the Medicare for All plan would be about $32 trillion of additional federal spending over a ten-year period. Blahous (2018) argues that proposed revenues would not fully cover the additional costs. Further, Blahous (2018) notes that the plan assumes that providers would be paid at Medicare rates, part of the savings of the plan. Apart from the resistance such a reimbursement rate would engender among providers, if rates were actually higher than so would be the costs. Blahous (2018) points out that others who made calculations, such as the Urban Institute, have come up with similar numbers. For example, an Urban Institute study (Holahan et al. 2016) cites an estimate that projected revenue increases under the plan would be about nearly $17 trillion below expenditures over a ten-year period.

One interesting point that can be seen in Balbous' (2018) report, pointed out by Scott (2018b), is that while costs to the federal government would increase, healthcare spending under the plan would be lower than projected under current law. Blahous (2018) presents a table showing projections through 2031. Here we will just look at the 2031 numbers. Projected personal healthcare spending under current law would be $6.494 trillion. Under the Sanders plan (Medicare for All or M4A), personal healthcare spending would be $6.406 trillion. Looking at overall healthcare expenditures, the current project for 2031 is $7.651 trillion; for M4A, the projection is $7.348 trillion. Of course, changing analytic assumptions, such as provider reimbursement rates, changes the projections.

Scott (2018b) points out the political implications of the analyses. For conservatives such as Blahous (2018), the new numbers are very high, and the role of government would expand, all good political talking points. For liberals, advocates of single-payer healthcare, the key is to emphasize that Americans as whole will save money.

Another variant of the Medicare for All-type proposals came from the liberal think tank The Center for American Progress (CAP) (CAP Health Policy Reform Team 2018). CAP begins its proposal by stating that healthcare is a right, that everyone should have access to healthcare. The plan, Medicare Extra for All, would first add benefits to Medicare. This includes dental coverage, hearing aids, better drug coverage, and a ceiling on out-of-pocket costs, vision care, and screenings for children that are available through Medicaid. Second, everyone would be eligible "regardless of income, health status, age, or insurance status" (CAP Health Policy Reform Team 2018). The CAP plan would allow employers to offer Medicare extra for All to their employees, or could make the CAP the employer plan. Providers would be reimbursed at rates similar to Medicare rates and Medicare would be allowed to negotiate drug prices with pharmaceutical companies.

Medicare Extra for All would leave in place all the other health insurance plans but allow options to join. Those turning 65 after the plan is enacted would be automatically enrolled in Medicare Extra for All.

The CAP plan, unlike the Sanders Medicare for All plan, includes cost-sharing features. Such features, including premiums, deductibles, and co-payments, would vary by income. Those at the bottom of the income scale would have no cost-sharing, while those at higher levels would bear some of the costs of the plan (CAP Health Policy Reform Team 2018).

Medicare Extra for All addresses Medicare Advantage. The plan recognizes the advantages of such plans, but also states that they have been overpaid. The CAP plan would change the name to Medicare Choice and then open up the program up for bidding by insurance companies. Medicare Extra would pay the plans at 95 percent of average beneficiary costs, taking the payments back to the 1997 Balanced Budget Act (CAP Health Policy Reform Team 2018).

The CAP plan envisions various ways to finance the program and achieve savings, similar to the Sanders plan. One, already referenced, would be provider-reimbursement savings. A second, also previously mentioned, would be negotiations over drug prices. A third is payment and delivery system reform. As one example of this, Medicare Extra for All would implement what are called site-neutral payments. This is an interesting part of the proposal, because the Centers for Medicare and Medicaid Services (CMS) under the Trump administration have enacted a rule for this. The problem this addresses has to do with hospitals buying doctor practices. If a patient sees a physician who is independent, not part of a hospital system, then the payment goes to the physician. If a hospital purchases the doctor's practice, the hospital raises the cost of seeing the physician, even if it is for the same medical issue and the patient is seen in the same doctor's office before the system bought the practice. The rule that CMS issued, and the CAP plan proposes as well, would pay physicians the same regardless of where the service takes place (Morse 2018). Of course, hospitals do not like the practice, arguing that they have additional costs that need to be covered. As a result, hospitals sued CMS over the rule (Luthi 2018). The CAP plan also assumed administrative savings, because there would be fewer health insurance plans to work with, no marketing, and no profits.

The Medicare Extra for All also calls for additional taxes. It assumes the repeal of the December 2017 tax cut (the Tax Cut and Jobs Act). It calls for higher taxes for higher-income people. It would curb the tax exclusion for employer-sponsored insurance. It would also include higher taxes on tobacco products and sugary drinks.

A related proposal is one offered by Jacob Hacker (2018). Hacker (2007) was an early advocate of using Medicare as the basis of healthcare reform. Hacker (2018), taking note of the attempts at healthcare reform and the obstacles reform faces, argues that Medicare as a program works and is simpler than the ACA. He also points out that Medicare is not a single-payer system because of the presence of Medicare Advantage (see Chapter 5), and that most countries, even those with universal health insurance coverage, are not single-payer systems. Hacker (2018) also observes that all those who currently have insurance will not look kindly on change. Because proposals such as Sanders' Medicare for All plan would require significant tax increases (even if they are replacing private spending) and a greater (federal) governmental role, that would also create opposition to change.

Hacker's (2018) plan is "Medicare Part E," where the "E" stands for everyone. The plan assumes that everyone is covered by Medicare, unless they enroll in a quality plan, which could include a good Medicaid program or an employer plan. Employers who do not have their own plan would be required to contribute to Medicare (what is known as "play-or-pay"). Hacker's (2018) plan would retain Medicaid because, as he sees, it has become a much better, more generous program over the years (see Chapter 4).

Those who enrolled in Medicare Part E would have to pay additional premiums, which would vary depending on income. Hacker (2018) gives a preliminary estimate of $300 a month extra for those at the higher end of the income scale. There would also need to be additional taxation, but the tax increase would be modest, again perhaps focused on higher-income people.

Medicare, under this plan, would be allowed to negotiate drug prices with pharmaceutical companies. Insurance companies would still play an important role in the healthcare system. Medicare Advantage plans would also continue to play its role within Medicare. Hacker's (2018) plan seems designed to meet many of the political objections to healthcare reform.

One of the more interesting set of reforms was offered by Wynne in a series of essays (2017a, 2017b, 2017c, 2017d, 2018a, 2018b, 2018c). Wynne (2017a) argues that the Affordable Care Act "stole" (his term) many good conservative ideas. These included the tax subsidies for purchasing private health insurance on the exchanges, the individual mandate, payment reforms, and flexibility in the states. All of these came about because of negotiations between Republicans and Democrats in 2008 led by the chair of the Senate Finance Committee Max Baucus (D-MT). Wynne was one of Baucus's staff members and labels the ACA as a "very moderate law."

Based on his experience, Wynne (2017b) believes that bipartisan reform is still possible and the only way to effect change. He then offers a four-step plan (Wynne 2017c).

The first is "enhancing the individual market." Here Wynne calls for a number of changes. Policies under this step include fully funding the cost-sharing subsidies, actively promoting the exchanges, and funding the risk corridor program (payments to insurance companies for keeping premiums down). Wynne (2017c) also suggests adding a copper plan for those who want a cheaper plan. The copper plan would be similar to a catastrophic health insurance plan, which covers costs after a high deductible (see the discussion below). Wynne (2017c) also suggests expanding the amount that insurance companies could charge to older beneficiaries from 3–1 to 4 or 5–1. Wynne (2017c) notes that with the subsidies, older recipients would not notice much change in their premiums. He also suggests cutting some taxes called for under the ACA and allowing markets and insurance companies to compete across state lines. As we will note below, many of Wynne's suggestions cross ideological lines.

The second step is to rationalize the employer market. One of his suggestions (Wynne 2017c) is to eliminate the "family glitch" discussed above. Other suggestions would be to allow small employers to utilize the exchanges and to find ways to limit the expenditures of employers, perhaps by some type of premium support: Give a fixed amount to employees and let them purchase their own insurance.

Wynne (2017c) also suggests that we need to look at "the tax exclusion for employer-sponsored insurance." Wynne (2017c) suggests either limiting the exclusion or doing away with it. One possible outcome of eliminating employer-sponsored insurance is that businesses may no longer want to provide health insurance as a benefit or, perhaps, keep the benefit but shift more of the costs to employees.

The third step is to "embrace Medicaid." Wynne (2017c) thinks all states should expand Medicaid, as called for under the ACA. He notes that states have new flexibility to design their Medicaid programs, particularly with the Section 1115 waivers (see Chapter 4).

The final step is to consider providers and patients. Here Wynne (2017c) suggests leaving providers alone. They have been strongly affected by regulations emanating from the ACA (and previous policies) dealing with payment systems, electronic health records, etc.

For patients, Wynne (2017c) suggests that we look at and perhaps change what he calls the "culture of health." Here he is writing about lifestyle issues, such as diet and exercise. He writes (Wynne 2017c): "Finally, it's worth noting that what the health care system does to our bodies is far less important than what we put in our bodies." For Wynne (2017c), the main problem is sugar.

In his next essay, Wynne (2017d) offers a comprehensive health reform proposal that he thinks will appeal to Democrats/liberals as well as Republican/conservatives. Wynne (2017d) writes:

> My goal with this post is to demonstrate that a "unified" (punchline: It wouldn't truly be single payer…), market-driven, federally regulated, privately delivered system need not possess any of these objectionable attributes. In fact, the parameters of such a system are all but staring us right in the face. I call it: Medicare Advantage Premium Support for All (MAPSA).
>
> While any flavor of single payer may be the last thing that comes to mind when contemplating bipartisan initiatives, just as the far left and far right share some libertarian (and other) commonalities, we may have indeed finally come full circle in this tiresome, so-far-futile debate. By combining two shots of conservative orthodoxy with one overflowing progressive one, and stirring slowly, it is not at all far-fetched to envision an endgame cocktail for our health care system that covers everyone, decreases costs, and can pass Congress. Cheers.

Without going into detail on the calculations (see Wynne 2017d), Wynne thinks that the financing of his plan would work with no new taxes and windfalls for both business and individuals. Individuals and households would be given a tax credit with which they could purchase either traditional Medicare or Medicare Advantage. Wynne (2017d) sees the plan as consumer-driven (see below for further discussion of consumer-driven healthcare plans) and the subsidies can be adjusted as needed. Wynne (2017d) also notes that some adjustments would have to be made to the Medicare package. For example, Wynne (2017d) writes that there are services that children receive under Medicaid that are not available in Medicare. That would be one change that needs to be made.

Wynne (2018a) writes that providers would likely favor such a plan. Under MAPSA (Wynne's proposal), providers would be reimbursed at Medicare rates. This is less than provider reimbursement through private insurance but more than Medicaid reimbursement rates. Taking out Medicaid and those without insurance would ease the pain of the lower reimbursement. Wynne (2018a) also suggests that providers would favor such a plan because the administrative burden would be considerably lower than it is now.

The various liberal/Democratic plans all have the same basic ideas: Cover more people, if not the entire population; limit patient costs; restrain provider costs; administrative simplicity; generous benefits; higher taxes, at least for some portion of the population; and an expanded role for government, especially the federal government. There are differences in details (Kliff and Scott 2018; Neuman, Pollitz, and Tolbert 2018), and the differences can be significant. But the overall thrust of all the proposals is the same.

CONSERVATIVE/REPUBLICAN PROPOSALS

Conservatives and Republicans have several problems with the liberal/Democratic plans. One is the cost of the liberal reforms, which would mean higher taxes. It is an inherent part of much of conservative ideology that high taxes are bad. The 41st president, George H. W. Bush, lost his reelection campaign in 1992 to Bill Clinton at least partly because he broke the promise he made at the 1988 Republican National Convention that he would refuse to agree to new taxes. We could go back to at least the Reagan administration, if not further, to see the anti-tax platform (President Reagan eventually agreed to tax increases but called them "revenue enhancers").

A related complaint about the liberal policies, seen mostly clearly in the Sanders "Medicare for All" proposal, is the enhanced role of the federal government, especially at the expense of states and the private sector. Rove (2018) refers to proposals such as "Medicare for All" as a form of socialism. The following quote summarizes the cost and federal role issue that conservatives find distasteful:

> Consider the arguments against "Medicare for All." Do voters really want to abolish private insurance? After watching the Department of Veterans Affairs bungle the treatment of the nation's warriors, do Americans want their personal health decisions made by the unwieldy, unresponsive federal government? Do they want the wait times, the decline in quality, and the slowing of innovation that would come with a takeover by a new federal bureaucracy? And how will the country pay the $32 trillion cost of the Medicare expansion? The average working couple already pay $158,000 in Medicare taxes over their careers. How would they like to see their taxes skyrocket and their care cut?
>
> (Rove 2018)

A third conservative critique of the liberal proposals is the underlying assumption of those proposals that there is a right to healthcare. A right is a claim to something (Stone 2012). In the abortion debate, both sides claim rights, a right to life on the conservative side and a right to choose on the liberal side. Other policy areas also make use of rights. For example, there is a right to a lawyer in a criminal case. Stone (2012, 331–333) distinguishes between two types of rights. One is "positive rights," which are backed by and derived from government. The other is "normative rights." Stone (2012, p. 332) summarizes the essence of normative rights:

> In the normative tradition, rights derived from something higher than man-made law—moral principles that exist before and separate from government. Different schools of thought find these moral principles in natural law, religious texts, rational thought, public opinion, social practices and institutions, and the idea of universal human rights.

Liberal thought, as embodied in the Affordable Care Act, asserts healthcare as a right. This can be seen from politics early in the twentieth century. In his State of the Union message in February 1944, President Franklin Roosevelt proposed a "second bill of rights," this time based on economic needs. Among those rights were "A right to adequate medical care and the opportunity to achieve and enjoy good health" (quoted in Nichols 2015).

For conservatives, healthcare is more of good than a right, a good not much different from other goods. Napolitano (2017), for example, argues that the healthcare is a good, one that a person can choose to have or use or not have or use and how much would be used. Napolitano (2017) says that the Constitution does not recognize healthcare as a right and therefore the federal government cannot create one. It can provide a good. In this case, Napolitano (2017) sees that as one way that Congress bribes voters to stay in office, giving "the rich ... bailouts, the middle-class ... tax cuts and the poor made-up rights to all sorts of things."

With that as the foundation of much (but not all) conservative thought about healthcare, conservatives tend to look for market-type solutions in healthcare as an alternative to what they see as government-imposed policy.

To summarize, for conservatives, healthcare is a good, taxes should be low, and governmental programs tend to be inefficient and infringe on rights. Controlling government spending on healthcare is also important.

We begin with Paul Ryan (R-WI). Ryan, the Speaker of the US House of Representatives, and his staff prepared a series of policy proposals for the 2016 elections, entitled "A Better Way" (Ryan 2016). The health plan is briefly described as follows:

> As this plan shows, there is another way—a better way—to provide all Americans with health care that is accessible, affordable, and sustainable. In this plan, innovative, market-based, patient-centered solutions replace Obamacare's one-size-fits-all, Washington-knows-best approach. This plan empowers patients with access to affordable, portable health care options. It provides every American with the freedom to pick a plan that best fits his or her unique health care needs—not coverage mandated by Washington. It protects those individuals with pre-existing conditions and promotes innovation to encourage health care competition, to lower costs, and to foster new cures for patients.
>
> (Ryan 2016, 37)

The plan begins by pointing out how Obamacare (the Affordable Care Act) has been a failure. People are facing higher premiums and higher deductibles. Consumers are finding they have fewer choices as plans narrow provider networks to control costs. The tax increases called for under the ACA were oppressive to those they were imposed upon. The plan complains about the increase, "swelling" in the report's language, of Medicaid enrollment. The report also states that Medicaid puts pressure on state budgets and does not give adequate access to the healthcare system for its enrollees. The report also complains about the expanded role of the federal government in healthcare and in healthcare decisions. Related to this point, the Ryan report lists 17 ways in which the Obama administration issued unauthorized executive orders.

The Ryan plan has eight parts. The first is to expand consumer-directed healthcare. This would give consumers (patients) more choices about what kind of plan they want, what kind of care they want, and which providers they want. The Ryan plan would make use of private exchanges, health savings accounts, and health reimbursement accounts. All of these would give consumers (patients) more choice.

The second part is to make coverage support more portable. The recipient would receive a payment every month (a refundable tax credit) that would help pay for health insurance. If the cost of the insurance were less than the financial assistance, the recipient would keep the difference. Those funds could be used to pay out-of-pocket costs. If it were more, the recipient would have to pay the difference.

The third part is the preservation of employer-sponsored insurance (ESI). But it would limit (put a ceiling on) the tax exclusion for health benefits. The Ryan plan argues that doing see could result in larger paychecks and lower premiums for employees, because the tax-free benefits would decline and employers would put the money into workers' salaries.

The fourth part is to allow the purchase of insurance plans across state lines. This would create a national market for insurance plans and create more competition. The added competition would result in more affordable plans.

The fifth part is to expand opportunities for pooling. What this means is that small businesses and non-profits could work together, form pools, to create their own health insurance plans, what are called association plans. This would give the businesses a large enough group to negotiate with health insurers for better plans and lower costs. The Ryan plan suggests that individuals could get together and form individual health pools (IHP), again, to have the bargaining power to negotiate with health insurers.

The sixth part is to continue wellness programs. The plan would allow financial incentives to employees to engage in healthier behavior.

The seventh part is to protect employers who self-insure. The employer assumes the risks and can craft a plan to meet the needs of its employees. Such employers also purchase stop-loss insurance plans, basically a form of catastrophic insurance, in the event that there are unusually high claims.

The final part of the Ryan plan is reform of the medical liability or tort system. Here the plan calls for the end of frivolous lawsuits and an incentive to practice defensive medicine. The plan would limit non-economic damages, excessive lawyer fees, and "ensure that patients can recover full economic damages" (Ryan 2016, 19).

The Ryan plan also calls for protections for people with pre-existing conditions, by forbidding the denial of coverage for such conditions. The plan would allow insurers to charge up to five times as much for premiums for older Americans as for younger Americans. States could adjust that ratio up or down depending on their needs and the needs of the population.

The plan calls for the creation and support of high-risk pools for those whose health conditions price them out of the insurance market. There would be a combination of federal and state funding for the pools.

The Ryan plan calls for protecting life and conscience rights. Here the plan is referring to abortion and contraception devices. It takes a very strong pro-life, pro-abortion stance, and allows employers and providers to refuse service if it violates their conscience.

Medicaid is also subject to the Ryan plan. The plan calls for federal Medicaid payments, which are currently based on demand for services, to be transformed either into a block grant to states or a per-capita grant (a fixed amount per Medicaid recipient). This would give states more flexibility and, at the same time, Medicaid would be become a fixed expense for the federal government.

Medicare also gets attention from the Ryan plan. The most important part of the Medicare recommendations is premium support. Beneficiaries would get a refundable tax credit that would be used to purchase a healthcare plan. As we saw in Chapter 5, the premium support plan goes back at least to the Clinton administration. As with block grants for Medicaid, this would provide the federal government with a budgeted item that would be based on the number of recipients rather than the demand for healthcare. The Ryan plan would also combine Medicare Parts A and B. It would give Medicare Advantage plans more flexibility in plan design. The Ryan plan would limit medigap policies that help beneficiaries pay for cost-sharing.

The Ryan plan, "Better Care for All," is an excellent place to start looking at conservative healthcare reform policies. It contains many of the conservative positions on healthcare reform: Repealing Obamacare, more consumer choice, state flexibility, block grants and premium support, less regulation, and a diminished role for the federal government. While other plans may add some proposals, the Ryan plan should be considered a centerpiece of conservative healthcare reform thought.

Competition is an important component of conservative healthcare reform policy, though elements of competition can be found in more liberal reforms. One of the oldest of such policies is managed competition, discussed earlier in the book. The concept of managed competition, though using different language, goes back to the 1970s, embodied in the Health Maintenance Organization Act of 1973. Alain Enthoven's (1980) consumer-choice health plan was one of the early proposals in this vein (see Chapter 8). Managed competition was an essential part of the Clinton Health Security Act. And it is embodied in programs such as medigap and Medicare Part D, in the California Public Employees Retirement System (CALPers) and the Federal Employees Health Benefits program, and the ACA exchanges.

In 2018, Enthoven and Baker (2018) published an article suggesting that managed competition could be an important component of health reform, based on experience with such systems in California. The tenets of managed competition include fully integrated healthcare systems, consumer choice between a number of plans, quality measurement and the publication of such measurements, and giving consumers\patients a fixed sum, essentially premium support, to help pay for health insurance plans. Enthoven and Baker (2018) write that the experience with Covered California, the state-run exchange under the ACA, has been very positive, showing that the managed competition concept is workable.

In 2017, President Trump issued an executive order asking the Departments of Health and Human Services, Treasury, and Labor (cited in-text as HHSTL) to produce a report suggesting how to reform the American healthcare system, making use of choice and competition. That report was issued in 2018. The sense of the report can be seen in the following quote (HHSTL 2018, 7):

> Economists generally accept that free-market competition produces the most efficient production and distribution of goods and services. When consumers have choices, the incentives and information needed to optimize value, firms have the incentive to improve quality and lower costs through innovation. Competitive market forces and the incentive to innovate typically raise quality and drive down prices, including quality-adjusted prices, for goods and services over time (features observed in many well-functioning sectors of the economy), but which are generally absent in the highly regulated healthcare market). However, when government policies and regulations suppress competition, producers may use their market power to raise prices, produce lower-quality goods and services, or become complacent in innovating. In other words, without competitive pressure, the incentive to lower prices, improve quality, and innovate diminishes. As the government share of healthcare spending has increased over time, the healthcare market has become increasingly vulnerable to rules and regulations that impede market forces.

The report then goes on to look at the traditional ways that healthcare markets fail, thus requiring government action to correct poor markets, and finds all of those criticisms to be wanting. Interestingly, the report argues, as do others (see, for example, Silver and Hyman 2018), that current health insurance policies provide poor incentives to both providers and patients. The third-party insurance system is administratively complex, and it provides incentives for patients to consume as much healthcare as possible (including low-value healthcare) and providers to provide as much healthcare as possible because they make more money for providing more services (even those of limited value). The report, and others, argues that insurance should only cover high-cost, unpredictable health needs (such as open-heart surgery) rather than everything, including the predictable (such as well-baby checkups). The report compares the situation to auto insurance, where insurance does not cover gas or routine maintenance (such as oil changes) but does cover most of the costs in the event of an accident. The report critiques the tax expenditure for employer-sponsored insurance for helping to cover the low-cost and predictable events. While the report takes a comprehensive look at the healthcare system, such as mergers, graduate medical education, and foreign-trained physicians, the basic reform proposed is competition.

Here the report advocates greater use of health savings accounts, health reimbursement accounts, and high-deductible plans (essentially catastrophic insurance). Both set of accounts can be used to pay for those services not covered under the catastrophic plan. The HHSTL (2018) report proposes loosening rules on both types of accounts so that more people can take advantage of them. The report also calls for greater price transparency so consumers (and providers) can make more value-focused choices and greater use of telehealth as a means of delivery services to patients.

Chen (2018, 1) argues that conservative reform will be based on a "state innovation model approach." Chen (2018) points out that conservatives disagree on a number of health reform issues (disagreement exists among liberal reform advocates as well).

The first disagreement is over universal coverage. Chen writes that for many conservatives, government, especially expanded government, is overly bureaucratic, inefficient, has too much regulation, etc. But others see the goal as one that conservatives should adopt (see discussion below about conservatives and universal care).

The second disagreement is over how and whether to make use of the federal tax code as part of reform. Chen (2018) observes that some conservative thinkers would make use of the tax code to equalize tax treatment of those with employer-sponsored insurance and those who buy insurance on the individual market. Others see something like this idea as a new federal entitlement that would also have a harmful impact on the country's fiscal situation.

The third disagreement is over how to control healthcare costs. Many conservatives (see the discussion of Goodman below) argue for a consumer-oriented reform, including elements such as high-deductible plans associated with health savings and health reimbursement accounts. Other conservatives do not believe that the consumer orientation is sufficient by itself to control healthcare costs. Related to that is disagreement over how much regulation there should be of the healthcare system.

The fourth disagreement concerns Medicaid. Conservatives, in general, do not like the program. But it has been shown to be popular among the public, especially during the attempts to repeal-and-replace the Affordable Care Act in 2017. Some Republicans, both in Congress and among governors, support the program.

Chen (2018) believes that a state innovation approach, which was not included in any of the 2017 repeal-and-replace plans, could be the foundation for a Republican-based reform. Such an approach puts heavy reliance on federalism and gives states a great deal of flexibility in designing programs.

Chen (2018) lists the goals of a state innovation approach:

> lowering costs, expanding access to nonstandardized coverage options, and giving state leaders the resources and flexibility to make decisions about how best to address the needs of their residents.

Chen (2018) writes that these are not the goals of the Affordable Care Act, but they are important ones for Republicans to embrace.

The basis for the state innovation approach is Medicaid block grants. That approach provides states with considerable flexibility for helping the low-income population. For example, block grants could be used to help low-income people purchase insurance on the private market. The grants could also be used to lower premiums on the individual markets. The block grants could also be used to equalize spending among states (Chen 2018).

Chen (2018) also writes that state innovation reform should address Medicaid recipients and those in individual markets. Such reforms should eliminate many of the ACA regulations, such as the limits on the medical-loss ratio (the percentage of insurance premiums that must be spent on benefits) and the employer mandates. Higher limits of risk rating (higher premiums for those who are more likely to use medical services) should be allowed. Chen (2018) argues that, because of its political popularity, protections for those with pre-existing conditions should remain.

One of the most influential conservative thinkers is John C. Goodman. Goodman, like all conservatives, supports a market-based healthcare system. His reform (Goodman 2017) is based on three planks.

The first is a "universal health refund" (Goodman 2017). The refund, which would go to everyone, would be paid for by eliminating tax expenditures or subsidies for health insurance, the subsidies used to help consumers pay for insurance on the exchanges, and funds used to help the poor. Goodman's calculations are that healthcare funding would stay about the same, but individuals would be free to choose their own plans and the federal government's (and state's) role would be limited. A family of four would have about $8000 a year to use to pay for health insurance.

Goodman (2017) considers what impact such a proposal would have on employer-sponsored insurance. He writes that employers could keep their plans, but the tax benefits would no longer be available. Employees would use the refund to purchase the employer's plan or purchase on the open market. In the case of Medicaid, Goodman (2017) thinks that states should encourage recipients to enroll in private plans. Recipients could use the health refund plus the state's share of Medicaid per person to purchase private insurance.

The second part of Goodman's (2017) plan is flexible health savings accounts. The accounts would be used to pay for patient's primary-care needs. Interestingly, Goodman (2017) writes that health plans could deposit money into such accounts for those with chronic conditions if the patient would engage in effective self-care.

The third part of the plan is to protect people who have lost their coverage, perhaps because they changed jobs. Goodman (2017) is careful to note that people should not "game" the system, buying coverage when they anticipate a major health event such as hip replacement surgery. He also does not want plans to "dump" the sickest of patients. Instead, he calls for plans to adjust premiums so that medical costs would be covered. This is known as "free market risk adjustment" (Goodman 2017; "Turning the Exchanges into Real Markets" 2016). Goodman (2014) would also set up high-risk pools for those with preexisting conditions. In his plan, such a person could leave the high-risk pool and there would be additional help for paying premiums for such persons.

Goodman (2014) notes that his type of market-based proposal is a defined-contribution plan. In such a plan, everyone gets the same tax deduction to help purchase a plan. He argues that the Affordable Care Act is a defined-benefits plan, where everyone gets the same benefits. The defined-contribution plan, Goodman (2014) asserts, is more egalitarian that a defined-benefits plan.

Goodman (2014) would limit government's (likely meaning the federal government) role to three things: Refundable tax credits, high-risk pools, and Medicaid. Goodman (2014) sees the last two as temporary help.

Goodman's ideas are part of a congressional proposal sponsored by Senator Bill Cassidy (R-LA) and Representative Pete Sessions (R-TX). Sessions, Cassidy, and Goodman (2017) describe the goals of their reform:

> We believe the health care system is desperately in need of reform. But the focus of that reform should not be the Affordable Care Act. The initial goal should be: making sure everyone has access to health insurance that is affordable and that gives them dependable access to medical care. Further, we believe that goal can be accomplished with money already in the system. We don't need any new taxes or any new spending programs.

The plan calls for a "health status risk adjustment," arguing that current policy has perverse incentives with the sickest subscribers raising premiums for all subscribers. It suggests a single tax credit available for the purchase of private insurance. There could be adjustments for age and location, and there should be at least one plan available to everyone that costs the amount of the tax credit. Sessions, Cassidy, and Goodman (2017) offer a related suggestion: Everyone gets the same tax credit, whether purchasing insurance on the individual market or employer-sponsored insurance.

Sessions, Cassidy, and Goodman (2017) propose that employees should have the option of choosing the employer-sponsored plan or an individual plan. Employers should offer health reimbursement accounts, which allow employees to keep their accounts, and therefore pay for insurance and for services, even if they change jobs (portability).

Another part of the proposal is the integration of Medicaid and private insurance. They would do this by allowing Medicaid to use the tax credits to purchase private plans. They note that a large percentage of Medicaid recipients are already enrolled in private plans and argue that insurers could offer the same plan on the individual market. An important advantage of this part of the proposal is that many Medicaid recipients go back-and-forth between Medicaid and the exchanges, depending on how their income changes. This part of the plan would reduce the churning and the administrative complexity that accompanies it.

The final part of their plan is to create what they call "an effective safety net" (Sessions, Cassidy, and Goodman (2017). If there are people who remain uninsured, a portion of the tax credit would go to the community in which they live and provide additional funding for safety-net hospitals. If the uninsurance rate goes up, so do the additional funds from the tax credit. If the uninsurance rate goes down, a portion of the unused tax credits would go to support private insurance markets.

Silver's and Hyman's (2018) very comprehensive study of the American healthcare system and the Affordable Care Act identifies five problems that the ACA did not address. The first is that the healthcare system is under political control. They note that every time the (federal) government became more involved in the system, spending went up. And to be unbiased, they also note that despite President Trump's decrying the high costs of prescription drugs, his initial plans did nothing about them.

The second problem Silver and Hyman (2018) point to is third-party payment. The massive increases in healthcare spending in the United States began when Medicare and Medicaid were passed. And as insurance covered more, consumers directly paid less. Indeed, their key paragraph about the problems and the basis for their reform sets the tone for the rest of the book:

> The fundamental cause of spiraling health care costs isn't aging, technology, defensive medicine, or any of the other causes that are commonly cited. It is that we too often let others buy medical treatments for us instead of paying for them ourselves. Worse, excessive reliance on third-party payers has convinced Americans that they cannot and should not pay for medical services themselves. Tens of millions of people who would never think of using insurance to pay their mortgages or their rent reflexively use their health care coverage to pay for doctors' office visits and other medical services that cost far less. To dig ourselves out of this hole, we have to learn to treat health care like everything else. We should pay for most medical treatments directly, the same way we pay for housing, transportation, electricity, water, food, and clothes. Insurance should be reserved for calamities.
>
> (Silver and Hyman 2018, 8)

Their third problem is that prices are too high. They write that it seems as if the function of the American healthcare system is to move as much money as possible into the health sector. They note this "function" explains the waste and fraud that exists in the system.

Their fourth problem focuses on quality. Here they are referring specifically to medical malpractice issues. Quality is not as important as moving money.

Their final problem, related to the previous one, is the lack of transparency, the opaqueness of prices. Because insurance covers so much of medical care, patients/consumers do not care how much procedures or medicine costs. And for hospital charges, it is difficult to figure out what things actually cost (see, for example, Brill 2015; Makary 2015).

Silver's and Hyman's proposals follow from their diagnosis of the problems. They argue that the healthcare sector should operate like the retail sector, here pointing out how clinics in retail stores have been offering low-cost healthcare services for years. They note that a knee-replacement surgery might cost $31,000, the cost of a new car. So, why not pay for the surgery the way one pays for a car (assuming hospitals and doctors will allow payments over, say, a five-to-six-year period on the loans).

Their three-legged stool for change is, first, purchasing catastrophic health insurance policies to cover large and unexpected events. The second leg is to have people pay for most healthcare directly, say, the knee-replacement surgery, which is an expected event and can be planned for. The third leg is to provide support, what they call a budgeted item, for those who are poor or otherwise deserving.

A counter-intuitive idea from the conservative side comes from Madar (2017). Madar argues that conservatives will eventually endorse a socialized system based on the single-payer model. Such a system would cost less than the current American healthcare system and produce higher-quality care. In this vision, health insurance companies would no longer be needed. Government would have the power to set prices and, based on the experience of other countries, prices would go down.

Another point that Madar (2017) makes, one implied by Silver's and Hyman's analysis, is that there is an assumption that if healthcare is totally free at the point of service, then it will be overused. Madar (2017) writes that that has not been the experience of other countries with single-payer systems.

Madar (2017) notes that President Trump has praised the Australian healthcare system, a single-payer system. And Madar (2017) points out that public opinion shows support for many of the portions of the Affordable Care Act, even if people did not like Obamacare. His preferred policy option seems to be a Medicare for All plan.

What criticisms can be made of the Republican/conservative market-oriented plans? We start with the higher cost-sharing that such plans advocate. The basic idea here is that asking consumers/patients to pay more for their healthcare would incentivize them to shop more carefully (staying with the consumer metaphor), resulting in a more efficient use of resources and saving money. Three arguments can be made about this point.

First, as we have noted in the chapters on the ACA, Medicaid, and Medicare, there is a phenomenon known as concentration of healthcare expenditures. This tells us that a small percentage of the population accounts for a very disproportionate share of healthcare expenditures. If we are looking to spend less, this is the group that should be targeted. Of course, as we have noted elsewhere in the book, some of the people in this group have expensive chronic health conditions, some are in the last year of their life, and some have a temporary but costly medical need, such as knee surgery. Focusing on this group means making these distinctions and adjusting policy accordingly.

Second, while high-deductible plans are becoming more prevalent, the public seems to be pretty unhappy about this. We know this because cost-sharing is one of the principle consumer complaints about the Affordable Care Act.

Third, we also know that a sizable portion of the population has limited funds for out-of-the-ordinary needs. Many cannot come up with an extra $400 if needed in an emergency. Increasing cost-shifting increases the financial pressure on this group.

Fourth, we have some experimental evidence about what happens when we charge people for ordinary healthcare visits. The evidence is in the form of RAND health insurance experiments ("40 Years of the RAND Health Insurance Experiment" 2016). The influential study, which ran from 1976 to 1982, had subjects enroll in insurance plans with different types of insurance plans. Some were fee-for-service plans, with coinsurance varying from 0 to 95 percent. A fifth plan was a health maintenance organization. The major results were two-fold. First, and most heralded, was that cost-sharing led to decreased use of services, thereby reducing healthcare expenditures. The second finding was that participants decreased their use of services, whether they were essential or inessential. Thus, one can argue, based on the results, that consumers/patients are likely to reduce their use of vital services if asked to pay.

Fifth, there are insurance policies that would pay for services before a catastrophic plan, an important feature of conservative proposals, would come in. For example, those in traditional Medicare (outside of Medicare Advantage plans) can purchase medigap plans to cover costs that traditional Medicare does not cover. Insurance plans are likely to be developed that would cover initial costs under a catastrophic plan.

Sixth, a related point is health savings accounts (HSAs). HSAs are often teamed up with high-deductible plans. Employees put money into the accounts (which earn interest or are invested in stocks) and then can use that money to pay for medical expenses prior to the insurance plan coverage. Employers can add money to the account or set up a health reimbursement account (HRA) that then become available to employees. HSAs are growing in popularity.

But there are issues with HSAs. Tepper (2018) notes that Americans are very bad savers and that the savings rate has decreased over the years. She cites two reasons for this: One is wages that barely keep up with the cost of living and credit card debt. Only about 67 percent of people with HSAs make contributions to them. Many of those who did make contributions have a balance of about $2000, not nearly enough to pay for medical expenses that often occur. While policies can be envisioned that would address these issues, HSAs remain a pretty good deal for the healthy, but not quite as a good deal for those who experience health conditions.

One other problem with the cost-sharing/catastrophic/HSA proposals: Once the deductible is met, then insurance coverage has the same problems advocates of such policies are trying to address.

Another issue revolves around high-risk pools for people with expensive medical conditions, sometimes called the "uninsurables" (Pollitz 2017). Conservative/Republican proposals often seek to segment out those with serious medical conditions into a separate insurance pool. Those in the regular pool would see their insurance premiums go down, because the costly beneficiaries are no longer there. The problem here is for those in the risk pools. The premiums to cover this group would dramatically increase (experience rating; see Chapter 7) because healthier people would no longer be in the same insurance pool, as called for under the ACA. But the high-risk premiums would be so high that those in the pool might not be able to afford the premiums. Government at the state and federal levels stepped in.

Prior to the Affordable Care Act, 35 states had such pools. The ACA also created a temporary federal version of high-risk pools until full implementation of the ACA took place. The experience was not a happy one. States would not enroll people with pre-existing conditions for up to a year, though the federal plan did not make this condition. The costs were high and states often imposed annual limits on how much they would pay for certain services, such as pharmaceuticals, and lifetime limits on how much they would pay overall. Plans often had high deductibles (Pollitz 2017). Ultimately, although the population served was relatively small (especially compared to the size of the population with pre-existing conditions), the costs were very high and not sustainable.

While other comments might be made of the conservative/Republican proposals, we will end this discussion with one more element. If competitive markets are to work in healthcare, there has to be competition. This is the idea behind, as we have previously remarked, programs such as Medicare Advantage, Medicare Part D, and federal and California employee pension programs. One of the criticisms of the exchanges under the Affordable Care Act is that insurers, because of the instability of the markets, have pulled out. Some counties have, at best, a single insurer to choose from in their marketplace.

One solution, offered by conservative plans, is to create a national health insurance market. Under present conditions, insurers have to be certified in each state to offer insurance in that state. To some extent, as we saw in Chapter 3, the ACA has created a regulatory framework at the federal level. But most of the regulations remains at the state level. A national market might address this lack-of-competition problem. Under such a proposal, insurers could offer their product in any state, thus opening up more markets to competition.

The problem is that in the health insurance industry, as is true of a good portion of the healthcare sector in general, there is consolidation of companies. Fewer large companies are available to offer plans, and smaller companies are not substantial enough to make much of a difference. We see this at the local and state levels. Companies like Anthem Blue Cross offer plans in many states (though they have to be certified in each state). In a national market, such a company could extend its reach, avoiding state regulation. But that might not produce more competition if the same companies compete nationally instead of state-by-state or county-by-county. Thus, it is not clear that a national market would achieve the goals conservatives and Republicans envision.

CONCLUSION: HEALTHCARE REFORM CHOICES

The Terminator movies had one major theme: Attempts to change the future by changing the past. Ultimately, all such attempts failed. But there was an important line in the third movie about the future: "The future has not been written. There is no fate but what we make for ourselves" (Terminator Wiki, n.d.).

That is what we face in the twenty-first century. The Affordable Care Act (ACA) has matured and remains despite attempts by congressional Republicans and the Trump administration to undermine it. A federal district court decision in December 2018 (*Texas v. Azar*) threatens the ACA, creating uncertainty.

The question then becomes what we should do. The future is at least partly determined by the choices that we make. Those choices are a function of values, interests, feasibility, economics, and politics.

Let us begin, again, with values. Here we can ask several questions. From a libertarian standpoint, we can ask whether healthcare is a policy that government should be involved in. The libertarian would so "No!" and that would end the discussion. But if the answer is yes, then we have more questions.

One such question is whether healthcare is a right or a good. If we think healthcare should be a right, as Democrats and liberals/progressives do, then that suggests an aggressive role for government. If we think of healthcare as a good, as Republicans and conservatives do, then that would mean more reliance on private markets. A related question is, if we agree that government should be involved, which level of government should that be? Democrats and liberals/progressives argue for an active role by the federal government; Republicans and conservatives assert that the states are the better venue, better able to meet the needs of their citizens.

A second element is interests. Here we look particularly at groups such as pharmaceutical companies and insurance companies and various types of providers. What role should insurers have in a future American healthcare system? For some Democrats/progressives, that role might actually disappear. Bernie Sanders' Medicare for All would remove most of the role of health insurance companies. Some Democratic proposals would maintain important roles for insurance companies. For Republicans and conservatives, insurance companies would continue to be vital parts of a healthcare system.

We could also ask what should happen to current programs, such as the ACA, Medicare, and Medicaid. Some proposals would replace them all. Others would focus on improving the ACA (depending on the outcome of the *Texas v. Azar* case). Others would eliminate it entirely, such as Sanders' plan and some of the Republican/conservative plans. Should we build upon the strengths of Medicare and Medicaid? Again, that varies by proposal.

Another, related consideration, is where employer-sponsored insurance (ESI) fits in. More people are enrolled in ESI than in any other program. Should we eliminate it, as some proposals do (both liberal and conservative)? Should we build on it? As with all alternatives, we should examine the costs and benefits of any action.

A third consideration is feasibility. Can the program actually be put in place and be implemented in such a way that it produces the results we are hoping for? We have experience with programs such as the ACA, Medicare, and Medicaid. The ACA exchanges, particularly on the federal level, had some initial difficulties that have been worked out. We can also look at the experience of other countries to see what kinds of things work.

The fourth consideration is economics. Making economic projections is always a tricky business. There is an old economics joke, attributed to the Nobel Laureate in Economics, Paul Samuelson, that economists (or the stock market) have predicted nine of the last five recessions. A related joke is that it always tricky to make forecasts, especially about the future.

But predictions, forecasts are made all the time. As we saw in Chapter 3, the Congressional Budget Office (CBO) made predictions about the impact of the ACA on the deficit and on how many people would gain insurance as a result of its passage. CBO undertook the same task for the repeal-and-replace bills in 2017.

The most expensive of the healthcare reform proposals is Bernie Sanders' Medicare for All. It will, according to various analyses, cost an additional $32 trillion dollars of federal spending over ten years, though spending on healthcare would be lower than projected under current policies during that same period.

A related point is to what extent new taxes are needed. The Democratic/liberal/progressive policies would raise taxes, often on those at the upper income levels. The Republican/conservative proposals might need new revenue, but not nearly as much as the progressive proposals. The question then becomes: To what extent are we willing to increase taxes to cover more people?

Finally, we come to the politics question. Is there the will to make changes that various proposals envision? Our current political configuration suggests that this will be difficult. While there is an active discussion of the increase in political partisanship in the media and within academia, the fact remains that the country is divided along a number of dimensions. Bipartisan policy on the part of Congress is not impossible. For example, Congress passed, and President Trump signed, an important criminal justice reform proposal in December 2018. But Republicans and Democrats disagree on fundamental issues about healthcare and healthcare reform.

This was certainly the case in the 2009–2010 period, yet the ACA was passed. But it passed under specific conditions. The Democrats controlled both houses of Congress with significant majorities, especially in the Senate, and the presidency. No Republican in either house voted for the ACA. While Republicans had a similar situation in 2017 and 2018, the Republican majority in the Senate was too slim to allow any repeal-and-replace legislation to pass.

Meaningful healthcare reform requires bipartisanship, cooperation between the two parties and Congress and the President. It also requires public support. We should examine the various reform proposals to see which of those is likely to meet the requirements of obtaining sufficient support for passage. Perhaps an incremental approach, for example, Hacker's (2018) Medicare Part E, would be most acceptable.

We come back to *The Terminator* movies. The future is malleable, unknown. Healthcare in the United States has changed dramatically from the founding of the country, and certainly in the twentieth and twenty-first centuries. That evolution will continue.

STUDY QUESTIONS

1. The text makes the argument that the American healthcare system is highly fragmented. In what ways is the system fragmented? What are the impacts of such fragmentation?
2. Having gone through the entire text now, what do you see as the major problems facing the American healthcare system? What, if any changes, would you like to see?
3. This chapter makes references to a series of quality studies that compares the US healthcare system to other Westernized, industrialized countries. How well does the US compare to those other countries? Do you think those comparisons are fair? Why or why not? Are there other countries' healthcare systems that you think the US might do well to emulate? Which ones, which parts, and why?
4. This chapter suggests the importance of values and ideology as an important part of healthcare reform. Which of the three values mentioned in the chapter (order, freedom/liberty, equality) do you think is most important in healthcare reform? Why?
5. Do you have a political ideology? One way, though not the only way, to find out what your ideology is would be to take the "World's Smallest Political Quiz." Before you take the quiz, think about what your ideology might be. After you take quiz, ask yourself whether your initial thoughts fit in with the results. You might also think about how your ideology, whether self-identified or based on the quiz, fits in with the values you identified as important in the previous question.

    The quiz can be found here: www.theadvocates.org/quiz/?gclid=Cj0KCQiAgf3gBRDtARIsABgdL3lea58yWmgfv19NHYXDgGfZqZhTRbp5TwiiiyY843ysXc40TD8_RVAaAisyEALw_wcB.
6. We have presented several sets of alternatives for healthcare reform in this chapter. These include strengthening the Affordable Care Act, progressive reforms, and conservative reforms. Which of these do you think we should try? Defend your answer.
7. From your perspective, what would the perfect healthcare system look like?

REFERENCES

40 Years of the RAND National Insurance Experiment. 2016. Santa Monica, CA: The RAND Corporation.
Anderson, David, Jodi Liu, and Mark Friedberg. 2018 "Medicare for All: Sounds Good, But What Does It Mean?" *Health Affairs,* November 19.
Atlas, Scott W. 2011. *In Excellent Health: Setting the Record Straight on America's Health Care.* Stanford, CA: Hoover Institute Press.
Blahous, Charles. 2018. *The Costs of a National Single-Payer System.* Arlington, VA: Mercatus Center, George Mason University.
Bodenheimer, Thomas. 2017. "A New Plan to Rescue the ACA: Medicare-at-55". *Health Affairs,* October 16.
Brill, Steven. 2015. *America's Bitter Pill.* New York: Random House.
CAP Health Policy Reform Team. 2018. *Medicare Extra for All.* Washington, DC: Center for American Progress.
Chen, Lanhee J. 2018. "Getting Ready for Health Reform 2020: Republicans' Options for Improving Upon the State Innovation Approach." *Health Affairs,* 37, no. 12 (December): 1–8.
Davis, Karen, Cathy Schoen, and Kristof Stremikis. 2010. *Mirror, Mirror on the Wall: How the Performance of the U.S. Health Care System Compares Internationally, 2010 Update.* New York: The Commonwealth Fund.
Demko, Paul. 2016. "Obama Defends Obamacare, Acknowledges Problems with the Law." *Politico,* October 20.
Enthoven, Alain. 1980. *Health Plan: The Only Practical Solution to the Soaring Cost of Medicare Care.* Reading, MA: Addison-Wesley.
Enthoven, Alain and Laurence C. Baker. 2018. "Managed Competition Still Seeks to Reform Health Care." *Health Affairs,* 37, no. 9 (September): 1425–1430.
Gianoli, Gerard J. 2016. "Medical Error Epidemic Hysteria." *American Journal of Medicine,* 129, no. 12 (December): 1239–1240.
Ginzberg, Eli 1977. *The Limits of Health Reform: The Search for Realism.* New York: Basic Books.
Glickman, Howard. 2017. "Fix the Affordable Care Act By Letting People 55–64 Buy into Medicare." *Forbes,* April 28.
Goodman, John C. 2014. *A Better Choice: Healthcare Solutions for America.* Oakland, CA: The Independent Institute.
Goodman, John C. 2017. "A Conservative Approach to Health Reform." *Forbes,* March 6.
Gur-Arie, Margalit. 2014. "Digging Deeper into the Commonwealth Fund Health Rankings." KevinMD. Online at www.kevinmd.com.
Hacker, Jacob. 2007. *Health Care for America.* Washington, DC: Economic Policy Institute.

Hacker, Jacob. 2018. "The Road to Medicare for Everyone." *The American Prospect*, January 3. Online at www.prospect.org.
Holahan, John, et al. 2016. *Sanders Single-Payer Health Care Plan*. Washington, DC: Urban Institute.
Institute of Medicine. 1999. *To Err Is Human: Building a Safer Health Care System*. Washington, DC: Institute of Medicine.
Jost, Timothy Stoltfzus and Harold Pollack. 2015. *Key Proposals to Strengthen the Affordable Care Act*. New York: The Century Foundation.
Kaiser Family Foundation. 2018. *Side-by-Side Comparison of Medicare-for-All and Public Plan Proposals Introduced in the 115th Congress*. Menlo Park, CA: Kaiser Family Foundation.
Klein, Ezra. 2018. "The 3 Decisions that Will Shape Medicare-for-All." *Vox*, December 17.
Kliff, Sarah. 2017. "Bernie Sanders' New Medicare-for-All Plan, Explained." *Vox*, September 13.
Kliff, Sarah and Dylan Scott. 2018. "We Read Democrats' 8 Plans for Universal Health Care. Here's How They Work." *Vox*, December 13.
Krugman, Paul. 2013. "I Have Seen the Future, And It is Medicaid." *The New York Times*, September 21.
Kurtzleben, Danielle. 2017. "Here's What's in Bernie Sanders' 'Medicare for All' Bill." *National Public Radio*, September 14.
Luthi, Susannah. 2018. "Hospitals Sue over Site-Neutral Payment Policy." *Modern Healthcare*, December 4.
Madar, Chase. 2017. "The Conservative Case for Universal Healthcare." *The American Conservative*, July 25.
Makary, Martin A. and Michael Daniel. 2016. "Medical Error—The Third Leading Cause of Death in the US." *BMJ* (May) 353: i21369.
Makary, Marty. 2015. *Unaccountable: What Hospitals Won't Tell You and How Transparency Can Revolutionize Health Care*. New York: Bloomsbury Press.
Morse, Susan. 2018. "CMS Finalizes Site Neutral Payment Rule." *Healthcare Finance*, November 2.
Napolitano, Andrew P. 2017. "Is Health Care a Right or a Good." *Fox News*, March 30.
Neuman, Tricia, Karen Pollitz, and Jennifer Tolbert. 2018. *Medicare-for-All and Public Plan Buy-In Proposals: Overview and Key Issues*. Menlo Park, CA: Kaiser Family Foundation.
Nichols, John. 2015. "Seventy Years On, Let Us Renew FDR's Struggle for an Economic Bill of Rights." *The Nation*, April 14.
Papanicolas, Irene et al. 2018. "Health Care Spending in the United States and Other High-Income Countries." *Journal of the American Medical Association*, 319, no. 10 (March 13): 1024–1039.
Pipes, Sally. 2018. "The False Promise of 'Medicaid for All'." *Forbes*, August 21.
Pollack, Harold. 2015. "Improve and Repair: Three Ideas to Strengthen the ACA." *Democracy: A Journal of Ideas*, no. 38 (Fall).
Pollitz, Karen. 2017. *High-Risk Pools for Uninsurable Individuals*. Menlo Park, CA: Kaiser Family Foundation.
Rainey, Michael. 2018. "Majority of Americans Support Medicaid for All." *The Fiscal Times*, August 30.
Rove, Karl. 2018. "Stopping the Socialist Resurgence." *Wall Street Journal*, November 28.
Rushefsky, Mark E. 2017. *Public Policy in the United States: Challenges, Opportunities, and Changes*. New York: Routledge.
Ryan, Paul 2016. *A Better Way: Our Vision for a Confident America; Health Care*. Washington, DC: US House of Representatives.
Sanders, Bernie. 2017. "Bernie Sanders: Why We Need Medicare for All." *The New York Times*, September 13.
Sanders, Bernie. n.d. "Options to Finance Medicare-for-All." Online at www.sanders.senate.gov/download/options-to-finance-medicare-for-all?i.
Schneider, Eric C. et al. 2017. *Mirror, Mirror 2017: International Comparison Reflects Flaws and Opportunities for Better U.S. Health Care*. New York: The Commonwealth Fund.
Scott, Dylan. 2018a. "Poll: Medicaid Is Overwhelmingly Popular, Even as Trump Looks to Cut It." *Vox*, March 1.
Scott, Dylan. 2018b. "Bernie Sanders $32 Trillion Medicare-for-All Plan Is Actually Kind of a Bargain." *Vox*, July 30.
Sessions, Pete, Bill Cassidy, and John Goodman. 2017. "How We Can Repeal the ACA and Still Insure the Uninsured." *Health Affairs*, January 18.
Silver, Charles and David A. Hyman. 2018. *Overcharged: Why Americans Pay Too Much for Health Care*. Washington, DC: Cato Institute.
Sparer, Michael. 2017. "'Medicare for All' is the Democrats New Rallying Cry. 'Medicaid for More' Would Be Even Better." *Vox*, August 23.
Stone, Deborah. 2012. *Policy Paradox: The Art of Political Decision Making*, 3rd edn. New York: W. W. Norton.
Tepper, Taylor. 2018. "The Problem with Health Savings Accounts." Bankrate, June 29. Online at www.bankrate.com.
Terminator Wiki. n.d. "There's No Fate but What We Make Ourselves." Online at www.terminator.wiki.com.
Turning the Exchanges into Real Markets. 2016. Dallas, TX: The Goodman Institute for Public Policy Research.
US Department of Health and Human Services, US Department of the Treasury, and US Department of Labor. 2018. *Reforming America's Healthcare System through Choice and Competition*. Washington, DC: US Departments of Health and Human Services, Treasury and Labor.
Wynne, Bill. 2017a. "Five Lessons from the AHCA Demise." *Health Affairs*, March 27.
Wynne, Bill. 2017b. "What Now: A Four-Step Plan for Bipartisan Reform." *Health Affairs*, April 4.
Wynne, Bill. 2017c. "Medicare Advantage Premium Support for All." *Health Affairs*, May 11.
Wynne, Bill. 2017d. "Creating Medicare Advantage Support for All, Part 2: Benefit Design." *Health Affairs*, October 23.
Wynne, Bill. 2018a. "Support for All, Part 3: Provider Considerations." *Health Affairs*, April 18.
Wynne, Bill. 2018b. "Creating Medicare Advantage for All, Part 3: Financing." *Health Affairs*, July 9.
Wynne, Bill. 2018c. "Support for All, Part 5: Which Proposal is Actually Medicare?" *Health Affairs*, August 15.

APPENDIX A

Important Health Policy-Related Web Sites and Resources

FEDERAL GOVERNMENT

Agency for Healthcare Research and Quality (AHRQ): www.ahrq.gov
(US Department of Health and Human Services)

Bureau of Health Professions: www.bhpr.hrsa.gov
(US Department of Health and Human Services)

Bureau of Labor Statistics: www.bls.gov
(US Department of Labor)

Centers for Disease Control and Prevention (CDC): www/cdc.gov
(US Department of Health and Human Services)

Centers for Medicare and Medicaid Services (CMS): www.cms.hhs.gov
(US Department of Health and Human Services)

Congressional Budget Office: www.cbo.gov
(US Congress)

Food and Drug Administration: www.fda.gov
(US Department of Health and Human Services)

Government Accountability Office: www.gao.gov
(US Congress)

Health Finder: www.healthfinder.gov
(National Health Information Center, US Department of Health and Human Services)

Health Resources and Services Administration (HRSA): www.hrsa.gov
(US Department of Health and Human Services)

Indian Health Service: www.ihs.gov/
(US Department of Health and Human Services)

Library of Congress: www.loc.gov
(US Congress)

Medical Expenditure Panel Survey: www.meps.ahrq.gov
(Agency for Healthcare Research and Quality; US Department of Health and Human Services)

Medicare Payment Advisory Commission: www.medpac.gov
(Independent Commission established by Congress in 1997 to advise Congress on Medicare program)

National Center for Health Statistics: www.cdc.gov/nchs
(Centers for Disease Control and Prevention)

National Institute on Aging: www.nia.gov
(National Institutes of Health)

National Institutes of Health: www.nih.gov
(US Department of Health and Human Services)

National Mental Health Information System: www.mentalhealth.samhsa.gov/
(US Department of Health and Human Services)

National Practitioner Data Bank: www.npdb-hipdb.com/search/index.html
(US Department of Health and Human Services; Substance Abuse and Mental Health Services Administration)

Office of Minority Health: https://minorityhealth.hhs.gov/Default.aspx
(US Department of Health and Human Services)

President's Council on Bioethics: https://bioethicsarchive.georgetown.edu/pcbe/index.html
State of Oregon—Physician-Assisted Suicide: http://oregon.gov/DHS/ph/pas/index.shtml (Provides annual reports on physician-assisted suicide)

Statistical Abstract of the United States: www.census.gov/statab/www
(National data book containing statistics on social and economic conditions in the US)

US Census Bureau: www.census.gov

US Congress: www.congress.gov/

US Department of Health and Human Services: www.hhs.gov/

US Food and Drug Administration: www.fda.gov/

US Government/Health: www.usa.gov/health

US National Library of Medicine: www.nlm.nih.gov/nlmhome.html
(National Institutes of Health)

US Supreme Court: www.supremecourt.gov/
(Supreme Court of the United States)

Veterans Health Administration: www.va.gov/health/
(US Department of Veterans Affairs)

STATE GOVERNMENTS

National Academy of State Health Policy: https://nashp.org/about-nashp/
(A non-partisan forum of policymakers throughout state governments)

National Conference of State Legislatures: www.ncsl.org/research/health.aspx

Scorecard on State Health System Performance: www.usa.gov/health
(The Commonwealth Fund)

PRIVATE SECTOR

American Association of Retired Persons (AARP): www.aarp.org
America's Health Insurance Plans (AHIP): www.ahip.org

Guttmacher Institute: www.guttmacher.org
(Excellent source for information/statistics dealing with women's health issues, including abortion, contraceptives, and pregnancy)

Moving Ideas: The Electronic Policy Network: www.movingideas.org
(A Project of American Prospect—progressive/liberal perspective)

National Association of Insurance Commissioners: www.naic.org/index.htm

THINK TANKS/RESEARCH ORGANIZATIONS

Brookings Institution: www.brookings.org

Center on Budget and Policy Priorities: www.cbpp.org

Center for Studying Health System Change: www.hschange.com

Urban Institute: www.urban.org/
(A non-partisan economic and social policy research organization)

ACADEMIC

American Indian Studies Center: www.aisc.ucla.edu/
(University of California Los Angeles)

Center for American Indian Health: http://caih.jhu.edu/
(Johns Hopkins Bloomberg School of Public Health)

Institute of Medicine: www.iom.org
(National Academy of Sciences)

Leonard D. Schaeffer Center for Health Policy & Economics: https://healthpolicy.usc.edu/
(University of Southern California)

Program for Health Systems Improvement: www.phsi.harvard.edu
(Harvard University)

State Health Access Data Assistance Center: www.shadac.org/
(University of Minnesota—funded by the Robert Wood Johnson Foundation)

UCLA Center for Health Policy Research: www.healthpolicy.ucla.edu/

FOUNDATIONS/NON-PROFIT ORGANIZATIONS

American Enterprise Institute: www.aei.org

Carnegie Foundation for the Advancement of Teaching: www.carnegiefoundation.org/

Cato Institute: www.cato.org

Children's Defense Fund: www.childrensdefense.org

Commonwealth Fund: www.commonwealthfund.org/
(Supports independent research on issues and provides grants to improve practices and policy)

Cover the Uninsured Week: www.covertheuninsuredweek.org
(A project of the Robert Wood Johnson Foundation)

The Heritage Foundation: www.heritage.org/research/healthcare/index.cfm
(A conservative voice in health policy)

Institute for Health Policy Solutions: www.ihps.org

Kaiser Family Foundation: www.kff.org/statedata

National Academy of Social Insurance: www.nasi.org
(Non-profit, non-partisan organization made up of leading experts on social insurance)

National Academy of State Health Policy: www.nashp.org/index.cfm
(Non-profit, non-partisan organization)

National Conference of State Legislatures: www.ncsl.org
(Bipartisan organization serving state legislators)

National Health Policy Forum: www.nhpf.org
(Non-partisan information exchange program)

Public Health Foundation: www.phf.org
(Non-profit organization that helps health agencies and community health organizations)

Robert Wood Johnson Foundation: www.rwjf.org/index.jsp
(Seeks to improve health of all Americans)

State Health Facts: www.statehealthfacts.org/cgi-bin/healthfacts.cgi
(Kaiser Family Foundation)

United States Pharmacopeia (USP): www.usp.org
(The official public standards-setting authority for all prescription and over-the-counter medicines, dietary supplements, and other healthcare products manufactured and sold in the United States)

CONSUMER HEALTH ADVOCACY GROUPS

American Health Care Association (AHCA): www.ahcancal.org/

Center for Health Care Strategies (CHCS): www.chcs.org/

Children's Defense Fund (CDF): www.childrensdefense.org/

Families USA: www.familiesusa.org/

Health Consumer Alliance (HCA): www.healthconsumer.org/

Society for Healthcare Consumer Advocacy (SHCA): www.shca-aha.org

PROFESSIONAL ASSOCIATIONS

Alliance Cost Containment: www.alliancecost.com/

American College of Emergency Physicians: www.acep.org/

American Hospital Association (AHA): www.aha.org

American Medical Association (AMA): www.ama-assn.org

American Nurses Association (ANA): www.nursingworld.org

America's Health Insurance Plans (AHIP): www.ahip.org

Medical Device Manufacturers of America (MDMA): www.medicaldevices.org

National Coalition on Health Care: nchc.org/
Pharmaceutical Research and Manufacturers of America (PhRMA): www.phrma.org

USA Managed-Care Organization (USAMCO): www.usamco.com/

Washington Business Group on Health: www.businessgrouphealth.org

INTERNATIONAL HEALTH

Global Health Reporting: www.globalhealthreporting.org
(Kaiser Family Foundation, provides global health data)

Health Canada: www.hc-sc.gc.ca
(Canadian government)

Organization for Economic Cooperation and Development (OECD) www.oecd.org/home/

World Health Organization (WHO): www.who.int/en/
(United Nations' specialized agency for health)

World Health Organization Statistical Information System (WHOSIS): www3.who.int/whosis/menu.cfm

PUBLIC OPINION POLLS

Harris Polls: www.harrisinteractive.com/Harris_polls

Gallup Polls: www.gallup.com/home.aspx

Polling Reports: http://pollingreport.com/

Real Clear Politics: www.realclearpolitics.com/epolls/latest_polls/

Rasmussen Reports: www.rasmussenreports.com/

Washington Post Polls: www.washingtonpost.com/politics/polling/

JOURNALS

American Journal of Public Health
Health Affairs
Health Services Research
Inquiry
International Journal of Health Services
Journal of Health Care for the Poor and Underserved
Journal of Health Economics
Journal of Health Politics, Policy and Law
Journal of Public Health Policy
Journal of the American Medical Association
Medical Care Research and Review
Milbank Quarterly
The New England Journal of Medicine

APPENDIX B

Chronology of Significant Events and Legislation in US Healthcare

1778 The first national pension law is passed for soldiers who fought in the American Revolution.

1797 The first recorded inoculation of an American Indian takes place.

1798 President John Adams signs into law an Act providing for the relief of sick and disabled seamen, which approved the establishment of the first Marine Hospital.

1799 The first Marine Hospital is established.

1811 The federal government authorizes the first domiciliary and medical facility for veterans.

1830 The Indian Removal Act is signed into law by President Jackson, authorizing him to negotiate with American Indians in the southern United States for their removal to federal territories west of the Mississippi in exchange for their homeland.

1832 Congress appropriates $12,000 to hire physicians to provide vaccinations to American Indians. This is the first large-scale smallpox vaccination authorized by Congress.

1847 The American Medical Association (AMA) is founded.

1849 The Bureau of Indian Affairs (BIA) is transferred to the newly created Department of the Interior. The responsibility for Indian healthcare is transferred from military to civilian control.

1863 The National Academy of Sciences is established to assist in caring for the Union Army.

1865 The United States Soldiers and Sailors Protective Society is organized to help veterans.

1866 The Grand Army of the Republic (GAR) is formed as a political group to lobby for veterans' benefits.

1870 The First Reorganization Act federalizes the Marine Hospital Service.

1872 The American Public Health Association (APHA) is founded. This organization is concerned with the social and economic aspects of health problems.

1878 Congress passes a National Quarantine Act for the purpose of preventing entry into the country of persons with communicable diseases.

1930 The National Quarantine Act is signed into law. This legislation is designed to prevent entry into the country of persons with communicable diseases.

1879 The Arrears Act specifies that veterans' benefits start from the time of discharge from the army and for dependents from the time of the death and not at the time of application, as was the case previous to the Act.

1899 The National Hospital Superintendents Association is created. It later becomes the American Hospital Association (AHA).

1904 The Council on Medical Education is established by the AMA.

1908 Congress passes the Federal Employers Liability Act, preempting state tort law, designed to govern the liability claims brought by employees against railroads operating in interstate commerce.

1910 The Flexner Report is published, calling for the adoption of the German model of medicine, with scientifically based training, the strengthening of first-class medical schools, and the elimination of a great majority of inferior schools.

Congress starts to formally appropriate funds for Bureau of Indian Affairs healthcare services.

1912 The US Public Health Service (USPHS) is formed from the Marine Hospital Service. The Sherwood Act awards pension to all veterans of the Mexican War and Union veterans of the Civil War.

1914 Congress passes the Harrison Act, which requires that cocaine and heroin be sold only as prescription medicines.

1921 The Sheppard-Towner Act is signed into law. It establishes the first federal grant-in-aid program for local child health clinics.

The Snyder Act provides formal legislative authorization for Indian healthcare and provides for regular congressional appropriations.

1928 The Sheppard-Towner Act is terminated.

1929 Blue Cross is established.

1930 The National Institutes of Health (NIH) are established for the purpose of discovering the causes, prevention, and cure of disease.

President Herbert Hoover establishes the Committee on the Cost of Medical Care.

President Hoover signs a law consolidating many separate veterans' programs into an independent federal agency called the Veterans Administration.

The Veterans Administration Agency is created by combining Veterans Bureau, The Bureau of Pensions, and National Homes for Disabled Volunteer Soldiers.

1934 The Federal Emergency Relief Administration (FERA) gives the first federal grants to local governments for public assistance to the poor, including financial support for healthcare.

The Indian Reorganization Act encourages economic development and provides for Indian tribes' self-determination.

1935 The Social Security Act is signed into law. The Act provides for unemployment compensation, old-age benefits, and other benefits.

1937 The National Cancer Act is passed by Congress, establishing the National Cancer Institute (NCI).

1939 The Murray-Wagner-Dingell Bill is introduced, proposing national health insurance.

1943 The US Supreme Court, in the first reproductive rights case, *Skinner v. Oklahoma*, strikes down vasectomies as criminal punishment and recognizes the right to have offspring as a sensitive and important area of human rights.

1944 The Servicemen's Readjustment Act, famously known as the "GI Bill of Rights," offers low-interest loans for veterans to purchase homes, farms, or small businesses, unemployment benefits, financial assistance for education, as well as healthcare and rehabilitation services.

1946 The National Hospital Survey and Construction Act (Hill-Burton Act) mandates the provision of federal funding to subsidize the construction of hospitals.

The National Mental Health Act is signed into law, providing federal grants to states for research, prevention, diagnosis, and treatment of mental disorders.

Congress passes, and President Truman signs, Public Law 293, formally creating the Veterans Health Administration (VHA) within the Veterans Administration.

1951 The Internal Revenue Service rules that employers' costs for healthcare insurance premiums are tax-deductible.

1952 The nongovernmental Joint Commission on Accreditation of Hospitals (JCAH) is established.

The Health Insurance Association of America (HIAA) is formed.

1954 The Transfer Act moves responsibility for Indian health to the Public Health Service, at this time part of the Department of Health, Education, and Welfare.

1955 The Indian Health Service (IHS) is established as an agency under the United States Public Health Service.

1956 The Dependents Medical Care Act is passed, providing the Department of Defense with the authority to provide civilian healthcare to eligible dependents of military service members.

1960 The Kerr-Mills Act (Medical Assistance Act) is signed into law, providing federal matching payments to states for vendor payments.

1965 Medicare and Medicaid are passed as amendments to the Social Security Act of 1935.

In *Griswold v. Connecticut*, the US Supreme Court recognizes that married couples have a constitutional right to use contraception within a "zone of privacy" that encompasses marital relationships.

1966 The Comprehensive Health Planning Act is signed into law. This legislation is an attempt to implement healthcare facility planning through the states.

The Civilian Health and Medical Program of Uniformed Services (CHAMPUS) is established for active-duty family members and is later extended to retired service members and their dependents.

1971 Ralph Nader's Health Research Group is founded.

Senator Edward Kennedy introduces the Health Security Act, which calls for a comprehensive program of free medical care.

1972 President Nixon, in response to Kennedy's plan, introduces the National Health Insurance Partnership Act.

The Professional Standards Review Organizations (PSROs) are created through the Social Security Amendments of 1972.

The Office of Technology Assessment (OTA) is established. This organization maintains, in part, a concern for medical technology assessment.

482   APPENDIX B

In *Eisenstadt v. Baird*, the US Supreme Court extends the right to use contraceptives to unmarried individuals.

1973 The Health Maintenance Organization Act is signed into law.

The US Supreme Court legalizes abortion in *Roe v. Wade.*

1974 The Congressional Budget and Impoundment Control Act is signed into law.

The National Health Planning and Resource Development Act is signed into law.

The Employee Retirement Income Security Act (ERISA) is signed into law.

1975 The State of California passes the Medical Injury Compensation Reform Act, which places a cap of $250,000 on jury awards for noneconomic damages.

The Indian Self-Determination and Education Assistance Act (ISDEAA) is passed.

1976 The Indian Health Care Improvement Act (IHCIA) is passed.

The New Jersey Supreme Court rules that Karen Quinlan has a constitutional right of privacy, which her guardian can assert on her behalf.

1977 In *Casey v. Population Services International*, the US Supreme Court strikes down New York State's ban on the sale of contraceptive to minors under 16 years of age.

1981 The Omnibus Budget Reconciliation Act (OBRA) is passed.

The Health Care Financing Administration (HCFA) grants waivers to states to pay for home healthcare.

1982 The Tax Equity and Fiscal Responsibility Act (TEFRA) is signed into law.

The National Center for Health Care Technology (NCHCT) is abolished.

1983 The Prospective Payment System (PPS), a mandate of the Deficit Reduction Act of 1982, begins.

1984 The Deficit Reduction Act requires Medicaid beneficiaries to assign to states any rights they had to other health benefit programs.

1985 Congress creates the Physician Payment Review Commission (PPRC).

Congress passes the Medical Malpractice Immunity Act (MMIA).

1986 The Omnibus Budget Reconciliation Act (OBRA) of 1986 gives states the option to extend Medicaid coverage to pregnant women and infants who are members of households with incomes as high as 100 percent of the federal poverty level.

Congress passes the Health Care Quality Improvement Act.

The Emergency Medical Treatment and Active Labor Act guarantees emergency medical treatment to anyone, regardless of legal status or ability to pay.

1987 The Omnibus Budget Reconciliation Act increases the income requirements of pregnant women and infants to 185 percent of the federal poverty level.

1988 The Medicare Catastrophic Coverage Act is passed.

The Pepper Commission Report is released.

The Women Veterans Health Program is established to streamline services for women veterans.

1989 President Reagan elevates Veterans Affairs to the cabinet-level Department of Veterans Affairs.

The Omnibus Budget Reconciliation Act requires provision of all Medicaid-allowed treatment to correct problems identified during early and periodic screening, diagnosis, and treatment (EPSDT).

The Medicare Catastrophic Coverage Act is repealed.

The Office of Health Technology Assessment (OHTA) is established.

The Agency for Health Care Policy and Research (AHCPR) is created.

The US Supreme Court, in *Webster v. Reproductive Health Services*, gives states the authority to regulate and thus restrict abortions in public clinics.

The Medicare Prospective Payment System is extended to physicians.

1990 The US Supreme Court rules that a competent person has a constitutionally protected right to refuse life-saving hydration and nutrition (the Nancy Cruzan case).

The Safe Medical Devices Act strengthens the FDA by controlling the entry of new products and monitoring the use of the marketplace.

1991 Harris Wofford wins a special senatorial election in Pennsylvania, firmly placing healthcare on the policy agenda.

1992 Congress enacts the Prescription Drug Use Fee Act.

Amendments to the IHCIA of 1976 reauthorize the Indian Self-Determination Act and provide for tribal self-governance demonstration projects.

The US Supreme Court, in *Planned Parenthood v. Casey*, adopts an undue-burden test for the right to abortion.

The Veterans Health Care Act provides authority for a variety of gender-specific services and programs to care for women veterans.

1993 President Bill Clinton unveils his Health Security Act.

The CHAMPUS program is renamed TRICARE.

1994 Congress fails to pass any health reform bill.

President Clinton issues an executive order to facilitate tribal involvement in the administration of Indian programs.

Oregon voters approve the Death with Dignity Act.

1995 The Medicare Hospital Insurance Trust Fund is projected to go bankrupt by 2002.

Republicans adopt the balanced-budget target of 2002, calling for reductions in spending for Medicare and Medicaid.

President Clinton announces the balanced-budget target of 2005, with smaller reductions in Medicare and Medicaid.

President Clinton proposes federal regulation of private insurance.

Congress passes the Federally Supported Health Centers Assistance Act (FSHCAA).

The Office of Technology Assessment is abolished.

The FDA gives its approval to OxyContin for marketing starting in 1996.

1996 Congress passes the Personal Responsibility and Work Opportunity Reconciliation Act, separating Medicaid from welfare.

Congress passes the Health Insurance Portability and Accountability Act (HIPAA).

Congress gives mental health the same status as physical health.

States begin passing patients' rights bills, regulating health maintenance organizations.

The Veterans Eligibility Reform Act is passed, expanding veterans' benefits.

1997 Congress passes the Balanced Budget Act, creating the Medicare+Choice program, and extends the prospective payment system to nursing homes, home healthcare agencies, and hospice agencies.

The Balanced Budget Act increases health insurance for children through the creation of the State Children's Health Insurance Program (SCHIP).

The Women Veterans Health Program Office is established.

President Clinton establishes the Advisory Commission on Consumer Protection and Quality in the Health Care Industry (also known as the Quality Commission).

Texas passes a patient's rights law allowing enterprise liability suits.

The Food and Drug Administration (FDA) declares that emergency contraceptive pills are safe and effective.

1998 President Clinton proposes to extend Medicare to those aged 55 to 64 who are uninsured.

The House passes a patient's rights bill. The Senate fails to act.

The number of uninsured in the United States exceeds 40 million people, almost 16 percent of the population.

Some HMOs drop out of the Medicare+Choice program, citing high costs and federal refusal to raise payments.

The Veterans Eligibility Reform Act goes into effect. It dramatically changes and reforms the VHA.

1999 The FDA approves the emergency contraceptive Plan B as a prescription drug.

The Agency for Health Care Policy and Research (AHCPR) is renamed the Agency for Healthcare Research and Quality (AHRQ).

2000 The FDA approves the use of mifepristone as a safe and effective medical method for terminating pregnancy.

2001 The President's Council on Bioethics is founded.

George W. Bush assumes the office of the presidency following the November 2000 presidential election.

President George W. Bush reinstates the Mexico City Policy by executive order, prohibiting the use of taxpayer funds to pay for abortions or advocate or actively promote abortions, either in the United States or abroad.

President George W. Bush, in a televised address to the nation, announces that he will allow federal funds to be used for research only on the 60-or-so existing stem cell lines where the life and death decision has already been made.

2003 President George W. Bush signs into law the Medicare Prescription Drug, Improvement, and Modernization Act.

The Florida legislature passes "Terri's Law," giving Governor Jeb Bush the power to issue a "one-time stay" of any court order directing the withdrawal of nutrition and hydration so long as certain conditions are met. Using this power, Governor Bush issues an executive order to reinstate the feeding tube in Terri Schiavo.

Congress passes, and President George W. Bush signs into law, the Medicare Modernization Act. The law adds Part D, often referred to as the prescription drug benefit plan, to Medicare, to go into effect on January 1, 2006.

President Bush signs the Partial Birth Abortion Ban Act into law. The law outlaws a specific abortion procedure medically called intact dilation and extraction (D&E).

President Bush proposes converting Medicaid from an entitlement to a block-grant program. The proposal fails to pass Congress.

2004 The Medicare drug discount card program begins.

The US Commission on Civil Rights publishes its report, *Broken Promises: Evaluating the Native American Health Care System*.

2005 Congress passes the Act of Relief for the Parents of Theresa Marie Schiavo.

2005 Judge George Greer issues a restraining order prohibiting the Florida Department of Children and Families (FDCF) from removing Terri Schiavo from the hospice or reinserting the feeding tube.

Terri Schiavo passes away.

The Base Realignment and Closure Commission (BRCC) recommends closing down the Walter Reed Army Medical Center in Washington, DC, and moving its staff and services to the US National Naval Medical Center.

2006 The Medicare prescription drug benefit begins.

The US Supreme Court, in *Gonzales v. Oregon*, upholds the state of Oregon's Death with Dignity Act. Massachusetts passes a health reform bill that becomes a model for the Affordable Care Act.

2007 The US Supreme Court, in *Gonzales v. Carhart* and *Gonzales v. Planned Parenthood*, upholds the constitutionality of the Partial Birth Abortion Ban Act of 2003.

2008 Voters in Washington State approve the public "Initiative 1000," which establishes the state's Death with Dignity Act. The law goes into effect in 2009.

Barack Obama, a Democrat, is elected to the Presidency, setting the stage for a major overhaul of the US healthcare system.

2009 Congress passes the Children's Health Insurance Program Reauthorization Act (CHIPRA).

President Barack Obama signs an executive order allowing federal tax dollars to be used for broadening federal support for embryonic stem cell research.

President Obama creates the Presidential Commission for the Study of Bioethical Issues.

The President's Council on Bioethics is abolished.

Washington State's Death with Dignity Act goes into effect.

The Supreme Court of the State of Montana gives the green light for doctors to prescribe a lethal dose of drugs for their patients for the purpose of assisted suicide.

President Obama signs an executive order that allows federal tax dollars to be used for significantly broader research on embryonic stem cells.

President Obama signs into law the Children's Health Insurance Program Reauthorization Act (CHIPRA).

Montana's highest court, in *Baxter v. Montana*, legalizes the practice of physician-assisted suicide. It rules that state law prohibiting assisted suicide does not apply to doctors who give lethal doses of drugs to dying patients.

2010 The Affordable Care Act (ACA) is passed.

The Federal Emergency Contraception Education Act funds a national campaign to educate women and healthcare providers about emergency contraception.

Congress passes, and President Obama signs into law, the Affordable Care Act (also known as the Patient Protection and Affordable Care Act).

Congress passes the Emergency Contraception Education Act of 2010, designed to fund a national campaign to educate women and healthcare providers about emergency contraception; the law is credited with increasing awareness of emergency contraception and its use.

2011 Walter Reed Army Medical Center is merged and integrated with the National Naval Medical Center and renamed Walter Reed Bethesda.

2012 The Obama administration creates a new program called Deferred Action for Childhood Arrivals (DACA), under which certain people who came to the United States as children and meet several key guidelines may request consideration of deferred action (removal of an individual from the US is deferred as an act of prosecutorial discretion) for a period of two years, subject to renewal, and would then be eligible for work authorization.

The US Supreme Court decides *NFIB v. Sebelius*; it rules that states do not have to expand Medicaid, as called for by the ACA. As a result, Medicaid expansion becomes voluntary.

2013 US District Court Judge Edward Korman rules that the FDA must remove all age restrictions on the sale of emergency contraception without a doctor's prescription.

The FDA extends the availability of the Plan B One-Step morning-after pill without a prescription to girls aged 15 and over.

2014 In *Burwell v. Hobby Lobby*, the US Supreme Court rules that closely held for-profit corporations do not have to provide contraceptive coverage for their employees.

Congress passes the Veterans Access, Choice, and Accountability Act. The Act provides new funding, authorities, and other tools to support and reform the VA.

Brittany Maynard, at home with her family and close friends, ends her life by taking a lethal dose of medication prescribed by a doctor under Oregon's Death with Dignity Act.

Seventeen states and the District of Columbia pass "Good Samaritan" laws that grant limited immunity to drug users who seek help. The basic idea behind the laws is that anyone who seeks help in case of an overdose cannot be prosecuted for possession of small amounts of drugs or drug paraphernalia. However, such laws do not grant immunity for other crimes such as drug trafficking. By 2016, 48 states would pass similar laws.

2015 In *King v. Sebelius*, opponents of the ACA unsuccessfully challenge federal tax subsidies on exchanges run by the federal government, as opposed to exchanges run by states.

The US Supreme Court, in the case of *Obergefell v. Hodges*, rules that the fundamental right to marry is guaranteed to same-sex couples by the Due Process Clause and the Equal Protection Clause of the 14th Amendment to the US Constitution. The ruling requires all 50 states to recognize the marriages of same-sex couples with all the rights and responsibilities of marriages of heterosexual couples.

Sam Quinones' book, *Dreamland: The True Tale of America's New Opiate Epidemic*, is published; it describes events that happened during the mid- to late 1990s that created the current epidemics of prescription opioid and black-tar heroin addiction.

2016 Three days after being sworn into office, President Donald Trump takes executive action to reinstate the Mexico City Policy, which prohibits international nongovernmental organizations (NGOs) from receiving US funding if they perform or promote abortions. During the Obama administration, the NGOs that performed abortion procedures were allowed to receive funding for non-abortion services they provided, such as access to contraceptives and post-abortion care.

In a world's first, a Chinese scientists injects a human with cells genetically modified to fight cancer. The scientists uses a controversial "cut-and-paste" gene editing technique known as CRISPR-Cas9, in which scientists cut out the inherited genes that might cause cancer from the cells and replace them with healthy genes.

Great Britain becomes the first country to allow a "three-parent" IVF technique.

The first three-parent baby is born in 2016 to a couple in New York after they undergo a new IVF procedure at a clinic in Mexico.

Congress passes the Consolidated Appropriation Act of 2016, which includes a rider that prohibits germline modifications; the Act undergoes regular review and is still in effect at the time of writing. The term germline modification includes all genetic engineering on eggs, sperm, or early embryos—modifications that could be passed down beyond a single generation.

The Missouri Court of Appeals rules that a divorced man and woman must mutually consent to use embryos that were frozen and stored while they were married. The court declares that embryos are marital property and not humans with constitutional rights.

In the case of *Whole Woman's Health v. Hellerstedt*, the US Supreme Court strikes down Texas's requirement that doctors who perform abortions must have admitting privileges at nearby hospitals and that health/abortion clinics have to meet hospital-like standards for outpatient surgery.

Congress passes the Twenty-First-Century Cures Act (Cures Act) designed to accelerate medical product development and to bring new innovations and advances to patients quickly and efficiently. The law establishes new expedited product development programs for Regenerative Medicine Advanced Therapy to expedite the process for some biologic products, and the Breakthrough Device Program to speed up the review of certain new innovative medical devices.

2017 The Tax Cut and Jobs Act lowers taxes for upper-income individuals and corporations and repeals penalties for failing to have health insurance imposed under the ACA.

President Trump signs an executive order establishing the President's Commission on Combating Drug Addiction and the Opioid Crisis, with a mission to study the scope and effectiveness of the federal response to drug addiction and the opioid crisis and to make recommendations to the president to improve the response.

The Trump administration declares the US opioid epidemic a public health emergency and directs the relevant executive agencies to use appropriate authority to fight the crisis.

The FDA approves three gene therapies to enter the market. One is Luxturna, which is a virus vector-based therapy for the treatment of patients with retinal dystrophy. The other two are CAR T-cell therapies, called Kymriah (to treat leukemia) and Yescarta (to treat lymphoma).

Congress makes several attempts to repeal and replace the Affordable Care Act.

The House of Representatives passes the American Health Care Act.

2017–2018 The Trump administration makes changes that seek to undermine the Affordable Care Act.

2018 In the November 2018 elections, voters approve ballot initiatives in the states of Idaho, Utah, and Nebraska to expand the Medicaid program under the ACA.

The US Supreme Court, in the case of *National Institute of Family and Life Advocacy v. Becerra*, rules in favor of opponents of abortion on free speech grounds. The court rules that the state of California may not require religiously oriented crisis pregnancy centers to provide information about abortion services and the state cannot co-opt licensed facilities to deliver its messages for it.

The President's Commission Combating Drug Addiction and the Opioid Crisis issues its final report with a series of recommendations to address the opioid crisis.

Congress passes the Opioid Crisis Response Act, designed to make it easier for states to expand access to addiction treatment.

Trustees estimate that the Medicare Trust Fund Part A will go bankrupt by 2026.

APPENDIX C

Important Concepts

Assimilation policy	This policy is based on the notion that the interests of AIs/ANs are best served by assimilating them into larger American society. It became formal federal Indian policy during the Eisenhower years. This policy has also been referred to as the policy of termination.
Biocrossing	Refers to "fertility tourists" from affluent countries crossing national boundaries and traveling to low-income countries for the purpose of achieving conception and childbirth. A variety of terms are used to describe this phenomenon, such as "cross-border reproductive care," "travel ART/travel IVF," "reproductive tourism," "fertility tourism," and "procreative tourism."
Breakthrough therapy	An FDA designation as "breakthrough therapy" expedites the development and review of drugs that are intended to treat a serious medical condition and where clinical data indicate that the drug may demonstrate significant improvement over available therapies. A drug with this designation is also available for fast-track designation.
Commercial surrogacy	Involves payments from intended parents to the surrogate mother and typically focuses on living and medical expenses and life insurance coverage.
Consumer-driven healthcare	Under this concept, patients take on the role of sophisticated consumers who use information and the Internet to comparison shop and to make informed choices about their own healthcare and tailor their own custom-made health benefit packages.
Cost-benefit analysis	A systematic analysis of both direct/indirect costs and benefits of a policy or program.
Cost-effectiveness analysis	Comparing several different intervention strategies (policy alternatives) using common units of costs and benefits to measure effectiveness of a public policy or program.
Cost-sharing	Requiring enrollees in health insurance programs to pay out-of-pocket expenses such as co-payments, coinsurance, and deductibles.
Cybernetic enhancement	Involves the transformation of humans into cyborgs or cybernetic organisms.
Divided government	A government in which one political party controls the presidency while the other party controls one or both houses of Congress.
Doctrine of discovery	Colonizing countries of Europe used the doctrine of discovery as a first step in obtaining the right to possession of land from the native population. Under this doctrine, the first discovering state had the right to control of the land it discovered.
Doctrine of conquest	This doctrine was used by European countries to remove natives who were not willing to move from their land. It claimed that when a nation defeats another nation in a war, it gains the right to the defeated nation's land and control of its people. The United States was born into this established legal tradition based on the doctrines of discovery and conquest.

Fast track	The FDA puts the approval of a new drug on a fast track based on promising data from animal or human clinical trials so that the drug gets to patients earlier than the time it would take to approve a new drug through a regular or normal approval process.
Federalism	A federal system of government is one in which the powers of the government are divided up between the national (central) government and its constituent units, that is, state governments.
Federal waivers	Federal government grants states exemptions from certain federal rules and regulations, giving state governments more flexibility/discretion in implementing a program, e.g., Medicaid waivers.
Gene editing	Gene editing is a method used by scientists to change the DNA of organisms including plants, animals, and humans.
Gene therapy	Therapy to treat and often cure a disease by introducing the functional or curative form of the gene into a host to improve the functioning of the existing mutated gene or by replacing it with a healthy gene.
Genetic enhancement	Refers to sex selection of offspring, exclusion of offspring with certain genetic diseases by parental screening, selective abortion, *in-vitro* fertilization, or embryo selection.
Germline gene therapy	Germ cells (sperm, eggs, or early embryos) are modified by introducing a functional gene that is integrated into a patient's genome. Under this method, changes made are heritable and would be passed on to later generations.
Healthcare power of attorney	An alternative to a living will is for an individual to assign a permanent power of attorney for healthcare to another person. In this scheme, another person (for example, a spouse, a family member, or a friend) is designated as a surrogate healthcare decision-maker in case a person is unable or incompetent to make decisions for herself/himself due to serious illness.
Health Savings Account	A type of savings account that lets consumers set aside money on a pre-tax basis to pay for qualified medical expenses. For example, consumers can use untaxed dollars in a Health Savings Account (HSA) to pay for deductibles, co-payments, coinsurance, and some other expenses to lower their overall healthcare costs.
Human Genome Project	An international research project designed to sequence the human genome.
Incrementalism	Rather than consider all possible alternatives in a comprehensive manner, policymakers concentrate only on marginal values or relatively limited alternatives that bring about marginal changes in existing policies.
Interest-group liberalism	Various interest groups exercising countervailing veto power in a pluralistic system with many channels of access.
Iron triangle	A small circle of participants, such as a couple of congressional committees (a few legislators), executive agencies (a few bureaucrats), and interest groups that become semiautonomous in policymaking in a particular policy area.
Issue networks	Composed of a large number of participants with variable degrees of mutual commitment or dependence on others in the environment.

IMPORTANT CONCEPTS 491

"Just Say No"	During the 1980s, under the Reagan administration, First Lady Nancy Reagan's simplistic "Just Say No" campaign focused on the "demand" side of the drug problem.
Living will	A legal document signed by a competent person in good health giving permission to his or her doctor to turn off life-support systems in the case of terminal illness or a permanent coma.
Managed care/competition	Strategies to reduce the federal role in healthcare and expand the private-sector role. These strategies recognized some role for the government in managing competition and care.
Moral hazard	Third-party payers insulate healthcare consumers from the realities of healthcare costs, leading to overconsumption. Economists refer to this problem as "moral hazard."
Morning-after pill	Emergency contraception designed to prevent pregnancy after a woman has unprotected sex or if she thinks that the birth control method failed to work.
Pay-for-performance (P4P)	Providing physicians, hospitals, and other medical groups financial incentives to achieve assigned quality goals. The most common financial incentives are bonuses or add-on per-diem rates.
Pharmacological enhancement	Includes stimulant drugs that can be used to ward off sleep, improve concentration, and blood doping by athletes to increase muscle endurance.
Police powers	State governments' power to protect the health, safety, and general welfare of their residents.
Policy cycle	The process of getting problems to be considered by government and agenda setting; policy formulation and legitimation; budgeting, implementation and evaluation of policy, and decisions about policy continuation; and modifications and/or termination of legislation.
Policy environment	A total matrix of factors that influence and shape the policy cycle, such as constitutional, legal/statutory requirements, institutional settings and rules, values and ideology, economy, elections, and the like.
Political polarization	A sharp division into opposing groups or factions based on political party affiliations, ideology, or opinion.
Priority review	Priority-review designation means that the FDA plans to take action on a drug application within six months compared to ten months under the standard review process.
Provider taxes	Also referred to as fee or assessment, provider taxes are authorized by state law and collected through revenue from certain targeted groups of providers such as hospitals. In most instances, states used this as a tool to generate new instate-funds for the Medicaid program and match them with a federal fund to receive additional federal Medicaid dollars.
Public philosophy	An outlook on public affairs shared by the majority of the population in a nation.
Political tribalism	Refers to a condition in which groups/factions like political parties turn into tribes that come to view each other as enemies exhibiting belligerence, hostility, and a capacity for destruction.
Regenerative medicine	Interventions to replace underdeveloped, faulty, destroyed, or degenerated tissues by actually regenerating tissues.

Risk-benefit analysis	Analysis designed to weigh the potential for undesirable outcomes and side-effects against the potential positive outcomes of a policy/program.
Somatic gene therapy	Genes are transferred into somatic cells of a patient. Here, the modification of the gene and its effects are restricted to the individual patient alone and will not be inherited by the patient's offspring or later generations.
Specialty pharmacies	Offer a full range of clinical and operational services that enhance the safety, quality, and affordability of specialty medications for patients; they also perform a variety of management functions.
Unified government	A government in which the same political party controls the presidency and both houses of Congress.
Unitary system	A system of government in which the national government possesses all the power and is sovereign in all matters.
War on Drugs	President Nixon's "War on Drugs" focused on the "supply" side by attacking the drug problem through beefed-up law enforcement and tougher sentences for users and dealers.
War on Poverty	Refers to the Lyndon Johnson administration's creation of a mix of legislative programs designed to address the problem of poverty in the United States.

APPENDIX D

Important Research Reports

America's Children in Brief: Key National Indicators of Well-Being. 2018. Forum on Child and Family Statistics. Washington, DC: US Office of Management and Budget.
Online at www.childstats.gov/americaschildren/index.asp.

America's Health Rankings, Annual Report 2017. 2018. Minnetonka, MN: United Health Foundation.
Online at https://assets.americashealthrankings.org/app/uploads/ahrannual17_complete-121817.pdf.

Assisted Reproductive Technology National Summary Report. 2015. Atlanta, GA: CDC, Division of Reproductive Health.
Online at www.cdc.gov/art/pdf/2015-report/ART-2015-National-Summary-Report.pdf.

Broken Promises: Continuing Federal Funding Shortfall for Native Americans. 2018. Washington, DC: US Commission on Civil Rights.
Online at www.usccr.gov/pubs/2018/12-20-Broken-Promises.pdf.

Broker Promises: Evaluating the Native American Health Care System. 2004. Washington, DC: US Commission on Civil Rights.
Online at www.sprc.org/sites/default/files/resource-program/BrokenPromises.pdf.

Controversies in the Determination of Death. 2008. Washington, DC: President's Council on Bioethics.
Online at https://repository.library.georgetown.edu/handle/10822/559343.

Denied Posttraumatic Stress Disorder Claims Related to Military Sexual Trauma. 2018. Washington, DC: Office of Inspector General, Department of Veterans Affairs. Veterans Benefits Administration. Report # 17–05248-241.
Online at www.va.gov/oig/pubs/VAOIG-17-05248-241.pdf.

Dying in America: Improving Quality and Honoring Individual Preferences Near the End of Life. 2015. Washington, DC: National Academies of Sciences, Engineering, Medicine.
Online at www.nationalacademies.org/hmd/Reports/2014/Dying-In-America-Improving-Quality-and-Honoring-Individual-Preferences-Near-the-End-of-Life.aspx.

Flexner Report: Medical Education in the United States and Canada. 1910. Carnegie Foundation for the Advancement of Teaching.
Online at http://archive.carnegiefoundation.org/pdfs/elibrary/Carnegie_Flexner_Report.pdf.

Fueling an Epidemic: Insys Therapeutics and the Systemic Manipulation of Prior Authorization. 2018. Washington, DC: United States Congress. Committee on Homeland Security and Governmental Affairs.
Online at www.hsdl.org/c/.

Fueling an Epidemic, Report Two: Exposing the Financial Ties Between Opioid Manufacturers and Third Party Advocacy Groups. 2018. Washington, DC: United States Congress. Committee on Homeland Security and Governmental Affairs.
Online at www.hsdl.org/c/.

Fueling an Epidemic, Report Three: A Flood of 1.6 Billion Doses of Opioids into Missouri and the Need for Strong DEA Enforcement. 2018. Washington, DC: United States Congress. Committee on Homeland Security and Governmental Affairs.
Online at www.hsdl.org/c/.

Fueling an Epidemic, Report Four: Inside the Insys Strategy for Boosting Fentanyl Sales. 2018. Washington, DC: United States Congress. Committee on Homeland Security and Governmental Affairs.
Online at www.hsdl.org/c/.

Healthy People. **2010**. Hyattsville, MD: National Center for Health Statistics.
US Department of Health and Human Services.
Online at www.cdc.gov/nchs/data/hpdata2010/hp2010_final_review.pdf.

Health, United States. **2017**. Hyattsville, MD: National Center for Health Statistics. US Department of Health and Human Services.
Online at www.cdc.gov/nchs/data/hus/hus17.pdf.

How has U.S. Spending on Healthcare Changed Over Time? 2018. Peterson-Kaiser Health System Tracker.
Online at www.healthsystemtracker.org/chart-collection/u-s-spending-healthcare-changed-time/.

Mirror, Mirror: International Comparison Reflects Flaws and Opportunities for Better U.S. Health Care. 2017. Commonwealth Fund.
Online at www.commonwealthfund.org/publications/fund-reports/2017/jul/mirror-mirror-2017-international-comparison-reflects-flaws-and.

National Healthcare Quality and Disparities Report. **2017**. Washington, DC: Agency for Healthcare Research and Quality.
Online at www.ahrq.gov/research/findings/nhqrdr/nhqdr17/index.html.

Oregon Death with Dignity Act: 2017 Data Summary. 2017. Oregon Health Authority, Public Health Division.
Online at www.oregon.gov/oha/ph/providerpartnerresources/evaluationresearch/deathwithdignityact/documents/year20.pdf.

Perspectives on Health Equity and Social Determinants of Health 2017. 2017. Washington, DC:
National Academy of Science.
Online at https://nam.edu/wp-content/uploads/2017/12/Perspectives-on-Health-Equity-and-Social-Determinants-of-Health.pdf.

Prescription for Change: The Guiding Principles and Strategic Objectives Underlying the Transformation of the Veterans Health Care System. 1996. Kenneth W. Kizer. Washington, DC: Department of Veterans Affairs.

Prescription Nation 2018: Facing America's Opioid Epidemic. Itasca, IL: National Safety Council.
Online at http://safety.nsc.org/prescription-nation-facing-americas-opioid-epidemic.

President's Commission on Combating Drug Addiction and Opioid Crisis. 2018. Washington, DC: President's Commission on Combating Drug Addiction and Opioid Crisis.
Online at www.whitehouse.gov/sites/whitehouse.gov/files/images/Final_Report_Draft_11-1-2017.pdf.

Report on the State of Women's Health Policy. 2018. Washington, DC: Planned Parenthood.
Online at www.plannedparenthoodaction.org/stateofwomenshealth.

Review of Alleged Patient Deaths, Patient Wait Times, and Scheduling Practices at the Phoenix VA Health Care System. 2014. Washington, DC: VA Office of Inspector General.
Online at www.va.gov/oig/pubs/vaoig-14-02603-267.pdf.

IMPORTANT RESEARCH REPORTS

Safety and Quality of Abortion Care in the United States. 2018. Washington, DC: National Academies of Sciences, Engineering, and Medicine.
Online at www.nationalacademies.org/hmd/Reports/2018/the-safety-and-quality-of-abortion-care-in-the-united-states.aspx.

To Err Is Human: Building a Safer Health System. 1999. Washington, DC: Institute of Medicine.
Online at www.nationalacademies.org/hmd/~/media/Files/Report%20Files/1999/To-Err-is-Human/To%20Err%20is%20Human%201999%20%20report%20brief.pdf.

Unequal Treatment: Confronting Racial and Ethnic Disparities in Health Care. 2008. Washington, DC: Institute of Medicine.
Online at www.nap.edu/catalog/10260/unequal-treatment-confronting-racial-and-ethnic-disparities-in-health-care.

Vision for Change: A Plan to Restructure the Veterans Health Administration. 1995. Kenneth W. Kizer. Washington, DC: Department of Veterans Affairs.

Vital Directions for Health and Healthcare. 2017. Washington, DC: National Academy of Medicine.
Online at https://nam.edu/wp-content/uploads/2018/02/Vital-Directions-for-Health-and-Health-Care-Final-Publication-022718.pdf.

APPENDIX E

Healthcare-Related Documentaries and Films

HEALTHCARE-RELATED DOCUMENTARIES

Why Is Health Care in the US so Expensive?

Dr. Sanjay Gupta explores the high cost of healthcare in the United States.

Source: CNN; 2 minutes, 15 seconds; 2017

www.cnn.com/videos/health/2017/09/19/why-us-health-care-so-expensive-orig.cnn.

Sick Around the World

T.R. Reid goes overseas in this Frontline documentary to look at healthcare systems in other countries and make comparisons with the United States. The countries include Great Britain, Taiwan, Germany, Switzerland, and Japan. Reid asks what the United States can learn from these other countries. This film was shown the year prior to the passage of the Affordable Care Act.

Source: Frontline; 56 minutes; 2009.

http://video.pbs.org/video/1050712790/.

Sick Around America

Another Frontline documentary, this time looking at the problems of cost and access in the US healthcare system. This film was also shown during the year prior to the passage of the Affordable Care Act.

Source: Frontline; 54 minutes; 2009.

http://video.pbs.org/video/1099857730/.

Chasing Zero

This is a documentary produced by the actor Dennis Quaid about medical errors and the harm they cause. Quaid made the documentary after a near-tragic error was made on his and his wife's newborn twins.

Source: Discovery Channel; 53 minutes; 2010

http://dsc.discovery.com/videos/chasing-zero-part-1.html.

http://dsc.discovery.com/videos/chasing-zero-part-2.html.

http://dsc.discovery.com/videos/chasing-zero-part-3.html.

http://dsc.discovery.com/videos/chasing-zero-part-4.html.

The Suicide Tourist

A *Frontline* video about physician-assisted suicide and a couple who travel to Switzerland seeking help about this decision.

Source: PBS; 55 minutes; 2010

http://video.pbs.org/video/1430431984/.

Bill Moyer's Journal: Debating Health Care Reform

Bill Moyer talks with Trudy Lieberman and Dr. Marcia Angell to discuss healthcare reform and looks at the hostile industry of "Shock Jock" media and the role it plays in healthcare reform.

Source: PBS; 54 minutes; 2009

http://video.pbs.org/video/1194651895/

Overpill: The Darker Side of America's Mental Health

This film looks at how the pharmaceutical industry pushes its products, especially for people with mental illness, leading to overprescribing of medications. The film introduces us to several ordinary people who are struggling with issues related to mental health, addiction, and grave uncertainties for their future.

Source: Top Documentary Films; 50 minutes; 2017

https://topdocumentaryfilms.com/overpill/

Fix It: Healthcare at the Tipping Point

Healthcare costs are high and increasing, including the cost of health insurance. This film looks at the impact of high and increasing costs on various sectors of the American population.

Source: Top Documentary Films; 58 minutes; 2016

https://topdocumentaryfilms.com/fix-healthcare-tipping-point/

Big Bucks, Big Pharma: Marketing Disease and Pushing Drugs

This film looks at how the pharmaceutical industry (Big Pharma) utilizes various marketing strategies to sell its products. This includes direct-to-consumer advertising.

Source: Top Documentary Films; 46 minutes; 2006

https://topdocumentaryfilms.com/big-bucks-big-pharma/

Oxycontin: Time Bomb

The United States is facing an opiod epidemic, largely among people suffering from chronic pain. This documentary focuses how the pharmaceutical industry has used marketing campaigns to push products such as OxyContin, creating addictive dependency among users. The documentary explores how we can emerge from this epidemic.

Source: Top Documentary Films; 42 minutes; 2014

https://topdocumentaryfilms.com/oxycontin-time-bomb/

The Oxycontin Express

This film looks at the opioid epidemic, focusing on southern Florida. It shows how there is a pipeline for products. The film features interviews with users, law enforcement personnel and prison inmates, blaming poor laws and enforcement for the problems.

Source: Top Documentary Films; 47 minutes; 2009

https://topdocumentaryfilms.com/oxycontin-express/

The Price of Life

Rationing of healthcare occurs in the United States, though it is not often talked about in those terms. One basis for rationing is cost. This film looks at the UK's National Health Service and the process of making a decision about whether to offer treatment of a very expensive medication. The NHS cannot afford to offer all treatments so it needs to make these kinds of decisions. In Britain, rationing is an overt process.

Source: Top Documentary Films; 59 minutes; 2009

https://topdocumentaryfilms.com/price-life/

The Marketing of Madness: Are We All Insane?

This video looks at the partnership between the field of psychiatry and pharmaceutical companies. It questions the validity of psychiatric diagnoses and the effectiveness and safety of drugs. As the title indicates, the marketing of drugs is a huge enterprise.

Source: Top Documentary Films; 3 hours; 2013

https://topdocumentaryfilms.com/marketing-of-madness-are-we-all-insane/

Antibiotic Resistance

The development of antibiotics is one of the greatest advancements in medicine. They have helped cure infections and disease. But the heavy use of antibiotics has led to resistant bacteria. This documentary looks at the rise of antibiotic-resistant bacteria.

Source: Top Documentary Films; 29 minutes; 2016

https://topdocumentaryfilms.com/antibiotic-resistance/

Rise of the Superbugs

Similar to the film above, this documentary examines the rise of antibiotic-resistant bacteria, or superbugs. It examines the problems that the rise of superbugs has created.

Source: Top Documentary Films; 43 minutes; 2012

https://topdocumentaryfilms.com/rise-superbugs/

The Coming Pandemic

This film looks at the possibility of the rise of viruses that can destroy nations, examining possible scenarious based on some semi-medical findings and studies.

Source: Top Documentary Films; 35 minutes; 2005

https://topdocumentaryfilms.com/coming-pandemic/

Here's to Flint

Flint, Michigan saw its water supply changed to a source that, it turned out, contained lead pipes. This film looks at this totally preventable and unnecssary water crisis, which remains a problem even in 2019, though the water source has changed. The film looks at how this crisis came about and its effects on both Flint citizens and the people who made this tragic decision.

Source: Top Documentary Films; 45 minutes; 2016

https://topdocumentaryfilms.com/here-flint/

The American Abortion War

This video looks at the battleground issue of abortion. Since abortion was legalized in 1973, states have passed increasingly restrictive anti-abortion measures. Pro-choice advocates argue that the anti-abortion movement is anti-women and aimed at reproductive rights as much as abortion. The video examines the reframing of this very divisive issue.

Source: Top Documentary Films; 25 minutes; 2013

https://topdocumentaryfilms.com/abortion-war/

Fast Food, Fat Profits: Obesity in America

Obesity among Americans has become an epidemic and is responsible for decreasing health among the population. Minorities are disproportionately affected by obesity. Jash Rushing suggests that the ready availability of fast food is an important contributory factor in the epidemic, along with desserts and highly processed foods.

Source: Top Documentary Films; 24 minutes; 2012

https://topdocumentaryfilms.com/fast-food-fat-profits-obesity-america/

Money Talks: Profits Before Patient Safety

This video looks at tactics employed by large pharmaceutical companies to sell their products to both doctors and the public. The video argues that pharmaceutical companies place a higher priority on profits than the safety of their overpriced products.

Source: Top Documentary Films: 2006; 50 minutes

https://topdocumentaryfilms.com/money-talks-profits-before-patient-safety/

Prescription for Disaster

This film focuses on Vioxx, an anti-inflammatory drug that relieves pain. It suggests that the Food and Drug Administration has experienced regulatory failure when addressing Vioxx (and other pharmaceuticals), though the drug was eventually pulled from the market. The video examines the interrelationships among pharmaceutical companies, insurance companies, regulatory agencies, lawmakers, lobbyists, etc., demonstrating the failures of the system.

Source: Top Documentary Films; 90 minutes; 2009

https://topdocumentaryfilms.com/prescription-for-disaster/

Street Medicine

The US remains the only industrialized country lacking universal healthcare. This video looks at local efforts to provide care to the uninsured and the homeless.

Source: Top Documentary Films; 30 minutes; 2008

https://topdocumentaryfilms.com/street-medicine/

Sicko

Filmmaker Michael Moore focuses on the underinsured portion of the US population—those who have insurance, but whose insurance is inadequate for their needs. Rounding up a small number of such people, Moore takes off to examine healthcare systems in other countries, including France and Cuba.

Source: Top Documentary Films; 123 minutes; Dog Eat Dog Films/The Weinstein Company

https://topdocumentaryfilms.com/sicko/

U.S. Health Care: The Good News

Another video by T.R. Reid, this one focuses on the healthcare delivery system in Grand Junction, Colorado. Reid asks why this area has been successful in deliverying high-quality care at a reasonable price and wonders if the results can be replicated elsewhere in the US.

Source: PBS; 30 minutes; 2012

www.pbs.org/program/us-health-care-good-news/

Escape Fire: The Fight to Rescue American Healthcare

This 2012 release was an official Sundance selection that year and debuted on CNN in early 2013. This documentary focuses on the incentives of the American healthcare system, which it argues are badly misaligned.

Source: Lionsgate; 99 minutes; 2012

www.amazon.com/Escape-Fire-Rescue-American-Healthcare/dp/B00BLSY592

The Waiting Room

This multi-part video looks at a safety-net, public hospital in Oakland California and shows how difficult it is to operate when its patients are mostly Medicaid and Medicare recipients.

Source: PBS; 81 minutes; 2012

www.youtube.com/watch?time_continue=59&v=NWIAjsf9Xq0

What the Health

This documentary focuses on the collusion between government and business and the corruption that accompanies. The documentary argues that the result is trillions of dollars of wasted spending and a population that remains less healthy than it might otherwise be.

Source: *What the Health*; 92 minutes; 2017

www.whatthehealthfilm.com/

To Err is Human: A Patient Safety Documentary

This film focuses on mistakes and waste in the American healthcare system. This documentary looks at the evidence for the large number of preventable deaths each year plus illnesses acquired by those in contact with the system. The film looks at how these problems are being addressed

Source: 3759 Films; 80 minutes; 2019

www.indiegogo.com/projects/to-err-is-human-a-patient-safety-documentary-film-medicine#/

HEALTHCARE-RELATED FILMS

The Doctor

Starring: William Hurt, Christine Lahti, Elizabeth Perkins
Released: 1991

The Doctor, based on a memoir, examines how a doctor learns to see patients as people when he becomes a patient suffering from throat cancer.

Patch Adams

Starring: Robin Williams, Daniel London, Monica Potter, Philip Seymour-Hoffman
Released: 1998

Patch Adams voluntarily commits himself to a mental institution. He begins to help other patients in very nontraditional ways. Adams decides to be come a doctor, but drops out because of how medical students are taught to treat patients. He sets up an institute to pursue his views, but is soon brought before a review board.

One Flew Over the Cuckoo's Nest

Starring: Jack Nicholson, Louise Fletcher, William Redfield
Released: 1976

The main character, Randle McMurphy, convinces courts that he is insane and spends time in a mental institution. McMurphy confronts a tyrannical nurse who terrorizes the other patients. The film is an indictment of the mental health system in the US.

Philadelphia

Starring: Tom Hanks, Denzel Washington, Joanne Woodward
Released: 1993

Based on a true story, the film the film follows a lawyer who is gay and develops AIDS. As a result, the lawyer, Andrew Beckett, loses his job and sues his old firm. The film was made near the beginning of the AIDS epidemic and demonstrates much about the attitudes that existed at that time.

My Own Country

Starring: Naveen Andrews, Glenne Headly, Hal Holbrook
Released: 2000

This movie tells the story of Abraham Verghese, an Ethiopian doctor who moves to eastern Tennessee at the beginning of the AIDS epidemic. Verghese practices in a rural city and, because of his compassion toward those with AIDS, soon becomes overwhelmed with AIDS patients.

Awakenings

Starring: Robert De Niro, Robin Williams, John Heard
Released: 1990

Robin Williams plays a doctor who uses a new drug, L-Dopa, to help revive catatonic patients. Williams' character tries to show that these formerly catatonic patients can become part of the world again. However, the drug does not have a permanent impact and patients return to their catatonic state.

And the Band Played On

Starring: Matthew Modine, Alan Aida, Ian McKellen
Released: 1993

The movie follows Dr. Donald Pinkston "Don" Francis right at the beginning of the AIDS epidemic. Dr. Francis studies those infected with the virus in San Francisco, Los Angeles, and New York, at a time when the fear of AIDS leaves him working without much support.

The Hospital

Starring: George C. Scott, Diana Rigg, Robert Walden
Released: 1971

This movie looks at a day in the life of the chief of medicine at a hospital in Manhattan. The chief, Dr. Bock, has suicidial thoughts, but puts his plans off because of unusual deaths at the hospital.

Awake

Starring: Hayden Christensen, Jessica Alba, Terrence Howard, Lena Olin
Released: 2007

A man undergoing heart transplant surgery discovers that his surgical team is trying to kill him.

Extreme Measures

Starring: Hugh Grant, Gene Hackman, Sarah Jessica Parker
Released: 1996

This movie is a thriller about a British doctor working at a New York hospital. The doctor starts an investigation after a patient who dies in the emergency room disappears. The investigation points to an eminent surgeon at the hospital, but the doctor finds that he is under threat from those who want to hide what has happened.

Shutter Island

Starring: Leonardo DiCaprio, Emily Mortimer, Mark Ruffalo
Released: 2010

In 1954, a US Marshal investigates the disappearance of a murderer who escaped from a hospital for the criminally insane.

Outbreak

Starring: Dustin Hoffman, Rene Russo, Morgan Freeman, Kevin Spacey
Released: 1995

This is one of a number of films about the outbreak of a deadly virus and the measures taken/needed to contain the epidemic.

John Q

Starring: Denzel Washington, Robert Duvall, Gabriela Oltean, Kimberly Elise
Released: 2002

John Quincy Archibald takes a hospital emergency room hostage when his insurance won't cover his son's heart transplant.

Dallas Buyers Club

Starring: Matthew McConaughey, Jennifer Garner, Jared Leto
Released: 2013

Matthew McConaughey plays a man who cannot get a drug to treat his AIDS because the drug has not been approved by the FDA and insurance companies will not pay for it. McConaughey successfully fights for the right to use the drug.

Critical Care

Starring: James Spader, Kyra Sedgwick, Helen Mirren
Released: 1997

This movie examines the question of the ethics of keeping alive people who are in a vegative state. The question addresses the quality of life, the right to life, and the profits made by keeping such a person alive.

The Rainmaker

Starring: Matt Damon, Dennis Hopper, Victoria Duffy
Released: 1997

This movie, based on a John Grisham novel, deals with two people who take an insurance company to court for its refusal to cover a family member who is dying from leukemia. The insurance company loses, but the movie shows the difficulty of challenging company policies.

Contagion

Starring: Gwyneth Paltrow, Matt Damon, Kate Winslet, Jude Law
Released: 2011

Contagion is another movie that focuses on attempts to stop an epidemic. The government works with private scientists to find a solution. The focus is on a public health issue and the process of working out a solution to a deadly epidemic.

The Constant Gardner

Starring: Ralph Fiennes, Rachel Weisz, Danny HustonReleased: 2005

A clinical trial in Nigeria in the 1990s goes wrong and the husband of a victim searches for answers to his wife's death.

Elysium

Starring: Matt Damon, Jodie Foster
Released: 2013

Elysium is a futuristic movie about a time where sickness has been eliminated by a machine that can diagnose a human and cure that human of any diseases he or she might have.

Gattaca

Starring: Ethan Hawke, Uma Thurman
Released: 1997

This movie, which came out around the time of multiple investiations into genomes, raises the question of what happens to those with defective genomes. The movie strongly suggests that society will become prepared for the opportunities and challenges of the genomic revolution.

Prometheus

Starring: Noomi Rapace, Logan Marshall-Green
Released: 2012

Robotics are becoming more important in surgery. *Prometheus* raises the question of what will happen when robots can conduct all surgeries without human intervention.

ABOUT THE AUTHORS

Kant Patel (PhD, University of Houston, 1976) is an Emeritus Professor of Political Science at Missouri State University. From 1977 to 2011 he taught Health Policy and Politics, Policy Analysis, and Intergovernmental Relations. He has published articles in journals such as *Evaluation and Health Profession, Health Policy and Education, Political Methodology, Journal of Political Science, International Journal of Policy Analysis and Information Systems,* and *Journal of Health and Social Policy,* among others. He is co-author (with Mark Rushefsky) of *Politics, Power, and Policy Making: The Case of Health Care Reform in the 1990s* (1998); *Health Care Policy in an Age of New Technologies* (2002); *The Politics of Public Health in the United States* (2005); and *Health Care in America: Separate and Unequal (2008).*

Mark Rushefsky (PhD, Binghamton University [State University of New York], 1977) is an Emeritus Professor of Political Science at Missouri State University. He has taught and written about American government, public policy, and public administration. He is the author of *Making Cancer Policy* (1986) and *Public Policy in the United States: Challenges, Opportunities, and Changes,* 6th edn (Routledge, 2017) as well as articles and chapters on healthcare and the environment. He is co-author (with Kant Patel) of *Politics, Power, and Policy Making: The Case of Health Care Reform in the 1990s* (1998); *Health Care Policy in an Age of New Technologies* (2002); *The Politics of Public Health in the United States* (2005); and *Health Care in America: Separate and Unequal (2008).*

INDEX

A

abortion
  and contraception, 268, 373–374
  court cases, 380–384
  George W. Bush Administration, 59
  healthcare reform, 91–92
  RU-486 and medication abortion, 378–380
  Trump Administration, 63
  see also reproductive health
abuse of system, impact on costs, 308–310
access to healthcare
  1960s social programs, 283
  Affordable Care Act, 96, 119, 120
  community health workers, 249
  disadvantaged groups, 82–83, 243
  health insurance, 82–83, 86, 154, 249–251
  healthcare reform, 453–454
  illegal immigrants, 272–274
  indigenous communities, 202–204, 206, 211–212
  legal immigrants, 271–272
  Medicaid, 110, 115, 132, 141, 145
  Medicare, 175
Accountable Care Organizations (ACOs), 106, 182
actors, 71–72
  consumers, 28–29
  employers, 28
  health policymaking, 4
  healthcare providers, 22–25
  interest groups, 30–32, 71–72
  third-party payers, 25–27
acute lymphoblastic leukemia (AAL), 429
Adams, John, 45, 64
addiction, opioid epidemic, 293, 407, 414
administration
  cost containment, 340–341
  spending on healthcare, 311–312
advanced practice nurses, 24
advertising, prescription drugs, 316, 320–321
advocacy groups, 32
Affordable Care Act (ACA), 56, 120–124
  administrative challenges, 113–115
  challenges to, 101–106, 111–115
  contraception, 103, 106, 266–267
  cost containment, 341
  coverage gap, 174
  'doughnut hole', 100, 174, 189, 424–425
  evaluation of, 115–120
  events leading up to, 81–87
  experience rating, 257
  federalism, 108–111
  health insurance coverage, 96–99, 104, 107, 274
  implementation, 106–108
  indigenous communities, 202–203
  legal immigrants, 271–272

  legislative challenges, 111–113
  legislative process, 87–96
  Medicaid expansion, 97, 109–111, 131–132, 140–146
  Medical Loss Ratio, 257
  Medicare, 176–177, 189–190
  Obama Administration, 60–61
  patient protection, 96–102
  pre-existing conditions limitations, 257
  price regulation, 328
  process of passage, 81
  rationing, 333
  reform, 81, 90–95, 455–457, 463, 469
  social determinants of health, 247
  Trump Administration, 62–63, 72
  veterans, 217–218
African-Americans, healthcare policy, 258–259
age *see* child health; elderly care
Agency for Healthcare Research and Quality (AHRQ), 293
aging population, 442–443
AIDS, 204, 260
Alaska Natives
  accomplishments of the IHS, 210
  challenges, 210–213
  health policymaking, 199–203
  health status, 206–210, 262
  historical context, 198, 199–202
  Indian Health Service, 68, 203–213
  legal and constitutional status, 198–199
  population characteristics, 196–198
alcohol
  addiction, 408
  Behavioral Health Program, 204
  indigenous communities, 206, 213
ambiguity of evidence, 339, 342
American Hospital Association (AHA), 24, 31
American Indian Movement, 201
American Indians
  accomplishments of the IHS, 210
  challenges, 210–213
  health policymaking, 199–203
  health status, 206–210, 262
  historical context, 198, 199–202
  Indian Health Service, 68, 203–213
  legal and constitutional status, 198–199
  population characteristics, 196–198
American Medical Association (AMA)
  historical context, 44, 64, 65
  national health insurance, 165–166
  as policy actor, 30–31
  public health, 48–49
American Nurses Association (ANA), 31
American public *see* public opinion
American Public Health Association, 64–65, 66
America's Health Insurance Plans (AHIP), 31, 86, 88
anesthesia, 44

508   INDEX

annual insurance limits, 257
anti-kickback, 310
antisepsis, 44
Arrears Act, 215
Arrow, Kenneth, 323, 325
artificial hydration and nutrition (AHN), 387–388
artificial insemination, 363, 371, 371–372, 372, 375
assisted reproduction, 363–373, 382–384
  see also reproductive health
assisted suicide, 384–398
association health plans, 113–114
Association of American Medical Colleges (AAMC), 288

B

bacteriology, 44
balanced billing, 314
Balanced Budget Act, 167, 191
bankruptcies, households, 296
Behavioral Health Program, 204
Beveridge model, 83
bill of rights
  GIs, 215–216
  Patient's, 56
bioethics, 362
biomedicine
  assisted reproduction, 363–373, 382–384
  cognitive biases, 340
  contraception, 375–378
  cost containment, 341
  courts and abortion, 380–384
  family planning, 372–375
  gene therapy, 427–437
  historical context, 46
  law, politics, religion, and ethics, 361–362
  Pharmaceutical Research and Manufacturers of America, 32
  public health emergencies, 66
  right-to-die and physician-assisted suicide, 384–398
  RU-486 and medication abortion, 378–380
  spending on healthcare, 300–304
  technological environment, 22
  twentieth century, 65
birth control see contraception
birth control pills, 265, 268, 376–377
Bismarck model, 83
Blacks, healthcare policy, 258–259
blindness, gene therapy, 433
block-grant program, 58
Blue Cross plans, 45
Blue Shield plans, 45
Boren Amendment, 156
Bouvia, Elizabeth, 386
budgets
  Affordable Care Act, 112
  Clinton Administration, 55
  cost containment, 341–342
bundled payments, 182
bureaucracy, institutional environment, 9–10
Burwell v. Hobby Lobby Stores, Inc, 103
Bush Administration *see* George H. W. Bush Administration; George W. Bush Administration
business, healthcare spending impacts, 297

C

Camp Lejeune Family Member Program (CLFMP), 222
Canada
  healthcare system, 83
  right-to-die, 385–386
cancer
  indigenous communities, 208–209
  lifestyle choices, 310–311
capitation system, 333–334
cardiovascular disease *see* heart disease
care *see* home caregiving; long-term care
Caregiver (veteran program), 222
Carter Administration
  costs of healthcare, 51
  price regulation, 328–329
Cassidy-Graham bill, 112
Catholic Church
  contraception, 265, 266
  physician-assisted suicide, 397
  stem cells, 57
caucuses, 9
census data, indigenous communities, 196, 197
Centers for Disease Control and Prevention (CDC)
  contraception, 58–59
  cost-benefit analysis, 21
  financing, 70
  model legislations, 67
  organization and functions, 68
Centers for Medicare and Medicaid Services (CMS), 460
centralization, federal system, 5–8
certificate-of-need (CON) legislation, 327
Chen, Lanhee J., 466
child health
  African-Americans, 259
  before CHIP, 137–138
  comparative analysis, 42–43
  dental care, 269–270
  paid leave programs, 265
  uninsured population, 252, 254–255
childbirth, African-Americans, 259
  see also pregnancy
Children of Women Vietnam Veterans (CWVV), 222
Children's Health Insurance Program (CHIP)
  benefits, 139–140
  Clinton Administration, 56
  cost-sharing, 140
  coverage and spending, 27
  eligibility, 139
  financing, 140
  Obama Administration, 60
  origins and evolution, 137–139
  pregnancy care, 254–255
Children's Health Insurance Program Reauthorization Act (CHIPRA), 60
chronic health conditions, 292–293, 342
citizens groups, 15–16
  see also interest groups
civil false claims, 310
civil rights, equality and equity, 244–245
civil service, institutional environment, 9–10
Civil War
  opioids, 293
  public health, 64
  veterans, 215, 216
Civilian Health and Medical Program of the Department of Veterans Affairs (CHAMPVA), 222
Clinton Administration
  costs of healthcare, 312

divided government, 16–17
  healthcare reform, 13
  healthcare system, 54–56
  Medicaid waivers, 149
cloture rule, 9, 12, 89
coalition-building, political environment, 17–18
cognitive biases, 340
colonialism
  healthcare system, 43
  indigenous communities, 198, 206
Committee on the Costs of Medical Care (CCMC), 130
community
  social determinants of health, 247
  Veterans Health Administration, 219
community health centers, 249
community health workers, 249, 439
Community Living Assistance Services and Supports (CLASS) Act, 107–108, 156
community rating, 256
comorbidity adjustments, 342
comparative analysis *see* international context
comparative effectiveness research, 340
competition *see* market competition
compulsory sickness insurance, 45
computed tomography (CT), 301–302
confirmation bias, 340
Congress
  consensus-building, 12
  gridlock and dysfunction, 20–21, 89–90, 122
  healthcare reform, 90–91
  institutional environment, 8–9
  vetos, 10
Congressional Budget Office (CBO)
  costs of healthcare, 110
  Medicaid, 102
  prescription drugs, 330
  repeal-and-replace legislation, 112–113, 470
  technological environment, 301
  tort reform, 308
consensus-building, 12, 17–18
Conservative/Republican reform proposals, 85–86, 462–469
Consolidated Omnibus Budget Reconciliation Act (COBRA), 252
constitutional system
  health policy environment, 5–8
  indigenous communities, 198–199
  right-to-die and physician-assisted suicide, 389, 390
  veterans, 214–215
consumer advocacy groups, 32
Consumer-Choice Health Plan (CCHP), 333–334
consumer-directed healthcare plans, 152–154
consumer-driven healthcare, 59
consumers
  overconsumption, 45
  as policy actors, 28–29
  surprise medical bills, 314
  see also public opinion
contraception
  and abortion, 268, 373–374
  abstinence-only programs, 58–59
  birth control pills, 265, 268, 376–377
  condoms, 58–59
  debates over, 265–268
  for emergencies, 59, 375–378
  unintended pregnancies, 372–373, 374, 380–382

Cooperative Action for Health Programs (CAHP), 66
cost containment
  Affordable Care Act, 341
  bending the cost curve, 323
  contemporary context, 337–342
  federal budget, 341–342
  fraud, waste and abuse, 308–310, 338–340
  historical context, 49–50, 51–52, 327
  Medicaid, 49, 342
  medical technology, 303
  Medicare, 49, 177–182, 340
  planning, 327
  price regulation, 328–330
  strategy for, 342
cost curve, 323
cost-benefit analysis, 21, 304
cost-effectiveness analysis, 21, 92–93
costs of healthcare *see* financing; premiums; spending on healthcare
cost-sharing
  Affordable Care Act, 189–190
  Children's Health Insurance Program, 140
  healthcare reform, 456
  Medicaid, 136
  Medicare, 169, 186
  as strategy, 336–337
  surprise medical bills, 314
cost-shifting *see* cost-sharing
Council of Economic Advisers (CEA), 293
courts
  abortion, 373, 379, 380–384
  Affordable Care Act, 101–105
  assisted reproduction, 365, 368–372
  emergency contraception, 378
  judiciary, 11–12
  right-to-die and physician-assisted suicide, 386–392
coverage gap, 174
crowdsourcing, 297
Cruzan, Nancy, 387
cultural context
  indigenous communities, 212–213
  individualism, 249
  opioid epidemic, 413–414
culturally competent care, 212–213
cybernetic enhancement, 435

D

Davis, Karen, 342
debt, households, 296
decentralization
  Congress, 8–9
  federal system, 5–8
  public philosophy, 14
deductibles
  cost-sharing, 336–337
  impact on households, 296
  underinsurance, 252–253
defensive medicine, 306–308
defined-contribution plans, 187, 466–467
Democratic reform proposals, 84–85, 457–462
demographics
  aging, 442–443
  concentration of expenditures, 290–293
  indigenous communities, 196–198
  opioid epidemic, 410–412

veterans, 214, 227–228
dental care, 269–270
Department of Energy (DOE), 427–428
Department of Health and Human Services (DHHS), 27
diabetes
    indigenous communities, 208, 209
    lifestyle choices, 310–311
diagnosis-related groups (DRGs), 52–53, 179
direct-to-consumer advertising, 316, 320–321
disabilities, in veterans, 228
disadvantaged groups
    challenges, 274–275
    dental care, 269–270
    equality and equity, 243
    geographical context, 247–248
    health insurance and community, 256–257
    health status, 257–258
    immigrants, 270–274
    low-income, 258–262
    minorities, 258–262
    personal responsibility, 246
    public health, 245–246
    social determinants of health, 246–247, 248–249
    uninsured and underinsured, 249–256
    women, 262–269
discrimination
    disadvantaged groups, 243
    healthcare workforce diversity, 441–442
    Minority Health and Health Disparities Research and Education Act, 66
    pregnant women, 264–265
Disproportionate Share Hospitals Program (DSH), 273
disproportionate-share hospital payments, 136, 255–256, 273
diversity, healthcare workforce, 441–442
divided government, 16–17
doctors *see* physicians
'doughnut hole', Affordable Care Act, 100, 174, 189, 424–425
drug companies *see* pharmaceutical industry; prescription drugs
durable power of attorney, 396

E

economic context
    health policy, 21–22
    healthcare reform, 470
    opioid epidemic, 412–413
egg donation (assisted reproduction), 364, 370
egg harvesting (assisted reproduction), 365–366
eggs from laboratories (assisted reproduction), 365–366
elderly care
    concentration of expenditures, 292
    end-of-life, 338, 384–398
    Medicare origins, 166–167
    residential care facilities, 25
    see also long-term care; Medicare; veterans
elections
    Affordable Care Act, 122
    electoral cycle, 13
    Obama's campaign, 13, 87
electoral ideological polarization, 19–20
electronic health records (EHR), 341
Ellwood, Paul, 333–334
embryo donation (assisted reproduction), 364, 371
emergency contraception, 59, 375–378

emergency departments (EDs)
    balanced billing, 314
    uninsured population, 253–254, 255–256
Emergency Medical Treatment and Active Labor Act (EMTALA), 255
employers
    Affordable Care Act, 96, 107
    health insurance provision, 26, 28, 249, 250–251
    impact of rise in healthcare costs, 295, 297
    insurance and healthcare reform, 464, 470
    as policy actors, 28
employment
    healthcare workforce, 437–442
    Medicaid work requirements, 154
employment retiree benefits, 170
end-of-life care
    costs, 338
    right-to-die and physician-assisted suicide, 384–398
Enthoven, Alain, 333–334
Environmental Protection Agency (EPA), 66
epidemics
    historical context, 63–64
    opioids, 63, 293, 407–420
epinephrine, 315
equality
    disadvantaged groups, 243–245
    healthcare values, 455
equity
    disadvantaged groups, 243–245
    health insurance, 256
    healthcare workforce diversity, 441–442
errors *see* medical errors
ethics
    assisted reproduction, 383–384
    biomedicine, 361–362
    end-of-life care, 338
    gene therapy, 433–436
    health insurance, 256
    physician-assisted suicide, 397–398
euthanasia, 384–398
evidence basis
    biomedicine, 339, 342
    opioid epidemic, 420
executive branch, institutional environment, 9–10
experience rating, 256–257

F

fairness
    Affordable Care Act, 257
    equality and equity, 243–244
family, healthcare spending impacts, 294–297
Family and Medical Leave Act (FMLA), 264
'family glitch', 456
family planning *see* contraception; reproductive health
family separation, Mexico-US migration, 274
feasibility, healthcare reform, 470
Federal Employees Health Benefits Program (FEHBP), 334
federal government
    historical context, 45–51, 64, 66
    indigenous communities, 199
    judiciary, 11
    Medicaid, 135, 141
    Medicare, 187
    opioid epidemic response, 416–418
    organization and functions, 67–68

price regulation, 328–329
prospective payment system, 179–180
role in healthcare system, 67–68
social programs, 286
spending on healthcare, 70, 297–298
federalism
    Affordable Care Act, 108–111
    as system, 5–8
fee-for-service
    Medicaid financing, 137
    Medicare, 175
    prospective payment system, 179–180
fertility market, 366–367
    see also assisted reproduction
financing
    Children's Health Insurance Program, 140
    federal government, 297–298
    healthcare reform, 459–460
    Indian Health Service, 205, 211
    long-term care, 155–156
    Medicaid, 135–137, 459–460
    Medicare, 168–169, 175–176, 185–186
    public health, 70, 288–290
    veterans' healthcare, 225–226
        see also cost containment; spending on healthcare
Flexner Report, 45
Food and Drug Administration (FDA)
    assisted reproduction, 367
    gene therapy, 429, 432–433, 436–437
    OxyContin, 409
    role of, 68, 321
    specialty drugs, 422–423
Founding Fathers, 5, 6
fraud, impact on costs, 308–310, 338–340
freedom, healthcare values, 455
Friedman, Milton, 325
future of healthcare, 5
    aging population, 442–443
    challenges facing, 407, 443
    gene therapy, 427–437
    opioid epidemic, 407–420
    role of the healthcare workforce, 437–442
    specialty drugs, 420–427
        see also healthcare reform

G

Gelsinger, Jesse, 429
gender
    Affordable Care Act, 116
    health status, 260, 262–269
    healthcare workforce diversity, 442
    opioid epidemic, 411
    reproductive health, 265–268
    uninsured population, 263
    women veterans, 219, 222, 225, 231
gender justice, 244
gene editing, 430, 433–434, 435, 436–437
gene therapy, 427–437
general-care physicians, 440
genetic enhancement, 435
genetically modified organisms (GMOs), 430
geographical context
    disadvantaged groups, 247–248
    opioid epidemic, 410–412
    uninsured population, 252

    workforce shortages, 440–441
George H. W. Bush Administration
    healthcare system, 53–54
    Medicaid waivers, 149
George W. Bush Administration
    divided government, 17
    emergency contraception, 376, 378
    healthcare system, 56–60
    presidential signing statements, 10
    right-to-die and physician-assisted suicide, 390–391
gestational carriers (assisted reproduction), 364
GI Bill of Rights, 215–216
Gingrich, Newt, 8–9
Ginzberg, Eli, 453, 454
Global War on Terror (GWOT), 224
globalization, fertility market, 366–367
Goodman, John C., 326, 466–467
government *see* federal government; local governments; public health; state governments
government healthcare programs, 4
government regulation *see* legal framework
go-very-slow approach, 435
graduate medical education (GME), 288
Great Depression
    interest groups, 15
    political environment, 13
Gross Domestic Product (GDP), healthcare spending as proportion, 3–4, 283, 288–290, 454
group-model HMOs, 335

H

Hacker, Jacob, 458, 461
halfway technology, 300–301
Hamilton, Alexander, 6
Hastert Rule, 9
Hayek, Frederich, 325
Health and Human Services, Treasury, and Labor (HHSTL), 465
Health Care Cost Institute, 312
Health Care Fairness Act, 66
Health Care Fraud and Abuse Control program, 310
health information technology (HIT), 341
health insurance
    Affordable Care Act, 96–99, 104, 107, 274
    Affordable Care Act outcomes, 115–117, 119
    children, 137–138
    Clinton Administration, 55–56
    consumer perspective, 28–29
    costs of, 26–27
    disadvantaged groups, 256–257
    the elderly, 166–167
    employer costs, 28
    healthcare reform, 55–56, 86, 453–456, 458–468
    interest groups, 31
    long-term care, 184–185
    prescription drugs, 321
    private sector, 25–26
    underwriting, 256–257
    veterans, 218, 223, 226
        see also public sector health insurance; uninsured population
health insurance exchanges, 97–98, 103–104, 108–109, 118
Health Insurance Portability and Accounting Act (HIPAA)
    Medical Savings Accounts, 152–154

passage of, 56, 137
Health Maintenance Organization Act, 332
health maintenance organizations (HMOs)
  costs of healthcare, 52, 331–332
  definitions, 334–335
  managed care, 335–336
  managed competition, 333–334
  Medicare, 167, 174–176
  origins, 50
health policy actors *see* actors
health policy environment
  Affordable Care Act replacement, 62–63
  changing political environment, 16–21
  constitutional system, 5–8
  economic context, 21–22
  institutional environment, 8–12
  political factors, 12–21
  technological environment, 22
health policy institutions *see* institutions
health policy issues, 3
health policymaking, 4–5
  Congress, 8–9
  indigenous communities, 199–203
  judiciary, 11
  presidents' role, 10
  Supreme Court, 11
  veterans, 216–218
    see also legal framework
Health Resources and Service Administration (HRSA), 441–442
health savings accounts (HSAs), 59, 152–154, 468–469
health status
  concentration of expenditures, 290–293
  disadvantaged groups, 257–258
  immigrants, 270–274
  indigenous communities, 206–210, 262
  low-income individuals, 258–262
  minorities, 258–262
  social determinants of health, 246–247, 248–249
  uninsured and underinsured populations, 253–256
  veterans, 222–225
  women, 260, 262–270
health status risk adjustment, 467
healthcare costs *see* costs of healthcare
healthcare providers, as policy actors, 22–25
healthcare reform, 453
  abortion, 91–92
  Affordable Care Act, 81, 90–95, 455–457, 469
  child health, 137–138
  choices, 469–471
  Clinton Administration, 54–55
  Conservative/Republican proposals, 85–86, 462–469
  George H. W. Bush Administration, 53–54
  goals, 453–455
  health insurance, 55–56, 86, 453–456, 458–468
  Liberal/Democratic proposals, 84–85, 457–462
  Massachusetts Model, 86
  Medicaid, 151–155
  Obama Administration, 60–61
  public health law reform movement, 67
  public opinion, 93–94
  values, 455
healthcare support workers, 439
healthcare system
  Clinton Administration, 54–56
  colonial times, 43
  comparative models, 41–43
  early twentieth century, 44–44
  federal government's role, 45–51
  George H. W. Bush Administration, 53–54
  George W. Bush Administration, 56–60
  historical context, 71–72
  models of, 83
  nineteenth century, 43–44
  Obama Administration, 60–61
  political transformation, 51
  Reagan Administration, 51–53
  Trump Administration, 61–63
healthcare workforce, role of, 437–442
  see also nurses; physicians
heart disease
  indigenous communities, 208
  lifestyle choices, 310–311
heroin, 407, 408, 409
HHS, federal government, 67–68
high-deductible health plans (HDHP), 59, 336–337
high-risk pools, 99, 102
Hill-Burton funds, 45–47, 49, 453–454
Hippocratic Oath, 304
Hispanic paradox, 261
historical context
  Clinton Administration, 54–56
  colonial times, 43
  early twentieth century, 44–44
  evolution of public health, 63–67
  federal government's role, 45–51
  George H. W. Bush Administration, 53–54
  George W. Bush Administration, 56–60
  healthcare system, 71–72
  indigenous communities, 198, 199–202
  nineteenth century, 43–44
  Obama Administration, 60–61
  political transformation, 51
  Reagan Administration, 51–53
  Trump Administration, 61–63
  veteran benefits, 214–216
HIV, 204, 260
home and community-based services (HCBS), 155–157
home caregiving, 183–184
homelessness, veterans, 223
homicides
  African-Americans, 260, 262
  indigenous communities, 207
  physician-assisted suicide, 391
Hoover Administration, 130
hospitals
  federal government's role, 47
  historical context, 44, 47
  Medicaid financing, 136
  Medicare financing, 168
  as policy actors, 24–25
  regulatory strategies on costs, 327, 328
  spending on, 303, 313
  uninsured population, 253–254
House of Representatives v. Price, 104
households, healthcare spending impacts, 294–297
Howe, Barbara, 387–388
human enhancement, 435–436
Human Genome Project, 427–428, 429
human rights, equality and equity, 244–245

Hyde Amendment, 91–92
hydrocodone, 408

I
ideological polarization, 19
ideologies
  interest groups, 30, 71–72
  political environment, 89
  public philosophy, 14–15
  socialized medicine, 48, 71–72
illegal immigrants, 272–274
imaging technology, 301–302
immigrants *see* migration
imperfect information, 325
in vitro fertilization (IVF), 363, 365, 369
income *see* low-income individuals; poverty
incrementalism, 12–13
Indian Health Care Improvement Act, 202
Indian Health Service, 203–213
  accomplishments, 210
  challenges, 210–213
  federal government relationship, 68
  funding, 205, 211
  health status and trends, 206–210
  organization and structure, 203–206
  origins, 201
  see also indigenous communities
Indian Removal Act (IRA), 200
Indian Reorganization Act, 201
Indian Self-Determination and Education Assistance Act, 201–202
indigenous communities
  accomplishments of the IHS, 210
  challenges, 210–213
  health policymaking, 199–203
  health status, 206–210, 262
  historical context, 198, 199–202
  Indian Health Service, 68, 203–213
  legal and constitutional status, 198–199
  population characteristics, 196–198
individual mandate, 96, 101–102, 104–105
individualism, 249
infant mortality
  Hispanic paradox, 261
  indigenous communities, 201, 206, 262
  public health, 65
  quality of healthcare, 454–455
infertility, 367, 382
  see also assisted reproduction
information
  government regulation, 324
  market competition, 325–326
inoculation *see* vaccination
Institute of Medicine (IOM), 66, 253
institutions
  Affordable Care Act, 121
  health policy environment, 8–12
  health policymaking, 4
insurance *see* health insurance
insurance underwriting, 256–257
interest groups
  Affordable Care Act, 87, 88
  healthcare reform, 470
  Kingdon's multiple streams model, 87
  lobbying, 15–16
  as policy actors, 30–32, 71–72
  public philosophy, 14–15, 30
  public vs. private, 15–16
interest-group liberalism, 14
international context
  comparative models, 41–43, 45–46
  cost drivers, 322
  opioid epidemic, 413–414
  quality of healthcare, 454–455
  right-to-die, 385–386
  spending on healthcare, 42, 294
intrauterine insemination (IUI), 363
iron triangle, 14–15
Islam, contraception, 265–266

J
Japan, opioid prescription, 414
Jefferson, Thomas, 6
Jiankui, He, 434–435
Johnson Administration
  Great Society programs, 130
  public health, 48
Judaism, contraception, 265
judicial appointments, 11–12
judiciary, 11–12

K
Kaiser Family Foundation (KFF), as policy actor, 32
Kennedy Administration, 48, 166
Kerr-Mills Act, 48, 130, 166
Kevorkian, Jack, 384
King v. Burwell, 103–104
Kingdon's multiple streams model, 81–87

L
language issues, Latinos, 261
Latinos, health status, 261–262
legal framework
  abortion, 373, 374–375, 379, 380–384
  Affordable Care Act, 87–96, 101–105, 111–113
  assisted reproduction, 364–365, 367–372, 383–384
  biomedicine, 361–362
  chronology of significant events and legislation, 479–488
  cost containment, 327–331
  differing interest groups, 4
  divided government, 16–17
  gene therapy, 436–437
  gridlock and dysfunction, 20–21
  justification in healthcare, 323–324
  Medicare revisions, 170
  opioid epidemic, 413
  right-to-die and physician-assisted suicide, 386–392
  and spending on healthcare, 323–324
  see also health policymaking
legal immigrants
  Affordable Care Act, 110
  obtaining healthcare, 271–272
legal status, indigenous communities, 198–199
leukemia, gene therapy, 429
liability *see* medical liability
Liberal/Democratic reform proposals, 84–85, 457–462

liberalism
  public philosophy, 14, 30
  vs. socialized medicine, 48
licensed practical nurses (LPNs), 23
licensed vocational nurses (LVN), 23
life expectancy
  comparative analysis, 42
  historical context, 67
  indigenous communities, 206, 210
  public health, 245–246
lifestyle choices, costs of healthcare, 310–311
life-support technologies, 386–392
lifetime insurance limits, 257
living wills, 396
lobbying, interest groups, 15–16
local governments
  administration, 27
  decentralization, 7–8
  historical context, 44, 46, 47
  illegal immigrants, 273
  maternal mortality, 269
  role in healthcare system, 69–70
  spending on healthcare, 49, 70
location *see* geographical context
Locke, John, 14
longevity *see* life expectancy
long-term care
  Affordable Care Act, 107–108
  Medicaid, 135, 156
  Medicare, 182–185
  relationship with spending on healthcare, 337–338
  transition from institutional to community-based/home care, 155–157
  veterans, 221–222
long-term care insurance, 184–185
long-term services and support (LTSS), 156–157
low-income individuals
  Children's Health Insurance Program, 142
  health status, 258–262
  impact of rise in healthcare costs, 295
  Medicaid, 131, 133, 142, 169–170
  social determinants of health, 246–247
    see also poverty

M

Madison, James, 14
magnetic resonance imaging (MRI), 301–302
malpractice, 306
managed care
  definitions, 334–335
  Medicaid financing, 137
  Medicare, 175
  spending on healthcare, 334–336
managed competition, 333–334
managed-care organizations (MCOs), 151–152
mandates, Affordable Care Act, 96, 101–102, 104–105
manufacturing sector employment, 251
marginal benefits, medical technology, 304
market competition
  as cost driver, 322
  healthcare reform, 464–465
  spending on healthcare, 324–326
Maryland's price regulation, 329
Massachusetts Model, 86, 102
maternal mortality, 268–269

Maynard, Brittany, 391, 393–395, 396
McCaughey, Betsy, 92
Medicaid
  Affordable Care Act expansion, 97, 109–111, 140–146
  benefits, 135
  cost containment, 27, 49, 342
  costs of, 27, 147–148
  coverage, 26, 27, 71, 132–135
  differences with Medicare, 130–131
  eligibility, 107, 113, 132–135
  enrollment, 131, 147–148
  expenditure, 283–286, 297–299
  federal system, 8
  financing, 135–137, 459–460
  healthcare reform, 466
  indigenous communities, 210–211
  introduction of, 130
  key facts, 131
  long-term care, 135, 156
  managed care, 335
  objective and structure, 132
  origins, 130
  Pay-for-Performance (P4P), 157–158
  pregnancy care, 254
  prescription drug benefit, 60
  price regulation, 328
  reform, 151–155, 457–458, 461–462
  services, 135
  veterans, 220
Medicaid buy-in, 169–170
Medicaid waivers
  Affordable Care Act, 110
  categories, 148–149
  Clinton Administration, 54
  George W. Bush Administration, 57–58
  meaning of, 148
  Reagan Administration, 52
  trends, 149–151
  work requirements, 154–155
Medical Assistance for the Aged (MAA) program, 130
medical assistants (MAs), 438–439
medical bankruptcy, 296
Medical Device Manufacturers of America (MDMA), 32
medical errors
  comorbidity adjustments, 342
  cost containment, 338–339
  spending on healthcare, 304–308
Medical Expenditure Panel Survey (MEPS), 293
medical home *see* patient-centered medical home (PCMH)
medical liability
  defensive medicine, 306–308
  George W. Bush Administration reforms, 58
  healthcare reform, 464
  malpractice, 306
Medical Loss Ratio (MLR), 256, 257
medical malpractice, 306
Medical Savings Accounts (MSAs), 152–154
medical technology *see* biomedicine
medical tourism, 296, 366–367
Medicare
  administrative costs, 311–312
  Affordable Care Act, 99–100, 189–190
  Affordable Care Act outcomes, 119
  cost containment, 49, 177–182, 340
  coverage, 26, 53, 71

coverage and spending, 27
differences with Medicaid, 130–131
eligibility age, 185, 188–189
expenditure, 283–286, 297
financing, 168–169
introduction of, 48–49, 130
long-term care, 182–185
managed care, 335
origins, 165–166
politics and policy, 190–191
prescription drugs, 60, 171–174, 314–315, 316–320, 330
program objectives and structure, 166–168
prospective payment system, 52–53
reform, 458–462, 464
specialty drugs, 424–425
supplementing, 169–170
transforming, 170–177, 185–189
underinsurance, 253
Medicare Advantage, 99–100, 167, 175–176, 190, 461
Medicare Catastrophic Coverage Act, 53
Medicare Extra for All, 460
Medicare for All, 458, 459–460, 462
Medicare Modernization Act
 Affordable Care Act, 100, 176–177
 costs of healthcare, 185, 334
 prescription drugs, 59
Medicare Prescription Drug, Improvement, and Modernization Act (MPDIMA), 171–174
Medicare+Choice, 175–176
medication abortion, 378–380
medigap policies, 170, 186–187, 468
mental health
 indigenous communities, 209–210
 veterans' adjustment to civilian life, 222–223
Merit-Based Incentive Payment System (MIPS), 182
Merriam Report, 201
methadone, 408
Mexico City Policy, 63
Mexico-US migration, 274
migration
 Affordable Care Act, 110
 health status, 270–274
 indigenous communities, 198
 medical tourism, 296
 obtaining healthcare, 271–272
military sexual trauma (MST), 225, 230
minorities
 geographical context, 248
 health status, 258–262
Minority Health and Health Disparities Research and Education Act, 66
misinformation campaigns, 92–93
mistakes *see* medical errors
Mitochondrial replacement therapy (MRT), 365
modified adjusted gross income (MAGI), 133
Moore, Michael, 83
morality, physician-assisted suicide, 397–398
 see also ethics
morning-after pills, 377
morphine, 407
 see also opioid epidemic
multiple streams model, 81–87
Munoz, Marlise, 389
musculoskeletal injuries, veterans, 223

N
nanotechnology enhancement, 435
National Cancer Act, 46
National Cancer Institute (NCI), 46
National Federal of Independent Business v. Sebelius, 101, 113, 133
national government *see* federal government
national health insurance (NHI), 29, 30, 47, 50, 165–166
National Institutes of Health (NIH), 68, 428
National Quarantine Act, 45
navigators, health insurance exchanges, 109
New York City Dispensary, 64
Nimmo, Robert, 228
Nixon Administration
 cost containment, 50, 51–52
 health maintenance organizations, 332
nonincremental policy changes, 9
non-partisan health foundations, 32
nontechnology, 300
nurses
 American Nurses Association, 31
 as policy actors, 23–24
 qualifications, 23–24
 workforce profile, 438–439
 workforce shortages, 440
nursing homes, 182–183

O
Obama, Barack
 Affordable Care Act reforms, 455–456
 election agenda, 13, 87
 immigrants obtaining healthcare, 271–272
 judicial appointments, 12
Obama Administration
 Affordable Care Act, 87–88, 106–107
 emergency contraception, 376–377, 378
 healthcare system, 60–61
 partisanship, 93–94
 veteran scandal, 229
Obamacare *see* Affordable Care Act
obesity
 comparative analysis, 43
 costs of healthcare, 310–311
Omnibus Budget Reconciliation Act, 155
Operation Enduring Freedom (OEF), 222
opioid epidemic, 63, 293, 407–420
order, healthcare values, 455
organ transplants, medical technology, 300, 301
out-of-pocket costs
 decline in expenditures, 288–290
 as healthcare model, 83
 impact of rise in healthcare costs, 294–295
 national expenditure, 29
 specialty drugs, 425–426
outpatient services, veterans, 220
outrage industry, 89
overconsumption, 45
overdosing
 opioid epidemic, 293, 408, 414
 prescription drugs, 316
overpricing, 312–314
overuse of medical procedures, 342
OxyContin, 407, 408, 409–410, 416

516 INDEX

P

paid leave programs, 264–265
pain relief, 293
  see also opioid epidemic
partisan polarization, 18–19
partisanship
  Affordable Care Act, 120–121
  Affordable Care Act replacement, 62–63
  Congress, 9
  healthcare reform, 93–94
  SCHIP, 138
party affiliation, 20
party unity, 89
patient protection, Affordable Care Act, 96–102
patient-centered medical home (PCMH), 182
Patient's Bill of Rights, 56
pay, for physicians, 23, 217, 313
Pay-for-Performance (P4P), 157–158
Peer Review Organizations (PROs), 52
perimortem sperm/egg harvesting, 366
personal responsibility, 246
personalized medicine, 300
Petzel, Robert, 229
pharmaceutical industry
  Affordable Care Act, 88
  direct-to-consumer advertising, 316, 320–321
  opioid epidemic, 414–415
  prescription drug prices, 315, 318–322
  scientific trials, 339
  specialty drugs, 420–427
  Trump Administration, 330–331
Pharmaceutical Research and Manufacturers of America (PhRMA), 32
pharmacological enhancement, 435
Pharmacy Benefit Managers (PBMs), 330, 331, 421
philanthropic foundations, 45
physician assistants (PAs), 438
physician-assisted suicide, 384–398
physicians
  defensive medicine, 306–307
  government regulation, 323–324
  Medicare financing, 169
  as policy actors, 23
  prospective payment system, 180–182
  public health, 65
  spending on, 288, 312–313
  Veterans Health Administration (VHA), 217
  workforce profile, 437–438
  workforce shortages, 439–440
Planned Parenthood, 268
planning
  cost containment, 327
  costs of healthcare, 50–51
pluralism, 14–15
pocket veto, 10
polarization
  Affordable Care Act replacement, 62–63
  Congress, 9, 20–21
  gridlock and dysfunction, 20–21
  political environment, 17–21, 89
policies stream, Kingdon's multiple streams model, 83–86
policy *see* health policy environment; health policymaking
policy actors *see* actors
policy cycle, 4

political context, 3
  biomedicine, 361–362
  changing nature of, 16–21
  health policy environment, 12–21
    see also individual named Administrations e.g. Trump Administration
political feasibility, 13
political ideology, 20
political power
  Congress, 8–9
  constitutional system, 5
  executive branch, 10
  federal system, 5–8
politics of science, 58
politics stream, Kingdon's multiple streams model, 87
pooling, 464, 469
population
  aging, 442–443
  concentration of expenditures, 290–293
  indigenous communities, 196–198
  opioid epidemic, 410–412
  veterans, 214, 227–228
positron emission tomography (PET), 301–302
posttraumatic stress disorder (PTSD), 224–225
poverty
  health status, 258–262
  indigenous communities, 206, 210
  pregnancy care, 254
    see also low-income individuals
power *see* political power
power of attorney, 396
pre-existing conditions limitations, 257
preferred-provider organization (PPO), 335
pregnancy
  African-Americans, 259
  discrimination against, 264–265
  insurance coverage, 254–255
  Latinos, 262
  unintended pregnancies, 372–373, 374, 380–382
    see also abortion; assisted reproduction; contraception; reproductive health
pregnancy rate, 263
premiums
  cost-sharing, 336–337
  disadvantaged groups, 256
  malpractice, 306
  managed competition, 333–334
  Medicare financing, 168–169
  Medicare reforms, 185–186
  prescription drugs, 173
  underinsurance, 252–253
premium-support program, Medicare, 187–189
pre-paid ambulatory health plans (PAHP), 151
prepaid group plans (PGPs), 332, 333
  see also health maintenance organizations (HMOs)
pre-paid inpatient health plans (PIHP), 152
prescription drug benefit, 59–60
Prescription Drug Monitoring Programs (PDMPs), 419, 420
prescription drugs
  Affordable Care Act, 100
  emergency contraception, 375–378
  Medicare, 60, 171–174, 314–315, 316–320, 330
  opioid epidemic, 408–410
  price regulation, 329–330
  spending on, 59–60, 288, 314–322

INDEX 517

Trump Administration, 330–331
presidential policymaking, 10
presidential signing statements, 10
presidential veto, 10
preventable adverse events (PAEs), 304–305
price regulation, 328–330
primary-care case management (PCCM), 152
primary-care physicians, 440
private interest groups, 15–16
  see also interest groups
private sector
  and the Affordable Care Act, 99
  as cost driver, 322
  health insurance, 25–27
  historical context, 65
  managed care, 151–152
  veterans, 231
problems stream, Kingdon's multiple streams model, 82–83
professional standards review, 327
Professional Standards Review Organizations (PSROs), 50, 179, 327
propaganda, 15–16
prospective payment system, 52–53, 179–182
Protestantism, and contraception, 265
provider reimbursements, Medicare, 186
provider taxes, Medicaid, 136
providers *see* healthcare providers
public health
  accomplishments and challenges, 70–71
  evolution of, 63–67
  life expectancy, 245–246
  national health insurance, 29, 30, 47, 50, 165–166
  organization and functions, 67–70
  spending and financing, 70, 288–290
  waste, fraud, and abuse, 309–310
Public Health Improvement Act, 66
public health law reform movement, 67
public interest groups, 15–16
  see also interest groups
public opinion
  Affordable Care Act, 87, 105–106, 120–121
  fraud, waste and cost control, 338
  healthcare reform, 93–94
  polarization, 19–20
  political feasibility, 13
  prescription drugs, 321
  right to die, 384–385, 395–396
  spending on healthcare, 299
  tax, 462
public philosophy, 14–15
  interest groups, 30, 71–72
  socialized medicine, 48, 71–72
public sector *see* public health
public sector health insurance, 27
  federal government's role, 45–47
  historical context, 45–51
  interest groups, 30–31
    see also Children's Health Insurance Program (CHIP); Medicaid; Medicare
punctuated equilibrium, 12–13

Q

qualifications, nurses, 23–24
quality of healthcare, 454–455, 467

quality-adjusted life years (QALYs), 427
Quill, Timothy, 390
Quinlan, Karen, 386

R

race
  indigenous communities, 196–197
  opioid epidemic, 412
  uninsured population, 252
  veteran benefits, 227
  Veterans Affairs, 231
  workforce diversity, 441–442
RAISE Family Caregivers Act, 184
RAND health insurance experiments, 468
rationing
  comparative effectiveness research, 340
  and managed care, 335, 336
  spending on healthcare, 332–333
Reagan Administration
  healthcare system, 51–53
  Medicaid waivers, 149
  presidential signing statements, 10
  prospective payment system, 179, 181
reconciliation, Affordable Care Act, 96
recruitment, healthcare workforce, 439–440
reform *see* healthcare reform; medical liability reform; welfare reform
regenerative medicine
  gene therapy, 431
  medical technology, 300
registered nurses (RNs), 23–24
regulations *see* legal framework
Reid, Harry, 12
relative-value scale (RVS), 181
religion
  Affordable Care Act, 103, 106–107
  assisted reproduction, 382
  biomedicine, 361–362
  contraception, 265–266
  physician-assisted suicide, 397–398
remote patient monitoring, 300
repeal-and-replace legislation, 61, 112–113, 115–116, 470
reproductive health
  abstinence-only programs, 58–59
  Affordable Care Act, 103, 106, 266–267
  assisted reproduction, 363–373
  biomedicine, 372–375
  debates over, 265–268
  George W. Bush Administration, 58–59
  Trump Administration, 268
    see also abortion
Republican/Conservative reform proposals, 85–86, 462–469
residential care facilities (RCFs), 25
retiree benefits, 170
Revolutionary War, 43, 63–64
rights
  Conservative/Republican understanding of, 463
  GI Bill of Rights, 215–216
  to healthcare, 244–245
  Patient's Bill of Rights, 56
right-to-die
  biomedicine, 384–398
  comparative analysis, 385–386
  as movement, 384–385

risk factors
  health insurance, 99
  health status risk adjustment, 467
  indigenous communities, 204, 206–210, 212
  opioid abuse, 408
  and prescription drugs, 318
  spending on healthcare, 337
    see also health status
risk-benefit analysis, 21
risky behaviors, 207–208, 224, 258
Robert Wood Johnson Foundation (RWJF), 32
Roe v. Wade, 91–92, 373, 374, 380–381
Roemer's law, 327
Roosevelt Administration
  political environment, 13
  public health, 47
  rights, 463
Roy, Avik, 325–326, 340
RU-486, 378–380
rural areas
  concentration of expenditures, 293
  dental care, 270
  health status, 247–248
  workforce shortages, 440–441
Ryan, Paul, 188, 463, 464

S

salaries, for physicians, 23, 217, 313
same-sex couples, assisted reproduction, 370–371
Sanders, Bernie, 189, 312, 340, 458–459
sanitation, historical context, 63–64
satisficing, 12–13
scans, imaging technology, 301–302
Schiavo, Terri, 388–389, 393, 396
science
  ambiguity of evidence, 339, 342
  pharmaceutical industry, 339
  politics of, 58
    see also biomedicine
self-determination, indigenous communities, 201–202
self-governance, indigenous communities, 201–202
self-insurance, 464
self-referrals, 310
Senate, judicial appointments, 11–12
Senate cloture rule, 9
service sector employment, 251
Servicemen's Readjustment Act, 215–216
severability, 104–105
severe combined immunodeficiency (SCID), 428–429
sexual abuse, in the military, 225, 230
Sherwood Act, 215
Shkreli, Martin, 415
single-payer systems, 468
Skilled Nursing Care Centers (SNCCs), 25
Skilled Nursing Facility (SNF), 25
skinny plans, 253
smallpox, historical context, 63–64
Smith, Adam, 324–325
smoking
  costs of healthcare, 311
  indigenous communities, 209
Snyder Act, 201
social benefits, historical context, 46–47
social costs, opioid epidemic, 412–413

social determinants of health
  African-Americans, 259
  disadvantaged groups, 246–247, 248–249
social justice, 243
social movements, 15
Social Security Act, 47, 166
socialized medicine, 48, 71–72, 83
somatic gene therapy, 431
specialty drugs, 420–427
spending on healthcare, 4–5
  administration, 311–312
  Affordable Care Act controls, 100–101
  Affordable Care Act outcomes, 117–118, 119
  business impacts, 297
  Clinton Administration, 55
  comparative analysis, 42, 294
  concentration of expenditures, 290–293
  drivers, 322–323
  to employers, 28
  federal government, 70
  gene therapy, 432–433
  George W. Bush Administration, 57
  government health insurance, 27
  government impacts, 297–299
  government regulation, 323–324
  health insurance, 26–27
  health maintenance organizations, 331–332
  healthcare reform, 454, 465–466
  historical context, 327–331
  household impacts, 294–297
  indigenous communities, 211
  lifestyle choices, 310–311
  long-term care, 182–183
  managed care, 334–336
  managed competition, 333–334
  market competition, 324–326
  Medicaid, 27, 147–148
  medical errors, 304–308
  medical technology, 300–304
  Medicare, 170–174, 180–182
  Medicare Modernization Act, 185
  overpricing, 312–314
  planning, 50–51
  prescription drugs, 59–60, 288, 314–322
  as proportion of GDP, 3–4, 283, 288–290
  prospective payment system, 179–182
  public opinion, 299
  public sector, 288–290
  rationing, 332–333
  Reagan Administration, 51–53
  rise in, 283–286, 299–300, 343
  social determinants of health, 246
  specialty drugs, 423–426
  by type of health service, 286–288
  veterans, 225–226
  waste, fraud, and abuse, 308–310
  wellness, 336
    see also cost containment; cost-sharing; financing; premiums; third-party payers
sperm donation (assisted reproduction), 364, 370
sperm harvesting (assisted reproduction), 365–366
Spina Bifida Health Care Program (SB), 222
spousal impoverishment, 135
stability, and incrementalism, 13
staff-model HMOs, 335

State Children's Health Insurance Program (SCHIP), 56, 60, 138
state governments
  administration, 27
  Affordable Care Act, 109–111, 114
  comparative analysis, 68
  consumer-directed healthcare plans, 153
  decentralization, 7–8
  federal system, 5–8
  Kerr-Mills Act, 166
  maternal mortality, 269
  Medicaid expansion, 141–146
  Medicaid financing, 135–137
  Medicaid waivers, 148–149
  opioid epidemic response, 418–419
  role in healthcare system, 68–69
  spending on healthcare, 49, 70, 298–299
state health departments, 69
state innovation approach, 465, 466
stem cells, 56–57
strokes, indigenous communities, 208
subgovernment concept, 14–15
subsidies
  Affordable Care Act, 98
  Affordable Care Act outcomes, 119
  Medicare, 174–175
Substance Abuse and Mental Health Services Administration (SAMHSA), 68
suicide rate
  indigenous communities, 209, 262
  women, 263, 412
supplemental medical insurance (SMI), 167
Supreme Court, 11
surprise medical bills, 314
surrogate carriers (assisted reproduction), 364, 368–372
sustainable growth rate (SGR), 181

T

tax
  Affordable Care Act, 117
  Affordable Care Act outcomes, 119
  cost containment, 337
  healthcare reform, 462, 465, 470
  Medicare financing, 168, 186
  provider taxes, 136
tax credits, 456
tax cuts, Trump Administration, 112
Tax Equity and Fiscal Responsibility Act (TEFRA), 179
Tea Party, 94
technological environment *see* biomedicine
terrorism
  public health emergencies, 66
  and veterans, 223–224
Texas v. United States, 104
third-party payers
  healthcare reform, 467
  historical context, 45, 46
  as policy actors, 25–27
three-parent IVF, 365
tort law, 306, 308, 464
town hall meetings, 94
Transfer Act, 201
traumatic brain injury (TBI), veterans, 224
Treaty of Cession, 199

tribalism, 17–18, 20
TRICARE, 220
Troubled Assets Relief Program (TARP), 93
Truman Administration, public health, 47
Trump Administration
  Affordable Care Act, 62–63, 72, 111–112, 113–115, 122–123
  CHIP, 139
  family separation policy, 274
  healthcare system, 61–63
  judicial appointments, 12
  opioid epidemic response, 417–418
  pharmaceutical industry, 330–331
  reproductive health, 268
  unified government, 72
  veteran scandal, 229
  work requirement policies, 154, 155

U

underinsurance, 252–256
underwriting, 256–257
unified government, 16–17, 72
Uniform Parentage Act (UPA), 368
uninsurables, 469
uninsured population
  Affordable Care Act, 117
  African-Americans, 258–259
  consequences of, 253–256
  disadvantaged groups, 249–256
  gender, 263–264
unintentional injuries, indigenous communities, 209
unitary systems of government, 6
universal coverage, 465
urban areas, health status, 247–248
urban Indian Health programs, 204–205
Urban Indian Organizations (UIOs), 205
US Agency for International Development (USAID), 59
uterus transplants, 365

V

VA Mission Act, 218
vaccination
  historical context, 43–44, 63–64
  indigenous communities, 200
veterans
  adjustment to civilian life, 222–223
  benefits and services, 221–222
  benefits historical context, 214–216
  challenges, 230–232
  eligibility for care, 220–221
  enrollment, 220–221
  family members, 222
  financing healthcare, 225–226
  health policy development, 216–218
  health status, 222–225
  indigenous communities, 210
  population characteristics, 214
  TRICARE, 220
  use of benefits and services, 226–228, 230
Veterans Administration (VA)
  health policy development, 216–218
  healthcare system, 220–222, 230–231
  leadership, 231
  origins, 215
  scandals at, 228

Veterans Benefit Administration (VBA), 225
Veterans Bureau, 216
Veterans Eligibility Reform Act, 217, 230–231, 232
Veterans Equitable Resource Allocation (VERA), 217
Veterans Health Administration (VHA)
  coverage, 222
  funding, 225–226
  mission, 219
  organization and structure, 219
  origins, 216–217
  reform, 217–218
vetos, 10
Vicodin, 408

W

waivers *see* Medicaid waivers

Walmart, 251
Walter Reed Army Medical Center, 229
war on terror, 223–224
waste, costs of healthcare, 308–310, 338–340
welfare reform, 55, 96
wellness, spending on healthcare, 336
women
  health status, 260, 262–269
  maternal mortality, 268–269
  reproductive health, 265–268
women veterans, 219, 222, 225, 231
Women Veterans Health Program, 222
work requirement policies, 154
World War I, 15, 46
World War II, 47, 66
Wynne, Bill, 461–462